Psychiatric and Mental Health Nursing
The craft of caring

Second edition

Psychiatric and Mental Health Nursing
The craft of caring

Second edition

Edited by

Phil Barker PhD RN FRCN
Honorary Professor, University of Dundee,
Scotland

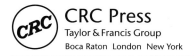

CRC Press
Taylor & Francis Group
Boca Raton London New York

CRC Press is an imprint of the
Taylor & Francis Group, an **informa** business

This book is dedicated to the memory of Mike Consedine (1940–2008) – psychiatric nurse, poet and psychodrama therapist.

Mike inspired many psychiatric nurses to embrace the most powerful kind of human helping in their work. Through his pioneering work in clinical supervision, he also helped nurses know themselves better, so that their true humanity might flower. It was my privilege to count him as a friend. There was nothing 'worth doing' that Mike would not do himself. Such 'living by example' will prove his enduring legacy as a teacher. I hope that readers of this book will discover the virtue of that same lesson in their own lives.

Contents

List of contributors

Trevor Adams MSc PhD RN Cert Ed
Lecturer, Faculty of Health and Medical Sciences,
University of Surrey, Guildford, UK

Jon Allen EN RMN BA (Hons) MSc MBA
Director of Nursing and Clinical Governance,
Oxfordshire, UK

Phil Barker PhD RN FRCN
Honorary Professor, University of Dundee, Dundee, UK

Ian Beech MA BA (Hons) RMN RGN PGCE
Head of Mental Health Division, University of Glamorgan,
Pontypridd, UK

Joy Bray RN RMN ENB650 RNT MA PhD
Mental Health Specialist Nurse, Cambridge University
Hospitals NHS Foundation Trust, Cambridge, UK

Nancy Brookes RN MSc(A) CPMHN(C) PhD
Nurse Scholar, Royal Ottawa Health Care Group, Ottawa,
ON, Canada

Poppy Buchanan-Barker
Director, Clan Unity International, Fife, UK

Philip Burnard PhD RN
Professor of Nursing, Cardiff School of Nursing and
Midwifery Studies, Cardiff University, Cardiff, UK

Mary E. Campbell RN MSN CS
Psychiatric Mental Health Clinical Nurse Specialist, Capital
District Mental Health Program; Adjunct Professor, School
of Nursing, Dalhousie University, Halifax, NS, Canada

Dave Carlyle RcompN PG DipHealSc
Lecturer, Department of Psychological Medicine,
University of Otago, Christchurch, New Zealand

Andrew Cashin RN MHN NP DipAppSci BHSc GCert PTT MN PhD
FACMHN
Associate Professor Justice Health Nursing, The University
of Technology Sydney, Faculty of Nursing, Midwifery and
Health, Sydney, NSW, Australia

Jon Chesterson RN MHN DipCPN BAppSc FACMHN MRCNA
Promotion & Prevention, Hunter New England Mental
Health, NSW, Australia

Liam Clarke DipNurs DipEd DipTheol DipMed Phil BA MSc MA PhD
Reader in Mental Health, University of Brighton,
Eastbourne, UK

Elizabeth Collier BSc RMN MSc PGCE
Lecturer in Mental Health, University of Salford, UK

Philip D. Cooper RN AdvDip MSc
Practice Educator, Suffolk Mental Health Partnership NHS
Trust, Education and Workforce Development, St Clements
Hospital, Ipswich, UK

Seamus Cowman PhD MSc FFNMRCSI DipN (London) RNT RPN RGN
Professor, Faculty of Nursing & Midwifery, Royal College
of Surgeons in Ireland, Dublin, Ireland

Sue Croom PhD MSc BA (Hons) RN HV PGCUTL
Senior Lecturer/Research Fellow, Northumberland and
North Tyneside Mental Health Trust, Berwickshire, UK

Marie Crowe RN PhD
Associate Professor, Department of Psychological
Medicine, University of Otago, Christchurch, New Zealand

John R. Cutcliffe RMN RGN RPN RN BSc (Hon) Nrsg PhD
David G. Braithwaite Professor of Nursing, University
of Texas (Tyler); Adjunct Dean Psychiatric Nursing,
Stenberg College, Vancouver, Canada; Visiting Professor,
University of Ulster, UK

Penny Cutting RGN RMN BSc (Hons) Nursing MA
Counselling and Psychotherapy Clinical Co-ordinator/
Women's Lead, Croydon Adult Integrated Mental Health
Services, Bethlem Royal Hospital, Beckenham, UK

Ruth DeSouza DipNurs Grad DipAdv Nurs Prac MA
Centre Co-ordinator/Senior Research Fellow, Centre
for Asian and Migrant Health Research, National Institute
for Public Health and Mental Health Research, AUT
University Te Wananga Aronui o Tamaki Makau Rau,
Auckland, Aotearoa/New Zealand

Dianne Ellis RMN PGCE MSc
Senior Lecturer Mental Health, Centuria Building, Teesside
University, Middlesbrough, UK

Mark Fenton RMN MA
Editor – Database of Uncertainties about the Effects
of Treatments (DUETs), James Lind Initiative, Oxford, UK

Cheryl Forchuk RN BA BScN MScN PhD
Professor, University of Western Ontario; Assistant Director
& Scientist, Lawson Health Research Institute, London, ON,
Canada

Paul French RMN PhD
Psychology Services, Mental Health Services of Salford, Manchester, UK

Ruth Gallop RN PhD
Professor Emeritus, Faculty of Nursing, University of Toronto, Toronto, ON, Canada

Lyn Gardner RMN PGCEA BSc MSc
Lecturer, School of Health Science, Swansea University, Swansea, UK

Evelyn Gordon MSc (Psychotherapy) MSc (Systemic Management) RPN
Lecturer in Mental Health and Psychotherapy, School of Nursing, Dublin City University, Dublin, Ireland

Alec Grant PhD MA BSc PGCTLHE Cert Res Meth RMN, ENB650 Cert
Principal Lecturer, University of Brighton, Eastbourne, UK

Chris Hart MA RMN RGN
Nurse Consultant in Liaison Psychiatry and Principal Lecturer, School of Nursing, Faculty of Health & Social Care Science, Kingston University & St George's University of London, London, UK

Yvonne Hayne RN BScN MEd PhD
Faculty of Nursing, University of Calgary, Calgary, AB, Canada

Michael Hazelton RN BA MA PhD FACMHN
Professor of Mental Health Nursing and Head of Nursing and Midwifery, The University of Newcastle, Newcastle, NSW, Australia

Anne Helm BEd
Consumer Consultant and Educator, Aorearoa/NewZealand

Steve Hemingway RMN V300 BA (Hons) MA (Couns) PGDE
Senior Lecturer in Mental Health, Department of Health and Human Sciences, University of Huddersfield, Huddersfield, UK

Agnes Higgins PhD MSc BNS RNT RPN RGN
Associate Professor of Mental Health Nursing, Trinity College, Dublin, Ireland

Colin A. Holmes BA (Hons) MPhil PhD
Professor of Nursing, School of Nursing Sciences, Midwifery & Nutrition, James Cook University, Townsville, QLD, Australia

Clare Hopkins RMN MSc MA
Primary Care Mental Health Worker, Newcastle Primary Care Trust, UK

Elsabeth Jensen RN PhD
Assistant Professor, School of Nursing, York University, Toronto, ON, Canada

Mami Kayama RN PHN MN PhD
Professor, St Luke's College of Nursing, Tokyo, Japan

Rachel A. Keaschuk PsyD Rpsych
Psychologist, Pediatric Centre for Weight and Health, Stollery Children's Hospital, Edmonton, AB, Canada

Tom Keen RMN RNT MSc
Formerly Senior Lecturer, University of Plymouth Institute of Health Studies, Exeter, UK

Richard Lakeman DipNsg BN BA (Hons) PGDip (Psychotherapy) Doctoral Candidate JCU
Lecturer, School of Nursing, Dublin City University, Dublin, Ireland

Philip Luffman RMN Dip Gp Psych
Hywel Dda NHS Trust, West Wales, UK

Hugh P. McKenna CBE PhD BSc (Hons) RMN RGN RNT DipN (Lond) AdvDipEd FFN RCSI FEANS FRCN
Professor and Dean, Faculty of Life & Health Sciences, University of Ulster, Coleraine, UK

Julie Mackenzie RMN CPN Cert Cert Family Therapy Dip Social Work and Social Policy MA in Systemic Practice
Nurse Consultant Crisis Service, Ravenswood Clinic, Newcastle upon Tyne, UK

Peter Morrall PhD MSc BA (Hons) PGCE RN
Senior Lecturer in Sociology and Health, School of Healthcare, University of Leeds, Leeds, UK

Mervyn Morris RN
Professor of Community Mental Health, Centre for Community Mental Health, Birmingham City University, Birmingham, UK

Erina Morrison RCpN BHSc MN
Clinical Nurse Director, Nursing, Mental Health and Addiction Health, Waikato, Hamilton, New Zealand

Eimear Muir-Cochrane BSc (Hons) RN RMN Grad Dip Adult Education MNS PhD FACMHN
Professor of Nursing (Mental Health Nursing), School of Nursing and Midwifery, Flinders University, Adelaide, SA, Australia

Lisa Murata RN BScN MEd CPMHN(C) CSFT
Clinical Nurse Educator, Royal Ottawa Mental Health Centre, Ottawa, Canada

Brendan Murphy MA RMN
South Trent Training Dynamic Psychotherapy, Department of Psychotherapy, Derbyshire Mental Health Service Trust, UK

Amanda S. Newton PhD RN
Assistant Professor and Clinician Scientist (Child and Adolescent Psychiatry), Department of Pediatrics, University of Alberta, Edmonton, AB, Canada

Anthony J. O'Brien RN BA Mphil
Senior Lecturer, Mental Health Nursing; Nurse Specialist, Liaison Psychiatry, School of Nursing, University of Auckland, Auckland, New Zealand

Mark Philbin RPN DipN (Lond) BSc MA
Lecturer in Nursing, School of Nursing, Dublin City University, Dublin, Ireland

Gary Platz
Strategic Advisor, Wellink Trust, Wellington, New Zealand

Nicholas G. Procter PhD Grad Dip Adult Ed BA RPN RGN CertAdvClinNsg (SACAE) MACMHN MRCNA FGLF
Associate Professor, School of Nursing and Midwifery, University of South Australia, Adelaide, SA, Australia

William J. Reynolds RN PhD
Former Reader in Nursing, University of Stirling, and Turku University of Applied Sciences; currently Freelance Educator and Researcher, Salo, Finland

Gary Rolfe RMN PGCEA PhD MA BSc
Professor of Nursing, School of Health Science, Swansea University, Swansea, UK

Denis Ryan PhD BSc RPN RGN CAC Cert BT Dip Prof Studies
Senior Lecturer, Department of Nursing & Midwifery, University of Limerick, Limerick, Ireland

Elaine Santa Mina RN BA BAAN MSc PhD
Associate Professor, Ryerson University, Toronto, ON, Canada

David Scarrott RGN RMN V300 BA (Hons)
Team Manager, Crisis Resolution and Home Treatment Team, Rotherham, UK

Angela Simpson RMN BA MA PGCE PhD
Lecturer in Mental Health/Research Fellow, University of York, York, UK

Mike Smith RMN BSc (Nurs) MA PhD
Director, CrazyDiamond, www.crazydiamond.org.uk

Shirley A. Smoyak RN PhD FAAN
Professor II at Rutgers, the State University of New Jersey; Professor, Continuous Education & Outreach, Edison, NJ, USA

Chris Stevenson RMN BA (Hons) MSc PhD
Chair in Mental Health Nursing, School of Nursing, Dublin City University, Dublin, Ireland

Margaret Tansey RN MSc(A) CPMHN(C)
Vice President Professional Practice and Chief of Nursing Practice, Royal Ottawa Health Care Group, Ottawa, Canada

Tracey Tully RN MSc PhD
Independent Consultant, Toronto, Canada

Paul Veitch RMN MSc
Team Manager and Senior Nurse, Early Intervention in Psychosis Service, Newcastle & North Tyneside Trust, Newcastle upon Tyne, UK

Martin F. Ward RMN DipNurs RNT Cert Ed NEBSS Dip Mphil
Independent Mental Health Nursing Consultant and Coordinator of Mental Health Nursing Studies, University of Malta, www.mwprof-development.com

Cheryl Waters RN BSc (Hons) PhD MACMHN MCN
Senior Lecturer, Faculty of Nursing Midwifery and Health, University of Technology, Sydney, Australia

Denise (Denny) Webster RN PhD CS
Professor Emerita, University of Colorado at Denver and Health Sciences Center, Denver, CO, USA

Irene Whitehill BSc PhD
Independent User Trainer and Consultant, Section 36, Northumberland, UK

Peter Wilkin RMN MA
Formerly Clinical Nurse Specialist with the Complex Cases Mental Heath Team in Rochdale, UK

Gary Winship PhD MA RMN Dip Gp Psych
Associate Professor of Human Relations, University of Nottingham, School of Education, Nottingham, UK

Jerome Wright MSc RGN RMN PGCE
Lecturer, Department of Health Sciences, University of York, York, UK

Stephen G. Wright MSc RN RCNT RNT DipN DANS RPTT FRCN MBE
Chairman and co-founder of the Sacred Space Foundation, Associate Professor, Faculty of Health and Social Care at the University of Cumbria, Carlisle, UK

The Cleansing has Begun

Chest deep in the Wainuiomata stream
Earth's energies combine with mine
Me the mighty super-conductor
Here to do God's will

Yes, the cleansing has begun

With Jehovah's name reverberating from the hills
Wainui's demons go screaming to the abyss
Ah Wainuiomata, New Jerusalem
River of life

The cleansing has begun

The cries of my disciples from the asylums of the world
Keep tearing at my soul
Hold on my followers, I'm coming

The cleansing has begun

Strapped to a sterile bed
Spiritual poison in my veins
Encrusting my heart, fogging my head
I'll keep fighting, my disciples

The cleansing has begun

Through days of haze
Hospital food
I keep sitting,
A god hunched
Looking for answers on the wall

Through days of haze
Hospital food
I see the answer
It's written in their eyes

I'm no god
Just a fool
Raped by heart and soul

The cleansing has begun

Then a power to be
Said you may go free
(I'll be tethered to him
With a chemical chain)
Oh try to get yourself a job

The cleansing has begun

Through days of haze
Timeless sleep
I lick my violated brain
Ah Wainuiomata

The cleansing has begun

Somehow I am much better now
I have taken that to be's advice
I'm searching the papers
Up dated my c.v.
Brought myself some shoes

Hey, wait a minute
You, out there
Do you have an opening
For a part time god

The cleansing has begun

Gary Platz

Gary Platz is Strategic Advisor, Wellink Trust, New Zealand. Gary has been involved in the service user movement since 1993. He is an advocate of peer services and has been successful in the setting up of several peer services including a peer recovery house, which is an alternative to acute hospitalization. He is a poet and writer of short stories.

The Space I'm in

Mike Consedine*

Recently, I have been privileged to sit in the small garden at the rear of our house nearly every day. It is warm and sheltered here, and a small rock pool provides the soothing sound of running water. Apart from the low hum of distant traffic nothing much else disturbs. So I can experience the flowers growing, the insects buzzing, the birds chirping, the cat sleeping, and of course the water. Such a special honour. This time to be with myself.

And in that time experiences buried deep have an opportunity to emerge, flooding my senses with feeling beyond expression: with life that had seemed lost forever. And I know again the passion I have for the experiences of being alive.

Sitting with this I see my social atom: the network of significant relationships both past and present, surrounding me. What riches! My wife, my former wife and our children, my brothers and sister, friends – relationships that have developed over many years, and colleagues with whom I have been intimately involved, as we strive to make a better world. All here, in my social atom.

And I know without doubt that this was all generated in my family of origin – my mother and father and the wider *whānau*.[a] And as I sit with this I feel the tears again: tears of gratitude for the good people they were/are. Not famous, just good. Doing what good people do; loving those around them and committing themselves without fuss to helping all.

These values are embedded in the current social atom which surrounds me and is my life. In this place I cannot fail. Like Jean Valjean I know who I am and that allows me to live with dignity, and the comfort of truth. I know that values, like most truths in life, are not taught, they are developed. They are developed through good doubling, mirroring, modelling, role reversal and discussion. Through these processes they are internalized and their life conserved. They are the cornerstones. They inform the roles we enact in the world.

Personality may be thought of as a series of roles and role systems. In a healthy individual life, development is always a work in progress. When I wept over my inadequacies as a parent, Harry, my old therapist, would always say 'every day is an opportunity to do it differently'. There is no need to keep on recreating the original social atom.

Poetry enables me to do it differently. Through it I am able to express myself fully in the world without self-aggrandisement, self-pity or harm to others. It's just the way things are for me at any given moment. It may express my delight and joy, or my sorrow anger and despair. The expression of who I am enables a full life. And I do want a full life.

Christchurch, New Zealand
3rd April 2007

*Mike Consedine was one of New Zealand's most respected psychiatric nurses. He had previously worked as a probation officer and then developed a successful career in psychodrama, operating an Independent Training Consultancy based in Christchurch, New Zealand. Mike was a past President of the Australian and New Zealand Psychodrama Association.

---

[a] Whānau (Maori): extended family.

Half dead

Sometimes he awoke
aware only that
he was half dead.

his body lay
side on
half buried in
the rubbish tip

his mouth and throat
were full of decay
seagulls circled
awaiting their turn
to feast.

the early morning light
boosted the smell
and the soft breeze
increased reflected light

half his head
was dead
and he did not
know what to do
except persevere.

Mike Consedine
March 2007
Christchurch, New Zealand

Preface to the second edition

George Bernard Shaw said 'The only man I know who behaves sensibly is my tailor; he takes my measurements anew each time he sees me. The rest go on with their old measurements and expect *me* to *fit* them.' The same is true of the world in which we live. It keeps changing, growing in some ways and shrinking in others. We, the inhabitants of that world, need to understand this, if we are to adapt ourselves to fit our changing circumstances.

There has been a lot of growth and perhaps some significant shrinkage, since we published the first edition of *The craft of caring*. Economics and its obsession with cost containment continues to dominate most services, and science and its fascination with evidence continues to tantalize us. What we would like to do, we cannot afford; and what we have been doing, apparently successfully, for a long time, we find has no proper 'evidence base'. What to do?

In the Western world, economics continues, ironically, to dominate the agenda, pushing the demand for more 'evidence' and a stronger scientific base for practice. In the rest of the world, we have finally woken up to the fact that everyone experiences the kinds of problems in living called 'mental illness' in the West, but we may call them by different names or give them a different significance. Slowly, we are beginning to ask how do people in war-torn or economically ravaged countries cope with such problems. And, where do nurses fit into this picture, if at all.

Although the catalogue of 'mental disorders' has grown, in leaps and bounds, since attempts were first made to classify 'insanity' a century ago, no 'new' forms of mental disorder have been added to the list in the past 15 years. However, all around us, 'mental health problems' appear to be on the increase, especially in affluent countries. We appear to have no end of resourcefulness in developing new ways of expressing misery and despair, fear and trembling. Is this to do with the pressures we impose upon ourselves, which we now call stress? Or is this to do with the sheer artificiality of our lives. Who knows? However, the more affluent a society becomes, the more miserable and angst ridden it also becomes. Little wonder so many seek the dream of a simpler life.

In this second edition, we have tried to reflect some of the changing world we see around us, not least within the field of nursing itself. All the original chapters have been revised and updated and we have added around a dozen new chapters, covering important new developments in mental health care or exploring areas of practice that represent a refinement of some of the key concepts in nursing practice.

We have extended our consideration of the naming of psychiatric disorders, trying to help the reader gain a sense of history but also an appreciation of what it might mean to receive a psychiatric diagnosis. In keeping with our core aim – to explore the concept of the craft of caring – we keep the focus on people and persons. How does diagnosis affect people?

The person with a diagnosis of autism has attracted a lot of public attention in the past few years, with a number of books written by people with different experiences of the autistic spectrum. Autism is a classic challenge for mental health nurses, since the people concerned have a very unusual concept of 'mind'. Mental health nurses could extend themselves greatly by exploring how to respond to people with autism.

We have also developed the section on services, by including liaison psychiatry, therapeutic communities, services for the older person, nurse prescribing and services for women. These represent exciting examples of how nurses are rising to the challenge of developing more innovative care, or trying to find new ways of ensuring that people too receive personally meaningful care, whatever their situation.

The focus on rights is developed further in a new chapter on the support of refugees and asylum seekers – two groups of people found now in every developed country on earth. The special problems encountered by these groups will stretch mental health nurses, and may also, in time, help them understand better the needs of people experiencing other forms of exclusion or marginalization.

We have also revised substantially the chapter on the law and mental health care, providing readers with not only a history of the development of 'mental health legislation' but also an appreciation of how this differs from one country to the next.

Finally, we have included a vital consideration of the concept of spirituality, conspicuously absent from the first edition. Given that the original mission of psychiatry was to study the *soul* or *spirit*, it seems fitting that nurses are finally turning their attention to this, the most abstract aspect of our common humanity.

This edition is significantly bigger than the first, but I hope, despite its size, that it retains a sense of human scale. It is all too easy to lose sight of the person, the family and the community of origin. It is all too easy to be overwhelmed by the sheer volume of concepts, theories, models, principles and various practices. I hope that you will find that the *person* makes an important appearance on every page of this book. Perhaps this anonymous person will become your guide, helping you to explore the text, with a view to clarifying your own concept of 'the craft of caring'.

Phil Barker
Newport on Tay, Scotland

Acknowledgements

Grateful thanks to Clare Patterson and Naomi Wilkinson at Hodder Arnold for all their support during the preparation of this second edition, and to all the authors for their commitment to the book and to the mental health field.

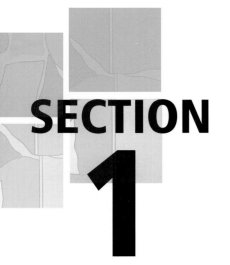

SECTION
1

THE NEED FOR NURSING

Preface to Section 1

When one isn't dominated by feelings of separateness from what he's working on, then one can be said to 'care' about what he is doing. That is what caring really is, a feeling of identification with what one's doing.

Robert Pirsig

The practice of nursing involves doing something that appears quite 'ordinary', in highly extraordinary settings and circumstances. Nurses care for people who, for different reasons, are unable or unwilling to care for themselves. In one sense, caring is hardly 'rocket science'. 'Anyone could do it' has become an increasingly popular cry, especially among economists and bureaucrats anxious to reduce the financial cost of caring. There is some truth in this. At least in principle, anyone could care for someone else. This often involves nothing more complex than giving one's time, sitting and talking with the person, sharing some of the load of the person's life. What could be simpler?

Like many things in life, the simple stuff often turns out to be the most complex. Nursing, as a professional discipline, differs greatly from the 'ordinary caring' provided by a friend or a relative. The difference is in the *context*. Caring for a friend or a relative is a moral duty or obligation, where the carer and the cared for are united by blood ties or the loyalty of love. Nurses often are required to care for people who have been abandoned by everyone else, or who may, for one reason or another, be difficult to care for, far less care *about*. Usually, nurses care for more than one person at a time, dealing with competing demands and often rapidly changing priorities. Such contextual challenges transform the ordinary *act of human kindness* into the *extraordinary discipline of human caring*.

In this section we begin with a consideration of the *nature of nursing* itself; how its meaning has changed over the years; and what is special about psychiatric and mental health nursing.

This leads, naturally, to a reflection on the challenges of 'getting personal'. How do nurses go about getting close to people in their care, getting to know them as persons and the nature of their unique human needs?

The profession of nursing, known by different names around the world, did not emerge out of a vacuum, but is merely the latest stage in the history of caring, which dates back centuries. We shall consider how things have changed down the years and what caring values remain intact.

Understanding the value of nursing, and the *evidence* that signals an appreciation of its worth, is central to current developments in the field. However, the nature of evidence has become a vexed issue, often confused by ideology or political bias. A *care*ful consideration of what evidence is and is not, will help the discipline clarify further its caring focus.

Debate has raged for at least a generation over whether nursing is an art or a science. This book raises an alternative perspective, the concept of nursing as *craft* is considered, and some critical thought is given to how we might *manage* the development of this craft in the complex world of practice.

Finally, we turn full circle to connect again with the *people* who might need nursing and who, given their status, might help nurses clarify the proper focus of their craft. These contributions are framed positively, emphasizing how nurses might aid and abet the recovery process, helping people to reclaim ownership of lives blighted or overtaken by mental distress.

The last two contributions in this section are the most important – reminding us of the *genuine purpose* of nursing. What – ultimately – is nursing *for*, if not to enable people to take back ownership of their lives and bid farewell to their professional carers?

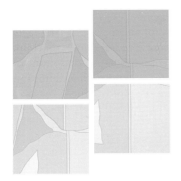

CHAPTER 1

The nature of nursing

Phil Barker*

Reflection

If you are a psychiatric or mental health nurse or are studying to become one, *ask yourself*:

- Why did I *want* to become a psychiatric–mental health (PMH) nurse?
- What did I *expect* that I would *do for* or *with* people as a nurse?
- To what extent are my original *expectations* of nursing, proving to be a reality?

If you are a member of another health or social care discipline, or someone with experience of mental health services, either as a 'patient', family member or friend, *ask yourself*:

- What is psychiatric–mental health nursing?
- What do these nurses do with or for the people in their care?
- In your experience, what do they *not* do that they *should* be doing?

WHY NURSING?

This is the most important chapter of all the chapters in this book. Not because it is the opening chapter, providing a 'way in' to the rest of the text, but because it invites you – the reader – to think about nursing.

- What is nursing?
- How do nurses do nursing?
- Why do they do this rather than anything else?
- How important is nursing to the welfare and recovery of people with any serious problem in human living?[a]

The answer to this last question is straightforward, if confusing.

- Psychiatric–mental health nursing is the *most important* discipline in mental health care worldwide.
- However, it is also the *least important*.
- Why the paradox?

NURSES: STILL INVISIBLE AFTER ALL THESE YEARS

When people have a 'mental breakdown', the Hollywood film drops them into the arms of a brilliant, humane and invariably caring psychiatrist.[1] Nurses, by contrast are invisible or, as de Carlo[2] noted, they occupy an 'aberrant, secret, and dangerous world' where their role is mainly that of 'custodial companionship'. If Nightingale was the icon for physical care nursing then, Nurse Ratched, from 'One flew over the cuckoo's nest', has become the mental health nursing icon (see http://en.wikipedia.org/wiki/Nurse_Ratched).[3]

Real life tells a different story. In hospital or community care, psychiatrists are few in number, and only fleetingly present at the care face.[b] In the 'real world' nurses are

---

*Phil Barker is a psychotherapist and Honorary Professor at the University of Dundee, UK.

---

[a] I use the term 'problem in living' since all forms of 'mental illness', 'psychiatric disorder' or other 'mental health problems' either *involve* or *result from* the person's *problem in living* with themselves, other people or life in general.
[b] Nurses often talk about the 'realities' of their everyday work as the 'coal face', implying that this is hard and dirty work. However, nurses have to 'get close' to the people in their care, becoming a recognizable face that the person comes to trust. In that sense, it might be more realistic to talk about the 'front line' of nursing as the *care face*.

the only caring constant.[3,c] Despite the media hype, when people talk about their 'recovery' from mental illness, they rarely name doctors, psychotherapy or even drugs. Instead, they talk about support, comfort, presence and other 'human' stuff,[4] which they believe sustained them on their recovery journey. They thank people who offered extraordinary human support, who nourished their souls. Apart from friends, families and other 'patients', invariably they thank *nurses*. This should not surprise us since 'psychotherapy' originally meant the 'healing of the soul (or spirit)', and nursing, originally meant 'to nourish'.

Some years ago, I had the privilege of spending time with Pat Deegan,[d] the famous American psychologist, survivor and key proponent of 'recovery' in mental health. We discussed her original 'breakdown', when she was diagnosed as a 'chronic schizophrenic' at 20 years of age and told 'not to hope for much'. Her recovery really began when she was discharged from hospital to a boarding house, where she roomed with 'a bunch of hippies'. This 'assortment of oddballs' supported her as she wrestled with her demons. 'They treated me like a person, not a patient', Pat recalled. Their caring acceptance appeared to kick start a process in which Pat began to care for, and also accept herself, for who she was. Although she went on to become a psychologist, rather than a nurse, her work emphasizes the social construct of nursing:[5] how to *support people* in facing life's challenges; how to help them *grow* and *develop as people*.

For Pat Deegan, what 'made a difference' was being accepted as 'just another human being', albeit with some problems in living. Those around her 'nursed' her in the most traditional manner, helping her to live and grow, from day to day. Ironically, this caring attitude was miles away from the kind of 'care' she had known as a hospital 'patient'. There are, however, many encouraging signs that nurses are beginning to reclaim 'genuine nursing' with all its human and social values.

WHAT IS PSYCHIATRIC AND MENTAL HEALTH NURSING?

In 2007, my colleague Poppy Buchanan-Barker and I tried to clarify the concept of psychiatric–mental health nursing and what it involved in practice.[6] We asked nurses from different countries: *'what is psychiatric and mental health nursing?'* and *'how do PMH nurses do nursing?'* To help them provide a brief answer we supplied examples of two-line definitions of medicine, psychology and social work, drawn from the Internet, and asked a range

of practitioners, leaders, researchers and professors – to *define* and *describe* their discipline in simple language. Most replied saying that they needed 'time to think about this'. Some needed weeks, others needed months, to come up with an answer. A few said such a definition *couldn't* be done, or, for various philosophical reasons, *shouldn't* be done. Almost all admitted that these were difficult questions.[e]

However, lay people were more forthcoming:

- Nurses *help* people;
- Nurses *relieve* a person's distress;
- Nurses help people *get through the day*, and *through the night*.
- Nurses help people '*deal with stuff … all sorts of stuff*'.[f]

However, behind these obvious, if not commonsense descriptions, lies a wealth of hotly disputed debate concerning what *is* (or is not) nursing; the *proper focus* of nursing;[7] and the often subtle difference between *care* and *treatment*. Maybe the nurses we involved in our study were trying to define psychiatric–mental health nursing as a *professional* idea, whereas the lay people described this as a human or social *service*.

Few of the nurses in our study referred to *caring* or *care*, except in very general terms – such as '*nurses give nursing care*', which is rather like saying 'doctors practise medicine'. However, one professor of nursing from the USA said that the field was divided into two 'camps'.

1 A subservient discipline and an extension of psychiatry's social control mechanism(s), for the policing, containment and correction of already marginalized people, which carried out a number of defensive, custodial, uncritical and often iatrogenic practices and treatments, based on a false epistemology and misrepresentation of what are, by and large, human problems of being, rather than so-called 'mental illnesses'.
2 A specialty craft that operates primarily by working alongside people with mental health problems; helping individuals and their families find ways of coping with the here and now (and past); helping people discover and ascribe individual meaning to their experiences; and exploring opportunities for recovery, reclamation and personal growth – all through the medium of the 'therapeutic relationship'.

> ### Reflection
>
> - How would you explain psychiatric–mental health nursing to a member of the public?
> - Which of the two groups described above do you belong to?

---

[c] The British psychiatrist, Albert Kushlick, once described everyone *except* nurses, as 'DC10s – offering direct care (DC) for only 10 minutes', before 'flying off' somewhere else.
[d] All the quotes here are taken from an interview with Pat Deegan, recorded in England in 1997. Available at: www.patdeegan.com.
[e] Further details of this study are available from the author at: phil.j.barker@btinternet.com.
[f] These are some of the replies we received when we asked a group of lay people 'what do nurses do?'

PSYCHIATRIC–MENTAL HEALTH NURSING: A DEFINITION

Of course, nursing was adequately defined over 50 years ago.[8]

> Nursing is a significant, therapeutic, interpersonal process. It functions cooperatively with other human processes that make health possible for individuals in communities … Nursing is an educative instrument, a maturing force, that aims to promote forward movement of personality in the direction of creative, constructive, productive, personal and community living.[9]

Peplau was defining what nurses focus on *doing*, and further developed this definition to represent nursing's *unique* focus:

> Nursing can take as its unique focus the reactions of the patient or client to the circumstances of his illness or health problem.[9]

Peplau was highly influential in the development of the *American Nurses Association's* definition of nursing:

> Nursing is the diagnosis and treatment of *human responses* to actual or potential health problems.[10]

The distinction between psychiatric *nursing* and psychiatric *medicine* was clear-cut for Peplau. The nurse's *primary* responsibility was to *nurture* and *aid* patients in their personal development through nursing services; helping 'guide patients in the direction of understanding and resolving their human dilemmas'.[11] The nurse's *secondary* responsibilities include cooperating with physicians who prescribe psychiatric treatments for patients.[11] Regrettably, in recent years, many PMH nurses have focused their attention on these *secondary* responsibilities. Some even assume that by emulating the work of their medical colleagues – e.g. by increasing their involvement in psychiatric diagnosis or prescribing of medication – they are 'advancing' the practice of nursing.

WHAT IS THE PURPOSE OF NURSING?

I have, for many years endorsed both the American Nursing Association (ANA) definition of nursing and Peplau's description of the 'proper focus' of psychiatric nursing. However, although the focus of nursing is clear, its *purpose* – what it was for – appeared less clear. Almost 20 years ago I tried to extend Peplau's original definition, by defining the purpose of nursing as *trephotaxis* – from the Greek, meaning 'the provision of the necessary conditions for the promotion of growth and development'.

- When nurses help people *explore* their distress in an attempt to discover ways of *remedying or ameliorating it*, they are practising *psychiatric* nursing.
- When nurses help the same people *explore* ways of *growing and developing*, as persons, exploring how they presently *live with* and might *move beyond*, their problems of living, they are practising *mental health nursing*.

These two forms of caring practice are closely related, with a highly fluid border separating them. The former might be seen as *problem focused* or situation specific, whereas the latter is more *holistic*: concerned with the person's life – how it is lived, along with its many inherent meanings.

By emphasizing the *purpose* of nursing, rather than its many different *processes*, more emphasis is given to the *developmental* and *educative* aspects of nursing, first described by Peplau. However, nurses do *not* 'make' people develop, far less 'change' them; *neither* do they 'teach' them anything directly. Instead, they provide the conditions necessary for the person to *experience* growth, development and change, and to learn something of significance from their own experience.[12]

Emotional rescue and psychiatric nursing

When people are acutely distressed, under threat – whether physical, psychological or spiritual – or presenting a risk to themselves or others, the high drama of the situation requires an equally dramatic nursing response. Here, the nurse might need to make the person and the environment as *physically safe* and *emotionally secure* as possible. This requires great skill and composure on the nurse's part. Such dramatic help is akin to the work of the lifesaver rescuing someone from drowning, or the fire-fighter delivering a person from a burning building. When people are suicidal or tormented by 'voices' they require just this kind of 'emotional rescue'. In such a situation the nurse provides the kind of *supportive conditions* that will reduce the experience of distress and prepare the way for a more detailed examination of what needs to be done *next*.

When nurses respond to people's distress by helping to contain it, delimit it or otherwise *fix* it, they are practising *psychiatric* nursing. Both the nurse and the person are locked in the present. The emphasis is on stemming the flow of distress, or keeping a watchful eye out for any signs of exacerbation of the original problem of living.

Growth and mental health nursing

As soon as the 'crisis' has passed, and the person – or their circumstances – appears to have calmed down, the focus turns to something more constructive and *developmental*. Once the 'drowning' person has been dragged ashore and is judged to be 'safe' the emphasis switches to 'rehabilitation': what needs to happen *now* to help the person return to normal living. If the person appears to have played a part in their own crisis – whether by accidentally falling or intentionally jumping into the river – the focus turns to an examination of the person's motives, or understanding of the risks involved. Of necessity, this will involve a more detailed, longer term enquiry, which aims to ensure the person's safety and well-being *in the future*. In such a situation:

The nurse tries to foster active *collaboration* – 'caring with' the person,[13] developing an active alliance, so that *together* they might develop an *understanding* of the problem, its personal meanings and relationship to the overall *life* of the person.

Such a careful, paced, developmental approach to clarifying the person's understanding of the *function* and *meaning* of her or his problems of living, and their possible solutions, is the substance of *mental health* nursing (www.patdeegan.com).

Nursing as a social activity

However, even if 'professional nursing' did not exist, people would still find 'ordinary nursing' in different areas of everyday life. People have been 'nursing' one another long before the birth of nursing, as a professional discipline. The most enduring example is the supportive care offered by parents to their children, which spans nations and cultures and is largely indistinguishable from the parenting found in the animal kingdom.

Being responsible for their offspring, parents shape the immediate physical environment of their young, ensuring that the 'space' is safe *and* will provide adequate room for growth. In the early stages of development, parental support is intimate and often very directive. As the child grows, the parents step back, allowing the child more opportunity to make decisions, *and mistakes*; helping the child towards autonomy and personal determination. If parents do not foster autonomy, they risk 'smothering' the child, suffocating its natural development. The ultimate aim of parenthood is *redundancy*: parents want their children to be able to survive without them. Nursing should embrace a similar ambition for redundancy.

Similar forms of 'ordinary nursing' are to be found in a variety of formal and loose-knit social groups, where members engage in mutual support, in an effort to develop resilience and encourage growth. The 'buddy system', made famous by Alcoholics Anonymous over 70 years ago,[14] inspired a range of other mutual-support and self-help groups. These do not try to control people, but to provide the kind of social support that might help members 'grow and develop', through and beyond their immediate problems. In many cases, the aim is to 'learn to live with' some problem, demonstrating that a full life is possible, despite the presence of a disability.

Reflection

- What groups have influenced how you think and feel about yourself and your life problems?
- How did the other group members influence you?

BACK TO BASICS: THE NATURE OF NURSING

The 'postmodern' problem

PMH nurses have struggled to *define* themselves and their work.[15] Some argue that the question of what nursing *is* 'has been "done to death" over the years, and we are no closer to a definition than we were fifty years ago'.[16] Other experienced and senior figures even question whether their discipline 'should be called "nursing" at all'.[17] Such comments are typical of the tortured self-examination found in the PMH nursing literature. Indeed, some contemporary authorities would argue that it is *impossible* to define PMH nursing as it involves a 'spectrum of roles, responsibilities and practices, defined by the economics, institutions and policies of the day'.[6] However, if nursing is simply to be whatever the 'economic, institutional and political' influences of the day demand, how do we avoid a repeat of the kind of 'nursing' that developed during the Third Reich.[18]

In these 'postmodern' times it has become unfashionable to attempt to 'define' things explicitly.[19] Some nursing academics argue that 'postmodernism considers reality to be subjective, not fixed or true and immutable'[20] and that 'postmodernism defies absolute definition because the words we use to describe it (or anything else) cannot be separated from the context in which those words are used'.[21] If we offer a definitive answer to a question, such as 'what is nursing?' we risk presenting our view as 'something special … another authorised version (grand narrative) of the nature of knowledge, from the academy'.[22] The problem with such postmodern debates, as Burnard argued, is that:

while they undermine any strong position, they also leave the commentator (or reader) unable to take any strong position for him or herself. Or, rather oddly, the reader can take any view. The writer's own view can, of course, always be undermined by another reading of that view. And so it all goes on, in a never-ending spiral that ultimately takes us nowhere particularly useful.[23]

Burnard seemed to be frustrated by *relativism*, which has been around for at least 2500 years.[24] However, when people say that their beliefs are 'true', do they mean 'just for me'? The philosopher, A. C. Grayling, does not think so, and offers a graphic example:

(Relativism may apply) in cases of taste or prefer-ence, and sometimes when there is known to be no way to settle a choice of view. But if I say that camels have humps, I do not mean to imply that it is simultaneously the case that camels have no humps just because someone else believes as much.[24]

This is the problem with so much 'philosophizing' in PMH nursing: it addresses 'things' in the abstract, but pays no attention to 'real things'.

I am uncomfortable with 'sitting on the fence' positions. I like to take a 'strong position' on issues that I consider to be important. In taking such a strong position, I have often found myself in conflict with received opinion, with trad-itional values and practices, and also with colleagues. So be it. If we believe that something needs changing, then dis-comfort may need to be part of the process of change.

Over a decade ago I wrote:

we need to forget how once we valued: competi-tiveness, domination, exploitation, fragmentation, blind reason and detached objectivity. (However) In these postmodern times, I remain comfortable declaring myself a humanist.[25]

It may be interesting, amusing and sometimes enlight-ening to see how people disagree about the nature of reality. However, if I was asked whether I could take a relativist view of nursing and say that *everyone's view* was *true*, my answer would be no.

- The people who sit in corridors, observing distressed people in their bedrooms, from a distance, may be called 'nurses' but *are not practising nursing*.
- The people who tell anguished people what is 'wrong with them' and then lecture them, however kindly, about the nature of their 'symptoms' may be called 'nurses', but *are not practising nursing*.
- The people who helped frail and disabled people to the gas chambers at Auschwitz may have been called 'nurses' but were *not practising nursing*.

One of my mentors (Annie Altschul) once said that 'a nurse is a person registered with the appropriate nursing council – there is no other definition'. This was, and still is accurate, but not particularly helpful. I want a defin-ition of nursing that 'works', that is more than just a label. Does it *do* what it says on the tin? If nurses *do not* 'provide the conditions necessary for growth and devel-opment', they may be doing something that is valued or approved by some professional body, but they are *not practising nursing* – as I understand it.

The nurses at Auschwitz were 'nurses'. We might excuse their actions on the grounds of 'just following orders', but could you describe their actions as 'nursing'?[g]

Common denominators

To gain any 'real' sense of 'nursing we need to deal with more basic issues. We need to grasp some fundamentals. Of course, 'nursing' will be different in different situ-ations, for different people, under different circum-stances, at different times. However, we need to put these 'differences' to one side and ask – what do these 'differ-ent' contexts have in common?

Despite the many different ways that nursing might be defined, there are some 'common denominators', which the philosopher might say represents some 'uni-versal truths'.

- People look after themselves, their family members and friends, animals, the environment, their prized possessions and a range of other 'things', in a way that might be called 'nursing'. They provide the conditions, under which the kinship, friendship, welfare or value of the person or thing will grow, develop or prosper.
- The athlete who sustains damage to a tendon or liga-ment is often said to be 'nursing an injury' – acting in such a way as to prevent the injury getting worse try-ing to promote healing.
- The seasoned drinker is often described as 'nursing a pint' – taking time over the consumption of a beer, savouring each mouthful, in a vain effort to prolong this enjoyable experience.
- The nurseryman, responsible for planting and overse-ing a new forest, 'nurses' his new shoots. The fragile new growth is sheltered from strong winds, and adequate drainage, irrigation and – most of all – *space* is made available, all of which are necessary if growth and devel-opment are to take place.[26]

In English, the words *nurse* and *nursing* have been used to represent fostering, tending or cherishing 'things' at least since the Middle Ages. PMH nursing stands in the shadow of those dictionary definitions, owing its very existence to ancient notions of the human value of tend-ing, and cherishing things, as part of our hopes to foster their growth and development.

THE CRAFT OF CARING

Blending art and science

Nurses have also debated whether nursing is an art *or* a science.[27] I believe that the practice of nursing requires both knowledge (science) and aesthetics (art), however these are blended to form a *craft*. Craft workers use their skills and knowledge to satisfy the demands or expect-ations of patrons or customers while satisfying their own aesthetic and technical ambitions.

---

g I chose this example for my mentor, Annie Altschul, *was* Jewish *and* a refugee from Nazi Germany.

Craftwork blends aesthetics and technique with the expectations of the patron. The craftsperson needs to know how to weave, dye or cut cloth; how much pressure silver will take without breaking; how high a temperature is needed to fire a piece of clay. This craft–science is augmented by some aesthetic – marrying shape, form and colour to suggest an unspoken, often culturally embedded message. The meaning and value attached to a wedding dress, a talismanic piece of jewellery or a pot, however, comes from the owner not the maker. Such value-making is invisible but transformative. Through such attribution, the crafted object becomes unique, if not magical; like no other, despite possible surface similarities.

The proper focus of nursing is the craft of caring. The value of care is defined by those who receive it.[13] How could it be otherwise? Yet, the nurse also brings value, expressed through carefulness and expertise. Knowing when to talk, what to say and when to remain silent while nursing a depressed, distressed or dying person takes great skill. This is not something that can be learned on a course, far less from books. It requires a lifelong apprenticeship, where the human tools of the trade are sharpened with every encounter.

The traditional image shows the craftsperson hunched quietly over the work, carefully, attentively and sensitively transforming the base material into something worthy of value. Genuine caring needs the same intimacy, quiet, care, attention and sensitivity to create the conditions under which the patient might begin to experience healing and recovery. In the clamour of the ward or clinic, nurses make a space – however metaphorical – for this to happen by being creative and resourceful, not by following protocols or national guidelines.

However, as health and social care has become increasingly organized, and subject to the influences of economics and the political philosophy of the day, this fundamental appreciation of nursing can become lost in a morass of policies, protocols and legislation.

However, although the term 'care' may have lost some of its original currency in nursing, 'caring' remains the universal, common denominator of PMH nursing. In the late twentieth century, many nurses grew dissatisfied with *caring*, exploring instead the idea of nursing as a *therapeutic* activity – in particular a behaviour change or psychotherapeutic activity. Of course, when nurses *care* effectively, what they do will be therapeutic – it will begin to provide the conditions under which the person can begin to be healed. As Nightingale observed: 'It is often thought that medicine is the curative process. It is no such thing; … nature alone cures. … And what [true] nursing has to do … is to put the patient in the best condition for nature to act upon him.'[28]

Psychotherapy originally meant the 'healing of the soul (or spirit)'. When nurses organize the kind of conditions

that help alleviate distress and begin the longer term process of recuperation, resolution and recovery, those activities become *therapeutic*, engendering the potential for healing.

Caring, sensitivity, attention to detail and respect

We should also value *caring* because it emphasizes the caution, attention to detail and sensitivity necessary when handling something precious. The archaeologist who seeks some long-lost treasure, may begin his work with strenuous and dramatic digging – excavating the site until there are signs that something of value might lie somewhere just below the surface. Then the powerful tools of excavation are exchanged for smaller tools, which can be used more sensitively. Finally, when a 'find' begins to emerge, these small tools are exchanged for brushes, used even more *carefully* to remove the earth and dust that hides the treasure.

The archaeologist's *careful* approach to unearthing and finally revealing a possible find suggests a *concern* and *respect* for the treasure. The team may have unearthed a relic from a bygone age, or they may simply have uncovered another stone. Either way, their work is characterized by *care, sensitivity* and *attention to detail*. These 'finds' are priceless – whatever their market value.

If a piece of pottery, buried in the earth a thousand years ago, is considered 'priceless', a person who is by definition unique should also be viewed as *priceless*. Respect for the person – irrespective of age, class, nationality, creed or colour, or the presumed nature or origins of their problems – lies at the heart of all the contributions in this book. If this is not a universal, defining characteristic of nursing, it should be.[29]

THE PURPOSE OF NURSING

This book considers the highly contested notion of 'mental health', which lacks any single, official definition.[30] However, this book is about *nursing* not about 'mental health'. In this sense, I hope that readers will discover in this book many examples of how, by *caring for people* diagnosed with one 'mental disorder' or another, they help those people to reclaim or attain the mercurial state known as 'mental health'. I hope that they will also discover how nurses might become social agents, in a much broader sense, helping families, communities and society at large to grow and develop, so that they might become healthy, meaningful and productive. Most of all, I hope that you will understand better what it is that nurses *do* in the name of nursing care, and why they do this rather than anything else.[31]

The progress of psychiatric and mental health nursing

In 2006 'reviews' of mental health nursing were published in England and Scotland.[32,33] One might have expected these reviews to talk, enthusiastically, about 'care' and 'caring'. Instead, the focus was on 'interventions', 'evidence' and 'technology'. Perhaps caring is no longer considered sexy, but science and technology is exciting! If the *craft of caring* is to make a difference in the world of mental health then nurses will need to embrace, carefully, both science and art, blending these together, to form a meaningful, practical reality – the *craft of caring*.

However, if a mental health 'revolution' is needed today, we need to ask to what extent *science* – in any form – will help make a significant contribution. History suggests that, however useful science in its various forms might be, it is not a necessary part of the 'mental health revolution'.

- Two hundred years ago, when the abolition of slavery began, this movement was not based on science or 'evidence' regarding the 'rights' or 'wrongs' of slavery, but on a *particular set of human values*.
- One hundred years ago, when the emancipation of women began, this movement was not based on science or 'evidence' regarding the 'rights' or 'wrongs' of votes for women, but on a *particular set of human values*.
- Fifty years ago, when the civil rights movement began in the USA, this was not based on science or 'evidence' regarding the 'rights' or 'wrongs' of racial equality, but on a *particular set of human values*.
- Thirty years ago, when the gay rights movement began to be taken seriously, this movement was not based on science or 'evidence' regarding the 'rights' or 'wrongs' of freedom of sexual expression, but on a *particular set of human values*.[34,35,h]

As Burnard[36] eloquently said, *caring* can give unselfish and even 'unrewarded' pleasure. Perhaps, the countless numbers of people who participated in the four 'revolutions' noted above, *cared* sufficiently to commit themselves – many at the expense of their health if not their lives – to make a change in their social world. It is difficult to imagine how those revolutions could have come about in the absence of caring.

Despite the absence of any solid 'scientific evidence', the significance of caring is obvious.

However it is viewed, it would seem that caring is an almost universal phenomenon and one linked to the very process of becoming and being a person … caring remains at the centre of the process of nursing, for whatever it is *not*, nursing is ultimately bound up with all aspects of the person.[36]

Reflection

- What does 'caring' mean to you?
- How important is 'caring' to PMH nursing?

NURSING THE WORLD

In 2007, the WHO and the International Council of Nurses published *Atlas: nurses in mental health*.[37] This reported that the number of skilled nurses was far too small to meet mental health service needs worldwide, and that basic and specialist training in mental health nursing was often absent or seriously deficient, even in more developed regions such as the European Union. In all continents, except Europe, there are fewer than three nurses in MH settings per 100 000 people.

Reporting these sobering statistics, Salvage[38] cited international mental health nursing expert, Ian Norman, as saying: 'the evidence base for MH nursing interventions is at its strongest for decades. Yet it is alarming that these interventions are not being delivered to patients in many parts of the globe because of inadequate training'. Professor Norman listed prescription and collaborative medication management; education and training of service-users to manage their illness; family psychosocial education; assertive community treatment; supported employment; and integrated treatment for people with mental illness and co-occurring substance use disorders as examples of the kind of 'evidence-based interventions' to which he was referring (I Norman, personal communication).

All these interventions are covered in later chapters, and may be good examples of mental *illness* services. However, if people in the more troubled and disadvantaged parts of the world are to realize their 'mental health' then something more radical will be necessary. They will need something more like the social actions that brought an end to slavery, opened the door to the emancipation of women, and guaranteed rights for 'people of colour' and gay and lesbian people.

If we are to 'make a difference' for people across the world, first of all, we need to care deeply about them and their plight. This intangible human value will fuel our advocacy, will sustain our interest in them and their problems of human living, and will foster the development of the range of innovative projects needed to

---

[h] Indeed, quite the reverse. Most 'contemporary science' supported slavery, the subjugation of women, segregation of 'coloured' people and the persecution of gay and lesbian people.

address the wide range of uniquely different social contexts.

If you are to make a real difference for the people in your village, city or community, you will need to *care about them*, as persons, so that you can begin to develop forms of collaborative support that will begin to address their unique problems of human living.

REFERENCES

1. Gabbard K, Gabbard GO. *Psychiatry and the cinema*, 2nd edn. New York, NY: American Psychiatric Press Inc, 1999.

2. De Carlo K. Ogres and angels in the madhouse: mental health nursing identities in film. *International Journal of Mental Health Nursing* 2007; **16** (5): 338–48.

3. Barker P. *The philosophy of psychiatric nursing*. Edinburgh, UK: Churchill Livingstone, 1999: 82.

4. Barker P, Jackson S, Stevenson C. The need for psychiatric nursing: towards a multidimensional theory of caring. *Nursing Inquiry* 1999; **6**: 103–11.

5. Barker P. Reflections on the philosophy of caring in mental health. *International Journal of Nursing Studies* 1989; **26** (2): 131–41.

6. Barker P, Buchanan-Barker P. What's the point? The death of vocation in the age of celebrity. Keynote address to the Conference: Health4Life Conference 2007 Thinking, Feeling, Being: Critical Perspectives and Creative Engagement in Psychosocial Health, Dublin City University, Ireland. www.dcu.ie/health4life/conferences/2007/resources/Health4Life2007_Keynote_Phil_Barker.pdf

7. Barker P, Reynolds B. Rediscovering the proper focus of nursing: a critique of Gournay's position on nursing theory and models. *Journal of Psychiatric and Mental Health Nursing* 1996; **3** (1): 75–80.

8. Peplau HE. *Interpersonal relations in nursing*. New York NY: Putnam 1952; reissued London: Macmillan, 1988: 16.

9. Peplau HE. Theory: the professional dimension. In: Norris CM (ed.). *Proceedings of the first nursing theory conference*. Kansas City, MO: University of Kansas Medical Center, 1969: 37.

10. American Nurses Association. *Nursing: a social policy statement*. Kansas City, MO: ANA, 1980: 9.

11. Peplau HE. Theoretical constructs: anxiety, self and hallucinations. In: O'Toole AW, Welt SR (eds). *HE Peplau selected works: interpersonal theory in nursing*. London, UK: Macmillan, 1994: 271.

12. Barker P, Buchanan-Barker P. *The tidal model: a guide for mental health professionals*. Hove, UK: Brunner Routledge, 2005.

13. Barker P, Whitehill I. The craft of care: towards collaborative caring in psychiatric nursing. In: Tilley S (ed.). *The mental health nurse: views of practice and education*. Oxford, UK: Blackwell Science, 1997: 15–27.

14. Alcoholics Anonymous. *Twelve steps and twelve traditions*, 38th edn. Center City, MN: Hazelden Publishing, 2002.

15. Cutcliffe J, Ward M. *Key debates in psychiatric and mental health nursing* [Editorial]. Edinburgh, UK: Churchill Livingstone, 2006: 22.

16. Clarke L. Declaring conceptual independence from obsolete professional affiliations. In: Cutcliffe J, Ward M (eds). *Key debates in psychiatric and mental health nursing*. Edinburgh, UK: Churchill Livingstone, 2006: 70.

17. Collins J. Commentary. In: Cutcliffe J, Ward M (eds). *Key debates in psychiatric and mental health nursing*, Edinburgh, UK: Churchill Livingstone, 2006: 46.

18. Berghs M, Diercks de Casterle B, Gastmans C. Practices of responsibility and nurses during the euthanasia programs of Nazi Germany: a discussion paper. *International Journal of Nursing Studies*, 2007; **44** (5): 845–54.

19. Holmes CA, Warelow PJ. Some implications of postmodernism for nursing theory, research, and practice. *Canadian Journal of Nursing Research* 2000; **32** (2): 89–101.

20. Williams R. From modernism to postmodernism: the implications for nurse therapist interventions. *Journal of Psychiatric and Mental Health Nursing* 1996; **3**: 269–71.

21. Stevenson C. Tao, social constructionism and psychiatric nursing practice and research. *Journal of Psychiatric and Mental Health Nursing* 1996; **3**: 217–24.

22. Stevenson C, Beech I. Paradigms lost, paradigms regained: defending nursing against a single reading of postmodernism. *Nursing Philosophy* 2001; **2**: 143–50.

23. Burnard P. Commentary. In: Cutcliffe J, Ward M (eds). *Key debates in psychiatric and mental health nursing*, Edinburgh, UK: Churchill Livingstone, 2006: 337.

24. Grayling AC. Grayling's question: How does one argue against a relativist? *Prospect Magazine* 2007: 133.

25. Australian Association for Mental Health (ANAMH). Keynote address. Life chances and mental health – forging ahead to the new millennium, 14 August 1997, Old Parliament House, Canberra. In: Barker P (ed.). *The philosophy and practice of psychiatric nursing*. Edinburgh, UK: Churchill Livingstone, 1999: 158.

26. Barker P. *The philosophy and practice of psychiatric nursing*. Edinburgh, UK, Churchill Livingstone: 1999.

27. Hirsch GA. Nursing: art or science. *Canadian Nurse* 1983; **79**: 4–5.

28. Nightingale F. *Notes on nursing: what it is, and what it is not*. New York, NY: D. Appleton and Company, 1860.

29. Barker P. Reflections on caring as a virtue ethic within an evidence-based culture. *International Journal of Nursing Studies* 2000; **37** (4): 32–6.

30. World Health Organization. *World Health Report 2001 – mental health: new understanding, new hope*, Geneva, Switzerland: WHO, 2001.

31. Barker P. Who cares any more, anyway? In: Wilshaw S (ed.). *Consultant nursing in mental health*. Chichester, UK: Kingsham Press, 2004.

32. Department of Health. *From values to action: the chief nursing officer's review of mental health nursing*. London, UK: DoH, 2006.

33. Scottish Executive. *Rights, relationships and recovery: the report of the national review of mental health nursing in Scotland.* Edinburgh, UK: Scottish Government Publications, 2006.

34. Szasz TS. *Insanity: the idea and its consequences.* New York, NY: Wiley, 1987.

35. Szasz TS. *Coercion as cure: a critical history of psychiatry.* London, UK: Transaction Publishers, 2007.

36. Burnard P. Why care? Ethical and spiritual issues in nursing. In: Brykczynska G (ed.). *Caring: the compassion and wisdom of nursing.* London, UK: Arnold, 1997.

37. *Atlas: nurses in mental health.* Available from: www.who.int/mental_health/en/index.html.

38. Salvage J. Ray of hope. *Nursing Standard* 2007; **22** (10): 18–19.

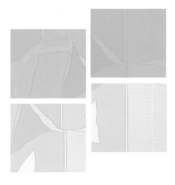

CHAPTER 2

Getting personal: being human in mental health care

Phil Barker* and Poppy Buchanan-Barker**

PEOPLE AND PROBLEMS OF LIVING

Making it personal

You are at work when the 'phone rings. A voice tells you that one of your loved ones has had a 'serious breakdown' and has been 'taken into care'. The exact nature of the 'breakdown' is not important. What is important is that someone – perhaps a parent, brother or sister, one of your children, a close friend, lover or partner – is in great difficulty. Perhaps they cannot fend for themselves. Perhaps they are acutely distressed. One thing is certain – they need help, otherwise they wouldn't be 'in care'.

Picture the scene. Put the 'loved one' who you are *most attached to*, right now, in this 'breakdown' situation. Let your imagination fill in some of the missing details.

Consider

- How might your loved one be feeling right now?
- What kind of things might she or he be asking for?
- What do you think could possibly have happened?

- What do you think is going to happen now?

Now, consider

- How are *you* feeling, right now?
- What thoughts are running through *your* mind?
- Does this mean that *you* are a 'carer' now?
- If so, what does that *mean*, anyway?

This 'imaginary' story may have happened to you and, therefore, is a 'real' memory. Few of us have not had 'bad news' such as this at some point in our lives. This imaginary scenario might well remind you of some of the feelings you have had before in your life.

When you feel sufficiently connected, *emotionally*, to this imaginary story ask yourself this simple, but critical question:

What would you *want to be done* for your loved one in the name of care?

Close this book *now* and take some time to think about this question.

---

*Phil Barker is a psychotherapist and Honorary Professor at the University of Dundee, UK.
**Poppy Buchanan-Barker is therapist and counsellor and former social worker. She is Director of Clan Unity International, the mental health recovery agency.

---

^a Attributed to a Scottish minister, John Thomson, who called his Edinburgh parishioners his 'bairns'.

We are a' Jock Tamson's bairns[a]

Poppy has asked this 'hypothetical' question, of literally thousands of workshop participants over the past 10 years, in different countries and across different cultures. Although people may speak a different language, or may be governed by different laws, or possess different cultural values, everyone gives much the same answer. Everyone wants *their* 'loved one' to be treated as a *person*: a unique, special, distinctive *human being*.

No one we have met is comfortable with the idea of their loved one becoming a 'patient' or 'client' or 'user' or 'consumer'. Instead, everyone wants the care team, who-ever they are, from whatever discipline, to recognize and respect the individuality – and difference – of their 'loved one'. The responses of these thousands of people to this simple question represent a powerful piece of human enquiry. In one way this is more significant than the results of any scientific survey or poll. The people in these workshops took time to reflect on what *they* would *want* for *their* 'loved ones'. They also discussed the question and their differing responses with everyone else present.

Interestingly, few were surprised that others also chose to focus on the 'human' situation of their loved one. Despite our ethnic, racial, cultural and social differences, people are very much alike 'under the skin'. In Scotland we say 'we are a' Jock Tamson's bairns': we are all part of the same human family. In a similar, but more formal vein, the American psychoanalyst Harry Stack Sullivan famously said: 'everyone is much more simply human than otherwise'.[1] Rather than discuss *psychopathology* Sullivan preferred to talk about people's 'problems in living'.[1,p.10] Today, we compliment ourselves for being 'person centred' or 'person focused'. Although probably not the first, Sullivan understood the importance of 'get-ting personal' over 80 years ago.

Where people are concerned, problems of living are always *human* problems, involving other *human* beings, or the everyday, and highly complex business of *human* living.

Human values for human services

In our work over the past decade we have tried to get back to the caring bedrock of human services.[2] We need to clarify what *exactly* are our professional values[3] if we are ever to escape the lunatic bureaucracy that bedevils all our talk about 'patients' and 'users' and their need for CBT (cognitive–behaviour therapy) or DBT (dialectical–behaviour therapy) or PSI (psychosocial interventions) or some other truncated form of 'therapy',[4] when per-haps what the person needs is *human helping*. What we would want for our 'loved ones' may be simple, but apparently not all that easy to assure.

The following points describe what we want from a caring service.

- *Do no harm*. This evokes the fundamental principle, found in the Hippocratic oath. Hippocrates said: 'As to diseases, make a habit of two things – to help, or at least to do no harm'. When charged with the responsi-bility of caring for someone we need to keep asking: what would be helpful? and how do we avoid doing harm?

- *Maintain dignity and respect*. When people become 'patients' or 'clients' they risk being treated as a 'thing' or an 'illness', and risk being exposed to all manner of humiliations and indignities. We need to cultivate an atmosphere where the *person's* human dignity is main-tained and the person is respected *as a person* in her or his own right. If we can manage this, we (the carers) will be more likely to be treated with dignity and respect in return.

- *Provide a safe haven*. Even if people are being 'cared for' in their own homes, they need to feel safe and secure – emotionally as well as physically. We worry a lot about people being physically injured. To what extent do we worry about their emotional security? People are precious. Indeed, people are priceless, and often need a place of sanctuary, where they can experience peace and quiet; feeling that they are pro-tected, and where the distress that rages within them is 'contained' by the caring team.

- *Accept people for who they are*. Every 'patient' is some-one's mother or someone's son, someone's best friend, or someone's lover. They are *special* to someone. People in need of care can often be 'difficult' to care for – for one reason or another. However, we do not have to *love* them as one of our own loved ones, neither do we have to *like* them as one of our friends. All we need do is accept them for who they are: a *person* special to some-one, who is presently experiencing difficulties.

- *Feed them well and keep them comfortable*. Food, drink and personal comfort cannot be rated too highly. Care settings often pay insufficient attention to these human essentials. Paying attention to special dietary needs and fancies, and trying to make eating, drinking and relaxing an enjoyable experience, may not resolve the problems that brought the person into care. However, this will help build their strength for the recovery journey that lies ahead.

- *Nurture an atmosphere of hope for recovery*. For a very small number of people, life is so difficult that they would happily settle for a life 'in care'. Most people, however, want to 'get over' or 'resolve' their problems of living as quickly as possible, so that they can return to their lives, and their own loved ones, again. Nursing is about nurturing an atmosphere within which the person can begin to imagine life beyond care, and begin to take the practical steps necessary to leave the care setting. (A similar set of values are described by our late colleague Loren Mosher.[5])

Reflection

Our values represent what we consider most *important* in life. What are your values?

The value of humility

We have spent over 40 years in the care field trying to work out what *exactly* we should be doing, if we are to help people and avoid doing them harm. We are not confident that we have found the perfect answer to this question, but we believe that we have found a good place to begin.

To work with a *person* who is experiencing some problem of human living rather than a *patient* with some illness, disease or disorder, we need to be modest, as well as respectful. We need to recognize that we know nothing of any real significance about this person. However, if we can be patient, and the person is willing to teach us, we might learn something about this person, and what ails them. In our view, *humility* is a key feature of caring.

To approach the person *respectfully*, we would ask the following questions.

- What do you believe are the problems or needs that brought you into our care?
- How big (or small) do you think these problems or needs are?
- What do you already have, or own, that might play a part in helping to resolve or meet these needs?
- What do you think needs to happen to bring about what you would call a positive change in your life?[2,p.103]

We discovered that our old friend Loren Mosher had used a similar set of questions during his time working at Soteria House in the early 1970s. He asked every new 'patient':

- Why are you here?
- What happened in your life that resulted in your coming (or being brought) to a psychiatric ward?
- What needs to be done to 'fix' the situation, and how can we help you with the 'fixing' process?[6]

We have long shared a common interest in *persons* who might need help rather than *patients* who need to be treated. As Robert Whitaker noted recently:

> If you read articles in medical journals on the merits of drug treatments, you'll find that they always discuss how the medications reduce *symptoms*. What you won't find in those reports is any sense of the *people* who are being so treated. There is no sense that we are talking about an individual with a life history, and that there was a path – most likely one filled with trauma – that led up to their psychotic breaks. Nor is there any discussion of how they are faring as human beings. Are they forming friendships, pursuing ambitions, able to feel the world?[7]

It is not *only* nurses who should be interested in 'patients' as persons. Whether we call them 'clients' or 'consumers' or 'service users', social workers, psychiatrists, psychologists and other therapists might benefit from expressing an interest in the person so named. However, given their close working relationship with the people in their care – involved in everything from listening to the stories of their distress to helping them use the toilet – nurses should have a greater interest in the 'personal' than any other health and social care discipline.

HUMANS, PERSONS, PROBLEMS

Personal illustration 2.1: Mary's story

People had noticed that Mary had changed over the past year – neighbours, friends and especially her family. She gets up during the night, ransacking drawers and cupboards, searching for precious things she has lost, that she believes have been stolen. She says that, sometimes, she comes downstairs to find the living room full of strangers. Their presence does not appear to disturb her, but she does wonder who they are and what they are doing there. Her oldest son, Archie, who visits his mother regularly, has never seen these strangers but is reluctant to suggest that they might be a figment of her imagination. Mary, who is in her mid-70s, has been widowed for over a decade and recently had to have her pet dog put down. Her family doctor is worried about her and decides to refer her to the local mental health service for older people for further assessment.

Personal illustration 2.2: Jake's story

Jake was bright but had trouble making friends. Arguably the smartest in his family, his grades started to slip in his mid-teens and he grew increasingly distant. Some nights his father would find him sitting naked in the garden, gazing at the stars. Last weekend he painted his whole bedroom black when his family went to visit his grandmother in hospital. His parents have separated twice before but always patched things up, for the sake of Jake and his two sisters. They argue a lot these days over Jake. His father thinks he is taking drugs but his mother says he is just a creative type. Sharon, his younger sister, is very close to Jake and he talks to her about some of the strange sensations he gets, like hands running over his body. Karen, the eldest, has a boyfriend who thinks Jake is 'seriously weird'. His teachers agree and he is referred to the school psychologist.

Mary and Jake are real people. We knew them both – one personally and the other professionally. We have disguised their names and some of the details of their story, but 'who' they are still shines through. We re-tell a tiny bit of their stories, for telling stories is the stock-in-trade of psychiatric and mental health nursing. When nurses meet the people in their care, all they can reasonably do is talk to them, and listen carefully to what they say. If they are lucky, the person will tell them a story about what has happened to them, or what has been happening for them, and what sense they make of this.

Often, the story might not make 'sense' – in any classic 'logical' manner. No one has actually seen the 'strangers' who Mary says fill her living room. Who are these people? Why not ask Mary? Certainly, they seem all too real to her.

Similarly, who really has any idea of what it is like to have 'hands running all over your body'? Well, Jake does, so why don't we ask him to tell us more about this?

Commonly, professionals don't ask Mary or Jake to talk, for the simple reason that they are thought to be demented or crazy, bereft of reason and unlikely to make any sense. Why bother?

Increasingly, we are encouraged to believe that people who are in the grip of one form of madness, or another, are having experiences that are the product of 'disturbed biochemistry' or 'over-large ventricles'. This may well be true. However, even a 10-year-old child would ask:

- Why does Mary *think* her house is full of strangers?
- Why does Jake *feel* hands running all over his body?
- Does everyone with disturbed biochemistry or over-large ventricles have *exactly* these experiences?
- If not, *why not*?

Even if these 'hunches' about the causes or origins of madness held water, a curious, empathic, compassionate human being would still ask:

- So what is it like for you (Mary or Jake) to have these experiences?'

If we do not ask these simple questions – the kind of questions a 10-year-old child would ask – we risk letting down the human side. We risk forgetting that they are human beings experiencing very special problems of human living. Further, we risk treating them as some kind of 'thing' other than a human being.

When people like Mary and Jake meet us, they reveal something of 'who' they are through their behaviour and they begin to reveal even more as they begin to talk about 'themselves'. Of course, no one reveals *all* of themselves. Very few of us *know* ourselves in any complete sense, so we cannot reveal everything. However, this process of revelation is important not only for the nurses, who gain some understanding of the person in their care, but also for the person, who may gain further insights into their human nature, and 'what' this might mean to others.

Hopefully, the nurses who encountered Mary and Jake would ask themselves some fundamental questions, such as: who exactly *is* Mary, and who *is* Jake? Hopefully, they also wondered about what, exactly, was going on in their lives? Only rarely do we get anything like a satisfactory answer, for these are provocative questions. We need to take a close look at the person, if we are ever to appreciate 'who' they are.

Our common fear of getting *too* close to people bred the psychiatric tradition of viewing people through the lens of diagnosis and classification, where they become *objects of study* – like plants or animals – somehow set apart from us. This objective approach is not entirely foolhardy, and some of the authors in this book will illustrate their belief in the value of choosing this approach to assessment. However, it seems clear that when viewed from a safe distance, or through the reverse telescope of diagnosis, which appears to *reduce* the complexity of the person, problems *seem* more distinct, tidy and intelligible. Things appear simpler from a distance. Viewing the person from a distance also often feels much safer. The closer we get, however, the less clear-cut and the more complex human problems become, and (invariably) the less comfortable we feel.

Through the psychiatric lens, Mary and Jake are classic examples of people at different stages of the development of different forms of 'serious mental illness'.[b] Traditionally, Mary's assessment would explore the possibility that she is depressed or developing a dementia. Jake might well just be a sensitive, creative type, but the psychologist will probably be looking for evidence of substance abuse or schizophrenia. Although such an *examination* of the 'patient' might be useful – either in the short or longer term – it is only one way of 'looking' at people in human distress. Even if we could state categorically, based on rigorous clinical examination backed up by laboratory tests, that Mary or Jake *had* a specific form of mental illness or psychiatric disorder, we would hope that nurses would still be primarily interested in knowing what the *experience* of dementia or schizophrenia was *like* for Mary and Jake.

> ## Reflection
>
> If you met either Mary or Jake for the first time what kind of questions would you want to ask them *as a person*, rather than a patient?

BEGGING QUESTIONS

This is a book about *people* like Mary and Jake. There will be various references to *clients*, *users*, *consumers*, *patients*, *survivors* and *experts by experience*. However, we hope that the reader does not lose sight of the human fact that

---

[b] Although in common usage, the term 'serious mental illness' is objectionable for several reasons, not least for the implication that some forms of 'mental illness' are trivial, or 'not serious'.

all are *people*, first and foremost. Different authors will approach psychiatric and mental health nursing from different angles. However, all are interested in the people who become the focus of nursing care and attention. Their differing perspectives reflect the different philosophical and theoretical perspectives associated with psychiatric and mental health nursing in the twenty-first century.

Despite the emphasis on developing person-centred *care*, we recognize that caring rarely can stand alone, and may even need the support or challenge of differing perspectives. We hope this book will show how these differing perspectives can be harmonized.

The various authors discuss how we might go about identifying what *exactly* might be going on in the lives of people like Mary and Jake, and how we – as a caring discipline – should respond.

- What is the *nature* of their present difficulties?
- How might we *support* Mary and Jake?
- How might our offer of help, whatever it entails, *fit in* with what other professionals might choose to do, or feel obliged to do?
- What will the *family* expect of us, as nurses?
- What will *Mary* and *Jake* expect of us?

The reality of human experience is that our *needs* are often subject to dramatic change. Sometimes we are like *this* and other times we are like *that*. The changeable nature of our experience – of ourselves, of others and the world in general – determines that a person's *needs* at any point in time are also subject to change.

Different authors will adopt different approaches to working out an answer to the question: what does the person need *now*? Some will begin, as we have done here, with part of someone's story, using this as a springboard for examining what might need to happen next. The author is trying to build a 'theory of the person' that might inform care. Others will begin from a formal theoretical perspective, using understandings about people *in general* to help us understand *this person* in particular. In our view, both approaches have different values but each, in the right context, is equally valid. Flexibility is one of the keys to opening the way to appropriate and, hopefully, enhanced human care. Hopefully the reader will come to appreciate, better, the need for flexibility of thought, as well as action, in the development of person-centred care.

There are very few answers to the problems that people experience in their lives. However, there are lots of interesting questions that we can ask, which might help us understand what might need to be done, now, to begin to address such problems. This book is dedicated to exploring these questions.

We hope that you – the reader – will become more inquisitive and respectful of the people you will meet who are placed in your care; we hope that you will never stop asking questions about what the person might need in the way of help; and we hope that you will never assume that what might be helpful for one person will, necessarily, be helpful for another.

People and persons

A hallmark of professional caring is the establishment of a close, confiding relationship. We need to get close enough to the person emotionally to begin to appreciate the human nature of their difficulties. Like lifesavers, we need to get into the water and get wet, if we are to begin to help the person. However, we need to avoid becoming so caught up in the person's experience that we 'drown' with them. When we cannot distinguish our feelings from those of the person, we risk exactly that kind of metaphorical drowning. This notion of getting close, but not taking over the person's experience, is a thread that runs through most, if not all, of the chapters in this book. We can never know another person's experience, but we can find out a little of what the person says that experience is *like*. Neither should we want to live the person's life for them.

We need to avoid smothering people with our care, advice and help. Instead, we offer people what they need right now – *and no more*.

Nursing is an interpersonal process, involving the establishment and development of complex relationships between nurses and the people in their care, their family and friends, as well as other health and social care disciplines. It also involves a complex of relationships between different aspects of the person who is the nurse.[8]

We should not forget that nurses too are people. They are women or men, who may be gay, straight or bisexual. They may have had multiple partners or may be celibate. They may be 'white' or 'black' or 'coloured', but on closer examination may be the product of a whole string of racial, ethnic and cultural influences. They may be the oldest or youngest members of a family, or have grown up in an orphanage. They may be the only child of a single parent, or the middle child of 13 siblings. They may be married, single, divorced, separated or widowed. They may be members of one of the traditional faiths – Christianity, Islam, Judaism, Hinduism or Buddhism; or belong to a little-known religious sect; or be an atheist, agnostic or 'fair-weather churchgoer'.

It goes without saying that nurses bring these dimensions of themselves to their relations with people in their care. On occasions, these personal aspects of the nurse may intrude into the professional aspects of the individual nurse. A key obligation of professional practice is to become aware of how such differing personal, social and cultural characteristics might influence our professional decision-making, and our relations with the person who is the patient or client.

Reflection

You are a person. If you met a friendly extraterrestrial from another planet, how would you explain what it meant to be a person? What would you tell ET?

Nursing as a human service

Nursing is, first and foremost, a human service: offered by one group of human beings to another. The extent to which one group (nurses) really differs from the other (patients or clients) is debatable. However, within the power dynamic of care, where one person has a *duty* to care for the other, the relationship is often artificially distinguished. Before we begin to consider how psychiatric and mental health nurses might develop the knowledge and skills that might allow them to help Mary and Jake, let us ask two simple, yet important, questions:

1 If you were Archie, what would you want for your mother? Why would you want *this*, rather than anything else?

2 In the same vein, if you were Sharon, what would you want for your brother, Jake? And why would you want this, rather than anything else?

We begin with these very *personal* questions since your answers will say something about you as a *person*, as distinct from you as a professional, whether you are a student or an experienced practitioner. Your answers will suggest some of the values, beliefs and prejudices – and perhaps even interpersonal problems – that have shaped you as a human being.

In most Western countries the first thing that might happen to Mary or Jake is that they might be admitted, perhaps against their will or wishes, to a psychiatric unit, or be obliged to receive a visit from a crisis team, or a member of a community mental health team. There, the problems Mary and Jake have been experiencing in their everyday lives will be examined by a whole string of professionals. Their problems will be subject to the highly unusual, and often frightening, spotlight of the psychiatric system. Perhaps you wanted your hypothetical mother or brother to be put 'under the spotlight', but we

doubt it. We suspect that you were thinking of something less harsh, and certainly a lot less threatening.

By putting ourselves, firmly, in the position of 'loved ones', we begin to appreciate why Mary and Jake, Archie and Sharon and all the family and friends that make up their close social circle, often feel let down by the services we offer. Because they are linked to Mary and Jake, in all sorts of ways, their view of what their 'loved one' needs, may differ markedly from our objective, often distant, sometimes wrongheaded, view of the person's needs. By reminding ourselves that the person who is the 'patient' or 'client' is someone's *mother* or *daughter*, *sister* or *brother*, *friend* or *lover*, we remind ourselves of the *human value* of the person. By focusing on the human being – the *person* – we remind ourselves of the potential weaknesses, or pitfalls, of what we might offer through a standardized professional service.

Various circumstances – such as inadequate funding, poor staffing, restrictive policies, or inter-professional disagreements – can appear to stop us delivering the kind of care, which we consider appropriate or necessary. However, such circumstances should not influence our judgement about what is really needed in the name of appropriate nursing care. When we view the need-for-nursing scenario[9] through the lens of our loved ones, all too often we can see the inappropriateness and deficiency of our nursing response writ large. It can offer a humbling, yet intensely revealing, perspective on the need for, and development of, individually focused care.

Mental health and human development

The relationship between people in need of nursing, and those who care for them, resembles the child–parent relationship. People who experience any one of the myriad threats to their personal or social identities commonly called *mental illness*, or *mental health problems*, experience a human threat that makes them vulnerable. For some, this vulnerability – which waxes and wanes – may last for a considerable time. Such people are not vulnerable every moment of every day. However, such is the nature of their difficulties, or their circumstances, that this perceived vulnerability casts a shadow over their lives; and often limits their opportunities for further human growth and development. For others, their vulnerability is more sharply defined, and the perceived threats to their physical safety or emotional security are more marked. Often described as 'acutely' mentally ill, such a person's degree of vulnerability may also fluctuate. However, when it does present itself, this may represent a formidable challenge to the person, often suggesting the need for some intensive or sophisticated support to address the emergent crisis.

Such physical, emotional and existential threats may, temporarily, disable or limit the person's capacity to operate, constructively, in the world. The greater the nature of the threat and concomitant vulnerability, the greater will be the person's perceived 'need for nursing'. In almost all societies, when a citizen's vulnerability or degree of concomitant incapacity is pronounced, provisions are made in law to detain the person in a safe and supportive environment until the threat has either abated or is, in some sense, 'under control'.

Such attitudes towards people experiencing a temporary or prolonged life crisis, reflect the moral scruples of society. Once regarded as the hallmark of a civilized society, the development of organized forms of care (and treatment) for people viewed as being 'mentally ill' reflects the moral values commonly associated with parents and their offspring. In much the same way as parents are (at least in principle) responsible for the safekeeping and physical, intellectual and emotional development of their children, so society adopts a similar role in relation to its members. Those who appear unable (or even unwilling) to care for themselves receive the kind of support that might meet their needs, either now or in the future.

However, many people reject or are never able to access the kind of support they believe they need to deal with their life difficulties. Consequently, the view of a caring society sketched above appears false or idealistic. We assume that readers are interested in advancing *mental health* care, so we assume that an idealistic stance is the best place to begin.

Through clarifying what, *exactly*, people need to live with, or begin to resolve, the problems of human living that affect them, nurses might begin to develop *mental health* services that are genuinely worthy of the name. This might be very different from the mental *illness* services – often focused only on the amelioration of distress, or the management of crises – that commonly operate under the wholly inappropriate title of 'mental *health* services'.

NAME CALLING AND LABELLING

> Sticks and stones may break my bones but names will never hurt me.

What we call people, and their various experiences, and the services that they receive – will play an important part in this book. As children, we both recall singing out the 'sticks and stones' lines whenever someone tried to taunt us; an example of children putting on a brave face, for in truth some names did hurt and they still do. Many of the everyday terms used already in this chapter – mental *illness*, mental *health*, *enduringly mentally ill*, *acutely mentally ill*, *patient*, *client* – are highly loaded, especially in terms of their emotional impact on people to whom they are applied. To complicate matters, they mean different things to different people. Indeed, mental

illness and mental *health* – two expressions that are fundamental to this book – possess no clear, accepted definition. However, they are used in everyday conversation *as if* their meaning is unambiguous.[10]

However, these linguistic confusions either do not matter or may even be helpful. If we are unsure of what, exactly, these terms mean, we might be more careful in using them. Alternatively, if we believe that the meanings are obvious, we can simply get on with dealing with 'illness' and promoting 'health'.

One of the key principles underlying the philosophy of this book is that nurses do *not* deal with illness, disease or disorder. This is something that we believe. However, as you will discover, some other authors might have differing views. Such 'differences of opinion' are important, as they may help you to work out what you believe – and why!

We believe that nursing is a special kind of human response to the problems of living that people experience when they are viewed as ill, disordered, diseased or dysfunctional. In that sense, nursing is focused on *human responses* to *human problems*.[11] Nursing may augment and complement the services provided by various other health and social care practitioners, but its unique focus is on providing a human response to some very special human problems.

Nurses are mainly involved in providing the kind of support that will help people to reduce the experience of distress, so that they might make decisions for themselves, act for themselves and live their lives as autonomously as possible, given their immediate circumstances. Given such a focus, quibbles over whether they are mentally ill or healthy will become redundant. Arguably, few people are fully healthy – if by that we mean 'whole'. Most people are, however, sufficiently healthy to be able to act for themselves and to influence, constructively, the direction of their lives. Perhaps this focus, on how people live their lives and their capacity to transfer their constructive choices and decisions into a meaningful reality, should be the focus of nursing care plans. Nurses do not heal or otherwise cure people of their various ailments – physical or mental, emotional or spiritual. When nursing does succeed in making a difference, however, the person is placed – as Nightingale famously remarked – in the right condition to be healed by Nature or by God.[12]

Reflection
What names have you been called that you found unsettling, offensive or demeaning?
Consider why these particular names affected you in the way they did.

Vive la différence!

In this book you will read the work of authors from different countries and different philosophical, theoretical and practice backgrounds. This diversity will result in some cases in different emphases being given within the chapters. These differing backgrounds influence our perception of the human problems that people bring to the field of mental health care; what might be the nursing response to such problems; and what this might mean for the development of the discipline of nursing. We hope that you will, like us, value such diversity, seeing it as a positive asset, reflecting the value of holding different, perhaps changeable, views of nursing – *what it is*, *how it works* and what it might *mean* for health care.

Given the complexity of twenty-first century mental health care, and the social and cultural worlds it inhabits, a single, monolithic, unchanging view of 'what needs to be done' seems as inappropriate as it does unlikely. We hope you will agree.

Persons and citizens

Over the past few years, debates have raged over what to call the people who use mental health services. In the UK the expression 'users' has become fashionable, although – given its older association with illicit drugs – the term is seen, by some, as problematic. In the USA and Australia, efforts to streamline health care along business lines led, indirectly, to the popularization of the term 'consumer'. However, the extent to which anyone who receives a mental health service has anything like the rights of the average 'consumer' is debatable, to say the least. The term 'client', well established in social work and counselling, has also enjoyed some popularity, arguably on the grounds that it acknowledges the independent status of the person using the service. The expression derives from the Latin *cliens*, which referred to a plebeian – a working-class person of low birth – who was supported by a patrician – or nobleman. The *cliens* offered the patrician loyalty and service in return for which he received support and security. To a great extent this reflects the power relationship between professionals and 'clients' in current mental health services, where much emphasis is given to compliance and the inherent wisdom of the professional. Although considered by many to be outmoded, the term 'patient' still has much to recommend it. Certainly people who receive mental health services often are required to exercise great patience as they await the outcomes of the deliberations of the nursing team, or as they wait, patiently, for nurses to recognize what are their true needs.

Our need to find ways of defining the people who receive mental health services has become something of a professional neurosis. It is not at all clear why we cannot simply call people who use nursing services, *people*!

We can recall arguing the case for 'persons' and 'people' over 20 years ago. Perhaps, the recognition that 'patients' are 'persons' (like us) is too uncomfortable: reminding us that they have the same rights as us, are just as valuable or precious as us, and (at least in principle) have the same human rights as us. So why do we need to call 'them' anything other than their name – or persons and people?

In the traditional world of health care – where the presumed 'illness' and its 'aetiology' were seen as all-important – the human dimension has often been neglected. It is easy to become so focused on the person's illnesses or presumed disorder that we risk forgetting the human dimensions of people like Mary and Jake. Some years ago, on a trip to New Zealand, we encountered the Maori expression:

What is the most important thing to the world?

It is the people, it is the people, it is the people.

Maori people recognize that *who* people are is very much a function of the family relations, culture and the heritage of the ancestors. This *people* focus offers a fitting frame for our consideration of what anyone might need by way of a nursing service.

- How might we help people to grow and develop, as human beings, so that they might become more aware of the *problems of living* they experience, which commonly are called mental illness or psychiatric disorder?
- How might we help people to address, deal with and perhaps recover from, or overcome, the *problems* and *difficulties* that distress them, or limit their ability to function effectively in the world?

The focus of nursing is to help *people* identify, name and begin to control, manage or live with, different problems of human living. In that sense, nursing has much in common with psychotherapy, where it has long been clear that the 'method' of therapy is not as important as the personal qualities of the helper/therapist.[13]

This 'person-meets-person' scenario is, arguably, the most challenging aspect of psychiatric–mental health nursing. In this era of evidence-based practice there exists a considerable risk that nurses might assume that there is some 'method', 'technique' or 'technology' that can be 'administered effectively' to all 'patients' with the same 'diagnosis'. The truth – dare we use such a powerful word – is simpler, yet more complex. Each person's problems may, superficially, be similar to those of another person, but this is the most dangerous of half-truths. As Allport[14] keenly observed – each person is like *every other* person, like *some other* people, like *no other* person. Once nurses realize that their most precious and valuable 'tool' is their personal selves, they might realise that their unique contribution to care rests within their personal uniqueness. As nurses they are no more or less unique than the people whom (hopefully) they serve.

Such realizations might spark interest in *creating* a novel caring response to a unique set of human problems – or at least what the person-patient believes are a unique set of circumstances. Now, caring can become interesting, challenging and potentially much more rewarding.

REFERENCES

1. Evans FB. *Harry Stack Sullivan: interpersonal theory and psychotherapy*. London, UK: Routledge, 1996: 18.

2. Barker P, Buchanan-Barker P. *The tidal model: a guide for mental health professionals*. Hove, UK: Brunner-Routledge.

3. Buchanan-Barker P, Barker P. The ten commitments: a value base for mental health recovery. *Journal of Psychosocial Nursing and Mental Health Services* 2006; **44** (9): 29–33.

4. Buchanan-Barker P, Barker P. Lunatic language. *Openmind* 2002; **115**: 23.

5. Mosher LR. Non-hospital, non-drug intervention with first episode psychosis. In: Read J, Mosher LR, Bentall RP (eds). *Models of madness: psychological, social and biological approaches to schizophrenia*. London, UK: Routledge, 2004: 351.

6. Mosher LR, Hendrix V. *Soteria: through madness to deliverance*. Philadelphia, PA: Xlibris, 2004: 298.

7. Whitaker R. Foreword. In: Mosher LR, Hendrix V (eds). *Soteria: through madness to deliverance*. Philadelphia, PA: Xlibris, 2004.

8. Peplau HE. *Interpersonal relations in nursing*. London, UK: Macmillan, 1987.

9. Barker P, Jackson S, Stevenson C. The need for psychiatric nursing. *Journal of Psychiatric and Mental Health Nursing* 1999; **6** (4): 273–82.

10. Stevenson C. Living within and without psychiatric language games. In: Barker P, Stevenson C (eds). *The construction of power and authority in psychiatry*. Oxford, UK: Butterworth-Heinemann, 2000.

11. American Nurses Association. *Nursing: a social policy statement*. Kansas, MO: ANA, 1980.

12. Barker P. Reflections on caring as a virtue ethic within an evidence-based culture. *International Journal of Nursing Studies* 2000; **37** (4): 32–6.

13. Bohart AC, Tallman K. The active client: therapy as self-help. *Journal of Humanistic Psychology* 1996; **36** (3): 7–30.

14. Allport G. *Becoming: basic considerations for a psychology of personality*. New Haven, UK: Yale University Press, 1955.

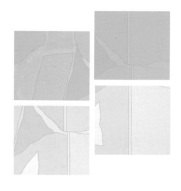

CHAPTER 3

The care and confinement of the mentally ill

Liam Clarke*

INTRODUCTION

In the beginning was Bedlam: at first it was called the Priory of St Mary of Bethlehem (but was later bowdlerized to Bethlem or Bedlam). In the thirteenth century it was the only lunatic enclosure in England. Indeed, it was England's original 'castle of fantasy' and at a time when the fantasy could be realized for the price of an entrance fee. Freak shows were the order of the day and Bedlam was the biggest show in town, way above the level of circus sideshow by virtue of its perceived philanthropy. Philanthropy aside, it was (at first) probably privately owned and being small (originally six patients) was unlikely to tax the strength of curious visitors.

Bedlam is important because much of psychiatry's reputation would rest on different perceptions of it and their reification over time. Superficially, we can see it as a place where the affluent paid to watch the 'antics' of confined, brutalized, terrified lunatics. The passage of time would canonize this image, perhaps as a contrasting backdrop against which the 'liberating' activities of Pinel in Paris or the Tukes in England could assume heroic form. Allderidge[1] notes that very little written about Bedlam derives from primary sources, resulting in easy-going

assumptions about the nature of its provision and money-making proclivities. The brutality of chaining and whipping, which lasted until the eighteenth century, is hardly denied but, as Allderidge shows, things are more complicated than has sometimes been portrayed. By 1677, for instance, Bethlem's rules stated that:

> None of the Officers or Servants shall at any time beat or abuse any of the Lunatics in the said hospital, neither shall offer any force unto them but upon absolute necessity for the better government of the said Lunatics.[2]

Force, in other words, while a real possibility, was not seen by the Bethlem authorities as ordinarily acceptable. Also, the existence of two wards for 'incurables' suggests that, for some patients, cure was not an unrealistic aspiration. In truth, the early asylums – built in the mid-eighteenth century – were known for their weird and wondrous attempts to cure insanity. A Doctor Cox,[3] for instance, suspended patients from the ceiling in a contraption that rotated them 100 times per minute; unsurprisingly, many hastily reported a marked improvement in their condition. As Peter Ackroyd[4] observes, 'You have to be brave to be mad'.

*Liam Clarke has worked as a lecturer for Brighton University, UK, for 12 years and has published widely on mental health and psychiatry. His interests include the history of psychiatric nursing and its relationship to the management of hospitalized patients and especially their confinement and containment. He is currently developing ways of increasing psychiatric user participation in undergraduate nurse training programmes.

Allderidge says that the practice of paying to watch lunatics lasted hundreds of years, implying that it had become custom and practice and not just a money earner; was there, perhaps, an element of almsgiving involved? In 1673, a new building, at Moorfields, took the place of the old Bethlem and although – like the later Victorian asylums – its outward appearance was grand, it was anything but inside. Inmates continued to be put on display, this time along two galleries, one above the other. In addition, 'on each floor a corridor ran along a line of cells, with an iron gate in the middle to divide the males from the females'.[4] This practice, the rigid separation of the sexes was to remain until the post-Thatcher closure of the mental hospitals.

Beyond Bedlam

After Bethlem, from the early eighteenth century other asylums sprang up mostly on the basis of individual local initiative. These constitute the first wave of public asylums in England beginning in 1751 with St Luke's, London, under the guidance of William Battie whose *Treatise on Madness* became influential. One of Battie's first actions was to ban asylum sightseers. St Luke's also broke with the past by accepting medical students. It seemed as if a new liberalism was about to dawn in English psychiatry. However, it was the invention of 'moral therapy' by a family of Quakers at York, which heralded a fundamental shift in how lunacy was conceived and managed. Following a suspicious death at the York asylum, heretofore an institution of good repute, the Tuke family opened their Retreat, also at York.

Perhaps its most significant departure was to recognize that communities of carers and patients, together, could be a force for good. Rather than following established practices of trying to break the lunatic's will, by medicine fair or foul, the patient was now gently coerced as a kind parent would 'inculcate' goodness in a child. The intent seems to have been to admonish, as well as praise, the behaviours of inmates so that they might recapture their dignity and acquire self-control. In her history of the Retreat, Ann Digby[5] records that this liberalism was not new but was premised on received ideas of ethical and rational justice coupled with the abandonment of physical restraints then becoming common.

Yet the Retreat exerted little direct influence on contemporary asylum practices, perhaps unsurprisingly given the uniqueness of its religious disposition. True, pockets of liberal treatment occurred throughout the early asylums and some of them showed commendable tolerance of their inmate's behaviour (see Chapter 10 in Porter[6]). But they could never rid themselves fully of their custodial function, the sheer 'bricks and mortar' density of their presence made liberalism extremely unlikely. For example, the perimeter walls of these asylums were 15 feet in height. Although this prevented the 'gaping at the lunatics' phenomenon, which, despite Battie's efforts, had continued into the early nineteenth century, they were primarily intended to prevent escape. The windows in these hospitals were small and set high up in their inner walls, a deliberate invitation to claustrophobic menace.

Smith[7] reminds us that the fine grounds were for walking in by fee-paying inmates only, and not for the pauper lunatics who had to take their exercise in airing yards. The frightening conduction of sounds, particularly at night, the poor diet, the bland hospital garb, the dead hand of routine, the bludgeoning of individuality and so on and on and on, all of this endured into the second wave of public asylums built by the Victorians.

Initial summary

The history of professional psychiatry begins with the separation of the mentally ill into institutions. Bethlem was hardly a prototype but – within the story of confinement – it set a metaphorical standard that influenced how subsequent developments would be seen. For Roy Porter,[8] 'the epic of English madness opens in the late 18th Century' and with 'psychiatric institutionalization as the key to this history'. From its beginnings, confinement represents the basic conundrum of psychiatry – an excruciating conundrum for nurses – that is the problem of reconciling custody and care.

At Bethlem, the natural impetus, for years, was to chain and punish. By the sixteenth century more enlightened minds prevailed and current opinion suggests that treatments as well as a measure of compassion were by this time becoming acceptable.[8,9] The unleashing of restraints at Hanwell (announced by John Connolly in September 1839),[10] although not an isolated act, represented a watershed mainly on account of the (large) size of Hanwell and Connolly's charismatic leadership. Leadership was needed, as attendants often required intense pressure to relinquish their attachment to chaining and other punitive measures.

By the mid-nineteenth century, however, dissatisfaction with custodialism and coercion was coalescing into a social push for change. In 1845, change came in spades with the passage of 'arguably the most significant mental health legislation of the century'.[7] This required county magistrates to establish pauper lunatic asylums and with a remit that they reflect Connolly's principles of care.

Porter has argued that nineteenth-century asylums did not follow on the back of an earlier century of neglect and cruelty: the pauper lunatics certainly suffered inside their seventeenth- and eighteenth-century institutions but no more than they would have done had these institutions not existed. What the nineteenth century represented was an unprecedented public-spiritedness: 'Victorian England was, after all, a time of great men, of great vision, of great achievement',[11] and with a disposition to attack problems with verve and tenacity. The Victorians did not invent compassion for the plight of mad people, and their asylums lasted a mere century. Nevertheless, theirs was an extraordinary optimism, and achievement, all the same.

MORAL STRICTURES

To what extent did moral therapy (at the Retreat) entail elements of moral *expectations*? And, did this constitute a more subtle form of restraint? Smith[7] observes that:

> Moral treatment comprised more than a gentle, considerate approach. There were also aspects which sought to alter inappropriate behaviour. By 1800, the conception was widely accepted that the doctor had to gain ascendancy over the madman, as a precursor to curative treatment.

This is important because even allegedly liberal psychiatric regimes can camouflage malevolent intentions. For example, therapeutic communities[12] have typically advocated principles of democratization, permissiveness, communalism and so on. However, these principles may cloak moral imperatives such that, if the workings of the community break down, more traditional forms of management will re-emerge to put matters right. Lindsay,[13] a resident in a therapeutic community, noted that whenever life became intolerable, conventional codes issued forth to redress imbalances and restore equilibrium.

The implication is that, ultimately, therapeutic communities only work when they have – at least during crises – conventional moral codes to fall back on. A more complicated overlap between public and institutional moralities is where hospitals evince progressive features – such as unlocking doors, patients wearing their own clothes, etc. – features that represent change and development at one level, but whose apparent liberalism is intended to make confinement more acceptable.

Michel Foucault[14] has much to say about confinement along these lines. He talks of the

> invention of a site of constraint, where morality castigates by means of administrative enforcement ... institutions of morality are established in which an astonishing synthesis of moral obligation and civil law is effected.

Although Foucault hurled his edicts at the York Retreat and its works (for example the abolition of physical constraints, instigating a generally caring milieu), his injunctions just as easily castigate confinement generally. Foucault sees the Retreat as an asylum where the free terror of madness is substituted with the stifling anguish of responsibility; fear no longer reigns outside the asylum gates, it now rages under the seals of conscience.

Rather than punish guilt, the asylum now organizes it, an illusion of therapy is created by a new age of rationality, which objectifies and distances the experiences of its inmates.

Insightful obeisance

Much of Foucault's work is premised on patients as unwilling or ignorant participants in their treatment when, actually, patients are often complicit in their treatment or even detention. For example, the first patients at the York Retreat were themselves Quakers and so probably did not experience their 'moral management' as irksome or unwarranted.

However, a libertarian agenda drives Foucault's writings and one suspects that his conclusions are not trustworthy reflections of available evidence. Contrary to Foucault, Digby's account[5] of the York Retreat *is* consistent with the high praise that its humanitarianism has traditionally warranted. One measure of its openness, for example, was that less than 5 per cent of inmates were restrained at any time and only if violent or suicidal. Most of its patients mixed freely with visitors; they dressed ordinarily, took tea with the governors and even, now and then, ventured outside the hospital walls.

However, Digby's version does support Foucault's assertions about moral control by listing the Retreat's implicit *threat* of restraint as well as its prevalent religious training and work regimes. The basic idea of the Retreat was to allow people to regroup or recollect their senses and faculties. The Tuke family were appealing to the unaffected faculties of its inmates, and were influenced, in this instance, by John Locke's assertion that insanity is a disturbance of *ideas*, not of the spirit, nor of the person. The problem with Foucault, however, is not his scepticism about the Retreat's achievements so much as the glib connections he makes between events, and the *wilfulness* he attaches to the medical colonization of thought and behaviour as he sees it. That a therapeutic community *might* elicit guilt from residents falling foul of its precepts is plausible enough; that this would preclude good therapeutic intentions as well sounds one-sided. Also, was it necessarily wrong to implant guilt in the minds of eighteenth-century pauper lunatics if what was intended was an improvement in their moral probity? Such an admission might raise eyebrows today, but in an eighteenth-century religious context? Hardly.

Separation

A central theme of Foucault's is that in the seventeenth century a grand confinement of society's rejects and misfits took place, eventually culminating in the building of the Victorian asylums. However, as Roy Porter[8] points out, seventeenth-century schemes of confinement were parochial in nature: much of the management of madness was in (often lucrative) private houses or in families (the latter classically realized in Bronte's Jane Eyre) and it was not until the early nineteenth century that a widespread separation of the mad was attempted.

Separation means new rules – different rules – distancing the separated from everyday life, an implication of moral inferiority and societal threat. The conventional view is that the 'asylum separation' was a positive result of political altruism, as well as medicine's growing confidence in its ability to manage the insane. Commenting on this, Andrew Scull[15] stated:

> The very language that is used reflects the implicit assumptions which for many years marked most historians' treatment of the subject – a naive Whiggish view of history as progress, and a failure to see key elements of the reform process as sociologically highly problematic.

Foucault's view of the pre-nineteenth-century world is that it is at ease with madness: in a sense, the village fool is indeed a fool 'but he's our fool': he possesses consensual worth because, as yet, no epistemology exists by which to debar him. Foucault postulates this so as to attack a psychiatric science, which he alleges objectifies patients, thus marginalizing them. He has a point, since the close of the eighteenth century sees the advent of philosophical and scientific rationalism with their offspring, sociology and psychology, when religious thought becomes superseded by humanist discourse. Psychiatry comes about because it invents a new concept of madness in which unreason is no longer considered virtuous.

According to Foucault, the 'madman' – combined roughly of two parts noble savage and village buffoon – moves from a primitive but socially viable status, to one of mental defective where, in the name of medical expertise, his social 'position' is severely thwarted.

According to Edward Shorter[16] this perspective is faulty. In the years before the asylums were built, people

> were treated with a savage lack of feeling … there was no golden era, no idyllic refuge from the values of capitalism. To maintain otherwise is a fantasy.

These are harsh words. However, in the sense of 'golden eras' they are true enough. That said, Foucault's point is not so much about how people treated one another – life was nasty, brutish and short for everyone – but that the mad were now confined on grounds of disease: the mad are now conceptually excluded by scientific advance.

THE PRINCIPAL ISSUE

An important issue is whether the asylums were a product of Victorian paternalism, or a result of increasing

medical power, coupled with an impetus to protect society from the criminal and/or eugenic propensities of the mentally ill. Edward Shorter provides a flavouring of the discussion:[16]

> To an extent unimaginable for other areas of the history of medicine, zealot-researchers have seized the history of psychiatry to illustrate how their pet bugaboos – be they capitalism, patriarchy, or psychiatry itself – have converted protest into illness, licking into asylums those who otherwise would be challenging the established order.

And Andrew Scull noted:[15]

> The direction taken by lunacy reform in the nineteenth century is thus presented as inevitable and basically benign – both in intent and in consequences – and the whole process crudely reduced to a simplistic equation: humanitarianism + science + government inspection = the success of what David Roberts calls the great nineteenth-century movement for a more humane and intelligent treatment of the insane.

The issue is the extent to which elements from one or other (or both) of these strands holds true. Nietzsche states that, ultimately, all argument represents 'a desire of the heart' and this is certainly an arena where 'evidence' feeds conflicting attitudes about the purposes of psychiatry. The interpretations of anti-institutionalists, intent on revising traditional accounts, have been more inspired, more creative. That said, their central point, that nineteenth-century reforms operated, not as noblesse oblige, outpourings of Victorian benevolence, but as attempts to corral troublesome citizens, is now without foundation.

Kathleen Jones[17], while acknowledging the second class status of asylum patients, their use as cheap labour, as well as the recurring violence, smell and abuse of rights, nevertheless states that asylums were humane and intelligent. She believes that much that has been written about asylums is biased: 'we must', she says, 'get beyond prejudice, both old and new, assessing the asylum movement in the context of its own day'. What this means is that given the conditions of nineteenth-century working-class life, both in the workhouses and in general, asylum admission may well have been a blessing. For Jones, removing mentally ill people to rural hospital outposts protected them from 'the pestilence and open cesspools' of urban living. It may have helped. Eerily, Peter Ackroyd[4] records that Bethlem had a fresh water supply from an Artesian well, which indeed provided a lifetime's freedom from cholera. But siting the asylums in rural areas was probably more to do with finance; the imperative to purchase building land in cheap non-urban settings.

So why did the Victorian asylums get built?

Certainly 'social control' cannot be discounted at a time of political concerns about public disorder. The asylums satisfied Victorian worries about the plight of lunatics: their secondary purpose to make the streets safe cannot however have been far from their minds. Neither can the good or therapeutic intentions of interested parties be set aside as lightly as some have done. In Walton's view,[18] it may have been the promise of 'cure' that forced the development of asylum psychiatry. Undoubtedly, *some* anticipation of psychiatric cure prevailed, for at least some mental states. However, the new 'mad doctors' (as they were first called) needed a medical arena in which to work and, with the building of the public asylums they got it.

Also, asylums became *the* places for working class people to send relatives whose behaviour had rendered them unsuitable for family living and at a time when market economics was leading to a separation of home and workplace. So long as the insane needed to be looked after at home, they threatened the practicality of cottage industries. For example, Scull[15] presents the *Lunacy Commissioners and Asylum Superintendents' Reports* for the 1890s, which show that asylums were populated by 'the impossible, the inconvenient and the inept'. Whereas the old madhouses had accommodated obvious cases of madness, the clientele of the Victorian asylums was much broader. Scull notes that in 1891 there were 15 853 institutionalized pauper lunatics in London but that this had increased to 26 293 by 1909. Since this sudden increase in hospital numbers could hardly reflect an increased incidence in mental illness the implication is that some form of 'social cleansing' was at play. The governing principle seems to be that whenever those in power restrict hapless, unproductive, people this probably represents some coercive intent. If this interpretation is unpalatable, you can always subscribe to traditional views whose governing principle is that a Victorian faith sought to return the mentally belligerent to normalcy through benevolence and the provision of mental hygiene training. Of course, both views can cohere: there are examples of powerful magistrates and doctors incarcerating people so as to maintain social order but, equally, there are examples of relatives supplicating for such action to be taken, presumably in the 'best interests' of their relatives.

The Nature of the beast

Although the nineteenth-century asylums contained many that would today be diagnosed 'schizophrenic', the variation in cases was remarkable. Walton[18] describes the case of 'Emma Blackburn, a 19-year-old, admitted to an asylum in 1871 after having been confined to Haslington workhouse for five months'. She was said to be suffering from 'political excitement' and the notes on her case are interesting:

> A fine healthy looking young woman, well nourished and of robust frame. Since admission has continued to shout and cry at intervals. Her countenance and eyes are much suffused. She does not occupy herself in any way and is occasionally quarrelsome. Frequently will not respond to questions put to her. Takes her food well but is restless at night.

Partly as a result of giving her morphine but also, I imagine, the sheer horror of her predicament, led to her deterioration and after 2 years she died. Such cases were hardly rare and although beliefs about women and madness varied across political and social dimensions (such as poverty), Elaine Showalter[19] states that:

> The prevailing view amongst Victorian psychiatrists as that … women were more vulnerable to insanity because the instability of their reproductive systems interfered with their sexual, emotional, and rational control.

Reflection

- Several issues can be weighed up at this point before moving into the 1950s and what can be called the modern era. For example, note the emphasis on female anatomy and vulnerability and how this increased in inverse ratio to women's demands for education – as well as growing assertiveness about their changing social roles. We universalize this point when we argue that psychiatric practice rarely fails to conform to prevalent social attitudes and mores.
- Also note how we are graduating slowly from the asylum as a building into its new designation as hospital and on to its fragmentation into 'services in the community'. It is at this point that we might ask whether change is necessarily superficial and designed to camouflage that which remains fundamentally the same. For instance, does the apparent sophistication (and rationales) of forensic systems ensure their continuance as forms of custodialism?
- Look especially at how different historians 'read into' events sometimes widely differing interpretations. To what extent do such interpretations influence contemporary perceptions of the profession and its varying activities? What kind of history does a profession require to further and underpin its ongoing designs and ambitions?
- Coming up to the present, for example imminent changes such as nurse prescribing, which historical accounts and rationales would prescribers favour as opposed to non-prescribers?
- Remember that history – as opposed to 'the past' – *happens now*: There are axes to grind and stories to tell: bear this in mind as you read on towards where we are now and beyond.

Skultans[20] agrees saying that:

> women's reproductive role [was seen as] precluding her from intellectual activity which she engages in at the risk of insanity.

THE 1950s ONWARDS

From the 1950s, psychiatry painstakingly got its medical act together: concepts of pauper lunatic were long gone and therapeutic zeal mushroomed. An eagerness to cure was shunted along two different fronts. One was social in nature and composed of two strands, namely therapeutic community 'proper' (typified by the work of Maxwell Jones at the Henderson Hospital) and a therapeutic community 'approach' reflected in less radical activities such as unlocking doors and minimizing regimentation.[21]

A second front was a single-mindedness to unleash physical treatments that would halt mental illness once and for all. These two fronts could be complexly linked. For example, William Sargant – doyen of physical treatment methods – insisted that the advent of phenothiazine drugs sounded the death knell of the asylums since their administration allowed previously troublesome, withdrawn or disturbed patients to return home. Thus begins the mythical 'phenothiazine revolution', the supposed 'real' reason behind the unlocking of hospital doors and other liberal moves. In fact, the post-war period was more intricate than this with changing hospital practices stemming, mainly, from changing attitudes towards mental illness and its causation. The sobering spectacle of soldiers going to war in (apparent) mental health and returning psychologically wrecked, suggested that mental illness need no longer be seen, *necessarily*, as a pathology of the nervous system. That mental illness could come about, or at least be mediated by, social events severely dented the traditional regard for mental distress as 'inborn and irredeemable'.

The shortfalls of benevolence

By the mid-twentieth century, the Victorian mental hospitals were becoming subject to criticism and review. David Clark (personal communication), medical superintendent at Fulbourn Hospital, had usefully separated them into three groups.

- The first, influenced by therapeutic community principles, achieved a good level of care for their patients.
- The second, much larger, group remained institutionalized but with a paternal/maternal approach and minimal punitiveness.
- The third group were 'the bins': large hospitals situated near cities and operating at a low point of restrictive and punitive care.

Martin's 'Hospitals in Trouble'[22] chronicles the failures of this last group as well as the abuses that they inflicted on patients. Writing in the 1950s, Johnson and Dodds[23] reported that:

> the attitudes of the hospital towards its patients is one of regarding them as unmitigated nuisances and undeserving malcontents. [cited in Porter[6]]

The problem was partly the hospitals themselves. As Gittins[24,p.5] observes, 'class, gender and categorizing illness were literally built into the hospital infrastructure'. Their architecture was closely linked to their function so that no matter how hard an enlightened staff might try to encourage good care the institutions themselves hobbled all that occurred within them (see Chapter 8 in Scull[15]). And, of course, we can add the abysmal overcrowding and a demoralized nursing staff saddled with the thankless task of trying to contain it all while paying lip-service to notions of care and treatment. It says a lot about human will that, amidst sometimes fanatical regimentation, there took place innumerable instances of companionship between nurses and patients.

Confinement had always meant separating the sexes: eugenic fears of the mentally ill reproducing with abandon were always strong. At first sight, therefore, the instigation of sexually integrated psychiatric wards always looked like progress. But it merely showed (again) how patients become a means of accomplishing (ostensibly liberal) professional ends. Notwithstanding the serial humiliations of older people now exposed to 'integration', this 1970s 'reform' went ahead anyway. It was well meant but, regrettably, the idea of asking patients what *they* might want was still some time off. That some of these old people, with attitudes rooted in an earlier age, might object to being nursed among the opposite sex, being too polite, too circumspect, to protest, was lost on a generation of mental health nurses.

Into the community

If, over the years, mental hospitals had weathered a growing liberal condemnation, it was, at least, criticism that stemmed from professional and ethical concerns. By the 1970s, however, liberalism had become fair game for Thatcherite economics and the closure of expensive hospitals in favour of community care. The grossly precipitous implementation of community care, however, could only mean a shortfall of actual or efficient care; in fact, the 'plight' of the mentally ill under 'care in the community' became a sorry conclusion to a century that had started with such high hopes. Cataloguing community psychiatric grief is beyond the scope of this chapter, so I will focus on one or two aspects only.

Smith's outline[25] of assertive outreach shows how its initial intentions have quickly coalesced around primary concerns with medication and the professional difficulty of 'non-compliance' by whatever name. In Smith's view there has been:

> a re-emergence of old institutionally based ideas of biomedical illnesses requiring control, containment and, in particular pharmacological treatments – the very issues that led to 'learned helplessness' for so many people in asylums.
> In effect, a spreading therapeutic bureaucracy ensnares patients, so that their continued monitoring by professionals – their continued membership of the community – becomes contingent on complying with medication.

Hemming et al.,[26] concerned that the restrictive functions of assertive outreach might take hold in the public imagination, tried to provide a definitive (warmer) account of it but which, in its detail, matches Smith's foreboding. Hemming et al. describe a world where patients are a problem per se. They typically fail to comply with their treatments and are in need of *clinical* supervision, especially in relation to risk assessment. Associating the mentally ill with concepts of risk is part of a process of fixing them within a neighbourhood in such a way as to sustain the policing role of community psychiatric nurses.[27] Just as Bethlem had insisted that those of its inmates begging in London's streets wear a tin badge fixed to their arm, so is this echoed in the maintenance of 'at-risk registers' of patients in the community, patients who may need to be quickly identified and treated either in their own abode or through reconfinement.

The Italian experience?

Beginning in the 1960s, a radical psychiatric movement called *Psychiatrica Democratica* (led by Franco Basaglia) forced an Italian government, in 1978, to legislate mental hospitals out of existence. The hospitals would be replaced by community services which replacement reflected a marked reduction (or abolition) of medical influence. Influenced by the British therapeutic community movement, the Italian reformers were more politicized, Italian psychiatrists being less likely to play down the political and economic implications of their trade. The impression created (in Britain) was that something truly radical had occurred in Italy and with much talk of its possible translocation to British hospitals.

The question quickly turned on what *had* occurred and how widespread the change was. Significantly, Professor Kathleen Jones[28] re-emerged to insist that the 'Italian Experience', as it had come to be known, was not all it seemed to be. The debate that followed revived much of the rhetoric and discourse of the past concerning the moral worth of psychiatry as a medical speciality. Professor Jones visited various centres in Italy and her reports contradicted those that had praised the Italian changes as revolutionary and widespread.[29] In fact, stated Jones,[28] the successful closure of mental hospitals had only happened at Trieste, with other centres only partially implementing community programmes because they were hindered by ongoing lack of resources. In some ways, Jones's account sobered up what had become accepted at face value, whereas what actually was happening in Italy was more piecemeal and problematic. But Jones's account was more than this. Stung by the criticism that she favoured mental hospitals, but, more so, dismayed that these Italians exulted in their hospital closures, Professor Jones went on to reiterate her lifelong contention that 'what matters is the quality of care, not where they are housed'.[28] This, of course, misses the point because it *does* matter where psychiatry is practised: the architectural environment of patients does encourage deterioration and development of stereotypical beliefs and behaviours.

Trieste was the natural home of the Italian reform and Jones praised it as a fascinating experiment in human relationships. She describes a carnival atmosphere combined with a refreshing rejection of professionalism with everybody on first name terms and everyday life replicated as far as possible. However, the problem, she believed, was that, by and large, the Trieste experiment was not replicated elsewhere other than in a half-hearted fashion. Also, some categories of patients, for example those with dementia, were excluded. As such, references to an *Italian* experience were, stated Jones, a misnomer. This is a fair point but is a mistake that Jones herself also makes as, for example, when she refers to Britain's 'open door movement',[28] which, as I have shown,[30] was patchy and hardly a widespread 'movement'.

In the long run, the ideas that propelled Italian radicalism are what matter, because a central criticism of psychiatry is its unacknowledged political intent. The role of psychiatric dissidence is to critique psychiatry's rationale as much as the vagaries and mishaps of its practice. This is why criticism is viewed as intolerable by the psychiatric establishment. So Professor Jones ends her commentary on Trieste with references to 'frolic radicalism' as well as its appeal 'to the non-rational side of the human mind'. There is a stern warning that the Italians are not above confusing politics with psychiatry, added to which is the admonition that 'in a country with a Catholic heritage, symbols and dogma still have a considerable power'. The implication here is that a dogma-free Britain – still unencumbered by symbols – is hardly the place for non-rational applications of psychiatric care. Granted, British practitioners would hardly align themselves with political parties or even claim that their work was directly political. Yet few would argue that mental illnesses are managed within conventional norms of what constitutes mental health; norms that closely match what counts as acceptable social behaviour.

Psychiatric practices probably do not travel well – as current difficulties with ethnic minority mental health patients demonstrate – and what works in Trieste might not go down well in Tunbridge Wells. Nevertheless, *Psychiatrica Democratica* reminded us that psychiatry can still be perceived as a malevolent force, particularly when it ignores the political and economic dimensions of mental distress.

ACCOMMODATING LOSS

As we try to accommodate losing our mental hospitals, combinations of legal restrictions and concerns with 'non-compliance' echo older desires to confine 'the mad', whether for their own or society's good. The Victorians believed that their lunacy mansions were a solution; we came to dislike their *form* while continuing to respect their function. But these hospitals were the visible reminder of *our* repressive impulses and so we needed to devise less obtrusive ways to manage insanity, to devise systems with the power to treat when required and even if objected to by patients. Such objections, in any event, are transformed by psychiatrists to a symptomology that can be over-ruled. To attribute legitimacy to such objections is seen as immoral and heartless; heartless, that is, not to treat the symptoms even when this requires preliminary confinement. Such confinement will henceforth rest more on community-processed restrictions, such as at risk registers, assertive outreach programmes and compulsory treatments. As psychiatry becomes ever-more medicalized and dependent on biotechnology, its self-assuredness may become less susceptible to incursions from non-medical thinking. To be fair, psychiatric radicals more often than not arise within psychiatry's own ranks but almost always as a reaction to psychiatry's capacity for, and inclination towards, reductionist thinking and benevolent coercion, respectively.

And yet the insistence (and optimism) of psychiatric nurses on working therapeutically with patients is undiminished. This insistence is not misguided, nor is it cynical. It is an aspiration that finds expression in a million and one encounters between nurses and patients. Regrettably, personal expressions of humanity have had to contend with a collective commitment which errs on the side of confinement if, in many cases, this is seen as a prerequisite to providing care. Even if, as has been argued,[27] a policing role is endemic to psychiatric nursing, it is the *regrettable and objectionable* necessity of that role that should govern its expression. In psychiatry, confining people has become an activity so lacking in moral wakefulness as to be almost

banal: the effect of a psychiatric diagnosis is to collapse any ethical doubts that might attend removing people's rights. Yet we know, from disparities in the diagnoses and confinement of ethnic minority groups, that diagnosis is hardly a scientific activity. Perhaps confinement is a necessary prerequisite to caring and treating recalcitrant patients? If so, is it not wise, therefore, to keep the Trieste flag flying, to continue to be wary of a profession that, although largely benign in its intentions, confirms the marginalization of people nevertheless and which historically has made the denial of human freedoms a highly respectable activity. It may be that I have been too effusive in my admiration of the humanizing and benevolent functions of nurses when, as I write, significant numbers of them appear willing – even enthusiastic – to take up the mantle of 'nurse prescribing'. Whatever one's views on the efficacy of drugs, this is a shift of epic proportions since it alters the relationship between nurse and patient. By prescribing, the nurse is circumscribed in how he/she now reacts to patient's opinions, reluctances, even negativities towards medication. To whom will patients now turn where there occur differences with the prescriber: who now will give that support and information necessary for them to come to terms with their (perceived) dispossession?

SUMMARY

1 The history of psychiatric care is grounded in ambivalence both in its intent and in its practice.
2 This ambivalence takes the form of a balance to be struck between therapeutics on the one hand and a perceived need for confinement and safety on the other.
3 Although the structures and frameworks of delivering care alter and change, from asylum to hospital, to community and outreach programmes, it is argued that these two fundamental themes of coercion and benevolence are sustained albeit in more subtle forms.
4 An important, if neglected, point is the denial, within British contexts, of the considerable political forces – typically played out in gender, class, and economic terms, that impinge upon the delivery of care in many of its aspects.
5 Many nurses have had to struggle (yielding contradictory results) against the odds of institutional care and ever ongoing social/political expectations of nurses.
6 This is reflected in current debates about nurse prescribing which, again, produces oppositional forces reflecting the ambivalences that continue to gnaw their way around mental health nurses and their problematic identity.

REFERENCES

1. Allderidge P. Bedlam: fact or fantasy. In: Bynum WF, Porter R, Shepherd M (eds). *The anatomy of madness: essays in the history of psychiatry*, Vol. II. London, UK: Tavistock Publications, 1985: 17–33.

2. Minutes of the court of governors of Bridewell and Bethlem. 30 March 1677.

3. Cox JM. *Practical observations on insanity in which some suggestions are offered towards an improved mode of treating diseases of the mind to which are subjoined Remarks on medical jurisprudence as connected with diseased intellect*, 2nd edn. London, UK: Baldwin and Murray, 1896.

4. Ackroyd P. *London: the biography*. London, UK: Chatto and Windus, 2000.

5. Digby A. Moral treatment at the Retreat 1796–1846. In: Bynum WF, Porter R, Shepherd M (eds). *The anatomy of madness: essays in the history of psychiatry*, Vol. II. London, UK: Tavistock Publications, 1985: 52–72.

6. Porter R. (ed.). *The Faber book of madness*. London, UK: Faber & Faber, 1991.

7. Smith LD. *Cure comfort and safe custody*. London, UK: Leicester University Press, 1999.

8. Porter R. *Mind-forg'd manacles*. Harmondsworth, UK: Penguin Books, 1990.

9. Andrews J, Briggs A, Porter R. *The history of Bethlem*. London, UK: Routledge, 1997.

10. Jones WL. *Ministering to minds diseased: a history of psychiatric treatment*. London, UK: William Heinemann Medical Books, 1983.

11. Winchester S. *The surgeon of Crowthorne: a tale of murder, madness and the Oxford English Dictionary*. London, UK: Penguin Books, 1999.

12. Jones M. *The therapeutic community: a new treatment method in psychiatry*. New York, NY: Basic Books, 1953.

13. Lindsay M. A critical view of the validity of the therapeutic community. *Nursing Times* (Occasional Papers) 1982; **78**: 105–7.

14. Foucault M. *Madness and civilisation: a history of insanity in an age of reason* (Trans. R. Howard). London, UK: Tavistock Publications, 1967.

15. Scull A. *The most solitary of afflictions: madness and society in Britain, 1790–1990*. London, UK: Yale University Press, 1993.

16. Shorter E. *A history of psychiatry: from the era of the asylum to the age of Prozac*. Chichester, UK: John Wiley, 1997.

17. Jones K. The culture of the mental hospital. In: Berrios GE, Freeman H (eds). *150 years of British psychiatry 1841–1991*. London, UK: Gaskell, 1991: 17–28.

18. Walton JK. Casting out and bringing back in Victorian England: pauper lunatics, 1840–70. In: Bynum WF, Porter R, Shepherd M (eds). *The anatomy of madness: essays in the history of psychiatry*, Vol. II. London, UK: Tavistock, 1985: 132–46.

19. Showalter E. *The female malady: women, madness and English culture, 1830–1980*. London, UK: Virago Press, 1987.

20. Skultans V. *English madness: ideas on insanity 1580–1890*. London, UK: Routledge and Kegan Paul, 1979.

21. Clark D. *Administrative therapy*. London, UK: Tavistock, 1964.

22. Martin JP. *Hospitals in trouble*. Oxford, UK: Blackwell Science, 1984.

23. Johnson D, Dodds N. *The plea for the silent*. London, UK: Christopher Johnston, 1957.

24. Gittins D. *Madness in its place: narratives of Severalls hospital, 1913–1997*. London, UK: Routledge, 1998.

25. Smith M. Assertive outreach: a step backwards. *Nursing Times* 1999; **95**: 6–7.

26. Hemming M, Morgan S, O'Halloran P. Assertive outreach: implications for the development of the model in the United Kingdom. *Journal of Mental Health* 1999; **8**: 141–7.

27. Morrall P. *Mental health nursing and social control*. London, UK: Whurr, 1998.

28. Jones K, Poletti A. The Italian experience reconsidered. *British Journal of Psychiatry* 1986; **148**: 144–50

29. Rotelli F. Changing psychiatric services in Italy. In: Ramon S, Giannichedda MG (eds). *Psychiatry in transition: the British and Italian experiences*. London, UK: Pluto Press, 1991.

30. Clarke L. The opening of doors in British mental hospitals in the 1950s. *History of Psychiatry* 1993; **iv**: 527–51.

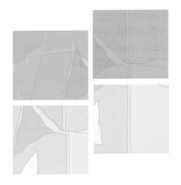

CHAPTER 4

Evidence-based practice in mental health

Hugh McKenna*

It appears strange that I should start this chapter by stating that the title is incorrect. Since the last edition of this text there have been a plethora of articles on evidence-based practice or its many derivatives (Evidence-based nursing, Evidence-based medicine, Evidence-based healthcare, etc.). However, the word 'based' implies an almost unquestioning belief in evidence. From my perspective, the term 'Evidence-*informed* practice' is probably more accurate. Nonetheless, evidence-based practice is a universal label and will be used here.

This chapter will deal with a number of issues regarding evidence-based practice (EBP), including an overview of terminology and definitions, exploring how evidence is derived and its philosophical roots. I will also outline the political implications of using best evidence and how this has encouraged rationing in some health services. Finally, I will discuss how mental health nurses can use evidence and when they can legitimately ignore what may be best evidence.

EBP emerged from what was originally termed evidence-based medicine (EBM).[1] As alluded to above, this has been extended to include other disciplines, e.g. evidence-based or evidence-informed nursing.[2,3] Moving away from a profession-specific position, evidence-based *health* (intended to indicate a comprehensive approach) has become a popular variation in the terminology. It is now even recognized that patients who nowadays participate much more fully in their treatment and care must be provided with adequate information – thus leading to the EBM offshoot, *evidence-informed patient choice*.[4]

The importance of basing practices on the best available evidence has now extended well beyond health, recognizing that policy and programme management issues must also draw upon the best available evidence. There is therefore a push towards such approaches; the term used in the UK is *evidence-based policy and practice*, promoted from Government level[5,6] and increasingly recognized in the wider academic, research and service delivery communities.[7–11]

To the uninitiated, the variety of terms is confusing. Nonetheless, one thing they have in common is aspiration towards the best *available* evidence. You will note here that the word *available* is highlighted, because for some practices the best available evidence may be very old or, indeed, there may be *no* evidence available at all!

There are many definitions of EBP. Here are three of them.

1 An approach to decision-making in which the clinician uses the best evidence available.[12]
2 Conscientious and judicious use of current best evidence in making decisions about the care of individual patients.[13]
3 An approach to health care that promotes the collection, interpretation and integration of valid, important and applicable patient-reported, clinician-observed and research-derived evidence.[14]

*Hugh McKenna is Professor and Dean of the Faculty of Life & Health Sciences at the University of Ulster, UK. He is currently involved in research programmes on young male suicide, depression services for adults, and support services for heroin users.

The last definition by McKibbon *et al.*[14] is the most comprehensive and includes as evidence the comments of patients and the observations of clinicians as well as research findings. This reflects what could be termed 'practice-based evidence'. Not everyone would sign up to this definition and the philosophical, political and practical reasons for this will be clarified later in the chapter.

In most instances when people refer to EBP they are implying that the evidence was research derived. For mental health nursing, this could be problematic. For example, suppose the Government issued an instruction stressing that mental health nurses should not undertake any clinical procedures unless they are based on up-to-date research evidence. The result would be that most nursing interventions would cease! This would not be unique to nursing; research studies have showed that many interventions undertaken by doctors are not underpinned by evidence.[15,16]

THE POLITICS AND ETHICS OF EVIDENCE-BASED PRACTICE

EBP has become a powerful political tool. One of the main reasons is that health care is becoming increasingly expensive. Therefore, if cash-strapped health service managers fund practices or expensive technologies that have not been proven to be effective, this would be a waste of scarce money, and could make patients' conditions worse.

When there is sound evidence to prove the effectiveness of interventions, some of these may be rationed for economic reasons. Recent UK cases included surgeons refusing to carry out costly heart operations on people who smoke tobacco, or liver transplants on people who continue to drink alcohol. There have even been stories that people who have schizophrenia have been refused expensive medical and surgical treatment because their future contribution to the economy would be small.

The ethical implications are obvious but I fear such rationing will not go away. For instance, it is estimated that 10 per cent of the UK and US populations have a serious mental illness like depression and a higher percentage will have less serious psychiatric illnesses. Recent figures show that 24 per cent of women and 17 per cent of men in Northern Ireland show signs of possible mental ill health. As a result, we can take it for granted that their close family members will also suffer from anxiety and stress. In addition, many people with serious physical problems will also have emotional problems. Therefore, in a population the size of the UK, there will never be enough therapists or mental health professionals to cope with the demand for therapy. In such cases, rationing of effective and evidence-based but costly and prolonged interventions will continue.

THE PHILOSOPHICAL ROOTS OF EVIDENCE

There are three main philosophical sources for the evidence that can underpin mental health care: rationalism, empiricism and historicism.[11]

Rationalism

Rationalism has its stem in *ratio* the Latin word for 'reason'. Charles Darwin stated that of all the faculties of the human mind, reason stands at the summit.[17] It is a philosophy of science which emphasizes the role that reason has to play in the development of knowledge and the discovery of truth.

Evidence is formulated here through mental reasoning (a priori reasoning). This 'armchair theorizing' has been ridiculed, mainly because of the absence of hard data. Nonetheless, the absence of data has not stopped people taking knowledge derived from rationalism seriously. For example, Freud[18] had very little data to support his theories on the Oedipus complex, or the id, ego and super ego. Furthermore, many well-known nursing theories were conceived through reasoning rather than research.

Rationalism as an approach to knowledge development can be traced to René Descartes (1596–1650), the seventeenth-century French philosopher and mathematician whose work influenced the development of knowledge for the next 300 years. Perhaps the best word to signify his contribution to the generation of evidence was 'Doubt'. He realized that to arrive at new knowledge you must doubt former opinions and experiences.

Most of our knowledge comes from our senses – our ability to see, hear, smell, touch and taste. However, Descartes noted that our senses can play tricks. For example, we may think something tastes sweet but when we try it, it tastes bitter, or something looks cold but when we touch it, it is hot. From this, Descartes encouraged himself to doubt all that he previously held to be true. He even began to doubt his own existence. However, he realized that there was one thing that could not be falsified. He reasoned that by thinking, he must exist or else he would not be able to think. Such reasoning led him to the one certain conclusion: *Cogito, ergo sum* (I think, therefore I am). Following this, he held that by means of reason alone, knowledge and certain universal self-evident truths could be discovered, from which evidence could then be derived.

Empiricism

In contrast to rationalists, empiricists believe that the data to underpin evidence are derived entirely from sensory experience. Rather than doubt our five senses, empiricists believed that if something cannot be perceived through the senses, it does not exist! As distinct from rationalism, empiricism denies the possibility of spontaneous ideas or a priori reasoning as a predecessor to the generation of evidence.

Reflection

Empiricism only recognizes knowledge derived from experience – that which is observed, sensed and where possible measured. Is this an attractive philosophy for mental health nursing?

John Locke (1632–1704) was the first to put forward empiricist principles. For Locke, knowledge was derived through the outside world writing on our minds through our senses. Therefore, he envisioned the mind at birth to be a blank slate or *tabula rasa*.[19] As the child develops, this slate is written on by experience.

Locke distinguished between primary and secondary qualities. Primary qualities are objective whereas secondary qualities are more subjective. For example, the primary qualities of schizophrenia could be the physical signs and symptoms and biochemical changes that can be observed and measured. Less important for empiricists would be the fear and distress that the schizophrenia causes for the person and the person's family. These would be labelled secondary qualities by Locke. Put very simplistically, from an empiricist perspective psychiatrists might be mainly concerned with the physical and biochemical manifestations of a mental illness, whereas nurses might be more concerned with the effect the illness was having on the person and his/her family. Neither may be right but the philosophies underpinning the education and training of these different health professionals may go some way to explaining these diverse perspectives.

Almost a century after Locke's death, the French philosopher Auguste Comte (1798–1857) gave empiricism a new twist. Comte used the term 'positive' knowledge to differentiate it from the negative knowledge that he believed underpinned woolly and metaphysical thinking. Adopting such a 'positivist' approach meant that through the use of robust scientific methods human problems would be solved and social conditions improved. To him scientists should focus on ordering confirmable observations in a rigorous manner and this alone should constitute human knowledge. Subjective approaches to knowledge development were not perceived as meaningful pursuits. Therefore, reflection and intuition as a basis for EBP would be shunned and denigrated by positivists.

Throughout his life, Comte had been plagued by mental health problems and on occasions he had attempted suicide. In his later years his mental illness returned and with it a softening of views regarding positivism. For instance, in some of his last writings he stated that the intellect should be the servant of the heart! Nonetheless,

it is for his earlier work on positivism that Comte will be best remembered.

It is evident how empiricism and positivism has influenced the development and perception of EBP and why people with a positivist perspective would not favour a definition that favours empirical research. Many mental health professionals, including some nurses, still believe that the 'gold standard' of evidence is the double blind randomized controlled trail (RCT), a research approach with its roots in this tradition. They like to build hierarchies of evidence with RCTs at the summit.

An example of this can be seen in Table 4.1. Muir Gray[12] believed that expert opinion, or clinical examples, are less important sources of evidence than RCTs or non-experimental studies. In fact, the views of patients, the experiences of nurses and the results of qualitative research studies or indeed audits are *not* perceived as sources of evidence at all!

An interesting way to view the tension between empirical research evidence and established belief is to take the example of Galileo Galilei (1564–1642). His invention of the telescope proved that the earth and other planets revolve around the sun, an assertion in opposition to the dominant Catholic church view of the earth as the centre of the universe. However, Galileo had hard empirical evidence to prove his case. He brought his telescope to the Vatican and asked the then Pope and his advisors to look through it and see the evidence with their own eyes. They refused, stating that there was no need to because they already knew the truth. When Galileo eventually published his evidence, he was tried before the Catholic Inquisition, forced to retract and imprisoned for the remainder of his life. To summon up empirical evidence to dispute faith was tantamount to heresy. It was not until 1990 (over 350 years later) that Pope John Paul II endorsed a Vatican church commission's finding that Galileo was wrongly convicted.

Another example of Galileo showing his support for physical proof was when he famously stated that we should 'measure what is measurable, count what is countable and what is not countable – make countable'. However, you will accept that there is much in mental health care that cannot be measured: how do you *count* compassion, *calibrate* empathy or *calculate* presence? Rationalist or empirical approaches cannot be applied to

TABLE 4.1 Hierarchy of evidence

Level I	Meta-analysis of a series of randomized controlled trials
Level II	At least one well-designed randomized controlled trial
Level III	At least one controlled study without randomization
Level IV	Well-designed, non-experimental studies
Level V	Case reports, clinical examples, opinion of experts

these phenomena, which brings me to the third type of philosophical source that could underpin the generation of evidence.

Historicism

So far we have dealt with evidence that is objective and can be perceived through the senses. Much of this can be checked through measurement. In contrast, historicism recognizes that everyone has a different life history and so we are all influenced by our different experiences, values and beliefs.

Reflection

The historicist perspective recognizes that our knowledge is constructed in contexts, and influenced by our past experiences and present circumstances. Is this a philosophy that you would support for understanding mental health care?

Consider the following example. Two nurses observe a patient self-administering his medication. However, they interpret what they see differently. One believes that the patient is dependent and in danger of giving himself the wrong drug or dosage and that he should not be allowed to do this. The other perceives the patient as gaining independence and is pleased that he is administering his own medication. These nurses observe the same phenomenon, yet past education, experience, reflection or intuition led them to understand and interpret it differently.

A number of philosophers are proponents of this type of thinking.[20–22] They challenged the positivist view and stressed the importance of history and perception in the development of knowledge. They rejected the idea of objective truths, arguing instead that the development of knowledge is a dynamic process and so there are no final and permanent truths.

Historicism underpins most qualitative research approaches, which in turn provide evidence generated from people's experiences, perceptions and beliefs. Edmund Husserl,[23] the founder of phenomenology, believed that science involved the exploration of perceptions, judgements, beliefs and other mental processes. Because of its refusal to count anything other than observable entities and objective reality, positivism was not capable of dealing with human experience.

In most textbooks on EBP, historicism as a basis for evidence has either a lowly status or indeed is not alluded to at all. This raises several important issues for mental health nurses. If only evidence, generated from 'gold standard' RCTs is supported by the health service and government, then evidence based on the intuitive, experiential knowledge and beliefs and values of mental health nurses has a lowly status. Such 'alternative' evidence is less likely to be supported, encouraged and funded.

McKibbon *et al.*'s definition of EBP respects both patient-reported and clinician-observed (historicism) evidence as well as research-derived evidence (empiricism). But here is another definition of EBP. I leave it to you to decide what philosophy of science it comes from:

A shift in the culture of health care provision away from basing decisions on opinion, past practice and precedent toward making more use of research and evidence to guide clinical decision making.[24]

HOW DO NURSES' KNOW AND HOW DOES THIS AFFECT THE EVIDENCE THEY USE IN PRACTICE?

Most psychiatric–mental health (PMH) nurses have long accepted that people undergoing care deserve interventions that are based on sound evidence. However, from the above you would agree that there is much confusion on whether evidence should have its foundations in rationalism, empiricism or historicism or all three.

Know *how* evidence and know *that* evidence

Two distinct types of knowledge have been described by Rhyl:[25] 'know *how* knowledge' and 'know *that* knowledge'. The former is skills based and involves knowing how to do something. For instance, you may know *how* to use a cash dispenser or how to mow the lawn. But you may know *that* the computer in a cash dispenser is *programmed* using FORTRAN or that the lawn mower is based on mechanical *theory*. In nursing, much of 'know how knowledge' is perceived as our 'art' and therefore has its roots in historicism. In contrast, 'know that knowledge' has its basis in empirical research and theory and is often perceived as our 'science'.

Categories of evidence

Pierce identified seven ways of knowing.[26] You can justifiably replace the word knowing with the word evidence:

- knowing (evidence) based on the word of an authority figure
- knowing (evidence) based on unverified hearsay
- knowing (evidence) based on trial and error
- knowing (evidence) based on past experiences (history)
- knowing (evidence) based on unverified belief
- knowing (evidence) based on spiritual/divine understanding
- knowing (evidence) based on intuition.

This covers the historicism and rationalism philosophies of evidence but not that of empiricism.

More recently, however, Kerlinger[27] addressed this, asserting that the way to verifiable knowledge is through rigorous experimental research. Here 'hard evidence' is required to be certain that something is or is not true. You will note that this reflects a positivist viewpoint. But Kerlinger also identified what he thought were 'less respectable ways of knowing'. These are 'tenacity', 'authority' and 'a priori'.

To illustrate Kerlinger's approach we could take the example of the knowledge that providing cognitive–behavioural therapy relieves anxiety in individuals with agoraphobia. Nurses may take this as evidence for practice because 'it has always been done this way' (tenacity) or the nurse lecturer told them so (authority) or that it is reasonable to assume that if a person gets such support they will be less anxious (a priori). We could also have identified Kerlinger's preferred positivist way of obtaining knowledge: nurses provide agoraphobic patients with behaviour therapy because this practice was proven effective through the collection of empirical data.

Reflection

Identify another nursing intervention that reflects Kerlinger's types of knowing. Which of the types do you believe is the most valid and why?

Like Muir Gray (see Table 4.1), physical scientists such as Pierce and Kerlinger feel comfortable building categories and hierarchies of evidence. In Kerlinger's scheme the empiricist method is supreme and intuitive knowledge occupies a lowly position. For a practice discipline like nursing this may be an incomplete way of viewing evidence.

ACCEPTING AND REJECTING GOOD EVIDENCE

Barbara Carper identified four patterns of knowing in nursing.[28] In her seminal paper the four patterns of knowing are: *empirics*, the science of nursing; *aesthetics*, the art of nursing; *ethics*, moral knowing; and *personal knowing*. For the purpose of this chapter I will again replace the word knowing with that of evidence. This will not alter Carper's original views.

Empirics

By now you can probably predict the type of evidence that 'empirics' would signify. According to Carper 'empirics' represents that which is obtained by rigorous observation or measurement. It provides evidence that is *verifiable, objective, factual* and *research based*. This is the type of quantifiable and objective evidence seen in

Levels 1 to 4 of Muir Gray's hierarchy and coincides with Kerlinger's empirical knowledge and Rhyl's 'know that' knowledge. The quantifiability of empirical data allows objective measurement that yields evidence that can be replicated by multiple observers.[29] On occasions nurses can ignore this type of evidence because it is superseded or contradicted by one or more of Carper's other types of evidence.

Aesthetics

Empirics is a rather narrow perspective and mental health nursing is also perceived as an art. *Aesthetics* gives us the evidence that focuses on the craft of nursing and is based on tacit knowledge, skill and intuition. It reflects Rhyl's 'know how knowledge' and has its roots in the philosophy of historicism. Aesthetic evidence is subjective, individual and unique. It enables us to go beyond that which is explained by existing laws and theories and accept that there are phenomena that cannot be quantified. Therefore, intuition, interpretation, understanding and valuing make up the central components of aesthetics.

Because of aesthetic *evidence*, nurses can ignore *empiric evidence*. For instance, there are many research-based scales that are used to assess and predict patients' risk of suicide. Nonetheless, the clinical judgement based on experience and intuition of an experienced nurse could overrule what the scales indicate. Similarly, research evidence may provide guidance on when patients can be discharged from a caseload but the intuitive expertise of the nurse regarding the patient's capability may justifiably override this.

Ethics

Ethics' provides us with evidence about what is right and wrong and what is good and bad, desirable and undesirable. It is expressed through moral codes and ethical decision-making. In everyday practice, nurses often have to make choices between competing interventions. These choices and judgements may have an ethical dimension, and to select the most appropriate position or action requires careful deliberation. For ethical reasons, some nurses may decide not to participate in a particular treatment even though the results from clinical trails or other studies (empirics) note that it is effective for some conditions. For example, some nurses will not participate in electroconvulsive therapy or the early discharge of patients. Ethical evidence may also be used to make decisions about the rationing of treatment described above.

Personal evidence

Like aesthetics, *personal evidence* is subjective yet is about us being aware of ourselves and how we relate to others. It represents knowledge that focuses on our own unique history, self-consciousness, personal awareness and empathy. If, as various theorists argue, caring is an interpersonal process[30] where interactions and transactions between people are central, then we must know our own strengths and weaknesses in order to be expert practitioners. Invariably, what mental health nurses have in their therapeutic arsenal is themselves and they use themselves therapeutically to make a positive difference to patients. Nurses often learn as much from a caring relationship as patients do and a good caring relationship will depend on their own self-regard. Therefore, personal knowing requires self-consciousness and active empathic participation on the part of the nurse.[29] You will note that here again, the influence of historicism is evident.

Nurses may reject empirical evidence because of what their personal evidence tells them. For example, consider the situation where a nurse is working with a patient experiencing a grief reaction. Despite research findings that suggest a linear movement through a number of grieving stages, the nurse's personal experience may indicate that not everyone has to go through all these phases or in the order suggested by the empirical evidence.

Experienced mental health nurses often use these four types of evidence interchangeably. For instance, they will be aware of the research and theoretical basis for providing medication by injection (empirics) and have the skills and intuition to ensure the patient understands the treatment and is as comfortable as possible while receiving it (aesthetics). However, the issue of withholding medication because of the severe side-effects and sometime poor results is a moral decision to be made with the patient (ethics). Finally, knowing themselves and their inner resources is important in the construction of an interpersonal therapeutic relationship with the patient so as to establish trust and confidence (personal evidence).

As you reflect on these four patterns of evidence you will note that the patterns are not mutually exclusive: there is overlap, interrelation and interdependence. By recognizing that there are legitimate types of evidence other than empirical evidence, Carper has made a valuable contribution to evidence-based nursing practice. Further, as outlined above it may be possible to reject empirical evidence because of the influence of one or more of the other types of evidence.

THE IMPORTANCE OF EVIDENCE-BASED PRACTICE FOR MENTAL HEALTH NURSING

I find it heartening that mental health nurses are beginning to accept and use types of evidence other than having a blind allegiance to the empiricist approach. This should have a powerful effect on identifying a body of evidence that has particular relevance to to those people who need mental health care.

Most mental health nurses have an earnest desire to provide individuals, families and communities with the highest possible standard of care within the resources available. It would be a waste of time and effort to implement care that was not based on the best available evidence. It would also be inefficient, ineffective and possibly detrimental to those receiving such care. Therefore, I hope this chapter has been helpful in outlining the different definitions of EBP and the different sources and origins of meaningful evidence.

It is important to distinguish between the different types of evidence. Do not get too enchanted by hierarchies and be aware that the so-called 'gold standard' can apply to approaches other than the favoured RCT. For example, if a psychiatrist wanted to test the effectiveness of a new drug or the biochemical activity in bipolar disorder then the RCT would be the gold standard. However, if he wanted to know what it is like to live with a person who has a bipolar disorder or experience such a diagnosis then in such cases a phenomenological approach would be the gold standard.

It is also important to remember McKibbon et al.'s definition of evidence-based nursing, where the views of patients and the experience of nurses are important sources of evidence. It would however be foolish to believe that such sources were always unbiased, just as the findings for empirical research studies may not always be unbiased.

The future of mental health generally and mental health nursing in particular is predicated on the public having trust in our judgements and practices. Basing care on questionable evidence or no evidence will simply move us from being perceived as professionals to being perceived as charlatans. Therefore, each mental health nurse has a responsibility and duty to search for the best available evidence to inform their practice. Such evidence will change with time and circumstance and therefore the search is a continual one. There are no reasons left why this should not be done – only excuses.

Reflection

Identify another nursing intervention that reflects Carper's four types of evidence. Show how the empiricist way of knowing can be countermanded by one or more of the others?

REFERENCES

1. Sackett DL, Straus SE, Richardson WS *et al. Evidence-based medicine: how to practice and teach EBM.* Edinburgh, UK: Churchill Livingstone, 2000.

2. Ingersoll G. Evidence-based nursing: what it is and isn't. *Nursing Outlook* 2000; **48**: 151–2.

3. McSherry R, Simmons M, Pearce P. An introduction to evidence-informed nursing. In: McSherry R, Simmons MP, Abbott P. (eds). *Evidence-informed nursing: a guide for nurses.* London, UK: Routledge, 2002: 1–13.

4. Entwhistle VA, Sheldon TA, Sowden A, Watt IS. Evidence-informed patient choice: Practical issues of involving patients in decisions about health care technologies. *International Journal of Technology Assessment in Health Care* 1998; **14**: 212–25.

5. Cabinet Office. *Modernising government.* London, UK: The Stationery Office, 1999.

6. Cabinet Office. *Better policy delivery and design: a discussion paper.* London, UK: The Stationery Office, 2001.

7. Pawson, R. *Evidence based policy: II. The promise of realist synthesis.* London, UK: ESRC UK Centre for Evidence Based Policy and Practice, University of London, 2001.

8. Pawson, R. Evidence-based policy: in search of a method. *Evaluation,* 2002; **8**: 2, 157–181.

9. OECD *Social sciences for knowledge and decision making.* Paris: Organisation for Economic Cooperation and Development (OECD), 2001.

10. Davies H, Nutley S, Smith P. *What works? Evidence-based policy and practice in public services.* Bristol, UK: Policy Press, 2000.

11. McKenna HP, Slevin OD. *Nursing theories, nursing models and nursing practice.* Oxford, UK: Blackwell, 2007.

12. Muir Gray JA. *Evidence-based healthcare: how to make health policy and management decisions.* New York, NY: Churchill Livingstone, 1997.

13. Sackett DL, Richardson WS, Rosenberg W, Haynes RB. *Evidence-based medicine: how to practice and teach EBM.* New York, NY: Churchill Livingstone, 1997.

14. McKibbon KA, Walker CJ. Beyond ACP Journal Club: how to harness Medline for therapy problems [Editorial]. *Annals of Internal Medicine (ACP Journal Club Supplement 1)* 1994; **121**: A10.

15. Gill P, Dowell AC, Neal RD *et al.* Evidence based general practice: a retrospective study of interventions in one training practice. *British Medical Journal* 1996; **316**: 1621–1622.

16. McColl A, Smith H, White P, Field J. GP's perceptions of the route to evidence-based medicine: a questionnaire survey. *British Medical Journal* 1998; **316**: 361–365.

17. Barnhart CL, Barnhart RK. *The Worldbook Dictionary* Chicago: Enterprises Educational Corporation, 1976.

18. Freud S. *An outline of psychoanalysis.* New York, NY: W.W. Norton, 1949.

19. Stokes P. *Philosophy: 100 essential thinkers.* London, UK: Capella, 2004.

20. Feyerabend P. Consolidation for the specialist. In: Lakatos I, Musgrave A (eds). *Criticism and the growth of knowledge.* Cambridge, UK: Cambridge University Press, 1977: 197–230.

21. Kuhn TS. *The structure of scientific revolutions,* 3rd ed. Chicago, IL: University of Chicago Press, 1977.

22. Toulmin S. *Human understanding.* Princeton, NJ: Princeton University Press, 1972.

23. Husserl E. *Ideas: general introduction to pure phenomenology.* New York, NY: Collier, 1962.

24. Appleby J, Walshe K, Ham C. *Acting on the evidence.* Research Report. London, UK: NAHAT, 1995.

25. Rhyl G. *The concept of the mind.* London, UK: Penguin, 1963.

26. Pierce CS. *Essays in the philosophy of science.* Indianapolis: Bobbs-Merrill, 1957.

27. Kerlinger FNB. *Foundations of behavioural research,* (3rd edn). New York, NY: Holt, Rinehart & Winston, 1986.

28. Carper BA. Fundamental patterns of knowing in nursing. *Advances in Nursing Science* 1978; **1**(1): 13–23.

29. Carper BA. Philosophical inquiry in nursing: an application. In: Kikuchi JF, Simmons H (eds). *Philosophic inquiry in nursing.* Newbury Park, CA: Sage, 1992.

30. Peplau HE. *Schizophrenia.* Conference Presentation, Annual Conference, University of Ulster, N. Ireland, 1995.

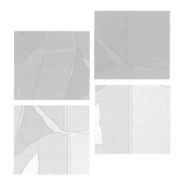

CHAPTER 5

The craft of psychiatric–mental health nursing practice

Peter Wilkin*

> You have made fair hands, you and your crafts! You have crafted fair!
>
> **William Shakespeare,**
> *Coriolanus, Scene VI*

INTRODUCTION

It is your first day on the ward. You are suddenly approached by a middle-aged man who, seconds ago, was a complete stranger to you. His face is fixed, creased with overwhelming concern. He addresses you, although his eyes do not, with the words: 'I did but taste a little honey with the end of the rod that was in mine hand, and, lo, I must die'.[a] Slowly, his gaze rises until it meets your own. His eyes project his pain, his hopelessness and his guilt. What do you say? What do you do? How can you engage him as he begins to turn away from you, already tried and convicted by the internal demons that persecute him? How do you craft your nursing response to this man who is hell-bent on scripting his own crucifixion?

The answer, of course, is that there is no right answer – although a thousand 'experts', if pressed, would undoubtedly offer a thousand possible responses, some remarkably similar, yet all slightly different. Such hypothetical dilemmas, neatly constructed within the black and white of the scholarly text, can only ever lift the curtain on any psychiatric episode. If such an incident were to unfold before your eyes as a psychiatric–mental health nurse it would be loaded with unique possibilities too numerous to imagine. This leads us to ask: how can any nurse hope to master a craft when the materials that make up each psychiatric situation are never the same?

Psychiatric–mental health nursing is primarily 'being' and 'becoming' with people who are suffering (either directly or indirectly as carers) the effects of mental *dis*-ease and distress. It does not – should not – involve working out people's problems and finding solutions for them. To do so would be to invalidate the person's experiences, robbing them of their right to navigate their own recovery.[1] For much of the time, psychiatric– mental health nursing is about 'not knowing' and tolerating the anxiety that this emptiness generates within us. It can be compared to what Keats[2] described as 'negative capability': an ability to tolerate 'uncertainties, mysteries, doubts, without any irritable reaching after fact and

*Peter Wilkin is an author and poet and was Clinical Nurse Specialist with the Complex Cases Team in Rochdale, UK, until 2007.

[a] In the bible Jonathan uttered this as a response to his father's, Saul, proclamation of death upon the person who had incurred God's wrath upon his army. (Following investigation, this turned out to be Jonathan himself, who had unwittingly broken the fast that his father had imposed.) It seemed to be an incredibly harsh sentence (which was, indeed, eventually revoked) passed out of bitterness for a very minor misdemeanour. 1 Samuel XIV: 43.

reason'. Your willingness to 'be' (to stay with), rather than 'do' (or flee) during such situations transmits a valuable message to the other. You are saying, non-verbally: I have the time, the patience and the commitment to journey with you through your distress; I am genuinely interested in you. The psychiatric–mental health nurse must function from within a developmental stage that never ends: they must become good enough to forge therapeutic alliances with most of the people, most of the time, and to tolerate and learn from those inevitable occasions when they do not.

With this vital premise constantly in mind, our brief passage together through this chapter becomes a journey of purpose. We shall gather together the raw materials that enable us, as psychiatric–mental health nurses, to practise our craft as lifelong learners and eternal students, being taught by those who always know better than us – our patients.[3,p.84]

CRAFTING OUR PRACTICE

Rather than explaining psychiatric–mental health nursing as an art or a science, Barker and Whitehill[4,pp.15–27] offer us a more relationship-based interpretation that echos Peplau's[3] philosophy of interpersonal relations. Truly collaborative caring, he believes, is based on an implied 'contractual relationship' between the psychiatric–mental health nurse and the person being nursed. It is a 'craft of caring' that focuses upon the human development of people in mental distress. Choosing to accept psychiatric–mental health nursing as a craft may imply that we must reject either scientific or artistic contributions towards the creation of our product (whatever that might be). That is not so. The psychiatric–mental health nurse 'needs to speak, however hesitantly, two different and yet related languages: the language of science and the language of art'[5,p.xiii] to form a feelings language – 'a language of the heart'.[5,p.15]

Any occupation that is predominantly relationship based must rely heavily on the social sciences to explore the human factors that might inform future practice (e.g. how do some people respond to a particular approach in a given situation?). Similarly, breaking down a particular therapeutic approach into structured stages of application helps the psychiatric–mental health nurse adopt this technology and achieve a level of competency in its application. The same can be said of art, whereby the nurse's artistic interventions figure prominently within the caring relationship. In the broadest sense, many psychiatric–mental health nurses have integrated the 'arts' into their practice as alternative pathways towards personal growth and emotional healing (painting, music, dance, drama, storytelling). And if we were to break down psychiatric–mental health nursing into its component parts, we would surely acknowledge the art of conversation, as we ' "spontaneously" choose words, expressions and gestures that express ... forms of feeling'.[5,pp.93–4]

Yet the application of science and technical skills, blended together with the creativity of conversational brush strokes, does not constitute the whole of our craft. Technical knowledge, or skill, must always be wrapped with ethical knowledge to deliver a response that fits each individual. The guiding principles that form our belief systems will always need to be modified to fit the unique circumstances that we, as psychiatric–mental health nurses, encounter. This process of application is even more complex when one realizes that every nursing intervention can be influenced by the history, tradition, race, culture, gender and faith of both the nurse and the other, who is the 'patient'. These are the incalculable 'ifs' that govern all our actions. Who will tell us, for example, that prudence may be the best nursing response at any given moment: where prudence may be a word, a gesture, a procedure – or even a retreat? Scientific theory and technical artistry may inform practice, but cannot deliver it. Only we, as psychiatric–mental health nurse practitioners, are capable of deciding 'where to go' in any given psychiatric situation. And it is only having reached a particular therapeutic destination (which always is unique) that we can say, in retrospect, how we came to be there.

The craft of caring involves a person-centred agenda that sits surrounded by a consideration of the 'whole'. The psychiatric–mental health nurse needs to view the psychiatric situation with maximum depth of field, while focusing sharply on the eyes of the other. It is a craft that relies heavily upon a pragmatic approach to caring akin to Bergson's *le bon sens*.[b] Rather than searching for explanations, a pragmatist tries to identify how best to cope with and respond to a particular set of circumstances.[6] Yet such pragmatism nestles safely beneath warming blankets of training, experience and a desire to do no harm. It is no 'bootstrap theory', but rather is a moving vehicle from which to see the situation from many different perspectives.

Every psychiatric moment begins for the nurse as they try to make some sense of a situation. It is a naive and muted picture that they see; a hastily drawn sketch that can only gain colour and form through the other – the experiences of the person who is the 'patient'. A genuine understanding of the other can only dawn through them and their view of the world. We must pay attention to the other and create conversations that are inspired through them. They are always the leader and the

---

[b] *Le bon sens* was a term used by the French philosopher Henri Bergson to describe a form of 'common sense'. Contrary to scientific dogma, *le bon sens* advocates a combination of tactfulness, morality and human relationship as the primary guiding principles towards human relating. It is cited in Gadamer H-G. *Truth and method*, 2nd edn. London: Sheed and Ward, 1989, p. 26. Unfortunately, the original paper is only available in French. Bergson H. *Écrits et paroles*. Paris: Presses Universitaires de France, 1957: 84–94.

instigator of 'the glory of discovery'.[7,p.135] They alone hold the key to the craftwork cupboard. Unless the nurse consults them and looks at life from their viewing gallery, they will fashion an object that is precious only to themselves. The craft of caring is always dependent upon the other, whose own personal growth becomes a catalyst for the incidental development of the nurse.

Creating conditions for growth and development

The concept of emotional or spiritual growth is ambiguous and difficult to measure. Unlike the fruit on the tree, the human being shows no external signs of psychological ripening. Yet the ethereal nature of personal growth is quantifiable beyond all reasonable doubt merely through verbal confirmation. People tell us, through their stories, of the growth taking place within them. If we listen 'actively'[c] we will hear those words that signify human growth and change. Such statements usually demonstrate greater understandings, clearer pictures, changed perspectives and a more positive sense of self. The craft of psychiatric–mental health nursing involves modifying the climate of the caring relationship to bring about 'the necessary conditions for the promotion of growth and development'.[4,p.20]

A woman once described to me her grief. It was 'paralysing' and made her feel 'dead inside'. When we finally parted company, she was feeling 'released' and 'able to get on with living'. This common theme of disablement surfaces in various guises, irrespective of the mental trauma. It is the part of the problem that enervates and pervades one's being as drizzling grey rain, lethal black ice or demoralizing mirages.

When these disabling emotions begin to subside, the person becomes able to channel their intent and energies outwards once more. The rutted winter months of distress begin to melt away and new shoots of purpose slowly begin to surface. This healing process – this period of growth by way of understanding and discovery of more fruitful ways of living – is all part and parcel of the nurse–other alliance. The opportunity to grow through and with the other is just as much an option for the psychiatric–mental health nurse as their partner. What a privilege to practise a craft that enables us to set sail each working day on a voyage of 'becoming with'.

Becoming with the other: a journey of togetherness

'Becoming with' means picking up the tempo of the other and joining with by joining in. It is a tune called and conducted by the other. The role of the psychiatric–mental health nurse is to identify the melody and harmonize accordingly. Sometimes, this is a conscious process, where the nurse pays attention to the messages being broadcast by the other. Guided by their feelings, they work out their best responses to the emotional pain and distress of the other.

From my own lived experiences as a psychiatric–mental health nurse, I find myself first enveloped by certain feelings during this process. These feelings, generated by the other, become my guiding light through a formulatory process that involves a conversation within myself. I begin to ask myself, if I were this 'other', I mean *really* were this particular other, what would I be feeling or believing now? Walsh[8] calls this process of understanding 'shared humanity': a 'being-in-the-world-with-patients' that 'makes the ordinary extraordinarily effective in helping patients'. Gradually, I begin to check out just how close I am to understanding with the other. I begin to put together a hypothesis that I can tentatively share: 'So, I'm not too sure, yet, but I wonder if …?' A furrowed brow, a considered sigh and a moment's hesitation all signify that I have further to travel before I can bathe in the warm glow of that shared understanding. Often, the response from the other is silent and deafening: the sudden eye contact that speaks louder than any words: 'Oh! You've touched my heart'; the rocking motion that says: 'You're getting close, too close right now – back off!'; the body that suddenly switches to a different frequency with inaudible voices that do not speak to me, is the body that transmits a signal telling me I have been tuned out.

At other times, the psychiatric–mental health nurse will become oblivious to their own otherness. They will have crossed the threshold of conscious separation and joined the other person in all but body. They will see no colour on the walls, no curtains at the windows, no features on the face of the other. They have temporarily ceased to be aware of their own existence and plunged into the wholeness of togetherness. In Buber's[9,p.41] terms, this has become an I–Thou moment: a potential space of exclusivity where man steps 'out of the glowing darkness of chaos, into the cool light of creation'. As the psychiatric nurse plies their craft, it is always *with* the other.

Those magic I–Thou moments are inevitably swathed in blissful ignorance – and can only be acknowledged by reflective after-light. I can recall my own such experiences of subliminal togetherness, best described, perhaps, as spiritual confluence, devoid of any doing – pure becoming. Such therapeutic closeness, to my mind, is artless metaphor untempered by and defiant of theoretical reduction. It is beautiful knowing that cannot be explained but can be completely understood through

---

[c] 'Active listening' was coined by Gerard Egan, and describes the total presence of the listener. As well as attending to the verbal content, active listening includes non-verbal behaviour, hearing the words in the context of the person's whole life situation and, finally, the 'spin' that the speaker puts on the story. Egan G. *The skilled helper: a problem-management approach to helping*, 6th edn. USA: Brooks/Cole, 1998

experience. As Keats[10] so elegantly wrote, 'Beauty is truth, truth beauty – that is all ye know on earth and all ye need to know'.

Collaborative healing

Somewhere within this I–Thou alliance exists the spiritual dimension of healing: a collaboration of the two 'others' that defies and always will defy any analysis. Indeed, the merest attempt to explain separates us from this process like the sudden roar of the outboard motor kills the joy of the tranquil loch. The only theoretical device capable of carrying the spiritual component of nursing is metaphor, which is born out of experience. When I grope and feel my way towards such experiences, which lie within my own nursing practice, I can recall heart-melting moments of spiritual togetherness. Hobson,[5,pp.279–80] in his own inimitable style, offers his own interpretation for those sublime, spiritual moments between two people in therapy: 'aloneness–togetherness … an imaginative activity which discloses the possibility of creating a kind of loving that lies within and between persons'.

Collaborative caring is the journey of two fellow travellers 'into the flow of life'.[11,p.127] Only when people step into the life-stream together are they able to make sense of what it is to feel hard pebbles under their feet, or the cool rush of noisy water against their skin. Making sense of things reduces fear and introduces new possibilities, new options and new ways of being. The road ahead is cleared of debris and despondency gives way to hope. Without hope, there can be no wind change and, indeed, no 'X' on 'the treasure map of the territory of care'.[11,p.119] When the chains of emotional distress prove just too heavy, it is the psychiatric–mental health nurse who offers the 'tender leaves of hope' by showing a genuine belief in the other.

To offer hope, the psychiatric–mental health nurse must trust and believe in the other without reservation. Perhaps this is their most challenging responsibility? Or perhaps not? Benner[12] suggests that 'Nurses establish a healing relationship and create a healing climate by mobilizing hope in themselves … and the patient'. Having faith in ourselves constitutes the very first step, as we journey through the rivers of distress with the other. Each subsequent step is taken in tandem with that other

person until the banks of the river are within reach. The psychiatric–mental health nurse becomes an emotional lifeguard, on hand to prevent the other from drowning. Should the other stumble and fall from their stepping stone, the likeliest consequence is that, despite becoming emotionally drenched, they will scramble back onto the stone themselves.[13,p.57] The most that we will have to do is offer a handhold, together with a message of support: 'Come on – I know you can do it'.

Emotional life saving,[14] however, is a final response that we rarely have to resort to. Most of the time we sit with the other and admire their resilience and commitment to survival. By far the greatest amount of time is spent being and responding, keeping apace as they choose which stepping stone to try next. As we approach the riverbank, we can drop back a step, enabling the other to reach dry land first. Through our relationship with the other, we are able to nurture a positive concept within them and reinforce their potential to become.[15] Depending on the depth and rapidity of the water flow, emotional river crossing can be a harrowing experience. If we are to engage in healing relationships, we must be willing to accept that we, too, are as susceptible to being emotionally wounded as any other is. If the psychiatric–mental health nurse is feeling emotionally fragile, irrespective of the reasons why, they need to put themselves first and tend to their own wounds. This may mean seeking extra supervision and support from their colleagues, engaging in some form of personal therapy or even taking time out for a while. It is perfectly acceptable for nurses to ask for help. Collectively, psychiatric–mental health nurses need to acknowledge the demanding nature of their role and be available for each other at all times.

As you read this text, my words may draw you into a shared understanding of the craft of psychiatric nursing. Conversely, they may sail past your heart like passing ships in the night. They may reflect pictures of psychiatric nursing that mimic images of your own. Or they may not. Look on these words as waves within the psychiatric ocean. Sail on them or sail past them. Like reading a book, the craft of psychiatric nursing involves constant searching for meaning with the other. It is a voyage of perpetual discovery. Do not become disheartened or disabled if you struggle to grasp the reasoning and supposition within this chapter. More importantly, each and every time you engage with the other you are living and learning your craft.

Personal illustration 5.1: George's story

Let us return to the beginning of this chapter, to the hospital ward where I first met George, tried and sentenced by his own internal judge and jury. Our paths first crossed in the dramatic fashion I described in the opening paragraph. Detained under a section of the Mental Health Act, he had been medically diagnosed and prescribed a hefty regime of psychoactive drugs to treat his mental illness. George had not worked for several years, although he had held an officer's commission in the Salvation Army until his recurrent mental ill health had caused him to take early retirement. A very knowledgeable man, with a degree in theology, much of his conversation was related to his religious beliefs.

Being heavily sedated, he would sleep for long periods during the day. During his wakeful moments he would sit with glassy eyes and spittled mouth, slowly and self-consciously raising both his cup and saucer to his lips, as his noticeable tremor caused the tea to flow over the brim. Little by little, George disclosed his persecutory beliefs to me. He believed that he had contributed significantly to the demise of Christianity and that he, alone, was responsible for the recent closure of a nearby church. God had spoken to him many months ago, telling him that it was his mission to boost the congregation and save the church. Alas, he had failed to do so.

Conversation with George was, sometimes, very one-sided. He would leave our conversational frequency and engage in dialogue with God. He would eventually join me once more and share with me what God had said to him. I would listen with the utmost respect and, at times, revel in the gift of his extensive biblical awareness. On such occasions, George and I would lose ourselves together as we wandered through the wilderness of his torment.

Six weeks after my privileged meeting with him, George began to emerge from the desolation of his psychosis. By now, I had come to know his wife and, during an evening visit to the ward, the three of us sat together drinking tea. We were making the final preparations for George's weekend leave, in preparation for being discharged home. I remember his wife suddenly turning to me and placing her hand on my arm. Sincerity shone in her eyes as she expressed her gratitude to me for 'being so nice to George and helping him get through everything'. I decided to ask George what it was that had helped him to survive and transcend his emotional ordeal. He responded by saying that he thought his medication had played a vital role in his recovery. His wife agreed and added that she had prayed continually for God to look after George and 'heal him'. George nodded his support and reflected for a moment. 'Yes', he smiled, 'Yet when I first came into hospital I thought He'd abandoned me'.

open door that led into his life; and, latterly, the conversations that decorated the borders of his road to recovery. Several months later I received a letter from George. It was a lovely surprise, particularly as it confirmed that he was feeling 'completely regenerated'. Towards the end of his letter, George made reference to a student nurse, Laura, who was on placement during his stay with us. 'Please tell her just how much I appreciated her kindness. I'm not sure if I saw her as a daughter figure, but she treated me as I imagine she would her own father. She seemed so genuine in her desire to do whatever I needed her to do in order to speed my recovery. She encouraged me to the breakfast table when eating had ceased to be a priority and she made the ward bathroom my own personal space in her attempts to rekindle my interest in myself'.

Finally, George turned to our relationship, as he wrote, 'At one stage, I thought I had entered hell. It was the most frightening experience of my life. I felt tormented and terrified. I just could not understand why you had followed me there, but you had. You were with me, Peter, and that's just where I needed you to be. Rather than trying to convince me that I was hallucinating (which would have been completely pointless, others tried and failed miserably) you chose simply to stay with me. And more than once. For that, I will be eternally and everlastingly grateful. I was in the lion's den – you dared to be there with me'.

George's letter is confirmation enough that I helped to sustain him during those awful psychotic episodes. It also bears witness to the most memorable psychiatric nursing interventions during his almost unbearable moments of madness: Laura's kindness and loving interventions and my willingness to be with him. The craft of our caring was cast in collaboration with George. Nothing was done for him, rather, he was engaged with: encouraged and spiritually (and, on occasions, physically) held through his emotional trauma. There were times when he was so troubled he did not know how he could be helped. There were no therapeutic skills to be employed, nor any clever words to interpret or console. During such times, the craft of psychiatric nursing practice is simply to be with in readiness to become with.

With George, both student nurse Laura and myself exercised our craft sensitively and productively. The craftwork that took place always involved George. On admission, he was trapped in and bedevilled by his psychotic experiences. With George's permission, we joined with him as often as possible as privileged wayfarers as he wandered through difficult terrain: two, sometimes three, sets of footprints all heading in the same direction. Time passed by and George reached a stage of development where he no longer needed our company. He would craft his own life once more from outside the hospital ward. The finished product of mental healthfulness was of the utmost value to George. The fact that he

Soon afterwards, George did, indeed, return home. For a week or so, I missed his presence: the intrigue and exclusivity of his divine experiences; the privilege of having an was able to enjoy the fruits of our labours together strongly suggests that I practised my craft well enough. Yet I know that, at times, I failed to respond as perhaps I should have. I failed to listen carefully, said the wrong thing; acted in my own interests rather than his; or acted out of impatience and anxiety, instead of waiting and being. Such second-class craftings are to be expected. They will always happen, even to the most experienced psychiatric nurse practitioner. When they do, they become golden opportunities for us to learn from and grow. The craft of psychiatric nursing can only ever be practised, never mastered.

EMPOWERMENT

Relationship as a gift

Over recent years, psychiatric nurses have introduced the word empowerment into their vocabulary.[16] In one respect it is a misnomer and detracts from the real craft of care. It implies that the psychiatric–mental health nurse must carry with them an agenda that includes 'giving' or 'handing over' chunks of power to psychiatric service patients. As power is an abstract construct, that is of course impossible.[13,p.78] A person can only ever feel to *have* power or *be* powerful. The science within the craft of caring is purely an awareness of, and belief in this. That willingness to be with the other leads both players to the edge of the water – only one step away from a significant shift of feeling from powerless to powered.

If the psychiatric–mental health nurse is to play any part in empowering the patient (other than by cheerful accident), they, themselves must feel empowered. Through the process of being with the other, the nurse is able to learn how to become in order to give their best response. If the patient has a need to be empowered, it is the patient who will have shown the nurse what needs to be done. The nurse will offer a response from this position of empowerment and, if the patient is ready, they will step into the pool – always slightly ahead in terms of knowing themselves better than the nurse knows them.

Once the other feels sufficiently supported and sustained to wade into the waters, there dawns the realization of the potential self. The psychiatric–mental health nurse has cultivated the conditions of growth by 'sustaining the other as a subject of action rather than attempting to negate' (him).[17,p.147] They have fostered the patient and (under their expert direction) utilized their potential to be and become. Whilst power is, indeed, at play here, the nurse learns how to become a 'channel for

the perspective of the other',[17] releasing them and enabling them to use their freedom productively.

Frequently, psychiatric–mental health nursing care is delivered through surveillance: either overtly under the watchful eye of the nursing sentinel or more covertly (and possibly more intrusively) through clinic appointments and home visits. Fox[18] describes this as the 'vigil of care', which he sees as 'the continual subjection of care's clients and increasingly, all aspects of the environment in which they live to the vigilant scrutiny of carers'.

Although the concept of 'community care' implies a less restrictive programme of interventions, it is always driven by legislation and policies that are often too opaque (the patient is not fully aware of the influential aims, objectives and recommendations of the care programme approach) and a medical model that is too powerful for the patient to reject or even question. The power of the 'healer' is still considered to be 'the central ethical problem in medicine'.[19]

When nursing practice is driven by vigilance, a heavy shadow is cast, which intimidates the other and blocks out sunrays of hope. It involves a nurse–patient relationship driven by a model of care based on sameness and repetition. The feelings of power predominantly belong to the nurse, as they use their badge of office to impose the controlling structure of the organization onto every patient. It is a relationship constructed on the foundations of power and knowledge that shape the interventions of the psychiatric–mental health nurse. According to Cixous,[20,p.87] it is a relationship that springs from within the masculine realm of what she terms the 'proper': a relationship that seeks to possess, to profit, to pleasure and to measure success in terms of 'return'. By contrast, Cixous offers the feminine relationship-as-gift, where she 'with open hands, gives herself – pleasure, happiness, increased value, enhanced self image' without ever trying 'to recover her expenses'.[20] Even within the most panoptical institutional setting, there is room for the individual to grow by way of their relationship with others.[21]

Each and every time care is gift-wrapped with kindness and consideration, a climate of possibility has been created between nurse and other. The other has been liberated enough to make choices rather than following the prescriptive route markers of a depersonalizing system. They have become 'deterritorialized': their quarantine has been lifted and new 'lines of flight'[d] drawn to wherever they choose. 'You are suffering from schizophrenia', 'You need to take this medication', and 'You need to stay in hospital for a while' may constitute professional recommendations delivered in the patient's 'best interests'. Yet they are really no more than paternalistic impositions

---

[d] In their seminal text *A thousand plateaus*, Deleuze and Guattari use the expression 'deterritorialization' to describe the process of breaking free from a restrictive or oppressive discourse (such as the disempowering consequences of a regime of psychiatry based upon subjugation). Deterritorialization is achieved by creating a new 'line of flight' – an escape route – towards becoming what Deleuze and Guattari term a 'nomad': free to travel 'beyond' and discover new, more liberating ways of being. Deleuze G, Guattari F. *A thousand plateaus*. London: Athlone Press, 1988.

and, as such, are loaded with control. There is no negotiation, no shared understandings and, often, no room for manoeuvre. They are interventions that carry the agendas and prejudices of the psychiatric provider and, as such, they negate the experiences of the other. The person who is patient remains unrecognized in their distress and, as such, is unable to live it and survive it.

Even when a person is emotionally distressed and presenting a serious risk to themselves or others, there is usually a (albeit sometimes very narrow) corridor available for shared conversations. 'You need to stay in hospital for a while' – although quite possibly an instruction borne out of necessity – can be opened out and rephrased to become more of a discussion point rather than a fait accompli. Having explained the rationale behind implementing a section under the Mental Health Act, the best response that one might hope for in this situation could be a declaration of relief from the sectioned person and a willingness to talk further.

However, we must acknowledge that the 'worst' outcome may be a violent and aggressive reaction that, in some way, needs to be physically contained. If this is so, it then becomes crucial that we nurses remain aware of the perceived power differentials between those controlling and the person being controlled. Our only agenda during any such acts of restraint must be one driven by safety: for the person being restrained, for any other people in the immediate area, for our colleagues and, of course, for ourselves.

Crafting nursing practice in such situations becomes difficult, as voluntary collaboration between the person and the nurse ceases to exist. There is still always an intersubjective relationship between the two people, in that the individual actions of each person will be reacted to by the other in some way (e.g. the patient may refuse to talk to the nurse or, perhaps, scream and shout at them – or the nurse and their colleagues may engage in some form of physical containing procedure). And, as the nurse and patient continue to interact (either verbally or nonverbally) with each other, there is still the potential for care to be crafted, though circumstances will dictate that such craftings are unequivocally carried out by the nurse from within an I-it[e] framework. Caring-with the person in this situation involves a safe resolution of the crisis, followed by a period of waiting and acceptance … until a safe space appears for the person to talk about the incident and their experience of being physically restrained. This may take hours, days, weeks … and in some instances, for whatever reason, the opportunity may never present itself.

After such an incident, even the most experienced nurse may have some residual feelings, such as guilt, anger, anxiety or relief. Experiencing these feelings is understandable and even desirable – we humans are driven by emotions and to not feel would be a way of denying and avoiding the issues generated by the incident. What is vital is that we talk them through as soon as possible in some form of supervisory forum, where we can make sense of such feelings and clear the ground for future craftings to take place.

At every given opportunity, the craft of psychiatric–mental health nursing embraces the act of offering what rightly belongs to the other. In order to survive an experience, a person must experience that experience as it is for themselves (and not as someone says it is for them). The craft of caring involves a decolonizing of the other by enabling them to reclaim their own territory. If the psychiatric nurse is to play any part in this returning home, it is merely to 'gently guide the tiller'[7,p.156] in response to the navigational prompts of the other. Each response needs to be blessed by 'a universal common sense'[22] that is always applied to the difference of the other. It is the way they say things that takes precedence over their need to influence outcomes. Their 'words (must) take their meanings from other words rather than by virtue of their representative character'.[23,p.368] Otherwise, genuine conversations will either degenerate into sterile inquiry or become distorted and meaningless for the other. The only acceptable nursing agenda 'is to keep the conversation going'[23,p.377] and the door open to brand new ways of being.

Reflection

What do you understand by 'empowerment'? How influenced are you by your organization's policies of vigilance and observation? To what extent are you able to 'care-with' someone and offer your caring unconditionally as a gift? How important are qualities such as kindness and genuine consideration to the crafting of your practice?

SUMMARY

Like any other craftsperson, the psychiatric–mental health nurse fashions a product to please a customer. As nurses, we have come to call our product 'care'. Unless we engage with those customers by asking questions and actively listening to their responses, our craftwork will become an artefact of our own design. It will be of no value to our customer. As Barker and Whitehill[4,p.21] so poignantly declare, 'If we are to develop a craft of care in psychiatric nursing, then we need to know what the experience of mental ill health *means* (author's italics) to the person who is "in" that experience'. The craft of our caring, then, must always follow a pattern fashioned by our customer – the person in need of our care.

---

[e]The concept of 'I-it' is the antithesis of what Buber[9] describes as I–Thou (see text). It describes the conscious separation between a person and an other, to the point where the other is seen as a separate object and empathy or any shared understanding becomes impossible.

As each new working day begins, we enter our workshop with the other knowing only that the material to be crafted will be familiar, but always will be different from that which we have previously encountered. We will be faced with interesting and challenging situations that materialize through the togetherness of the nurse–patient relationship. Because the psychiatric–mental health nurse can never be sure what their craft-mate will bring, they will always need to improvise. Although they will, by necessity, have their tool bag to hand full of interventions, they must first engage the other as the primary director of their care. This may take time and patience and involve lengthy periods of rejection and not knowing for the psychiatric–mental health nurse. Accepting this and showing a genuine willingness to wait and still be available is a crucial component of our craft. It is only when the other person feels secure enough within the caring relationship that the conditions can sustain that person's growth and recovery.

Psychiatric–mental health nursing is an occupation that carries a salary, enabling us to pay our mortgages and feed our families. We are employed by an organization to practise our craft. Yet, without a steady stream of customers, we would be redundant. I find it sobering that our world is constructed in such a way that we, as psychiatric–mental health nurses, rely upon the psychological suffering of others to pay our wages. It would be crass, therefore, to say that we choose to nurse by way of a 'calling' and nothing more: there is *always* something more in it for the psychiatric–mental health nurse. Yet, as far as the 'other' goes, we really should expect nothing from them, only 'the common wages'[f] that all relationships are capable of yielding.

Although this comprehensive textbook will, hopefully, become your constant companion throughout at least the formative years of your career in psychiatry, you can only ever learn your craft with the other. Paradoxically, the emotionally disabled person who turns to you for succour will become your most reliable guide and teacher. Follow their lead and resist any desire to forcibly re-describe their experiences – for those experiences are their only proof that they exist.

REFERENCES

1. Chamberlin J. The medical model and harm. In: Barker P, Campbell P, Davidson B (eds). *From the ashes of experience: reflections on madness, survival and growth*. London, UK: Whurr Publishers, 1999: 171.

2. Keats J. Letter to George and Thomas Keats, 21 December, 1817. In: Barnard J (ed.). *John Keats: the complete poems*, 3rd edn. London, UK: Penguin Books, 1988.

3. Peplau H. *Interpersonal relations in nursing*. Basingstoke, UK: Macmillan Press, 1988.

4. Barker P, Whitehill I. The craft of care: towards collaborative caring in psychiatric nursing. In: Tilley S (ed.). *The mental health nurse: views of practice and education*. Oxford, UK, Blackwell Sciences, 1997: 15–27.

5. Hobson RF. *Forms of feeling: the heart of psychotherapy*. London: Tavistock Publications, 1985.

6. Menand L. An introduction to pragmatism. In: Menand L (ed.). *Pragmatism: a reader*. New York: Vintage Books, 1997: xi–xxxiv.

7. Barker P, Kerr B. *The process of psychotherapy: a journey of discovery*. Oxford, UK: Butterworth-Heinemann, 2001: 135.

8. Walsh, K. Shared humanity and the psychiatric nurse–patient encounter. *Australian and New Zealand Journal of Mental Health Nursing* 1999; **8**: 7.

9. Buber M. *I and Thou*. Edinburgh, UK: T. & T. Clark, 1958.

10. Keats J. (1820) Ode on a Grecian urn. In: Barnard J (ed.). *John Keats: the complete poems*, 3rd edn. London, UK: Penguin Books, 1988.

11. Barker P. *The philosophy and practice of psychiatric nursing*. Edinburgh, UK: Churchill Livingstone, 1999: 127.

12. Benner P. *From novice to expert: excellence and power in clinical nursing practice*. Menlo Park, CA: Addison-Wesley, 1984: 213.

13. Watkins P. *Mental health nursing: the art of compassionate care*. Oxford: Butterworth-Heinemann, 2001: 57.

14. Barker P. The Tidal Model: the development of personal caring within the chaos paradigm. 8 pages, The Tidal Model, Internet, 25th May 2001. Available from: http://members.nbci.com/_XMCM/drphilbarker/Phil_Barker~2/Tidal_paper.html.

15. Graham IW. Seeking a clarification of meaning: a phenomenological interpretation of the craft of mental health nursing. *Journal of Psychiatric and Mental Health Nursing* 2001; **8** (4): 335–45.

16. Barker P, Stevenson C, Leamy M. The philosophy of empowerment. *Mental Health Nursing* 2000; **20** (9): 8–12.

17. Crossley N. *Intersubjectivity: the fabric of social becoming*. London, UK: Sage, 1996: 147.

18. Fox NJ. *Beyond health: postmodernism and embodiment*. London, UK: Free Association Books, 1999: 81.

19. Brody H. *The healer's power*. New Haven, CT: Yale University Press, 1992: 36.

20. Cixous H. Sorties: out and out: attacks/ways out/forays. In: Cixous H, Clément C (eds). *The newly born woman*. London, UK: Tarris, 1996; 87.

21. Wilkin PE. From medicalization to hybridization: a postcolonial discourse for psychiatric nurses. *Journal of Psychiatric and Mental Health Nursing* 2001; **8** (2): 115–20.

22. Gadamer H-G. *Truth and method*, 2nd edn. London, UK: Sheed and Ward, 1989: 17.

23. Rorty R. *Philosophy and the mirror of nature*. Oxford, UK: Blackwell Publishers, 1980: 368.

[f] A line from Dylan Thomas's aptly named poem *In my craft or sullen art* refers to the spontaneous and esoteric rewards that relationships yield: solidarity, rapport and, perhaps most importantly, an acceptance of individual limitations. *The Dylan Thomas omnibus*. London: Phoenix Giants, 1995.

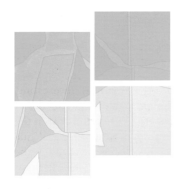

CHAPTER 6

Leading developments in the craft of caring

Angela Simpson*

INTRODUCTION

Since the end of the 1990s the 'modernization' of health services and demands for 'cost-effective care' have emphasized the need for the effective management of nurses. This chapter discusses how, historically, nurses have worked within organizational cultures characterized by autocratic and hierarchical management. This bureaucratic approach is contrasted with leadership, which is underpinned by a more responsive, creative and trusting way of working with people. This leadership approach has been recognized as being a more productive form of organizing staff and developing clinical services, by organizational and nursing theorists alike.

Leadership is different from management. It hinges on strong communication, mutuality and respect. It emphasizes a more participatory and interactive way of working. This chapter discusses the softer focus of leadership in more detail, and will examine in detail the skills of transformational leaders. Research has demonstrated that transformational leadership skills can be learned and developed like any other.[1,2] Transformational leadership has also been positively linked with enhancing clinical services and developing nursing practice.[3]

NURSING AND MANAGEMENT

Nursing has a well-documented history dating back to the turn of the twentieth century. At this time, men strictly controlled the position of women in society. This was also the case within nursing, led by the male-dominated medical profession, which managed hospitals and was the powerful decision-maker. Nurses with management responsibilities at this time were from the upper classes. It is perhaps due to this factor that autocratic management became the accepted norm. Rawdon[4] observed that the class divisions present within nursing contributed to a climate of subservience and noted that nursing was influenced as much by its own class divisions as it was by the sexist attitudes present at that time. These combined influences contributed to his view that nursing became a rigid profession with its ultimate control firmly in the grip of predominantly male medical staff.

*Angela Simpson is course leader for the post-graduate diploma in Mental Health Nursing and a Research Fellow at University of York, UK. She has worked extensively in mental health nursing over a 20-year period and has a particular interest in nursing practice development in acute in-patient admission settings. Her recent research focused the management of depression in primary care settings and recovery from self-cutting.

Nursing still retains some aspects of this early sub-servience to and dependence upon medicine. These are best observed within the routines of task-orientated practice, where nurses engage in clinical roles without questioning their purpose or timeliness.[5] Today, it would appear that nursing is still attempting to free itself from its past. Although nurses are predominantly female, beyond first-line (clinical) management, nursing continues to be disproportionately managed by men.

Although management styles within nursing have remained fairly static, over the years the environment within which nurses work has changed greatly. The modernization of health services in the UK, driven by a desire for high-quality, cost-efficient health care, has necessitated a reorganization of clinical services. Consequently, nurses face a new and challenging organizational culture that appears highly competitive, fast moving and constantly changing. Traditional management styles involving hierarchy underpinned by bureaucracy are inappropriate within such a climate. Their inherent inflexibility results in work environments that are slow to adapt and change. However, abandoning the tradition of autocratic management represents a huge cultural shift for nursing. This shift can be better understood when we differentiate between the skills of managers and the skills of leaders.

DISTINGUISHING MANAGEMENT FROM LEADERSHIP

Management in the context of nursing has been identified as involving the use of delegated authority within formal organization settings to organize, direct and control responsible subordinates.[6] This illustrates the distinguishing characteristics of managers. They are *appointed* to, and occupy, formal positions of organizational authority, and use legitimatized power to *command*, *reward* or *punish* the workforce. Leaders on the other hand tend to *emerge* from within the workforce and attract followers. In contrast to managers, leaders often possess little power with which to influence the actions of colleagues. Leaders are people who are able to communicate and resonate with their followers despite the absence of formal 'position power'.[7]

Kouzes and Posner[1] suggested that the root meaning of the words *manager* and *leader* help to distinguish them. 'Manage' originated from the word meaning 'hand'. Thus *managing* is about *handling* or organizing things while also maintaining order. In contrast the root meaning of the word leader refers to 'going or travelling', suggesting that the constant movement towards achieving new objectives might be of greater interest to leaders than the ultimate destination. The metaphor of the leadership journey is described by Nelson Mandela in *Long walk to freedom*:[8]

a leader is like a shepherd. He stays behind the flock, letting the nimble go ahead, whereupon the others follow not realizing that all along they were being directed from behind.

The notion of 'leading from behind' is interesting. Although those who follow might perceive the leader to be in front, leaders themselves are to be found within the pack steering and guiding those around them. While adopting this position, leaders are closely involved in the primary roles and functions of core tasks. Perhaps because of this leaders tend to be viewed by followers as possessing legitimate expertise. Leaders lead by example and are expert *role models*. They are acutely aware of the delicate relationship of *influence* over *authority*, recognizing that meaningful change cannot be forced, and will happen only at its own speed.

The leader pays close attention to the movement of the workforce on the journey towards its agreed destination often encouraging novel or creative approaches to traversing this new territory. Where leaders differ most from managers is in their intense interest in the journey itself (as opposed to possessing an overwhelming desire to achieve the goal for its own sake). Leaders recognize that by the time the goal is achieved it is already likely to be past its 'sell-by date' and the next goal will already have emerged. Change is the only constant. Leaders understand what motivates people, and are concerned with finding out how to support and promote that forward movement. They know that this is highly valuable for a maturing workforce. Hence, leadership is a broader and more interpersonal concept than management, and hinges upon personal relationships. Over the years theorists have attempted to identify the distinguishing characteristics of leaders, recognizing that the leadership styles of men and women vary significantly.

> ### Reflection
>
> Think about a clinical leader with whom you are involved.
>
> - What qualities of leadership distinguish her/him from a manager?
> - How does the leader communicate with team members? How does this differ from the way that a manager relates to staff?
> - Think about the balance of power, trust and respect evoked by the leader and contrast this with hierarchical management.

LEADING LADIES: THE GENDER AGENDA

Rosener[9] recognized that men and women describe leadership attributes very differently. Men frequently describe using *power* and *authority*. Typically, men viewed management performance in terms of transactions, utilizing the traditional skills of command and control. Women's descriptions of leadership differed and placed greater emphasis on getting other people to support the task. Conflict avoidance was recognized in women's desire to find *win–win* solutions. Also, women who described themselves as *feminine* or *gender neutral* reported higher levels of 'followership' among women workers, than those who describe themselves in masculine terms. Thus people who adopt these more feminine leadership traits are viewed as *transformational*. They adopt a leadership style that:

- is interactive and participative
- validates other people
- delegates authority
- shares in the decision-making process.

Although women were found to have a natural orientation towards the transformational leadership qualities described above, it is also possible for men to adopt similar leadership behaviours. The term 'feminine' leadership illustrates the softer focus of this approach and distinguishes it from more traditional power base management.

The feminine approach to leadership has a softer, more creative focus. This is highly desirable within organizations that face persistent change.[10] However, such skills are often not regarded highly within traditional organizations with a dominant masculine or *macho* culture resulting in the commonly held belief that only by adopting typically masculine traits can one be perceived as competent.

Although nursing has been slow to embrace the potential of feminine leadership, many businesswomen have adopted this style with great success. The late Anita Roddick, founder of the Body Shop, based her business around feminine principles[11] defining these as:

> principles of caring, making intuitive decisions, not getting hung up on hierarchy, having a sense of work as being part of your life, not separate from it, and putting your labour where your love is.

Transformational leadership has been recognized as holding great potential in the further development of nursing.[3] Indeed adopting a feminine or transformational approach to leadership especially at the ward or clinical team level might be the creative release necessary to advance the craft of psychiatric caring. Pearson[12] suggested that nurses must 'confront' the ever-present, dominant masculine ideology that underpins modern health care. However, it is questionable if 'confronting' anything or anyone fits with this softer focus. The best way forward is for nurses to adopt a feminine style of clinical leadership aiming to creatively explore the therapeutic nature of nursing through active/constructive 'doing'. Developing nursing practice hinges on constructive action not confrontation.

TRANSFORMATIONAL LEADERSHIP: THE ART OF EMPOWERING PEOPLE

Transformational (feminine) leadership emphasizes strong interpersonal communication, mutuality and affiliation. The transformational leader:

- gets to know staff, taking an active interest in them and their development;
- seeks to empower the workforce, delegating tasks and giving praise;
- seeks to promote excellence beyond mere tasks;
- encourages employees to become ideas orientated and solution focused.

Bass and Avolio[13] identify transformational leaders as those who can:

- stimulate interest among followers to view work from a fresh perspective;
- generate an awareness of a vision, towards which the team is headed;
- develop followers to higher levels of ability and potential;
- motivate followers to look beyond their own interests, towards those that will benefit the group.

Thus transformational (feminine) leaders go far beyond mere task attainment. For them, work is a developmental opportunity, within which the leader and followers are motivated to produce higher levels of performance. Transformational leaders steer their course away from hierarchy and rules nurturing a culture in which others might become empowering leaders themselves.[14]

Transformational leadership is not, however, a magical quality possessed by a few. It is an observable set of core behaviours that can be learned and developed.[1] Further, nurse leaders in nursing development units appeared (naturally) to adopt transformational styles of leadership in practice.[3]

Reflection

Identify a transformational leader that you have worked with.

- What does the transformational leader do to encourage and support you?
- How does the transformational leader make you feel?

Kouzes and Posner[2] suggested seven lessons in leadership that guide the process of transformational leadership. Each of the seven lessons is described and discussed in the context of developing nursing practice.

LESSON 1: LEADERS DON'T WAIT

Leadership is an adventure requiring a pioneering spirit.[2] In nursing this begins with a shift in attitude. Capturing this pioneering spirit involves swapping the cynicism or despair that frequently inhibits clinical environments, for the belief that things have the potential to be better. Changing attitudes does not necessarily involve additional resources. Rather, success hinges on the leader's ability to view the world differently. Typically this will involve 'letting go' of the constraining attitudes and beliefs present in everyday practice. How easy (or difficult) this will be depends on each individual team and its motivation to do so. An Indonesian story illustrates this.

> Hunters setting traps for monkeys, cut holes in coconuts that are just the right size for a monkey to put his hand through. The hunter then secures the coconut to the bottom of the tree, places a banana inside and hides in wait. The monkey sees the banana and places his hand through the hole to take hold of it. The hole however is crafted so the monkey can pass his open hand through it, but when he clenches his fist round the banana, he cannot withdraw his hand. The solution is simple. To free him self, all the monkey has to do is to release hold of the banana. Most monkeys however, do not let go. And so, they are trapped!

Many nurses are clutching a (metaphorical) banana, in the shape of some aspect of practice that does not work for them, their clientele or both. They find it hard to engage in the creative, 'break-through thinking' needed to advance practice.

Break through thinking is often subtle and grounded in the everyday practice of nursing, rather than located in some complex organizational reconfiguration, or the latest government guidelines. The word 'innovation' often conjures up the notion of far-reaching change. This need not be the case. Indeed, truly creative approaches to nursing practice might be 'blinding' only in their relative simplicity. Meaningful change is often small scale and subtle but, nevertheless, makes a significant contribution towards improving care and developing practice.

Leading a new venture within a turbulent organizational climate is often seen as overwhelmingly difficult. We often believe that positive change can only occur within stable conditions. However, much of the stress involved in change is a function of our human need to control or resist it. A more constructive view is to accept the pace of change. Instead of resisting, we should take an active interest in change. Learn to roll with it rather than against it. Nurse leaders serious about developing nursing practice recognize that textbook conditions never apply in practice. They don't wait for favourable organizational conditions. Instead they understand the need to make progress, often in small steps or stages, accepting that the journey will involve as much fair weather as foul. The famous organizational management theorist Tom Peters[15] understands that modern organizations face constant change. He observed that 'if you sense calm, it's only because you are in the eye of the hurricane!'

LESSON 2: CHARACTER COUNTS

Personal qualities like courage, conviction, honesty and being forward looking are all powerful leadership attributes.[2] These result in the leader being viewed as a credible source of information, who is viewed as 'standing for something' tapping into a value system. Their work assumes a moral, rather than simply a professional focus. Decisions become based around a belief or value system that makes sense to followers. Thus work assumes a moral rather than simply a professional focus. As decisions become based around a belief or value system there is added stability through predictability (even within chaotic organizational conditions) because decisions hold true to certain fundamental principles or values. Leaders are closely in touch with their own values but more importantly involve others in developing a set of shared beliefs. This fosters a philosophical approach to practice. Burns[16] viewed transformational leaders as taking the team to a higher moral level. At the highest stage of moral development persons are guided by near-universal ethical principles of justice such as equality of human rights and respect for individual dignity. These philosophical principles match those required when making genuine attempts to develop the craft of psychiatric–mental health practice.

LESSON 3: LEADERS HAVE THEIR HEADS IN THE CLOUDS AND THEIR FEET ON THE GROUND

It is important to recognize that attracting followers involves being viewed as credible. Because of this, leaders work from within the pack, often performing the routine aspects of the work. They also have a strong sense of personal direction, which others feel inspired to follow. They do this by creating an uplifting picture of the future and inviting others to join the journey.[2]

Psychiatric–mental health nursing needs to consider where it is *now* and where it wants to *go*. Currently, nursing appears constrained, perhaps with good reason. Inadequate resources play a significant part in demoralizing nurses. There is however a real danger that by succumbing to these factors nursing might allow its very spirit to become imprisoned in a self-imposed claustrophobia, within which nursing loses its will to determine its own future. The best way of re-engaging nurses with a totally clinical nursing agenda is to identify ways at the clinical interface in which the most mature and senior clinical nurses are able to engage in the 'hands on' practice of nursing. The modern management culture has often worked against this, resulting in skilled nurses managing resources at a distance from people in care rather than leading nursing practice developments.

LESSON 4: SHARED VALUES

People have a tendency to drift when they become unsure or confused about what they should be doing. It is however possible to stabilize teams facing constantly changing environments. This involves articulating shared values that dovetail with wider organizational objectives. Where this consistency exists there are benefits for both employee and the organization: strong feelings of personal effectiveness and reduced levels of job stress and tension.[1,2] Transformational leadership is 'values' leadership.[17]

Identifying and sharing core values within the nursing team is only a useful exercise if the core principles are 'alive' at ward level or within the clinical team. Reducing this task to a dry philosophy statement pinned to the office wall isn't enough. Significant meaning can be derived from this invisible code through the development of a practice philosophy clearly articulated within core beliefs. These beliefs need to become a touchstone for the entire team. This might best be achieved within clinical supervision, for example where critical incidents are explored in relation to core team values. Nurses are then able to discuss and self-assess how close they are in the clinical context to the values they aspire to practise.

LESSON 5: YOU CAN'T DO IT ALONE

There is no leadership without a team. The collective efforts of the whole have greater value than any one individual. Leaders seek the active involvement of those around them to achieve mutually agreed goals. Competition between group members is counterproductive. Leaders seek the collective will of all involved.[2] Nurse leaders often go beyond their own locality for personal inspiration. Developing this 'outsight' involves establishing contact with other leading clinicians, or well-established nurse academics. The Internet has made such contact easy to accomplish. You might link your clinical team, for example, with a similar one in another continent, exchanging experiences of different approaches to care, stimulating further debate and interest among your colleagues.

LESSON 6: THE LEGACY YOU LEAVE IS THE LIFE YOU LEAD

People are moved by deeds. It is actions that count, talking is never enough.[2] Effective leaders *walk the talk* performing the deeds consistent with the shared values of the team. In leading nurses, involvement and participation are the keys to success. In a work environment that is constantly changing, leaders bring stability through behavioural predictability. Leaders do what they say they will do.

LESSON 7: LEADERSHIP IS EVERYONE'S BUSINESS

The idea that leaders are born not made is a myth. Leadership is not a magical quality possessed by a lucky few, it is an observable set of practices that can be learned.[1,2]

Those who are most successful at bringing out the best in others are people who set achievable goals that stretch both themselves and the people involved in achieving them.[2] Leaders hold a fundamental belief in their ability to develop the talents of others. Leadership is 'the process that ordinary people use when they are bringing forth the best in themselves and in others'.

Reflection

Think about the different managers and leaders that you have encountered.

- What attitudes values and beliefs underpin transformational leadership?
- Identify philosophical values that you think might best lead the development of genuine caring.
- How might nurse leaders share their vision of developing clinical practice?

IN SEARCH OF TRANSFORMATIONAL NURSING

Historically nursing has been influenced by its religious and military backgrounds. These influences contributed to a culture in which formal structures and autocratic hierarchy became the organizational norm. These background conditions strongly influenced the culture of nursing which has, by and large, struggled to break free and develop new ways of working that truly enhance nursing care. The need for nurses to trade in stability and tradition and replace this with new and effective ways of caring for people has probably never been greater, but developing the practice of caring within modern turbulent organizational conditions is a challenging task. This chapter has emphasized how the use of leadership skills can nurture and develop staff at all levels. Nursing has a long humanistic tradition. The conditions that support the potential for growth for people in care are also the conditions that support the growth and developing maturity of nursing. In Peplau's[18] original words nursing is 'a maturing force'. Just as people in care need trust to be placed in them, so that they may examine their circumstances and choose future directions, so nurses also need trust to be extended to them, so that they might experiment with creative approaches to developing practice. Transformational leadership is one way that nurses can potentially bring stability to a currently destabilized ward or clinical team environment. Where the skills of transformational leadership are applied nurses might be released to take constructive action in the development of their discipline. There is some evidence that this might result in nurses enjoying more open and creative thinking, and lead to significant advances in the craft of psychiatric caring.[3]

REFERENCES

1. Kouzes JM, Posner BZ. *The leadership challenge: how to keep getting extraordinary things done inside organisations.* San Francisco, CA: Jossey-Bass, 1995.

2. Kouzes JM, Posner BZ. Seven lessons for leading the voyage of the future. In: Hesselbein F, Goldsmith M, Beckard R (eds). *The leader of the future.* San Francisco, CA: Jossey Bass, 1996: 99–110.

3. Bowles A, Bowles NB. A comparative study of leadership development in nursing development units and conventional clinical settings. *Journal of Nursing Management* 2000; **8**: 69–76.

4. Rawdon R. *Managing nursing.* London, UK: Baillère Tindall, 1984.

5. Walsh M, Ford P. *Nursing ritual research and rational actions.* Oxford, UK: Butterworth-Heinemann, 1989.

6. Yura H, Ozimek D, Walsh MB. *Nursing leadership: theory and process.* New York, NY: Appleton Century Crofts, 1981.

7. Adair J. *Effective leadership.* London, UK: Pan, 1988.

8. Mandela N. *Long walk to freedom.* London, UK: Abacus, 1994.

9. Rosener JB. Ways women lead. *Harvard Business Review* 1990; **Nov–Dec**: 119–25.

10. Aburdene P, Naisbitt J. *Megatrends for women: women are changing the world.* London, UK: Random House, 1994.

11. Helgesen S. *The female advantage: women's ways of leadership.* New York, NY: Doubleday, 1990.

12. Pearson A, McMahon R. *Nursing as therapy.* London, UK: Chapman and Hall, 1991.

13. Bass BM, Avolio BJ. *Improving organisational effectiveness through transformational leadership.* London, UK: Sage, 1994.

14. Manley K. A conceptual framework for advanced practice. In: Rolfe G, Fulbrook P (eds). *Advanced nursing practice.* Oxford, UK: Butterworth-Heinemann, 1998.

15. Peters T. *The Tom Peters Seminar: crazy times call for crazy organisations.* London, UK: Macmillan, 1994.

16. Burns JM. *Leadership.* New York, NY: Harper and Row, 1978.

17. Fairholm GW. Values leadership: a values philosophy model. *International Journal of Value Based Management* 1995; **8**: 65–77.

18. Peplau H. *Interpersonal relations in nursing.* London, UK: Macmillan, 1988.

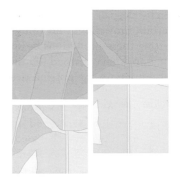

CHAPTER 7

Recovery: a personal perspective

Irene Whitehill*

> I realized I was free to take one of the many attitudes towards the situation, to give one value or another to it. ... I had the clear, pure perception that this was entirely my own affair; that I was free to choose any or several of these attitudes
>
> **Roberto Assagioli**[1,p.14]

SURVIVING THE SYSTEM

Recovery has become one of the 'buzzwords' in contemporary mental health nursing,[2,3] although it has been around for at least 70 years.[4] To put recovery into context I shall take a brief look at my own psychiatric career.

I have used psychiatric services for over 25 years, having my first hypomanic episode in 1981 while writing up my doctoral thesis. I heard voices and thought I was the Virgin Mary. I was hospitalized for 3 months during which time I was given the label of 'manic depressive disorder' and prescribed lithium carbonate. This was the first of many such psychotic events over the years; years that led to hospitalization.

My reaction to that first episode changed the whole direction of my life. I determined that I wanted to gain more information about mental health issues and become involved with people who had gone through similar experiences. I joined a local MIND group (the National Association for Mental Health in the UK) and soon became a representative at regional and national levels. At the same time I became a founder member of MindLink, MIND's consumer network. This involvement with fellow service users formed the bedrock upon which 'my journey to recovery' was founded. Following a career in further education, I retrained in health promotion before moving into the voluntary sector in 1988. For the past 13 years I have worked in advocacy and user involvement, setting up my own consultancy, Section 36, in 1993.

Between 1981 and 1998 I experienced one psychotic episode each year. The early episodes were extremely traumatic and reflected my initial 'spiritual crisis'. I believed I was Emily Pankhurst and Wayne Sleep and was sectioned on four occasions. In 1999 I experienced my worst event and was hospitalized for 3 months. I had both physical and psychiatric symptoms. I recall that I first brought my Emily Pankhurst persona to life at a striking miner's rally in Yorkshire, when I leapt on to a table and tried to rally the miners' revolutionary fervour. On another occasion, I danced down the street, in full Wayne Sleep ballet mode, despite having no dancing ability to speak of. On reflection, these personas, which my psychiatrists perceived as 'delusional states', reflected aspects of my personality that had lain buried for years. My great compassion for my fellow human beings had found its voice in Emily Pankhurst, and my great need to free myself from the past found shape in Wayne Sleep's inimitable ballet dancing.

---

*Irene Whitehill was writing up her doctoral thesis in biology when first diagnosed with manic depression and has endured a further 15 episodes during the past 20 years. She became a lecturer, but later retrained in health promotion and set up advocate and user/carer involvement projects in the voluntary sector. Since 1993 she has worked as a User Trainer and Consultant offering training and research skills to a wide variety of agencies across the Northern Region of England.

I view my periods of hospitalization as a form of 'containment' rather than a therapeutic process. Service users are just expected to sit in the lounge, watch television, sit in the smoking room, play pool or go to occupational therapy. When I am in hospital I focus on *surviving* the experience. I just try to live by the rules and keep my head together. In my own way I try to adopt the Buddhist concept of just 'being'.

On leaving hospital my self-esteem and self-confidence are always severely undermined. Although I may well be pining for the sanctity of my own home, the most difficult task is to start rebuilding my life once I have been discharged. This was particularly difficult following the severe episode I experienced in March 1999. I felt extremely vulnerable, shell-shocked, emotionally wounded and lacking in energy. I cried myself to sleep most nights throughout the first 6 months after discharge. I was grieving for all the major losses in my life – the cot death of my younger brother at 2 months; the incarceration of my mother into a large psychiatric hospital for 10 years; broken family ties; the death of both my parents; the emigration of my brother; my hysterectomy; being without a partner; failed relationships; having to give up my consultancy – Section 36; the trauma of 15 psychotic episodes. It took 3 months before I felt physically and emotionally resilient enough to attend a creative writing course for women, and 6 months before I was able to start work again, in a voluntary capacity.

Thankfully, I have not experienced a psychotic event for over 3 years. Most days my mood is stable and I feel extremely positive about life. However, twice a year I go into a depressive phase which lasts for 3 weeks. Fortunately, my self-management skills enable me to survive these phases, safe in the knowledge that I will come out the other end. Emotionally, I often feel extremely vulnerable, but these periods do not last forever and I am learning to deal with my emotions more effectively.

I wrote this chapter because I believe that mental health nurses have a key role in helping people make their 'journey to recovery'. I base these observations on my various roles as service user, project manager and user consultant.

Meanings of 'recovery'

Before considering the effect nurses can have upon the recovery of service users let me define exactly what I mean by the term. The definition of 'recover' in *Chambers 20th Century Dictionary*[5] is 'to cure'.

In the context of mental health, 'recovery' means something quite different and is not synonymous with 'cure'. Recovery does not mean that all suffering has disappeared, or that all symptoms have been removed, or that functioning has been completely restored.[6] Dr Pat Deegan,[7] a clinical psychologist with a late childhood diagnosis of schizophrenia recognized that 'recovery' was

not a 'cure' but sees no reason for despair. Being in recovery means I know I have certain limitations and things I can't do. But rather than letting these limitations be an occasion for despair and giving up, I have learned that in knowing what I can't do, I also open up the possibilities of all I can do.[8]

In contrast, Dan Fisher,[9] from the National Empowerment Centre, in the USA, has developed an empowerment model for 'recovery', believing that people can fully 'recover' from even the most severe forms of mental illness. However, it is accepted that people need time to heal emotionally:

I do not feel totally 'cured' of manic depression, and still experience minor mood swings a few times a year. The emotional pain bubbles up to the surface when I am least expecting it. Most days, however, I feel a sense of 'well-being'. I have developed a greater insight into my condition and learnt how to self-manage my highs and lows more effectively. I now recognize the importance of being able to have more control over my emotions. I have been teaching myself to consign them to the 'left luggage', so to speak, until I feel able to deal with them. These behavioural changes cannot be achieved overnight. Recovery is not so much an event, as a process. For many people, including myself, this may well be a lifelong quest.

Acceptance is a key factor in the recovery process. As, Pat Deegan[10] has noted:

> … an ever-deepening acceptance of our limitations. But now, rather than being an occasion for despair, we find our personal limitations are the ground from which spring our own unique possibilities. This is the paradox of recovery … that in accepting what we cannot do or be we begin to discover what we can be and what we can do … recovery is a process. It is a way of life. It is an attitude and a way of approaching the day's challenges.

After a great deal of soul searching, I have been able to accept that although my journey to recovery may last a lifetime, I can still value myself and get back into the driving seat of my life. I accept that:

- I really do have infinite self-worth.
- I can confront my own vulnerability without feeling inadequate.
- I am worthy of love and friendship.
- I need to be able to ask for support from both professionals and friends, without feeling embarrassed or inadequate.
- I need to acknowledge that I can be as much of a friend as my friends have been to me.
- I am not a failure because I had to give up my business and am now working in a voluntary capacity and living on disability benefits.

- I subjected myself to too much stress and turned into a 'workaholic'. Too much of my 'persona' was tied up in my work.
- I have a great deal of expertise and practical skills that will enable me to put something back into the community and enjoy a good life.

Over a decade ago I thought that I was 'stuck' and would never be able to get my life back together, let alone move forward. However, I learnt to develop my self-management skills. By adopting the concept of *being your own scientist* I have found that it is possible to become more aware of my moods and how to manage them (P Barker, personal communication). More recently, I attended a self-management training course organized by the Manic Depression Fellowship (2001), which consolidated a great many of the issues I had discussed with my colleague Professor Phil Barker.

However, despite the improvement in self-management skills the pace of my life was too fast and I still found it impossible to balance work, socializing and time for myself. I found it very difficult to relax. I was labelled a 'workaholic' but no one was offering me any solutions. Finally, after 18 years in the system, I was referred to a psychotherapist. At first I was very sceptical, but as the weeks went by I realized what a luxury it was to meet with someone on a regular basis, who listened to me without being judgemental. We have worked together for the past 3 years. During that time we have focused upon the following themes that I have tried to integrate into my daily life:

- *Balancing* – getting the balance right between work, socializing and time alone.
- *Pacing* – learning to live my life at the pace that suits me.
- *Boundary setting* – letting things or people into my life that are acceptable to me.

Trust soon developed and we have developed a good working partnership. Therapy is not an easy option. I have had to work in the gaps between the sessions and sometimes it has been extremely painful. Further down the line, I know that it has been a life-changing process.

The path to recovery also relies upon positivity. Over the years, I have read a great many books on positive thinking, self-help and personal development. I have not always found my reading very profitable. It is one thing to read a book but another to put its message into practice. However, one book, which I have found particularly helpful is *You Can Heal Your Life* by Louise Hay.[11] She believes that developing a positive attitude to daily life can overcome any disease. I was very fortunate to participate in a 1-day training course that promoted her thinking. On the day I developed my own set of 'positive affirmations' a copy of which I have tacked to the wall in my office and refer to them every day:

Irene's affirmations

- You are a unique and independent woman. You choose not to compare yourself with other people.
- You are in 'control' of your life and approve of yourself.
- You are capable of handling everything you choose to do and stay well at the same time.
- You let go of other people's business and look after yourself.
- You enclose yourself in a protective bubble and feel peaceful.

The psychotherapy sessions and training in positive thinking have helped me to redefine who I am. It's as if I have reinvented myself. There has been a distinct change in my 'self'. Simon Champ, a prominent Australian mental health activist, also views recovery as a lifelong process, requiring important changes in 'self':

> I have come to see that you do not simply patch up the self you were before developing schizophrenia, but that you have to actually recreate a concept of who you are that integrates the experience of schizophrenia. Real recovery is far from a simple matter of accepting diagnosis and learning facts about the illness and medication. Instead, it is a deep searching and questioning, a journey through unfamiliar feelings, to embrace new concepts and a wider view of self. It is not an event but a process. For many, I believe it is a lifelong journey.[12]

These changes have been painful at times but have brought with them great periods of personal growth. Anthony has written:

> Recovery is described as a deeply personal, unique process of changing one's attitudes, values, feelings, goals, skills, and/or roles. It is a way of living a satisfying, hopeful and contributing life, even with limitations caused by the illness. Recovery involves the development of new meaning and purpose in one's life as one grows beyond the catastrophic effects of mental illness.[13]

I try to live 'one day at a time'. Most days I experience a sense of well-being and feel good about myself. I am learning to live my life at a pace that suits me and to appreciate the simpler things – such as my morning walk to the local shops; watching cloud formations from the bus window; walking along the beach; the arrival of the first daffodils; rediscovering a favourite piece of music; trying out a new recipe. I have different priorities. I work hard to ensure that my voluntary work does not envelop me completely! I need time for my hobbies, seeing friends and time for myself. Most days I feel in a state of equilibrium, safe in the knowledge that if I did experience a mood swing I could deal with it myself or, if necessary, seek out the appropriate professional support.

complain. Socially, I have a habit of picking up leaflets, reading notice boards and getting myself on arts and music mailing lists. I may not be able to afford to go to everything I used to, but I can have interesting conversations with friends who have been to a particular play etc!

BLOCKING THE RECOVERY PROCESS

There is always a downside. Some things and people have conspired to block my recovery process.

* *Friends* – Friends can be overprotective. They don't believe that I should be moving on in a particular direction. I have felt hindered sometimes because they do not approve of me 'getting back into the driving seat'.
* *Relatives* – My brother fails to understand why I work in mental health and believes that it would be far better for my health if I worked in a flower shop, for example. Although I appreciate his concern, I will not let my diagnosis limit my life-style. I do not wish to feel as if the sword of Damocles is hovering over my head. If I cannot take risks, even experience failure, I may as well be institutionalized.
* *Stigma* – I have frequently experienced the stigma and prejudice associated with mental illness. On meeting people for the first time I have had to gauge when and how much to disclose. I baulk against this because I am not ashamed of who I am. However, when you are in the early stages of recovery it can be very painful to be faced with rejection because of your health status. Quite often people have spoken to me as the 'label' and not the 'person'. My own sister-in-law thinks that anyone labelled with a mental illness should be 'carted off to the funny farm'. Many service users only have professionals or fellow service users as friends because they are frightened of being stigmatized if they 'come out'. They find it very difficult to socialize outside of user groups. I am fortunate in that once I have recuperated I have enough confidence to join an evening class, for example, and make friends outside mental health.
* *Benefits trap* – Service users need to have good budgeting skills to exist on benefits for long periods. It is very difficult to make that leap from living on benefits back into employment. Many service users do not feel able to take the risk in case they cannot get back onto benefits should they need to.
* *Impatience* – On occasions I do get extremely frustrated when I think of the possibilities of me ever getting back to paid work. However, I recognize that I need to practise the art of patience and live each day to the full rather than hankering after something I may never achieve.

Reflection

Pat Deegan said that recovery involved 'accepting our limitations'.

* What are your limitations?
* How have you gone about 'accepting' them?

MENTAL HEALTH NURSES AND RECOVERY

Mental health nurses are the key personnel working with service users on the ward and in the community. They have an essential role in supporting service users in their journey to recovery. I list below just some of the critical aspects of their relationship with the service user, from admission to discharge.

* *Service users as 'people' not 'labels'* – Many mental health nurses are prejudiced towards people in their care. There is a tendency for mental health nurses to relate to the diagnosis and not the person, especially when the service user has been admitted on several occasions (the 'revolving door' patient). Quite often mental health nurses have limited expectations of people in their care because they know very little about their lives outside of hospital. Some mental health nurses are frightened of giving up their power by relating to service users on an equal level, while others have been trapped in the office doing paperwork for so long that they have forgotten how to relate to service users as ordinary people.
* *'Caring with' not 'caring for'* – The mental health nurse forms a partnership with the service user to support them through the recovery process.[15,16] The trustworthy nurse acts as an ally and brings to the relationship both ordinariness and professionalism. The attitudes, beliefs and expressed needs of the service user should be accepted at every stage, and the user knows that the advice of the nurse may not necessarily be accepted.
* *On admission* – A mental health nurse needs to be present on admission to make the process less threatening and to add a sense of continuity when the service user moves on to the ward.
* *Assessment* – A mental health nurse needs to carry out the initial assessment with the service user. The assessment should be carried out in such a way that service users feel comfortable about expressing their views. All experiences should be accepted as 'true' and not dismissed as 'hallucinations' and added to notes without discussion. What does the service user feel caused their admission and what do they feel they need to address these problems?
* *Aids/blocks to 'recovery'* – A mental health nurse needs to work with service users to identify things/people, which might aid or block recovery.

- *Skills assessment* – A mental health nurse needs to work with the service users to identify skills that are required to promote recovery. Service users may not feel able to identify skills or join in any self-management/recovery groups. There is a right time for everything and service users must be allowed to dictate the pace of their own recovery.
- *Facilitating self-management/recovery groups* – Specifically trained mental health nurses facilitate a selection of groups informed by the skills assessments carried out with service users. Contents could include assertiveness, decision-making, building self-esteem and self-confidence, self-presentation, self-management skills, dealing with psychosis, living with voices, mental health promotion; self-medication, complementary therapies, etc.
- *Nurse training* – All mental health nurses need to undergo training in 'positive images' and 'user involvement' facilitated by an 'independent user consultant' or representatives from a local 'user group'. Specific preparation in one-to-one and group work is necessary, so that nurses might be more effective in working with individual service users and facilitating self-management/recovery groups.
- *Acting as a 'link'* – The mental health nurse needs to act as a link with other professionals involved in the individual's package of care: acts as the user's voice within multidisciplinary team meetings. If acceptable, the mental health nurse make links with carers/friends/advocate to ensure that they are kept informed of an individual's progress and to ascertain what role they will play when the service user is discharged. If appropriate, the mental health nurse introduces the service user to the on-site welfare rights officer.
- *Promoting social inclusion* – The mental health nurse needs to make links and collect information about appropriate agencies (housing, benefits agency, employment, job clubs, skills centre, self-help groups, social groups, women's groups, play groups, adult education classes) operating within the hospital's catchment area. Prior to discharge, the mental health nurse should work with service users to consider their needs once they have moved back into the community. The nurse then contacts the agencies to ensure that they do indeed meet the needs of the service user. A CPN is appointed who can support the service user once they have moved back into the community. The mental health nurse informs the CPN about the service users' progress on their path to 'recovery' and feeds back the information gleaned from the agencies that they have contacted.
- *Discharge* – Prior to discharge, the service user meets with the CPN to discuss their expressed needs and how the CPN can support them now that they are moving back into the community.

> **Reflection**
>
> Nurse are now talking a lot about recovery
>
> - What is your experience of helping a person in care to begin to recover?
> - What did you *do* that appeared to enable the person's recovery?
> - What do you find difficult or challenging about adopting a recovery approach in your work?

THE CHALLENGE FOR MENTAL HEALTH NURSES

Three main challenges face mental health nurses in the twenty-first century:

1 A paradigm shift is needed to move properly from 'containment' to 'therapeutic experience'. Mental health nurses need to break out of the mechanistic routine, which restricts their dialogue with service users. This ranges from giving orders – 'come down to the dining routine it's time for meds'; 'It's Tuesday, put clean sheets on your bed' – to relating with service users as people.

Nurses often base themselves in the office doing paperwork and only come out at specific times, to take out the drugs trolley, serve the meals or periodically observe different service users. The people who spend most time talking with service users are nursing assistants and domestic staff. In the 20 years I have been using services, I have found the quality of nursing to be based more upon the intrinsic personal qualities of particular nurses – *compassion, empathy, active listening, ordinariness* – rather than specific nurse training.

2 Mental health nurses must be prepared to undergo specific training that would enable them to 'care with' not 'care for' service users. There is a need to put the person at the heart of the 'caring' process, focusing on the possibility of recovery, for everyone.[16]

3 Having taken the leap from containment to therapeutic experience it would be counterproductive if an attempt was not made to promote 'social inclusion' when service users move back into the community. Mental health nurses will need specialist training so that they may form a bridge between service users and community services.

Above all, mental health nurses must be bearers of hope and believe in the 'recovery' of service users no matter what particular path they have had to follow.

I agree with Gillian Stokes when she says:

> We may not all be blessed with as sanguine an approach to life as Assagioli but he makes his points well. We create our own heaven and our own hell by how we interpret events.[1,p15]

I have always been an optimistic person but over the past year it has been difficult to regain hope for the future. I try to practise 'thinking one day at a time' and each getting better. I also try to practise patience and the Buddhist practice of just 'being'. The watch word is 'try'.

REFERENCES

1. Stokes G. *Contentment: wisdom from around the world.* London, UK: MQ Publications, 2002.

2. Department of Health. *From values to action: the Chief Nursing Officer's review of mental health nursing.* DoH, London, UK, 2006.

3. Scottish Executive. *Rights, relationships and recovery: the report of the national review of mental health nursing in Scotland.* Edinburgh, UK: Scottish Government Publications, 2006.

4. Buchanan-Barker P, Barker P. Clarifying the value base of recovery: the 10 tidal commitments. *Journal of Psychiatric and Mental Health Nursing* 2008; **15**: 2.

5. MacDonald AM (ed.). *Chambers 20th century dictionary.* London, UK: Chambers Harrap, 1978.

6. Repper J. Adjusting the focus of mental health nursing: incorporating service users' experiences of recovery. *Journal of Mental Health* 2000; **9** (6): 575–87.

7. Deegan PE. Recovery as a journey of the heart. *Psychiatric Rehabilitation Journal*, 1996; **19** (3): 91–7.

8. Deegan PE. Recovering our sense of value after being labelled mentally ill. *Journal of Psychosocial Nursing* 1993; **31**: 7–11.

9. Empowerment model of recovery from severe mental illness: an expert interview with Daniel B. Fisher, MD, PhD. *Medscape Psychiatry & Mental Health* 2005; **10** (1). Available from: http://www.power2u.org/articles/recovery/expert_interview.html.

10. Deegan PE. The independent living movement and people with psychiatric disabilities: taking back the control of our own lives. *Psycho-social Rehabilitation Journal* 1992; **15**: 3–19.

11. Hay L. *You can heal your life.* London, UK: Eden Grove Editions, 1988.

12. Champ S. A most precious thread. In: Barker P, Campbell P, Davidson B (eds). *The ashes of experience: reflections on madness, survival and growth.* London, UK: Whurr Publishers, 1999: 113–26.

13. Anthony WA. Recovery from mental illness: the guiding vision of the mental health service system in the 1990s. *Innovations and Research* 1993; **2**: 17–24.

14. Barker P, Jackson S, Stevenson C. What are psychiatric nurses needed for? Developing a theory of essential *nursing* practice. *Journal of Mental Health and Psychiatric Nursing* 1999; **6**: 273–82.

15. Barker P, Whitehill I. The craft of care: towards collaborative caring in psychiatric nursing. In: Tilley S (ed.). *The mental health nurse: views of practice and education.* Oxford: Blackwell Science, 1999.

16. Barker P, Buchanan-Barker P. *The tidal model: A guide for mental health professionals.* Hove, UK: Brunner Routledge, 2005.

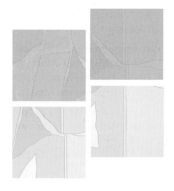

CHAPTER 8

Recovery and reclamation: a pilgrimage in understanding who and what we are

Anne Helm*

THE UNIVERSALITY OF THE TASK

Recovery has become the 'in' word of psychiatric practice. As a long-time user of the mental health system I find the word ambiguous in its resonance and meaning. The importance of understanding that 'nothing ever stays the same' is, I believe, a given. We who are service users can rebuild our lives, defined by us in terms of quality. More so, you (the reader) and I (the service user) are, from birth to death, in a constant process of 'recovery'. The complexity of early relationships provides in itself much for some of us to recover from. Add to that the difficult adolescent voyage towards self-identity and the uncertainty of adult life and it could be asked of anyone reading this chapter, has she recovered? Recovery is not a destination, but the journeying task of making sense of life itself, and I ask the reader to accept the universality of the task. We are all in recovery. There are no *patients* to seek recovery for, no *nurses* to map the waterways and guide the boats on the voyage. We are all fellow wayfarers, who can share experiences and insights from our own lives, thereby facilitating each other's progress.

Humanness, in the twenty-first century, means we are constantly called to make sense out of our experience and incorporate it into our lives. For those of us with the experience of mental illness, making sense and giving value to that experience can be likened to doing a jigsaw puzzle with no picture to work from. In doing the task, we often discover several different puzzles have been placed within the same box. For me, some of my puzzle pieces may always be missing. In some instances specific treatments have created black holes in linear memory. The challenge to understand who and what I am is always a constant. However, I do get more of an integrated sense of self as I get older, and wellness accompanies that. My quest for wellness was amidst the experience of horrific practices that are thankfully outmoded and relegated to psychiatric nursing history. My journey has therefore been mostly an internal one and my contributions to this chapter will reflect that.

*Anne Helm is a service user leader who works as a consultant educator in New Zealand.

MY BACKGROUND OF MOVING FROM SURVIVAL TO RECOVERY

I had my first experience of psychosis at the age of 19. My struggle for sanity and understanding through it took place in the context of nursing in the late 1960s onwards in New Zealand. This was a time when lock-ups, seclusion cells, narcosis sleep therapy and the threat of electroconvulsive therapy as a means of control were common. This was a time when wards of the forgotten were housed, fed, watered and medicated and sometimes strapped to their beds. The nursing staff came from the surrounding countryside by night and day and drove back along the long, sealed driveways to their lives on the outside. They brought their gossipy news of their socialized lives to share with each other, excluding us from their conversations as if we were inanimate objects. We, the crazed, were removed from the community and placed in institutions with sadly ironic names like Cherry Farm and Sunnyside. There was no flow-through traffic from the wider community and many of us – abandoned by families who were unable to deal with the shame or cope with the insanity of their kin – were placed daily in front of television to work out where we were in time and place, with no human reference points.

The reflections I have about it now are of a period when body and thoughts were dulled by heavy anti-psychotic medications. Lack of interest was the all-pervading, emanating characteristic of the trained nursing staff, as heavy roll-lock keys swung and jangled at the jailers' sides. My last long-term hospitalization was in 1979. Lake Alice Hospital had branded my being to the core. In one way it 'worked' – I had gained a slight but smouldering sense of self that would never allow my being to be placed in an institution again, and I never did.

While within that place I developed a theory about who was helpful and who didn't give a damn. Almost without exception the more stripes on the shoulder and medals that swung from the breast the less caring and humanly interactive the staff became. The first time I was bathed after the barbarity of seclusion, a young, dark-haired endorsed nurse (one step above a nurse aid) gently washed my hair, touching my scalp with delicate massaging fingers. The simple experience of that act of caring was immensely powerful, as human touch had been so long denied me. I lay in the bathtub and as I looked up at her I felt I was in the presence of a different kind of human being altogether. She was an angel, and goodness was in existence again in my world.

THE SIMPLICITY OF THE SOLUTION

I have read much about the principles of the recovery focus in mental health. Words like partnership, acceptance, empathy, respect, building on strengths, hope and compassion are to be found there. The task of rebuilding my life feels for me like a much more solo-navigated journey, as much of it had to be done out of isolation – away from what *was* my life. I do know though, that the stars that shone upon my craft came in the form of simple acts of human kindness from people such as the nurse I have just mentioned. Write as many words about recovery as you wish, one word fits all. It is of course *love*. This is the essential healer. Poets, musicians and spiritual leaders tell, and retell us. What counts *was* love, *is* love and *will always be* love.

Coming through a period of psychiatric institutionalization, where the act of loving in caring practices was the exception, made me hold on to those drops of nourishment, which helped restore my own sense of dignity and enabled me to begin the journey of reclamation.

In spite of the anguish of my struggle, I know from rubbing shoulders with certain gentle, humble people of this world that healing is possible and life can be fully and joyously lived amidst the crisis events of our lives, and in spite of diagnosis.

HEALING RELATIONSHIPS

The importance of realness in relationships

I was held by a long-time committal in that hospital and so began to look for quality relationships within its walls. I sought out the nurse aids, gardeners and cooks for real conversations about their lives and they listened with interest to the fragments of what I could tell them about mine. Practical down-to-earth people with their own struggles and openness in sharing helped give me a frame of reference to reflect my own life against. This place was a wasteland of the rejected, where the institution existed to support the needs of the staff who ran it. Meaningful caring was not part of the ethos. The less trained were different. Simple acts of human kindness – like kitchen staff putting boiled water aside for me at morning tea time so I did not have to drink the mass-served, lukewarm, highly sweetened milky tea – became a sign of my own individual worth.

One or two special events stick in the memory and had a profound effect. The following is one of them.

I was very sensitive to sound of any kind. I am after all a musician. Unable to deal with the noise of socialization, I had been constantly returned to a barren, bed-less seclusion cell. I had broken this pattern to progress to a locked, but more pleasant room, with a bed and a cabinet. One evening in a talent quest I had found my voice to sing and stunned the hall into silence. I carried my little green vase, given to me as the winner, back to the villa and placed it on the cabinet. Medicated and locked in for the night I thought how strange it was that this little vase was all I amounted to at that time. In the morning

I awoke to an abundance of velvet red roses in bloom beside me. One of the aids, an older man who I had often dragged out of his reticence into conversation, had gone home and cut them for me from his much-loved garden. I learnt much from that quiet, retired seaman. He is prominent in the league of the gentle, humble angels to whom I owe pure, deep gratitude.

Many of the unqualified aid staff were fine people. It was the aids who took me during their lunchtime to the swimming pool so I could use the pool alone, diving deep like a dolphin, swimming underwater to find my sense of aliveness and weightless freedom. And it was the aids who would unlock my room and the day room, at dawn before shift change, so my fingers could find their way over a piano again.

Authentic relationships and commonalities

Nowadays we have fewer stories of long institutional lives unlived, and yet within the community care model, patronizing attitudes of mental health professionals who '*know*' and the recipients of their 'help' who '*don't know*' still prevail.

Much is now written about the 'therapeutic relationship' in nursing practice. However, I still have to ask, what the hell is that? I have used the psychiatric district nurse system here in New Zealand and the best relationship I have had is with a nurse who battled with her own family alienation issues because of her sexual orientation. This nurse and I had parallel issues about stigmatization, and our relationship, as a result, was gritty and real. Whether any of us function or do not function depends on our self-concepts as we live among the wider community, and that is universal. Effective relationships are, as Mary Auslander, the American consumer advocate says, about 'looking for the commonalities amongst us rather than the differences we discern from diagnosis.'[a]

The most therapeutic happenings in my journey have been with people who share of their own lives.

Seeing us as other

If the nurse sees us as 'other' – observing behaviours as symptoms of the illness – barriers are erected to relating, and to understanding what is going on for us. Some behaviour is hard to see beyond, yet I do believe that whatever is presented, a process of searching lies within it. Here is a challenging example.

A young woman in manic scattered psychosis has been placed in a barren seclusion cell. Naked except for an ill-tying gown, she has a rough blanket for sleeping on, and a plastic bucket for her toileting. The practice of the day meant she had been given initial sedation of paraldehyde, which left her struggling like a wounded animal to even pick up her body from the cold lino floor. Heavy brown brogue shoes of fat-calved charge nurses periodically pushed food in plastic bowls towards her. No one spoke, no one told her where she was, and the only touch given to her was the prizing open of her jaw to pour the thick brown anti-psychotic syrup down her throat. She was left for days. In psychosis she did not experience 'delusion' as clinicians had said. In fact her psychosis had much beauty and a sense of connectedness to the world. Her awareness of the emotions of the human condition had been sharply intense. She had witnessed in many faces extremities of despair, anguish and human angst, being contrasted with the sheer joy and lightness of the simple act of smiling and giving of affection. Her world has sparkled. In that cell, all perceptions of her universe were boxed in and removed. Drugs took over. Any interaction with her now was as a jailer to a beast. New thoughts formed as she tried to make sense of her incarceration and where she was. Perhaps she really had lost the plot and had gone mad. Trying to make sense out of what was happening, she thought in her madness she must surely have killed a child, something dearly loved and innocent. Only an act such as that could warrant the disdain with which she was treated. She pleaded with her inner god that it had not been so and with the blanket wrapped around her, rocked and crooned for days, struggling to find a section of her mind that would assure her she had committed no crime. Weeks passed.

One day she changed things in her world. She held the only material available in her hands and painted the walls of the cell, fingers and palms exploring the texture and flowing designs. In the timelessness of day into night into day again, and left without human interaction, she had found a minute speck of something of herself and within herself: creativity. This act of doing and creating was the beginning of piecing herself together again. Discovering the primal urge to fashion something with the only material available was the beginning of her recovery. To 'do' after all is to be human. Who would ever understand this behaviour? This after all was an act of regression, an act of faeces smearing.

I understand. I was that young woman. We are the experts of our own experience.

CONSUMER-DEFINED RECOVERY

Definition of self

Recovery is a self-defined process. To me recovery means just getting on with life. 'Getting over it', as my children would say. It means incorporating the experience into the fullness of all my living. How can someone 'get over' mental illness when the severity and complexity

---

[a] Mary Auslander, quoted by Tregoweth J, *Awhi Tautoko Aroha. Celebrating recovery-focused mental health workers.* Wellington New Zealand: Mental Health Commission, 2001: 23.

of reasons for diagnosed conditions are so variable? Does it mean the successful suicide has failed to get over it? How do I write of recovery and believe I am well down that path, when I still have 'a diagnosis' and an occasional visit to the psychiatrist, and am at present on maintenance medication? Services are beginning to understand that recovery is not a place to get to but a process. The starting point of this process is a belief in one's own value.

To some of the people I work with, recovery is seen as a confusing term associated with an illness being 'cured'. The medical profession looks to return the patient to the not-ill state. But people have mental illness as an experience, not an objective reality. It is woven into the fabric of who and what they are. Sometimes recovery is expressed as 'learning to live with it'. This feels similarly disempowering to me. My 'it' is part of me and always has been. I am more than the sum of my genetics and have tried to avoid subscribing to the brain disease/ chemical imbalance medical focus to describe my reality. I would have remained in an institution without the healing power of bare feet upon wet grass if I had believed these constructs were all I amounted to.

Recovering what?

Recovery indicates gaining something that was lost, but the depth of the journey is much richer than that. I would say it was finding something of my explicit uniqueness and wonder as a human being along the way. It is a voyage towards integration of the self. Who am I? and what am I? are questions we all ask ourselves from time to time. Those of us with mental illness are probably called upon to ask the question more often. The challenge of my journey has been whether I will weave the experiences of 'illness', my psychotic state, into an integrated sense of self, or regard the 'illness' as being part of an 'otherness'. This is the challenge, and as long as nursing practice focuses on the 'otherness' our self-perception and fragmentation is affected. If recovery is 'a state of mind' as has been said, making sense of who I am, as experienced through my mind, can be difficult.

Actualizing wellness

The recovery journey then comes from an internal desire for wellness. It should have no clinical definition, as it is the service user who must define what the outward display of that means for himself/herself. On one level there may be functional abilities to recover – such as the ability to concentrate to read and keep the hand steady enough to write, to converse without the slurring of the heavy-medicated tongue and fogginess of the mind. Oftentimes, medicated sedation and their side-effects are the greatest hindrance to this basic reclamation. As we move into clearer functioning we wish to claim the

functions of the wider community, like the right to drive a car, work, make love and have children. Then there are the more external things to realize and recover. Our illness will always put us on the back foot economically. Returning to education, establishing a home base, restoring old friendships and building new ones, and finding our place again within our families of origin, can be an overwhelming challenge. For some of us the returning to our families of origin can never be part of our wellness plans, as our madness was born out of them. Some families have been mystified and hurt by the nature and consequence of the illness experience and see it in terms of a sad reality and deficit for their family member. Recovering with such surrounding attitudes can be counterproductive and difficult for everyone.

The individual internal journey lies at the core of reclamation. Courage, self-responsibility, realizing we are more than our illness, feeling good about ourselves and finding peace in the integration process, are just some of the elements that we have to find for the work required.

Integrating into community

Other people are essential to confirming our wellness. Our sense of who we are is often fragmented. Some of us have lost our work place and therefore have no definition by our jobs. If abandoned by family and friends we have no human context from which to glean a sense of the self, and no reflectors or interactions that will tell us we are OK people. As we bridge back into our local communities we meet hesitation and uncertainty in the eyes of people who know we have a mental illness. Fear of the unknown and therefore the 'dark' nature of mental illness is a reality, and our group's coverage in the media does nothing to allay such fears. In such an environment, working out our self-identity as other than 'the mentally ill' takes much weaving, discarding many threads and choosing others. The choice will be affected by the affirmations of people around us.

Responding to people's needs within the community, as we do today, rather than removing them from the context of their life into inpatient settings, does much to assist people to remain connected to their total lives. However, attitudinal response to the individual remains a powerful influence on self-concepts and feelings of worthwhileness necessary for healing.

CARING NURSING PRACTICE

My wellness came as a result of many simultaneous processes at work. I have spoken at length about the internal processes, and hope this sharing is helpful. There are obvious attitudes and behaviours that are not helpful to the rebuilding work we have to do. I came through a period of 'care' that exemplified many of them. Among these were belittlement, lack of human respect and the loss of human dignity; lack of validation of the 'patient's' experience and our accompanying emotions; seeing us only as a set of behavioural deviants. And then there was the distant expert psychiatrist who seldom entered into conversations with the patients but knew what was 'best' for us and kept institutions functional for staff by his decisions. (Historically these 'experts' were almost always men.) Even now as a consumer worker, I meet health professionals who, with superior attitude, know more about my 'illness' than I do myself, and who can jettison my sense of wellness and sense of place, although experientially I understand more than they ever will about the reality and impact of madness.

The fine-tuning required to strike an empowering attitude of care is a delicate thing. 'Do-gooders' with a sense of helping the unfortunate, although nobly motivated, can be a pain in the proverbial arse. By its nature, this model means that the professional occupies a state of the 'more' to the 'less than' in what is, undeniably, a patronizing relationship.

What really helps is the acknowledgment of our own resourcefulness and innate talents and capabilities. What is needed for such real relationships to happen is a certain humility. I return to my opening paragraph about the universal nature of making sense out of life, or 'recovery', if you like. Sharing what *you* know and what *I* know needs to ebb and flow between us. The reward for relatedness is that we learn from each other.

CONTINUAL RECOVERY AND ANGELS ON THE JOURNEY

I have thought a lot about this word *recovery* and how it resounds within me. Part of my early story involved recovery from addictive substances. This proclivity did nothing for my already ignited disposition towards mania. Contextually that part of my life was real journeying both in the mind and on foot! I was dealing with the death of my mother, the loss of my family home, and a broken late-adolescent marriage and the subsequent removal of my first child. Trying to nullify the pain by self-medication and seeking psychedelic experiences seemed a good way to go. On reflection, I can see a young woman trying to work out where she was going and who she was in the midst of all this.

The continuing search for identity

My first baby was born amidst young relationship dysfunction and I entered a period of deep grieving for my mother, made complex by my own sense of maternal inadequacy and anxiety. I had postnatal depression they said, and when my anxieties became manifest as the crying voice of my own baby I was 'crazy again'. Baby and

mother were separated and hospitalizations followed. There were no family members who could extend support to me in my maternal role. I had lost contact with my university friends and lived in a depressive flat above an early-morning drinkers' pub overlooking the city gas works. Motherhood was a foreign experience to me. I remember lacing up my white roller-skating boots I had from childhood and skating around the wooden floor of the old disused 1920s ballroom at the back of the flat in an attempt to hold onto something of the person I was and had known. Now there was a small helpless little baby girl dependent on me and on me alone. I was overwhelmed by the intensity of the responsibility. The baby's father was only a teenager himself but he was a young man going places. He worked long hours and I befuddled my way through days of confusion and displacement in the grime of my surroundings. The music enthusiast, classical singer and student once so enthusiastic about life and living had gone. I battled with my task of caring for my child until one day, knowing I was not mother enough, and fearing the snapping of my own sanity, I locked the baby's door, filled a bath, and slit my wrists after overdosing on as much as I could find. Providence – in the form of the pub sandwich-maker needing to use an unblocked toilet – meant I survived that act, an act I had chosen with such clear certainty. In a strange sense, another angel had been put my way.

The ebb and flow of the journey

I see the journey towards wellness as an upward spiral motion. Sometimes the bottom of the spiral touches the base line of where we have been before, but it is often moving in an ebb and flow motion.

The climb back to finding life worth living again was a very long haul. I was encouraged to play the piano again. At one stage I had a considerate doctor, another angel, who would bring in the music of his favourite arias for me to learn and place them beside my bed. When it came to group activities he would just say 'Anne will not be involved, she will be at the piano again'. I began to experience the joy of singing again and slowly over a period of time regained a sense of centre from which to rebuild. Placing motherhood within my life was complex, and few believed in my own capacity to do so. My baby was placed elsewhere and my husband took off up north in an exciting career move. The feeling surrounding my baby's removal and the subsequent effects are part of the weave of my life. The day she was taken, I gave my bridal veil to a young kid in the street for dressing up and started self-medicating the pain of accumulated loss.

Drugs and hitching on the side of the road where the traffic was heaviest became my way of life. Drifting among the carefree days of the 1970s, thinking I was doing the hippie thing and living amidst the glorious drop-out people, eating home-made bread and dropping acid until life was like a series of psychoses, was both wonderful and frightening. Intuitively I knew I was on a road to burnout and possible death. I gradually sought a new group of people with hippie values and a life code without drugs.

I was well on the road to recovering my sobriety when the universe provided that ultimate sanity tester. I fell deeply in love with a poet. The beauty of the universe sparkled sublime as I entered my mania. Weeks of road travel, singing with the planets and taking no food but the air I breathed, placed me in a detox unit. I was after all an 'addict in recovery' but there is no detoxification process for love. I was taken 'crazy' to one of the most notoriously feared institutions in New Zealand, incarcerated and certified. Much of the experience of this narrative occurred in this dreaded place. This was an irony. I had recovered from drugs only to be smitten by the most powerful drug of the gods themselves. What was I to recover from now?

In conclusion: a return to the simplicity of the solution

No singular action or interaction within the institution's walls could have been the pivotal catalyst for recovery. Days and nights came and went, as did the seasons. I needed someone to validate my human worth. It came in the form of a music tape sent to the hospital. A musician friend had composed a series of songs for me, and in Cat Stevens-like cleverness sang of our friendship and his caring. I sat hour upon hour playing and replaying it on the small tape recorder in the corner of the bleak day room in the geriatric villa. I was so removed from the outside world and yet now so connected to it. There was a refrain at the end of one song: 'and if a friend can say that he loves you, that's all there is to be said'. It kept floating through my mind. My family had given up on me, the friends of my Faith had visited once but, embarrassed by the asylum nature of the place and unable to relate to it – or me – had never come back. My uniquely poetic and special boyfriend of that time had bowed to the pressures of his family who were against our marrying because of my schizophrenic diagnosis, and he left the area. I had sat for months amidst the long-term abandoned geriatric senile/mentally 'ill', embarrassed by mass bathing practices, spoon-feeding and my own menstruation. I was 28 years old and the idea that I was OK could not be realized without outside intervention. That tape gave me life. My dear musician friend died young but he holds the special ranking of humble angel closest to my heart. His songs were the turning point in recovery. 'Love' in a caring response after all, is all there is to be said.

ADDITIONAL REFLECTIONS: ON REPONSES THAT ARE JUST

Realizing a place of peace with one's life path is often very hard work. It is especially difficult when the response by services has added to trauma and shattered self-concepts. Response to this thing we call illness continually needs to be challenged as does the positions of power people have over the journeying pathway of the person deemed to have an illness or disease.

Much time has passed since first writing this chapter. The last 2 years I have been a panel member for the New Zealand government in a redress process for people, including family and staff, who had experiences of services prior to the New Zealand Mental Health Compulsory Assessment and Treatment Act 1992. This process was called the Confidential Forum for Former Inpatients of Psychiatric Hospitals. With regard to that work, time, place and context of the day can never make acceptable much of what we were told in the Forum hearings. The work is most grave. In the midst of it however panel members experienced the participants' dignity, strength and immense courage, time and time again. Goodness recognizes goodness and the ignited light flickers with hope in the darkness wherever it is found. This also was part of the stories we were privileged to hear.

The resilience and strength of the human spirit to rebuild and recreate is profound. For a clinician the ability to tap this essence lies at the core of assisting the healing process. Giving any response to distress either by attitude or treatment that cuts across the individual's sacred place of healing is profane. That place is the same in all of us. If empathy is the alchemy of life's experience, we only have to tap into the learnings within our own lives to reach out meaningfully to others. Though I still hold that the most important attitude to respond with in the art of caring is from a position of love, I also know that there is a requirement to act justly. Working in mental health is complex. No matter what side we sit on in the clinical/consumer divide it is only a conceptual barrier to real relationships. Real relationships that can heal. To 'do justly and to love mercy'[b] has been given to us by texts of the religious. It would be a good adage to steer the course of true responses to those who come to you in distress and confusion.

I work alongside many exceptional people in clinical and consumer roles who constantly press for improved responses and environments of care. Continual dialogue and reciprocity of exchange will create the healing of both the legacy of our system and improvement of current-day practice.

---

[b] Micah 6: 8 He hath shown thee, O man, what is good; and what doth the Lord require of thee, but to do justly, and to love mercy, and to walk humbly with thy God?

Final salutations

Sometimes on reflection one can point to significant events that changed the journey. My struggle to make sense of my life and who I am has and is happening internally and with the kindness and honesty of others.

I urge health professionals to find an openness of heart that can offer meaningful, simple acts of caring kindness, and to carry out their actions with fairness. Those of us who walk this journey from illness to recovery will confirm the status of humble, gentle angel upon you. May many of you be found in the humane practices of your profession, and in sharing with us may God speed you on your own journeying of self-discovery.

SECTION 2

ASSESSMENT IN PRACTICE

Preface to Section 2

The simplest way to find out about people is to ask them questions. Properly handled, *curiosity* is the key to all knowledge. By owning up to our ignorance, we lay the way open to learning something about other people and the world they inhabit.

The heart of nursing practice lies in asking very particular questions, which help us to explore the person's experiences – of pain, loss, hurt or loneliness, for example. We are trying to answer a simple question – who is this person? – as a step towards identifying what this person might need, to begin to resolve the different problems, which currently unsettle the person's life.

Assessment represents the bookends of care. The story that slowly emerges as part of the narrative of care is tightly wedged between the first, fumbling questions the nurse asks, in an effort to get to know the person; and the final, more sophisticated line of enquiry that leads to discharge. However, assessment – in various forms – appears on every page of the story of care, as nurses try to judge the effect caring is having on the person or the family.

Section 2 begins with a discussion of the place of assessment in nursing practice, locating it as the key building block in the development of nursing care.

We explore the kinds of methods that nurses commonly use to develop different kinds of pictures of the people in their care and the problems of living that they experience, and explore in detail the interview – undoubtedly the simplest, but potentially most challenging form of assessment.

The importance of engaging the person in care, and the person's family where appropriate, in the assessment process is now widely accepted. Collaborative assessment provides openings to a wide range of different caring approaches, which although challenging, hold the promise of more mutually satisfying nurse–patient relationships.

Of course, few problems of living do not involve the family in one way or another. The assessment of people and their problems within the context of their family groups is rarely easy, but offers the promise of a more realistic picture of the person, set in the often chaotic, but intensely natural, habitat of the 'real world'.

Finally, we address some of the commonest sources of information about 'who we are' – found in examples of thought, feelings and beliefs, which are drawn from our private, internal world of experience. Although often difficult, if not emotionally painful to talk about, thoughts, feelings and beliefs *signal* the person more than any other form of information. Often, it is the nurse's singular privilege to be granted access to these vital secrets of personal experience.

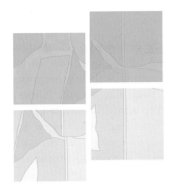

CHAPTER 9

Assessment: the foundation of practice

Phil Barker*

INTRODUCTION

Assessment, in its various forms, is the fundamental basis of any practice. Before we can begin to think about any planned action, we must ask: what needs to be done? This applies just as much to repairing machinery as it does to caring for people, only with people the process is much more complicated and potentially much more risky. If we do not complete a very *careful* assessment of the person and the person's situation in the beginning, we risk damaging the machinery or the person and the person's life.

As nursing is a social activity, the very heart of nursing assessment involves asking questions – trying to find out what has happened to the person,[a] and what the person is experiencing *now*, so that we might begin to work out what needs to be done in the name of care that is appropriate to this particular person at this time. Assessment can be seen as representing the 'bookends' of nursing care. The story of care is written in the various nursing practice records. This begins with the first, preliminary assessment undertaken when the person enters care, and ends with the final assessment, which maps out how the person might be discharged, appropriately, from the service. The story of the person's journey through the caring experience is tightly wedged between the initial, exploratory assessment and the final assessment for discharge. In that sense, the 'bookends' of assessment represent the beginning and endpoint of care, and support all the stories of the experience and delivery of care.

In recent years nursing has begun to move away from its traditional position of 'caring for' or otherwise 'looking after patients'. Increasingly, nurses emphasize the importance of engaging the person (who is the patient) in the whole caring process. That engagement begins with the nurse's attempts to involve the person (collaboratively) in the whole assessment process. Collaborative assessment[1] provides openings to a wide range of caring interventions, which offer challenges to nursing practice but also hold the promise of more mutually satisfying caring relationships.

Although we shall emphasize the assessment of the individual person in this chapter, we recognize that few problems of living do not involve the family in one way or another. The assessment of people and their problems within the context of their family groups is rarely easy, but offers the promise of a more rounded picture of the person in the often chaotic, but intensely natural habitat of the real world.

*Phil Barker is a psychotherapist and Honorary Professor at the University of Dundee, UK.

[a] The experience of becoming a 'patient' is often 'depersonalizing'. To emphasize that we are talking about individual people, rather than 'patients' in general, we shall use the term 'person' throughout, to refer to the 'person in care', i.e. patient/client.

WHY ASSESS?

Although of vital importance to the whole process of care, assessment can often be a very ordinary activity. In everyday life, people assess themselves and their surroundings almost without thinking about it. We ask:

- What are the chances of our soccer team winning their next match? or
- Will our son pass his next school exam?

Such questions involve a consideration of *probabilities*. To what extent is something likely to happen? To what extent will it 'probably' occur?

To answer such questions we need to assess various *factors*, any of which might influence the outcome. However, although assessment may be informed by scientific principles, by definition, it is more an art form than a scientific endeavour, at least where people are concerned. The commonest answer people might give to the two questions above is, it depends! The chances of our favourite team wining the next game 'depends' on whether or not all the players are fit; on how good the other team is; on the weather; on the support offered by the crowd; on the referee's decisions, and so on.

When we assess people in mental distress, we are interested to know, what is going on *within* them as a person (e.g. what are they thinking and feeling?) that might have an impact on what they might do next. We also will be interested in what is going on *around* them (the influence of other people, such as family, friends or staff), their physical state (fitness, health, how their body is 'working'), and so on. Indeed, there are so many possible factors at work, within the person and within the person's physical and social environment, that even the very best piece of assessment must be no more than a calculated guess. If there is a scientific equivalent of psychiatric assessment it is probably meteorology (weather forecasting), which often can be wildly inaccurate.

In mental health care, people's lives are upset by what is commonly called 'mental illness'. However, mental 'illnesses' are not like cancer, diabetes or even hypertension. There are no blood tests, highly sophisticated scans or X-rays in routine practice that will confirm the existence of depression or schizophrenia, for example. Most often, all we have to guide us is what people *say* about their experience – thoughts, feelings or beliefs – or how they behave towards themselves or other people. By observing people, whether formally or informally, or interviewing them alone or with their family members, we begin to build up a picture of what we think 'might' be happening within their world of experience. Such 'assessments' are the basis of psychiatric diagnosis and nursing practice.

The key purpose of nursing assessment

We need to remember that the person who is in distress will probably also be asking similar questions. Many people are bewildered and bemused by their experiences and commonly ask: what is happening to me? Nurses, like everyone else, can never know, *exactly*, what is happening to the person, far less what it might *mean*. So, a key aspect of our assessment becomes focused on caring *with* the person, exploring and considering all the available information or experiential evidence, which might help the person come to understand, better, what is *happening* – and what it might *mean* on a personal level. Nursing assessment is mainly involved in clarifying our understanding of what is happening *now*, so that the nursing team might plan how to respond in a way that meets the person's immediate needs.

Increasingly, Western countries prize 'evidence-based' health care,[2] which assumes the existence of 'effective' ways to deal with specific health-related problems[3] (see Chapter 4). We shall return to this idea later, when we discuss specific forms of assessment 'technology', which have developed from research, or have been widely tested in practice. However, we should not forget that the most valuable form of 'evidence' at our disposal in mental health care is the person's *experience*: what people are able to tell us about what is happening within their private world (e.g. their thoughts, feelings, values and beliefs) and what they believe this might 'mean' within the wider story of their lives.

> **Reflection**
>
> What would you tell a layperson who asked you, what exactly are you trying to do when you assess someone?

ASSESSMENT AND MAKING JUDGEMENTS

Assessment lies at the core of the nurse's function. Nurses cannot offer valid and reliable forms of nursing care without valid and effective assessment. Invariably, people present with a wide range of problems of living, which often require very different forms of attention. Even where people share the same diagnosis, their problems of living and their experience of their common 'illness' might differ greatly.

Assessment may identify the characteristics that different people have in *common* (*nomothetic*), e.g. people with a diagnosis of depression often report feeling 'low in spirits' or say they are 'tired and lethargic'. However, assessment can also help us *distinguish* one person from another: helping clarify what makes *this* person's experience unique (*idiographic*).

Most dictionaries offer a fairly restrictive definition of 'assessment'. Traditionally, this referred to taxation, where an assessor fixes the value of something. More recently we have come to understand the term as having something to do with estimating the character of something or someone. This seems more relevant to psychiatric and mental health nursing. We are interested in making careful judgements about the people in our care, in terms of *who* they are and *what* they might become in the immediate future. People are, quite literally, priceless and this meaning emphasizes the inherent worth of a person.[4] This *idiographic* view contrasts with traditional medical diagnosis, which seeks to identify the nature of the pathology of the patient: looking for what is wrong with the person. Although people may appear to be having similar experiences when they are in mental distress, their experience is unique – framed by the unique context of the person's life history. One of the great challenges of nursing assessment is to make sense of this unique phenomenon. As Hilda Peplau[5] noted, the key focus of any assessment – observation – is transformed by interpretation into a meaningful explanation.

Assessment is linked strongly to *evaluation*, which involves judgements concerning something's 'value' or 'worth'. A judgement (evaluation) of a work of art differs little from an evaluation of our children's performance at school. Information is collected, which is then used to comment upon what we have observed. Few such evaluations are done for their own sake, but are undertaken with a view to some future action.

This suggests that there are, at least, two important kinds of assessment.

- *Exploration or description*: We can assess a situation to 'find out' what is going on. Most forms of assessment in mental health care involve such 'explorations' or 'examinations' of the person's experience of self and others.
- *Measurement*: We can assess a person, or their situation, to establish how 'big' or 'small' are their problems; how 'many' difficulties they are experiencing; or whether these appear to be 'improving' (getting better) or 'deteriorating' (getting worse).

Assessing people not 'patients'

In recent years nurses have begun to move away from the strict use of a medical–diagnostic model in favour of an assessment of the worth of the individual. Since the early 1970s, the nursing process movement[6] has urged all nurses to show concern for the person behind the patient label, reminding us to look for 'worth' amid what might seem like insurmountable problems. Today, there is a risk that nursing might drift back into a reductionist approach to care delivery, using medical diagnosis as the primary determinant for the design of care[7] (see Chapter 16). Private healthcare insurance companies in the USA will not authorize care and treatment unless the person is accorded a medical psychiatric diagnosis, and some advanced nursing practitioners are now authorized to make a psychiatric diagnosis. To some extent this reinforces the view that the diagnosis is central to the planning and delivery of 'care', rather than merely an economic necessity.

Hilda Peplau, commonly referred to in the USA as the 'mother of psychiatric nursing', recognized that although diagnosis represented a useful way of talking about groups of people, with similar problems, it was largely irrelevant to the consideration of what any individual might need in terms of nursing care. We can answer that question only by exploring the widest possible personal context, which will allow us to gain some insight into what is meaningful for this particular person, as opposed to what might be considered 'appropriate' for a group of 'patients'.[8]

Towards the end of her life Peplau noted that nurses increasingly had made the claim that:

> consideration of (the patients) their needs and interests as persons having dignity and worth, are primary values inherent in the design and execution of nursing services. These values should be implicit in a nursing approach for the care of patients having a diagnosis of schizophrenia. In keeping with these claims, it would behove nurses to give up the notion of a disease, such as schizophrenia, and to think exclusively of patients as persons.[9]

Perhaps Peplau was speaking for many nurses who recognized that psychiatric nursing was concerned, first and foremost, to address the person's *human response* to problems involving his relationship to himself or others.[10] In that sense, we can make a distinction between nursing and medical assessment. Doctors commonly assess, 'the atypical, socially unacceptable behaviours which are called symptoms, and view them as indicators of disease.'[9] Nurses, by contrast, are focused on understanding how the person *reacts to* or is *affected by* the phenomenon called illness or disease.

If nursing assessment involves making any kind of judgement, it is the judgement or evaluation of the person's *human responses* to general or specific mental health problems that is most important. When nurses ask the simplest of questions – how are you doing? – by implication they are asking:

> What is your human response, now, to whatever is happening to and for you now, in the wider context of what has been happening to and for you recently?

FORMS OF ASSESSMENT

Any assessment may be formal or informal. In a *formal* assessment the organization and structure is apparent, e.g. using checklists, questionnaires and rating scales, or a specific interview plan. In an *informal* assessment the information is collected in a less structured manner and might appear quite haphazard.

An interview may be formal or informal. In both cases the person is asked questions and the replies are written down. However, in a formal interview questions will be prepared carefully in advance. The informal interview lacks this structure. The nurse merely asks the questions she considers important at that time, in the way she thinks appropriate.

Although both informal and formal assessment methods are in common use, formal systems will have important advantages over less structured methods. The rules, guidelines and specific procedures that are established in a formal system may help us to assess all the people in our care in more or less the same way. As a result, our own prejudices and idiosyncrasies are reduced. This means that the outcome of the assessment is likely to be similar, irrespective of the nurse involved. The same cannot be said of more informal methods, where our prejudices, opinions and other 'value judgements' influence the conduct of the assessment. Such factors can have a big influence on the kind of information collected.

Key assessment questions

Any nursing assessment looks for information about the *nature* (description) and *scale* (measurement) of the person's problem.

- What is the person's problem or difficulty?
- To what extent does it distress the person?
- To what extent does it interfere, and in what way, with everyday living?
- To what extent is the person able to exercise any kind of control over the problem?

In some situations the choice between formal and informal methods is determined by the person. Where someone is talkative, intelligent and anxious to communicate, the nurse may gain most of her information from open-ended conversations. Where the person is less amenable, or less articulate, a more focused assessment of how the person 'appears' might be the best place to begin. This might be followed by use of standardized rating scales, rather than casual interviewing, and will be more formal as a result.

WHAT SHOULD WE ASSESS?

The kind of problems of human living that people experience when they are diagnosed with a mental illness will vary from one person to the next. However, all such problems, and their consequences, will be expressed on one or more of the person's *levels of living*.[4] These become the focus of the assessment. Here we gain an appreciation of 'what is happening' for the person and what resources might be needed to begin to resolve the problem (Figure 9.1).

Levels of living

People function across a range of levels of human experience. These can be characterized as inter-related but distinct levels of the human 'self' (see Figure 9.1).

- We function at a *physiological* level (or self). Although we are not aware of this, the most fundamental level of living, what happens here is vital to the stability of our lives and our physical survival. This molecular or biochemical level of functioning is clearly the most basic level of our lives, but supports the function or expression of all the other levels of living.
- At the next level lies our *biological* self. Here, our various organs work constantly to maintain the outward

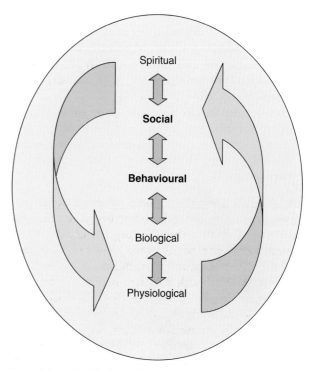

Figure 9.1 Levels of the human being

appearance of 'life', supported by our complex muscular and skeletal system, of which we have only the crudest awareness. Usually, we only become aware of this level of experience when we experience pain from injury or through exertion.

- At a third level is our *behavioural* self, which attracts most attention in mental health care. At this level the person *acts* out the story of his or her life. How people *think* and what they *feel* has a major effect on how they behave, and such thoughts and feelings are also influenced by the person's *beliefs*, about themselves and the world in which they live. By the same token, only a small proportion of our behaviour is not a function of thought and emotion. Consequently, the nursing assessment usually pays a lot of attention to *how* these four distinct aspects are interconnected.

- At the fourth level lies our *social* self. This is characterized by our relationships with the many people who make up our world. Some are close to us, such as family and friends. Others are simply the rest of 'humanity'.

- The final level might be called our *spiritual* self. Here we live in the very private world of our hopes, dreams and the 'meaning' or 'sense' we make of our experience of being alive, or in pain. Here we experience views of ourselves, and of the world around us. Often our experiences at this level are obscure, symbolic or vaguely defined. The very nature of our spiritual self might suggest that it is impossible to define. Many of the more unusual experiences associated with mental distress are located at this level of living: loss of identity, waking-dream states, and many of the powerful realizations about ourselves and the meaning of our lives.

The real challenge of any assessment is to decide which of these levels of living should be the focus of the assessment. A further challenge exists in working out how the 'picture' that emerges of one aspect of the individual might be related to some other aspect of their overall 'selfhood'.

The life story

All people are storytellers. Some tell more exciting or interesting stories than others, but everyone expresses their 'lived experience' through story. The key aim of any nursing assessment is to get a *whole* sense of what is happening for the person, and what might need to be done to address this. Although it is often practical to focus on one or more of the levels of living – how the person *feels*, what the person *thinks* etc. – the person's experience is always a *whole* or *complete* experience. Feelings are a part of thinking, which is related to beliefs, which are expressed through behaviour, which is expressed through biological functioning, which ultimately is dependent on

deep physiology. Although we cannot gain direct access to this 'whole lived experience' we can view it indirectly – through the person's story.

People know who they are and they become more knowledgeable about themselves, their lives and their problems, by talking about themselves. In Hilda Peplau's insightful words: 'people make themselves up as they talk' (HE Peplau, personal communication). This illustrates the storytelling nature of people. Three hundred years ago, Enlightenment philosophers, like David Hume and John Locke, tried to account for our human identity solely in terms of psychological states or events. Regrettably, much the same tradition continues today, with oversimplistic neuroscientific or cognitive explanations of 'how people work'. These accounts fail to take account of the background to human identity: the stories that people are *born into*, and *become part of*, through the telling of their own story.

Narrative: making up the story

Just as history is not a simple catalogue of events, or a long list of characters, so the story of a person's life involves more than the events that the person experiences. The philosopher MacIntyre suggested that:

> It is through hearing stories about wicked step-mothers, lost children, good but misguided kings, wolves that suckle twin boys, youngest sons who receive no inheritance but must make their own way in the world, and eldest sons who waste their inheritance on riotous living and go into exile to live with swine, that children learn or mislearn what a child and a parent is, what the case of characters may be in the drama into which they have been born and what the ways of the world are.[11]

Although such background stories vary from one country and culture to another, the power of story is universal. For this reason it is vital that the nursing assessment tries to get some sense of the background stories that frame the developing script of the story of the person, here and now.[12]

When nurses begin an assessment they are obliged to ask: *who* is this *person*?

This is very different from asking: what is *wrong* with this *patient*?

In so doing, they cannot divorce the person (and their story) from all the stories that helped the person become who he/she is. According to MacIntyre, if we deprive children of stories we may 'leave them unscripted, anxious stutterers, in their actions as in their words'.

This philosophy carries a profound message. If we are to understand the *people* who are in our care, we need to listen to the stories of their lives. I am the story that I tell about myself – or that sometimes is told about me.

This is also, obviously, true for the people in my care. In MacIntyre's words:

> I am the subject of a history that is my own and no-one else's, that has its own peculiar meaning. When someone complains – as do some of those who commit suicide – that his or her life is meaningless, he or she often and perhaps characteristically complaining that the narrative of their life has become unintelligible to them, that it lacks any point, any movement toward a climax or telos.[11]

MacIntyre's use of the Greek word *telos* signifies how life is in constant flow towards some endpoint, whether we are aware of it or not. Viktor Frankl[13] would have argued that the person whose life has lost its meaning has simply lost his or her awareness of the presence of meaning. One of the aims of assessment is to help people describe, explore and come to appreciate more where they are on their life path and what they think all of this might mean for them. In this sense, the assessment heralds the possibility that the intimate, constructive relationship between the nurse and the person-in-care will lead to the re-authoring of the person's own story, which they will eventually name *recovery*.

THE PROBLEMATIC CONCEPT OF NORMALITY

The traditional Western view of madness[14] was inherently pessimistic, predicated on the assumption that something 'abnormal' was occurring within the person. Modern psychiatry and psychology developed this view with their emphasis on 'abnormal psychology',[15] which led to the development of the various diagnostic systems for identification of different forms of psychopathology.[16] The concept of 'abnormality' assumes, of course, that there is such a thing as 'normality'. Although there are various statistical ways to define 'normality' it is, essentially, a mathematical concept. The normal distribution (or Gaussian curve[17]) accounts for the majority of any population: the normal range. However, all people who are, for example, *exceptionally* intelligent, creative, strong or tall lie on the perimeters of this curve of distribution and are, by definition, all 'abnormal'. Highly intelligent people are as 'abnormal' as people deemed to be 'intellectually disabled'. However, as societies tend to value intelligent (or creative, athletic, 'useful') people over those with more limited powers of reasoning, the concept of 'abnormality' tends to be restricted to people with low levels of any such 'quality'.

However, many of the 'norms' associated with human behaviour are not fixed. Fifty years ago many women who did not conform to the social stereotype of the 'housewife' or 'mother' risked being diagnosed as mentally ill. Thirty years ago it was unusual (i.e. abnormal) for women to wear trousers to work. Now, this is part of the everyday dress code of many women, especially those in business roles. If 'female trouser-wearing' has not become normal, it has at least become commonplace.

However, society does not try to treat, fix or otherwise contain tall, creative, intelligent or strong people – or women who wear trousers – because we assume that their attributes are valuable – to them, us or society at large. Madness in its various manifestations is often seen as a social problem not because it is abnormal, but because it has no social value. However, some of the experiences associated with 'serious' forms of madness – like hearing voices, or seeing visions, or descending to the depths of despair – have been used by people down the ages as the basis for creative experiments in art, literature and even the sciences.[18] The critical issue appears to be *how* do people respond to the experience of mental distress. If they can use this constructively as part of the development of their life story, it may be distressing, but is still of value. If people cannot make sense of, or otherwise learn from, the experience, then it is deemed to be worthless, and people will wish to get rid of an experience (like emotional pain).

However, there is no genuine 'gold standard' for normal/abnormal behaviour or experience. Indeed, social definitions of normality have been changing down the centuries. In our own lifetime, sexual preference and drug use are two examples of behaviour patterns that once were deemed illegal, immoral or symptomatic of some psychological disturbance but are now accepted as examples of 'personal choice' or 'freedom of expression'. Homosexuality was classed as a 'mental illness' until the mid-1970s. However, heterosexuality is not so much normal as commonplace.

Reflection

What is your definition of 'normality'? Can you summarize it in a few words?

Cultural influences

Nurses are mainly interested in assessing people through studying what people say, do, think, feel, etc. However, although it may be easy enough to collect information about these phenomena, it is much more difficult to answer the question: what does it all mean? How do we go about judging whether the behaviour we have witnessed is *normal* or *abnormal*? How do we determine whether or not such behaviour is a problem? More importantly, does it really 'matter'? Arriving at such a decision is rarely easy, since normal behaviour can vary from one person to the next, from one culture to another, and can be influenced by different laws even within the same country.

Human behaviour is influenced most by the culture within which the person lives.[19] Most of our behaviour is learned: human beings appear to be poorly supplied with instincts, unlike our animal and insect relations. Even infants of only a few weeks old have already begun to learn how to respond to their environment: their behaviour is not established before birth. We have no instincts to help us to tie shoelaces, cook food, order a beer, comb our hair, catch a bus or open a window for fresh air. These mundane behaviours are acquired through learning and are all part of the culture to which we belong. Were we to move to a different culture such as an underdeveloped country or a hospital ward, such behaviour might be redundant or might even be discouraged. Those features of our behaviour that are at present normal might become 'abnormal', deviant or at the very least unusual.

The idea that all human behaviour is either 'normal' or 'abnormal' is overly simplistic. What is accepted as 'normal behaviour' appears to be defined by cultures. Even within one culture, discrete subcultures may determine different patterns of behaviour. Society may view gang members as 'anti-social' and 'abnormal' but within the subculture to which they belong, violence and criminal activity are completely 'normal'. In most Western countries scantily dressed women are viewed as fashionably 'normal'; however, such modes of dress are often deemed highly unacceptable (abnormal) by Islamic societies, or even by Muslim people living within Western countries.

There are few, if any, universal norms as far as behaviour is concerned. One might assume that murder, incest and child abuse would be viewed as unacceptable by all societies and cultures. Sociologists would argue that this is not the case. Many cultures, admittedly some of them 'uncivilized' by Western standards, will tolerate, even encourage, such practices under certain conditions. Even exceptional behaviour, such as the experience of hallucinations is relatively common in some cultures. Romme and Escher's Dutch research into the prevalence of 'hearing voices' – what psychiatry calls an auditory hallucination – illustrated that sizeable proportions of 'non-patient' groups reported hearing voices. Such findings question some of our established beliefs about the nature of 'madness', many of which are culture bound by the Western tradition.[20,21]

Romme and Escher's work is merely the latest chapter in what could be called the demythologizing of madness. Over 40 years ago researchers showed that one-third of a random sample of Zulu women had reported visual and auditory hallucinations involving 'angels, babies and little short hairy men' and more than half of the women engaged in 'screaming behaviour', often yelping for hours, days, even weeks.[22] Such behaviour would be viewed as grossly abnormal in the West, yet few of these women showed any other signs of mental disorder. Within their own culture their hallucinations and screaming were legitimate. Similarly, over 20 years ago African psychiatrists began to recognize that persecutory delusions were more frequent in African, Jamaican and Caribbean subjects than in any other groups, something which is now widely accepted. They explain this finding by attributing the delusions to beliefs in witchcraft and voodoo common to these cultures.[23] The beliefs (which are commonly called delusions) held by West Indians diagnosed as psychotic appear to be the same as those held by 'normal' West Indians. The only difference between the two groups appears to be the abnormal reaction (or behaviour) of the so-called 'psychotic' person to these beliefs.

ASSESSMENT: AN EDUCATED GUESS?

In any assessment it is incumbent on the nurse, not merely to record and measure what is seen and heard, but also to interpret this in a sociocultural context. We might add that it is important to avoid 'pathologizing' (i.e. medicalizing) everything that appears 'odd'. In another context, this 'odd' behaviour might well be adaptive, meaningful or otherwise 'normal'.

In this chapter I have tried to emphasize the *ordinariness* of assessment. It is different only in quality and importance from assessing how much seed will be needed to cover the bare patches on the lawn, or how we might undertake a trip around the world. Anyone can make a wild guess as to what these exercises might involve. There is no substitute, however, for the 'educated guess' made by the keen gardener or the regular traveller – someone who really cares about the garden or the journey. Such calculations, by a genuinely interested party, are based upon knowledge and experience. Later (Chapters 10 and 11), I shall discuss some of the specific approaches to assessment. However, knowing *how* is never a substitute for knowing *why*.

Mark Twain famously said, 'give a man a hammer and he will treat everything as if it were a nail'. Knowing *how* to complete a checklist, fill out a rating scale or conduct an interview is a valuable skill. However, it is only valuable if we have first established *why* such a 'tool' is appropriate for the job in hand. The hammer used by the silversmith is quite different – in form and function – from the hammer used by the blacksmith. We can do a lot of damage by using the tools of assessment inappropriately. The silversmith and the blacksmith are both focused on *hammering*. The crucial differences are:

- *how* they use the hammer (sensitivity);
- the *nature* of the hammer itself (tool);
- their purpose in *selecting this* tool over any other (rationale).

Asking people questions can seem like a fairly innocuous activity. We assume that even if it does not deliver anything of value, at least it will not harm the person. This is one of the myths of psychiatric practice. The inappropriate administration of anything – from distant 'observation' to close-up, in-depth interviews – can do great damage to the vulnerable person on the receiving end. Our motto should be 'seek first to understand'.

- To begin to understand the person in care we must first understand fully what are our options – how might we explore and examine the situation with the person, their *experience* of what is happening.
- Then, we must understand why we have chosen one approach over another. (Why have we chosen to use this tool, in this particular way?) In a very real sense, nurses must understand themselves – their feelings about those in their care, and the motives underlying their attitude towards them. But most of all, nurses need to understand how little they really know about the people in their care.

A well-planned and carefully executed assessment may help the nurse learn something of value, about the person and their experience. In so doing, this will rid the nurse of some of the ignorance that often bars the way to the delivery of personally appropriate care in mental health. If the nurse is fortunate, a well-planned assessment might pave the way for the re-authoring of the person's own life story.[24]

REFERENCES

1. Keen T, Kenn, J. Developing collaborative assessment. In: P Barker (ed.). *Psychiatric and mental health nursing: the craft of caring.* London, UK: Arnold, 2003: Chapter 11.

2. Straus SE, Tomlin A, Price J, Geddes J. *Practising evidence-based mental health.* Abingdon, UK: Radcliffe Medical Press, 1999.

3. Dicenso A, Guyatt G, Ciliska D. *Evidence-based nursing: a guide to clinical practice.* St Louis, MO: Mosby, 2004.

4. Barker PJ. *Assessment in psychiatric and mental health nursing: in search of the whole person,* 2nd edn. London, UK: Nelson Thornes, 2004.

5. O'Toole AN, Welt SR (eds). *Hildegard E. Peplau. Selected works. Interpersonal theory in nursing.* Basingstoke, UK: Macmillan, 1984.

6. Habermann M. *The nursing process: a global concept.* Edinburgh, UK: Churchill Livingstone, 2005.

7. Hayne YM. Experiencing psychiatric diagnosis: client perspectives on being named mentally ill. *Journal of Psychiatric and Mental Health Nursing* 2003; **10** (6): 722–9.

8. American Nurses Association. *Nursing: a social policy statement.* Kansas City, MO: American Nurses Association, 1980.

9. Peplau HF. Another look at schizophrenia from a nursing standpoint. In: Anderson CA (ed.). *Psychiatric nursing 1974–94: a report on the state of the art.* St Louis, MO: Mosby Year Book, 1995.

10. O'Toole A, Loomis M. Classifying human responses in psychiatric and mental health nursing. In: Reynolds W, Cormack D (eds). *Psychiatric and mental health nursing: theory and practice.* London, UK: Chapman and Hall, 1990.

11. MacIntyre A. The story-telling animal. In: Bowie L, Michaels MW, Solomon RC (eds). *Twenty questions: an introduction to philosophy.* London, UK: Harcourt Brace Jovanovich, 1988.

12. Barker P, Kerr B. *The process of psychotherapy: the journey of discovery.* Oxford, UK: Butterworth-Heinemann: 2000.

13. Frankl V. *Man's search for meaning.* London, UK: Hodder and Stoughton, 1964.

14. Foucault M. *Madness and civilization.* London, UK: Routledge, 2006.

15. Kring AM, Davison GC, Neale JM, Johnson SL. *Abnormal psychology,* 10th edn. New York, NY: Wiley, 2006.

16. Hersen M, Turner SM, Beidel DC. *Adult psychopathology and diagnosis.* New York; Wiley 2007.

17. Bell, ET. The prince of mathematicians: Gauss. In: *Men of mathematics: the lives and achievements of the great mathematicians from Zeno to Poincaré.* New York, NY: Simon and Schuster, 1986: 218–69.

18. Barker P. *The philosophy and practice of psychiatric nursing.* Edinburgh, UK: Churchill Livingstone, 1999.

19. Burr A, Chapman T. Some reflections on cultural and social considerations in mental health nursing. *Journal of Psychiatric and Mental Health Nursing* 1998; **5** (6): 431–7.

20. Romme M, Escher S. *Making sense of voices: a guide for mental health professionals working with voice-hearers.* London, UK: Mind Publications, 2000.

21. Bentall RP. *Madness explained: psychosis and human nature.* London, UK: Allen Lane, 2003.

22. Lee SGM. *Stress and adaptation.* Leicester: Leicester University Press, 1961.

23. Ndetei DM, Vadher A. Frequency and clinical significance of delusions across cultures. *Acta Psychiatric Scandinavica* 1984; **70**: 73–6.

24. Barker P, Buchanan-Barker P. *The tidal model: a guide for mental health professionals.* New York, NY: Brunner Routledge, 2005.

CHAPTER 10

Assessment methods

Phil Barker*

INTRODUCTION

How we collect the information is the assessment *method*. When nurses try to establish a format of assessment that is *reliable*, irrespective of who undertakes assessment, and which will provide *valid* information about the actual people and their problems of living, the *methodology* they will use will – in one way or another – be *scientific*.

Information about people can be collected in two ways. The most obvious, and realistic way to assess a person is to invite a *report* on his/her situation. We can ask the person questions, or ask them to complete some kind of a record of his or her experience. Either way, we need to be confident that the person is *willing* (motivated) and *able* (competent) to provide such subjective reports. We also need to be assured that the person has no reason for wishing to mislead us. If we are not confident that the information we shall obtain will be accurate, it may well be worthless.

Alternatively, we might ask other people to make observations on the person. Family members might use their proximity to the person to report on him or her from close range. Where the person is in care, members of the care and treatment team can provide differing kinds of 'observation' from their various vantage points in relation to the person in care. However, in both cases such observations are bedevilled with practical and ethical problems.

However, in every case, the aim of assessment is simple, yet complex. We want to answer the question:

> What is really *going on here*, and how will this help us work out what we need to do by way of a caring response?

INFORMATION SOURCES

The methods discussed in the next section involve *subjective* or *objective* reports. Wherever possible, information should he obtained *direct* from the person, either in the form of some kind of 'self report' or via observation. The ideal form of assessment is *collaborative*, where the nurse and the person explore the problem together. 'Second-hand' observations, obtained from fellow professionals, family or friends come a very poor second in this respect. We should be aware, however, that in some cases the person may be unwilling or unable to provide the information needed, requiring the nurse to fall back on the reports provided by others.

However, other people's comments and observations may be important as they involve information known only to them, corroborating or contradicting the story offered by the person. This is particularly important where the person is in care. Junior staff members often have more contact with the person than senior staff. The person may also behave differently with staff they assume to be of a more junior status, perceiving them to be less threatening by dint of their inexperience or lack of authority. Often, people confide in junior staff because they feel closer to them than to more senior staff or other specialist therapists. Paradoxically, therefore, less-experienced staff may be a more useful source of information or access point for assessing the person in care.

The views of 'significant others' – family, or friends who know the person well – are also invaluable in helping to develop the 'bigger picture'. Even if their perspective appears to contradict the story offered by the person him

*Phil Barker is a psychotherapist and Honorary Professor at the University of Dundee, UK.

or herself, ultimately this can be useful – if only in illustrating how different parties have different views on the problem or its inherent nature.

Collecting information from the person, or 'significant others', usually involves some *informal* method of assessment. Highly structured (*formal*) assessments can make people uncomfortable and may prejudice the chance of gaining accurate information. By contrast, information supplied by staff will probably be more formal, involving the use of some standardized method of observation or recording. The specific *aim* of the assessment, and the particular people involved, will determine which form of information *source* is selected.

- If we need to know how the person *thinks* or *feels*, or if we need to identify the person's values or beliefs, we need to *ask the person*.

- If we need to know what *other people* think, or feel, or believe about the person, we need to *ask those other people*.

- If we need to know how the person behaves under certain conditions, either we ask the person to observe or reflect on their own behaviour, or we ask someone else to observe the person. (These two options may, of course, provide completely different reports.)

PSYCHOSOCIAL ASSESSMENT

Given that people are highly complex, it is important to assess the person across a wide range of dimensions. The primary focus of nursing assessment is, however, on what might be called the psychosocial plane. The term *psychosocial* refers, simply, to one's psychological development in and interaction with a social environment (see http://en.wikipedia.org/wiki/Psychosocial). In everyday nursing practice, every interaction between a nurse and a person in care (who is conscious) *must* be a psychosocial interaction, since it involves the nurse's interaction with the person – both at the level of their existing psychological development. Regrettably, the term has been reduced to mean a delimited programme of 'psychological *intervention*', often with specific psychiatric populations,[1] rather than the exploratory encounter of one person with another.[2]

Nurses can, and often do, participate in the physical examination of the person: through collection of body fluids and their analysis; undertaking routine physical assessments; or supporting physicians undertaking more complex diagnostic assessments such as computerized axial tomography or positron emission tomography scans. These biomedical assessment activities are often a critical part of the diagnostic process for some people, and may represent a valuable contribution to determining appropriate medical intervention. However important these

functions may be, arguably, they do not represent the 'proper focus' of nursing.[3] Nurses focus upon, address and subsequently become involved in the person's *interaction* with their environment, which includes other people, groups, organizations and aspects of the expressed culture which lie within that environment. Given this focus, psychiatric and mental health nursing assessment methods emphasize this psychosocial world.

The term *psychosocial* includes consideration of a wide range of personal and interpersonal factors. These include *psychological* and *biological phenomena*:

- functional (behavioural) performance
- self-efficacy;

and ecological factors, including:

- relationships within the family
- relationships with the wider social environment
- interpersonal communication
- social resources.

In any genuinely *psychosocial* nursing assessment the encounter would focus on what the nurse experienced: how what the person said and did affected the individual nurse. It seems axiomatic that the *effect* will differ, depending on the emotional, psychological or spiritual maturity of the nurse who is present. Regrettably, much of the literature pays little heed to the relative 'maturity–immaturity' of the professionals concerned.

> ### Reflection
>
> What is the difference between assessment and diagnosis? How important is assessment for the development of appropriate nursing care?

THE FOUR MAJOR ASSESSMENT METHODS

Each of the main methods of assessment has a different function, producing different kinds of *data* – or information – from the others. Most assessments involve a mix of these different approaches.

Interviewing

During an interview the nurse asks the person about feelings, thoughts, beliefs or specific views of the person's behaviour. These questions may relate to life in general or may be specific to particular problems of living or aspects of care and treatment. An interview can simply involve 'sitting down and chatting with the person'. In other contexts the interview may involve asking the person to answer yes or no to a series of questions.

These represent the extremes of highly *unstructured* and *structured* formats. Somewhere between the two lies the *semi-structured interview.*

In the *semi-structured interview* the person is asked a range of *exploratory* questions on various topics. The answers usually generate additional questions that need to be answered before moving on to the next topic. By contrast, wholly unstructured 'chatting' may be too rambling to lead to any useful conclusions. The rambling nature of the enquiry might even make the person uneasy, feeling that the conversation isn't going anywhere. At the other extreme the highly structured 'quizzing' of the person may seem impersonal and officious. Where the nurse uses a fixed *interview schedule*, there is very little room for manoeuvre, as all the interactions are determined by the questions on the paper.

The *semi-structured* format is a common preference in most situations as the developing conversation is orderly, without being too regimented. There is room to break off at tangents, as appropriate, without losing the place. This allows the conversation to flow, affording both nurse and the person some security.

The success or failure of any interview is dependent on the nurse's behaviour. Problems in interviews are most often associated with the nurse's relationship with the person, and less often with the person him or herself.

The importance of the relationship
The success of the interview depends on the nature of the relationship established between the nurse and the person. Interviews should always be undertaken in a relatively quiet and relaxed setting. Although this need not be a formal interview room, privacy and comfort are essential. The purpose of the interview should be explained at the outset, in language that is appropriate to the intellectual and emotional status of the person. Following this, the nurse should begin with general questions, aiming to achieve rapport and put the person at ease.

Example of dialogue:

Nurse: I am really pleased to meet you. I would like to talk about what is happening for you right now. I would like to begin to work out what you might need right now. I have a few questions that I would like to ask, but please stop me if you want to ask me something. I would like this to be more of a conversation than an interview. How do you feel about that?

The importance of motivation
Some people are threatened by the prospect of the interview and may feel inclined to deny, minimize or exaggerate their problems of living. Consequently, it is important to encourage the person to complete the interview fully and accurately. Often, this can best be achieved by linking the interview to the care planning process that follows.

Example of dialogue:

Nurse: What we talk about here will help us work out what kind of care you need right now and maybe also over the days ahead. So I'd like you to take your time with this. We can come back to any things that you are not sure of later, if you like. Is that OK?

The nurse's attitudes
Before beginning the interview, the nurse should consider, carefully, her *attitudes* towards the person and the problems of living that are likely to emerge. If the interviewer feels uncomfortable, or negatively predisposed towards the person, this may prevent the person getting fully involved in the interview. Where the person's problems generate some attitudinal conflict for the nurse, this should be addressed as part of the nurse's ongoing clinical supervision.

Recording the interview
Some kind of record of the interview must be made and, ideally, this should be done during the interview, clarifying the person's responses before committing anything to paper. Recording an interview after it has been conducted is fraught with difficulties, not least remembering what exactly was said, coupled with the risk that the interviewer's interpretations of what has been said will dominate.

The role of the interviewee
The manner in which the interview is conducted can have a profound effect on the person being interviewed, influencing what they say and how the person might feel, about the interview and the interviewer. The time of day can be crucial, especially where the person is affected by time-related variations in mood or energy levels. When the interview is over, the person should always be offered an opportunity to discuss it with the nurse.

Advantages
The interview has several advantages over other methods.

- *Interviews are popular because they appear simple.* Many nurses can 'converse' with the person with little or no training. Of course, they might converse a lot better if they were properly trained. The interview may be most appropriate where the person is unable to use any kind of self-assessment. This is especially the case where the person has literacy problems, or is able to speak the common language but finds it difficult to express this in writing. This may be the case where the person belongs to an ethnic minority population.
- *Interviews allow the nurse to check the person's understanding.* If the person appears hesitant or puzzled she can rephrase the question, or amplify it in some way,

to help the person answer. This is not possible where the person is left to fill in a questionnaire or rating scale unaided.

- *Interviews allows the person to provide as much detail as necessary.* The semi-structured format allows the person to develop a theme, which seems on reflection, important. This is rarely possible by any other means. Of course this is only possible if the nurse has the ability to recognize that something significant has been said and can encourage the person to pursue this, so amplifying the response.
- *Interviews usually allow the nurse to design the rest of the assessment.* Interviews are often the first port of call in the assessment process. The preliminary interview gives us the clues regarding what might be important aspects of the person and/or the person's life, which might be explored further through other interviews or other forms of assessment.

Disadvantages

There are, however, some disadvantages.

- *Interviewing can be time-consuming.* In a difficult (or badly handled) interview, much time may be spent for little reward. A successful interview may be equally costly: a lot of time is spent preparing the ground, asking general questions, probing the details and recording the person's replies. A further issue is the time that may be wasted exploring 'dead ends' or issues that appear to lead nowhere in particular.
- *Interviews are very dependent on the expertise of the interviewer.* Many nurses are obliged to assess the people in their care, often with little or no training. Where the person is very confused or otherwise distressed we must challenge the wisdom of such a practice, not to mention the ethical problems involved. Where the person is not manifestly distressed, but is anxious to resolve his problems, this may also tax the expertise of the nurse. Highly intelligent and articulate people can be as demanding as those who find it difficult to communicate because of an intellectual impairment or limited vocabulary. In both cases nurses need a lot of skill to cope with the person's difficulties or expectations. One way to resolve this problem is to allow junior staff to develop their interviewing skills gradually, beginning with the highly structured 'quiz', which usually greets the person on admission to the service, working gradually towards a more semi-structured format.
- *The interview may have a negative effect upon the person.* Some people become anxious during interviews, especially when they are uncertain about the aims of the interview or find it difficult to supply the answers. They may also be anxious about how their replies might be interpreted. Similar anxieties may be present when someone is asked to fill in a form. However, interview anxiety often stems from being looked at,

when the person may feel that he or she is being scrutinized or put under the spotlight. The intense, interpersonal nature of the interview may cause problems for some people.

Diaries, logs and personal records

Many people use diaries, logs or other personal notes to record aspects of their daily life. Reading published diaries gives us an insight into the personal identity of the author. By inviting the person to reflect on his or her experience, staff can gain a similar insight into the person's experience of their illness or care and treatment. This can be done in several ways, all of which involve recording details of behaviour, feelings or thoughts *as they occur*, during the course of everyday activity or soon afterwards.

A *log* or a *diary* will provide details of the person's experiences while engaged in different activities with different people. The diary may be completed once a day, such as in the evening. Or the person may complete the log or diary as events occur, or at prescribed points in the day – lunchtime, at the end of the afternoon, before retiring. There are no rules of what constitutes a log or a diary. Ideally, the person should choose his or her own format and also should choose how to complete it. However, the nurse needs to let the person know what kind of information would help the team, but beyond that the form of the log or diary needs no boundaries – and may include drawings, poems, pictures or other accumulated 'scraps' of information that communicate something of the person's lived experience.

Advantages

The main advantage is simplicity. It can also be seen as cost-effective, since it can reveal a wealth of information for minimal staff time. This information can be 'qualitative' – focused on stories, notes or other reflections on experience; or 'quantitative' – recording discrete information regarding how *often* or for how *long* the person engaged in a particular form of behaviour (such as hand-washing or social interaction). Where the person is already a diary keeper, these notes may be seen as a simple extension of the routine 'self-study', which is already part of everyday life. Where the person is less confident about committing experiences to paper, it may be necessary to tailor the recording format to suit the person, perhaps even helping the person design the kind of recording format that would be most appropriate. For example, if a person described a feeling of anxiety that came and went throughout the day, it might be helpful to monitor this. If the anxiety appeared to prevent him or her from doing things, the nurse might suggest recording

- any activity that was *disrupted*
- *when* the anxiety began and ended
- the *severity* of the feeling of anxiety.

Such information not only provides more details about the presenting problem, but can be used to evaluate progress at a later date.

When used appropriately, the self-study nature of the log or diary can have an inbuilt therapeutic effect, and may reduce the scale of a problem even before treatment begins. In many cases, the use of the diary or log becomes an integral part of the subsequent therapy.[4]

Disadvantages

There are, however, several disadvantages.

- Although diary formats require little investment of nursing time to complete, they can be costly in terms of *analysis*, especially where the person commits a lot of information to paper.
- If the nurse asks the person to study only one area of life experience, this may prejudice the person's observations, resulting in a failure to be open to the *wider context* of the problem.
- If the person is advised to record every instance of a particular problem – such as hearing voices or becoming anxious – the person may develop an *increased awareness* of the problem, appearing to enlarge the scale of the problem. This is commonly called 'observer effect', and equally applies to staff observations of the person's behaviour.
- By 'looking for' instances of particular problems, the person may experience a *heightened emotional awareness*, potentially increasing the sense of 'emotional burden'.
- Alternatively, if the person is asked to record the number of times they drank to excess or lost their temper, the person may record less of these, given their awareness of their 'undesirable' nature.
- Since such notes, diaries or logs are so *ordinary* and commonplace, the person may simply forget to complete them. If this is the only information being collected then the assessment of the person can be delayed considerably. For this reason any such diaries or logs should be designed to suit the person, rather than using standardized formats that may have no personal meaning.

Questionnaires and rating scales

Questionnaires and rating scales are designed to gain very *specific* measures of some problem area. Usually they are developed from research projects, or are designed to support scientific research. Commonly, drafts of the questionnaire or rating scale are tried out on a sample population and revised and modified, depending on its success. When the research is complete, the questionnaire or rating scale should provide a reliable and valid measure of a specific problem for the minimum amount of effort.

A vast assortment of such methods has been developed to assess various psychiatric phenomena, e.g. depression,

dependency, disorientation or 'social competence'. However, each problem is a '*construct*' rather than a reality. Each problem comprises various behavioural, emotional or cognitive 'problems'. The questionnaire or rating scale provides only a crude estimate of its severity.

Questionnaires

If the nurse wishes to assess only one aspect of the person's functioning, a questionnaire might help this to be done for little effort. Some questionnaires require only yes/no answers, generating a total score for a particular construct – such as 'assertiveness' or 'obsessionality'.[5] This allows a judgement to be made of 'how assertive' or 'obsessional' the person is compared with available group norms. Other formats might use 'true' or 'false' answers.[6] Such questionnaires can be completed by the person alone, or as the basis of a structured interview.

Although such forms of questionnaire are *simple*, the information gained is usually equally limited.

Rating scales

The rating scale may also specify a problem area, but the person is asked to rate the *severity* of a problem or to rate their *performance*; or to indicate the extent to which they *agree* or *disagree* with certain statements. In principle, the rating scale may assess any area of human functioning. Particular patterns of *behaviour* may be assessed, e.g. How often do you brush your teeth? Never (1) through to More than three times a day (5). Alternatively, the scale may focus on measures of *belief*: success in life depends on luck – I *agree* strongly (1) through to I *disagree* strongly (5).

Although there is considerable variation, all rating scales end in a numerical score. This score will reflect the extent to which some emotion is *felt*, some behaviour is *performed*, some thought is *experienced* or some belief is *held*.

The Likert scale

Many rating scales are described as 'Likert' scales after the originator of this scaling method. Likert found that the best results were achieved by using five categories of response.[7] Typically a rating scales will use a scale extending from:

0 = Not present or Not at all or Never

5 = Extreme or All the time or Maximum.

In principle, the Likert scale can be used to measure anything, and might also be used to measure 'change'. For example:

0 = No change

5 = Significant improvement.

Advantages of questionnaires/rating scales

There are three main advantages.

- *Standardized methods generate a quantifiable 'measure' of a problem for the minimum investment of time.* Whereas we might spend 20 minutes interviewing the person about how they feel, the rating scale may require only a few minutes' explanation and a further few minutes' completion, and might generate a more manageable body of information about the person's feelings.

- *Since the same facets of the problem are assessed, comparisons can be made between one person and another.* Published questionnaires and rating scales include 'norms', reflecting the range of scores obtained from the study of different populations – e.g. hospitalized patients or 'normal subjects'. It is possible therefore, to compare the person's score with the available norms. It is possible to say that, for example, this person is very dependent, depressed, lonely, anxious. Such judgements are not opinion but are made in the light of available knowledge regarding how people (in general) function.
- *Standardized methods usually break problems into component parts.* This may help both team members and the person-in-care to appreciate what the problem involves. A scale measuring depression (for example) might cover aspects of the person's motivation, mood, libido, appetite, etc. An anxiety scale might measure a range of anxiety-related factors: feeling tense, panic attacks, sweating, urge to pass urine, etc. These are not simply whimsical exercises. The various items on the scale or questionnaire have been arrived at through careful study and experimentation. They refer to the phenomena experienced or exhibited by *most* people who are described as suffering from anxiety, depression, etc. These methods are the psychosocial equivalent of the measuring tape or thermometer.

Disadvantages

However, there are at least three disadvantages.

- *Their rigid and structured nature prevents the nurse from responding, flexibly, to the person.* The person may gain the impression that he or she is being 'processed', and that we are only interested in parts of them and their problems, rather than in them as 'whole people'.
- *Many people find it difficult to express themselves using a structured format.* Where the questionnaire demands a yes/no response, the person may want to answer, sometimes or just in the morning. The scale, however, may make no concession to these varieties of experience. Where ratings are involved the person, again, may feel compromised if asked to choose between 'agree' or 'disagree' categories. The person may say that sometimes this rating applies but at other times another rating is more accurate. This may frustrate or even infuriate the nurse, who might think that the person is simply being difficult. Such a difficulty, however, may only illustrate the uncertainty of their experience.
- *Some people are unhappy with the written format, even when this is completed by the nurse.* The demands of the exercise may unnerve them completely, adding to

their distress. For this reason it may be necessary to be selective where questionnaires or rating scales are involved.

For a detailed list of such assessment instruments see the chapter 'Assessment in psychiatric and mental health nursing' in Barker[3] and the *Handbook of assessment and treatment planning for psychological disorders.*[8] Many of the most popular instruments in common usage are, however, copyright, requiring a licence to use in practice.

Observation

Although 'observation' is used commonly in nursing practice, often this involves little more than 'watching' the person and making notes about their behaviour or 'presentation'.[9] This relatively simple approach can, however, be used in a more rigorous and methodical manner. Perhaps by virtue of the rigour required, observation is often the least practised of the four methods discussed here.[10]

Observation may be carried out in several ways:

- by the person themselves ('self-monitoring')
- by members of the staff team
- less frequently, by members of the person's family.

The principles behind self-monitoring and observation by others are very similar.

Self-monitoring

Self-monitoring is an extension of the diary/log format discussed above. However, here the self-assessment is made more formal. The person is helped to identify specific targets for self-observation, which are defined clearly and unambiguously, so that some kind of *measure* can be taken across time. The person may self-monitor any aspect of their experience, but in practice specific *behaviours*, discrete *thoughts* and clearly defined *feelings* may be appropriate targets.

Following the initial assessment the nurse discusses with the person the specific problems of living or aspects of problems that might be most appropriate for self-monitoring. Then a decision can be made regarding the kind of measure that might be appropriate. Usually this involves an estimate of how often the person engages in a pattern of behaviour, or has a particular experience *(frequency)* or how long the behaviour or experience lasts *(duration)*.

In self-monitoring *frequency* the person might record how often they

- experienced a panic attack
- drank alcohol
- spoke to a stranger
- lost their temper.

The only requirement is that each incident should be broadly similar in size or severity to the others. Before beginning, it may be appropriate to ensure that the person can distinguish (for example) between 'anger' and 'jealousy' or even 'annoyance'. The simplest way to ensure this is to ask the person to say what they might *do* or *say* when angry, jealous, annoyed, etc.

In some instances the definition can be quite specific:

* 'drinking alcohol' can be defined in terms of *units* of alcohol consumed, rather than glasses of beer or gin and tonic;
* 'speaking to a stranger' might be defined in terms of the sort of interaction that might be involved, and could also include some 'exclusion criteria', such as saying hello to a passer-by.

The best targets for a *frequency count* are those with a clear beginning and end. The person might record each time they:

1 drink 1 unit of alcohol
2 swear at their partner
3 smoke a joint
4 think 'I'm a failure'
5 turn down a request
6 hear the voice of their dead mother.

These 'self assessments' could help the person evaluate at least one facet of their drinking (1), bad temper (2), drug-taking (3), self-esteem (4), assertiveness (5) or hallucinatory experience (6).

For other behaviour patterns, it may be more helpful to measure *how long* the person spends *engaged* in the action (*duration*). This is indicated where the action may be short-lived (shouting for a few seconds) but for others it may last much longer (e.g. a violent argument lasting 20 minutes). Instead of counting the number of times the person loses their temper, washes their hands, checks the doors and windows or has a conversation with a workmate, they are asked to note roughly how long they spent engaged in the activity.

In a few cases a slightly different kind of time measure may be appropriate. Where the person is particularly slow at doing something, such as summoning up the courage to say 'hello' to someone or making decisions, they might measure how long they take to complete these actions. The person might record how *long they take* to:

1 get up in the morning
2 get dressed
3 answer a question
4 choose what to wear
5 answer the telephone.

These were all problems for one person, who described these problems as:

1 I can't be bothered getting up
2 I can't decide what to wear
3 I can't think of anything to say

4 I can't make up my mind
5 I'm frightened who might be on the line.

Using a traditional psychiatric approach, these problems might be described variously as:

1 apathy
2 indecisiveness
3 insecurity
4 obsessionality
5 anxiety.

All these problems have a common denominator: the person took a *long time* to complete any of these actions.

However simple the measurement system that is selected, there can be no guarantee that the person will continue with the self-monitoring. Unless they already are an avid 'self-watcher' – such as a diarist – they are is likely to tire of the chore. Consequently it is necessary to provide regular boosts of encouragement or offers of alternative ways of collecting the information. Otherwise the exercise may simply become another problem on top of many.

Some nurses think that their 'patients' would not be capable of such apparently complex forms of self-observation. Although the methods outlined above may appear complicated, depending on the context, they may be simplicity itself. The issue here is not so much the method as the degree of collaboration with the person-in-care. Self-monitoring is particularly useful in a rehabilitation setting, where there is intensive nursing support and the aim is to develop independence and a degree of self-reliance in the person.

Advantages of self-monitoring
The major advantages are:

* the person is intimately *involved* in the process. The person, therefore, retains *ownership* of the problem;
* the method may be *simple or complex*, this being determined by the capabilities and preferences of the person concerned;
* the number of ways self-monitoring might be *recorded* are potentially infinite – from using standardized checklists through to making notes on the back of a cigarette packet;
* with the advent of various public health education programmes, many people will be aware of the concept of 'self-monitoring' and may already have some experience of using this form of 'self-assessment'.

Disadvantages of self-monitoring
The major disadvantages are:

* any form of 'self-monitoring', whether simple or complex, requires considerable *motivation*. Many people can *begin* to study their behaviour – e.g. monitoring their smoking, eating or drinking – but few can *sustain* this for any length of time;

- the data generated by this form of assessment represent a behavioural 'outcome' – i.e. what the person 'does'. It provides no information on what *might* be the person's 'problem' in a more holistic sense, far less any information as to 'why' this is a problem for the person.

Staff monitoring

Observation is used most commonly by staff members where they describe how the person

- *presented* at interview
- *behaved* during the course of a period of inpatient assessment
- *behaved* during a family meeting or in a group.

Such observations are focused on what can be 'seen' or 'heard'. Regrettably, professionals rarely keep objective records of behaviour, or fastidious notes on presentation, preferring instead to make judgements on the significance (perceived or actual) of what they have witnessed.

In nursing, 'observation' often becomes a dedicated process for the management of people at risk of suicidal, self-harming or violent behaviour.[11] Nurses have a legal responsibility to document various aspects of the care they deliver, including making notes on the presentation of those in their care. Such records should be as objective and free of unnecessary interpretation as possible. Irrespective of the situation – inpatient ward, rehabilitation unit, group therapy session, outpatient clinic appointment, family meeting – the nurse should record only *observable* facts: what she *saw* and *heard*. This objective information can be supplemented with a range of information, which can be drawn from other sources:

- from the person themselves
- from family members and friends (where appropriate)
- from other therapists or team members.

All assessment is focused on answering the question, what is really going on here? These people will provide their own perspective on what they believed was *really* going on, if only from their own perspective.

Although there is a great emphasis on the importance of evidence for health in routine psychiatric practice there is often a surfeit of opinion, judgement and conjecture. In asking different people for their differing perspectives on 'what is going on here', the ultimate aim is to separate solid, reliable information from mere opinion or conjecture.

Advantages of staff (or family) observation
The key advantages are:

- this provides an *alternative perspective* on the 'problems' (which may complement or contradict that of the person/patient).
- staff may be expected to be highly adept in conducting objective observation. Consequently, they should be able to provide reliable and valid reports on the person's presentation across time.

- observations from staff or family members may help to develop a 'bigger picture' when used to augment the person/patient's own perspective on the problem.
- independent observations might highlight contradictions – e.g. between staff and patient views of the 'scale' of the problem – leading to more focused, critical assessment.

Disadvantages of staff (or family) observation
The key disadvantages are:

- this reinforces the 'paternalistic' model of 'looking after' the patient;
- such observations are the product of the perceptions of the observer (whether staff or family member) and are influenced by the observer's values and beliefs about the 'problem', and especially by the observer's 'attitude' towards the person/patient;
- the information from such observations may contribute to a conflict of 'opinions' – between 'patient', staff and/or family – regarding the nature or even existence of the problem.

Reflection

What forms of assessment do you use most commonly in your practice?
Why do you use these methods rather than any other?

The focus of assessment

All assessment is potentially complex. We open our bag of assessment tools looking for the one tool that will unlock our understanding of the person's problems. We do so in the hope of developing, with the person, a shared understanding of what is happening within their world of experience, so that we might work out what might need to be done to meet the person's immediate human needs.

However, any assessment rarely involves only *one* function. We might assess people:

- to find out *who they are* – as in the life profile;
- to describe and measure specific 'problems of living' – as in the problem-oriented interview; or
- to describe their assets and personal and social resources – as in the strengths assessment.

At the same time we might try to assess the *scale* of these problems or *assets*; here assessment doubles as *evaluation*, judging whether problems (or assets) appear to be diminishing, increasing or remaining at the same level. Common to all these areas is the hope that through assessment we might grow to understand the *meaning* or *human significance* of the person's problems.

Because of its roots in medicine, psychiatry has tended to view the 'patient's' *presentation* or behaviour as merely *symptomatic* of some greater distress, or something below the surface of life. Increasingly, the assorted psychiatric 'problems of living' are seen as a function of some bio-chemical anomaly or genetic influence. However, although nursing can help people deal with their 'illness', a more specific function of nursing is to help people live from day to day, which explains nursing's general interest in 'activities of daily living'.[12] In the mental health field it is axiomatic that nursing should be focused on helping people (who are 'patients') understand better what is happening to them, so that they might work, collaboratively, with the nursing team, to begin to address these problems of everyday living.

ASSESSMENT STAGES

All 'assessments' usually develop through a series of interconnected stages.

1 *The simple sketch*: An unstructured interview will elicit a vast amount of information about the person, their interactions with others, their beliefs, ambitions and hopes and dreams. Most of this information will be non-specific and general and characterized by its fuzzy outline. A structured interview will begin the process of defining the person and their situation more clearly. Interest in the person's stream-of-consciousness may begin to wane as we start to narrow our focus – looking for more specific answers to increasingly more focused questions. Naturally, the person's freedom to talk begins, also, to be reduced. By the end of the structured interview we should have identified the areas of the person and their life that need to be addressed, to develop appropriate care.

2 *The detailed portrait*: We may now wish to describe these significant aspects in more quantifiable terms, perhaps beginning by asking the person to summarize aspects of their life, their behaviour or their beliefs (their thoughts) through rating scales or questionnaires. These may produce a quantifiable measure of some specific construct – e.g. anxiety, social interaction, independence, depression. These will reflect either how the person sees themselves or how they are perceived by others. These are only indirect measures. They are based upon the person's *perception* of themselves. At a stage slightly beyond this lies the perception of the person held by others, e.g. staff, family or friends.

3 *Putting the picture in context*: At the next stage, we could narrow the focus further by assessing the discrete patterns of behaviour that have been highlighted through the more indirect forms of assessment. By studying what the person *does*, and *where, when* and *with whom* they engage in such behaviour, we can begin to quantify in greater detail the nature of the person and their problems, that we see before us. Staff or family members might (for example) record how often, or for how long, they engage in certain patterns of behaviour, under different circumstances. This would bring us closer to understanding 'what is really going on'.

4 *Bringing the picture to life*: This is finally achieved when the person can study themselves closely under a range of conditions. Using logs, diaries, self-ratings or any one of a number of creative, yet simple self-monitoring techniques, the person can begin to describe what is really happening for and to them in different life settings.

These methods may represent a form of 'personal science'[13] where the person might study themselves in much the same way as a naturalist might study a butterfly or bird. The person-in-care has an advantage over the naturalist, as they can assess thoughts and feelings as well as their patterns of behaviour.

> ### Reflection
>
> - Recall the first assessment you undertook in practice. What kind of feelings did you have about the assessment?
> - How well prepared were you to undertake that assessment?
> - How might you have been prepared better?

SUMMARY

Nursing assessment is not a single thing but an approach to understanding people and their worlds of experience. Like a toolkit, each assessment tool has a different function, but taken together all the tools are used to better understand the person and their problems.

The single, most important *purpose* of any assessment is to clarify what is happening within the *personal* and *interpersonal* world of experience of each individual 'patient'. This is rarely easy. Given the complexity of the person's experience different methods are often needed to begin to assess the person, or their predicament.

Great emphasis is given, rightly, to the need for *valid* and *reliable* assessment as part of the 'evidence base' of health care. However, we should not forget that we need to be *creative* in finding ways to assess the wide range of people *and* situations encountered in everyday care. Wherever possible, assessment should be *collaborative*. Even in the early stages of crisis care, nurses are helping the person take the first steps in rehabilitation or to begin their recovery.

Any understanding of the person's present problems should be *shared*, as part of the empowering aspect of health care. Nurses should *care with* people: exploring, examining and evaluating their experiences. Through such collaboration general principles can be used to inform the development of more personally appropriate forms of assessment, which in turn might inform the development of personally appropriate care and treatment.

REFERENCES

1. Harris N, Williams S, Bradshaw T. *Psychosocial interventions for people with schizophrenia: a practical guide for mental health workers*. London, UK: Palgrave Macmillan, 2002.

2. Evans ME. Using a model to structure psychosocial nursing research. *Journal of Psychosocial Nursing and Allied Mental Health Services* 1993; **30** (8): 27–32.

3. Barker P. *Philosophy and practice of psychiatric nursing*. London, UK: Elsevier, 1999.

4. Barker P, Kerr B. *The process of psychotherapy: the journey of discovery*. Oxford, UK: Butterworth Heinemann, 2000.

5. Cooper J. The Leyton obsessional inventory. *Psychological Medicine* 1970; **1**: 261–96.

6. Watson D, Friend R. Measurement of social-evaluative anxiety. *Journal of Consulting and Clinical Psychology* 1969; **33**: 448–51.

7. Likert RA. A technique for measurement of attitudes. *Archives of Psychology* 1932; **140**: 140–55.

8. Barlow DH, Antony MM. *Handbook of assessment and treatment planning for psychological disorders*. New York, NY: Guilford Press, 2002.

9. Jones J, Jackson A. Observation. In: Harrison M, Howard D, Mitchell D (eds). *Acute mental health nursing: from acute concerns to the capable practitioner*. London, UK: Sage, 2002.

10. Haynes SN, O'Brien WH. *Principles and practice of behavioral assessment*. New York, NY: Springer, 2000.

11. Cutcliffe J, Barker P. Considering the care of the suicidal client and the case for 'engagement and inspiring hope' or 'observations'. *Journal of Psychiatric and Mental Health Nursing* 2002; **9** (5): 611–19.

12. Roper N, Logan WW, Tierney AJ. *The elements of nursing*. Edinburgh, UK: Churchill Livingstone, 1980.

13. Mahoney MJ. Personal science: a cognitive learning therapy. In: Ellis A, Grieger RM (eds). *Rational-emotive psychotherapy: handbook of theory and practice*. New York, NY: Springer, 1977: 352–66.

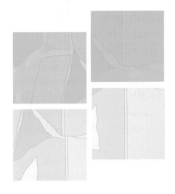

CHAPTER 11

The craft of interviewing

Phil Barker*

INTRODUCTION

The simplest way to learn about people is to talk with them. The interview is a way of talking with people: very simple but potentially highly complex. The interview in a psychiatric mental health context differs little from any other, such as a job interview. Both involve an *imbalance of power* and may involve 'open' as well as 'hidden' agendas. Only the questions and format will differ. The common aim is to build up a picture of the person through conversation – albeit a fairly one-sided one.

Interviews usually involve a face-to-face *meeting* between two people. Interviews may be conducted over the telephone but usually only in special situations. The meeting is focused on finding out something. The interaction between interviewer and respondent is highly specialized. We need no special qualification or training to be an *interviewee* – when, for example we are applying for unemployment benefit or a bank loan. By contrast, the *interviewer* needs special training to handle the potential complexity of the interview situation.

The golden rule

Inadequate assessment will result in inadequate care. To see the person as a whole, the nurse needs to avoid *assuming* too much. Problems need to be seen against the 'backdrop' of the person's whole experience. However, we can never find out *everything* about a person, or even about a specific problem. Neither should we want to. Interviews need to be thorough, but we should avoid

examining areas of the person's experience that are either irrelevant or unnecessary for our needs.

It has been estimated that three-quarters of the material covered in a psychiatric interview could be omitted without any appreciable loss, since it plays little or no part in the plan of treatment.[1] Such interviewing is not only inefficient but raises an ethical issue: what right have we to subject aspects of the person-in-care's life to needless enquiry? Interviews need to be planned carefully. By engaging in idle chatter we may end up exploring aspects of the person's life that are of no relevance to care or treatment. The *golden rule* is:

find out everything you need to know and no more.

Idle curiosity has no place in a professional interview.

THE RELATIONSHIP

Interviewer characteristics

The goal of interviewing is to shine a light upon the person and their problems. To do so the nurse needs to collect as much *relevant* information as possible by the shortest route. First, what should be *avoided*?

- *Avoid appearing abrupt, rude or officious*. You will be unpopular *and* ineffective as an interviewer.
- *Avoid appearing cold or indifferent*. You will not generate the trust needed to allow talk about delicate or highly personal material.

*Phil Barker is a psychotherapist and Honorary Professor at the University of Dundee, UK.

- *Avoid appearing surprised.* People will discuss things that, in ordinary life, might appear shocking:
  - suicidal intent
  - sexual practices
  - past misdeeds that have inspired guilt
  - material considered bizarre or 'crazy'.

These may unsettle the novice interviewer. Any expression of surprise, astonishment, reproach or even stunned silence will stifle any further admissions or self-examination.

By contrast, aim to appear warm, friendly and accepting. Your intention is to help the person think: here is someone I can talk to; here is someone who understands me, and who is not sitting in judgement over me.

The questions, and how they are asked, are of equal importance. Aim for accuracy, objectivity and organization. At the same time, display signs of warmth, empathy, genuineness and unconditional positive regard (see Truax and Carkhuff[2] for a detailed discussion; see also Chapters 36 and 37 by Bill Reynolds). This will encourage the person or the family to tell their stories.

The need for accuracy

It is not enough to obtain information. This should be accurate and should be reliably recorded for future reference. Some nurses have tried to resolve this problem by writing down everything the person-in-care says in a verbatim transcript. Although rarely used in practice it emphasizes some important principles.

First of all, inaccuracies can develop even when interviews are written up as soon as they have taken place. Even if we set aside time to record the interview as soon as it has taken place, we are bound to get some of this 'reporting' wrong. This may have something to do with the demands of having to record so much information in a short period of time. An alternative is to summarize the interview. However, when we condense the interview we may isolate and report upon certain items that are relatively unimportant; and we neglect others that are crucial. Clearly, some kind of compromise is needed as far as writing up the interview is concerned. In the *Tidal model*,[3] all assessments are recorded with the person in situ, using the person's own language and where appropriate, helping the person to record a summary of the conversation.

Some nurses tape-record interviews, using this as a memory aid when writing up their notes. However, this may be too time-consuming. Perhaps the simplest procedure is to decide in advance upon the focus of the interview, in the form of headings, to which we can append brief notes during the interview. These can then be extended into longhand (if necessary) as soon as possible after the interview. We must accept that we are likely to make mistakes in reporting our conversations. The reporting process that we finally adopt should attempt to reduce the risk of mistakes.

The idea of a verbatim transcript is interesting. We write down *word for word* what was said. We do not report what we *thought* the person meant, only what was said. In the early stages of any assessment there is a great advantage in describing the events of the interview. Our aim in writing a report is to have something to reflect upon, reminding us of what took place, so that we can give more thought to what was said. When we are in the heat of the interview – trying to listen attentively, making brief notes, thinking of the next question – it may be difficult to digest what has been said. For this reason we need a verbatim account of what the person actually did say. We can then study these notes, recollecting how certain comments were made, and come to some conclusion about what it all means for the care planning process.

The other advantage of the verbatim account is that we can discuss with other members of the care team what the person said. Instead of saying: 'I interviewed John today and felt that he was very depressed; almost suicidal', we can tell our colleagues that 'I interviewed John today and this is what he said'.

Reflection

- What do you think are the most important objectives of an interview?

BELIEFS, VALUES AND ATTITUDES

Interviewers need to be non-judgemental. Often, the person-in-care's life-philosophy, values and attitudes towards themselves and others may conflict with those of the nurse. It is important to avoid appearing narrow-minded, especially where the person is describing material that might be viewed as bizarre, irrational or unorthodox. It is important to accept the person's value system, even where it conflicts with that of the nurse. We are not being asked to agree or disagree. We are not being asked to join their life, far less to live it. We are simply being asked to acknowledge who and what the person *is*.

Nurses should keep their own selves out of the relationship. This raises the criticism that the so-called 'collaborative relationship' is somewhat one-sided. This seems only appropriate, since it is not the nurse who is in need of care. Consequently, the focus is very much upon the person. The nurse may act as an important model during psychotherapeutic treatment, during which they might disclose feelings or thoughts of their own, to help the person identify with them. However, there is little room for such disclosure within the assessment. Discussion of the nurse's views, experiences or problems serve only as distractions.

The need for patience

Few interviews are without difficulties. The person may appear uncooperative, uncommunicative or inarticulate, resulting in a lengthy, and possibly frustrating, interview.

Some people are unwilling to talk about any aspect of their lives. They may feel that they have been over the same ground repeatedly with other members of the healthcare team. The person needs an explanation of why *this* interview is important and *different*. The person also needs time to find out about the interviewer, and time to change their attitude towards the interview process.

Others may find it difficult to answer questions, what they want to discuss being too distressing. Or they may find it difficult to find the 'right words'. Again, patience is essential.

In other cases the person may appear to be skirting around the subject, going off at tangents, taking a long time to answer a question or avoiding answering at all. This may be an indication of difficulty. Again the person needs time, not criticism – whether overt or veiled. Avoid showing signs of impatience.

Keeping to time

One way of dealing with time constraints is to ask the person to 'keep time'. Not only might this 'empower' the person, but will allow the nurse to give the person full attention. By asking: 'How much time do we have left?' or 'How are we doing for time?' the nurse offers the person a degree of control over the process of the interview.

Resolving conflicts

Few nurses like everyone that they meet in the course of their work. Some people exasperate us, others have 'histories', personalities, attitudes or values that we find repugnant. However, we do not need to like or approve of people to be able to offer them help. We simply need to *accept the person* as a fellow human being. In developing the craft of caring we should take care not to

- argue with the person
- belittle the person
- blame the person for their failings.

In general, we need to avoid being moralistic. Many people-in-care have had more than their fair share of conflict already. What they *have been* or what they *are* may be in conflict with what they would *hope to become*. Avoid adding to that conflict.

The collaborative relationship

Interviews frequently pose significant problems for the person-in-care. Interviews are not natural conversations. This is especially true for most people who enter the psychiatric system. At least nurses have a chance to become

'natural' through practice. The unusual nature of the interview may cause much anxiety. The person may be unaware of why they are being interviewed, or may simply feel uncomfortable when questioned closely about the private corners of their life. This is only natural. Most of us feel uneasy when under such 'direct fire'. The nurse should be sensitive to this, even when the anxiety is not obvious.

Many people disguise their discomfort, displaying their uneasiness indirectly through hesitant answers, short replies or apparent 'striving to please' – always answering yes, or agreeing with everything the nurse says. Appropriate questioning may reduce this. The interview should always begin by addressing non-threatening material; simple questions about the person, where they live, etc. These should be phrased to allow very short answers. Avoid asking for opinions or 'self-analysis' in the early stages as it is too demanding. If the interview has progressed beyond this stage and the person again becomes anxious, postpone questions that appear upsetting. If the person becomes manifestly distressed it may even be appropriate to return to more mundane topics, allowing the person to regain composure. The interview can return to the 'threatening' material gradually, allowing the person to regain confidence through active participation.

It may be appropriate to ask the person directly if they are ready to return to a particular line of questioning:

> We spoke earlier about … do you feel ready to return to that? If you don't want to discuss it just now, just say so.

Giving the person a chance to influence the direction of the interview is crucial. This fosters a sense of partnership and reduces feelings of being manipulated by the interviewer. This partnership should begin early. The nurse's first responsibility is to tell the person what is the plan for the interview, what is the rationale for this process and what will be the person's role in the whole proceedings.

The simplest question is most often the one that might get to the very nub of the issue by the shortest possible route. It also offers the person the greatest room for manoeuvre.

- What have you brought along with you today?
- What brings you here?
- So … how would you like to use this time?

Such questions hold no obvious 'hidden agenda' but represent the simplest forms of enquiry. The last question is perhaps the most sensitive, and offers the person an opportunity to control the proceedings. This kind of question may well help build the kind of confiding relationship that the nurse most desires.

Another important question that should be asked at the outset is:

> Do you want to ask anything before we begin?

This may be the best guard against anxiety, since it removes much of the threat of the unknown.

The person may not be keen on being interviewed. This is often true when people are first admitted into care. The person may already have seen a long line of such interviewers and may be irritated by the prospect of another. The nurse should acknowledge that such irritation or annoyance is natural and appropriate. The nurse should acknowledge how the person might be feeling. Indeed, it is useful to emphasize exactly how *this* interview will be different and also how important the person is to the development of the interview. Indeed, the nurse should spell out clearly how the person will be helping the nurse through the telling of the story. The person should be placed firmly *in the driving seat*.

Traditionally, psychiatric professionals employ the concept of *resistance* to explain difficulties in the interview process. However, instead of blaming the person for their poor cooperation, try to see the interview from the person's angle, so that we may prevent such resistance developing.

Some people may be unhappy about being grilled or cross-examined. This seems only reasonable. Why need the interview be so unpleasant? It must be something to do with the line of questioning or the way that questions are being asked. We should not assume that the person does not want to answer our questions. The interview should be designed to encourage participation. Even where people are not resistant they may not be overly enthusiastic. Again, this may be a reflection of the interview format. Are we rushing through a routine checklist, ticking off answers, looking as if we have done this a hundred times before, and have a lot more pressing work ahead of us? If this is so, the person may feel that this is not very important, and may be disinclined to 'work' at the interview. There is great value in trying to make each interview a stimulating prospect, for the person and interviewer alike. Even if this is the hundredth interview this month, we should try to tailor the interview to suit the person: making it something personal and special. The focus of the interview is the person's life. How can it *not* be special?

> ## Reflection
>
> - How would you describe your interview 'style'?
> - What are your strengths in interviewing?
> - What aspects of your interviewing skills do you want to develop?

OVERVIEW OF THE INTERVIEW

Phrasing the question

Questions are the central feature of the interview. The first priority is to avoid confusing the person who may already be confused or at a loss.

Be specific

The first priority is to avoid ambiguity. Avoid questions that may have more than one meaning. Focus the question so that it will draw information on *one* aspect of the person's life or experience. If you don't get the answer you expected, you may not have asked the question you meant to ask.

Keep it short

Brevity is also important. Avoid long rambling questions. Avoid making general observations about the person or their situation, where a question is hidden somewhere among your comments.

Don't ask

You were saying earlier that you feel pretty tense all the time … that must be pretty awful. I can see that you are tense right now. You're sitting all sort of hunched up … is that what you mean? Like you said a moment ago, I mean … is that how you feel … all tense, anxious, nervy, like you said. Is it?

Do ask

> You said a moment ago that you often felt tense. [Pause]
>
> Tell me more about that. [Await reply]
>
> When you feel tense … what does that mean for you? [Await reply]
>
> So … how do you feel right now? [Await reply]
>
> You are sitting sort of hunched up. Is that how you usually are when you feel tense? [Await reply].

If the question is not specific, it is more difficult to answer and may increase the person's anxiety. The same is true of the string of questions. Ask one question at a time, unless you have very good reasons for acting otherwise.

Sharpen the time focus

Be specific about time. For instance, 'How do you feel *now?*' or 'How have you been feeling over the past *2 or 3 days?*'

Where the time-scale needs to be vague, you might ask:

- Can you tell me what sort of *things* you were able to do *when you felt you were well?*
- How did you *feel* when you were well? Following up the reply by asking
- And how *long ago* was that?

Be aware that when distressed many people feel that they have 'always' been like this. Help them sharpen the time focus.

Open and closed questions

There are two kinds of question: those that elicit a *short* reply and those that require *fuller* answers.

- Are you still feeling depressed?
- Your husband left you. Do you think that made you depressed?
- Do you hear voices a lot?

All these *closed* questions can be answered *yes, no* or *don't know.*

- How are you feeling today?
- How did you react to your husband leaving you?
- You say that someone is talking to you, in your head. Tell me more about that.
- Can you give me an idea of how you are feeling right now.

All these *open* questions provide people with an opportunity to talk at length, should they wish to do so.

Closed questions may be appropriate in the initial stages of the interview as they put fewer demands on the person. They are also appropriate when the person is very distressed or withdrawn. Open questions will, however, provide more information about what it is like to *be the person*, providing more information about the person's experience.

The value of reflection

When the person says something that appears interesting or significant, try to develop this theme, or gain more information. The simplest and least intrusive way to do this is to *reflect* – or bounce back – the reply.

Person: I get so confused sometimes I just don't know whether I'm coming or going.

Nurse: Coming or going?

Person: That's right. I mean … I just don't seem to be able to cope with things. I feel so useless all the time.

Nurse: I see … so tell me more about how you feel useless.

Give emphasis to certain words to show that you are phrasing a question, and not simply repeating what the person has said. However, reflection needs to be used with discretion. If the nurse repeatedly reflects the person's answers they might think that they were answering the questions badly, or that the nurse was poking fun.

Reflection can be taken a stage further by using the person's actual phrasing to frame another question:

You say that you don't know whether you are coming or going. Can you tell me what you mean by that?

Reflection involves giving the minimum amount of guidance. The flow of the conversation is interrupted, no more than is necessary, making for more efficient interviewing. More importantly, it helps the person talk as much as possible, without losing the necessary structure.

Threatening questions

Some questions are bound to be disturbing. Avoiding such questions is not a solution. Instead, questions about sensitive or distressing subjects should be framed carefully to reduce their impact. It is not possible to list all possible threats, since these will vary from one person to another. However, even in today's liberated society detailed questioning about sex is often perceived as a threat. The same is true of domestic violence and sometimes psychotic states.

Don't ask
- How often do you and your partner have sex?
- Do you ever hit the kids?
- How long have you been having these auditory hallucinations?

Do ask
- You talked about you and your partner … how do you feel about your relationship?
- What happens when you lose your temper at home?
- What can you tell me about the voices?

If the person feels threatened they may simply deny the existence of any problem. By taking a more oblique line of questioning the 'glare' of the searchlight is reduced, making it easier for the person to admit to problems of which they might be ashamed.

The need for a framework

An interview needs a structure, which can be rigid or flexible depending on the demands of the situation. Structure most commonly refers to the order and nature of the questions asked. For example, a typical interview might begin with very *open-ended* questions:

Would you like to tell me what's bothering you at present?

Gradually, more specific queries can be introduced:

How often has this happened?

Eventually, the person's perception of the problem can be narrowed down to finer detail:

So how bad would that be just now, say on a scale of 1 to 10?

These stages – *beginning, middle* and *end* – show how the interview begins with very broad concerns and gradually sharpens the focus on one or two problems. The first interview might be devoted entirely to drawing up a list of the person's problems. Subsequent interviews might take individual problems as topics, devoting the time to trying to understand each one better through closer analysis.

A flexible framework, where the line of questioning is developed within the interview itself, is best left to the highly expert interviewer. Most of us need a simple framework to provide some security, so that we don't get lost for words. Our aim is to have a conversation with the person, so we want to talk as normally as possible. A general outline of the questions we want to ask, or the areas we want to explore, may help us – and the person – feel more comfortable (see Romme and Escher[4] for an example of the use of a specific structure to elicit information about hearing voices).

Troubleshooting

Interviews rarely turn out the way we plan. Prepare for problems.

Failure to respond

The person may find it difficult to give the information you want, especially at the first interview. How far should you press them? Should you press them at all? If the person fails to answer to your satisfaction perhaps the question was badly phrased. Try presenting the question from a different angle.

Poor question

When there is conflict within the family, what kind of coping strategies do you employ under such conditions? (No answer try again.)

Alternative

Well, as you say … when there's an 'atmosphere' at home, how do you deal with that?

Difficult to answer

The person may answer, but not to their satisfaction. Offer some words of encouragement, helping the person to find the words needed to express themselves. Beware, however, of putting words into the person's mouth. Instead, try to help shape up the answer through discreet feedback.

Nurse: So how did you feel when that happened?
Person: Oh, I don't know. Just lost … sort of … eh … I … oh, I don't know.
Nurse: Uh-huh, you felt 'lost': *lost* in what way?
Person: Lost, yes. Didn't know what to do … what to say.
Nurse: Lost for words?
Person: Yes … lost for words. Didn't know what to say to her. Felt powerless. No, that's not right. Can't seem to think straight.
Nurse: You were lost for words. You didn't know what to say to her – or you felt that you couldn't tell her how you felt?
Person: Well, maybe that's true. I knew how I felt, but I just couldn't face her. Yeah, I guess I couldn't bring myself to tell her how I felt.

Dealing with refusal

Sometimes the person may not answer at all – which is an answer of sorts. Silently, the person is saying, I am not willing (or ready/able) to answer.

What should we do?

- Rephrase the question?
- Try to nudge the person gently?
- Or simply respect the person's wishes, leaving this issue for another time, or another place?

The last solution is probably best, although there are always occasions when it might be appropriate to try the others. If we choose to 'postpone' a question, however, we should let the person know why we have done so.

- You don't seem to be too happy with that question. (Pause)
- Maybe it was the way I put it. Or maybe you don't feel ready to discuss that with me just yet? (Pause)
- Maybe we could come back to it some other time, when you think you're ready. OK? (Pause)
- We were talking a moment ago about …. (Move on to the next topic)

Going off at tangents

Rarely do we get all the answers to our question in a single interview. Ideally, one question leads to another and may span several interviews. In practice, however, one question usually produces a number of answers, some aspects of which are relevant, others less so. The nurse must decide whether or not to follow up such 'tangents' or to stick to the core question. If you decide to deal only with some of the person's replies make it clear that you are doing this.

Nurse: You were talking yesterday about going shopping in town.
Person: Oh, I don't know. I get terribly tense in the crowds. Then there's my Henry, I should have rung him. He doesn't really manage well on his own. I worry about him ever so much … and I promised to take Johnny – he's just 11 … to the game on Saturday. I keep letting him down. He can hardly look at me. It's all so pointless.
Nurse: Uh-huh. I see. Your family obviously mean a lot to you. That's why you worry about them. Maybe we need to spend some time just talking about that. Do you want to talk about that now, or do you want to carry on discussing the shopping trip you planned?

The nurse had a decision to make: either to follow the person or stick to the interview agenda. By turning the decision over to the person, the nurse empowered the person's decision-making. No agenda is ever fixed. The interview may follow any course that is deemed appropriate. However, we need to gauge the flow of the conversation carefully.

The interview setting

The interview is a 'formal' conversation, the outcome of which is crucial to the person. Interviews need not, however, be structured in a formal manner. Sometimes it may be appropriate to interview the person in their bedroom on the ward; the sitting room at home; a consulting room off the ward; or an interview room at a clinic. It may be just as practical, however, to interview the person in the hospital grounds or while walking the dog in the park. The important consideration is:

Will this place be private, peaceful and quiet?

The person is unlikely to discuss personal problems within earshot of other people and may become distracted if there are repeated interruptions. In some cases, walking in the park may feel more private and distraction-free than a consulting room, where people may be heard talking through the wall.

The setting is also important for putting the person at ease. A distressed person may feel more comfortable chatting over a cup of coffee in the corner of the hospital cafeteria or when walking in the fresh air. The restrictions of a small interview room may make the person more anxious, making conversation more difficult. However, sometimes it is appropriate to pick an awkward setting. If the person has identified a situation that appears to trigger a problem, it may be appropriate to conduct the interview there. We might take someone with social anxiety out into the street. If the person was suffering from a grief reaction, we might take them to a setting that evoked special memories of the loved one. The setting selected might trigger certain emotions, thoughts and memories, which might be less evident in a more formal interview setting.

The power of ordinary communication

Some people do not like being interviewed. This may stem from bad experiences at the hands of over-efficient, cold or insensitive interviewers. In addition to being warm, empathic, genuine and non-judgemental, it is also important to talk to the person in language they understand. The longer any professional spends in the field, the harder it can be to talk in plain English. We should strive to speak plainly, avoiding jargon and technical language that might strain the person's understanding. Sometimes, it may help if you can speak to the person in dialect. This may strengthen rapport.

Nurse: You're looking pretty down today, Derek. Is there something troubling you?

Derek: Oh, I'm just proper … scunnered, like. Been like this for weeks.

Nurse: You feel scunnered (emphasis). What … with everything?

Derek: Yeah, just sick of everything. But especially myself.

Nurse: Tell me more about that.

By picking up on the person-in-care's use of the expression 'scunnered'– meaning sick or tired of – the nurse develops rapport. The person may think, 'this person is someone I can *really* talk to'. The nurse need not actually know the exact meaning of the key words picked up

and reflected back. By using Derek's language the nurse encourages him to amplify the point he is making. The more he is encouraged to express himself, the more information he gives and the more the nurse can build up a picture of 'what it is like to be this person'.

The power of respect

It is also worth picking up the use of more technical terms – like 'depressed', 'anxious', 'alienated', 'paranoid', 'hostile'. These have very special meanings in professional language, but have become part of the vernacular. We should not assume that because they are in everyday use their meaning remains the same. Where the person uses such technical expressions we need to ask them to clarify their meaning.

It is also important to avoid translating the person's words into our own convenient shorthand.

Nurse: Tell me more about how you feel.

Jane: Oh, blue.

Nurse: You mean that you're depressed.

Jane: [Sighs] I guess so.

This is a missed opportunity. If Jane had intended to say she was depressed, she would have said so. By translating her use of 'blue', the nurse devalues it. The person knows their experience better than anyone. By valuing the words the person uses, we value the person.

In some situations it may be appropriate to encourage the person to talk about the problem without even naming it. Where the problem is a source of embarrassment, or the person does not feel prepared to trust the nurse, talking about the problem in the abstract may be a solution.

Nurse: I get the feeling that you are not ready to talk about this situation yet. In fact … there is no need to tell me about this … whatever it is. Not until you are ready to. What about if we just called it X? Maybe you could tell me how X is a problem for you?

Alternatively, the nurse could ask:

- How does X make you feel? or
- How long has X been a problem for you? or
- When did X first become a problem for you?

Providing that this is acceptable to the person, the nurse can explore the problem fully without ever asking the person to define 'X' specifically. Where the person is discussing some taboo (like a sexual abuse scenario) or an experience that is normally considered implausible (like being possessed by demons), they might feel empowered by the opportunity to disguise the issue in this manner.[5]

Reflection

- When was the last time you felt *comfortable* when being interviewed?
- What did the interviewer *do*, which helped you feel comfortable?

THE PRESENTATION OF THE INTERVIEW

Preparation

Before beginning, the nurse should clarify:

- the aim of the interview
- how best to conduct it
- how much time is available.

Aims vary from one interview to another. Some preparation is necessary to ensure that you cover all the points you wish to cover. A general outline is helpful for the following reasons.

- It acts as a guide to the line of questioning, guarding against being unduly sidetracked.
- It helps foster a logical, sensitive line of questioning, beginning with non-threatening material building up gradually to more sensitive material.
- It guards against duplication of lines of questioning.
- It guards against taxing the person's concentration (e.g. by being unduly long).
- It guards against time-wasting (e.g. by spending too much time on general issues) before reaching the key questions.

Plan to conclude the interview at least 10 minutes early, thus allowing the person time to regain composure or to ask any further general questions.

The plan

In considering the various ways of phrasing questions, it is helpful to distinguish between *higher* and *lower* order questions.[6,a]

Lower order questions
There are four main kinds of lower order question.

1 The first involves the *recall of information*. The person might be asked:

> Have you ever felt this bad *before*? – to which they can answer yes or no.

Alternatively, they might be asked to recall *more* information:

> When did you *last* feel this bad?

2 The second kind involves *rephrasing* or rewording certain concepts or ideas:

> Can you tell me, in your own words what you mean by 'helpless'?

3 In the third class the person is asked to *compare* or *contrast* situations or experiences:

> In which *situations* do you normally feel worst?

Can you tell me, then, *where* you would feel OK?

4 The last class invites the person-in-care to present *alternatives* to what they have done in the past:

> How could you handle that differently?

> Given what we have just discussed, how would you tackle that situation in the future?

Higher order questions
These questions involve more complex replies, inviting the person to *analyse a situation*, giving some indication of why they believed that something happened. These motives or causes cannot, of course, be drawn simply from memory; the answer needs to be more 'creative' and is therefore more difficult.

- Why do you think your wife stopped talking to you? or
- How do you think you came to be depressed?'

This class also contains questions that invite the person to make *predictions* or to discuss *complex ideas*:

- What would happen if you did that? or
- What would be so bad about that?

Ideally, the interview should begin with lower order questions, inviting the person to dip into memories or provide simple problem-solving answers. As the person becomes more comfortable, more complex questions, relying on complex reasoning, may be introduced.

Seating

Classically, interviewers sit behind a desk, with the interviewee facing. Such a job interview arrangement is inappropriate, as it gives strong messages about who holds the power and is in control. Where two people face each other *directly*, it may appear confrontational. Where a desk is used it may appear to represent a shield (suggesting that the interviewer wishes to remain at a distance) or barrier (placing the interviewee at a disadvantage).

The height and design of chairs are also important. If the interviewer sits on a higher chair, this will confer an advantage. If the person is given a stiff, high-backed chair while the nurse sits in an easy chair, again this might represent an advantage; the nurse appearing more relaxed and comfortable. Ideally, both people should sit on the same kind of chair, at roughly 60 degrees to one another. This allows easy eye contact and orientation, as found in most normal social interactions (see Argyle[7] for a detailed review). Where matching chairs are not available the nurse should offer the person first choice. Where the nurse visits the person at home they should ask where the person would like the nurse to sit.

---

[a]Format quoted in the text is adapted from this work.

The seats should be close together, registering the privacy and intimacy of the conversation. If they are far apart, this may be interpreted as a gulf that is difficult to bridge. As with other aspects of the interview, check with the person that such arrangements are acceptable before beginning.

Where the person has a disability, or is from a different cultural or ethnic background from the nurse, it is important to explore how best the interview should be convened, to acknowledge the importance of such issues.

Opening

Begin by advising the person of the aims of the interview, asking if they have any queries or objections.

- Hello Mr Jackson. My name is Jacqueline and I am responsible for your care while you are here. This all might seem strange to you and you may still be trying to get your bearings, but I would like to spend a little time, getting to know you a bit better. [Pause]
- I'd like to talk with you about what led up to you coming in to hospital. [Pause]
- That will help me get an idea about what kind of care you might need while you are here. At the same time, if you have any questions for me, I hope that you will feel OK about asking me. Is that OK with you?

The nurse makes it clear who they are and what they want to do. They also try to acknowledge how the person might be feeling, trying to make the interview as non-threatening as possible. They pause briefly throughout their introduction, giving them time to speak, or to allow their words to register. This kind of opening may reduce the person's natural anxiety. The emphasis upon collaboration – *talk with you* – may also enhance the person's self-esteem.

The interview core

The structure should emphasize the beginning and end of each section with summaries where appropriate.

Example

1 'To begin, I'd like you to tell me a bit about yourself.' This may be followed immediately by a series of specific queries, e.g. Do you live on your own? Who does your shopping for you? Where did you work before you retired?
2 'Good. Maybe we could talk a bit about how you came into hospital? Now you said that you lived alone …' Having recapped on some of the points already covered in (1) the nurse moves on to more open-ended questions: When did you first feel that you needed help? Who did you discuss these problems with? How did you feel about being on your own?
3 'That's fine. I have found that very helpful. Perhaps we might discuss some of the problems you have mentioned

in more detail? Are you ready for that just now?' If the person agrees, further questions of a who, where, when, what and how variety might be asked: Where did that first happen? Were you on your own at the time? What would be so bad about that? In what way is that a problem for you?
4 'From what you have said a number of things appear to be a problem just now. These voices appear to be distressing you a lot. Am I right?' The information collected can now be summarized briefly. At the same time the nurse can check that their interpretation of the 'facts' is correct.

Promoting responses

The nurse's key role is to encourage the person to tell a story that will help in the development of appropriate care. The non-verbal aspects of the interview also are important.

The 'good' interviewer expresses their skills most often through non-verbal behaviour. Or rather, the person is likely to perceive the nurse positively or negatively on the basis of how the nurse *stands, sits, uses gestures* and *looks at the person*. The following is a 'rough guide' to the importance of body language.

Spatial behaviour

Sitting close to the person, suggests intimacy and being on an equal footing. This also suggests the absence of status. If you wish to 'control' the other person, you try to look down at them or sit behind a desk. Sitting side-by-side will probably communicate your liking for the person, or at least acceptance, and may give reassurance.

Posture

Try to appear relaxed and comfortable, communicating self-confidence. At times, a change of posture will enhance the conversation – leaning forward if the person is discussing confidential material or is distressed, or settling back in the chair if the person appears to want to talk at some length. These postural changes communicate confidentiality or a willingness to listen. In general sitting turned slightly towards the person – leaning slightly in their direction – is most helpful in facilitating conversation.

Facial expression

Our faces provide a regular commentary on our speech, as we flash our eyebrows, smile, frown or grimace. Try to follow the person's conversation by displaying appropriate facial expression. However, this should always be controlled naturally, otherwise it may look theatrical and insincere. Partner the person, showing that you appreciate the meaning or significance of what is being said.

Eye contact

We look at other people to pick up non-verbal cues. However, gaze has another function: it adds emphasis to our speech and can be used to 'reply' to the other person. Although the amount of eye contact varies from one situation to another, we rarely gaze constantly at others, except when madly in love or enraged with anger. Normal gaze patterns involve looking and quickly looking away. If we give more than around 70 per cent of gaze contact time we may appear confrontational (although this varies greatly across cultures and subcultures). Alternatively, we may look embarrassed, ashamed or suspicious if we do not give sufficient eye contact for the given situation.

Reflection

If you are interviewing a person who uses a wheelchair:

- How would you arrange the interview setting?
- How would you involve the person in beginning the interview?
- What other issues might you need to take into consideration?

SUMMARY

Conversation helps us gain insights into the unique world of another person, discovering something of their experience of 'being-in-the-world'. All interviews need to be adapted to suit the person's age, sex, cultural background, values, beliefs and presentation. This will influence the structure of the interview: what we do and say, how long it lasts, where it takes place and how we record the outcome.

The interview has no single purpose apart from gaining information. Instead, it may be used for many purposes, from learning about the patient as a person, to evaluating how things are changing. However, some basic principles remain constant.

- The interview is a *two-way* process. The person should be encouraged to take part, informed regularly of progress, and wherever possible told *in advance* of 'what is coming next'.

- The person should *play a part in controlling the interview*, perhaps being asked to decide when they are ready to discuss certain topics, or to 'keep time'.
- The interviewer must be *unbiased*, isolating any preconceptions or prejudices that might influence the conversation that will develop.
- The person's value system should be *accepted*, although this need not mean that it is given active approval.
- The person's perception of his world and himself is used as the vantage point from which the assessment will develop. The interviewer tries to *see the world through the person's eyes*, at least for the time being.

The interview is a highly sophisticated interaction and often can be therapeutic. If handled properly the person may discover things of which they were unaware. Sometimes, however, these revelations can be traumatic and the person may require support afterwards.

A 'good interview' should benefit the person. Even a difficult or distressing interview will yield some fruit. However, the nurse should never use their status to manipulate the person. Collaboration is central to the development of purposeful care.

REFERENCES

1. Peterson DR. *The clinical study of social behaviour.* New York, NY: Appleton Century Crofts, 1968.

2. Truax CB, Carkhuff RR. Towards effective counselling and psychotherapy training and practice. Chicago, IL: Aldine Press, 1967.

3. Barker P, Buchanan-Barker P. *The tidal model: a guide for mental health professionals.* Hove, UK: Brunner Routledge, 2005.

4. Romme M, Escher S. *Accepting voices.* London, UK: Macmillan/Mind, 1993.

5. Barker P. *Assessment in psychiatric and mental health nursing: in search of the whole person.* Cheltenham, UK: Nelson Thornes, 2004: 245–6.

6. Hewit FS. Communication skills: questions and listening. *Nursing Times* 1981; 25 June: 21–6.

7. Argyle M. *Bodily communication.* London, UK: Routledge, 1988.

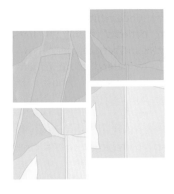

CHAPTER 12

Developing collaborative assessment

Tom Keen*

INTRODUCTION

Psychiatric assessment, or diagnosis, is essentially an attempt to attribute a person's suffering to an underlying illness, and thereby identify appropriate treatment. Insofar as psychiatric nurses assist psychiatry, nursing assessment may be understood as a part of this diagnostic process.[1] Assessment is conducted by observation, interviewing (the patient and significant others) and measuring (using tests, questionnaires, etc.). Objectivity, benevolent neutrality, professional knowledge and expertise are assumed. The psychiatric nurse is a scientist, armed with knowledge of psychiatric classification and psychopathology; psychological processes; and an understanding of potential pathogenic stressors. At the end of the process, a comprehensive assessment should be reducible to concise care plans, consisting of a few briefly specified goals and accompanying plans of how they will be attained – what the patient will do, and how psychiatric treatment and nursing care will help. The virtues of this approach may be summarized as professional unity, objectivity and, paradoxically, simplicity. People generally understand how to be a patient in relation

to illnesses, doctors and nurses. If they accept both this status and a medical perspective on their lives, then their compliance with the service enables unambiguous treatment prescription and goal selection. Proponents of psychiatrically subordinate nursing emphasize the empirical evidence-based strength of close allegiance to well-researched medical practice.[2] However, if formal psychiatric approaches are applied too rigidly, the service risks inducing excessive dependence, negativistic hostility or passive aggressive behaviour because various routine assessment procedures, clinical cultural styles or staff attitudes may be perceived as personally invalidating, patronizing or even oppressive and threatening.[3–6]

However, it is possible to construe mental health nursing otherwise – as primarily concerned not with the identification and treatment of disease, but with understanding and helping people to overcome *their* real-life problems, fulfil *their* needs and achieve desirable, realistic *personal* goals. These may be socioeconomic, spiritual, intellectual, psychosocial or physiological in nature. From this perspective, assessment becomes not an objective task at all, but rather a more open-ended and uncertain process in which

*Tom Keen was a Lecturer in Mental Health at the University of Plymouth for many years, previously working as a nurse, therapist or manager in a variety of settings across the south of England.

the nurse attempts to gain insight into the person's own subjective experiences and aspirations.[7]

HOW COLLABORATIVE IS COLLABORATIVE?

The concept of collaboration is not as straightforward as may be assumed. When used to denote a working relationship with patients, little operational distinction is made between 'collaboration', 'involvement', 'consultation', 'participation', 'alliance' and 'partnership'. It may be thought of as simply an expression of politeness or courtesy to patients, so that they feel respectfully involved and decently treated.[8] It may function as a euphemism for paying lip-service to patient involvement.[9] This may be achieved by having a tick-box on an assessment form labelled something like 'Level of patient consultation: (if appropriate)' or asking patients to sign their care plans. Such half-hearted attempts at collaboration may arise from a belief that therapeutic partnership may be at best an unrealistic ideal or at worst clinically abusive for people considered seriously mentally disordered. Gamble and Brennan[10] suggest that seriously mentally ill users can at least be involved in their assessment by having an opportunity to discuss the results of formal tests before care plans are drawn up. These authors go on to suggest that 'using and choosing appropriate assessments is the foundation on which successful collaborative intervention is built'.[10,p.83] Other authors describe 'the semi-structured interview' as the basis for collaborative care and emphasize the importance of establishing rapport and having patients feel involved in their care.[11] Cognitive–behavioural therapists generally refer to Beck's concept of a collaborative relationship, but differ as to the relative significance attached to its development during assessment. Some emphasize 'working from the patient's perspective' and explicitly advocate allowing time and working flexibly,[12] whereas others describe the early use of formal batteries of tests.[13] Some practitioners are clearly prepared to meet their clients halfway in formulating treatment, although the strictures imposed by modern 'managed care' often place unrealistic pressures on staff to complete assessments rapidly, and provide excessively brief emollient treatment.[14]

However, collaboration in its fullest sense implies a fundamentally different relationship between nurses and patients than commonly found in the tightly managed and basically medical culture of most modern psychiatric services.[15] It may also require fundamental shifts in the relationships of 'services' to 'patients', along the lines often indicated by radical critics and service-users' movements[16–18] and require staff to defend more patient, flexible, client-centred assessment practices against organizational demands for a brisker clinical tempo.[14] Nurses are certainly challenged to find ways of achieving genuine collaboration within a service geared more explicitly to coercive social control[19,20] and may argue that a more authoritative approach is essential for effective risk management. Morgan[21] however insists that service users should be deeply involved in both assessing and planning how to manage any risks they pose to themselves or others. Collaborative risk assessment is not only ethically sound, it is also less disempowering and more effective than making actuarially informed guesses from a position of detached professional isolation.[22]

There has been little authoritative exploration or clarification of the preferred nature and extent of collaboration. Perkins and Repper[9,23] insist that it is not sufficient simply to take account of patients' views. Rather, the 'patients' themselves must be fully involved and their views and choices should be central to the whole process of care. Too often patients' views are subordinated or ignored completely while care and treatment are reduced to whatever results from the impact of competing professional ideologies upon the supposedly collaborative multi-disciplinary team.

ASSESSMENT AS EXPERIENTIAL RESEARCH

The process of assessment can be understood as a form of research – a single case study where the experimenter is in close and constant interaction with the subject (person) of enquiry. 'New paradigm' research models such as 'collaborative inquiry' and 'experiential research methodology'[24] provide conceptual and operational frameworks that translate readily to the assessment process. The assessor understands that the clinical environment, process of assessment and the nurse themselves are part of the interactive reality being assessed, not phenomena that exist in isolation from the person as object of study.[25,26] The problems, needs or goals being assessed are not assumed to be aspects of categories predefined by the psychiatric service, whether conceptualized as disease process, behavioural deficits or excesses, inappropriate cognitions, unconscious conflicts or emotional tensions.

The issues may be initially defined within the patient's frames of reference, and elaborated dialectically with those held by the assessing nurse.

Traditional assessment is based on an underlying, often unconscious, paradigm (amounting to a psychiatric and nursing schema) in which the assessor has ownership of interpretation, meanings, attributions, categories and hypotheses. Conceptual frameworks and clinical decision-making come within the ambits of professional knowledge (e.g. symptomatology), belief systems (e.g. diagnostic categories) and organizational imperatives (e.g. risk assessment formats). This ownership has consequences in terms of the power balance within a supposedly caring relationship. Not only the kind of knowledge, but the justification for knowing it, the methods of acquiring it, the right to and means of challenging or disputing any of those things are all within the control of the professional services.[27] Apart from the obstacles this situation poses to the development of trust and a therapeutic relationship, there are issues about the authenticity, validity and reliability of the information collected by such means. Such knowledge is at best narrow and exclusive, at worst artificial, sterile and inapplicable to everyday realities. Collaborative, relatively loosely structured assessment may produce much richer information, which is closer to the reality of the person being assessed.[28,29] Collaborative assessment should concentrate on the meanings of experiences and behaviours within their social context, which can include the clinical situation and the assessment dyad itself, as well as the family and wider socioeconomic environments. Thus, collaborative modes of assessment address people's reality, and privilege 'objective difficulty' aetiological explanations over 'personal defectiveness', or disease model, attributions (see Smail[30]). The emphasis should be upon sharing and interaction, in which both parties discuss the meanings attributed to specific behaviours and experiences, rather than their becoming clues to the allocation of diagnoses. The assessor accords especial priority and significance to the patient's own terminology and interpretations, so that subjective data become the central focus of the assessment inquiry.[31] This perspective displaces and relegates the supposedly more real objective material. In doing so collaborative assessment upends conventional hierarchies of evidence, and privileges single case study as the 'gold standard' for mental health nursing over the highly structured objective randomized control trial – the gold standard of the medicopsychiatric paradigm. Hypotheses and formulations emerging from collaborative assessment are not intended or likely to readily generalize to whole diagnostic classes of people. The collaborative analysis should conform to inductive, rather than deductive processing. That is, theories, explanations, hypotheses are searched for *within*, and allowed to emerge *from*, the information uncovered, rather than the assessor using the data revealed to confirm pre-existing hypotheses (e.g. diagnoses, schema modes or behavioural

deficits). This enables unexpected or unaware concerns to be discovered. Creative solutions can be explored more confidently.[31] Beck's term 'collaborative empiricism' implies a similar inquisitive fascination with the shared discovery of meanings to help create therapeutic alliances.

A young man dressed in an oddly anachronistic and colourful fashion approached a senior nurse who entered his ward and struck up a conversation. Although the two had never met before, the young man stood very close to the nurse and stared straight into her eyes as he carefully enunciated: 'Hello, who are you? I hope you don't mind my talking to you. The staff say that I'm too nosy and that I put people off by my eye contact.'

Nurse: Well, you are standing very closely – does that help your nose to make sense of me?

Patient: I've got to go to pottery soon. I enjoy pottery, but I'm much more interested in archaeology. Would you like to see my pots?

Nurse: Are they ancient pots or modern ones?

Patient: They're modern of course, but they might become ancient, if they live longer than me. How old are you?

Nurse: Forty-five. You know, to me all these things about you seem connected.

Patient: Well they're all part of me, aren't they, and I'm connected?

Nurse: Yes, I suppose so. Archaeology is all about finding out about what once happened and has become hidden; staring closely at people might help you know what thinking is happening but is hidden; and pottery is about finding out what might be hidden within some clay, that you could make happen in the future. How much do you like to find out about what might be hidden, and maybe how to effect what happens?

The terminology and concepts used in assessment summaries should be uniquely tailored to the individual because it has emerged from their experience and has employed their own language and experience as both enzyme and substrate. The use of 'ordinary, poetic and picturesque language' is also emphasized in accounts of therapeutic change as a process of rewriting one's life story, rather than being a participant in the medical elimination of problems. Such a process necessarily begins at the very beginning – the assessment. 'A therapy situated within the context of a narrative mode of thought would privilege the person's lived experience … and encourage a sense of authorship and re-authorship of one's life and relationships.'[32,p.83]

By taking seriously the sense-making constructs that patients use, collaborative assessment challenges the potential falsification or narrowing of real-life experience. Such phenomenological constriction is a possible outcome of confining assessment to predetermined structural formats, questionnaires, etc.[31] In traditional modes of assessment, self-reportage is restricted to replies to questions previously determined by professionals. Without full collaboration, patients' realities are explored using only the system of knowledge and tools possessed and authenticated by the assessing professional service. (It is like a walk through a landscape by two people – the person who lives there and a visiting expert on one or more, but probably not all, of various admittedly relevant subjects. These may include botany, zoology, geology, meteorology, history, painting, photography, poetry, etc., but will exclude intimate local knowledge. The conversation during the walk is controlled by the expert who chooses the various subjects that will be discussed during the walk and poses questions to the subordinated local whose home terrain is under investigation.)

Nurses trained to be the dominant figure during assessment may fear being suckered – duped by tall stories spun by mischievous, confused or deluded patients. After all, although it is important for people to feel believed or see that their relative is treated respectfully, it may feel equally important not to find that the key-worker is a fool.

Nearing the end of a formal initial assessment after admission to a rehabilitation hostel, a young man of limited intelligence suffering from schizophrenia was asked a specified question about future employment:

Nurse: What work would you like to do when you leave here?

Resident: I'm going to be a racing driver.

Nurse: Oh really? What attracts you about being a racing driver?

Resident: I want to be like David Coulthard.

Nurse: So what do you admire about him?

Resident: He's got lots of money, and he's always with beautiful women.

Nurse: Yes, that's true! What other things do you like about him?

Resident: He's really confident and sure of himself – you have to be to go that fast.

Nurse: So how confident are you? Are you confident enough to become a racing driver?

Resident: Not now.

Nurse: Did you use to be more confident then?

Resident: Yes, but I lost it.

Nurse: How did that happen?

Resident: When I was on a training scheme. They used to laugh at me a lot and make me do things I didn't want to.

Nurse: So would it help if we tried to get your confidence back while you're living here?

Would we be in danger of discrediting professionalism, and appearing credulous idiots, to premise assessments on such a respectful, believing attitude? Although we may find ourselves apparently accepting fantastic rubbish, how much worse might it be, from a user's perspective, to reject the truth as madness? Effective collaborative assessment is not in a sense simple detective work, where the professional strives to uncover absolute truth. It is often more important to help the person clarify their personal story or narrative. Life needs to make sense if people are to confidently take control of their personal affairs again. A recovery focus may require that eventually people confront and accept the truth of their situation, but in the early stages of rescue, probing for literal truth may be less important than other therapeutic aims, such as:

- containing and clarifying underlying emotions;
- exploring meanings through metaphorical elements of personal storytelling devising plot-lines or narrative threads that may suggest desirable future possibilities.

ASSESSING NEEDS, PROBLEMS OR SOLUTIONS

Bradshaw[33] addresses the question of how *needs* are defined, and whose definition is given priority. He distinguishes four categories of need: *normative need*, which is professionally defined; *felt need*, which is the subjective dissatisfactions experienced by individuals; *expressed need*, which refers to the explicit demands made of the service by clients; and *comparative need* which is the prioritized, permitted needs identified during assessments. A needs-based collaborative assessment in effect requires the nurse to suspend their preoccupation with professional formulations of need and hold in abeyance the tendency to make judgements based on clinical categories, diagnoses and psychopathological aetiologies. The next step is to enable users to contact, explore and express felt needs, and arrive at a formulation which expresses in positive terms what life would be (and is) when each need is met. Then the partnership studies the desirability, achievability and ecological impact (on others, and other aspects of the person themselves) of each identified aspiration. This process takes time, and certainly cannot be completed in an hour on the day of admission – it is an ongoing process (see Johnstone[5]).

Perkins and Repper[9,23] advocate such alliances, and point out that 'needs-led' assessment may be little different from 'problem-based' assessment unless professionals pay attention to their own attitudes and beliefs, the mystifying effects of clinical language,[34] and the partnership forged with users. 'Needs-led assessment' does not necessarily constitute a real shift from 'problem-based' assessments while professional definitions of problems and service-led priorities hold sway. As one influential report on overcoming engagement difficulties with mistrustful patients states: 'Specialist mental health staff must be needs-led in their approach and allow the users' priorities to set the agenda'.[35,p.58]

Arabella was a young woman diagnosed as having a borderline personality disorder. She cut her arms and breasts daily, and frequently burned her hands with cigarettes. The staff's clinical priorities were that she stopped this mutilating behaviour and concentrate on helping them to find some suitable supported accommodation. Arabella thought that she needed to spend much more time with her pony, Jasper. She felt sure she could get back her work as a stable-girl, and would happily sleep in the stable loft for accommodation. It took 6 months' sojourn in an admission ward to convince her key-worker and consultant psychiatrist that she did not self-harm when with her beloved Jasper.

Recently, solution-focused and narrative forms of conversational, client-centred therapy have claimed considerable success.[32,36–38] Hoyt summarizes some significant differences between such approaches and conventional psychiatric attitudes.

Possibility versus certainty

Fascinated curiosity and the identification of possibilities typify collaborative approaches, whereas formal assessment is predicated on discovery of fact or based on an assumption that there is a truth to be uncovered – the problem, disease diagnosis or unmet need. The often intensely audited economic strictures imposed on modern clinical services create pressures not only to discover the truth (what it is that's wrong) quickly, but to do something effective about it just as quickly. If certainty cannot be achieved, then humans tend to devise temporary formulations or hypotheses as working models (heuristics) to explain the phenomena under investigation. These heuristics often become reified and frozen into professional quasi-scientific certainties (e.g. see Dorothy Rowe[39,40] on 'self-esteem' or Pilgrim[41] on 'personality disorders'). Collaborative assessment practice should insist that such hypotheses are explained and discussed with the user, and abandoned or reformulated if unacceptable. These seemingly innocent heuristic devices, which in truth may be no more than metaphorical constructs, easily assert their grip on professional thinking, and nurses can become convinced of their reality and applicability.

Egalitarian versus expert

Nurses (and other clinicians) should not allow their possession of clinical knowledge, technical skills and

therapeutic attitudes to delude them into believing they have life-changing expertise. Having some insights into human conditions does not bestow absolute authority of wisdom about *The human condition*, and certainly doesn't imply intuitive comprehension of the condition of the individual human being assessed. Patients are potentially disempowered by such professional hubris, and prefer the sense of partnership they derive from feeling understood and equal.[42] Treatment is more likely to be effective when the patient shares ownership of the plan with the professionals.[43,44] This is best achieved by a collaborative conversation between equals. Professionals use terms like 'consultation' to describe situations where one partner begins by being apparently more competent. Collaboration is a different process.

Competency versus pathology

Collaborative assessment is characterized by the nurse being solution focused (see De Shazer[36,37]) and strengths based.[30] The primary interest is to establish what the patient wants and what skills and abilities they have or need to achieve their goals. Even when faced with very deranged, disturbed or distressed behaviour, a collaborative assessor will retain a respectful belief that the person has disguised, hidden or temporarily misplaced competence, and seek to elicit it. Mills[45] recognizes that collaboration can be scary for both professional and patient, but stresses the importance of 'the person with psychosis working alongside the professional ... Both parties have a role to play in the development of new understandings and coping methods'.[45,pp.129–30] On the other hand, Morgan[46] discusses strengths-based assessment and emphasizes how much 'fun' can be had for client and practitioner. Conventional assessment procedures tend explicitly or subliminally to explore aspects of pathology (defect, deficit or weakness) even when couched in the recommended rhetoric of 'needs' rather than 'problems'.[16,23]

Systemic versus unilateral thinking

By focusing on the patient's experiences and constructs, a nurse undertaking a collaborative assessment would be led to embrace wider perspectives than narrowly focused individual pathology. This systemic gaze could involve exploring the reverberating interactions occurring in someone's family[47,48] or getting to grips with the reality of someone's social and economic stressors.[49] Working with problems embedded in family belief systems and communication matrices requires a fundamental shift in how nurses construe interpersonal aetiology. In order to sensibly understand the repetitive patterns of interaction within families, it helps to distinguish between *linear* and *circular* causality. A circular, reciprocal view of problem formation and maintenance stresses how the action of each person influences the other, whose behaviour in turn influences them. This is fundamentally different from linear explanations, which presuppose that one person's behaviour simply determines how another thinks, feels or acts: as though one person *makes* another do something, who then forcibly influences a third, in a sort of inter-psychic pecking-order.[48] A second, even wider systemic perspective requires nurses to take account of the openness and vulnerability of individuals and families to political, economic and cultural influences on behaviour, thought and feeling. Sadness, anxiety, anger and obsessive weirdness may have roots in threatening, absurd or alienating world events and situations, just as much as in defective neurosignalling processes.[49] However wide or variously targeted the systemic gaze is, it takes full account of the 'fundamental attribution error' in not overestimating individual dispositional causes of difficulties (which an illness focus may very easily entail) or underestimating situational, environmental factors.[50] This includes of course the impact on the patient of the clinical environment, of which the personality, attitudes and behaviour of the nurse assessor and the internal relationships between them and the rest of the clinical team are significant components.[51]

USER COLLABORATION AND INTEGRATION WITH OTHER POLICY THEMES

Increased collaboration is just one of several themes in recent mental health policy. Indeed, Rogers and Pilgrim[52] argue that user collaboration is a policy that may already have climaxed, and is destined to be relegated against other policies, such as public safety. Currently, user collaboration is augmented, balanced, contradicted or undermined by other policy themes.

- Strengthening the social control function of psychiatric services, and developing more effective means of compelling people to accept either treatment or behaviour management.[53,54]
- Basing treatment and care on effective methods that have been reliably demonstrated or 'evidenced-based practice'.[55,56]
- Establishing more effective communication between professional disciplines and integrating practice within multiprofessional care planning using a synthesis of clinical models, usually under the aegis of psychiatric conventions.[57–59]
- Using more formal assessment tools to improve evaluation of effectiveness and enhance communication between agencies and disciplines[15] (see also Gamble and Brennan[10] and Tunmore[60]).

Policies often appear to be in conflict or tension, as when users, who otherwise agree their needs have been properly assessed, do not feel that their strengths and abilities were taken into account.[16] Nurses also frequently experience dilemmas when prioritizing clinical policies.[23] The clinical virtue of enabling a person to plan their own care is often weighed uncertainly against a managerial risk avoidance imperative, e.g. when working with personality-disordered people or people with paranoid feelings that may lead to withdrawal, violence or self-harm. Similarly, there is often a tension between wishing to enhance autonomy or develop a trusting relationship by preserving confidentiality, instead of feeling obliged to share intimate revelations with other professionals.[61]

Increased use of formal assessment tools may conflict with the goal of full collaboration, if not with the step of enhanced user participation. Psychiatric nursing has prioritized concise, cogent and communicable formulations of patients' needs and risks[15] and emphasized the use of structured interview processes, rigorous observation schedules and formal assessment tools.[10] These emphases are sometimes softened by employing concepts like 'holism' to differentiate nursing assessment from medical examination[62] or referring to 'the semi-structured interview' as a means of involving patients.[11]

The variety of tools used within a service reflects the range of treatment models on offer. Each model of care or treatment develops its own assessment measures, designed to determine problems or needs as defined within the particular treatment paradigm, whether biomedical, cognitive–behavioural or nursing models are favoured. These models are not simply the treatment preferences of otherwise open-minded professional helpers. They also reflect the professionals' ideas about human nature, and specifically the nature and causes of human distress or disturbance.[63] The person undergoing assessment may well entertain quite different notions about human nature and their specific personality, needs or preferences. While the professional continues to view the person through the lens of their particular clinical world view, then sapiential authority has been unilaterally imposed upon an already unbalanced power relationship. The professional has both statutory and structural authority and therefore potential power over the patient. The imposition of sapiential authority, via predetermined and unnegotiated models of pathology and allied assessment measures, completes the patient's invalidation and may lead to either oppositional conflict or excessively compliant dependence. Speedy[64] claims that in the absence of an already established alliance, nurses' use of psychiatric concepts and language invalidates the users' experiences and renders them powerless. It certainly jeopardizes the attainment of a collaborative working partnership,[34] even though nurses may attempt to involve patients in negotiations about treatment decisions.[65]

Although some use of formal tools may be a necessary response to clinical or managerial imperatives,[15] a richer picture, or a thicker narrative, may be obtained by synthesizing such methods with a collaborative, conversational approach. Embedding formal assessment tools within the matrix of a previously established, genuinely collaborative relationship is likely to enhance the clarity, accuracy and relevance of the results gleaned from assessment tools.[60] Patients are likely to feel more cooperative, more attentive and less anxious or mistrustful of the assessment procedure once they have been involved in determining and agreeing their use.[3,12,66]

People entering mental health services as patients, clients or customers often express a wish for less formal, more empathic processes of exploration of their difficulties and discovery of solutions.[67,68] They would like to be involved, but commonly feel excluded from the whole assessment process, despite evidence that when there is collaboration, or at least participation, quality of care improves and satisfaction with the service increases.[16,55,59] People needing nursing care experience such complex, subtle difficulties and conflicting or unrealistic aspirations that more informal, exploratory and responsive processes are necessary to enable shared understanding of their struggles to develop within an essentially conversational relationship.[69,70]

Full collaboration requires that not only formal assessment measures but also formal professional thinking are understood and engaged with willingly by the patient. This can only happen if the *model* from which a tool derives, and whose concepts and categories it has been designed to measure or classify, has also been discussed, however minimally, and accepted, however uncertainly. A person whose mental health is being assessed may be experiencing potentially disabling cognitive difficulties or emotional distress. In traditional assessments, if a model of treatment or care is to be discussed, the onus is on the professional to not only present concepts clearly and accessibly, but also relate them to the individual's experiences.[5] Collaborative assessment would relegate the proposal of a tool and the explanation of underlying theory (if it should happen at all) to some point after the user's perspective has been fully explored. Collaboration begins with the professional nurse attempting to set aside personal or professional prejudice; suspend clinical or philosophical certainties; and reach out to experimentally embrace or contain the patient's current way of experiencing the world, however deranged that may seem. Then *negotiation* can truly begin, rather than the *imposition*, however subtly managed, of the professional, clinical perspective. 'Imposition tends to generate opposition.'[14,p.3]

Marsha Linehan[71] explores this stance of empathic acceptance in relation to working with people diagnosed as borderline personality disordered. She refers to such deep validation as a 'core strategy': 'The essence of validation is this: The therapist communicates to the patient that her responses make sense and are understandable within her current life context or situation. [The nurse] takes the patients responses seriously and does not discount or trivialise them.'[76,p.222] The initial adoption of a professional 'one-down' respectful stance may give the therapeutic

alliance a working chance especially when there is a high degree of defensive sensitivity. However, collaboration is not thence best achieved by the worker simply switching conventional roles with the 'good patient' and transforming into a compliant pussycat. The energy needed to transfigure a cosily collusive relationship into a dynamically effective working partnership may well derive from the dialectical tensions that result from the juxtaposition and sustained interaction of opposing points of view. When both perspectives are recognized and validated at the same time, resolution can occur with the emergence of a third possibility that may resemble a compromise, or be some apparently entirely unrelated possibility.

Reflection

How well does your service balance the use of *formal assessment tools* with the development of *effective therapeutic alliances*?

SUMMARY: COLLABORATION AND ASSESSMENT, ANCIENT AND MODERN

Prior to the prescribed introduction of a highly structured version of *the nursing process*[72] into care in the 1970s, many patients in mental hospital acute wards and day centres were nursed to recovery without any formal nursing assessment at all. Medical diagnosis was the sole form of assessment in most clinical situations. Despite the well-documented abuses prevalent in many mental hospital situations, there were wards and units where enthusiastic, caring staff worked imaginatively and with sustained goodwill to try to understand and help people. These individuals and teams had no formal assessment procedures or standardized tools. They simply tried to work with their patients' distress and hopes. Recovery came about largely because nurses and patients conversed and socialized together during long periods of each day. Within these relationships, patients' psychic pains were contained, and new versions of reality co-created. Through well-attuned conversation and therapeutic activities nurses helped people to reconstruct their past experiences; reappraise their present plights; and envision new future possibilities. Arguably, before the emergence of *narrative therapy* as a theory and practice, nurses and patients intuitively collaborated to 're-author the narrative' of peoples' lives.

Whether people are subjected to an assessment process or not, on entry to a mental health service they primarily subjectively want real *help* (not necessarily either nursing *care* or medical *treatment*). This need for help precipitates people more deeply into a state of mixed distress and expectation, which has existential roots in the earliest state of infantile dependency. Whether conscious of this or not, patients and care-givers are participating in the most fundamental form of responsive collaboration: attachment relationships.[73,p.291] The attachment bond is characterized by containment of emotion, and internalization (on the infant's part) of the care-giver's responses and the interpersonal relationship itself to co-create an internal model of reality. This internal model is then used as a template to observe, appraise, experience and react or respond to the outside world.[74,p.71] The model persists into adulthood and is acutely reactivated in times of distress and need. The adult-to-adult interactions of nurses and patients are inextricably intertwined with infant-with-care-giver experiences, and their emotional and cognitive resonances in the present. As Peter Watkins[70] asserts, these rich conversations form the basis of not only negative or destructive outcomes, but also effective collaboration and successful care.

> I do not much care for the term *assessment*. It symbolizes for me the power differential in helping relationships, where one person who has the expertise and knowledge assesses a client who has limited or no knowledge of what their distress means and little expertise to help themselves … I visualise it much more as a collaborative dialogue in which the clients story unfolds and is filled out in the context of a developing relationship[70,p.50]

During a collaborative assessment process, when both parties are deeply attuned to each other, at times a state of contemplative reverie occurs, which can feel pleasantly trance-like or disturbingly uncomfortable (or both) depending on the nurse's personality, self-awareness, therapeutic skill, and the quality of supervision available. It is these reveries that most strongly imitate good positive attachment and provide restructuring opportunities for the patient. Reverie is not achieved by tight formally structured clinical relationships, question lists or standardized assessment tools. Clinical objectivity probably militates against collaborative attunement; and in many services nowadays, any nurses allowing themselves to enter into states of reverie with patients would be accused of 'over-involvement' and probably be disciplined for unprofessional conduct. Nevertheless, effective collaboration entails interpersonal attunement, which makes reverie more likely, which in turn leads to deeper collaboration, emotional containment and co-creation of alternative realities.

Johnstone[5] describes some of the difficulties, such as defensiveness, mistrust and breakdown of communication, created by 'the contrast between service users' desire for a psychosocial understanding of their difficulties and the primarily medical model of the professionals'. However, nurses who adapt and incorporate deep collaborative processes into their assessment practice may find that their nursing relationships move from polite formalism, grateful subordination, negativistic opposition,

> I remember in my third year as a student nurse a quiet Sunday evening spent in the homely small lounge of an admission ward while the sunlight filtered through the dust motes, and a budgie chirped in a background cage, sharing the rare peace with a newly admitted young homeless lad, an Irishman, and a stranger to the town and the service. He was unknown and had been very untalkative, and undisclosing. I fell into a pleasantly comfortable reverie, and found myself wondering about the boy sitting quietly with me. After some time, he just started speaking, and I just listened. I cannot remember the details of his monologue, but I remember it was about his parents and their death. I reported it to the staff nurse, who made a note in the ward report book. The next afternoon I was told that Dennis's notes had arrived from Ireland, and that he was nothing but a simpleton (subnormal was probably the term used) and a schizophrenic. Much mirth prevailed during the handover at the idealistic berk who thought the village idiot was a sage; but I hadn't dreamt it; he'd spoken sensitively, intelligently and with feeling.

Reflection

How freely and deeply do you allow yourself to converse with patients?

How confident are you of your ability to attune to others within conversations? How fearful are you of the consequences of intimate conversations?

stagnation or helpless dependency to productive dialectic. The happy virtue of full collaboration may often not be achieved in practice. Many people are perhaps initially far too damaged to participate much in their own care. That is however no reason not to keep full collaboration in mind as the gold standard of decent mental health nursing care, and to constantly strive to move nursing practice from imposed formulations and coercion through compliance, consultation, negotiation, participation, to collaboration and, finally, professional redundancy.

REFERENCES

1. Ritter S. *Bethlem Royal & Maudsley Hospital manual of clinical psychiatric nursing principles and procedures*. HarperCollins, London, 1989.

2. Newell R, Gournay K. Introduction. In: Newell R, Gournay K (eds). *Mental health nursing: an evidence-based approach*. Edinburgh, UK: Churchill Livingstone, 2000: 1–7.

3. Barham P, Hayward R. The lives of 'users'. In: Heller T, Reynolds J, Gomm R *et al.* (eds). *Mental health matters*. Basingstoke, UK: Macmillan Press and Open University, 1996.

4. Lindow V. Survivor-controlled alternatives to psychiatric services. In: Newnes C, Holmes G, Dunn C (eds). *This is madness: a critical look at psychiatry and the future of mental health services*. Ross-on-Wye, UK: PCCS Books, 1999.

5. Johnstone L. *Users and abusers of psychiatry*, 2nd edn. London, UK: Routledge, 2000.

6. Faulkner A. *Strategies for living*. London, UK: Mental Health Foundation, 2000.

7. Barker P. *Assessment in psychiatric and mental health nursing*. Cheltenham, UK: Stanley Thornes, 1997.

8. Sugden J. The process by which nursing intervention is facilitated. In: Sugden J, Bessant A, Eastland M, Field R (eds). *A handbook for psychiatric nurses*. London, UK: Harper & Row, 1986.

9. Perkins R, Repper J. *Working alongside people with long-term mental health problems*. London, UK: Chapman & Hall, 1996.

10. Gamble C, Brennan G. Assessment: a rationale and glossary of tools. In: Gamble C, Brennan G (eds). *Working with serious mental illness: a manual for clinical practice*. London, UK: Baillière Tindall, 2000.

11. Fox J, Conroy P. Assessing clients' needs: the semi-structured interview. In: Gamble C, Brennan G (eds). *Working with serious mental illness: a manual for clinical practice*. London, UK: Baillière Tindall, 2000.

12. Fowler D, Garety P, Kuipers E. *Cognitive behaviour therapy for psychosis*. Chichester, UK: Wiley, 1995.

13. Kingdon DG, Turkington D. *Cognitive-behavioural therapy of schizophrenia*. Hove, UK: Psychology Press, 1994.

14. Hoyt MF. *Some stories are better than others: doing what works in brief therapy and managed care*. Philadelphia, PA: Brunner-Mazel, 2000.

15. Standing Nursing and Midwifery Advisory Committee. *Addressing acute concerns*. London, UK: Department of Health, 1999.

16. Rose D. *Users voices*. London, UK: Sainsbury Centre for Mental Health, 2001.

17. Lucas J. Multi-disciplinary care in the community for clients with mental health problems: guidelines for the future. In: Watkins M, Hervey N, Carson J, Ritter S (eds). *Collaborative community mental health care*. London, UK: Arnold, 1996.

18. Newnes C, Holmes G. The future of mental health services. In: Newnes C, Holmes G, Dunn C (eds). *This is madness: a critical look at psychiatry and the future of mental health services*. Ross-on-Wye, UK: PCCS Books, 1999.

19. Howell V, Norman I. Steering a steady course in an era of compulsory treatment: taking mental health nursing into the millennium. *Journal of Mental Health* 2000; **9**: 605–16.

20. Morrall P. *Mental health nursing and social control*. London, UK: Whurr Publishers, 1998.

21. Morgan S. *Clinical risk management: a clinical tool and practitioner manual*. London, UK: Sainsbury Centre for Mental Health, 2000.

22. O'Rourke M, Bird L. *Risk management in mental health: a practical guide to individual care and community safety*. London, UK: Mental Health Foundation, 2001.

23. Perkins R, Repper J. *Dilemmas in community mental health practice: choice or control?* Oxford, UK: Radcliffe Medical Press, 1998.

24. Reason P, Rowan J (eds). *Human inquiry: a sourcebook of new paradigm research*. Chichester, UK: J. Wiley, 1981.

25. Rowan J, Reason P. On making sense. In: Reason P, Rowan J (eds). *Human inquiry: a sourcebook of new paradigm research*. Chichester, UK: J. Wiley, 1981: 113–37.

26. Rowan J. Research ethics. *International Journal of Psychotherapy* 2000; **5** (2): 103–11.

27. White M. Deconstruction and therapy. In: Gilligan S, Price R (eds). *Therapeutic conversations*. New York, NY: W.W. Norton, 1993.

28. O'Hanlon WH. Possibility therapy: from iatrogenic injury to iatrogenic healing. In: Gilligan S, Price R (eds). *Therapeutic conversations*. New York, NY: W.W. Norton, 1993.

29. May-Stewart V-D. Working single mothers and stress: a collaborative inquiry. *Dissertation Abstracts International: Humanities and Social Sciences* 2000; **60** (7-A): 2708.

30. Smail D. *The origins of unhappiness: a new understanding of personal distress*. London, UK: Constable, 1993.

31. Coolican H. *Research methods and statistics in psychology*. London, UK: Hodder & Stoughton, 1994.

32. White M, Epston D. *Narrative means to therapeutic ends*. New York, NY: W.W. Norton, 1990.

33. Bradshaw J. The conceptualisation and measurement of need: a social policy perspective. In: Popay J, Williams G (eds). *Researching the peoples' health*. London, UK: Routledge, 1994.

34. Johnstone L. 'I hear what you're saying': how to avoid jargon in therapy. *Changes* 1997; **15**(4): 264–70.

35. Sainsbury Centre for Mental Health. *Keys to engagement: review of care for people with severe mental illness who are hard to engage with services*. London, UK: Sainsbury Centre for Mental Health, 1998.

36. De Shazer S. *Keys to solution in brief therapy*. New York, NY: Norton, 1985.

37. De Shazer S. *Clues: investigating solutions in brief therapy*. New York, NY: Norton, 1988.

38. Gilligan S, Price R (eds). *Therapeutic conversations*. New York, NY: Norton, 1993.

39. Rowe D. *Guide to life*. London, UK: Harper Collins, 1995.

40. Rowe D. Self-esteem – buy now while stocks last. *OpenMind* 2001; **110** July/Aug: 7.

41. Pilgrim D. Disordered personalities and disordered concepts. *Journal of Mental Health* 2001; **10** (3): 253–65.

42. Burns D, Auerbach A. Therapeutic empathy in cognitive-behavioural therapy: does it really make a difference? In: Salkovskis PM (ed.). *Frontiers of cognitive therapy*. New York, NY: Guilford Press, 1996.

43. Ryle A. *Cognitive-analytic therapy: active participation in change*. Chichester, UK: John Wiley, 1990.

44. McGinn LK, Young JE. Schema-focused therapy. In: Salkovskis PM (ed.). *Frontiers of cognitive therapy*. New York, NY: Guilford Press, 182–207.

45. Mills J. Dealing with voices and strange thoughts. In: Gamble C, Brennan G (eds). *Working with serious mental illness: a manual for clinical practice*. London, UK: Baillière Tindall, 2000.

46. Morgan S. *Community mental health: practical approaches to long-term problems*. London, UK: Chapman & Hall, 1993.

47. Proctor H, Pieczora R. A Family oriented community mental health centre. In: Carpenter J, Treacher A (eds). *Using family therapy in the 90s*. Oxford, UK: Blackwell, 1993.

48. Dallos R, Draper R. *An introduction to family therapy: systemic theory and practice*. Buckingham, UK: Open University Press, 2000.

49. Smail D. *How to survive without psychotherapy*. London, UK: Constable, 1996.

50. Ross L, Amabile T, Steinmetz J. Social roles, social control and biases in social perception. *Journal of Personality and Social Psychology* 1977; **35**: 485–94.

51. Goodwin I, Holmes G, Newnes C, Waltho D. A qualitative analysis of the views of in-patient mental health service users. *Journal of Mental Health* 1999; **8** (1): 43–54.

52. Rogers A, Pilgrim D. *Mental health policy in Britain*, 2nd edn. Basingstoke, UK: MacMillan Press, 2001.

53. Department of Health. *Review of the Mental Health Act 1983: report of the expert committee (The Richardson Report)*. London, UK: Stationery Office, 1999.

54. Department of Health. *Reforming the Mental Health Act*. London, UK: Stationery Office, 2000.

55. Department of Health. *Modernising mental health services: safe, sound and supportive*. London, UK: HMSO, 1999.

56. Department of Health. *Treatment choice in psychological therapies and counselling: evidence-based clinical practice guideline*. London, UK: DoH, 2001.

57. National Health Service Executive and Social Service Inspectorate. *Effective care co-ordination in mental health services: modernising the care programme approach*. London, UK: Department of Health, 1999.

58. Department of Health. *Building bridges: a guide to arrangements for inter-agency working for the care and protection of severely mentally ill people*. London, UK: HMSO, 1995.

59. Ramon S. Contextualising innovation: macro and micro issues. In: Ramon S (ed.). *A stakeholders' approach to innovation in mental health services*. Brighton, UK: Pavilion Publishing, 2000.

60. Tunmore R. Practitioner assessment skills. In: Thompson T, Mathias P (eds). *Lyttle's mental health and disorder*, 3rd edn. Edinburgh, UK: Baillière Tindall, 2000.

61. Liese BS, Franz RA. Treating substance use disorders with cognitive therapy. In: Salkovskis PM (ed.). *Frontiers of cognitive therapy*. New York, NY: Guilford Press, 1996: 470–508.

62. Maphosa W, Slade M, Thornicroft G. Principles of assessment. In: Newell R, Gournay K (eds). *Mental health nursing: an evidence-based approach*. Edinburgh, UK: Churchill Livingstone, 2000.

63. Messer SB, Winokur M. Ways of knowing and visions of reality. In: Arkowitz H, Messer SB (eds). *Psychoanalytic therapy and behaviour therapy: is integration possible?* New York, NY: Plenum Press, 1984.

64. Speedy S. The therapeutic alliance. In: Clinton M, Nelson S (eds). *Advanced practice in mental health nursing*. Oxford, UK: Blackwell Science, 1999.

65. Castillo H, Allen L, Coxhead N. The hurtfulness of diagnosis: user research about personality disorder. *Mental Health Practice* 2001; **4** (9): 16–19.

66. Tarrier N. Management and modification of residual positive psychotic symptoms. In: Birchwood M, Tarrier N (eds). *Psychological management of schizophrenia*. Chichester: John Wiley, 1994.

67. Beeforth M, Conlon E, Grayley R. *Have we got views for you: user evaluation of case management*. London, UK: Sainsbury Centre for Mental Health, 1994.

68. Sainsbury Centre for Mental Health. *Pulling together*. London, UK: Sainsbury Centre for Mental Health, 1997.

69. Hulme P. Collaborative conversation. In: Newnes C, Holmes G, Dunn C (eds). *This is madness: a critical look at psychiatry and the future of mental health services*. Ross-on-Wye, UK: PCCS Books, 1999: 165–78.

70. Watkins P. *Mental health nursing: the art of compassionate care*. Oxford, UK: Butterworth-Heinemann, 2001.

71. Linehan MM. *Cognitive-behavioral treatment of borderline personality disorder*. New York, NY: Guilford Press, 1993.

72. Carlson S. A practical approach to the nursing process. *The American Journal of Nursing* 1972; **72** (9): 1589–91.

73. Symington N. *The analytic experience: lectures from the Tavistock*. London, UK: Free Association Books. 1986.

74. Siegel DJ. *The developing mind: how relationships and the brain interact to shape who we are*. New York, NY: Guilford Press, 1999.

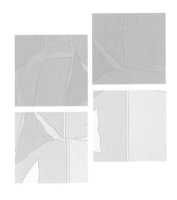

CHAPTER 13

The context of family assessment

Evelyn Gordon* and Chris Stevenson**

Jack feels Jill is greedy
because Jill feels Jack is mean
Jill feels Jack is mean
because Jack feels Jill is greedy[1]

This chapter outlines an approach to mental health assessment within the wider context of the family, professional and social networks. This form of systemically oriented assessment is viewed as a holistic approach that enables the emergence of rich information within the assessment process, facilitating relevant treatment planning. Assessment and intervention are viewed as both independent and interconnected endeavours: information gained from assessment guides intervention, whereas new information emerges in the intervention phase, which enriches hypotheses expressed in the initial assessment.

FOCUS: INDIVIDUAL OR SYSTEM OR BOTH?

Within mental health there has been a shift in understanding in relation to causality of and response to mental health problems. During the twentieth century, psychiatry has been predicated on linear cause and effect explanations. It has been underpinned by the idea that biological, psychological and/or social pathology leads to mental distress. Until fairly recently, psychiatric mental health nursing has been based on similar assumptions. General system theory (GST), articulated by von Bertanlanffy[2] during the 1940s, offered a different way to account for phenomena that did not seem to lend themselves to traditional linear ideas of cause and effect, instead advocating circular or systemic causality. According to Walrond-Skinner[3] a systemic approach to understanding the world seemed to:

> … provide a unifying theoretical framework for both the natural and social sciences, which needed to employ concepts such as organisation, wholeness and dynamic interaction, none of which lent itself easily to the methods of analysis employed by the pure sciences.

According to GST, we can identify a system or bounded group of units, the system's environment or supra-system, and the system's components or sub-systems. From this position, linear cause and effect do not fully encapsulate the system as a whole and its dynamic nature. For example, it is viewed as overly simplistic to think that someone becomes depressed because of a social loss. In GST, causality is seen as a circular process. It has no beginning or end but can be punctuated at different points, which give rise to multiple ways of looking at and explaining the activities of the system. From this perspective depression might be seen as emerging from a

*Evelyn Gordon is a lecturer in Mental Health Nursing and Psychotherapy in Dublin City University, Dublin, Ireland. Her doctoral research is in suicidology.
**Chris Stevenson is Chair of Mental Health Nursing at Dublin City University, Dublin, Ireland. Her doctoral research focused on the processes inherent in family work.

context where the person has suffered a loss (their job) in a family context where employment defines status and at a point in time where they were struggling to negotiate independence from the family. Now they must instead resume a childlike and powerless role, or re-engage in a less hopeful independence 'battle'.

GST is often illustrated with reference to a thermostat. The thermostat is a mechanism that monitors the ambient temperature (for example of a room). If the temperature drops to below a certain point, the thermostat responds by switching on the heating system. If the temperature rises, the thermostat responds by switching off the heating. Thus, it operates on both positive and negative feedback to produce a steady state (homoeostasis). When this concept is applied to individuals and families it highlights the struggle between stability and change which is frequently an issue that arises in mental health assessment and treatment; the recursive influence between the parts of the family system and the supra-system; and, the complexity of the relationships among those operating in and between the family and wider social systems. A child displaying temper tantrums may be seen by the family as the cause of their distress. However, the temper tantrum may be a response to the mother's strictness, which is a response to father's more easy-going attitude. The stricter mother becomes, the more temper tantrums erupt. The more temper tantrums erupt, the more easy-going father becomes, the stricter mother becomes, and so on. Thus, 'symptoms' serve a positive or negative feedback function in maintaining the balance or stability of the family system, influencing it in much the same way that a thermostat adjusts the temperature, in response to positive and negative feedback.

With such circular causality the 'here and now' becomes a primary focus as problem behaviour is actively maintained in the present, while links are also drawn between the historical development of events and relationships, the present situation and future possibilities. Although the balance achieved by the family may not be satisfactory, in terms of personal development of those concerned, it may be perceived (consciously or unconsciously) by family members, as preferable to the unease, such as family break up, which imbalance could trigger. For example, the temper tantrums may be a way of sidetracking the parents from their own marital disagreements, which might ultimately end in separation and divorce. Yet, the tantrums are not a pleasant experience for the child or other family members.

Although this systemic approach was initially applied to psychotherapeutic practice in the family therapy field, it has more recently been incorporated into the work of other disciplines. Thus, a challenge that exists in mental health assessments is to make sense of the system and the person's place within this while also attending to the individual patient's (IP's) intrapsychic needs. This chapter is however primarily concerned with the former; therefore, the assessment and intervention theories and practices outlined below emphasize this approach.

ASSESSMENT

Although there are differences in systemically oriented 'schools', there are some unifying ideas. It is worthwhile clarifying where commonalties lie, as the suggestions for assessment that follow are based on these common assumptions rather than being related to specific approaches.

Relationship

Most systemic approaches set the 'pathological' individual in a system of inter-related players. For example, Laing and Esterson[4] state:

> … we are interested in what might be called the family nexus, that multiplicity of persons drawn from the kinship group, and from others who, though not linked by kinship ties, are regarded as members of the family. The relationships of persons in a nexus are characterised by enduring and intensive face-to-face reciprocal influence on each other's experience and behaviour.

As symptoms are embedded in social life, some family therapists, notably Jay Haley, refused to meet with 'incomplete' families. However, as Gorrell-Barnes[5] notes, different forms of family organization are increasing, and no clear boundaries exist to define what constitutes the 'family unit'. This, along with the idea that there is a ripple effect on the entire system when change occurs, has led some family therapists to be less attached to the idea of assessing 'whole' families. Thus, there are many ways to complete a systemic assessment; for example, meeting some family members together or inviting the family to decide who should participate.

Context

Most systemic therapy approaches agree that individual and family systems are influenced by wider social and cultural narratives and practices. These historical and contextual stories and norms influence their view of themselves and their interaction with the 'outside' world. The 'identity' of the family is further shaped by unique events that they experience, such as bereavement. For example, a family who value independence and view themselves as strong may perceive an attempt to engage with professional helpers as a sign of weakness on the part of the family, as they have failed to 'sort themselves out'.

Meaning and information

Most systemic approaches share the view that problems and their solutions should be explored in relation to the patterns of information exchange, or communication, that occurs between family members, which defines the nature of relationships. For example, Gregory Bateson and colleagues[6] explored paradoxical communication within double bind communications. They noted that all communication has two levels, a report level, which is the content or information that is being conveyed, and a command level, or meta-communicative level. This level is concerned with conveying a message *about* the information. The two levels may be matching and therefore convey a clear message, or clashing, thereby conveying a confusing, or paradoxical, message to the recipient. The report level is usually based in words, whereas the command level is usually non-verbal. For example, the nurse who tells the patient that it is no problem to fetch some clean towels while looking exasperated at being disturbed in the midst of report writing is simultaneously presenting conflicting messages. Another example from family life might involve a mother who goes shopping and buys her teenage daughter two T-shirts, one blue and one red. The girl is delighted with them and rushes upstairs to try them on. She comes down stairs wearing the red T-shirt. Her mother looks and says: 'Oh, so you didn't like the blue one'. The innocuous words (content) are accompanied by a higher level communication of criticism. The girl is trapped in a no-win situation. She cannot wear two garments at once; therefore, regardless of which she chooses she can be 'accused' in this manner by her mother. Bateson *et al.*[6] did not think that isolated incidents of this kind could cause schizophrenia (as popular fallacy has often argued); however, they did believe that sustained paradoxical communication could lead to psychological distress and perhaps 'breakdown'.

In summary, it can be seen that family theorists share an interest in the relationship dynamics and communication patterns between family members and between the family system and others, and in the historical and social context of the family. Therefore, from a systemic perspective it is of paramount importance to explore these with the client/patient and family so that the practitioner can formulate hypotheses about the family system that will guide intervention.

Box 13.1 outlines some key areas of family assessment. You may wish to take a moment to reflect upon how you address the areas outlined when you are routinely conducting a mental health assessment.

EXPLORING THE FAMILY

From the above discussion it can be seen that family assessment can be clustered under the following three

Box 13.1: Key areas of family assessment

- Boundaries: lines of demarcation between sub-systems and system and suprasystem.
- Hierarchy and power: allocation of decision-making power within the system.
- Roles: allocation and balance of responsibilities in system functioning.
- Communication: style, level and patterns of information exchange within the system.
- Relationships: generational patterns of family regulation and cohesion.
- Functioning: adjustment and adaptation skills, coping mechanisms, strengths and vulnerabilities.
- Life cycle: system developmental stage, expected and unexpected life events and challenges.
- Beliefs, myths and legacies: assumptions underlying family patterns of interaction and functioning.
- Problem perceptions: shared and unique ideas about the problem and its resolution, attempted solutions.
- Treatment expectations: perception about and expectations of treating professionals, desired level of involvement in treatment process.

key areas: historical and contextual factors that have influenced the family identity and its beliefs and position vis-à-vis other systems; relationships between individuals and sub-system members that influence role and boundary formation, which in turn influence patterns of crisis response; and communication skills, style and patterns that influence practices such as problem-solving. Some methods of exploring these structures and processes are described below, including conversational practices, exploratory exercises for enhancing these and the use of psychometric scales, all of which are designed to help the family offer their understandings. As stated, it is not possible to entirely separate the assessment and response process; therefore, these methods are equally applicable within assessment and ongoing therapeutic work.

Conversational practices

Much of the work conducted with the client/family is based on developing therapeutic conversations that facilitate the exploration of key issues related to the person/family distress; therefore, some central systemic conversational techniques such as circular interviewing, externalizing the problem and the use of metaphor are outlined below.

Circular interviewing

Ann Rambo and colleagues[7] suggest that the best therapists are those who have a natural curiosity, since being curious is an attribute that can be translated into the ability to ask interesting questions. Most staff with training in psychiatric mental health nursing can make a distinction between open and closed questioning. Both of these types are useful in working with people, as techniques for opening up or closing down conversation. However, there is a specific form of interviewing used in working systemically that seeks to invite different or new information about the processes within the entire system. This is called circular interviewing, which focuses on relationship and circular causal patterns rather than individual traits and linear cause and effect patterns. This form of interviewing relies heavily on the use of circular questions and feedback loops that are created between members of the therapeutic system (client/family, interviewer and treatment team).

Circular questioning is a system of questioning developed by the early Milan family therapy group that helped them to explore hypotheses generated by the team from referral information and initial assessment.[8] Linking questions to hypotheses can create a purposeful and coherent interviewing pattern that reveals new information and people's different perceptions of the problem and potential solutions. How this information is discussed becomes the basis for ongoing work.

Circular questions seek relational connections; therefore, they are based on dyads and triads. People are asked to comment on their own or others' thoughts, behaviours and relationships with each other or with a specific event or idea. Circular questions can be grouped for convenience into eight rough categories that have some overlap: specific interactive sequence questions; comparison/before and after questions; problem-solving attempt questions; classification/ranking questions; mind-reading questions; hypothetical questions; relative influence questions; and targeted questions. Each of these is discussed below.

1 Specific interactive sequence questions involve more than one person and attempt to track a repetitive sequence of interactions and/or events, for example:

  When Ann (mother) is depressed what do father and daughter do?

  When father is angry with son, what does mother do?

2 Comparison/before and after questions track changes that indicate a significant shift in behaviour and/or meaning before and after an event, for example:

  Did your sisters get close to each other before or after your mum died?

3 Problem-solving attempt questions enquire about previous attempts to address the presenting problem, i.e. what has been tried, what worked or did not work, what and who helped, or did not help, and how. For example:

  When Jane's mood last became low what was the most helpful advice she got?

  Sometimes the strategies people use to rid themselves of the problem actually become the problem;

for example, where a person constantly tries to 'cheer up' someone describing themselves as depressed. Therefore, it is worthwhile enquiring if and how these attempted solutions are helping.

4 Classification/ranking questions put people, events and explanations in hierarchies according to specific criteria, in terms of importance, concern, etc. For example:

  Who in the family is most upset when X happens?

  Between A, B and C, who do you think is closest to D?

  Of the explanations given by mother, which one do you think dad agrees with most?

5 Mind-reading questions can reveal differences of opinion between people over important issues. For example:

  If your sister were alive today, what do you think she would say?

  In a moment I'm going to ask your brother whether he agrees or disagrees with your sister's view. What do you think he will say?

6 Hypothetical questions enquire about past/current/future situations, ideas or explanations that invite people to imagine alternatives outside of their 'reality'. The most famous of these is the miracle question, which is a future-oriented hypothetical question:

  If a miracle were to happen tonight while you were asleep and tomorrow you awoke to find this problem was no longer a part of your life, what would be different? How would you know that this miracle had taken place? How would other people be able to tell without you telling them? How would you act to try and maintain the new situation?

7 Relative influence questions invite two different descriptions of family members' association with the problem. The first is a question about the influence the problem has in their lives (directed to all family members). For example:

  When Tom is hearing voices, how does the family find itself operating differently? (This is passive influence.)

  The second is a description of the influence of family members in the life of the problem (active influence). For example: When Tom is hearing voices, what do the family members do to try to make the voices go away or be less of a nuisance for Tom?

8 Targeted questions seek to explore specific issues pertinent to the system being interviewed such as gender. These questions can be used to explore intergenerational beliefs about men's and women's roles, for example:

  Did either of your parents have a hard time meeting their parents' expectations about femininity/masculinity?

You may have noticed that some questions combine well together; however, the use of these kinds of questions requires practice. Try to use some in your next therapeutic conversation to gain a deeper understanding of the position the person occupies in the system and the concerns they have about this.

Externalizing the problem

Externalizing the problem refers to the process of separating the problem from the person. This is in contrast to other accounts, which are frequently 'problem-saturated' descriptions of the person in distress and family life. It is an approach used by Michael White[9] when working with people who feel entangled with a problem that is negatively influencing their lives. Externalizing the problem has several potential benefits.

- It encourages people to objectify and sometimes personify the problems they are experiencing.
- It is useful when the problem is thought to be inherent to the person and is seen as permanent.
- It offers a new story that can free people from the fixed and dominant story they have about a problem.

We have broken down the approach into three phases, which is a less sophisticated version than that described by White. We have found this method useful in practice and offer some practice illustrations:

Phase 1: get a picture of the relative influence between the person and the problem

This can be achieved by inviting two different descriptions. As described above one enquires about the influence the problem is having on the life of the person and the other enquires about the influence the person is having on the problem.

Phase 2: gain a definition of the problem to be externalized

This can be done by using the person's description to begin and gradually introducing alternative descriptions that are more fluid and temporary, less professionally laden and not located in the person. The definition of the problem may change over time as people struggle to describe their experience, as they move from the general to the specific. For example, sometimes people say, 'I have schizophrenia'; however, over time they may say, 'I have the experience of hearing a voice which torments me by telling me that I am a pervert'. A consultant psychiatrist who was not attached to diagnosis as a helpful means of understanding people's distress was asked by the family what a diagnosis meant. He replied: 'Personally, I don't find it useful to describe someone's reality disagreement as schizophrenia. There is a lot of negativity attached to that name. I prefer to find a way to describe what has been happening for you all and beginning to think about how we can address some of the issues.'

If necessary, use characters/personifications. Many practitioners do this naturally, for example, they might ask a patient: 'How are the voices today?' However, here is a more conscious use of personification that has been helpful. Jane was constantly taunted by past experiences,

which were referred to as 'skeletons in the cupboard'. It became possible to talk about how these skeletons in the cupboard had somehow escaped and needed to be reconfined.

Phase 3: find unique outcomes

This can be done by identifying a time when the problem is/was not present, or dominant, or is/was constructively managed. These 'unique outcomes' may relate to the past, present or future. They can be explored by asking 'comparison questions', which may need to be persistent in order to identify the non-problem-saturated situation. For example, in Jane's case the skeletons could not come out of the cupboard when she was reading the Bible.

Start with current unique outcomes that are present as you meet with the person; for example, responding to the person who says 'I am always afraid of speaking about the problem' with 'You are here speaking with me today'. If you cannot find a unique outcome in the present go to the past. For example, sometimes a patient will say, 'I'm too anxious to be able to think'. In this case, you might say 'When you were getting married, how did you conquer your nervousness?' Future unique outcomes involve the person's plans to escape the problem. Ask 'What can you do to salvage your life?', or the 'miracle question', followed by, 'What will you do to help the miracle to occur?'

In these searches for unique outcomes, you are making a presupposition that something different is possible. This is a means of promoting hope that things can change. When people identify unique outcomes, of necessity, they alter their relationship to the problem. They recognize they can resist the problem, it becomes external to them, and they can refuse to submit to the problem and its effects. Therefore, the problem becomes less constraining and the person begins to become more in charge of it and its effects on their life.

Metaphor

It is sometimes difficult for a person to speak directly about a problem or concern; therefore, the use of metaphor can assist with distancing the problem in a way that allows it to be spoken about indirectly. Coale[10] uses an approach she calls 'costumes and pretend identities' in order to help co-create new meanings with family members in therapy. Dressing differently or adopting a different (pretend) identity can allow different kinds of relations and behaviour to occur. She provides the following example:

> A young woman complained of always being put upon at work. She was the older sister of a chronically dysfunctional 'schizophrenic' brother and felt some guilt that she had escaped the mentally ill position in the family. Since she was a history/literature major, I asked her what character in history she felt most like and she promptly responded 'Joan of Arc'. I then asked her to identify all of the 'Joan of Arc' things she did and, with alacrity, she gave me a profile of her self-abnegating behaviours. I asked her if she would be willing to go

to work each day for a week, acting like Joan of Arc and wearing some clothing that, to her, symbolized Joan of Arc. She decided how to do this and, after a week of Joan of Arc behaviours, started acting more assertive with both co-workers and family. With the help of her pretend identity to immerse her intentionality into her martyred behaviour, she had become tired of being put upon.[10,p.50]

Exploratory exercises

All of the above therapeutic methods are based on direct conversation between the client/family and practitioner; however, it is sometimes difficult to create different meanings in relation to the shared situation through dialogue alone. In these circumstances, it can be useful to develop a more playful approach that serves to engage the client/family in a different relationship to the therapeutic work. Exercises such as genograms and sculpting are described below.

Genograms

The 'genogram' is a form of enhanced family tree that can map information on family structure, relationships and functioning. One way of breaking the ice with a family is to collaboratively draw their family tree, which is especially useful if there is someone in the family who is nervous and with families where children are involved. One family member may be elected to be the 'scribe' to increase the level of involvement. A family tree, which has been completed earlier can be used to rejoin with the family; for example, to assess whether there have been any changes in family life following involvement in family assessment and planning meetings. You can also invite the family to reflect on the genogram and to note any obvious and/or previously unidentified connections. This process opens space to share and compare different reflections.

Within family work the genogram charts structural information such as family membership, age and occupation; relational information such as levels of closeness and distance; functional information such as engagement in substance misuse or patterns of illness in response to stress; and significant family events. Never assume that events that are talked about are not significant – record them anyway. A common set of symbols is used to map a genogram (see Figure 13.1). Sometimes, with families, it is easier to use colours and a large flip chart, as family organization is not always simple!

Figure 13.2 represents the Dinsdale family. You might like to write a short paragraph about the impressions of the family that you have gained through 'reading' their genogram. Think about the family structure and what questions might be interesting to explore with the family around that.

Sculpting

Sculpting is a technique that re-creates family relationships *in space*, through the formation of a physical tableau.

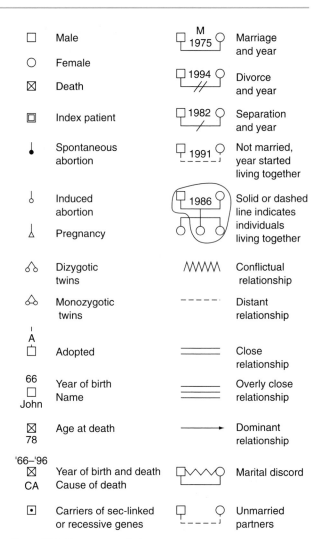

Figure 13.1 Genogram symbols

This symbolizes the emotional position of each member of the family in relation to others. The interviewer may ask the family to 'try out something a little different', emphasizing that it will involve everyone. If the interviewer is enthusiastic enough it will help to overcome any initial reluctance and shyness.

The interviewer invites a family member to act as the sculptor. The remainder of the family is the 'clay' that the sculptor has to mould. The rationale for whom is chosen as the sculptor is variable. For example, the identified patient may be selected because they are is already responding to perceived issues in family life; or a family member who seems less connected to the family may be offered the role as a way of making them more included. Once the sculptor is selected, the interviewer asks the rest of the family to stand up and to move into whatever position the sculptor suggests to them.

The interviewer moves into an observing role when the sculptor starts to move the family members around. They may ask the sculptor questions about what is happening. For example, enquire whether the family member has

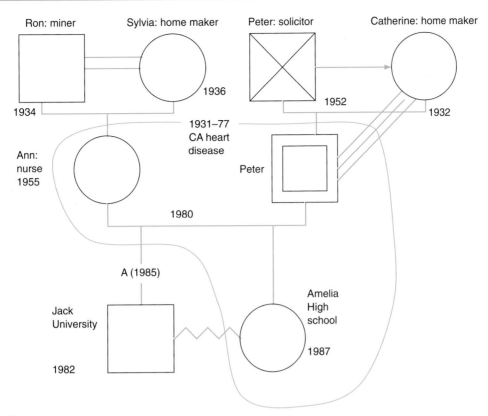

Figure 13.2 Family genogram

moved close enough to another family member; or invite them to describe what each position is meant to represent. The family members who are being positioned may be asked questions also; for example, how they are feeling at that precise moment in terms of their physical position. Sculpting can be a powerful intervention and people often use emotion-laden words like 'being put down'; or 'feeling pushed out'. When the sculpting is complete, the interviewer may ask the sculptor to find a place for themselves. As well as representing the present, the sculptor may be asked to position family members in relation to how things were in the past, for example when grandma died, to how things would change in a particular future, to how different degrees of closeness might have ripple effects in other family relationships.

With young children, small pebbles or dolls can be used to represent family members. Children are asked to position the dolls in relation to one another with reference to different scenarios or events. For example, how they see the family now and then how they would like to see the family in 6 months' time; or how the family members' positions would change if someone left or became more prominent in family life. The level of engagement in the task helps younger children to speak freely and spontaneously and not to follow pre-scripted responses, even when there is a parent present.

These spatial descriptions are often reflections of the emotional positions that family members occupy in

relation to each other. It is not difficult for the family to make connections between relationships, communication and family issues, without this being explicitly discussed.

Flexibility and Cohesion Evaluation Scale

Finally, assessment can also be enhanced through the use of psychometric scales such as Flexibility and Cohesion Evaluation Scale (FACES IV). Psychometrics can be helpful is some situations, for example, if family members cannot overtly state their perceptions in case of upsetting others, or they are unable to put their concerns into words. FACES IV is a well-validated and reliable family assessment tool.[11] It was originally developed by Olson et al.[12] for family members aged 12 and over. It measures four aspects of family organization and functioning: cohesion, flexibility, communication and satisfaction.

Cohesion and flexibility measure the degree of family balance with high scores being healthier. Within the cohesion scale are two dimensions, disengagement and enmeshment, and within the flexibility scale two dimensions, rigidity and degree of chaos. These dimensions refer to family imbalance and high scores on these dimensions are problematic. The scores can be plotted and compared against specific family types: balanced, rigidly cohesive, mid-range, flexibly unbalanced, chaotically disengaged and unbalanced. From the scale scores, a balanced and unbalanced ratio score can be calculated for each family member in relation to cohesion and flexibility. A total ratio score provides a summary of a family's balanced (health) and unbalanced (problem) characteristics in a single score. A ratio score of zero indicates the most unbalanced system, and the higher the ratio score the more balanced the system, with scores above 1 as indicative of a more healthy system. In addition, FACES IV includes scales to measure family communication and satisfaction[13] and categorize them, for example 'the family are generally happy about their family'. Family measurement is useful in that it allows the practitioner to develop hypotheses or narratives about the family that can be explored in engagement with the family. However, family psychometrics are not a substitute for clinical assessment when a richer account of family life can be constructed.

It might be worthwhile thinking about your own preferred ways of engaging with people in the assessment and therapeutic process; for example, through conversation or the use of other methods, using formal or informal assessment tools, involving members of the system together or separately.

SUMMARY

When nurses begin to think about assessing and working with wider systems they may feel inadequately prepared and/or skilled in this area. This chapter has outlined some basic assumptions and made some practical suggestions that can aid the nurse and family in exploring patterns of relationships, communication and response to events, which fosters a more holistic approach to mental health assessment and intervention. We have often been impressed by the tolerance of families when one is groping to find the next question in interviews and worried that the questioning might in some way 'make things worse'. With the benefit of practice experience, we are assured that this is rarely the case. We end, therefore, by encouraging nurses to experiment with the methods and techniques presented here. Be transparent with the families you meet, tell them that you are new to a systemic approach and do not be afraid to take a prompt sheet with you. When invited into collaborative exploration together clients/families are generally very helpful and keen to contribute.

REFERENCES

1. Laing RD. *Knots*. New York, NY: Pantheon Books, 1970: 51.

2. von Bertanlanffy L. *General systems theory*. Harmondsworth, UK: Penguin, 1968.

3. Walrond-Skinner S. *Family therapy: the treatment of natural systems*. London, UK: Routledge and Kegan Paul, 1976: 12.

4. Laing RD, Esterson A. *Sanity, madness and the family*. Harmondsworth, UK: Penguin, 1964: 21.

5. Gorrell-Barnes G. *Working with families*. London, UK: Macmillan, 1984.

6. Bateson G, Jackson D, Haley J, Weakland J. Toward a theory of schizophrenia. In: Jackson D (ed.). *Human communication, I*. Los Angeles, CA: Science and Behaviour Books, 1968.

7. Rambo A, Heath A, Chenail RJ. *Practising therapy: exercises for growing therapists*. New York, NY: Norton, 1993.

8. Pallazzoli MS, Boscolo L, Cecchin G, Prata G. Hypothesising–circularity–neutrality: three guidelines for the conductor of the session. *Family Process* 1980; **19**: 3–12.

9. White M. The externalising of the problem and the re-authoring of lives and relationships. *Dulwich Centre Newsletter*, Summer, 1998/89, reprinted in M. White *Selected papers*. Adelaide, Australia: Dulwich Centre Publications, 1989: 5–8.

10. Coale HW. Costume and pretend identities: a constructivist's use of experiences to co-create meanings with clients in therapy. *Journal of Marital and Family Therapy*, 1992; **11** (1): 45–55.

11. Gorall DM, Tiesel J, Olson DH. *FACES IV: Development and validation*. Minneapolis, MN: Life Innovations, 2004.

12. Olson DH, Portner J, Bell R. *Family adaptability and cohesion evaluation scales (FACES)*. Unpublished manuscript 1978.

13. Olson DH, Wilson M. Family satisfaction. In: Olson DH *et al.* (eds). *Families: what makes them work*. Newbury Park, CA: Sage Publishing, 1989.

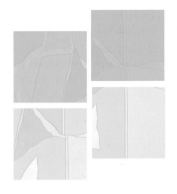

CHAPTER 14

The assessment of feelings, thoughts and beliefs

Mark Philbin*

For mental health nurses, assessment represents an attempt to 'get to know' people-in-care. Of course, there is a limit on the extent to which any person can know another. Human beings are complex, constantly changing and always capable of surprises. Furthermore, people are selective in what they notice about others and so nurses' knowledge of people-in-care is always partial. Nonetheless, it is important that nurses make a serious effort to comprehend and appreciate the people they are trying to help. Such effort is necessary for a number of reasons.

1 Nurses have a better chance of helping people when they know those people as individuals and have a sense of what they are experiencing.
2 Nurses' attempts to gain such understanding can help people-in-care to develop a different, perhaps more useful, understanding of their own situation. When nurses ask questions about particular experiences or issues, they may encourage people-in-care to examine and reflect upon what is happening within their lives. This might in itself help people to develop a clearer perspective on their situation, work out why certain experiences have occurred or notice something else that is significant.
3 People-in-care learn important lessons about nurses from the way and the extent to which nurses make an

effort to get to know them. For example, they often make judgements about nurses' levels of interest, courtesy, sensitivity and competence. In other words, nurses are assessed by the people they assess! This is significant because it is at least plausible that positive outcomes are more likely when people-in-care view the personal qualities and professional capabilities of nurses in positive terms. In the psychotherapy field, there is research evidence suggesting an association between these kinds of positive perceptions and positive outcomes.[1]

Given the potential benefits associated with getting to know people-in-care and trying to understand their experiences, how might this be achieved? This is difficult to answer comprehensively, but should at least partly involve an assessment of how they *feel*, what they *think* and what they *believe*. In this chapter, then, the focus is on how and why mental health nurses assess each of these matters as well as the inter-relationship between them.

ENQUIRING INTO FEELINGS

A *feeling* is a physical sensation, an emotion or a combination of the two. There is a range of ways in which nurses can approach the assessment of feelings.

*Mark Philbin is a lecturer in nursing at Dublin City University, Dublin, Ireland with an interest in strengths-based perspectives in mental health care. His current research is in the area of psychosis and the self.

Talking with people who identify feelings as a problem

Often, people-in-care are very aware of how they feel and consider 'feeling bad' as a major aspect, perhaps the most important aspect, of their problems. This can be a useful starting point for an 'assessment interview' as an examination of the following excerpt from an interaction illustrates:

Person-in-care:	I've been feeling really down for the past month.
Nurse:	What's it like when you feel down?
Person-in-care:	It's like a dark cloud has descended on me. I'm gloomy and I don't feel like doing anything. Everything is such an effort.
Nurse:	What else do you notice about yourself when this dark cloud descends?

Here, the person-in-care defined their problem in terms of how they feel and the nurse encouraged them to elaborate in more specific detail on what this feeling involves. If this were continued, the nurse would gain a clearer sense of what 'feeling down' meant for this person and might also display their commitment to understanding this. To pursue this line of enquiry further, the nurse might encourage the person to talk about the following kinds of things.

- A specific example of a *time* when they were feeling 'most down' – what they were *doing*, the nature of the *situation*, the involvement of *other people*, what they were *thinking*, what *happened afterwards*, a *rating* of how bad the feeling was.
- The course of the problem – the timing of the initial onset, when they felt better, when they felt worse, factors that seem to be associated with feeling better or worse.
- The implications of the negative state of feeling – for their level of activity, for their relationships with other people, for their view of the future, for their enactment of social roles and responsibilities.
- The events in their life – what changes have occurred in their life circumstances, the relevance of such changes to how negatively they feel, things that are happening in their life that are somehow problematic.

As well as contributing to a clearer picture of people's experience of their problems, conversation about these kinds of issues can help nurses to begin to understand why people are feeling so bad. For example, it might become apparent that there is a connection between a person's negative feelings and certain kinds of situation such as an argument with relatives. On recognizing such a connection, a nurse has an indication of one issue that might usefully be focused upon in trying to help this person. Furthermore, this kind of connection might usefully be made by a person-in-care. For example, some stressful event might have occurred before the onset of a problematic feeling but may not have been identified as significant. Through discussion, the person may come to view this event as relevant and therefore be helped to understand why the problematic feeling is being experienced. If people-in-care are helped to view their problems as explicable in this way, this in itself can be helpful. Often, people need to understand the reasons for their problems as a basis for believing they can be resolved. This need for explanations is often emphasized in first-hand accounts of mental illness such as those of Ken Steele[2] and Kay Jamison[3] as well as research into the experiences of family members of people with serious mental illness.[4]

Searching for feelings

Some helpful consequences can emerge from enabling people to talk in detail about feelings they consider problematic. However, there are other scenarios in which mental health nurses assess feelings. One involves nurses in looking for feelings they assume to be significant even when this may not be immediately evident to people-in-care. This is illustrated in the following excerpt from an initial interview between a community mental health nurse and a woman whose baby had died 4 weeks before:

Nurse:	How have you been since your baby died?
Person-in-care:	[Smiling] Fantastic. I'm doing really well. My doctor referred me here because he knows I've had psychiatric problems in the past but there was no need. I've been flying. My family are really pleased with me because they feared the worst, they thought I wouldn't be able to cope but I'm fine. Things are going really great, I have that feeling you have when you're on holiday.
Nurse:	What happens to holiday feelings after a holiday? [pause]
Person-in-care:	They disappear when you have to face reality [starting to cry]. I've got a really long way to go, haven't I?

In this situation, the nurse made an assumption about the feelings that are appropriately associated with the experience of grief. One reason for this assumption was a familiarity with the bereavement literature and the idea of a 'grieving process', developed by people like Colin Murray Parkes[5] and John Bowlby.[6] Although the idea of a grieving process that is universally appropriate is questionable,[7,8] the nurse was concerned by the person-in-care's assertion that she 'felt great'. The nurse quickly suspected that this might be a sign of 'denial' and that the person needed help to express feelings associated with the reality of her loss. Although the concept of denial is criticized in the grief literature[9] in this situation it informed the nurse's efforts to sensitively prompt emotional expression. From that point onwards, it was possible to discuss with the person the circumstances of her bereavement and her experiences of grief.

This represents one example of how nurses can search for people's feelings as part of an assessment. There are, of course, other ways.

Nurses often *observe* the behaviour of people-in-care and make *inferences* about whether they are feeling angry, sad, happy, anxious, contented and so on. These observations and inferences can be a basis for useful dialogue with people-in-care and can highlight, for example, inconsistencies between how they appear and how they feel 'inside'. Some people feel anxious and assume that their anxiety is highly visible to others. Indeed, this assumption can in itself be a source of greater anxiety. A nurse might observe a person, in this situation, and suggest that they appear a good deal calmer than they actually feel. Discussion of this observation can encourage the person to evaluate and even challenge the original assumption that others can see how he or she feels. Furthermore, observations of, and inferences about, feelings can help nurses to recognize sequences or patterns in people's behaviours and modes of relating to others. For example, a nurse might notice that an apparent feeling of agitation recurrently precedes a particular kind of behaviour such as violence towards another person. This recognition could then inform an early intervention to diffuse the impetus towards such behaviour. For Peplau,[10] such observation and recognition of problematic patterns of interaction were central to the assessment role of nurses.

Other methods of assessing feelings

Some people-in-care find it difficult to put their feelings into words. Observational approaches to assessment can take on an additional importance in such circumstances. However, there are some other methods of assessing feelings that can also be appropriate. Creative activities such as art, drama, storytelling and writing can give some people-in-care an opportunity to express feelings that have been difficult to verbalize. Indeed, one of the benefits of these approaches is that they often enhance people's ability to articulate what they are feeling. Questionnaires can also be helpful in this respect. There are a number of self-report questionnaires that are designed to assess things like anxiety, agoraphobia and depression. A number of these have been reviewed by Phil Barker.[11] Although these questionnaires are often used for diagnostic purposes, many of the individual items relate to statements about feelings. After people have completed such questionnaires, it can be useful for nurses to read each item that has been rated because they might discover information that has not arisen in the course of their discussions with people-in-care.

Only negative feelings?

When people discuss a particular way of feeling, they often re-experience that feeling in talking about it. This could be a positive thing because a person might, for example, have experienced traumatic events like sexual abuse and have been denied a proper opportunity to express how he or she feels. In this kind of a situation, a person might meet a nurse, as part of an initial assessment, and use the opportunity to re-experience and discharge feelings that he or she has 'contained' for a long period of time. This kind of emotional discharge is often called 'catharsis'. Although the value of catharsis is under-researched,[12] some people-in-care talk about the relief that they feel as a consequence of 'getting things off their chest'. The possibility that people can gain such relief is another reason that nurses should focus on people's negative feelings, and encourage their expression as part of an assessment. However, there is a question of whether mental health nurses should only focus on people's negative feelings, rather than any other kind, during an assessment. The concept of catharsis is relevant to a consideration of this question.

Referring back to the idea of catharsis, a nurse could make an enquiry about a person's childhood and, in response, be told that it was an unhappy one. On making this reply, a person might also begin to look a little upset. The nurse might notice this and ask what is upsetting about the memory of childhood. In response, the person might become still more upset and tearfully recount memories of parental neglect or abuse. With each question the nurse asks, the conversation might focus in more detail on the person's unhappy memories and, in so doing, amplify the feelings that are associated with those memories in the present moment. As mentioned, the person might gain some relief from this and the nurse might gain some understanding. However, what this example suggests is that if nurses continuously attend to people's negative feelings then they might encourage people-in-care to do the same. In other words, if nurses only enquire into what is wrong with the way people are feeling this might prompt people to feel worse on an ongoing basis and therefore prove unhelpful.

In the light of this danger that nurses can *over-assess* negative feelings, they also need to pay attention to positive feelings. Nurses need to enquire into the detail of such feelings and the circumstances in which they occur. Such enquiry might serve to amplify people's experience of 'feeling better' and expand their awareness of their own ability to do things that are associated with feeling good. Furthermore, this kind of enquiry can help nurses to develop a broader understanding of people-in-care. This involves an awareness of people's strengths, abilities and successes as well as their problems, traumas and setbacks. In a range of professional fields, practitioners are increasingly cognisant of the need to recognize and encourage the positive achievements of people they help. This is reflected in the emergence of a range of strengths-based approaches like solution-focused brief therapy,[13–15] narrative therapy,[16] strengths-based case management[17,18] and positive psychology.[19,20]

> **Reflection**
>
> Recall a recent situation in which someone talked about 'feeling bad' and another situation in which someone talked about 'feeling better' or 'feeling good'. In each situation, what further details could you have sought about their feelings and why?

ASSESSING THOUGHTS

Thoughts consist of the words that people say to themselves in their own minds (what some cognitive–behavioural therapists call 'self-talk') and the images that pass through their minds. One reason that mental health nurses should assess what people think is that people's problems are often, in part, problems of thinking. If mental health nurses want to understand such problems then they need to give careful attention to what people are thinking and how this relates to how they are feeling.

Problems of thinking

Sometimes, people-in-care identify their thoughts as the principal feature of a problem. For example, a person might describe a nagging thought about the possibility of some kind of awful event occurring, which cannot be defused by recognition that such an event is unlikely. On the other hand, many people may not be so clear about the role of thoughts in their problems and may be preoccupied by their feelings or some other kind of issue. In both these scenarios, nurses should enquire into the specific details of thoughts that are involved in experiences that are problematic. This is because thoughts are an important element in any experience and so a full picture of any problem that a person experiences has to include the thoughts that were, or are, involved.

In addition, knowledge of what people are thinking at a given moment is often the key to making their feelings or behaviours intelligible. For example, it might become apparent as part of a discussion of a person's panic attacks that these experiences involve feeling a particular sensation (like a pain in the chest), interpreting that sensation as a symptom of an impending heart attack and then feeling increasingly panic-stricken. The person's panic becomes understandable when it is clear that he or she thinks that death is imminent from a heart attack that is signalled by chest pain. Furthermore, it might become apparent that the person has a systematic tendency to interpret bodily sensations (that are associated with anxiety) as a sign of serious illness and, still more widely, that he or she has a habit of expecting the worst possible things to happen.

So, problematic experiences can be particularly associated with nxegative thoughts that occur in given patterns. This insight is especially emphasized in the cognitive–behavioural therapy literature. One highly influential figure within that literature is Aaron Beck,[21,22] who detailed the various kinds of thoughts that are associated with particular emotional problems and who gave a number of examples of the patterned ways in which people can negatively interpret themselves, their experiences and their futures. One question that arises for nurses from all of this is how these negative thoughts can be identified.

Identifying negative thoughts

Of course, the simplest way to find out about negative thoughts is to ask people about them. Often, this involves focusing on a particular situation where a person experienced a problem and asking for details of what specifically he or she was thinking at the time. This is illustrated in the following example of an interaction:

Person-in-care:	I get these pains in my stomach and I get convinced that I have cancer.
Nurse:	Tell me about the most recent time you had these pains.
Person-in-care:	Just this morning, after breakfast, I was sat in this chair and feeling really uncomfortable in my stomach. I started to think that it was stomach cancer.
Nurse:	What exactly passed your mind, when you were thinking this?
Person-in-care:	I was thinking about dying.
Nurse:	Dying?
Person-in-care:	Yes, I imagined myself on my deathbed and I could see my family stood around me looking upset. Then I thought to myself that it's only a matter of time before this will be happening.
Nurse:	How much did you believe that thought?
Person-in-care:	Oh, I believed it.
Nurse:	Out of 100, how strongly would you rate this belief at the time that you were thinking it.
Person-in-care:	I'd say maybe 98%.

By focusing on a particular situation in which pains were experienced, the nurse was able to gain an impression of some of the actual thoughts that were associated with having cancer. However, it is not always as straightforward as this because people can sometimes have considerable difficulty in specifying these kinds of thoughts. Instead, people may talk in a generalized way in terms of what they were thinking about rather than what they were actually thinking. This can be because of difficulties to do with recall and the way that memories of an experience can quickly fade. Alternatively, people may find such memories distressing and may be reluctant to 'revisit' a disturbing thought. Or they might be concerned about what nurses might think of them if they were to acknowledge certain kinds of thoughts, especially ones that might be thought bizarre.

David Clark,[23] identified each of these potential difficulties in the recall of specific thoughts and has suggested some ways of helping people to overcome them. These include the use of role-play or imagery to relive a particular experience and therefore gain more immediate access to the thoughts that were involved. Alternatively, there are times when it seems apparent that a person's emotional state has suddenly changed and that, for example, he or she has become noticeably more anxious. On these occasions, it can be helpful to notice this emotional change and enquire into what the person is thinking at that moment. Nurses can certainly use either of these approaches as part of an assessment. Furthermore, nurses can suggest assignments in which people are asked to monitor their emotional state and to identify thoughts that are associated with negative feelings. These kinds of assignments, and their use by nurses, have been discussed by Phil Barker.[11] One approach involves people-in-care keeping a written record on a form that is divided into three columns.

- In the first column, a person describes the details of a situation in which negative feelings were experienced.
- In the second, the person identifies those negative feelings and rates their severity.
- And in the third column, the person specifies the thoughts that passed through his or her and mind and rates the extent to which these thoughts were believed.

Through these different methods, people can be assisted to notice and specify their negative thoughts. Something that nurses need to consider is the helpfulness of such assistance as part of an assessment.

The value of noticing thoughts

When a person is asked to notice negative thoughts that are associated with particular negative feelings, this can be helpful in at least two ways. First, the person may find it helpful to establish that there is a link between their thoughts and feelings. People can sometimes be bewildered by the way that they are feeling and they often view their problems as more explicable when they recognize the ways in which their thoughts shape their feelings. Second, nurses can devise ways to help people once they are aware of the particular thoughts, and patterns of thoughts, that are associated with particular difficulties. If, for example, nurses discover that a person is preoccupied by the possibility of a terrible event that, objectively, is unlikely to happen then it might follow that this

person can be helped by encouraging them to pay realistic attention to the probabilities of that event.

Although these positive consequences can stem from helping people to notice their negative thoughts and their relationship to negative feelings, it does not follow that this is the only kind of attention to thoughts that nurses should promote. Just as nurses can be too preoccupied with negative feelings, this can also be said about negative thoughts for the same reasons. In addition, some people can become quite demoralized by the idea that their thoughts are a 'problem' because they view thinking as an automatic thing that cannot be consciously controlled or changed. Partly for these reasons, it is often valuable for nurses to encourage people to attend to thoughts that are not part of their problems but that instead are a part of 'exceptions' to problems.

For example, it can be useful to ask people to identify what they were thinking on an occasion when they were coping most effectively. Such a request encourages people to focus on their experiences of success and can promote a belief in the possibility of further success. Another potentially useful enquiry that nurses can make about thoughts concerns what people *would be* thinking if their problems had disappeared. This can be helpful as part of a discussion of how people would like their lives to be different and might encourage them to selectively attend to signs that a preferred scenario is developing or that it has already developed in some sense. These kinds of enquiries, and their empowering possibilities, are usefully explored in solution-focused brief therapy literature[13–15,24,25] and that of related strengths-based approaches.[26,27]

> ## Reflection
>
> When asked about their thinking in a particular situation, people-in-care often describe what they were thinking *about* rather than the specific content of their thoughts. How can you help people to be specific in accounting for their thoughts?

ASSESSING BELIEFS

Beliefs are what people accept as true and incorporate implicit assumptions that people make as well as what they explicitly and consciously profess to believe. Nurses are often taught to respect people's beliefs but the implications of this idea are not always fully explored. One such implication is that mental health nurses need to identify which beliefs should be respected.

Beliefs to respect

Nurses have always made routine enquiries about people's religious beliefs. These enquiries are focused on some details of a person's religion such as the particular practices and outlooks that are involved and the extent to which the person observes them. One purpose of these enquiries is to provide information that will enable nurses to manifest respect for people's religious beliefs. And manifesting this kind of respect involves recognition that such beliefs are potentially important for a range of reasons. For one thing, people's religious beliefs can be an important factor in their resilience and ability to cope with adversity.[28] One reason for nurses to respect religious beliefs is that this can lend support to people's ways of coping.

Hence, as part of an assessment, nurses often enquire about people's religious beliefs because these can be a positive factor in people's ability to 'get by' in life. However, there are many other kinds of beliefs that are relevant to how people cope, so nurses have to be broad in their understandings of beliefs they should respect. For example, people have beliefs about themselves in relation to:

- their abilities to succeed
- their capacity to find ways of achieving their goals
- how much control they have over their lives
- how attractive they are to others, how loveable or valuable they are.

The importance of such beliefs is well recognized in the field of psychology where they are expressed in concepts like self-efficacy,[29] hope,[30] locus of control[31] and self-esteem.[32] Sometimes, the positive implications of these kinds of beliefs are clearly expressed by people-in-care, as the following interaction illustrates:

| Nurse: | You've told me that, over the years, you had a lot of torment from voices in your head and you had to deal with some really weird and awful things. Yet you've had very little contact with psychiatric services. |
| Person-in-care: | Yes, that's right. It's 18 years since I was in a psychiatric hospital. I don't really like having contact with doctors and nurses. I try to stay away from them. I don't need them. I can get by in life – I look after my flat, I pay my bills, I have a boyfriend, I don't hassle anybody and nobody really hassles me. I don't want to depend on psychiatrists and the drugs that they give me. |

As this conversation progressed further, it became increasingly clear that this person valued her own independence and believed in herself as a person that could 'stand on her own two feet'. This belief seemed justified in the sense that she was able to attend to the everyday aspects of living even though, from the nurse's perspective, she was experiencing psychosis for much of the time. Importantly, this ability to cope appeared to be founded on her belief that she could do so.

In this situation, then, the nurse was able to identify beliefs that 'worked' for a person-in-care. However, this person's beliefs involved a rejection of the nurse's conventional way of working that involved administering and monitoring medication as well as visiting people, in her caseload, on a frequent basis. Yet the nurse developed an approach to this person that showed respect for her beliefs. She kept a certain distance, signalled her availability and provided help with certain practical matters, like repairs to her council flat, when the person asked for it. Of course, the nurse could be criticized for failing to assert the value of medication to this person because of evidence that people with her diagnosis benefit from such medication. Yet there is also some evidence that people tend to benefit from care and treatment that accommodates their beliefs.

Priebe and Gruyters[33] undertook a small randomized controlled trial of day hospital treatment for people with a diagnosis of schizophrenia. They found that positive outcomes were more associated with tailoring treatment to people's wishes than with the provision of a standardized service. In other words, people made greater progress when they received help that was consistent with their belief about the kind of help that they needed.

Although this study was small and its results should be viewed with a degree of caution, it does highlight the possibility that a service that reflects a respect for people's beliefs may also be effective in meeting their needs. Hence, mental health nurses need to assess people's beliefs and understand their positive implications as a basis for such a service. However, beliefs can also have problematic implications and this also needs to be a focus for assessment by mental health nurses.

Problem beliefs

There are times when people hold beliefs that are manifestly false, but this in itself is not very significant. What is significant is a situation in which a false belief has problematic consequences, such as emotional distress or harmful behaviour. For example, a person might be terrified because of a false belief that their neighbours want to kill them. This belief might preoccupy them to the extent that they are monitoring the behaviour of their neighbours and tending to interpret their actions as indicative of their murderous intentions even though, objectively, they are just going about their daily business. In this kind of situation, people's beliefs are clearly a prominent part of their difficulties. Perhaps less obviously, people hold beliefs that are not blatantly untrue but are somewhat unrealistic. For example, a person might believe that decent parents never lose their temper or get impatient with their children. If this belief is strongly held, the person might be very self-critical for shouting at their children on a particular occasion and might therefore feel excessively guilty about falling below their standards of parental behaviour. Beck[21] observed a range of ways in which these kinds of unrealistic beliefs shape patterns of negative thinking that give rise to negative emotions.

Hence, people's beliefs are often an important aspect of the problems they experience. Both nurses and people-in-care therefore need to identify the beliefs that are associated with a problem in order to understand it. Furthermore, by identifying such beliefs, a basis can be created for challenging and changing them.

How to find out about beliefs

So, nurses and people-in-care often need to identify problematic beliefs as well as those that should be respected. Furthermore, such beliefs need to be explored in terms of their consequences, the extent to which they are firmly held and perhaps also their relationship to the person's wider biography. This can be relatively straightforward when the focus is on beliefs that the person consciously espouses. However, many important beliefs are implicit assumptions that people rarely or never reflect upon. In assessing these kinds of beliefs, it will probably be insufficient for a nurse to simply ask, for example, 'what are your beliefs about yourself?'. Instead, a nurse can often detect themes in a person's actions or in his or her accounts of various issues. One such theme is perfectionism and this can reflect a person's belief that he or she must always get things right and never fail. Of course, such themes can also often be identified by people-in-care themselves once they have the opportunity to reflect upon their own situation and upon the questions posed by nurses.

Reflection

Identify an occasion where you met a person-in-care whose beliefs 'worked' for him or her in some sense but did not fit with the expectations of professionals. How could this person's beliefs have been accommodated in a process of assessment?

SUMMARY

Assessment is a process in which mental health nurses and people-in-care are active participants. The idea that assessment is something that nurses do *on* or *to* people-in-care should therefore be discarded. Instead, the assessment of what people feel, think and believe should be approached with a view to the benefits that can be gained by both nurses and people-in-care from processes of *enquiry* and *discovery*. These processes are ongoing and are not confined to any 'stage' in a person's nursing care. Assessment is an ongoing endeavour and the information generated can only ever be provisional as people change

and new things are discovered. Indeed, the very notion of assessment should be a developing one and subject to continuing refinement and alteration.

- Assessment can be helpful in itself for people-in-care.
- Assessment is a never-completed process.
- Feelings, thoughts and beliefs should be assessed in specific detail.
- Feelings, thoughts and beliefs have negative and positive aspects that should be assessed.

REFERENCES

1. Asay TP, Lambert MJ. The empirical case for the common factors in therapy: quantitative findings. In: Hubble MA, Duncan BL, Miller SD (eds). *The heart and soul of change: what works in therapy.* Washington, DC: American Psychological Association, 1999: 33–56.

2. Steele K, Berman C. *The day the voices stopped: a memoir of madness and hope.* New York, NY: Basic Books, 2001.

3. Jamison KR. *An unquiet mind: a memoir of moods and madness.* London, UK: Picador, 1996.

4. Karp DA. *The burden of sympathy: how families cope with mental illness.* New York, NY: Oxford University Press, 2001.

5. Parkes CM. *Bereavement: studies of grief in adult life.* London, UK: Tavistock, 1972.

6. Bowlby J. *Attachment and loss.* Vol. III. Harmondsworth, UK: Penguin, 1980.

7. Wortman C, Silver RC. The myths of coping with loss. *Journal of Consulting and Clinical Psychology* 1989; **57** (3): 349–57.

8. Dent A. Supporting the bereaved: linking theory to practice. *Healthcare Counselling and Psychotherapy Journal* 2005; **5** (3): 16–9.

9. Karl GT. A new look at grief. *Journal of Advanced Nursing* 1987; **12**: 641–5.

10. Peplau H. Pattern interactions. In: O'Toole AW, Welt SR (eds). *Hildegard E Peplau, selected works: interpersonal theory in nursing.* London, UK: Macmillan, 1994.

11. Barker PJ. *Assessment in psychiatric and mental health nursing: in search of the whole person.* Cheltenham, UK: Stanley Thornes, 1997.

12. Kettles AM. Catharsis: an investigation of its meaning and nature. *Journal of Advanced Nursing* 1994; **20**: 368–76.

13. de Shazer S. *Clues: investigating solutions in brief therapy.* New York, NY: WW Norton, 1988.

14. Sharry J, Madden D, Darmody M. *Becoming a solution detective: a strengths-based guide to brief therapy.* London, UK: Brief Therapy Press, 2001.

15. O'Hanlon B, Rowan T. *Solution-oriented therapy for chronic and severe mental illness.* New York, NY: WW Norton, 2003.

16. White M, Epston D. *Narrative means to therapeutic ends.* New York, NY: WW Norton, 1990.

17. Rapp CA. *The strengths model: case management with people suffering from severe and persistent mental illness.* New York, NY: Oxford University Press, 1998.

18. Barry KL, Zeber JE, Blow FC. Effects of strengths model versus assertive community treatment model on participant outcomes and utilization: two-year follow-up. *Psychiatric Rehabilitation Journal* 2003; **26** (3): 268–77.

19. Seligman MEP. Positive psychology, positive prevention, and positive therapy. In: Snyder CR, Lopez SJ (eds). *Handbook of positive psychology*. New York, NY: Oxford University Press, 2002.

20. Snyder CR, Lopez SJ, Edwards LM *et al*. Measuring and labeling the positive and the negative. In: Lopez SJ, Snyder CR (eds). *Positive psychological assessment: a handbook of models and measures*. Washington, DC: American Psychological Association, 2003: 3–12.

21. Beck AT. *Cognitive therapy and the emotional disorders*. Harmondsworth, UK: Penguin, 1989.

22. Beck AT, Rush AJ, Shaw BF, Emery G. *Cognitive therapy of depression*. New York, NY: Guilford Press, 1979.

23. Clark DM. Anxiety states: panic and generalized anxiety. In: Hawton K, Salkovskis PM, Kirk J, Clark DM (eds). *Cognitive behaviour therapy for psychiatric problems: a practical guide*. Oxford: Oxford University Press, 1989.

24. Sharry J. *Solution-focused groupwork*. London, UK: Sage, 2001.

25. de Shazer S. *Words were originally magic*. New York, NY: WW Norton, 1994.

26. Duncan BL, Hubble MA, Miller SD. *Psychotherapy with 'impossible' cases: the efficient treatment of therapy veterans*. New York, NY: WW Norton, 1997.

27. Duncan BL, Miller SD. *The heroic client: doing client-directed, outcome-informed therapy*. San Francisco, CA: Jossey-Bass, 2000.

28. Canda ER. The significance of spirituality for resilient response to chronic illness: a qualitative study of adults with cystic fibrosis. In: Saleeby D (ed.). *The strengths perspective in social work practice*, 3rd edn. Boston, MA: Allyn and Bacon, 2002.

29. O'Brien KM. Measuring career self-efficacy: promoting confidence and happiness at work. In: Lopez SJ, Snyder CR (eds). *Positive psychological assessment: a handbook of models and measures*. Washington, DC: American Psychological Association, 2003.

30. Snyder CR. Hope theory: rainbows in the mind. *Psychological Inquiry* 2002; **13** (4): 249–75.

31. Fournier G, Jeanrie C. Locus of control: back to basics. In: Lopez SJ, Snyder CR (eds). *Positive psychological assessment: a handbook of models and measures*. Washington, DC: American Psychological Association, 2003.

32. Heatherton TF, Wyland C. Assessing self-esteem. In: Lopez SJ, Snyder CR (eds). *Positive psychological assessment: a handbook of models and measures*. Washington, DC: American Psychological Association, 2003.

33. Priebe S, Gruyters T. A pilot trial of treatment changes according to schizophrenic patients' wishes. *The Journal of Nervous and Mental Disease* 1999; **187** (7): 441–3.

SECTION
3
THE STRUCTURE OF CARE

Preface to Section 3

When ideas fail, words come in very handy

Goethe

The language of 'madness' has been around for centuries but has, in the past century, evolved from a limited number of forms of 'insanity' into several catalogues of 'mental disorder' or 'mental health problems'. Today, we talk more to one another, through more different media, than ever before. Not for nothing have educated people been described as the 'chattering classes'. However, it remains unclear to what extent all this 'communication' is meaningful, or merely an attempt to fill the emptiness of our lives.

Although we talk a lot about 'mental health problems' and have developed hundreds of ways of naming, or labelling, these phenomena, to what extent do we understand 'madness' better, than our ancestors?

Section 3 begins with a review of the history of psychiatric diagnosis, providing a summary of the most commonly used formats for classifying 'mental disorders'.

Of course, a diagnosis is a 'label', whether we admit this or not, and it can have a profound effect on the person labelled. Drawing upon some powerful stories, we discover something of the effect of living with a psychiatric diagnosis.

For over 30 years, the nursing process has provided the basis for defining the structure of care. Nursing diagnosis was proposed as an adjunct to medical diagnostic systems, aiming to broaden the approach to classifying human problems. Nursing diagnosis is not, however, without its problems, both methodological and practical and some of these are addressed here, as we ask 'what is the most appropriate way to frame problems of living, from a nursing perspective?'

The importance of recognizing that 'patients' are not lone individuals, but often are part of a complex social unit, to which nurses need to relate if they are to offer meaningful care. In the final chapter in this section we address the complexities of working collaboratively with families, the traditional social support group of the person in care. What part can families play in supporting the care planning process and how might nurses enlist the support of family members as part of the therapeutic effort?

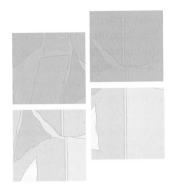

CHAPTER 15

Psychiatric diagnosis

Phil Barker*

'What's the use of their having names', the Gnat said, 'if they won't answer to them?' 'No use to *them*' said Alice, 'but it's useful to the people that name them, I suppose.'

Lewis Carroll
Alice Through the Looking Glass[1]

THE NEED FOR CLASSIFICATION

The language of disorder and therapy

Fifty years ago, the concept of 'mental health' was in its infancy, and the field of psychiatry was based, almost exclusively within 'mental hospitals'. Today, the concept of 'mental health' is used in an increasingly liberal fashion, especially in providing an umbrella concept for various health and social care services, and a variety of charitable and voluntary sector projects. Additionally, many sections of the general public read about and discuss 'mental health' in a manner that once would have been viewed as morbid or unseemly. At least at the level of *talk*, much has changed in 50 years.

However, if we consider how much *authority* any of this talk possesses, we would be obliged to say, 'not much'. The 'proper' language of 'mental health' remains distinctly medical. People may talk about suffering from a 'mental health problem', or their search for 'mental well-being', but few, if any, get help to address such problems or to attain such a state of well-being. Instead, these problems will be translated – or codified – as one 'mental illness' or 'mental disorder' or another. Their need

for 'mental well-being' will, at least in most professional settings, be translated into an 'outcome measure', the final destination on a 'clinical pathway'.

Certainly, there has been a 'softening' of the language, with the creation of intentionally vague expressions, such as *'mental health problems'* or *'mental health difficulties'*. However, like most other illustrations of political correctness, these expressions mean 'all things to all people', embracing everything from 'occupational stress' to 'suicidal despair'.

However, the shift towards more 'politically correct' ways of discussing people's 'mental' problems is irrelevant – at least at the level of access to services, whether publicly funded or privately purchased. To receive formal care and medical treatment, a person needs to be *diagnosed* with one of a range of psychiatric disorders. In most countries a person cannot receive 'treatment' – whether medication or psychotherapy – without first having a diagnosis. Or rather, insurance companies or other funding bodies will refuse to pay for the therapy without details of the 'condition' requiring treatment.

The situation appears less black and white in the voluntary sector, where people (rather than patients) are viewed primarily as needing help and social support as opposed to medical treatment. However, even here, the language of psychiatric medicine is all pervasive. One of the biggest mental health charities in England – Rethink – was originally called the National Schizophrenia Fellowship (NSF). It is still registered under that name, and its sister organization in Scotland still uses the NSF title. Rethink and NSF (Scotland) feature prominently details

*Phil Barker is a psychotherapist and Honorary Professor at the University of Dundee, UK.

of 'mental illness' and 'disorders' on their websites (www.rethink.org/about_mental_illness/mental_illnesses_ and_disorders/index.html), acknowledgement, perhaps, of the importance of such concepts for members of the public.

Reflection

Do members of the public think there is a difference between a 'mental health problem', a 'mental illness' and a 'mental disorder'?

The diagnosis of mental disorder

In simple terms, a 'mental disorder'[a] refers to any state where a person displays or experiences one or more emotional or behavioural problems that interfere with aspects of their everyday functioning. The states called 'mental disorders' have been described throughout the ages, but, with the increasingly successful treatment of many forms of serious physical illnesses, 'mental illness' has been identified as a more noticeable cause of human suffering. Increasingly, the public – especially in affluent countries – expects the medical profession to help it improve its quality of life in both the 'mental' as well as the physical terms. The growth of both drug and psychological therapies has also raised public expectations that the attainment of 'mental well-being' is not simply possible, but a human right. (Some organizations – such as the UK mental health charity MIND – promote a more responsible attitude: 'Good mental health isn't something you have, but something you do. To be mentally healthy you must value and accept yourself.' www.mind.org.uk/Information/Booklets/How+to/How +to+improve+your+mental+wellbeing.htm).

There is no universally accepted definition of mental disorder because different cultures have different ideas regarding what constitutes an 'abnormal' pattern of behaviour or 'mental state'. Here, psychiatry deviates sharply from conventional medical practice.

Signs of illness

To make a diagnosis, the physician observes the body through a physical examination. This may reveal unusual *signs* (e.g. raised blood pressure and clubbing of the fingers), which may or may not be accompanied by subjective observations made by the patient (*symptoms*) who complains of 'fatigue' or 'breathlessness'. These objective and subjective observations are then checked against the results of laboratory tests, radiological reports, etc. Few physicians would make a *clinical diagnosis* solely on the basis of symptomatic presentation, in the absence of manifest signs of disorder. As Szasz noted: 'The physician

observes signs not diseases; the latter is an inference drawn from the former'.[2,p.77] In linguistics, the *indexical* sign functions 'through a causal connection: smoke is a sign of fire and fever a sign of infectious disease. In the *iconic* class belong signs that acquire their sign function through similarity. For example, a photograph is a sign of the person in the picture'.[2,p.76]

The physician attempts to distinguish between *indexical* and *iconic* signs, 'by ascertaining whether the sign is "given" by a person or "given off" by him. Iconic signs resemble conventional signs: both are manufactured, more or less deliberately, by an agent, that is a person, whereas indexical signs are given off passively by an organism or thing'.[2,p.77] *Chronic fatigue syndrome (CFS)* is a contemporary example of a 'condition' that most patients believe to be a physical disorder. However, in the absence of manifest signs or supportive laboratory indications of pathology, many doctors describe CFS as a psychological problem.[3] The physician suspects that the 'signs' of illness are, however unwittingly, being manufactured by the patient, not emanating from the body itself.

Symptoms of distress

In psychiatry, there are no standard laboratory tests which might confirm the presence or absence of any form of 'mental disorder'. Even autopsies fail to demonstrate any pathology that might explain the 'mental disorder' previously experienced by or attributed to the deceased. (The reader might suggest that some forms of dementia present pathological findings at autopsy. However, it seems more accurate to define cerebrovascular dementia, for example, as a physical disorder, with some 'mental' symptoms, rather than a mental disorder per se.) Research involving positron emission tomography (PET) scans have suggested that specific brain abnormalities may be associated with schizophrenia and or bipolar disorder. The Mayo Clinic website even suggests that 'doctors may also use a PET scan to detect memory disorders and certain mental health disorders, such as schizophrenia and depression'. However, they add that: 'Such uses are currently being investigated' (www.mayoclinic. com/health/pet-scan/CA00052). Interesting though this research may be, it may only demonstrate how the brain changes as a function of life experience and behaviour. (The neuropsychologist Ian Robertson has likened the brain to a muscle. How we use it affects the way it grows and develops.[4])

A popular fallacy is that some forms of 'mental disorder' are the result of a 'chemical imbalance'. Depression and bipolar disorder are commonly attributed to this 'imbalance'. There has never been any evidence of such a 'chemical imbalance'. Indeed, if such an 'imbalance' had existed then a test would have been developed to

---

[a] I use scare quotes for the term 'mental disorder' throughout this chapter, as there is no significant agreement as to what this term means.

confirm the diagnosis. Rowe[5] noted that even the world-famous Institute of Psychiatry (IOP) at the Maudsley Hospital in London had bid 'farewell to chemical imbalance'. The IOP website (www.iop.kcl.ac.uk/apps/depression/introduction.aspx) stated that:

> Depression cannot be described any longer as a simple disorder of the brain, but rather as a series of behavioural and biological changes that span mind, brain, genes, body – and indeed affects both psychological and physical health.

The identification of all 'mental disorders' is the result of behavioural observation, by the diagnostician and self-observation, or reporting of symptoms, by the patient. (Physical examination of the patient and laboratory analysis of blood, tissue, etc., serve only to rule out a physical illness.) The UK National Health Service website NHS Direct (www.nhsdirect.nhs.uk/articles/article.aspx?articleId=302) advises new patients:

> When you first see a psychiatrist, they will assess your mental and general condition. This could involve asking you questions about your life and thoughts and taking information from other sources such as your GP, relatives, and social workers.

Despite the wide range of interview schedules, self-report measures, rating scales and other forms of 'psychosocial assessment', the core method involved in making a diagnosis is talking: professionals talk with the patient, or talk to other people about the patient. The resulting information forms the basis for making a judgement as to the presence/absence of 'mental disorder'. The most common form of such information are 'symptoms' – where the person reports a subjective experience of something 'abnormal' or 'distressing', or family and friends report their subjective feelings and thoughts about the patient and or the patient's behaviour.

Reflection

Think of someone you know, who has a specific psychiatric diagnosis.

How was that person diagnosed?

What other diagnoses were considered before a decision was made?

FORMS OF CLASSIFICATION IN MENTAL HEALTH

The two main forms of classification in psychiatry aim to distinguish groups of patients with the same or related clinical symptoms, as a first step towards the provision of appropriate care or treatment, or the prediction of the prospects of recovery for any individual member of that group. However, as McGorry et al.[6] have noted:

> Diagnosis in psychiatry increasingly struggles to fulfil its key purposes, namely, to guide treatment and to predict outcome.

The two forms of classification of psychiatric disorders discussed here are the *International statistical classification of disease and related health problems*[7] (ICD-10) published by the World Health Organization (WHO), and the *Diagnostic and statistical manual of mental disorders*[8] (DSM-IV), published by the American Psychiatric Association.

The ICD-10

The origins of the statistical classification of diseases dates from the nineteenth century, with important contributions made by the early medical statistician William Farr[9] (1807–1883) and later by Jacques Bertillon (1851–1922), who gave his name to the *Bertillon classification of causes of death*. Using Farr's principle of classifying diseases by site, Bertillon's classification was widely adopted in 1893 and further revised in 1900, 1910 and 1920 as the *International list of causes of death*.[10] In 1900, the French government arranged the first international conference for what became known as the *International classification of causes of death*. It was decided to revise the classification every 10 years, and responsibility for the classification was taken over by the WHO in 1948, at the time of the sixth revision, when *causes* of morbidity were included for the first time.

Renamed the *International classification of diseases and related health problems* the ICD is used to classify diseases and other health problems on health and vital records, such as death certificates and hospital records. The ICD enables the storage and retrieval of diagnostic information for both treatment and epidemiological purposes. WHO member states also use ICD to compile national mortality and morbidity statistics.

ICD-10 comprises 22 chapters, ranging from 'Infectious and parasitic diseases' to 'External causes of morbidity and mortality'. Chapter 5 addresses 'Mental and behavioural disorders'. Table 15.1 shows the list of 10 disorder groupings in the ICD classification, plus an 'unspecified' diagnostic category.

Each discrete disorder within each category is coded. The *Neurotic, stress-related and somatoform disorders* cover Codes F40 to F48. Within this grouping are, for example, *Generalised anxiety disorder* (F41.1) and *Depersonalization, derealization syndrome* (F48.1). Each disorder is defined in a short description, and – where appropriate – advised about exclusion criteria. *Generalised*

TABLE 15.1 ICD-10 mental and behavioural disorders

Code block	Type of disorder
F00–F09	Organic, including symptomatic, mental disorders
F10–F19	Mental and behavioural disorders due to psychoactive substance use
F20–F29	Schizophrenia, schizotypal and delusional disorders
F30–F39	Mood (affective) disorders
F40–F48	Neurotic, stress-related and somatoform disorders
F50–F59	Behavioural syndromes associated with physiological disturbances and physical factors
F60–F69	Disorders of adult personality and behaviour
F70–F79	Mental retardation
F80–F89	Disorders of psychological development
F90–F98	Behavioural and emotional disorders with onset usually occurring in childhood and adolescence
F99	Unspecified mental disorder

anxiety disorder is defined (www.who.int/classifications/apps/icd/icd10online/) as:

> Anxiety that is generalized and persistent but not restricted to, or even strongly predominating in, any particular environmental circumstances (i.e. it is 'free-floating'). The dominant symptoms are variable but include complaints of persistent nervousness, trembling, muscular tensions, sweating, light-headedness, palpitations, dizziness, and epigastric discomfort. Fears that the patient or a relative will shortly become ill or have an accident are often expressed.

The DSM-IV

The *Diagnostic and statistical manual of mental disorders DSM-IV is* probably the most widely consulted classification system in psychiatry. The DSM's dedicated focus on 'mental disorders' has ensured its popularity among not only psychiatrists, but other clinicians and researchers from a wide range of disciplines in the mental health field. The DSM provides a system for the classification of all 'mental disorders', including differential diagnosis, with a coding system for each 'disorder' for record-keeping purposes. The manual is designed to:

* guide diagnosis in clinical practice;
* facilitate research and improve communication among clinicians and researchers; and
* serve as an educational tool for teaching psychopathology.[11]

Although used widely among different professional groups, the authors of the DSM refer repeatedly throughout

the manual to the 'Cautionary statement'. This includes the following 'warning':

> The specified diagnostic criteria for each mental disorder are offered as guidelines for making diagnoses, because it has been demonstrated that the use of such criteria enhances agreement among clinicians and investigators. *The proper use of these criteria requires specialized clinical training that provides both a body of knowledge and clinical skills* [emphasis added][11,p.xxxvii]

This represents a clear reminder to the reader that the 'manual' is not intended for 'casual' use.

Reflection

Consider your own education in relation to psychiatric diagnosis.

Who taught you about diagnosis and classification?

Which classification systems were used in the teaching programme?

History of the DSM

The origins of the DSM, like the ICD, lie in the mid-nineteenth century, when the US Census department began to count the number of people detained in asylums. In 1849 the idea of developing a uniform system for classifying 'madness' was proposed at a meeting of the Association of Medical Superintendents of American Institutions for the Insane (which became the American Medico-Psychological Association in 1892 and the American Psychiatric Association (APA) in 1921). Similar proposals were made at the beginning of the twentieth century, but it was not until 1918 that formal data were collected, this information having been made a requirement by the Federal Bureau of the Census.[12] By 1950 the compilation of statistics had become the responsibility of the National Institute of Mental Health established in 1949. The first version of the DSM was published by the APA in 1952. (Table 15.2 details the revisions to the DSM.)

DSM-I (1952)

At the end of the Second World War, four different classification systems were in competition: the original system developed by the APA in 1932 and systems developed separately by the US Army, Navy and Veteran's Administration.[13] Military psychiatrists were dissatisfied with the existing diagnostics system, developed by the APA. In their view this under-represented 'less severe and psychosomatic disorders'. The first version of the DSM was heavily influenced by Adolf Meyer's 'psychobiological' approach. Meyer understood 'mental illness' as a reaction of the personality to psychological,

TABLE 15.2 Development of the diagnostic and statistical manual of mental disorders

Year	Version	Length	Number of disorders
1952	DSM- I	130	106
1968	DSM -II	134	182
1980	DSM- III	494	265
1987	DSM- III-R	567	292
1994	DSM-IV	886	297
2000	DSM-IV-TR	943	297

TABLE 15.3 DSM-IV five levels (axes) of psychiatric diagnosis

Axis I	Clinical disorders: e.g. *anxiety disorders, mood disorders, schizophrenia and other psychotic disorders, developmental and learning disorders*
Axis II	Underlying *personality disorders and mental retardation*
Axis III	*General medical conditions and physical disorders* including, for example, those diseases or disorders that might affect mood or functioning
Axis IV	*Psychosocial* and *environmental factors* contributing to the disorder: e.g. family, educational, housing, financial, social environment or occupational problems; and other problems (war, disaster etc).
Axis V	*Global Assessment of Functioning* (GAF): aimed at developing and evaluating the effects of a treatment plan. Three other specific 'global' scales measure 'Social and Occupational Functioning', 'Defensive Functioning' and 'Relational Functioning'

social and biological factors. Meyer's[14] concept of 'reactions' was used to define most of the 'mental disorders' in this first edition.

DSM-II (1968)

The second version of the manual aimed to have no dominant theoretical framework and was designed to be compatible with the mental disorders section of the ICD-8. Although this version moved closer to a Kraepelinian approach to diagnosis, symptoms were not defined in any great detail for each of the disorders. Instead, a disorder was seen as reflecting broad underlying conflicts or maladaptive reactions to life problems, illustrating the continued influence of psychoanalysis.

DSM-III (1980)

Work began on this revision in 1973 and introduced a major shift away from the first two editions. First of all, the APA introduced detailed descriptions of symptoms, removing all reference to possible aetiological factors. In abandoning the whole concept of 'cause' DSM-III moved firmly in the phenomenological arena. This version also abandoned the distinction between 'neurosis' and 'psychosis', the concept of 'neurosis' being dropped altogether. Taking the place of this distinction was the *multi-axial system* of symptom evaluation (see Table 15.3).

The diagnostic criteria used in DSM-III were influenced greatly by the Research diagnostic criteria[15] and by the leadership of Robert Spitzer, who in addition to reinforcing the reliability of diagnosis, wanted to define mental disorders as a subset of medical disorders. The DSM Task Force decided on a much vaguer definition: each mental disorder was conceptualized as a 'clinically significant behavioral or psychological syndrome'.

Two significant developments occurred with DSM-II.

1 The diagnosis of homosexuality as a mental disorder had been withdrawn from DSM-II in 1973. Although there continues to be dispute over the reasons for this[16] the consensus is that the APA decided to withdraw homosexuality from its classification following sustained lobbying of its annual conference by gay rights activists.[17] The rest, as the saying goes, is history. Homosexuality, once integral to the psychoanalytic construction of 'mental illness' was 'declassified' and became 'normal behaviour'.

2 The so-called 'St Louis group' of psychiatrists had developed 'research diagnostic criteria' for schizophrenia. They were mainly identifying 'markers' for schizophrenia that would allow the disease to be studied accurately at other research sites. As a result, a tool developed originally for research purposes became a diagnostic method applied to all mental disorders. The proponents of this change in emphasis were all biological psychiatrists, keen to dismiss all terms and theories associated with hypothetical or explanatory concepts from the manual. This shift from an *explanatory* to a *descriptive* (phenomenological) approach continues to the present day, and often is called the 'neo-Kraepelinian revolution'.[18] The term *empirical* also began to be used, emphasizing the reliance on experience or experiment alone, without the need for theories or hypotheses.[19] This move towards a more detailed, reliable means of achieving a diagnosis was undoubtedly influenced by the scandal that followed the publication of the Rosenhahn study,[20] where he demonstrated that psychiatrists could not discriminate between 'real' patients and 'pseudopatients' who told the admitting doctor that they heard the sounds 'thud' and 'crunch'.[21] Rosenhahn's study appeared to demonstrate the inherent weakness of DSM-II, where individual doctors made diagnostic judgements based more on theoretical ideology than empirical observation of specific diagnostic criteria.

DSM-IV (1994)

Under Spitzer's leadership, the task force reviewed DSM-II in the mid-1980s, and in 1987 published a revision (DSM-III-R). This included the renaming and reorganization of categories, and changes to some diagnostic criteria.

Controversial diagnoses such as *pre-menstrual dysphoric disorder* and *masochistic personality disorder* were considered but eventually rejected.

By the early 1990s, most DSM-III diagnoses were supported by a growing body of published studies involving their use. These publications were reviewed as preparation for the publication of DSM-IV. The National Institute of Mental Health, along with two drug and alcohol abuse agencies, supported field trials of DSM-IV, comparing the diagnostic criteria published in DSM-III, DSM-III-R and ICD-10 with the new diagnostic criteria proposed for DSM-IV. These trials recruited subjects from different ethnic and cultural backgrounds as part of a concern for cross-cultural relevance. This phase of development also included much closer cooperation with the WHO and the designers of ICD-10.

The most recent version of DSM-IV (the 'text revision' published in 2000 – DSM-IV-TR) continued this emphasis on gaining widespread approval. The APA acknowledged that 'more than 1000 people (and numerous professional organizations) have helped in preparation of this document'[11,p.xix].

The multi-axial system

In 1980 DSM-III introduced a new system of five 'axes'. This *multi-axial system* was designed to provide a more comprehensive picture of the patient, especially where complex mental disorders were concerned or where more than one disorder could be attributed. This multi-axial system was also meant to promote use of the *biopsychosocial* model across all settings in which DSM might be used. Reference to Engel's original alternative to the traditional 'medical model', was clearly significant, showing that DSM-IV-TR *did not* support any specific 'school' or theoretical tradition regarding the causes of mental disorders. The five axes and the diagnostic categories, therefore, represent no particular theory about the sources or fundamental nature of mental disorders, and at least in principle, could be used by clinicians and researchers of any theoretical persuasion.

The atheoretical nature of DSM-IV-TR also carried legal implications, especially in the forensic context. The APA note that the questions that concern the law are not the same as those raised concerning a clinical diagnosis. The diagnostic categories within DSM-IV do not meet the forensic standards required to define 'mental defect' or 'mental disability'. DSM-IV-TR advises legal professionals specifically *against* the use of DSM diagnostic categories in making any decisions about a person's criminal responsibility or competence.

The five axes of DSM-IV are shown in Table 15.3. A clinical diagnosis is attributed under Axis I. The other axes identify underlying 'personality disorder' or 'mental retardation' (II), concurrent general medical conditions (III), the possible effects of psychosocial or environmental factors (IV) and finally the overall 'functioning' of the person is measured (V).

Diagnostic categories

Within Axis I the range of possible clinical disorders are represented by 15 categories (see Box 15.1). All these categories are symptom based, what the manual describes as 'criteria sets with defining features'.

Each diagnostic category features: a coding (e.g. 300.62); a general description of the disorder; a detailed list of 'symptoms' or presenting features, observable to the diagnostician or others; a list of 'associated features'; and a list of disorders to assist 'differential diagnosis'. All categories include disorders NOS (not otherwise specified). The APA noted that:

> Because of the diversity of clinical presentation, it is impossible for the diagnostic nomenclature to cover every possible situation. For this reason, each diagnostic class has at least one Not Otherwise Specified (NOS) category and some classes have several NOS categories. Four situations in which an NOS diagnosis may be appropriate are:

1 the symptom picture is atypical;
2 the symptoms lead to a symptom pattern not included in the DSM-IV;
3 there is uncertainty about aetiology (i.e. whether the disorder is caused by a medical condition, a substance or is primary);
4 there is insufficient opportunity for complete data collection.'[11,p.4]

Box 15.1: Axis I: clinical disorders, other conditions that may be a focus of clinical attention

Disorders usually first diagnosed in infancy, childhood, or adolescence
Delirium, dementia, and amnestic and other cognitive disorders
Mental disorders due to a general medical condition
Substance-related disorders
Schizophrenia and other psychotic disorders
Mood disorders
Anxiety disorders
Somatoform disorders
Factitious disorders
Dissociative disorders
Sexual and gender identity disorders
Eating disorders
Sleep disorders
Impulse control disorders not elsewhere classified
Adjustment disorders

Illustration

In some 'disorders' the classification is complex. For example, the 'Mood disorders' category includes:

- Major depressive disorder single episode
- Major depressive disorder recurrent
- Dysthymic disorder
- Bipolar I disorder
- Bipolar II disorder
- Cyclothymia
- Mood disorder due to medical condition
- Substance-induced mood disorder
- Mood disorder NOS.

To allocate, for example, a diagnosis of 'bipolar I disorder' the diagnostician must have evidence of at least one 'manic' or 'mixed' episode, but there may be evidence of episodes of 'hypomania' or 'major depressive disorder'. Consequently, the distinct diagnostic codes specify:

- Bipolar I: single manic episode
- Bipolar I: most recent episode hypomanic
- Bipolar I: most recent episode manic
- Bipolar I: most recent episode mixed
- Bipolar I: most recent episode depressed
- Bipolar I: most recent episode unspecified.

The 'biopsychosocial model'

DSM-IV acknowledges the importance of the 'biopsychosocial model', attributed to the influence and work of George Engel.[22] In the 30 years since Engel first made his radical proposal, much has changed. Borrell-Carrió et al.[23] noted:

> Since Engel first proposed the biopsychosocial model, two new intellectual trends have emerged that could make it even more robust. First, we can move beyond the problematic issue of mind–body duality by recognizing that knowledge is socially constructed. To some extent, such categories as 'mind' or 'body' are of our own creation. They are useful to the extent that they focus our thinking and action in helpful ways (e.g., they contribute to health, well-being, and efficient use of resources), but when taken too literally, they can also entrap and limit us by creating boundaries that need not exist. By maintaining what William James[24] called 'fragile' categories, we can alter or dispose of categories as new evidence accumulates and when there is a need to engage in flexible, out-of-the-box thinking.

Despite its move towards use of the 'biopsychosocial' model, arguably the key weakness of DSM-IV-TR is its continued medicalization of problems of living as 'mental disorders'.[5] DSM's use of terms like 'psychopathology', 'mental illness', 'differential diagnosis' and 'prognosis' all derive from medical practice. This is of note, given the criticisms of the 'medical model' in psychiatric practice, especially in the latter part of the twentieth century, and the rise of alternative theoretical and philosophical conceptualizations of 'mental illness/disorder'.

In his proposal of an alternative model of 'interactive dualism', the Australian psychiatrist McLaren largely dismissed the biopsychosocial model:

> Since the collapse of the 19th century models (psychoanalysis, biologism and behaviourism), psychiatrists have been in search of a model which integrates the psyche and the soma. So keen has been their search that they embraced the so-called 'biopsychosocial model' without ever bothering to check its details. If, at any time over the last three decades, they had done so, they would have found it had none. This would have forced them into the embarrassing position of having to acknowledge that modern psychiatry is operating in a theoretical vacuum.[25]

Reflection

Which classification system is used in the services in which you have worked?
In what way does diagnostic classification help (or hinder) you in your work as a nurse?

CRITIQUES OF DIAGNOSTIC CLASSIFICATION

The criticisms of the role and function of diagnostic classification in psychiatry are multiple and wide-ranging.[26–30] They include the following, commonly observed, criticisms.

- Diagnosis reduces people to one-dimensional sources of 'data' and obstructs any attempt to care for the 'whole person'.
- By medicalizing complex problems of human living, a diagnosis of 'mental disorder' perpetuates social stigma.
- The use of symptom-based criteria, in the absence of any classic 'signs' of disease or disorder, has resulted in a seemingly endless multiplication of the original number of 'mental disorders'. Within 30 years the DSM has grown from 134 to 943 pages.
- The politics, and inherent values, of the criteria for inclusion and/or exclusion of disorders is self-evident. 'Post-traumatic-stress disorder' was included following lobbying from trauma victims, and homosexuality was dropped following lobbying from gay rights groups. A similar scenario could never be envisaged in relation to genuine physical illnesses and disorders.
- Diagnostic criteria within both DSM and ICD imply, but do not state directly, the notion of psychological 'well-being'. However, the extent to which so-called

'disorders' represent unexceptional deviations from the 'normal' state of well-being, is not addressed. The idea of retrospectively (and blindly) 'diagnosing' famous people from the past began with Freud and his 'analysis' of Leonardo da Vinci.[31] Today, the absurd practice of 'genius/celebrity profiling' has become commonplace.[32]

- The current classification systems display an obvious bias in terms of the kind of disorders addressed. Despite the obvious presence of anger, hostility and aggression as sources of social unrest and interpersonal harm, only one DSM-IV disorder explicitly addresses this area (intermittent explosive disorder). By contrast, entire categories are devoted to 'depression' and 'anxiety'.

- Perhaps of greatest importance is the effect of diagnostic classification in the 'medicalization of everyday life'.[11] The implicit biological underpinnings of the diagnosis of 'mental disorders', expressed through the widespread borrowing of medical language from general medicine, contributes greatly to the popular belief that problems of human life can be solved by taking medication.

ALTERNATIVES TO DSM AND ICD

The holistic model

The year after the publication of DSM-IV Ross and Pam took the whole diagnostic exercise to task, arguing that it:

> ... arises from the reductionist philosophy of late twentieth century North American psychiatry ... psychiatric disorders are largely treated as separate entities, consistent with the hypothesis that there is one gene for schizophrenia, a gene for depression, and another separate gene for alcoholism. Although there are groupings of disorders, and various exclusion rules based on the pressure of other disorders, the main purpose of the system is to sort patients out into discrete categories. The way in which diagnoses are placed in categories, rather than being phenomenologically based, is highly determined by historical artefacts, the residual effects of Freudian theory, and political turf disputes among different subcommittees.[33]

The American community psychiatrist, Dan Fisher (www.power2u.org/who.html) has used his own experiences – and diagnosis of schizophrenia – to promote a more holistic approach to mental disorders. He wrote:

> I do not find the neurobiological theory of mental illness as helpful to my recovery because it deprives me of any sense of self-determination and responsibility. When I think that I am a group of chemical reactions,

> each with its own scheme and plan, I feel dehumanised and powerless. I feel that I am thinking, feeling and acting at the whim of those chemicals, not through any effort or responsibility of my own.[34]

The model of recovery developed by Fisher and his colleagues at the National Empowerment Center in Boston (www.power2u.org/articles/recovery/expert_interview.html) represents a distinct alternative to the 'pathological' approach implied, if not actually accounted for, by DSM-IV. Fisher and his group set out a bold strategy focused, first of all, on *understanding people*, rather than 'diagnosing patients'. Such understanding is integral to the development of the different forms of support that people might need to address the problems in their lives.

The essential or perspectival model

Arguably the most complex alternative model emerged from the medical curriculum at Johns Hopkins University. This model identifies four broad 'essences' or perspectives that can be used to identify the distinctive characteristics of mental disorders. The authors argue that the present *categorical classification* obscures these 'essences'.[35]

Four discrete 'perspectives' are included in the Johns Hopkins model: disease, dimensions, behaviours and life story. According to Kaminsky *et al.*,[36] this model has been

> the backbone of the resistance, resilience, and recovery paradigm. Briefly, the Hopkins' 'perspectives' provide a framework for understanding the essential natures of and substrates underlying clinical disorders, trauma related and otherwise. Rather than adopt one worldview for elucidating psychopathology, the Hopkins approach employs four distinct but overlapping perspectives. Each of these assessment viewpoints drives a set of exploratory propositions.

These 'overlapping perspectives' address:

- *what* the person 'has' (biologically based disease and physical illness);
- *who* a person 'is' (graded dimensions of temperament and disposition);
- *what* a person 'does' (purposeful, goal-directed behaviour);
- *what* a person has 'encountered' (their life story and the meaning that has been given to those experiences).[36]

In the Johns Hopkins model, each 'perspective' has its own approach to treatment: the *disease* perspective seeks to cure or prevent biological disorders; the *dimensional* perspective attempts to reinforce any constitutional weaknesses; the *behavioural* perspective seeks to address any problematic behaviours helping patients find alternatives; and the life story perspective offers help in 'rescripting' a person's life narrative.

SUMMARY

Classification of people and their 'mental disorders', in one form or another, has been around for a long time. The medical language of diagnosis is now firmly established as a part of everyday conversation. To impress the laity, physicians began to adapt Greek or Latin words to describe the body and its various diseases. As Szasz has noted:

> they called inflammation of the lung 'pneumonia' and kidney failure 'uraemia'. The result is that people now think that any Greco-Roman word ending in *ia* – or with the suffix *philia* or *phobia* – is a bona fide disease. This credulity would be humorous if it were not tragic.[11,p.101]

A century ago there were only a handful of forms of 'insanity'. Today, there are literally hundreds of forms of 'mental disorder'. In general medicine, diagnosis provides an economical means of communicating clearly and precisely about the presence of *actual* bodily disease, or the presence of actual organic or functional disorder. Medical diagnosis gives a name to a process that is evident within the body itself.

The 'madness classification industry' associated with psychiatry is quite different. Psychiatric diagnoses represent a naming of complex patterns of *behaviour* and or *subjective experiences*, which are 'given off' – or *exhibited* by people, interpersonally or socially. The very same behaviour, occurring or exhibited in private or alone, is excluded from diagnostic consideration. For example, masturbation – once viewed as a key cause of 'insanity' – is a completely amoral act when practised in private, but may be classed as a criminal offence if performed in a public space. More importantly, a person who seeks sexual gratification by rubbing himself against another person in public might be prosecuted for indecent assault, but could also be *excused* on the grounds of suffering from the 'mental disorder' of *frotteurism* (DSM-IV – 302.89).

As noted earlier, *homosexuality* was long considered not simply a vice, but a serious form of 'mental illness'. Now, it is merely a 'sexual preference'. Szasz has noted that the practice of 'celibacy' long recognized by the Catholic Church as a:

> virtue, a 'gift from God', even though celibacy is at least as 'abnormal' as homosexuality, which the church continues to define as a grievous sin – an 'intrinsic evil'. ... Regardless of how unnatural or socially destructive a pattern of sexual behaviour might be, if the church declares it to be virtuous – as with celibacy or abstinence from non-procreative sexual acts – psychiatrists do not classify it as a disease. Thus a religion's moral teachings shape what is ostensibly a scientific judgement.[11,p.96]

This is another clear illustration of the 'politics of diagnosis'. Szasz adds another, pointed example:

> Psychiatrists diagnose the person who eats too much as suffering from 'bulimia' and the person who eats too little as suffering from 'anorexia nervosa'. Similarly the person who has too much sex suffers from a 'sex addiction', while the person who shows too little interest in sex suffers from 'sexual aversion disorder'. Yet psychiatrists do not consider celibacy a form of mental illness; celibate persons are not said to suffer from 'anerotica nervosa'.[11,p.96]

On one level, DSM and ICD are benign – merely bureaucratic – systems for classifying the states people find themselves to be in, or are viewed by others as occupying. Classification 'opens the door' to offers of help, care or treatment for the said 'mental disorder'.

However, the situation becomes malignant when the person does not seek such a classification, or especially when the person wishes to avoid such care or treatment. Those who deny that they have a 'mental disorder' are either 'in denial' or 'lack insight'. The more they protest, the more 'seriously' their 'mental disorder' is viewed.

Thirty years ago, the American psychiatrist Loren Mosher established an innovative and highly successful project for people with a diagnosis of 'schizophrenia'. When he met with the 'patient' for the first time, he did not engage in the complex, diagnostic interviewing process in which he had been trained (at that time DSM-III). Instead, Mosher[37] said:

I asked each patient a simple series of questions:

- Why are you here?
- What happened in your life that resulted in your coming (or being brought) to a psychiatric ward?
- What needs to be done to 'fix' the situation, and how can we help you with the 'fixing' process?

All those involved in the mental health field, but perhaps especially nurses, might ask themselves *what else*, apart from Mosher's three questions, do they need to ask a person – at least for 'starters' – to begin the helping/caring process. They also might ask:

> How would a diagnostic interview be 'better' *for the person concerned*, than Mosher's simple, personal approach?

REFERENCES

1. Kirk SA, Kutchins H. *The Selling of DSM: the rhetoric of science in psychiatry* [Cited in the Preface]. New York, NY: Aldine de Gruyter, 1992.

2. Szasz TS. Hysteria as language. In: *The medicalization of everyday life*. Syracuse, NY: Syracuse University Press, 2007: 77.

3. Fulford KWM. Commentary. *Advances in Psychiatric Treatment* 2002; **8**: 359–63.

4. Robertson I. *Mind sculpture: your brain's untapped potential.* London, UK: Bantam Books, 2000.

5. Rowe DA. Farewell to chemical imbalance. *Openmind* 2007; **143**: 15.

6. McGorry PD, Hickie IB, Yung AR *et al.* Clinical staging of psychiatric disorders: a heuristic framework for choosing, earlier, safer and more effective interventions. *Australian and New Zealand Journal of Psychiatry* 2006; **40**: 616–22.

7. World Health Organization. *The international classification of disease and related health problems – 10th revision.* Geneva: WHO, 1992.

8. American Psychiatric Association. *Diagnostic and statistical manual of mental disorders,* 4th edn, *Text revision (DSM-IV-TR).* Washington, DC: APA, 2004.

9. Dunn PM. Dr William Farr of Shropshire (1807–1883): obstetric mortality and training. *Archives of Disease in Childhood. Fetal and Neonatal Edition* 2002: **87**: 67–9.

10. World Health Organization. History of the development of the ICD. In: World Health Organization. *International statistical classification of diseases and related health problems. 10th revision,* Vol 2, Ch 6. Geneva: WHO, 1993.

11. American Psychiatric Association. *Diagnostic and statistical manual of mental disorders,* 4th edn, *Text revision (DSM-IV-TR)* Washington, DC, APA, 2004.

12. Grob GN. Origins of DSM-I: a study in appearance and reality. *American Journal of Psychiatry* 1991; **148**: 421–31.

13. Figert E. *Women and the ownership of PMS.* Hawthorne, NY: Aldine de Gruyter, 1996: 29.

14. Mazure CM, Druss BG. A historical perspective on stress and psychiatric illness. In: Mazure CM (ed.) *Does stress cause psychiatric illness?* Arlington, VA: American Psychiatric Publishing Inc, 1995.

15. Williams JB, Spitzer RL. Research diagnostic criteria and DSM III: an annotated comparison. *Archives of General Psychiatry* 1982; **39**: 1283–9.

16. Spitzer RL, The diagnostic status of homosexuality in DSM-III: a reformulation of the issues. *American Journal of Psychiatry,* 1981; **138** (2): 210–5.

17. Boorse C. Homosexuality reclassified. *The Hastings Center Report* 1982; **June**: 42.

18. Compton WM, Guze SB. The neo-Kraepelinian revolution in psychiatric diagnosis. *European Archives of Psychiatry and Clinical Neuroscience* 2005; **245** (Special Issue 4/5): 196–201.

19. Kirk SA, Kutchins H. *The selling of DSM: the rhetoric of science in psychiatry.* New York, NY: Aldine de Gruyter, 1992.

20. Rosenhahn T. On being sane in insane places. *Science* 1973; **179**: 250–8.

21. Barker P. *Assessment in psychiatric and mental health nursing: in search of the whole person,* 2nd edn. Cheltenham, UK: Nelson Thornes, 2004: 290–1.

22. Engel G. The need for a new medical model: a challenge for biomedicine. *Science* 1977; **196**: 129–36.

23. James W. *Pragmatism: a new name for some old ways of thinking.* New York, NY: Longmans Green, 1907.

24. Borrell-Carrió F, Suchman AL, Epstein RM. The biopsychosocial model 25 years later: principles, practice, and scientific inquiry. *Annals of Family Medicine* 2004; **2**: 576–82.

25. McLaren N. Interactive dualism as a partial solution to the mind-brain problem for psychiatry. *Medical Hypotheses* 2006; **66**: 1165–73.

26. Pilgrim D. Psychiatric diagnosis: more questions than answers. *The Psychologist* 2000; **13**: 302–5.

27. Boyle M. *Schizophrenia: a scientific delusion?,* 2nd edn. London, UK: Routledge, 2002.

28. Kutchins H, Kirk SA. *Making us crazy: DSM – the psychiatric bible and the creation of mental disorders.* New York, NY: The Free Press, 1997.

29. Bentall RP. *Madness explained: psychosis and human nature.* London, UK: Penguin, 2003.

30. Caplan PJ, Cosgrove C. *Bias in psychiatric diagnosis.* New York, NY: Rowman and Littlefield, 2004.

31. Anderson WV. *Freud, Leonardo da Vinci and the vulture's tail.* London, UK: Karnac Books, 2001.

32. Gold K. The high-flying obsessives. *Guardian* 12 December 2000.

33. Ross CA, Pam A. *Pseudoscience in biological psychiatry: blaming the body.* New York, NY: John Wiley & Sons, 1995.

34. Fisher D. Hope, humanity and voice in recovery from mental illness. In: Barker P, Campbell P, Davidson B (eds). *From the ashes of experience: reflections on madness, survival and growth.* London, UK: Whurr, 2000: 127–33.

35. McHugh PR, Slavney PR. *The perspectives of psychiatry,* 2nd edn. Baltimore, MD: The Johns Hopkins University Press, 1998.

36. Kaminsky M, McCabe OL, Langlieb AM, Everly GS. An evidence-informed model of human resistance, resilience, and recovery: the Johns Hopkins' outcome-driven paradigm for disaster mental health services. *Brief Treatment Crisis Intervention* 2007; **7**: 1–11.

37. Mosher LR, Hendrix V. *Soteria: through madness to deliverance.* Philadelphia, PA: Xlibris Corporation, 2004; 298.

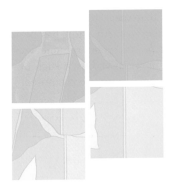

CHAPTER 16

Psychiatric diagnosis: living the experience

Yvonne Hayne*

INTRODUCTION

Paralympian Paul Rosen had spent years intensely labouring in training to participate in the 2006 Paralympic Games in Turin, Italy. All that had paid off in one of the proudest moments of his life, as bearer of the prized gold medal. But then, 'in the blink of an eye …' it vanished! While out celebrating, Paul had placed the medal on a table, 'turned around to get something, turned back and the medal was gone'.[1] Disconsolate in his search for the cherished gold icon, only the counsel of his wife brought him a measure of peace. 'The medal is inside you', she insisted, 'and that will never disappear'. Unwittingly she had declared the strength of symbolism and the location of meaning.

Representations can embody enormous power. For Paul, that power was encased in a gold medal. Other representations might reside in official statements such as, 'I now pronounce you husband and wife!' or, 'Guilty as charged!' Medical terminology can be especially consequential, as it was for Jeff who 'trembled' at the words of his diagnosis.[a] Jeff describes the immense power of the label handed him that he had long successfully evaded. Five years into treatment, still Jeff had no recall of having ever been directly told:

> My mother was told, and my wife was told. And even some of my friends were told. And I learned about what I had through them; in kind of round-about ways. But in all those years no explanation about what it was ever came from a medical person. They never actually sat down and talked to me about my diagnosis.

But the distinct moment did finally happen, precipitated by an incident that made *it* evident:

> I decided to seek 'forgiveness' from my student loans and that required medical forms to be filled out. I was in the doctor's office and I watched him write it down there. Then he handed the form back to me. And there it was in black and white: 'paranoid schizophrenia'! I looked at it and … everything else sort of disappeared. Then after a time … I picked up the pen and wrote my own name on the form where I needed to sign.

In that moment, the actuality of *it* on paper forced a new experience for Jeff. Now, he had a *diagnosis*! It was the instant of a *'some thing'* to be reckoned with, and that reckoning was distinctly different from that required of the illness itself.

DIAGNOSIS AS 'SCIENTIZED' SELF

The language of science as an existential reality 'has so permeated our everyday living that our human existence, our

*Yvonne Hayne is a member of the faculty of nursing at the university of Calgary, Calgary, Alberta, Canada. She has extensive history in nursing instruction, preceded by diverse experiences in general-duty nursing, public health and nursing administration. Her main interests are in psychiatry and mental health care, and her scholarship is founded on a spectrum of nursing related to that specialty.

[a] This chapter incorporates findings from a phenomenological study conducted by the author. Participant drawings, quotations and anecdotal notations (per pseudonyms) are directly cited from Hayne Y. *To be diagnosed – the experience of persons with chronic mental illness*. University of Alberta, Edmonton, AB, Canada: Unpublished Dissertation, 2001.

experience of the world and of our selves, has become sci-entized'.[2] Nowhere, perhaps, is this more pronounced than in the areas of health and illness where personal profiles are graphed by bleeps that bounce across screens, scans digitize colourful images of 'our' internal organs and numbers churn out a detailed codified status to situate persons in all but 'virtual' states of existence. Specialized technicians set coordinates to 'beam' into common worlds of diagnostic terminology. And so, persons are summed into distillations as to their state of *being*. Peering through the eyes of science into one's 'core' can be unnerving to say the least. Indeed, it can be an experience fraught with ambiguity particularly if the diagnostic pronouncement targets 'one's' state of mind. How does one incorporate a medicalized statement that holds the power to threaten one's notion of *self*? In one sense, a 'being' is a delicate thing! In another sense, it is most stable in that it cannot be conceived and reconfigured on a whim. This 'chapter' addresses the lived experience of psychiatric diagnosis (herein *diagnosis*), an intimate and personal encounter with scientific terminology that obvi-ates the reality of 'illness' and can threaten a person's per-ception of self and being. The power of *diagnosis* is examined and all care practitioners are called on to be aware of that power in their duty of care.

THE NATURE OF PSYCHIATRIC DIAGNOSIS

Dr William Chester Minor,[3] a notable contributor of the *Oxford English Dictionary*, spent much of his adult life in a mental asylum diagnosed with monomania. The term eventually came to be replaced by dementia praecox and, more recently, schizophrenia. It seems most fitting that the illustrious Dr Minor, committed as he was to accurately defining dictionary terms, was spared the daunting diagnosis of modern psychiatric terminology. The reality of countless revisions to that terminology has led to a proliferation of diagnostic descriptions that some would charge overextends reasonable professional juris-diction. Diagnosis reaches into our courts, schools, social agencies; seeps into our theatre and other art forms; and merges into the very fabric of our everyday language to make judgements on all facets of life and living, and quite literally 'making us crazy'.[4] And so, the drive to diagnose is not without controversy!

Within counselling professions, however, the conceptu-alization of an 'accurate' diagnosis is a prelude to treat-ment. Consequently, diagnosing is promoted and becomes the primary intention for mental health therapists.[5] Currently, the *Diagnostic and statistical manual of mental conditions* (DSM-IV-TR) prevails as the most widely used formula for defining mental disorders in acute as well as community care centres, affecting a flourishing population of persons carrying labels of acute and chronic mental dis-orders. To recognize the need to attend the dilemmas this poses for individuals, this chapter includes a range of

individual *personal* accounts that speak to the nature of the persons' experience of *diagnosis*. An effort has been made to 'let the words speak', to retain genuine vital meanings. Amidst understandings derived from such dis-closures appropriate ways of caring might be prompted.

DIAGNOSIS: LIFEWORLD PHENOMENON

The term *lifeworld* captures the notion of lived experi-ence within one's being.[6] Lifeworld is distinguished from a theoretical attitude in that it is recognized as a more primordial state of *being*. It represents a person's 'natural' and instant attitude to some *happening*, before the per-son has come to reflect, critically, upon that event. In my phenomenological study, descriptions of *diagnosis* were noted to both deify and vilify the experience. The data analysis established both *incidental* and *essential* themes. Incidental themes existed in some but not all experi-ences of diagnosis. Essential themes were fundamental to the lived experience of *diagnosis*.

Incidental themes

For Julia, *diagnosis* was the key that held promise of release from inner confinement. She felt driven to have a declared statement of what was wrong with her. Only with that did she see possibility for self-affirmation and prospect of her future reality. In her words:

> If someone could say, 'This is what you have, then I could come to the treatment experience knowing what the disorder was, what the implications of the treatment were; what the medications were for. … It speaks to the reality of who I am!'

Even so, coming *to know* was anything but painless for Julia in that now it was also '*to know for certain*' the grim reality of her childhood; one marred by unspeakable abuse (Figure 16.1). Still, Julia needed to validate for herself if all the sordid memories that pulled at her con-sciousness were in fact real:

> … around the fact that our parents did this, … that it was my life … that I never really had the kind of caring parents. … It is a tremendously difficult thing. The diag-nosis represents all of that ugliness … that that's what really happened. … I mean, that is my reality.

There are some similarities between Julia's account of *diagnosis* and Teresa, who had also pursued *diagnosis* for years and alleges it was intentionally withheld from her. Teresa experienced being denied self-knowledge until she inadvertently happens on her elusive diagnosis by eyeing old charts left in her view:

> The first thing on that page of my file is [the diagno-sis]. I looked at that sheet and I went, 'They knew … twelve years ago they knew what was wrong with

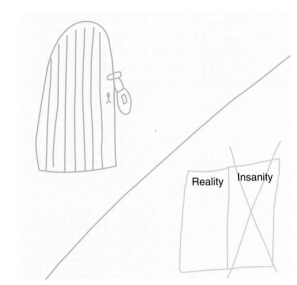

Figure 16.1 *Diagnosis*: Julia before and after

me and they didn't do anything'. Its like, 'you came into the hospital with a broken leg.' And they look at it and go, 'hmm, we don't treat broken legs … but we're not going to tell her, her leg is broken 'cause heaven forbid she should go somewhere else and get it set.' And that's the way I felt.

Teresa resents a perceived 'cover-up' of her diagnosis, which she asserts has denied her the prospect of reintegration. However, when Evelyn is readily told of her diagnosis, she experiences a devastation of self-integration. Evelyn said:

I'd always felt like I knew who I was and then all of a sudden I didn't … I felt like my identity was taken away and, I didn't have a clue who I was. … The Self I thought I was isn't … [with] the question [now] of … who I am.

Even so, with the added knowledge of *diagnosis*, Evelyn realizes a barrier is partially lifted, making possible her future goal of 'reintegration'.

Clearly, the participants in this study share similar as well as divergent experiences in acquiring *diagnosis*. On the one hand are perceived benefits. Yet they also talk about an unsavoury dimension. Perhaps the most acrimonious experience is expressed by Kevin, who has been besieged by mental demons taunting him since his mother's abandonment of him in early childhood. Years later, Kevin finds no relief in hearing the word of diagnosis from his doctor. Indeed, by his description all optimism for life vanishes at that point:

If you're told you're schizophrenic it's like breaking a glass. It shatters. It damages. It hurts. … I thought I'd been injured a lot in life. … And giving me a label like that … I couldn't take it. It seemed to me, you know,

after all what happened to me – it sounded like he [the doctor] was adding insult to injury.

Cathy, too, feels traumatized in her experience of being diagnosed. That sense of 'being renamed' devastated the person she recognized as 'self'. Cathy speaks of a terrorizing ordeal, of frantically evading *diagnosis* that threatened to unleash a lifetime of sordid abuses that would destabilize her:

I didn't want it to have a name. I knew that … giving it a name meant that in all probability the memories that I was having were not false memories. They really had happened and I had been severely traumatized and I had a lot of stuff to work through. … I had wanted something a five-minute prayer would cure.

For most, however, having *diagnosis* is reportedly preferable to the mystery of not knowing what 'it' is. Ultimately, declares Jean, '… the Lithium said it!'

Instantly I knew that it was the right drug. … It was almost like a moment of truth. It was the difference between waking up in the morning and being able to take a deep breath and actually feel the air coming in, as opposed to being restricted with that gray weight on my chest.

Still, it shook her sensibilities to hear the doctor say: 'bipolar disorder!' Jean said: 'It was clinical! It was cold!' and it was the chronic piece that jarred the most:

It's in your face. It's big. It's not going to go away. It's not fatal, but it's not going to go away … hearing it in audible sound says something about who you are. … 'You have bipolar disorder' therefore, you are mentally ill … . We know that right now nine hundred milligrams of Lithium a day keeps me stable. We don't know if that will happen next month … . You know it's not going to get better.

There is unshakable permanence of her mental illness signified in that diagnosis with considerable uncertainty about a progressively deteriorating future which Jean writes about in her personal journal. Then one day she devises a way of purging it all:

And so I thought that if I put it [the diary] all on fire then I would cleanse it all from me. But it kind of goes with you … because it's got a label.

In Susan's story, the permanence of *diagnosis* is weakened by the hope of regaining a 're-instated self'. For Susan, having 'manic depression' confirmed by the doctor drove home a stunning realization but also summoned her courage:

I'm one of them now!' … Suddenly I was a permanent psychiatric case … . I'm one of the crazies, one of the loonies … one of those people, the rejects of society? The feared diagnosis … just said chronic things to me … it was like a knife was being thrust in my chest … . But I had some knowledge about myself now … and I'm like, 'okay, fine! I'll deal with this – this beast'.

Through *diagnosis* Susan recognizes the value of *that* knowledge in the interest of her own health management. Her experience is not unlike Gary's who admits his initial reaction was: '*Oh, I better watch my neck now!*' For Gary, the diagnosis was:

… kind of an offensive statement that brought to mind my own perceptions of what the mentally ill were about. Before I ever was ill I used to have these biases and thoughts about mass murderers and all of this. It really was quite ignorant when I think of it now.

But *diagnosis* was 'gaining self-knowledge' and that established, in Gary, a sense of determination. His motto: 'Cassandra(s) not welcome!' gives his experience a positive spin.

And so, a montage on the experience takes shape through select incidental themes of *diagnosis*. Rather like stumbling in the dark, different parts of 'the elephant'[7] are touched to acquire semblance as to the nature of *diagnosis*. Its essential nature, however, still recedes into the shadows. More definitive understanding is supplied through four essential themes which assemble a distinct structure to *diagnosis* as an existential phenomenon.

Essential themes

Four stories illuminate the fundamental nature of *diagnosis*. First, through Matt, we come to the essence of '*diagnosis*' as '*A Knowing that Knows*'. Matt's story holds strong tones for the theme of 'knowingness'. His life had raced out of control: '*like being on a fast runaway train*' and he had desperately wanted to see it 'normal'. But acquiring the diagnosis did not fulfil this wish. Anything but 'psychotic' he thought! Why not '*bizarre experience*' or something more benign? But psychotic! Matt had long been unsettled with his genetic bloodline to 'insanity' and he shuddered at the prospect of being diagnosed (Figure 16.2).

Insanity is personal baggage to Matt, 'a secret he held to himself about himself'. Now the diagnosis threatens exposure of that which he embodies. He trembles at the knowing of what he was born into; forced into the self-proclaimed notion: 'I *am* flawed! *Not*, I *have* a flaw, but I *am* flawed!' Etching a facial profile he haloes hair quality in a 'foreboding hue' by his interpretation. There is no evading *that* knowledge that now reveals him. In time, though, Matt comes to a reckoning with that fact. In a second image he replaces that colour with, brighter hair which he interprets as *hopeful*. That, he says, signifies the '… *self-acceptance*' he eventually has come to.

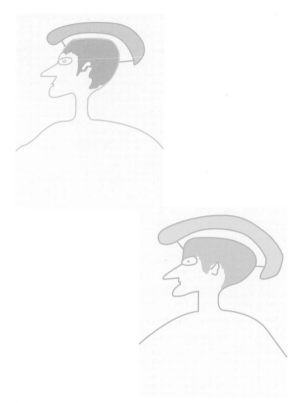

Figure 16.2 *Diagnosis*: Matt before and after

A second essential theme of '*Making Visible the Invisible*' emerges from Cheryl's experience of *diagnosis*. Cheryl wonders whether her wedding plans touched-off the illness. That was the point in time when everything changed and the '*me*' just slipped away, she says, '*behind a curtain or something*'. Six weeks into treatment, the doctor revealed a diagnosis of schizophrenia leaving Cheryl '*dumbfounded*'. Cheryl desperately looked for someone to say, '*Look, its OK! You will get better. And, you can participate in your life again.*' But none of that happened; no information, no explanation no hope of restoration! Just the horrifying verdict: '*schizophrenia*'! The anonymity of a broken mind is irrefutably lifted. It is clear to her now! The enemies of her deluded thought were not '*out there*'. They were absolutely and without doubt '*in here*', '*in my head*' she says. Cheryl's entire world suddenly gets absorbed in that one word of diagnosis. She is left seeing herself a 'phantom' floundering in a 'sea of illness' from whence she must retrieve a semblance of hope.

A third essential theme – '*(Destructive) Gift of Difference*' – emerged from Steven's experience. Through the scope of his diagnosis, Steven now understands how his historical life choices were motivated. '*When you're manic you think fast. And when you think faster you process more. So, I was just always processing more information quicker*', he says. And this accelerated rate of *being* served him well for a good many years. He was so full of energy and creative ideas that worked in his behalf. And, when things did collapse, the diagnosis simply confirmed to Steven his '*near genius capacity*'. It was *that* which had enabled his tremendous social and financial success until it all spun dramatically out of control, and his world came crashing in. Personal and business bankruptcy foreshadowed his hospitalization and eventual diagnosis. This rendered Steven different and, by his assertion, '*a case to be treated*'.

Steven's gift, '*… the ultimate high*' he historically revelled in, had become reconfigured through *diagnosis*; a naming that occluded the gift and magnified the *disorder*. '*If I wasn't diagnosed … I could be considered to be off the wall, or inventive or gifted, but the minute the diagnosis enters in, then, all the other positive traits that could be associated with the condition are removed and, "you now have an illness!".*'. Steven's narrative reveals *diagnosis* as, at one and the same time, a confirmer *and* destroyer of *being*.

A fourth essential theme to diagnosis – '*Making Knowledge Knowledgeable*' – lay in Jim's experience. 'It was a five minute visit [by the doctor] at tops … . You've got this thing called panic disorder … . Here's some pamphlets. *Go home. Take these pills. And I'll see you in a month*.' That was what transpired and to Jim it was just so many empty words, and that '*blew me away*'. In this, Jim's experience seems more one of context than of content for, indeed, the message of diagnosis was rather bereft of content. Jim heard the diagnosis as brief and shallow and trivializing. It minimized the horror of his 'pain'. How could something of such enormity to him be reduced in 5 minutes to the proportion of a '*sneeze*' a '*cold*' a '*hangnail*'?

Uneasy misgivings about himself were transmitted because of '*the five minute thing*'. This shows how the 'word' of diagnosis can be the enemy of treatment if it is simply a 'word experience' rather than a relational experience.[8] A process in which true knowledge ability is acquired must rightfully be linked to knowing the 'knower' of diagnosis. That appears to be what evaded Jim.

This assortment of *essential* and *incidental* themes offers a representation of what it is to have *diagnosis*. This offers a glimpse of a phenomenon with benefits and drawbacks, all of which must be considered to more fully appreciate the reality of what it is to bear a *diagnosis*.

DIAGNOSIS: LIVING THE AFTERMATH

'Living the aftermath' involves recognizing how complex everyday life can become for people, after being named mentally ill through *diagnosis*. To the bearer of *diagnosis*, the realities of conducting life are impacted, with a range of benefits and barriers or drawbacks.

Benefits

Many life aspects contribute to a sense of personal identity. That identity may, in part, be derived from one's body and its appearance but, personal identity is also an extension of other criteria such as one's history and nationality; an outcome of the roles one assumes in work and play; one's social and financial status; and how one is regarded by others. All this gives shape to our thoughts, feelings, beliefs and values, and to imagining and actualizing one's possibilities. 'However, such an identity is forever at the mercy of events; forever vulnerable, and forever in the need of protection and support. If anything on which our identity depends changes, or threatens to change, our very sense of self is threatened'.[9]

Diagnosis seems such a lifeworld *thing*! For most it provokes initial grief and a crisis of identity that, with time and support, can resolve. *Hope* seems vital to this process of stabilization. With hope individuals traumatized by *diagnosis* can become experts on matters related to their disorder. In the interest of their own mental health, they can become aware of intuitive insights that may help them resolve a range of health obstacles. They can learn about their medication and how to manage potential side-effects; set health patterns for sleep, exercise and nutrition; and balance their social life. Becoming knowledgeable about their typical signs and symptoms may be empowering and that may bring accomplishments not possible before gaining the diagnosis. Indeed, knowing what is now conveyed by *diagnosis* may actually relieve significant long-standing distresses. Certainly, it may help explain some of the chaos that may have existed before diagnosis. Now, commitment to a treatment regime may result in symptom control to the extent that new ways to move forward are identified, and the person can take charge in establishing, at long last, an elusive 'quality of life'. In effect, a major benefit can be realized by 'living wellness'.[b]

However, it is worth recognizing the great diversity within the 'mental health' population overall, *where* people may be situated anywhere on the continuum of 'high' to 'poor' health/illness stabilization. For those whose personal resources are more compromised, forces within the word of diagnosis may identify their eligibility for follow-up supportive programmes.

Averting recurrence of acute illness is a principal intent for stabilization programmes. Although access to urgent or emergency care may be foremost, supportive care is increasingly recognized as the more cost-effective alternative. Services with applicable mandates may therefore be assertive in engaging persons for rehabilitation and health maintenance. Such operations provide information related to community mental health clinics, wellness programmes and recreational opportunities. Outreach

[b] The author gratefully acknowledges commentary by Jennifer Finley, Street Outreach & Stabilization, Canadian Mental Health Association; Balbinder Atwol, CARNAT Centre, Calgary Health Region; Michelle Missiurelli and members of Partnership, Outreach & Unsung Heroes Programs, Schizophrenia Society of Alberta Calgary Chapter.

provides information about social supports, advocacy groups and primary healthcare resources; housing referrals, approved or group home programmes, may be addressed as an essential need presenting to this population. Supplementary income sources may be facilitated through 'systems navigation' assistance. Needs related to employment, personal development and skills of basic citizenship are all objectives of programmes such as 'Community Extension and Treatment', 'Independent Living Skills' and 'Assertive Community Outreach'. Beyond treatment aims is social awareness of the need for base funding and sponsorship of community resources in the interest of health maintenance for those living with *diagnosis* aftermaths.

Barriers

Unique challenges are known to present in the aftermath of *diagnosis*. The bearer lives more in the shadows of *illness* than in the light of *wellness*. The myths and stigmas of mental illness held in the label of diagnosis impose real world dilemmas. Much testimony confirms this as the case. Significant drawbacks are posed, as shown in Steven's before and after drawings of the *diagnosis* experience (Figure 16.3).

> Before diagnosis, I had a business, a home, a wife, children, and friends! The sun shone in my world. After diagnosis, there was just me. I lost the business, my home and, my friends. My wife thought she married a gifted person, not a mentally ill person. She took the kids and left.
>
> **Steven**

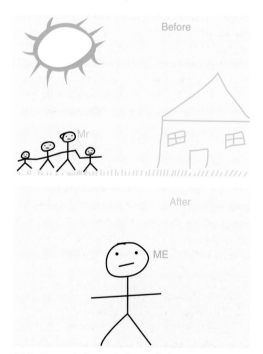

Figure 16.3 *Diagnosis*: Steven before and after

Like Steven, many acquiring *diagnosis* come to realize innumerable losses. Others have commented on the 'aftermath' as follows:

- I was prevented from continuing my work as a computer programmer.
- I can't travel outside of Canada without a psychiatrist's letter/I had difficulty getting a passport/My travel insurance was turned down.
- I was denied life insurance/I am excluded from mortgage disability insurance/My car insurance costs are higher.
- I was rejected as a volunteer/I was denied a bank account.
- I now need an annual medical to keep my driver's licence.

Regular reports of *under-employment* surfaced; a disturbing recognizable precursor to poverty and ultimately homelessness. Many described being screened out of job opportunities by information requested about medications, or having to explain gaps in employment history due to hospitalization. To evade employment discrimination, some elected to ignore identifier questions and not tell employers their diagnosis. One person said:

> I just didn't say I have schizophrenia so that 'he' doesn't make assumptions about my performance or my mood or treat me like I have a disability or exclude me from work or associations with others.

By far the most common barriers were interpersonal, with stories of abandonment by friends and subtle messaging, such as: 'I feel like they share a secret or attitude that I am excluded from'.

Diagnosis as a lifeworld phenomenon with aftermath particularities is an example of 'where knowledge alone can profoundly change people's lives'.[10] Barriers do not result from manifesting symptoms of illness but are the outcome of 'word signification'. The diagnostic term itself seems to actualize 'a something' into being: seeding the suspicion; introducing an uncertainty; inducing a fear! *That* word bears impact; it brings to the foreground an unusual realness about *the* illness it signifies. In sum, the diagnostic term foreshadows the person, and steals true personhood.

When people say: 'You're looking tired these days!', most people would take this as a welcome show of concern, and resolve to get more rest! But, to the bearer of *diagnosis* it can touch on a sense of vulnerability and be unusually troublesome. They might start asking themselves: 'Has *it* come back?' A subtle internal tremor triggers menacing questions to everyday life. Moving in and out of foreground, *it* can factor into most major life decisions. Thoughts seep in about a self now experienced as '*damaged goods*', leading to worrying questions, such as:

- 'What career can I endure?'
- 'Who will want to marry me?'

- 'Can I have kids?'
- 'Should I have kids?'

And so it goes! Susan described her sense of 'tentativeness to life' as *'feeling like a glass ball'*. This causes a wistfulness to just *'simply be normal'*; to not know what *diagnosis* has brought to light.

IMPLICATIONS FOR CARE

It has been said that 'knowledge is power'. Together nurses and patients 'have a great collective knowledge about caring'.[11] A reciprocal contribution to knowledge, and therefore a powerful force for quality care, is realized when nurses allow themselves to become informed through partnering those in their care. Knowing of *diagnosis* is imparted through the voice of those living the experience, setting a basis for 'practical wisdom'.[12] This can translate to discerning ministrations by practitioners to persons living *that* experience. Invoked is the therapeutic use of self in the *healing* of *the being* and personhood. At issue is the *caring* as distinct from the *curing*. 'Curing is an event … while healing is an internal process that draws on the patient's own resources.'[13] Healing requires the active participation of 'the' person in care, and it is here, soliciting that participation specifically in person-centred care, that nurses can recognize a principle role.

Power within the word of *diagnosis* has been seen to significantly impact one's lifeworld with sequelae[14] of induced brokenness. This plays out as *broken sense of self* and as *broken sense of self-sufficiency*. Healing in both domains is nurtured through hope and practitioners have a vital role in promoting this by exploring with individuals' their personal strengths, and helping them fortify their coping strategies.[15] In the territory of *self*, healing is thereby promoted as the person is supported in the process of finding answer to: 'Who am I?' With shattered *self-sufficiency*, the hopeful person is mobilized to regain a sense of personal legitimacy, achieved through assuming control over life and health. Knowledge with *caring* can be instrumental to inspiring a hope whereby persons feel empowered and healing in both realms of brokenness can be realized.

Few were more committed to the notion that persons exceeded the sum of their illness than Hildegard Peplau. A true advocate of person-centred and holistic care approaches Peplau invoked use of *self* in therapeutic engagement with clients.[16] She may have been especially disposed to instrumental *caring* in situations of *diagnosis* for she proposed that nursing:

> … must reject the notion of packaging people and their care according to medical diagnostic criteria …. The focus of nursing is … [not] in people's diseases or their health for that matter; nurses are interested in people's relationships with their illness, or with their health.[17]

It would seem Peplau's emphasis to tend the person in distress would readily have picked up the challenge to facilitate people's move beyond the confines of their diagnosis. Feeling *'put in a box'* (Irene) describes such a sense of being designated. In being diagnosed, Irene gained the impression the box assigned her was a medical convenience. It was comfortable for 'them' but it left her feeling abandoned through assignment:

> It didn't seem to give any answers other than that I was in a box that they named … . But they couldn't tell me how long I would be in the box. Whether I'd get out! Whether I'd be back in and out of the box! They couldn't tell me any of that. So the box just seemed like an empty shell as opposed to something that would help me better understand the experience or to find meaning in the experience. (Irene)

Once consigned to the box of diagnosis Irene, the person, felt imperceptible. She was 'therapized' but not 'seen'. She wanted to shout: 'Where are you looking? Don't you understand that you're trying to find me in that little 4 × 4 square and this is where I am?' And so Irene is left to 'the box' and discerning care evades her.

Jeff, on the other hand, experiences discernment and caring interventions. He depicts this in before and after drawings of *diagnosis* and stories the scarecrow as depicting himself pre-diagnosis (Figure 16.4):

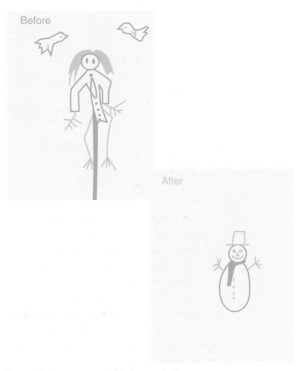

Figure 16.4 *Diagnosis*: Jeff before and after

(Before diagnosis) ... forgotten in a field somewhere; in disarray, just stuck there on a pole! I'm not going anywhere ... . The scarecrow is blue because ... life was very cold. I didn't put a smile on it at all ... the pole is holding the scarecrow up. It's hung there not touching the ground ... . (After diagnosis) the snowman has a smile ... . He has cold hands but that's just physical ... . I'm there in the snow, but it's not cold. Obviously somebody is melting up some snow with their hands to build me and fill me up ... . I was re-built ... . Someone cared enough to build me. Snowmen don't have legs. They don't need to run away. They just are! And the arms are outstretched ... happy arms.

Jeff's words are expressive, showing the elements of the caring that gave him shape and helped rebuild his sense of being. For Jeff, to be diagnosed was '... to have the comfort of a battle-plan as a basis for living'. In his portrayal is clear sense of mending, both to 'sense of self' and to 'sense of self sufficiency'.

In sum, it is well to emphasize that scientized terms of diagnoses go well beyond nomenclature and on to an absoluteness of knowledge. Perhaps nowhere more than in psychiatry is their subjective power felt. Particularly here generates a 'lifeworld phenomenon' with a consequential 'aftermath' of benefits and drawbacks to those who wear the label. While care providers value the explanatory and predictive propensities of diagnostic knowledge they must be mindful that receiving a diagnosis alters the landscape of a person's life. In spite of all that becomes apparent to caregivers through diagnosis, experientially for the recipient there may be a sense of knowing nothing at all.

SUMMARY

Review of this chapter will prompt the reader to:

* consider the symbolism that inheres in medical terminology;
* appreciate the particular power of diagnostic terms and their subjective impact;
* note *diagnosis* as the lifeworld phenomenon of receiving a psychiatric diagnosis;
* recognize distinctions between incidental and essential themes that describe *diagnosis*;
* become sensitized to an array of benefits and barriers induced by *diagnosis*;
* anticipate the aftermath of *diagnosis* to persons and implications for 'care'.

REFERENCES

1. Rosen P. *Gold medal stolen from Canadian paralympian.* Available from: www.citynews.ca/news/news_6907. aspx. Accessed 17 January 2007.

2. van Manen M (ed.) Scientized experiences. In: *Writing in the dark: phenomenological studies in interpretive inquiry.* Ontario, Canada: The Althouse Press, 2002: 179.

3. Winchester S. *The professor and the madman.* New York: Harper Collins, 1998.

4. Kutchins H, Kirk SA. *Making us crazy.* New York: The Free Press, 1997.

5. Gerig MS (ed.). Employment settings: where mental health and community counselors work and what they do. In: *Foundations for mental health and community counseling: an introduction to the profession.* Upper Saddle River, NJ: Pearson Education, 2007: 108–37.

6. Husserl E. *The crisis of European sciences and transcendental phenomenology.* Evanston, IL: Northwestern University Press, 1970.

7. Arberry AJ. http://en.wikipedia.org/wiki/Blind_Men_and_ an_Elephant# note-Saxe. Retrieved 22 January, 2007.

8. Cousins N. *Belief becomes biology.* Victoria, Canada: Shaw Cable Television, 1997.

9. Russell P. *From science to god: a physicist's journey into the mystery of consciousness.* Novato, CA: New World Library, 2002: 79.

10. Hayne Y. Experiencing diagnosis. In: van Manen M (ed.) *Writing in the dark: phenomenological studies in interpretive inquiry.* Ontario, Canada: The Althouse Press, 2002: 181.

11. Hakesley-Brown R, Malone M. Patients and nurses: a powerful force. *The Online Journal of Issues in Nursing* 2007; **12** (1): 1–16.

12. van Manen M. *Researching lived experience: human science for an action sensitive pedagogy.* Ontario, Canada: The Althouse Press, 1990: 156.

13. Curtin L. This I believe ... about the care of human beings. *Nursing Management* 1996; **27** (12): 5–6.

14. *Merriam-Webster's medical desk dictionary:* Revised edition. Springfield, MA: Mirriam-Webster, 2005: 753.

15. Hayne Y. Experiencing psychiatric diagnosis: client perspectives on being named mentally ill. *Journal of Psychiatric and Mental Health Nursing* 2003; **10**: 722–9.

16. Videbeck SL. Foundations of psychiatric mental health nursing. In: Videbeck SL (ed.). *Psychiatric mental health nursing.* Philadelphia PA: Lippincott Williams & Wilkins, 2004: 9.

17. Barker P. The eye of the needle: Research and the proper focus of nursing. In: Barker P (ed.). *The philosophy and practice of psychiatric nursing.* Edinburgh UK: Churchill Livingstone, 1999: 46.

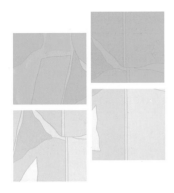

CHAPTER 17

Nursing diagnosis

Dianne Ellis*

INTRODUCTION

Imagine for a moment that someone has entered into your life making a judgement about some aspect of it – your thoughts, appearance or behaviour. How might you feel? Perhaps you will feel relieved that at last someone has acknowledged, explained or named an issue that has been troubling you for some time. Alternatively you might feel different from other people, not whole or not perfect. You might be angry at his or her impertinence. You may simply disagree and want to discuss it further. Whatever your reaction it will be unique because it will be your own.

As a psychiatric–mental health nurse you will frequently enter into the lives of other people to help them. This chapter focuses on how and why you would make a *nursing diagnosis*, bearing in mind the possible feelings that can emerge during this process? Both the value and the disadvantages of this process are given an appraisal with discussion about how you can respond to the individual's experiences and opinions? This chapter examines various approaches to nursing diagnosis internationally and in the UK. It considers the huge amount of mental health nursing knowledge, considering how nurses decide what aspects of this body of knowledge to apply. Finally, it considers the potential negative impact nursing diagnosis can have upon people discussing the benefits of collaborative working.

Personal illustration 17.1: Samantha has a case of 'the blues'

The 'blue' feelings experienced by Samantha following the birth of her daughter became progressively worse. Feeling very distressed she sought help from her general practitioner and was referred to a consultant psychiatrist. An assessment was subsequently completed and the reported symptoms and observed signs were compared against the Diagnostic Statistical Manual for Mental Disorders (DSM) classification system. After ruling out physical illness the psychiatrist reached the following conclusions:

- changes from a previous level of functioning were noted;
- distress, social impairment and occupational impairment, all were noted;
- symptoms of depression weight loss, insomnia, and feelings of guilt and fatigue were evident;
- this appeared to be a singular episode;
- the onset was between 2 weeks and 12 months after delivery (post-partum);
- a global assessment of Samantha showed a functioning level of 60 (moderate symptoms of disturbance);
- using these data, the psychiatrist made the following diagnosis, using the DSM-IV – (296.22f) single episode, post-partum major depressive disorder with moderate symptoms.

*Dianne Ellis has worked within Adult Mental Health Services as an RMN since 1985 with much of her experience as a community nurse. She completed an MSc in Mental Health and Psychiatric Nursing at Newcastle University, where her research dissertation focused upon collaborative care, examining how nurses interacted with people receiving care. Dianne is a Lecturer at Teeside University, UK.

DIAGNOSING DIAGNOSIS

The historical development of nursing as a profession highlights the importance of nursing theory in relation to the organization and delivery of patient care. Since the 1950s the nursing process has been the vehicle for such theoretical application by nurses internationally,[1] enabling nurses to deliver systematic care through individualized

1 assessment
2 planning
3 implementation
4 evaluation.

In the USA the nursing process has evolved into a six-step model incorporating 'diagnosis' as the second step following assessment.[2] Diagnosis is more commonly associated with medicine; however, other professions such as teaching and engineering also use this decision-making process.[3] The term originates from the Greek word *diagnoskein*, meaning to discern – 'Perceive clearly with the mind or senses. Make out by thought or by gazing or listening'.[4] The process of diagnostic reasoning involves the nurse forming a hypothesis in relation to the person's problem and its cause, following assessment, which enables the nurse to then decide what else needs to be known or understood in order for a diagnosis to be made.[5] Assessment is a continuous process and like a kaleidoscope the diagnostic picture can change at every turn. To maintain a well-informed understanding of the person's needs it is essential to listen to the patient and fully take on board his/her opinion.[6] Being too focused upon the 'diagnosis' can prevent a nurse from actually hearing what the person has to say.[7]

The information made known during the assessment is compared against a diagnostic framework so that a decision – in the form of a statement – can be made about the nature of those needs. It should:

* be a short and clear statement of the health problem;
* offer a concise description of the diagnosis;
* include the factors that support this diagnosis;
* include the factors that are causing, influencing or maintaining it.

As such, diagnosis refers to:

1 a *process* by which nurses
2 determine knowledge from
3 a classification system.

Reflection

What are the responses of your colleagues when they hear a particular diagnosis or problem – e.g. this lady has been referred with postnatal depression?

CLASSIFYING CLASSIFICATION

In mental health, there is a vast amount of knowledge available that might inform practice nursing. The process of classification is used to group together and order information making it more accessible to nurses. This arrangement of knowledge has been used to create a range of models, frameworks and taxonomies.[8] Classification in health care has a multitude of functions, for example:

* to order phenomena to enable communication among professionals;
* to categorize information from research;
* to facilitate literature reviews;
* to develop theory;[9]
* to develop diagnostic systems.

As many characteristics are involved, the task of classifying is problematic. Given the uniqueness and complexity of human nature, classification in health care is intricate, unlike, say, the traditional classification systems of mathematics,[10] particularly in relation to mental health care with regard to people's thoughts, feelings and behaviour.

Standardized classification systems are taxonomies of knowledge, which are intended for universal application. For example, for decades the Diagnostic Statistical Manual for mental disorders (DSM) published by the American Psychiatrist Association and the International Classification System (ICD) developed by the World Health Organization[11] have been used by psychiatrists to diagnose mental illness. The two systems share a unified theoretical belief that mental illness is the result of behavioural, psychological or biological dysfunction.[12]

From the medical perspective underpinning diagnosis, post-partum depression is used to describe a *pathological* reaction, a symptom, syndrome, disorder or illness. For Samantha (Personal illustration 17.1), this had a major impact upon her self-concept, marital relationship and future care. Because post-partum depression heralds a bipolar disorder requiring immediate medical treatment[13] the diagnosis became the focus of further assessments and treatment plans. She was prescribed antidepressant medication and was referred to a day hospital for a comprehensive nursing assessment and medication/symptom monitoring/support.[14]

It has long been argued that nursing should have its own standardized classification system to provide a precise, universally recognized language for nurses.[15] In 1994 the *International Nursing Review* reported that this system would describe specifically what nurses do (nursing interventions) in response to differing patient conditions (nursing diagnosis) with what effect (nursing outcomes). In the 1970s the *Nursing Diagnosis Movement* was initiated in the USA and in 1973 the first *Nursing Diagnosis Conference* took place, aiming to develop a classification system for nursing.[16] Such standardized systems either

TABLE 17.1 An example of the NANDA nursing diagnosis based upon Samantha's assessment so far (medical diagnosis: post-partum blues; NANDA nursing diagnosis: impaired adjustment)

NANDA definition	Rationale	NANDA outcomes
Inability to modify lifestyle/ behaviour in a manner consistent with a change in health status	Failure to take actions to prevent further health problems, failure to achieve optimal control, low state of optimism, lifestyle change, lack of motivation to change	Samantha will: Accept change in lifestyle State personal goals for dealing with change Alter behaviour to adapt to change Accept help in dealing with change in lifestyle

Interventions
Assess Samantha's perceptions about being a mother
Assess level of support available to her
Allow Samantha adequate time to express her anxieties
Discuss resources and opportunities available to her

relate specifically to one theoretical viewpoint (for example, the medical model discussed above) or employ a more flexible umbrella system, which can work alongside various theoretical positions. The *North American Nursing Diagnostic Association* (NANDA) developed a system in 1973 based upon human response patterns to diseases or conditions.[17,18] This is an amalgamated system aiming to ensure that nurses pinpoint the areas that they treat and can then therefore measure the achievement of outcomes successfully. When this system was reviewed in 1992 there were over 100 diagnoses available – all described as based on research and, following audit, shown to be valid and reliable.

NANDA defines diagnosis as:

a clinical judgement about individual, family or community responses to actual and potential health problems/life processes, which provides the basis for the selection of nursing interventions and outcomes for which the nurse is accountable.[19]

Had Samantha been referred to a day unit in North America or many European countries her care plan would have been developed using the NANDA system (Table 17.1). The care plan is adapted from a standard format based upon her medical diagnosis and additional information about her current situation, i.e. being a new mother.[20]

Although nursing diagnosis has become the cornerstone of nursing practice in the USA, where the standardized NANDA system is very much part of nurse training, and in some European and Asian countries, it has never fully established itself in the UK. The nursing process has remained a four-stage model where assessment incorporates problem identification.[21] Despite differences of opinion within the nursing literature[22] it can be argued that both processes provide a statement about the person's nursing needs following an assessment. The diagnostic process in the UK in not linked with a standard taxonomy such as NANDA. Rather, nurses from various fields of nursing and practice settings access a range of theoretical frameworks to plan patient care.

Reflection

- Do you think all nurses should use a standardized classification for nursing?
- How do you think such a system would impact upon your nursing practice?
- How do you think it would affect a client's experience?

Samantha attended a day hospital where the nursing practice was guided by the principles of the nursing theorist Sister Callista Roy (Table 17.2).[23] Roy's Adaptation Model offers a typology of commonly recurring adaptation problems and a typology of indicators of positive adaptation. The model itself is not discussed here, but it is an example of a conceptual nursing model that tells nurses how to observe and interpret phenomena.[24]

Because of the success of cognitive–behavioural approaches[14,25] in the treatment of depression, a referral was made to see a psychologist. During this assessment period the psychologist learned that not only was George (Samantha's husband) unsupportive, but that he was also emotionally and physically violent towards her. (People involved, long-term, in family violence have higher levels of depression and self-contempt.) During pregnancy, 15–25 per cent of women suffer violence[26] Owing to the psychologist's diagnosis of family violence, her psychotherapy became orientated towards them as a couple, with George's behaviour the focus. Samantha was introduced to a community psychiatric mental health nurse for additional support. At this point in her life Samantha and her family were viewed as 'dysfunctional' (Table 17.3).

Although Samantha found her medication and therapy very helpful, she found elements of her care plan unhelpful and this caused frustration. Day care was a burden because of having to make child care arrangements. This was ironic given that Samantha's main anxieties were:

- returning to work and leaving her baby at home;
- finding someone who she could trust to look after her baby.

TABLE 17.2 A nursing diagnosis based on an assessment of Samantha's needs using Roy's Adaptation Model

Nursing diagnosis	Supporting data	Outcome criteria	Short-term goal
Nutrition less than body requirements	Unable to take a balanced diet Has lost weight since birth of daughter outside of normal range for build	Samantha will resume her usual appetite She will gain weight to that appropriate for her height	Complete a teaching programme about maintaining a healthy diet Complete a nutritional assessment Weigh weekly
Inadequate pattern of activity and rest	Reports poor sleep pattern and worrying thoughts	Samantha will resume her usual sleep pattern	Education programme about relaxation Involve in daily activities Attend one activity session per day
Ineffective pattern of aloneness and relating. Avoids friends and work because of how she feels	Samantha does not want to return to work, or to spend time with friends	Resume usual relationships with family and friends Initiate social activities	Discuss two other ways of dealing with the need to withdraw socially

TABLE 17.3 An example of a nursing diagnosis based upon a dysfunctional family model

Short-term goal	Intervention	Rationale
Samantha will state that violence has decreased by (date)	Continual assessment of violence and abuse Emphasize need and strategies maximize safety Discuss emergency and crisis services and contact numbers	Validates seriousness of situation and
Samantha will be free from self-harm	Continually monitor self-harm potential Identify other options and contacts	Because of potential towards self-harm
Samantha will make decisions about her future by (date)	Encourage Samantha to examine situation and alternatives Reinforce the use of problem-solving skills	When in a dependent situation people find decision-making difficult
Samantha will have made two behavioural changes by (date)	Explore ways to make changes Assist in decision-making regarding her future	Directs assessment towards positive areas and can improve self-esteem
Samantha will identify resources and supporters that are important by (date)	Assist by discussion and activities	Identification of support and active support from nurse will help coping

Nursing diagnosis: dysfunctional family system.

Rationale: inappropriate use of aggression causing negative thinking and helplessness.

Supporting data: violence and aggression between husband and wife – depression, social anxiety, poor sleep/diet and weepy.

Expected outcome: to have definite plans in order to change her current situation.

When the psychology appointments began with George she had been relieved, but soon Samantha felt 'pushed out, as her needs were not being met'. This illustrates how assessment and diagnosis direct care rather than contribute to it. Consequently, important issues may be missed.

Scientific knowledge should not be taken as absolute fact. What constitutes the 'truth' has been the subject of philosophical debate for centuries.[27] The theory of knowledge, or epistemology, constitutes many opinions about how we understand or know what is true (or untrue) about our world and ourselves,[28] and all diagnoses incorporate theoretical frameworks based upon philosophical and ethical assumptions.[29] Such frameworks encompass the systems of classification through which our lives (and problems of living) are examined (and hopefully understood). This situation is analogous to the work of a microbiologist. The laboratory slide represents the *problem* being examined, the microscope the diagnostic tool and the lens the *theoretical viewpoint*. We cannot forget, however, that the microbiologist

TABLE 17.4 An example of collaborative nursing diagnosis

Person's diagnosis	Person's goals	Nursing plan	Rationale
I have difficulty sleeping	I will get some sleep each night	Education about relaxation Teach techniques to use Encourage activity Discuss Samantha's anxieties weekly	Sleep is easier when the body and mind are relaxed
I have little energy – not eating	I will gain energy and feel less tired	Education about high energy foods Prescription for high energy drinks Keep a check of weight	With no appetite small high energy foods will help
I am afraid about the future because of work and my daughter	I will feel supported with this problem	Listen to me when I am scared Help me to think of solutions Help me to get sick pay until things are sorted out Reduce my day hospital attendance because child care is difficult to manage	Practical help and support
I don't know what to do about George Can George change?	I will know what to do about George	Listen to my feeling about the psychology appointments Help me to make sense of what is happening	Need support to deal with what she is learning about her relationships

brings individual characteristics, attitudes, other forms of knowledge and experience, all of which can influence the *interpretation* of what is seen through the lens of the microscope.

The Tidal Model[30] recognizes, through researching the views of people who use mental health services, that nursing needs to strike a balance between the 'ordinary' and the 'professional' nurse.[31] Nursing should deal with the 'person's description of their own immediate needs'. Care should gradually extend outward into the wider world of the person's experience.[32] It is important, therefore, to ensure that people like Samantha are involved within the diagnostic process. Collaborative working ensures that both nurse and individual influence the decision-making process. Here, if you like, the lens, or theoretical viewpoint, is that of the individual (Table 17.4) and it is important that the nurse uses critical reflection in order to manage personal influences impacting upon the interpretation of the assessment.

Nursing diagnosis *should not be*:

- an *essential* requirement of nursing but rather should be one method of approaching nursing;
- *restricted* to one method, since there are numerous approaches to the diagnostic process;
- *the end-product* of care, but an element in the process of care.

- *a static statement*, because any nursing diagnosis made will continue to evolve in response to new information and the individual's changing needs.

Nursing diagnosis *should be*:

- a *statement* about the person's health problem;
- based upon information gained from *assessment*;
- based upon a problem that *requires nursing care*;
- *validated* by the person.

Samantha's brief experience of the psychiatric system illustrates the diversity of nursing assessment and diagnostic systems available. Each one corresponds to a particular set of theoretical assumptions about psychiatric mental health nursing. The nurse's difficulty is to decide which one to use. How does a nurse determine which body of knowledge to apply to a particular set of circumstances? In most areas of medicine, the theory, which supports medical diagnosis is common to practitioner and patient. However, when those judgements are about thoughts, feelings and actions, conflict between the practitioner and patient can occur. In particular, diagnoses, applied to human relationships, have the potential to cause harm to the individual.[33] An important consideration therefore when using any diagnostic system is to consider how the diagnosis will affect, both positively and negatively, the individual receiving care.

- Which theory underpins your nursing practice?
- How does this relate to assessment and care planning?
- How do you ensure that the client is actively engaged in the process?

UNRAVELLING THE DIAGNOSTIC KNOT

One finger in the throat and one in the rectum makes a good diagnostician.

Sir William Osler (1849–1919)

Diagnoses are very similar to knots in that they can both be useful and annoying. Children often harass their parents with laces riddled with knots and yet rock climbers would be on dicey ground (or mountains) without them. Likewise, a diagnosis can steady a person who is dealing with mental distress but it can also create obstacles on the path of recovery. For many people with mental health problems, being given a diagnosis can have a negative impact upon their lives. The degree of this negative impact is often underestimated and yet these experiences can be used to inform the wise application of nursing diagnosis so that nursing might help people to feel safe and secure but not bound and gagged.

- People who disagree with a diagnosis that has been made about them can feel misunderstood and alone.[34] When such disagreement is vocalized often individuals are labelled as being difficult, anti-social, non-compliant or as having no insight. This can then affect the way in which other people behave towards them.[35]
- Nursing diagnosis can lead to the stereotyping of a person. Describing the depersonalization, disempowerment and isolation that he experienced as a result of being given a diagnosis, Coleman stated: 'Two years ago I gave up being a schizophrenic and decided to be Ron Coleman'.[36]
- Once a person has received a diagnosis, often, all aspects of their lives then become subject to assessment. This can create a situation where an individual is fearful of discussing the nature of their experiences, and so important information is withheld.[37]
- Often very practical problems in relation to housing or finance for example can emerge because of a diagnosis.
- In 1986 a cross-national study revealed significant differences between American and British psychiatrists' diagnoses when using the DSM. Anthropological research has also revealed cultural differences in relation to perceptions of mental illness. It is essential to keep individual and cultural difference in mind when making a diagnosis.[38]

- Not all nursing theories are compatible with the diagnostic process. Those with a focus upon problem/needs (such as Orem's Self-care Model, which categorizes the activities of daily living) fall neatly into a diagnostic process. However, models such as that developed by Rosemarie Rizzo Parse (Human Becoming Theory) state that nurse–client interactions are not limited by prescriptions.[39]
- Not all nurses are orientated towards problem-solving approaches and the controlling of human behaviour. Indeed, some nurses are orientated towards accepting, understanding and being with the person. The issues of judging another person can cause tension for the nurse with such ideals.[40]
- Diagnosis can encourage a focus upon problems constructing a negative view of mental health with pessimistic treatment goals. For example, schizophrenia can be viewed as a chronic condition with a poor outcome. It could be argued that by focusing upon illness, other aspects of the person (including strengths) are missed.[41]

The level of control that a theory has and the rigour with which it is applied are significant issues in relation to the individual receiving care. If diagnosis is acknowledged as being the exercise of power of one person over another, then the potential to dominate an already vulnerable person becomes more apparent. It is a nursing responsibility to have this awareness and to avoid the unhelpful effects of the diagnostic process by respecting the individual's opinions and feelings.

How can you eliminate or minimize the negative aspects of nursing diagnosis, while maintaining structured and evidence-based nursing care?

SUMMARY

We take a handful of sand from the endless landscape of awareness around us and call that handful of sand the world.[42]

Robert Pirsig described how the knife of classification could separate the sand into categories of colour, size or texture, and how this process could go on and on because ultimately each grain is unique in some sense. This analogy demonstrates how the process of classification has the potential to be both creative and destructive.

Some nursing diagnoses can help aid understanding, providing a concise account of a person's health needs and the beginnings of an approach to offering a nursing response. Following assessment, a succinct statement defines the nursing purpose guiding the interventions and determining the outcomes. The diagnostic process

TABLE 17.5 A sense of balance

The nurse prescribes care	'Balance' negotiated care	The patient prescribes care
Always use diagnosis	Use diagnosis when appropriate and helpful	Never use diagnosis
There is one standardized classification system, which informs practitioners	There is no one universal truth about mental health and so nurses should be flexible, creative and responsive to the varying needs	Each person is unique and so information about mental health should never be ordered/classified
Diagnosis is central to and drives the care planning process	Diagnosis is a narrative device to help make sense of what is happening	Diagnosis serves no positive purpose It rules out all possibilities towards understanding the person's problems
Diagnosis identifies the cause and treatment of the person's problems	By formulating and naming person's problems that person can benefit from the order brought into a chaotic life but if presented as the absolute truth can cover up reasons	Giving the person a label is stigmatizing and it disempowers people

aims to 'improve accuracy in relation to the classification of disease states.'[43] Several typologies can be used to complement a theoretical viewpoint and the diagnostic process can support the production of well-organized care plans. So, nursing diagnosis may benefit nurses, managers and auditors. But what about the people receiving care? The individual may benefit from a well-informed and designed care plan but, as noted, the diagnostic process can also be stigmatizing.

Nursing diagnosis can affect a person's self-concept, liberty and life. The divide between the individual and the nurse can widen when it should be being bridged. Being labelled as 'one of 57 varieties' can create distance.[44]

Despite its implementation in America at some point during the 1970s, nursing diagnosis has not been fully integrated into nursing practice in other countries.[45] Concerns have been raised regarding cultural influences, and not being able to provide accuracy from a list of options and difficulties measuring multiprofessional outcomes.[46]

Table 17.5 observes the 'black and white' thinking that can exist in relation to nursing diagnosis. The two viewpoints are extreme and, to be successful, nurses might opt for a more 'balanced approach'. Open-mindedness and creativity are essential ingredients to ensure that nursing assessment and diagnosis are to be framed by the individual.[47] With sufficient thought and skill, people who receive psychiatric mental health nursing needn't be reduced to labels that describe them as 'dysfunctional'. The road to recovery can be difficult enough without generating more obstacles.

REFERENCES

1. Seaback W. *Nursing process: concepts and application*, 2nd edn. Canada: Thomson Delmar Learning, 2006.

2. Townsend MC. *Psychiatric mental health nursing: concepts of care in evidence-based practice*, 5th edn. Philadelphia, PA: F.A. Davis Company, 2006.

3. *The Collins English dictionary*. London: HarperCollins, 1998.

4. *The Oxford English dictionary*. Oxford: Oxford University Press, 1996.

5. Chase SK. *Clinical judgment and communication in nurse practitioner practice*. Philadelphia, PA: F.A. Davis Company, 2004.

6. Barker PJ. *The tidal model: theory and practice*. Unpublished. Newcastle: University of Newcastle 2000.

7. Rambo A, Heath A, Chenail R. *Practising therapy: exercises for growing therapists*. New York, NY: Norton, 1993.

8. Crowe M. Constructing normality: a discourse analysis of the DSM-IV. *Journal of Psychiatric and Psychiatric-Mental Health Nursing* 2000; **7**: 69–77.

9. Vincent KG, Coler MS. A unified nursing diagnostic model. *Image Journal of Nursing Scholarship* 1990; **22**: 93–5.

10. Hogston R. Nursing diagnosis and classification systems: a position paper. *Journal of Advanced Nursing* 1997; **26**: 496–500.

11. Sartorius N. *The ICD-10 classification of mental and behavioural disorders: clinical descriptions and diagnostic guidelines*. Geneva: World Health Organization,1992.

12. Trubowitz J. Mental health: theories and therapies. In: Varcarolis E. (ed.). *Foundations of psychiatric psychiatric-mental health nursing*. New York: Saunders, 1998: 29–64.

13. Stuart GW. Emotional responses and mood disorders. In: Stuart GW, Laraia MT (eds). *Principles and practice of psychiatric nursing*. St Louis, MO: Mosby, 1998: 348–82.

14. National Institute Clinical Excellence. *Depression: management of depression in primary and secondary care*. London, UK: NICE, 2004.

15. Mills C, Howie A, Mone F. Nursing diagnosis: use and potential in critical care. *Developments in Practice* 1997; **2**: 11–16.

16. Griffiths P. An investigation into the description of patient's problems by nurses using two different needs-based nursing models. *Journal of Advanced Nursing* 1998; **28**: 969–77.

17. Taptich B, Iyer P, Bernocchi-Losey D. *Nursing diagnosis and care planning*. Philadelphia, PA: Saunders, 1989.

18. Farland GKM. *Nursing diagnosis and interventions*. St Louis, MO: Mosby, 1993.

19. Carpentio LJ. In: Griffiths P. An investigation into the description of patients' problems by nurses using two different needs based nursing models. *Journal of Advanced Nursing* 1998; **28**: 969–77.

20. Ackley BJ, Ladwig GB. *Nursing diagnosis handbook: a guide to planning care*, 7th edn. St Louis, MO: Mosby Elsevier, 2006.

21. Martin, EA. *A dictionary of nursing*, 4th edn. Oxford, UK: Oxford University Press, 2004.

22. Hammers JPH, Huijer Abu-Sad H, Halfens RJG. Diagnostic process and decision making in nursing: a literature review. *Journal of Professional Nursing* 1994; **10**: 154–63.

23. George JB (ed.). *Nursing theories: the base for professional nursing practice*, 4th edn. New York: Appleton and Lange, 1995: 251–79.

24. Alligood RM. Introduction to nursing theory: its history, significance, and analysis. In: Tomey AM, Alligood MR (eds). *Nursing theorists and their work*, 6th edn. St Louis, MO: Mosby Elsevier, 2006.

25. Varcarolis EM. Depressive disorders. In: Varcarolis EM (ed.). *Foundations of psychiatric psychiatric-mental health nursing*, 3rd edn. Philadelphia, PA: Saunders, 1998: 552–88.

26. Smith-Dijulio K. Families in crisis: family violence. In: Varcarolis EM (ed.). *Foundations of psychiatric psychiatric-mental health nursing*, 3rd edn. Philadelphia, PA: Saunders, 1998: 387–416.

27. Harrison-Barbet A. *Mastering philosophy*. London, UK: Macmillan, 1990.

28. Morris T. *Philosophy for dummies*. USA: IDG Books Worldwide, 1999.

29. Bracken P, Thomas P. Post modern diagnosis. *Post psychiatry: Openmind* 2000; **106**: 19.

30. Barker P, Buchanan-Barker P. *The tidal model: a guide for mental health professionals*. New York, NY: Brunner Routledge 2005.

31. Jackson S, Stephenson C. What do people need psychiatric and psychiatric-mental health nursing for? *Journal of Advanced Nursing* 2000; **31**: 378–88.

32. Barker PJ. Mental health: it's time to turn the tide. *Nursing Times* 1998; **94**: 70–2.

33. Mitchell GJ. Nursing diagnosis: an ethical analysis. *Image: Journal of Nursing Scholarship* 1991; **23**: 99–103.

34. Crawford P, Nolan PW, Brown B. Linguistic entrapment: medico-nursing biographies as fictions. *Journal of Advanced Nursing* 1995; **22**: 1141–8.

35. Tilley S, Pollock L. Discourses on empowerment. *Journal of Psychiatric and Psychiatric-Mental Health Nursing* 1999; **6**: 53–60.

36. Coleman R. *Is the writing on the asylum wall? Power to partnership*. Gwynedd, UK: Handsell, 1995.

37. Reed A. Economies with 'the truth': professional's narratives about lying and deception in mental health practice. *Journal of Psychiatric and Psychiatric-Mental Health Nursing* 1996, **3**: 249–59.

38. Trubowitz J. Mental health: theories and therapies. In: Varcarolis E (ed.). *Foundations of psychiatric psychiatric-mental health nursing*. New York, NY: Saunders, 1998: 29–64.

39. Hickman JS, Rizzo Parse R. In: George JB (ed.). *Nursing theories: the base for professional nursing practice*, 4th edn. New York: Appleton and Lange, 1995: 335–54.

40. Mitchell GJ. Nursing diagnosis: an ethical analysis. *Image: Journal of Nursing Scholarship* 1991; **23**: 99–103.

41. Morgan S. *Helping relationships in mental health*. London, UK: Chapman and Hall, 1996.

42. Pirsig RM. *Zen and the art of motorcycle maintenance*. London, UK: Corgi, 1986.

43. Bennett M. Nursing diagnosis: in the beginning. *Australian Journal of Advanced Nursing* 1986; **4**: 43–6.

44. Barker P. *The philosophy and practice of psychiatric nursing*. London, UK: Churchill Livingstone, 1999.

45. Mason G, Webb C. Nursing diagnosis: a review of the literature. *Journal of Advanced Nursing* 1993; **2**: 67–74.

46. Chambers S. Nursing diagnosis in learning disability nursing. *Journal of Advanced Nursing* 1998; **7**: 1177–81.

47. Watkins P. *Psychiatric-mental health nursing: the art of compassionate care*. Oxford, UK: Butterworth Heinemann, 2001.

CHAPTER 18

Collaboration with patients and families

Tom Keen* and Richard Lakeman**

INTRODUCTION

Mental health policy, standards and vision documents in most Western countries aspire to a world where users of mental health services, families and carers work together in the provision of mental health care and the development of services. In several Australian States 'Carers Recognition' legislation mandates that carers must be included in the assessment, planning, delivery and review of services that impact on them. There is consistent evidence that mutually respectful collaborative alliances between professionals and patients are of central importance in determining the outcome of any therapeutic strategy, regardless of specific treatment modality.[1–5] Service users, however, report disappointing levels of involvement in their own personal care and treatment, as well as in the planning and development of services.[6,7] Similarly many families and carers of service users continue to report feeling excluded from decision-making, care and treatment processes[8–10] and feel blamed for the plight of their diagnosed relatives.[11]

Traditional assumptions about sickness and medical treatment derive from notions about the doctor as expert, nurses as kindly healers and the patient as needing to accept treatment and care. These concepts dictate service structure; define appropriate relationships between sufferers and professionals; and shape expectations about how health-related decisions ought to be made. However, health and welfare reform in North America, Europe and Australasia has been shaped by a discourse of consumerism that has shifted the relationship between the state, professions and citizens. This movement based on citizens' claims to self-determination (or individual autonomy) is concerned with improving consumer participation in decision-making, challenging professional power and encouraging people to take more responsibility for their own health and well-being.[12] There are tensions between the traditional dependent relationships of the patient, and expectations for people to be consumers of health services, or actively involved in healthcare-related decisions as empowered 'users'. Although many people may be content to acquiesce to the advice of health professionals, it is increasingly accepted that at the very least people have a right to make choices about their own health and health care, and receive full information about treatments, alternatives, risks and benefits in order to inform their choices.

It may be sensible when suffering from an uncontroversial medical ailment to forgo collaborative equality

*Tom Keen was a Lecturer in Mental Health at the University of Plymouth for many years, previously working as a nurse, therapist or manager in a variety of settings across the south of England.
**Richard Lakeman is Lecturer in Mental Health, Dublin City University, Ireland. He has worked across the spectrum of mental health service settings, most recently setting up a homeless outreach team and a clinical nurse consultant on a mobile intensive treatment team in North Queensland, Australia. Currently he has a general interest in helping people to realize recovery and how people live with extra-ordinary experiences such as hearing voices and suicidal.

and adopt the sick role – trusting the professionals' unclouded judgement and greater wisdom, expertise and psychological fitness (albeit at the risk of iatrogenic regressive dependency and compromised recovery). But psychiatric diagnoses are rarely aetiologically simple, frequently controversial and often the subject of conflicting therapeutic approaches.[13] The majority of service users have very complex needs, which should entail the abandonment of professionally imposed, rigid formulations of care, treatment, cure or rehabilitation.[14] There is some evidence that people do not benefit from and may be harmed by the attribution of a specific diagnosis and associated treatment protocols,[15] even if the award of an identifying diagnosis provides initial relief for both sufferers and staff.

Diagnosis provides clear treatment structure and direction, but such clarity may be gained by oversimplification of the patient and family system's complex dynamics, and by discounting individuals' unique characters, temperamental strengths, aspirations and resources. Mental health patients most highly value opportunities to discuss and make sense of their symptoms, rather than passively receiving structured services and medication.[16] As Perkins and Repper[17] assert, mental health service users generally prefer 'alliance, not compliance'. Full collaboration with patients and families is based on the establishment of partnerships, or therapeutic alliances,[18] not dependence on professionals, however benign or well meaning their presentations of themselves and their service.

COMPONENTS OF COLLABORATION

Hoyt describes three factors considered essential components of effective collaboration.[19]

Alliance

Being able to sublimate one's own professional concerns within a genuine partnership; being prepared to work *with* the other person's goals, formulations, preferences, etc., not labouring *on* their symptoms or social deficits; nor aiming interventions *at* their illness. A meta-analytic survey of 24 separate studies identified three characteristics of effective therapeutic alliances.[20]

- The client believes in the relevance of the shared problem formulation and the effectiveness of suggested treatment options.
- The client and professional agree on both the necessary and likely short- and medium-term expectations of care.
- An affective component: a warm relationship based upon a professional ability to appear caring, sensitive and sympathetic.

The therapeutic alliance is thought to account for up to 30 per cent of variance in outcome in psychotherapy research.[5] It is among the strongest predictors of dropout in residential drug treatment,[4] and is considered essential to rehabilitation in brain injury.[21] In schizophrenia it is considered necessary to enable psychotherapy to take place[22] and is the most reliable and consistent predictor of adherence to medication advice.[23] In the treatment of depression, therapeutic alliance points directly to positive outcome regardless of the treatment provided,[2] and in bipolar disorder it has been described as a mood stabilizer.[3] There are few things that a mental health professional can do that are more useful to others than developing good working relationships with people.

Evocation of resourcefulness

Being mindful that the person (however much apparently disabled by events or symptoms) has acquired abilities, intelligence, experience, skills and positive attributes. Nurses should attempt to mobilize and maximize these abilities, rather than risk colluding with patients' disowning their worth. To simply fulfil people's regressive needs for dependency may satisfy nurses' needs for approval, respect, etc., but may not be in service users' best long-term interests. From a nursing point of view, this factor suggests it is unhelpful to inculcate in users a sense of passivity – being subjected to treatment and control – rather than an expectation of active participation. We should establish clinical cultures wherein people feel they are *working* with staff on their problems, rather than being treated, trained and restrained.

Achievable therapeutic goals

Ideally *we* (the professionals) should be in search of *their* (the users') solutions. Psychiatrically defined clinical outcomes may be appropriate for drug trials, but often bear little relevance to the demands of ordinary life. For many people, complete loss of symptoms or absolute cessation of problem behaviour may be impracticable. The *solution-focused* approach to problem-solving[24] represents one practical example of effective collaborative goal-setting. Each goal should be something that matters to the individual, not simply to the treatment team. Goals should be small enough to achieve, and stated in clear, operational terms, so that the person will know when they have achieved their intention. Each goal should be checked against other aspects of the person's private life or social ecology, lest an apparently desirable gain in one area of personal functioning causes a corresponding breakdown in some other significant relationship. More recently, 'goal striving' has been incorporated into recovery-congruent 'evidence-based' packages, which include collaborative working and motivational enhancement.[25]

In mental health nursing the 'Tidal Model' incorporates elements of all the above three factors.[26] The 'Tidal

Model' advocates an essentially curious and undogmatic stance towards people's problems that privileges the user's own account of distress; personal meanings derived from their subjective experiences; and preferred solutions to their difficulties over 'off-the-shelf' psychiatric formulations. It also presupposes that people's situations are fluidly dynamic, and that problem status changes frequently – often several times in the course of a day, especially when enjoying or enduring active, collaborative care. This means that rigid or stagnant 'care plans' that conventionally remain unchanged for weeks or months are little use. The nurse–patient partnership should collaboratively review and rewrite care plans as often as understanding of the person's difficulties and potential solutions changes.

Personal illustration 18.1

Joan was diagnosed as suffering from a schizo-affective disorder and deemed by her psychiatrist and the ward staff to be deluded as she insisted that she was being poisoned by the medication she was being compelled to take. Joan distrusted electroconvulsive therapy because she believed that the anaesthetic and muscle relaxant were also poison. One nurse thought Joan's claims made sense, and that she may be suffering from unsettling side-effects. The staff discounted the idea of using a tool like LUNSERS (Liverpool University Neuroleptic Side Effect Rating Scale) as they deemed Joan too disturbed to answer the questions properly. The dissenting nurse thought that Joan's agitated, anxious restlessness may well be a form of akathisia and despite her colleagues' scorn, requested a visit from the pharmacist. He confirmed that Joan was suffering from medication side-effects and recommended a more suitable prescription.

Personal illustration 18.2

Mrs Chidgey was a middle-aged lady from a superficially jolly and supportive farming family who regularly if infrequently broke down and was well known to staff as a 'relapsing paranoid schizophrenic'. One of the symptoms of her illness was her belief – identified by staff as a recurrent delusion – that her husband and daughter (aged 19) slept together whenever Mrs Chidgey was away. This lady's illness had for many years been only partly effectively treated by neuroleptic medication of various kinds until the family moved and came under the clinical responsibility of a clinical team that advocated family-based approaches to all clinical referrals. After a few sessions of therapy, it transpired that members of the family often shared the parents' large bed when either spouse was alone, and especially when mum was in hospital and the family felt distressed. To the rest of the family, it had never been a secret, nor even an issue, but had never previously been clinically broached.

Collaboration is an integral part of a *therapeutic alliance*. Zetzel[27] coined this term, analogous with nursing's more customary *therapeutic relationship*, 5 years after Carl Rogers'[28] classic account of *client-centred therapy* gave the humanistic creed its clearest clinical formulation: that empathic understanding, genuineness (congruence) and acceptance (warmth or unconditional positive regard) are not only essential components of caring, but also sufficient conditions of care and treatment for people to begin to recover or change.[29] Rogers' connection between *acceptance* and *change* is echoed by recent strategies for working with seriously personality-disordered people. Marsha Linehan[30] identifies 'acceptance versus change' as one of the key paradoxical tensions or *dialectics* that professional staff need to maintain in their work with damaged personalities. Linehan uses the term 'validation' to refer to the professional's deeply held conviction that a patient's pathological, self-damaging or aggressively sabotaging behaviour should be responded to by understanding it as making sense from within the person's current situation, emotional status and belief system. Last century, the psychologist George Kelly[31] insisted that humans are essentially personal scientists, who attempt to create hypotheses or constructs that make sense of their experience, and behave accordingly. Following Kelly's insights, systemic family therapy teams have long embraced the idea that people's apparently pathological behaviours could be interpreted as 'attempted solutions' to underlying psychological, interpersonal or socioeconomic problems.[32]

Personal illustration 18.3

Mrs Smith was referred to the Day Hospital diagnosed as suffering from an obsessional–compulsive disorder. In the words of her psychiatrist, she 'exhibited trichotillomania'. Mrs Smith spent hours each day trying to achieve absolute symmetry by plucking single hairs from two almost perfectly circular bald patches she had created above her forehead. Despite his wife's obvious distress, Mr Smith would leave home each day for work, and Mrs Smith's mother would usually come around to help her daughter settle her anxiety by measuring the diameter of the bald patches. Sympathetic and curious nurses at the Day Hospital soon learnt that Mrs Smith had felt lonely and unloved for many years; was terrified of going out alone; and felt unable to discuss her feelings with her rather taciturn husband. Her hair-pulling, far from worrying or annoying her husband seemed to have gained some pity, perhaps confirming his sense of masculine superiority and role of provider. It also led to a rare agreement between Mr Smith and his mother-in-law, and re-established a strong supportive bond between daughter and mother, who would otherwise have also been at home alone.

Reflection

- Consider the different people whom one needs to consult and collaborate with in planning care for a person. What roles and responsibilities do these people have in the person's care and recovery? How might differences of opinion be resolved?
- What factors contribute to a good working alliance? Consider an occasion when you were involved in a genuine collaboration: what was going on for you, the other person(s) and between you that made this event collaborative?

IT'S NOT ALL IN THE MIND

Psychiatric custom and practice tends to locate the source of difficulties primarily within the patient. In attempting to accurately attribute the causes of illness behaviour, traditional psychiatric formulations may overstate personal, individual, internally located factors (such as genetic defect, constitutional weakness, personality type or organic pathology) and underestimate the significance of situational, objective, externally located causes (such as social deprivation, economic difficulty, interpersonal abuse or cultural alienation). There is for example compelling evidence that many people diagnosed with schizophrenia have a history of childhood abuse and adult trauma which has continuing residual and often profound impacts on people's lives.[33] Preoccupation with speculative biogenetic explanations obstructs the exploration of psychosocial factors that contribute to people's well-being.

Collaborative nursing can help to correct this imbalance by not discounting a person's own perceptions, understanding of their circumstances and by deeply validating their struggles to cope with life's very real pressures and stressors. Professionals can resist imposing their own clinical priorities and problem definitions, but instead work with clients to identify and prioritize their own, often more mundane, needs and aspirations. By practical collaboration and liaison with other professionals and agencies, nurses can help people with important practicalities such as benefits, accommodation difficulties, neighbourhood disputes, etc. The psychologist David Smail employs this kind of argument to substantiate a rigorous critique of specific models of psychotherapy. Smail[34,35] claims that people need effective, practical assistance to deal with the very real difficulties they encounter in life. Whenever psychotherapeutic care seems effective, it is because individuals indirectly obtain three important resources:

- comfort
- clarification
- encouragement.

Comfort refers to the therapist offering support and personal validation – aspects of what Hoyt[19] refers to as 'alliance'; Linehan[30] believes vital to effective helping; and Rogers[28] calls 'unconditional positive regard' and warmth – two of the 'necessary and sufficient conditions for change.' In nursing terms, a collaborative relationship requires the nurse to care *about* as well as *for* the person. This is not always easy to maintain, and certainly cannot be achieved simply by reciting a nursing creed of moral imperatives to be kind at all times. It requires the nurse to confront his or her own emotional needs, and clarify reactions and responses to patients and clinical interaction through deep personal reflection and supervision.

Clarification refers to some explanation of how the person's problems originated and developed. Such explanatory theories of psychopathology or life difficulties exist but differ in every school of psychotherapy, regardless of effectiveness. People need a story about their life that makes sense, and especially a narrative thread that could suggest a pathway out of their current difficulties. Some highly collaborative forms of therapy for psychosis based on narrative exploration and reconstruction exploit this insight, which lends itself readily to conversational application by mental health nurses.[36]

Encouragement refers to the ongoing support, confrontation, guidance and reinforcement that needs to accompany an individual's attempts to dare to be different or attempt another way of behaving, either specifically or in general, once problem maintenance factors and potential solutions have become clearer. Equally, encouragement may be needed to help people tolerate or cope with socioeconomic circumstances that remain stubbornly immune to practical efforts to improve them.

COLLABORATIVE CONVERSATIONS: BEING USEFUL WHEN PEOPLE WANT TO TALK

Peter Hulme[37] has outlined a useful framework for developing collaboration within a normalizing conversational approach to mental health nursing. Hulme criticizes the potentially oppressive rigidity of many conventional psychiatric formulations and expands Smail's notions about the importance of 'clarification', 'solidarity' and 'encouragement'. Both mental health professionals and distressed people in need of care often become too psychologically inflexible and rigid. Psychiatric beliefs, behaviours and attitudes are sometimes just as obstinate and unhelpful as so-called delusions, compulsions or depressions. Hulme uses the phrase 'collaborative conversation' to describe the context in which fixed beliefs, habits and feelings on both sides can begin to be dissolved away and replaced with more expansive possibilities (Table 18.1). There are three elements of such *collaborative conversations*:

- reflection, not drowning
- relativism, not dogmatism
- relatedness, not disowning.

TABLE 18.1 Elements of collaborative conversation

Rogers' 'necessary and sufficient conditions for change'[29]	Smail's 'components of psychotherapy'[35]	Hulme's 'aims of collaborative conversation'[37]
Unconditional positive regard and warmth 'A non-possessive caring acceptance of the client, irrespective of how offensive the person's behaviour might be. Unconditional positive regard helps to create a climate that encourages trust.' 'Conditional regard implies enforced control and compliance dictated by someone else' 'Non-possessive warmth springs from an attitude of friendliness, is liberating and non-demanding.'[56]	*Comfort (or solidarity)* 'The comfort to be derived from sharing your deepest fears and most shameful secrets with a "valued other" who listens patiently is one of the most potently therapeutic experiences to be had.' 'Comfort does not cure anything. The provision of therapeutic comfort is not unlike administering short-acting tranquillizers – it works, is addictive, but it will have to be withdrawn sooner or later.'[35]	*Reflection (not drowning)* 'When we are drowning in our experiences we are unable to separate ourselves from them. They govern us completely.' 'Reflection is the capacity to separate consciousness from its contents. We can step back, inspect and think about our experiences. We become capable of changing our relationship with them and altering their meanings for us.'[3]
Genuineness (congruence) 'The degree to which we are freely and deeply ourselves and are able to relate to people in a sincere and undefensive manner.' Genuineness encourages client self-disclosure, whilst appropriate therapist disclosure enhances genuineness.[56] Genuineness entails meaning what you say and do. It does not necessarily entail revealing all that you think. Paul Halmos wrote about being 'a vessel of honesty floating on a sea of concern.'[57]	*Clarification* 'The point of establishing how you got to be the way you are is to disabuse yourself of mistaken explanations, not the least of which is that you are responsible for it.' 'People are often mystified about the causes of their suffering, and an important aspect of their coming to understand what they can and cannot do about their predicament is to be demystified'[35]	*Relativism (not dogmatism)* 'Dogmatism is to beliefs what drowning is to experiences.' 'In the absence of doubt there is little incentive to change one's mind about anything: we do not hesitate to put our beliefs into immediate action when the situation seems to demand it.' 'The antidote to dogmatism is relativism ... We acknowledge that we have no monopoly on the truth, that we understand and experience the world at best imperfectly from a particular viewpoint or perspective.'[37]
Empathy 'The ability to step into the inner world of another person and out again.' Empathy is trying to understand another's thoughts, feelings, behaviours and personal meanings from their own internal reference frame.' 'For empathy we have to respond in such a way that the other person feels understood, or that understanding is being striven for.' 'Empathy is a transient thing. We can lose it very quickly.' 'Literally it means "getting alongside" '[56]	*Encouragement* 'Nothing will ever change the need for human solidarity, whatever form it comes in.' 'The courage needed for a tiny powerless organism to take a chance on the nature of its reality must be colossal, and can only be acquired through a process of encouragement, in which loving recognition of the uniqueness of the baby's perspective is central to the nurture and instruction offered.'[35]	*Relatedness (not disowning)* 'When we disown aspects of our experience they do not necessarily cease to influence what we feel think and do. We disown experiences that would otherwise engulf us. We disown conclusions that conflict with cherished beliefs.' 'Relatedness is the capacity to consciously acknowledge and relate to what we are experiencing. Without the capacity to own and reflect we remain helpless victims of our own inner life.'[37]

Reflection, not drowning

Rather than experience themselves 'drowning' in overwhelming difficulties, people need to be able to separate themselves temporarily from their lives; to separate their consciousness from chaotic experience; and learn to *reflect* upon their situation. Collaborative conversation aims to help people feel a sense of rescue, so that the absolute (and usually apparently awful) nature of truth and reality can be considered more calmly and other possible meanings and perspectives explored. Distressed people can be aided to achieve this by experiencing the reflective calm of their potential rescuer. Sometimes, especially when faced with chaotic acting-out or threatened violence, it may be necessary for professional nurses to 'act-as-if' and non-verbally feign such confident detachment, while verbally acknowledging the apparently extreme mess that their dependent partner is experiencing.

Relativism, not dogmatism

It helps if both nurse and patient cease to rely upon deeply engrained certainties or 'dogmatism', and challenge their own beliefs or assumptions about themselves and their world. Nurses can help people generate alternative explanations and even point out unusual beliefs that might initially uncomfortably challenge previously unshakeable world views. Paradoxically, the emerging possibility of doubt can be a step towards greater autonomy, freeing people from the usually unhelpful rigidity that has previously characterized their personalities. The development of such doubt and the consequent *relativism* helps dissolve unhelpful beliefs in the same way as reflection helps us to cope with difficult experiences.

Relatedness, not disowning

People often blame others for their difficulties long after any original damage may have been done to them. They deny any destructive, defective or negative attitudes on their own part; or simply refuse to face up to consequences, connections or causes. People need help to discern and accept the connections, patterns or relationships between external events and their internal feelings and thoughts. They also need to learn how their subsequent behaviours are interpreted or construed by others and how these constructs then determine reciprocal behavioural responses that may in turn generate further hurt and misunderstanding, or elicit other negative emotional reactions. This *relatedness* is the undermining challenge to 'disowning', and brings denied problems or solutions back into focus, and thence into possible reconstruction and resolution.

Reflection

Consider someone who may have an experienced a prolonged low mood (perhaps yourself, a family member or someone you know).

- How did the person's relationships contribute to the perpetuation and resolution of the low mood?
- How did the person relate to others differently during the period of low mood and subsequently?
- How did the person's thinking about the world change?

BETTER THAN COLD WAR: THERAPEUTIC COMMUNITIES AS COLLABORATIVE ENVIRONMENTS

A common emphasis in psychiatric nursing is to identify and locate problems *inside* people, rather than within relationships (*between* people) or between people and real life (*around* people). This emphasis can create obstacles to progress and personal growth, if that includes coming to terms with *relatedness* and the reciprocal effects of emotion, thinking and behaviour within relationships. Shared clinical environments, whether residential units or day centres, can usefully provide opportunities for socially reinforced learning, provided that people are allowed

some scope for expressing their difficulties and supported in receiving feedback from others about their behaviour. Patients can be helped to collaborate with each other's efforts to gain personal control and work towards recovery, rather than simply accept treatment passively from the professionals. This is after all what goes on informally and often surreptitiously within the subcultures of dormitory and smoking room. Nurses sometimes feel excluded from this community, and mistrust it, or feel unable to incorporate its potential benefits into the formal matrix of care.[38]

Outside of conventional psychiatric service organization, with its emphasis on one-to-one nurse–patient or psychotherapeutic relationships, perhaps the best example of shared collaborative responsibility is found within the various *therapeutic community* models of treatment. This model of recovery-based mental health care grew from the military hospitals caring for soldiers damaged by the stress of the Second World War. Hierarchies of patients and professionals were abandoned and replaced by a communal, democratic model of organization, planning, decision-making and problem-solving. In most models of therapeutic community practice, staff as far as possible abandon their clinical authority (although they do not entirely abdicate it, but rather hold it in abeyance) until forceful prescriptive interventions are essential to prevent serious harm. Staff and patients alike are expected to both support and confront people with observations and interpretations of ordinary, everyday acted-out behaviour, so that social, interpersonal and intra-psychic learning is maximized and opportunities to avoid the implications of dysfunctional or damaging personal traits all but disappear. Responsibility for all aspects of day-to-day functioning are shared, and the community becomes in effect a sociopsychological clinical laboratory for clarification of problems and a testing ground for more constructive behaviour.[39] This model of care thrived during the 1960s and 1970s, but shrank considerably during the 1980s and 1990s as the political climate in the UK and overseas swung from cooperative communal, social or municipal models of progress to embrace more competitive, individualistic ideals. The use of so-called 'community meetings' on some clinical units represents a vestigial survival of therapeutic community practice. Unfortunately, modern management procedures, confused treatment ideologies and rigid clinical hierarchies often mean that these meetings are shorn of their full democratic status. Instead of being a forum for dynamic problem-solving and collective decision-making, the community meeting's purpose often seems more a symbolic means of enforcing staff authority than an exercise in therapeutic liberalism. It has become a mechanism for staff announcements, ordering meals and complaining about food and apportioning blame or punishment for overnight acting-out. Recently, however, the drive to develop effective methods of helping people with severely disordered personalities has brought therapeutic community philosophy and practices back into political favour. The same principles could reinvigorate community-based acute and rehabilitation units.[40]

THE SICK SELF AND OTHERS: COLLABORATING WITH FAMILIES

Personal illustration 18.4

An on-call nurse in a community mental health centre received a 'demanding' phone call from an angry father 'You'd better get round here now and sort my daughter out – she's gone mental'. The nurse was refused permission to talk to the daughter herself. After their GP was contacted and made a referral, the family were offered a daytime appointment but instead turned up at the community mental health clinic (CMHC) that evening when only the Crisis Team remained on duty. The daughter, a 17-year-old schoolgirl, seemed distraught, and collapsed when told that the family should keep the appointment they had been offered. A nurse from the team took the girl, Lisa, away and spoke to her alone for over an hour, while a colleague interviewed her parents.

Lisa was a bright highly achieving A-level student but confessed to being 'totally at the end' and unable to stay at home 'It's doing my head in'. She'd been thinking about suicide, and yesterday had cut her arms superficially and packed a case to leave home – thus prompting the phone call to the CMHC from her father. Lisa described an atmosphere of constant hostility between her father and mother, with father bearing the brunt of mother's frequent violent rages, supposedly to stop her beating her own daughter. She was unable to identify a just reason for this rage, except that mum had had a 'terrible childhood – full of sexual abuse and that'. Dad had begged her never to leave home, as 'that would kill your mother' and he himself would be broken hearted. Lisa felt that she had to stay at home to prevent real harm coming to either parent, but at the same time dreaded staying for her own psychological and physical health.

When working with families collaboration becomes even more problematic, multidimensional and full of potential pitfalls. Even when working individually, in an ecological sense, nurses are usually, and often unaware of, working with the front-end of at least one family – a complex human system of friends and relatives. Families of people needing psychiatric services are rarely harmonious collectives. Behind each individual referral, there is usually a long history of grief and worry, emotional and social difficulties, pain and disappointment or conflict and recriminations. How can nurses collaborate with every part of an internally conflicted system?

If working collaboratively with an individual is easier said than done, families present even more complex and potentially painful difficulties. It is often helpful to work with a partner or co-worker, for various reasons:

- A single worker can be overwhelmed and drown in the emotional complexity or intensity of any family's intricate social system. A supportive partner will help share the emotional burden, clarify confused affective responses and enable improved objectivity, as well as increasing the intellectual resource available for identifying potential solutions, strategies, etc.
- Two people can more easily operate with the complex balance of shifting pairs, pacts and alliances between individual members, by being able to support opposing factions at the same time, facilitate stronger alliances and other means of prospering equilibrium and negotiation.
- Two workers who have a good relationship can help model or demonstrate (either explicitly or covertly) better ways of functioning by their unafraid discussion and resolution of disagreements or uncertainties.

It helps to have a clear objective structure or cognitive framework of family functions, in order to help clarify the multifarious behaviours and patterns of interaction that might otherwise simply bewilder the most well-intentioned workers. A clear map of family functioning will help to provide a normative overview when trying to identify areas that may be causing difficulties, or exploring potential routes to improved functioning.

Although various models of healthy family functioning have been developed, tried and tested, none has achieved general acceptance, and all may be subject to cultural or theoretical bias. Nevertheless, the need for a practical conceptual model persists and the McMaster model of family functioning[41] has proved its worth over nearly three decades. The model proposes six broad areas of function: communication, affective responsiveness, emotional involvement, problem-solving, behaviour control and allocation of roles and responsibilities. The model can be used with any family as a shared lens to scrutinize behaviour and enhance insight, or a tool to explore tunnels of unawareness and construct new pathways to change. Such a model can also be used as a professional tool to attribute pathology or reach a sociopsychiatric diagnosis. Then obviously the goal of collaboration will have been submerged, as so often, beneath the expediency of objective pseudo-science and the arrogance or security of assumed expertise.

Communication: how the family exchanges information. Everybody may be in the family's network or perhaps someone or others are excluded; pairs and sub-groups may exist. The model distinguishes between practical, *instrumental* material – news, plans, ideas, proposals, etc., and emotional or *affective* matters. Families often communicate much better about cool, factual issues, while having difficulty with more highly charged emotional stuff.

The model further distinguishes between *clear* and unclear or *masked* communication, and *direct* or *indirect* messages. The *clear/masked* continuum enables a collaborative study of the overall clarity of communication in general, or of specific messages or channels. Is the message clear (both to sender and intended receiver) or is it muddled, vague, disguised? The *direct/indirect* scale invites consideration of whether messages are sent to the person they are intended for or are ostensibly about. Alternatively, perhaps there is excessive secrecy, collusion or triangular, third-party deflection?

Affective responsiveness: how wide is the family's range of permitted, established or recognized emotions? How well or poorly does the family as a whole or individuals within it respond to the whole spectrum of human emotions? Perhaps there are blind-spots or prohibitions; prescribed or obligatory feelings; frozen or stagnated emotional states; flat, grey emotional landscapes; separation and allocation of feelings to various individuals as guardians or keepers. Some families are all right with joy and awful at anger; some cannot handle shame or disgust; others insist on pride and refuse to permit guilt (and vice versa). Joy, calm contentment, surprise; sadness, anger, fear, disgust; love (and lust); guilt, shame, pride, embarrassment, envy and jealousy: each and every one may be present, absent, exaggerated or denied, a potential source of conflict in the family's emotional repertoire. Sometimes, emotions seem to have been parcelled out: one member has the job of facing sadness and despairing at life, whereas another is the family's eternal optimist; yet another is critically angry with both, enabling a lucky fourth to carry the burden of calm serenity.

Affective involvement: how integrated, warm and balanced is the family's emotional interest in the activities, interests and aspirations of its members? The McMaster system distinguishes six levels of this dimension:

- *Lack of involvement*: the family seems detached, disengaged and isolated from each other, sharing a living space and perhaps a history but apparently little else.
- *Involved but without feelings*: apparently emotionally indifferent, showing little interest until it is demanded or extorted by acting-out or other means.
- *Narcissistic involvement*: members may feel that others in the family may only be interested in them for what they themselves may attain as a result.
- *Empathic involvement*: the most effective level, and an ideal to be aimed for, where members feel emotional investment in what something means for the others.
- *Over-involvement*: Over-intrusive, over-protective, overly enthusiastic behaviour: obviously all subjectively judged, but inferred by the statements, behaviour or revelations of those involved.
- *Symbiotic involvement*: sometimes referred to as *fusion*, there seems to be no personal boundary, or at least a very blurred one between individuals. People respond as one, claiming to know how the other is feeling, even better than they do themselves, and often reply for each other.

Problem-solving: a problem is any issue from within or outside the family that seems to threaten or compromise the healthy functioning of any member, or the whole system. Good problem-solving may require shared or well-led expertise at all stages of dealing with problems:

- *Identification of the problem*: Who sees it? How clearly? Is it a projection or displacement of other difficulties? Are emotional difficulties redefined as operational ones, or vice versa?
- *Communication*: Is it discussed with appropriate people both within and outside the family? Who decides, and how? What discussions and debate occur?
- *Generating alternative solutions*: Does the family grasp at the first idea for an action plan? Is it the same as usual? Is there any consideration of ideas from others, or always the same person?
- *Deciding on a suitable action*: Were other ideas seriously considered? Is there a single authority, or flexibility in decision-making, or pseudo-democracy? Do they rush to act, act chaotically with no coordination, procrastinate? Are any of these options appropriate?
- *Action*: Does the family do what it decided to do? Does it do anything at all, or get stuck in a frozen cycle of decision-making or denial? Does each individual play their part, or is there sabotage? Do some members feel disabled from participating in active solutions? Are they?
- *Monitoring and evaluation*: Does the family keep a check on the problem and whether it's being resolved or not? Or do they forget all about it until the next time something similar occurs? If they perform this function, how is it managed?

Behaviour control: what patterns have the family adopted for responding to actions in various situations: danger; expressing emotions, desires or biological needs; socializing within and outside the family. This dimension includes not only adult authority over children, but also how the adults conduct themselves in relation to the children, each other and the world. What standards have evolved? How much flexibility is there?

The McMaster system recognizes four broad styles of behaviour control:[41]

- Rigid control is characterized by strict authority, with tightly defined (even if unclear) standards and little scope for adaptation to circumstances (including maturational change).
- Flexible control allows for age-appropriate negotiation, and change according to context or development.
- Laissez-faire control describes those families where authority is absent or abdicated in favour of free choice, regardless of risk, judgement or maturity.

- Chaotic control is attributed to families that apparently randomly veer from the rigid to laissez-faire ends of the spectrum.

Roles: how do individuals within the family carry out specific desirable (or problematic) functions? Are vital roles achieved and is there a sense of security and confidence in the people fulfilling essential functions? What other roles seem to be being performed (or not)? Who decides on the nature or desirability of these jobs? How is their achievement or ongoing desirability monitored?

Vital roles include providing essential food, warmth and shelter; nurturing and sustaining development; preserving the family security and boundaries. Other roles can develop that may be useful or not, destructive or creative, subversive or caring. These roles may include sacrificing ones of well-being to keep the peace, or becoming ill to deflect attention from some other denied conflict.

Families that manage their own problems and seem to require little outside help demonstrate clear, direct communication patterns. When members of healthy families need to express their feelings, or achieve a particular task, they generally seem to understand what role they and others have in the situation, and speak directly to involved relatives in a lucid, unambiguous manner.[42] After years of traumatic stress, families with difficulties often manifest the opposite characteristics – they have fragile, permeable or impenetrable personal boundaries; show limited abilities to deal responsively with each other's emotions; and can tolerate only a restricted range or intensity of feelings. Fractured, unclear or indirect communications characterize their interactions. People make faulty assumptions about the meaning of other people's behaviour. They impute thoughts, feelings or motives that mismatch each other's beliefs about themselves, and then react to each other on the basis of these erroneous assumptions, thus establishing self-fulfilling spirals of distorted attitudes and interactions which over time become deeply engrained. The 'bow-tie' method of graphically depicting communication circularities is a simple heuristic devise that can sometimes dramatically clarify apparently bafflingly complex family interactions[43] (see Figure 18.1). Nurses can help families to consider each other's thoughts and behaviour differently, and identify new possibilities for tolerance, shared feelings or problem-solving, by helping them to clarify vague or mismanaged communications between individuals.

Nurse:	So Lisa, when you see Mum being so wild with Dad, what do you think, or how do you feel?
Lisa:	I feel angry with her, frightened for him, and I feel so stuck, I want to die.
Nurse:	And what do you actually do then, when you feel all that?
Lisa:	I usually go to my room, and cry.
Nurse:	How does Lisa's withdrawal and tears affect you, Mrs Jones?
Mrs Jones:	I feel guilty, of course I do, but it seems unfair as well – I get even angrier with John.
Nurse:	And what do you do when you feel guilty?
Mrs Jones:	I try to talk with Lisa about my frustration and tell her I'm sorry, but I always end up going off at her again.
Nurse:	What's that like, Lisa?
Lisa:	I'm sure she wants me dead, or different, but I can only be me.
Nurse:	Mr Jones – do you think that your wife wants Lisa dead or different?
Mr Jones:	I know she doesn't, but it must seem that way to Lisa.
Nurse:	A diagram of how this works out between you might make it clearer to me. Would you mind if we

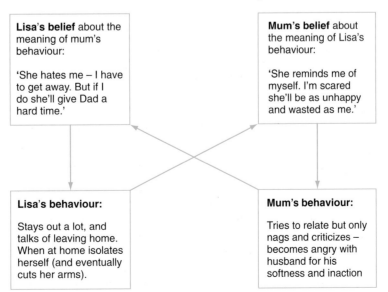

Figure 18.1 A's belief about B governs A's behaviour, which justifies B's belief about A, which governs B's behaviour, which justifies A's belief, which …

sketched it on paper? So, Lisa how does mum's nagging affect you again?

Lisa: I think she hates me, and I want to get away – but I worry about dad [see Figure 18.1].

Nurse: That's really very sad. How can you help each other with this fear that Mrs Jones is no good, and Lisa could become like her?

Reflection

Reflect on how your own family functions. Consider how your family communicates with each other, how feelings are expressed and controlled, how problems are solved, behaviour moderated and the allocation of roles and responsibilities.

Family education

'Family interventions' have been developed that aim to reduce the stress/distress of families, improve their coping and teach them about illness and its management. This kind of broad psycho-educational approach with families is almost considered a universal component of any integrated care package in schizophrenia and has been highly formalized in terms of training for health professionals. These programmes emphasize medication compliance strategies, educating people about relevant psychiatric diagnoses, enhancing people's preferred coping methods, teaching and applying problem-solving techniques and altering family communication patterns. Well-crafted packages have been found to contribute to a reduced frequency of relapse, reduced hospital admissions and improved social functioning.[44] Kuipers[45] concludes that it is important to '… replace the stress, anxiety and criticism in some families with calmer, more tolerant, more effective reappraisal and problem-solving, while trying to improve carer's coping and self-esteem'. The most important elements of successful programmes relate to improving communication between family members, reducing stress and reducing over-involvement.[46]

Reflection

Spend time with a family exploring their viewpoints regarding what is happening, habitual patterns of dealing with problems and their ideas about what might help improve the well-being of their family.

On giants' shoulders: paying one's clinical dues

Many collaborative strategies for working with families pre-date the development of 'psychosocial intervention packages'. Early pioneers stressed the necessity of making good relationships not only with the family as a whole, but also with each individual member. Salvador Minuchin[47]

described the processes of 'joining' and 'accommodation' that professionals need to negotiate successfully when engaging with families. 'Joining' a family involves accepting its unique organization and blending with its cultural style. Nurses should adjust their own self-presentation (or 'accommodate') to achieve effective joining. Maintaining a formal, stereotyped, professional image is less important than gaining the families trust and being allowed to experience their pain, pleasure and possibilities at first hand. Nurses should consciously allow spontaneous, natural imitation of communication (or 'mimesis') to help facilitate accommodation, and follow (or 'track') family conversational threads and themes, rather than stick doggedly to pre-set questioning or interview formats. Minuchin also felt it essential to maintain 'balance' within the therapeutic system, so that whenever he supported one member over a particular issue, he would seek an early opportunity to ally with other members who might have felt their point of view disregarded. Nurses can adapt such techniques within their unique professional matrix to therapeutically transform the kind of social, conversational or more formal, organizational role-bound interactions that many have with patients and their relatives.

Jay Haley[48] outlined a structure for conducting first and subsequent meetings with families. He emphasized the importance of beginning the session with a *social phase* during which the professional can make contact and engage with each member in turn by being genuinely interested in positive aspects of their life and personality, separate from any discussion of the family's problems. This phase is followed by a *problem* stage in which each family member is invited to contribute their perspective on the family's difficulties and his or her preferred outcomes. Nurses need to be respectful of each person's contributions, and firm enough to conduct the session by facilitating other family members' listening while each person speaks. During the third *interaction* stage the family is encouraged to talk together to share observations on a specific issue, understand each other's perspectives or behaviour and start to identify shared viewpoints or resolutions. Nurses need to be ready to intervene during this stage to maintain balance, prevent 'scape-goating' or other damaging interactions and ensure that family members continue to listen to their relatives. During the final *goal-setting* stage, nurse and family collaborate to identify, clarify and plan behavioural tasks and contracts involving all relevant family members in constructive change or support. Haley's framework offers nurses a structure to make more productive use of family meetings in both residential and sessional environments.

Collaborative conflict

Even with very careful attention to joint engagement, professionals can develop distorted perceptions of family processes, determined not only by their clinical orientation, therapeutic belief system and working practices but their own personality development and family experiences. Any unexplored or disowned aspects of self, personality rigidity, or prejudicial narrowness in professional education or cultural background may predispose a clinician to non-collaborative practice of one kind or another. Similarly, defensive interpersonal behaviours may stimulate emotional reactions in either nurses or clients, and unmet emotional needs may result in parataxic or projective distortion of working relationships. Regular personal supervision and staff sensitivity or support meetings are necessary if nurses are to avoid being disabled by unresolved needs or negativity.

Just as families (and individuals) are often internally riven with conflict, so also the history of working clinically with families demonstrates considerable theoretical and methodological dispute. Some forms of family therapy have been accused of 'blaming' families for the plight of a sick member, whereas family management practitioners have been indicted for unnecessarily pathologizing vulnerable members and hypocritically deceiving relatives.[49] The diagnosis of schizophrenia has been an especial focus of disagreement[50] and fraught with mixed messages and paradoxes. For example, families and health professionals have campaigned to reduce the sense of blame that has often been apportioned to or felt by families in relation to schizophrenia. However, high 'expressed emotion' of relatives (a combination of criticism, hostility and over-protectiveness) has consistently been found to be psychonoxious to relatives diagnosed with schizoprenia.[51] Furthermore, many people who are diagnosed with schizophrenia have suffered various forms of abuse, sometimes at the hands of family members.[33] It is reasonable that families and individuals experience mixed emotions and exhibit complex dynamics in keeping with their complex and multifaceted histories. Good family work requires the facilitation of conditions whereby families feel safe enough to ask questions and search for answers that make sense to them.[46]

As mentioned above, a useful concept deriving from early family therapy theory involves construing all family members' apparently pathological or unhelpful behaviours as 'attempted solutions' to perceived or underlying problems. The strangeness of a young schizophrenic may be interpreted as the result of efforts to escape the stifling conformity of a rigidly judgemental family culture,[52] or simply but stubbornly create a different culture more suited to the individual's emerging personality. Violent tantrums, bizarre behaviour, withdrawal or suicidal acts may all serve the purpose of detouring conflict – focusing attention and concern onto an apparently disturbed individual and away from unexpressed or unresolved conflict between other family members[43] Equally, a family's displays of strongly judgemental criticism or hostility may reveal evidence of ambivalent grief or frustrated

weariness, developed after years of ineffectual care and concern for a sick relative. Their well-meaning efforts may have been reacted to by resentment or rejection. They may have failed to dissuade an unwell relative from reckless deviance, unhappily odd preoccupations or dangerously careless behaviours. The family may desperately want to persuade the unwell member to conform to social or behavioural codes they sincerely believe to be better for their relative's welfare.[53]

All kinds of interpretation can fit the complex dynamics of a family in crisis. They are not mutually exclusive or contradictory. However, it is precisely this kind of difference in perspectives that has resulted in recrimination between clinicians from different schools of professional family work. *Family therapy* theories construe families as complex organic systems. Diagnosed pathology in an individual may be understood as the result of chronic pressure or conflict within the whole family system revealing itself by breakdown of the most vulnerable family member. *Family management* theories view the situation from the other end, and assume a priori the existence of disease in one individual. The unwell family member's relatives experience chronic stress, anxiety, frustration or grief. This in turn induces weariness, compassion fatigue or unhelpful responses such as excessive criticism, hostility or emotional over-involvement.[54] Bennun[55] provides a brief exploration of issues around these dichotomous approaches. In both cases, however, therapeutic progress is made by helping the family to change some aspect of its structure or function, either because the family itself is seen as the primary unit of pathology or because it has become less than optimally beneficial for all its members and ineffectively supportive as a caring network.

Whatever psycho-pathological perspective a clinical team works from, nurses should work to ensure that families experience a user-friendly service. Nurses can establish more informal, responsive relationships with both patients and relatives and avoid the arrogant dogmatism and technical excesses that have bedevilled various schools of family work. Nurses can use their relationships with both diagnosed individual and family relatives to work towards helping family members collaborate more with each other. Alternatively, there is a risk that nurses who remain unmindful of or insensitive to significant family dynamics may develop relationships with either diagnosed patients or family carers that mimic the debilitating effects of high expressed emotion. They may themselves become hostile critics, over-involved and emotionally invasive, or ally with one part of the family against another.

REFERENCES

1. Howgego IM, Yellowlees P, Owen C et al. The therapeutic alliance: the key to effective patient outcome? A descriptive

review of the evidence in community mental health case management. *Australian and New Zealand Journal of Psychiatry* 2003; **37** (2): 169–83.

2. Zuroff DC, Blatt SJ. The therapeutic relationship in the brief treatment of depression: contributions to clinical improvement and enhanced adaptive capacities. *Journal of Consulting and Clinical Psychology* 2006; **74** (1): 130–40.

3. Havens LL, Ghaemi SN. Existential despair and bipolar disorder: the therapeutic alliance as a mood stabilizer. *American Journal of Psychotherapy* 2005; **59** (2): 137–47.

4. Meier PS, Donmall MC, McElduff P *et al.*, Heller RF. The role of the early therapeutic alliance in predicting drug treatment dropout. *Drug and Alcohol Dependence* 2006; **83** (1): 57–64.

5. Bambling M, King R. Therapeutic alliance and clinical practice. *Psychotherapy in Australia* 2001; **8** (1): 38–43.

6. Rose D. *Users' voices: what works for whom?* London, UK: Sainsbury Centre for Mental Health 2001.

7. Healthcare Commission. *No voice, no choice: a joint review of adult community mental health services in England.* London, UK: Commission for Healthcare Audit and Inspection, 2007.

8. Jakobsen ES, Severinsson E. Parents' experiences of collaboration with community healthcare professionals. *Journal of Psychiatric and Mental Health Nursing* 2006; **13**: 498–505.

9. Prince JD. Family involvement and satisfaction with community mental health care of individuals with schizophrenia. *Community Mental Health Journal* 2005; **41**: 419–30.

10. Hodgson O, King R, Leggatt M. Carers of mentally ill people in Queensland: their perceived relationships with professional mental health service providers: Report on a survey. *Australian e-Journal for the Advancement of Mental Health* 2002; **1** (3): 1–15.

11. Corrigan PW, Miller FE. Shame, blame, and contamination: a review of the impact of mental illness stigma on family members. *Journal of Mental Health* 2004; **13**: 537–548.

12. Newman J, Kuhlmann E. Consumers enter the political stage? The modernization of health care in Britain and Germany. *Journal of European Social Policy* 2007; **17** (2): 99–111.

13. Coppock V, Hopton J. *Critical perspectives on mental health.* London, UK: Routledge, 2000.

14. Keene J. *Clients with complex needs.* Oxford, UK: Blackwell, 2001.

15. Read L, Mosher LR, Bentall RP (eds). *Models of madness: psychological, social and biological approaches to schizophrenia.* London, UK : Routledge: 2004: 349–64.

16. Mancini MA, Hardiman ER, Lawson HA. Making sense of it all: consumer providers' theories about factors facilitating and impeding recovery from psychiatric disabilities. *Psychiatric Rehabilitation Journal* 2005; **29** (1): 48–55.

17. Perkins R, Repper J. *Dilemmas in community mental health practice: choice or control?* Oxford, UK: Radcliffe Medical Press, 1998.

18. Watkins P. *Mental health nursing: the art of compassionate care.* Oxford, UK: Butterworth-Heinemann, 2001.

19. Hoyt, MF. *Some stories are better than others: doing what works in brief therapy and managed care.* Philadelphia, PA: Brunner-Mazel, 2000.

20. Horvath AO. Relation between working alliance and outcome in psychotherapy. *Journal of Consulting and Clinical Psychology* 1993; **38**: 139–49.

21. Schönberger M, Humle F, Teasdale TW. The development of the therapeutic working alliance, patients' awareness and their compliance during the process of brain injury rehabilitation. *Brain Injury* 2006; **20** (4): 445–54.

22. Miller R, Mason SE. Cognitive enhancement therapy: a therapeutic treatment strategy for first-episode schizophrenia patients. *Bulletin of the Menninger Clinic* 2004; **68** (3): 213–30.

23. Weiss KA, Smith TE, Hull JW *et al.* Predictors of risk of nonadherence in outpatients with schizophrenia and other psychotic disorders. *Schizophrenia Bulletin* 2002; **28** (2): 341–9.

24. De Schazer S. *Clues: investigating solutions in brief therapy.* New York, NY: Norton, 1988.

25. Oades L, Deane F, Crowe T *et al.* Collaborative recovery: an integrative model for working with individuals who experience chronic and recurring mental illness. *Australasian Psychiatry*, 2005; **13** (3): 279–84.

26. Barker P, Buchanan-Barker P. *The tidal model: a guide for mental health professionals.* London, UK: Brunner-Routledge, 2005.

27. Zetzel ER. Current concepts of transference. *International Journal of Psychoanalysis* 1956; **37**: 369–76.

28. Rogers C. *Client-centred therapy.* Cambridge, MA: Riverside Press, 1951.

29. Rogers C. *On becoming a person: a therapist's view of psychotherapy.* London, UK: Constable, 1967.

30. Linehan MM. *Cognitive-behavioral treatment of borderline personality.* New York, NY: Guilford Press, 1993.

31. Kelly G. *A theory of personality: the psychology of personal constructs.* New York: Norton, 1963.

32. Watzlawick P, Weakland L, Fisch R. *Change: principles of problem formation and problem resolution.* New York, NY: Norton, 1974.

33. Read J, Os J, Morrison AP, Ross CA. Childhood trauma, psychosis and schizophrenia: a literature review with theoretical and clinical implications. *Acta Psychiatrica Scandinavica* 2005; **112** (5): 330–50.

34. Smail D. *The origins of unhappiness: a new understanding of personal distress.* London, UK: Constable, 1993.

35. Smail D. *How to survive without psychotherapy.* London, UK: Constable, 1996.

36. Lakeman R. Adapting psychotherapy to psychosis. *Australian e-Journal for the Advancement of Mental Health* 2006; **5** (1).

37. Hulme P. Collaborative conversation. In: Newnes C, Holmes G, Dunn C (eds). *This is madness.* Ross-on-Wye, UK: PCCS Books, 1999.

38. Griffiths P, Pringle P. *Psychosocial practice within a residential setting.* Cassell Monograph No. 1. London, UK: Karnac, 1997.

39. Hinshelwood, RD. *Thinking about institutions.* London, UK: Jessica Kingsley, 2001.

40. Barnes T. The legacy of therapeutic community practice in modern community mental health services. *Therapeutic Communities* 2000; **21**: 165–74.

41. Epstein NB, Bishop D, Ryan C *et al*. The McMaster model view of healthy family functioning. In: Walsh F (ed.). *Normal family processes*. New York, NY: Guilford Press, 1993: 138–60.

42. Beavers R. *Successful families*. New York, NY: Norton, 1990.

43. Dallos R. *Family belief systems, therapy and change*, 2nd edn. Milton Keynes, UK: Open University Press, 1994.

44. Pharoah F, Mari J, Rathbone J, Wong W. Family intervention for schizophrenia. *Cochrane Database of Systematic Reviews* 2006; Issue 3, Art No: CD000088.

45. Kuipers E. Family interventions in schizophrenia: evidence for efficacy and proposed mechanisms of change. *Journal of Family Therapy* 2006; **28** (1): 73–80.

46. Aderhold V, Gottwalz E. Family therapy and schizophrenia: replacing ideology with openness. In: Read L, Mosher LR, Bentall RP (eds). *Models of madness*. London, UK: Routledge, 2004: 338–47.

47. Minuchin S. *Families and family therapy*. London, UK: Tavistock, 1974.

48. Haley J. *Problem-solving therapy*. San Francisco, CA: Josey-Bass, 1987.

49. Johnstone L. Family management in 'schizophrenia': its assumptions and contradictions. *Journal of Mental Health* 1993; **3** (2): 255–69.

50. Keen T. Schizophrenia: orthodoxy and heresies. *Journal of Psychiatric and Mental Health Nursing* 1999; **6**: 415–24.

51. Wearden AJ, Tarrier N, Barrowclough C *et al*. A review of expressed emotion research in health care. *Clinical Psychology Review* 2000; **20**: 633–66.

52. Laing RD, Esterson A. *Sanity, madness and the family*. London, UK: Tavistock, 1964.

53. Atkinson J, Coia DA. *Families coping with schizophrenia*. Chichester, UK: Wiley, 1995.

54. Leff J, Vaughan C. *Expressed emotion in families*. New York, NY: Guilford Press, 1985.

55. Bennun I, Family management and psychiatric rehabilitation. In: Carpenter J, Treacher A (eds). *Using family therapy in the nineties*. Oxford, UK: Blackwell, 1993.

56. Stewart W. *An A–Z of counselling theory and practice*, 2nd edn. Cheltenham, UK: Stanley Thornes, 1997.

57. Halmos P. *The faith of the counsellors*. London, UK: Constable, 1978.

SECTION 4

SPECIFIC NEEDS FOR NURSING

Preface to Section 4

Nurses claim that advocacy for patients, and consideration of their needs and interests as persons having dignity and worth, are primary values inherent in the design and execution of nursing services. These values should be implicit in a nursing approach for the care of patients having a diagnosis of schizophrenia. In keeping with these claims it would behoove nurses to give up the notion of a disease, such as schizophrenia, and to think exclusively of patients as persons.

Hildegard E. Peplau

The range of problems that people might encounter during the course of their lives is potentially infinite, given that the meaning and significance of any 'problem' varies enormously from one person to the next. However, it is interesting how similar our different problems become, when we can step back from them. In developing his theory of 'interpersonal relations', Harry Stack Sullivan famously said that people really had only two kinds of problems: they had problems relating to themselves and problems in relating to other people.

There was great wisdom in Sullivan's observation. All the problems that are described as 'mental disorders' are either experiences that people *complain* about, or complaints or criticisms made about the person by other people. This may be another way of illustrating Sullivan's idea that problems are either *intra*personal or *inter*personal.

It is also clear that, wherever we go in the world, the human problems that people complain about are much the same. Some of the detail may be modified depending on social or cultural conventions, but in general people have problems with themselves, and their 'private' experiences, or else they have problems in their relationships with friends, family, colleagues or neighbours.

Although any human problem that ends up being classified as a 'mental disorder' can have implications for the family or wider society, that problem is always, first and foremost, a personal crisis – a personal tragedy.

As the mental health field becomes increasingly influenced by research and socioeconomic models of service provision, we risk losing sight of the *person* who is the *human point* of the whole endeavour.

In this section, we introduce examples of some of the more common forms of problems in living, which present very different needs for nursing. It is all too easy to find ourselves discussing various *disorders*, *patient types*, *conditions* and *cases*, when we really need to be talking about the *people* who are the source or substance of these professional stories.

In this section, I have chosen examples of the kind of problems of living that either present nurses with most difficulty or are viewed as particularly problematic by society at large. Although all the 'people' included in the chapters are fictitious, they are all drawn from the authors' knowledge of considerable numbers of people with these kinds of problems. I have asked the authors to hold the *person* in sharp focus, using the features of the person's *condition* or *diagnosis* only in a supporting context.

We begin with the person who experiences anxiety – a problem that is understood by everyone, including nurses themselves, and which probably forms a part of many of the other problems of living in the psychiatric canon. Then we consider some of the most common problems in living that nurses are called upon to help people address. We end with a consideration of the person with a diagnosis of autism. Although not always considered to be a 'mental health' problem, the person with autism represents a complex problem of 'mind', which may well justify describing this group of people as among the most challenging that nurses might encounter in practice.

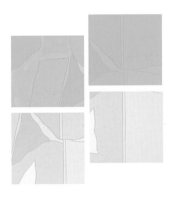

CHAPTER 19

The person who experiences anxiety

Eimear Muir-Cochrane*

... her chest tightened, she fought for breath and she trembled. She felt pain in her chest and arms and experienced tunnel vision. She thought she was having a heart attack and would die.[1,p.201]

INTRODUCTION

Anxiety is one of the most common treatable mental disorders. Effective treatments include cognitive–behavioural therapy (CBT), relaxation techniques and, occasionally, medication to control muscle tension.[2] Anxiety disorders range from generalized feelings of uneasiness to immobilizing bouts of terror.[2] Here, we shall discuss the most common anxiety disorders:

- generalized anxiety
- phobias
- obsessive–compulsive disorder (OCD)
- post-traumatic stress.

It is vital that, to be of use to those in their care, nurses reflect upon their own experiences of events that invoke anxiety and learn how to manage these feelings usefully.[3] Anxiety can be transferred interpersonally. For example, you arrive ready for an examination and find your fellow students extremely anxious. Although you felt quite calm, now you find your anxiety levels increasing dramatically.

Today, enough is known about anxiety to develop early intervention and prevention programmes. To that end, this chapter adopts a self-development approach so that nurses can develop their own anxiety-management skills, with a view to helping patients facilitate their own anxiety management. Remember, if people in your care recognize your anxiety, this will elevate their own.

THE IMPORTANCE OF RELAXATION

It is appropriate to approach the management of anxiety disorders by reflecting on our own anxiety. If nurses can use basic self-relaxation techniques, they may be more effective in helping people in their care to recognize tension and learn to relax and manage uncomfortable feelings and symptoms that interfere with their normal functioning.[4]

Reflection

Think of a time when you felt extremely tense. Make notes about your thoughts, feelings and sensations at the time. Then, think of a time when you were extremely relaxed and make notes accordingly. What do you notice that is different?

*Eimear Muir-Cochrane was Associate Professor at the University of South Australia, where she recently implemented a new postgraduate multidisciplinary mental health programme. In early 2008, she was appointed Professor and Chair of Mental Health Nursing at Flinders University, South Australia. Her research interests include the use of seclusion, absconding, the mental health needs of homeless young people and the involvement of consumers in postgraduate education.

Relaxation training

Relaxation training involves the deliberate release of tension, whether *physical* (e.g. muscle tension or stomach cramps) or *psychological* (e.g. excessive worrying). When someone relaxes, the nerves in the muscles send messages to the brain that are distinctly different from those sent when someone is anxious, tense or stressed. These different signals incur a general feeling of calmness in the person.[5]

Muscle relaxation has an effect on the nervous system, manifested in physical and psychological ways, and is extremely useful in helping to deal with feelings and experiences that disrupt everyday living. Relaxation training can help people who have been under stress for long periods of time, and who may have forgotten what it is like to relax and release their tension. Daily practice can help restore physical and psychological balance (equilibrium)[5] and reduce tense feelings that include being jumpy, irritable and nervy, as well as physical manifestations of tension (e.g. stomach complaints, diarrhoea or constipation, and backache). Learning to relax can enable the control of uncomfortable levels of anxiety and tension in stressful situations.[5]

To help people in your care learn to relax, it is vital that you examine and assess your own tension and anxiety (Box 19.1). Tension is *necessary* physically to help us move about or to exercise vigorously, and psychologically to keep us alert to respond to a situation such as a job interview. However, a lot of the tension we feel is *unnecessary*, and this can be determined by reflecting on the relationship between the level of tension and the activity involved, such as when the tension is not serving a useful function or when the level of tension remains high after the alerting situation has passed.[3]

Box 19.1: Assess your stress[2]

Use the following questions to assess your own stress levels:

- Where do I feel tension? (e.g. in my chest, back, jaw)
- What are the characteristics of the tension? (e.g. fatigued muscles, soreness)
- Which kinds of things lead to an increase in tension? (e.g. anger, loneliness, impatience, boredom)
- What external factors increase your tension? (e.g. loud noises, having to wait to be served, traffic, your relationships)

Progressive muscle relaxation

Like most things, relaxation training takes practice to be really effective. Encourage patients to persevere when they say 'I'm too tense to relax' or 'this is not for me, it's not doing me any good' (Box 19.2).

There are two core components to relaxation training: *recognizing tension* and *relaxing*. Progressive muscle relaxation training involves tensing and relaxing muscles in a

---

Box 19.2: Relaxation guide[4,p.629]

- First of all, clear your mind of any worrying thoughts. Let your mind be calm.
- Practise breathing in – holding your breath for a few seconds – and breathing out again. Try and control your breathing until it flows smoothly. Imagine that the tension in your body is flowing down and outwards, like water, every time you breathe out.
- Now it is time to relax your body, starting with your hands. For each muscle group, tense the muscles for 10 seconds, then let go and relax.
- Hands: curl your hands into fists and relax.
- Arms: tense the muscles in your arms and relax. Be aware of your biceps and the difference between tensing and relaxing them.
- Shoulders and neck: shrug your shoulders up to your ears, hold for 10 seconds and relax.
- Face: raise your eyebrows, hold and relax. Scrunch up your eyes, hold and relax.
- Jaw: clench your teeth (not too tightly) hold and relax.
- Chest: breathe in deeply – hold and relax.
- Back: lean your head and back forward – hold and then relax.
- Bottom: tighten your buttock muscles and then relax.
- Legs: push your feet firmly on the floor – hold and then relax. Lift your toes off the ground towards your shins and relax.
- Feet: gently curl your toes up – hold and then relax.
- Stay sitting quietly for a few minutes enjoying the sensation of being relaxed. Take some slow deep breaths, pay attention to your breathing. Try and practise every day; this will help your body to relearn how to relax and minimize tension building up.

---

repetitious fashion, moving from the hands to the shoulders, neck and head, and then down through the stomach and back to the buttocks, legs and feet – tensing and relaxing alternately for about 10 seconds each time, usually over a 20- to 30-minute time period. The best position is sitting comfortably with back straight, feet flat on the floor. It is generally advised not to lie down, as there is a good chance of falling asleep. Sitting upright in a quiet warm place is a good option.

Some people find other ways to achieve the same relaxation effect through exercise, meditation, yoga or ta'i chi. All provide an opportunity for self-reflection and letting go of the unnecessary stress we all carry, to varying degrees. If, as nurses, we can master the art of relaxation, we can model a relaxed and open demeanour to those around us. This, in turn, will increase the opportunity to build rapport and trust with our patients to explore how they view their concerns in a practical way and to reduce the amount of unnecessary and uncomfortable anxiety in daily life.[6]

THE NATURE OF ANXIETY

Anxiety is a normal part of the human condition, experienced by everyone to varying degrees. Anxiety is usually a transitory response to threat or danger. Most people experience a knot in the stomach over mounting bills or just before a job interview. Certain experiences and memories provoke anxious feelings, spurring us on, for example, to finish the essay that is due tomorrow. Nervousness in anticipation of an event is normal. However, the experience of anxiety can lead people to question how much choice and emotional control they have in their lives.[3] If people become preoccupied with unwarranted worries for longer than a short period, or the feelings cause the person to avoid everyday activities, they may be described as having an anxiety disorder.[7] Anxiety disorders can have an underlying biological cause (e.g. hyperthyroidism[7]) and frequently run in families.

Anxiety is also one of the most treatable mental disorders. It is characterized by a feeling of dread or uncomfortable anticipation with physical, psychological, behavioural and cognitive features. Nurses are likely to encounter people in their care showing a variety of anxious responses to their situation. In general hospitals, many patients are anxious about their medical condition, impending surgery or the experience of hospitalization itself. In mental health settings, most people receiving care will demonstrate some anxiety, with a smaller number being so severely affected that they cannot function normally in relation to work, family responsibilities, and interpersonal relationships.[5] With such people, specific interventions, including medications, are usually required.

Prevalence of anxiety

Between 8 and 12 per cent of the population experience a pervasive level of anxiety that impedes their daily lives; 5.3 per cent of the population experience an anxiety disorder.[8] Anxiety is the most prevalent single psychiatric disorder of the modern era with 80 million days per year worldwide lost because of mental illness.[9] Loss of productivity from the paid and unpaid workforce has profound implications for the fiscal and social capital of nations. The World Health Organization suggests that the three most productive things to invest in to reduce lost work productivity are migraine, anxiety and depression.[9] Women were more likely than men to have experienced anxiety disorders (12 per cent compared with 7 per cent). Of the 12 per cent of women experiencing anxiety, 2.2 per cent are most commonly referred to psychiatrists for generalized anxiety disorders (GADs), 1.9 per cent are referred for phobia/compulsive disorders anxiety and 1.3 per cent for post-traumatic stress anxiety disorders. For the 7 per cent of men experiencing anxiety-related issues, 3.5 per cent are referred for generalized anxiety and 1.2 per cent for post-traumatic stress anxiety disorders.[10]

Aetiology and contemporary treatments

Several theories purport to explain anxiety disorders.

- The biological view holds that anxiety disorders may have a genetic element, particularly OCD, and are associated with alterations in cerebral serotonin[7]. As with other psychiatric conditions, receptor sites in the brain have now been located for the action of benzodiazepines (anti-anxiety medication), in the medial occipital cortex, supporting the usefulness of these drugs in the reduction of symptoms of anxiety.[7]
- Learning theory supports the concept that anxiety is a conditioned response to specific environmental stimuli and has a biological survival value. The standard 'flight or fight' response – and the associated increase in heart rate and alertness – prepare the person for danger.[7] Over time, how a person acts in response to a stressful event is often the result of learning. If too many stressors occur in a short time period, the person may experience acute anxiety and exhibit maladaptive behaviour.[7] An example of maladaptive behaviour may be an increase in alcohol consumption after the loss of a loved one through death or separation. Some theorists believe that social and cultural factors will determine how personality develops and how a person responds to stress.[4] For example, a person with a low self-image is more likely to have problems coping with an unexpected problem in their daily life than someone with a very positive self-image.
- Cognitive–behavioural theory embraces a range of learning theories that view the way we feel, think and behave as inextricably linked.[1] Thus, a person with a poor self-image may have a disagreement with someone and conclude 'That person does not like me', feeling anxious and sweaty and deciding to avoid social situations in future. CBT is a relatively short-term treatment plan (2–20 sessions[1]) which aims to teach a person how to relax and to recognize and cope with their anxious thoughts and feelings. CBT aims to help people become aware of their thinking style, replacing or reframing this with more positive ways of thinking, which can lead to an increase in self-confidence, problem-solving ability and reduced associated anxiety.[1] The assumption behind CBT is that dysfunctional behaviours are the presumed underlying problem. CBT applies well-established learning principles to eliminate the unwanted behaviour and replace it with more constructive ways of thinking, feeling and acting. The major focus in CBT is to help the person examine and understand the world (their cognitions) and to experiment with new ways of responding (their behaviour). In this way, the client can be helped to be future focused and to behave more adaptively.[1]

Much has been learned in the past two decades about the treatment of anxiety disorders. Recent developments in neuroimaging techniques have led to better understanding of the biology of OCD and the brain circuits that may be involved in the production of symptoms. The most effective treatment approach appears to be CBT,[7] consisting of exposure and response prevention and specific medications. Pharmacotherapy for anxiety is recommended usually in combination with CBT in the following circumstances:

- where there is co-morbidity, such as depression
- when CBT is unsuccessful
- when symptoms are severely disabling.[7]

Recent research has demonstrated a shift in the type of medications being prescribed for the treatment of GAD from exclusive benzodiazepine treatment to a combination of benzodiazepine treatment and antidepressant treatment.[7] In future, more invasive and controversial techniques such as neurosurgery and neurostimulation may hold some promise.

THE MANIFESTATION OF ANXIETY

The material in Box 19.3 will help you to explore the various dimensions of anxiety.

Box 19.3: Physiological (physical) symptoms of anxiety[2,p.278]

- Shortness of breath
- Dizziness
- Choking sensation
- Palpitations
- Trembling
- Sweating
- Dry mouth
- Decreased appetite
- Nausea
- Diarrhoea
- Elevated blood pressure
- Affective (mood)
- Fear
- Terror
- Dread
- Sense of impending doom
- Apprehension
- Behavioural
- Exaggerated startle reflex
- Motor tension (foot tapping, restlessness)
- Irritability
- Nail biting
- Altered sleep pattern (too much, too little, difficulty going to sleep or waking up)

Refer to the notes you made about being tense and anxious. Allocate your thoughts, feelings and sensations to the categories here.

In children, several other symptoms may be observable or reported by parents who may not recognize these behaviours as being anxiety related. Nurses are frequently in contact with adults and children receiving care or who are family members of the sick person. Children often demonstrate anxiety symptoms as a response to the stress. Symptoms include irritability, marked self-consciousness, overconcern about the future and past events, a constant need for reassurance, unrealistic and excessive worry and distress on separation from parents. Children and adolescents with pervading anxiety require expert assistance through specialist intervention.

Relief behaviours

Hildegard Peplau[11] identified four relief behaviours commonly occurring as an uncomfortable reaction to the experience of anxiety. Learned over time, these are the physical manifestations of unconscious mechanisms and help the person cope with their feelings. Some of these behaviours prevent us from learning how to manage our emotions usefully and result in a reduced ability to learn new ways of coping. A constructive pattern of relief behaviour such as *realistic problem-solving* refers to the individual converting anxiety into useful energies, such as exercising to reduce tension and anxiety, resulting in the development of useful coping skills. The following three relief behaviours are not constructive, and once learned are often difficult to unlearn.

1 *Acting out* refers to impulsive behaviours such as shouting or self-harming in which the person displaces emotions from one situation to another. Acting out often distresses people witnessing the behaviour but the individual may not be as distressed or upset.[11]
2 *Somatizing* refers to the physical manifestation of anxiety into a condition or sensation such as paraesthesia or palpitations.[5]
3 *Withdrawal* involves removing oneself from situations that are perceived to be threatening.[11]

It is highly likely that these relief behaviours will be manifest when people are under duress. Nurses need to be aware of their function to respond calmly and with compassion.

Reflection

What relief behaviour are you aware of having used to manage your own anxiety?

THE EXPERIENCE OF ANXIETY

At a low to moderate level of anxiety we experience a narrowing of perception. With increased muscle tension (jitters), our speech rate increases, with mixed feelings of challenge, confidence, optimism and fear. At a physiological level, anxiety activates the sympathetic nervous system with an increase in blood pressure heart rate and respiration, pupillary dilation and peripheral vascular constriction.[2] Moderate levels of anxiety serve to improve performance, and even high levels of anxiety are often consistent with the demands of the situation.

However, high anxiety can disable people to the extent that they find it difficult to perform everyday activities. It is normal to experience anxious thoughts, but it is the extent to which these thoughts render the individual able to carry out their normal activities that determines their disabling effect.[2] Anxious thinking is often distorted thinking – anticipating that things are not going to turn out well and feeling unable to cope (Box 19.4). This can increase anxiety and lead to depression if it persists. For example, you see someone you know in the supermarket but he or she does not acknowledge you. An anxious thought may be 'That person does not like me'. A more realistic thought may be 'Oh, she has not seen me' or 'He may be preoccupied'. CBT aims to help people understand their negative self-talk and to develop more positive and realistic patterns.[1]

Box 19.4: Activity

Think of times when you have been anxious, listing the anxious thoughts you had then. Beside each 'anxious thought' write an 'alternative' thought that might reduce the feeling of anxiety.

ANXIETY DISORDERS

Anxiety can be disabling. The dysfunctional aspects are marked by three major components:

1 behavioural avoidance
2 catastrophic cognition
3 autonomic hyperarousal.[2]

None of these components differentiates between normal and pathological anxiety. The only criterion is the level of interference in personal, occupational or social functioning. It is also incorrect to say that *abnormal anxiety* is just a matter of being too anxious at a time when others are not. People with anxiety disorders have recurring irrational and specific fears that they recognize as being unrealistic and intrusive.

People with a generalized anxiety disorder experience chronic exaggerated worry and tension that is more intense than the reality of the situation. A diagnosis is made if the person has spent at least 6 months worrying excessively about everyday problems.[7]

Generalized anxiety disorder

An elderly woman was admitted after her daughter became increasingly concerned about her deteriorating physical activity and social isolation. The patient was bereaved 9 months ago. Since then she has become disinterested in activities she previously enjoyed. She says that she has gripping chest pains, often feels as if she cannot catch her breath and that her heart is pounding so loudly that other people can hear it. She is observed wringing her hands constantly and making multiple visits to the toilet.

Panic disorder is characterized by a white-knuckled, heart-pounding terror that strikes with the force of a lightning bolt, without warning. Some people feel like they are going mad, devoured by fear, or dying of a heart attack.[1] Because they cannot predict these attacks, many experience persistent worry that another could overcome them at any time. A significant number of people (50–60 per cent) also experience major depression.[7] Most panic attacks last only a few minutes but could last up to an hour in rare cases. With appropriate help, between 70 and 90 per cent of this group respond within six to eight sessions of CBT. CBT combined with medication – such as high-potency anti-anxiety drugs (e.g. alprazolam) and several classes of antidepressants, such as paroxetine and the older tricyclics and monoamine oxidase inhibitors (MAO inhibitors) – is considered to be the 'gold' standard.[7] Sometimes a combination of therapy and medication is the most effective approach to helping people manage their symptoms.[4]

Panic disorder

A 20-year-old student is admitted with a 6-month history of panic attacks. She has become unable to attend university regularly owing to overwhelming and disabling feelings of choking, vomiting and difficulty in breathing. She failed her first year of study after she experienced 'blocks' during examinations. Since then her anxiety has worsened to the extent that she is extremely uncomfortable in public places, has difficulty swallowing and thinks she is losing her mind.

Phobias are the most common form of anxiety disorder, affecting between 3 and 5 per cent of the adult population worldwide.[12] Phobias occur in specific forms. A specific phobia is an unfounded fear of a particular object or situation, such as being afraid of dogs yet loving to ride horses or avoiding flying on aeroplanes but being able to drive on busy highways. There is virtually an unlimited number of objects or situations that a person can be afraid of.

Commonly, people have phobias of snakes, spiders, open and/or closed spaces, dirt, blood injuries and needles. Many of the physical symptoms that accompany panic attacks (e.g. sweating, racing heart and trembling) also occur with phobias. Formal diagnosis is made when people experience extreme anxiety when exposed to a given situation or object yet recognize that the fear is excessive or unreasonable but are unable to change the feeling, with the result that normal routines, relationships and social activities are significantly disrupted.[5] CBT has the best track record for helping people overcome phobic disorders. The goals of this therapy are to desensitize the person to feared situations and to teach the person to relax and to recognize and cope with anxious thoughts and feelings. Anti-anxiety agents or antidepressants may also be used to minimize symptoms in the short term. There are differing views about the combination of medication and CBT. Some would use a combination, but others advocate that the symptoms need to be treated not suppressed by drugs.

OCD is one of the 10 leading causes of disability worldwide, representing a major worldwide health problem.[9] There are two main clinical features to this condition. An obsession is a persistent, intrusive and unwanted thought or emotion that the person cannot ignore. A compulsion is a behavioural manifestation of the obsessive thought, resulting in the performance of a repetitious, uncontrollable but seemingly purposeful act.[5] For example, a person may have obsessive thoughts about cleanliness and the associated compulsive behaviour of repetitive handwashing, perhaps to the point of having excoriated skin on the hands from excessive washing. The compulsion becomes disabling when the person cannot carry on his or her normal daily activities because

Obsessive–compulsive disorder

A married man, Peter, who is 35 years old with two children under 5, is admitted with OCD. Two years ago he developed the obsessive thought that the chemical used to treat his roof was poisoning his children. He began washing his hands and clothes excessively to the extent that he was in danger of losing his job because of the time it took to repeatedly carry out these cleansing rituals. On admission, he was noted to be of low mood with an anxious presentation. He told the nurses that he was on the verge of going mad and was worried his wife would leave him. Peter was offered a mild antidepressant and a programme of CBT that involved exposing him gradually (systematic desensitization) to stimuli that triggered the anxiety, at the same time helping him to voluntarily refrain from hand washing.

of preoccupation with obsessive thoughts and compulsive acts.[7]

It has been acknowledged only recently that anyone with experience of a traumatic event may experience *post-traumatic stress disorder* (PTSD), especially if the event was life-threatening.[2] In the past, PTSD most commonly referred to victims of war who had experienced heavy combat. Common PTSD experiences include kidnapping, aeroplane crashes or other serious crashes, rape, natural disasters and war. If the person is traumatized seriously by the event, the resulting psychological damage causes a significant impairment in the ability to maintain previous functioning – such as working or maintaining relationships. Symptoms can range from constantly reliving the event to a general emotional numbing. Persistent anxiety, exaggerated startle reflex, difficulty concentrating, nightmares and insomnia are common. Typically, people with PTSD avoid situations that remind them of a situation as it triggers intense emotion and distress.[2] For example, a person trapped on a road during a flood may deliberately avoid driving on that section of the highway.

Research in this area has increased in recent decades as individuals have developed PTSD after being involved in natural disasters such as bushfires in Australia and floods in Europe. Depression is often experienced in PTSD, as is the use of prescription and non-prescription drugs and alcohol to dull emotional pain. Psychotherapy, CBT, medication such as antidepressants and anxiolytics, support from family and friends and relaxation techniques form the basis of treatment programmes for these patients.[2]

NURSING THE PERSON WHO IS ANXIOUS

The care of people with disabling levels of anxiety involves being with individual patients and offering them time to, as Barker[6] calls it, 'name their distress', i.e. what meaning the patient places on his or her experience. The loss of control patients feel because of their disabling anxiety is often an extremely important component of their distress, and therefore gaining control is a common goal. To that end, the role of the nurse and structured programmes of therapy such as CBT involve creating a situation in which patients feel able to exercise choice about their future and how they think and feel about it. The relationship the nurse has with an anxious patient is extremely important if any interaction is to be meaningful.[6] Carl Rogers[13] describes warmth, genuineness, empathy and unconditional positive regard as core dimensions of the nurse–patient relationship. If a nurse does not present a genuine demeanour or exhibits anxiety towards the patient, it is more difficult to be helpful. Nursing strategies can best be related to the level of anxiety a person is experiencing (mild, moderate or severe), rather than the diagnosis of the disorder itself.

Box 19.5: Nursing interventions during an episode of panic[4]

- Stay with the person and encourage him or her to sit down.
- Take some deep breaths yourself and then begin to speak to the person in short sentences.
- Reassure the person that this episode will pass.
- Provide external control by being firm but caring.
- Encourage the person to breathe in and out slowly into a paper bag to reduce hyperventilation.
- Maintain a safe and quiet environment to reduce external stimuli.

Box 19.6: The value of 'being with'[2,pp.293–5]

Reassure the person that the anxiety will pass. Accept the person without judgement. Be available so that the person can approach you when the need arises.

- Listen attentively to what he or she is expressing and encourage such ventilation. Answer queries honestly and briefly.
- Meet with the person at the beginning of the day to assist with planning daily activities that act as a diversion and that are part of the treatment programme.
- Set daily and weekly goals that are agreed by both nurse and patient. Encourage the person to identify what the goals are to be.

Box 19.5 illustrates some simple strategies that might be used if the person is in a state of high anxiety or panic. These emphasize the need to remain with the patient and for the nurse to present a calm demeanour.

Working with anxious patients requires an initial assessment phase to gain a holistic picture of the person's situation and his or her potential and readiness to make positive changes.[6] Gentle discussion of how the person makes sense of being in hospital or coming to community health services for assistance will provide useful contextual information. Asking 'What brought you here today' can allow patients to begin to ventilate and make sense of what is happening to them.[6] From this beginning point the nurse can start to explore coping resources with the patient by gentle enquiry into the patient's perceptions of his or her social supports, economic circumstances, health status and cultural and spiritual beliefs.

Particular attention also needs to be paid to the person's interpersonal resources, social skills, positive relationships with family and friends and what Sperry[14] calls intrapsychic resources, including positive motivation, drive, and personal and professional ambitions, value systems and self-esteem. The way that people have coped with stress in the past is also a good indicator of their coping mechanisms. As has been previously discussed, people using relief behaviours over time generally find that they are not useful in adapting to expected or unexpected change and result in the person becoming cut off emotionally and often socially isolated. Effective coping skills include tackling the problem in a useful manner by, for example, seeking help. Stuart[2] also identifies cognitive coping mechanisms of searching for meaning, problem-solving and evaluating how realistic personal expectations may be and readjusting some goals.

For each of the clinical cases in this chapter, brainstorm nursing interventions that can assist these individuals while they undergo treatment. Compare your list with the principles listed in Boxes 19.6 and 19.7.

Box 19.7: Educative interventions[2,p.294]

- Relaxation methods: for example, controlled deep breathing and relaxation tapes. Group and individual relaxation sessions after visiting time on the ward can be well timed as many patients find this to be a vulnerable time.
- Encourage the use of a reflective journal on a daily basis to share thoughts and feelings.
- Identify the patient's strengths and useful coping strategies and support persons.
- Conduct group and individual sessions about the range of normal physiological responses to anxiety and how to identify warning signs of increasing stress.

ISSUES AND SOLUTIONS

It is not uncommon for people receiving treatment to develop a lowered mood, which prevents them from being able to undertake or complete aspects of their treatment, such as relaxation or CBT activities. The role of the nurse is vital in completing regular holistic assessments to recognize early warning signs of depression. If the person is depressed, treatment without medication is more difficult.[1]

Patients with OCDs may initially find it very difficult to complete the suggested tasks and to practise the relaxation methods they have been encouraged to use. They may complain of being too tense or develop further anxiety about the prospect of changing 'useless' behaviours, such as repetitive counting, checking and hand washing. If patients are admitted to hospital, it is not unusual for their compulsions to lessen dramatically in the first few days of hospitalization. However, once patients have familiarized themselves with their new surroundings the problematic behaviour re-emerges. Further, once the effects of treatment are manifest in a reduction in compulsive acts, different compulsions may emerge as the person's defence against anxiety. Understanding and support are vital to help patients deal with these eventualities.

Being relaxed and having an open and compassionate demeanour are skills that have to be learned over time, and which may not come easily, particularly for nurses who are naturally anxious. Witnessing relief behaviours – such as acting out – can be very stressful and clinical supervision and opportunities to debrief, beyond the immediacy of the event, are important support strategies in the workplace. Often, individuals experience more stress some time after experiencing some form of critical incident. Expressing personal judgement about a patient's problems may be a sign that the nurse is under stress and might benefit from clinical supervision or mentoring. It is also common for healthcare staff, particularly nurses, to avoid people who are highly anxious. Recognizing the potential for such avoidance and seeking the support of more experienced staff in working through such feelings can facilitate and enhance personal and professional growth.

SUMMARY

Nurses need to develop both personal and professional awareness of stress and anxiety if they are to care successfully for people with anxiety disorders. Today, various interventions are helpful in the management of disabling anxiety. However, being with anxious patients requires compassion and self-awareness, and understanding of the effect anxiety has on people's lives. Using different strategies, nurses, in a variety of healthcare settings, can help people to take control of their problems that are related to the experience of anxiety and manage them successfully.

REFERENCES

1. Westbrook D, Hennerley H, Kirk J. *An introduction to cognitive behaviour therapy: skills and applications*. London, UK: Sage Publications, 2007.

2. Stuart G. Anxiety responses and anxiety disorders. In: Stuart G, Laraia M (eds). *Principles and practice of psychiatric nursing*, 7th edn. St Louis, MO: Mosby, 2001: 274–98.

3. Langeland E, Wahl AK, Kristoffersen K, Hanestad BR. Promoting coping: salutogenesis among people with mental health problems. *Issues in Mental Health Nursing* 2007; **28** (3): 275–95.

4. Carson B (ed.). *Mental health nursing: the nurse–patient journey*, 2nd edn. Philadelphia, PA: WB Saunders, 2000.

5. Beary T. Anxiety disorders. In: Peate I, Chelvanayagam S (eds). *Caring for adults with mental health problems*. Chichester, UK: John Wiley & Sons, 2006: 87–102.

6. Barker P. *Assessment in psychiatric and mental health nursing: in search of the whole person*, 2nd edn. Cheltenham, UK: Nelson Thornes, 2004.

7. Collin Abrams A, Barnett Lammon C, Smith Pennington S. *Clinical drug therapy: rationales for nursing practice*, 8th edn. Philadelphia, PA: Lippincott Williams & Wilkins, 2007.

8. Australian Institute of Health and Welfare. *Mental health services in Australia 2004–05*. Mental Health Series no. 9. Canberra, Australia: AIHW, 2007.

9. Harnois G, Gabriel, P. *Mental health and work: impact, issues and good practices*. Geneva, Switzerland: World Health Organization, 2002.

10. Australian Institute of Health and Welfare. *Mental health services in Australia 2000–01*. Mental Health Series no. 4. Canberra, Australia: AIHW, 2003.

11. Peplau H. Interpersonal theory in nursing practice In: O'Toole A, Welt S (eds). *Selected works of Hildegarde Peplau*. New York, NY: Springer, 1994.

12. Somers JM, Goldner MD, Waraich P. Prevalence and incidence studies of anxiety disorders: a systematic review of the literature. *Canadian Journal of Psychiatry* 2006; **51**: 100–13.

13. Rogers C. *Client-centred therapy*. Boston, MA: Houghton & Mifflin, 1965.

14. Sperry L. Case conceptualizations: the missing link between theory and practice. *The Family Journal: Counseling and Therapy for Couples and Families* 2005; **13**: 71–6.

CHAPTER 20

The person who experiences depression

Ian Beech*

Depression is awful beyond words or sounds or images; I would not want to go through an extended one again. It bleeds relationships through suspicion, lack of confidence and self-respect, the inability to enjoy life, to walk or talk or think normally, the exhaustion, the night terrors, the day terrors. There is nothing good to be said about it except that it gives you an experience of how it must be to be old, to be old and sick, to be dying; to be slow of mind; to be lacking in grace, polish, and co-ordination; to be ugly; to have no belief in the possibilities of life, the pleasures of sex, the exquisiteness of music, or the ability to make yourself and others laugh.

INTRODUCTION

The opening quote above, from Kay Redfield Jamison's book *An Unquiet Mind*,[1] gives us some small idea of what the world is like for someone who is experiencing depression. This chapter will consider what it is the medical profession refers to when it talks about depression. There will be, therefore, some discussion of diagnostic criteria, but it should be borne in mind that it is not the remit of the nurse to diagnose a person as depressed. Neither is it the role of the nurse to prescribe antidepressant medication. These both remain the role of the doctor. The role of the nurse is something different. It is about *being with* a person who may feel guilt, shame, hopelessness and worthlessness. It is about being with that person for perhaps longer periods of time than any other professional. At the same time, it is not the role of the nurse to be the 'neighbour over the fence' or the 'friend in the pub'. People experiencing depression expect nurses to provide something more than either a sympathetic shoulder to cry on or an exhortation to 'pull yourself together'.

Neither is this chapter about how to provide psychotherapy to people experiencing depression. Although I will draw upon some aspects of different psychotherapies (e.g. cognitive therapy[2] and logotherapy[3]), the nursing approach suggested here does not sit exclusively within one theoretical approach, for the following four reasons.

1 'Therapy' traditionally and culturally (but not of necessity) takes place in 1-hour sessions under structured conditions. People live their lives 168 hours per week.[4] Nurses working with people experiencing depression come into contact with them (depending on the clinical context) for some, most, or all of those 168 hours, often in unstructured situations and often when emotions are raw. So nurses are *doing nursing* rather than practising psychotherapy.
2 In the same way that physical explanations of depression can suggest that a person with depression is somehow 'faulty', implying that the person needs fixing, so too can many psychotherapeutic approaches.[5]

*Ian Beech is Head of the Mental Health Division at the University of Glamorgan, Pontypridd, UK, and is researching a history of Cardiff City Mental Hospital.

3 To work exclusively with a single approach might be appropriate for someone with many years of experience in a particular therapy but, as many readers will be less experienced, it would be inappropriate to be too prescriptive about using any single approach.

4 When nurses think in terms of one linear explanation for the problems that people experience they risk forgetting the many other approaches that may be helpful, which lie beyond the model they learned in whichever 'therapy class' they attended.

When nurses start to work with people experiencing depression a number of issues can leave them floundering:

- 'What if I make things worse?'
- 'What if I say something that causes someone to kill him/herself?'
- 'What do I say?'

All such questions arise when nurses first encounter depression. Some may adopt the attitude that depression is a physical condition of the brain that can be treated physically. So long as nurses prevent the person from committing suicide, these physical treatments will do the trick.

Some may undertake a protracted training course to become a 'nurse therapist', working exclusively within one model of psychotherapy or another.

Most, however, will be somewhere in the middle, especially if they are relatively inexperienced. As a nurse, you will probably be involved in the administration of medication *and* in talking to people. This chapter is a journey through some of the theories that try to explain depression and some of the treatments that commonly are offered to people who are depressed. After a brief stop at each of these waystations, the journey will take us to our destination: a description of *nursing* approaches that might be helpful, both for someone experiencing depression and for the nurse who is trying to help that person.[a]

Reflection

Consider some of the people with depression with whom you have worked.

What feelings do you have about people considered to be depressed?

WHAT IS THIS THING CALLED DEPRESSION?

Barker[6] tells us that depression may be thought of in three forms. The first is where the person experiences depression suddenly and for a short period of time following an event such as loss of a job, or loss of belongings. This depression usually lifts as the person begins to rebuild after the event. The second is short-term but fairly serious in nature – following the death of a significant other, the breakdown of a relationship or some traumatic experience. In both of these forms of depression the person may experience a period of abject misery and may require the help of friends, family and possibly professionals to get through the problems. However, the majority of people encountered by nurses are those in Barker's third group: people whose depression endures and the distress either becomes long-term or keeps returning.

Depression may also be thought of as primary or secondary. In *primary depression* the problems associated with the person's mood are the central problems. In *secondary depression* the emotional problems are associated with other problems such as neurological and brain diseases, e.g. Huntington's disease, Parkinson's disease, dementia and endocrine disorders such as thyroid, parathyroid and diabetes, or as a side-effect of medication such as steroids, anti-malarial drugs, phenothiazines.

The American Psychiatric Association in its *Diagnostic Statistical Manual IV Text Revision* (DSMIV-TR)[7] provides the medical criteria on which a diagnosis of a major depressive episode is made. From the following list, either number 1 or number 2 has to be present along with at least four from numbers 4–9 to give a total of the presence of *five or more* in a 2-week period, representing a change in what is 'normal' for the person.

1 Depressed mood most of the day, nearly every day.
2 Diminished interest or pleasure (anhedonia) in almost all of the activities of the day, nearly every day.
3 Significant weight gain or loss when not dieting (more than 5 per cent of body weight in 1 month), or decreased or increased appetite nearly every day.
4 Insomnia (not sleeping) or hypersomnia (sleeping too much) nearly every day.
5 Abnormal restlessness (psychomotor agitation) or a drop in physical activity (psychomotor retardation) nearly every day.
6 Fatigue or loss of energy nearly every day.
7 Feelings of worthlessness or excessive or inappropriate guilt nearly every day.
8 Diminished ability to think, concentrate or make decisions nearly every day.
9 Recurrent thoughts of death, or recurrent suicidal thoughts without a specific plan; or a suicide attempt; or a specific plan for committing suicide.

In a similar vein, the World Health Organization[8] provides a list of symptoms and severity to guide diagnosis.

While these criteria give us some indication of the sort of symptoms psychiatrists look for when they are diagnosing depression, they neither give us an indication of

---

[a] During this chapter I will refer to nurses and people experiencing depression. It should not be assumed from this that the two groups are mutually exclusive.

what might be the explanation for a person experiencing depression nor do they tell us what the subjective experience of depression is like for the person.

To have an idea of what depression is like we either have to have experienced it ourselves or listen to those who can tell us. The description above by Redfield Jamison and the following description by Lewis Wolpert[9] offer some insight:

> It was the worst experience of my life. More terrible even than watching my wife die of cancer. I am ashamed to admit that my depression felt worse than her death but it is true. I was in a state that bears no resemblance to anything I had experienced before. It was not just feeling very low, depressed in the commonly used sense of the word. I was seriously ill. I was totally self-involved, negative and thought about suicide most of the time.

A QUESTION OF CAUSE

Traditionally,[10] nurses learned that depression could be divided into two types:

- one with a readily identifiable cause, i.e. one or more adverse life event (this type was known as reactive and neurotic);
- one that had no readily identifiable cause and that seemed to emanate from within the person (endogenous and psychotic).

This way of thinking about depression has become discredited for two reasons. First, people's experiences do not fit such neat stereotypes. Some experience long-term life-threatening depression as an apparent reaction to what might be seen as a fairly mundane life event, while others might experience a short period of depression with no apparent cause. Second, both of these ways of thinking about depression present problems for the patient. Thinking about depression as being reactive encourages people to think of themselves as weak in some way. They are experiencing depression, whereas others, faced with similar life events, have not become depressed. Thinking about depression as being endogenous, on the other hand, is no more helpful because this encourages the person to think that he or she must have some weakness of character that brought on depression for no apparent reason.

Explanations for the cause of mental distress abound. Each theory of psychotherapy puts forward its own formulation of how the mind works and what causes it to work in ways that distress us. Here, we consider some common theoretical explanations:

1 biological
2 psychodynamic
3 interpersonal
4 cognitive
5 social.

A personal illustration might help us to appreciate how each explanation might conceive of the experience of depression.

Personal illustration 20.1

Joan is a woman who has experienced depression for most of her adult life. She recounts how her parents used to beat her when she was a young child. When she left home she got married and had two children, only to find that her husband had a conviction for child abuse of which she was unaware. In an accident one night her youngest child was killed.

Over the next few years, Joan had attempted suicide on a number of occasions and had undergone a variety of different psychotherapies, had various admissions to hospital with changes to medication but constantly felt guilty about the death of her child, constantly felt worthless, had difficulty sleeping and thought about suicide.

It's all in the brain

The biological theory of depression asserts that the brain's balance of certain chemicals becomes disturbed, perhaps because of stress or genetic predisposition or a combination of factors. As a consequence of the imbalance the person experiences depression. Which chemicals exactly are implicated is subject to some debate.

Whether the same chemicals are implicated in all cases is also subject to discussion among scientists. The usual suspects in such matters are serotonin and norepinephrine. The rationale behind antidepressant drug therapies is that the drug redresses the imbalance in the brain chemical and therefore alleviates the depression. So in Joan's case a biological explanation for her depression might claim that the serotonin and/or norepinephrine levels in her brain are disturbed, possibly triggered by some of the events in her life, and that antidepressant therapy might redress the imbalance and help to alleviate her distress.

However, antidepressant drugs can be inconsistent in their effectiveness. *Different* people experiencing depression respond to *different* drugs in *different* ways. Some people find their depression lifts after taking medication, some find that they have to try a number of drugs or combinations and some find that the depression remains even after taking medication. Consequently, the purely chemical view of depression has some problems associated with it. Could it be that there are a number of different events happening in people's brains that give people experiences that society knows as depression? Or are the drugs we presently use too broad in their focus so that they are not 'smart' enough to pinpoint the exact neurochemical nature of depression? In either case, people usually find that while drugs may be helpful to many they are usually not the whole story of recovery.

It's all in the mind

Psychodynamic explanation

The psychodynamic explanation[11] proposes that, as a child, the person has experienced a highly significant loss and/or developed the belief that being loved was dependent on pleasing others. As a result, the child develops a distorted self-image. In adulthood, the person experiences a loss or difficulties with relating to events in life and associates this with feelings about the childhood loss or interpersonal relationships. This association of feelings about the current situation and the childhood memories often includes anger. The anger is internalized back into the person and this increases and intensifies feeling of guilt and lack of self-worth. In Joan's case the physical abuse suffered at the hands of her parents and the subsequent loss of her child could be explained as the dynamic processes which led to her depression.

Interpersonal explanation

Interpersonal theory[6] puts forward the view that a person develops a depressive way of being as a result of negative interpersonal relationships and the lack of positive reinforcement in life. In Joan's case the criticism and hostility shown to her by her parents might have led to her developing a depressive way of being.

Cognitive explanation

The cognitive explanation[2] of depression considers that depression results not from what is happening in the world of the person but in how the person thinks about what is happening in the world. In other words, the person interprets events in a negative way, which brings about negative responses and depressive feelings that cause events to become more negative and a spiral of depression ensues. For Joan, a cognitive explanation would focus on her negative schemata (ways of thinking) about herself, i.e. her feelings of guilt and worthlessness.

Social explanation

The social model[12] holds the view that depression in women arises out of social vulnerability, particularly in four areas: early loss of a mother; involvement in care of young children; absence of a confiding relationship; lack of a job. When stresses occur depression arises as a result of vulnerability in these areas failing to shore up the person. Joan did not physically lose her mother but did lose the nurturing parental relationship, which was replaced with abuse. She has no significant relationship, she cares for her children alone, she is female and she has no job. In other words, she shows patterns of vulnerability that the social model would lead us to expect to find in women who experience depression. Although such 'social' explanations emphasize the importance of the external world, it also acknowledges how the world of

experience is internalized in what might be called 'the mind'.

Joan's case can be viewed in terms of any of the theories explained. This demonstrates that no theory is *the* truth. They are all useful theoretical frameworks that professionals employ to help underpin their approaches to helping people.

Reflection

What, in your experience, do you consider to be the major causes of depression?

TREATING THE PERSON EXPERIENCING DEPRESSION

Medication

The drugs used in depression can be thought of in terms of groupings:

- drugs that inhibit the reuptake of serotonin into nerve cells
- drugs that inhibit the reuptake of serotonin and norepinephrine into cells
- tricyclic antidepressants
- monoamine oxidase inhibitors (MAOIs)
- others.

All drugs are chemicals that have effects on the body. When the effect is desirable we call it the *therapeutic* effect. When it is undesirable we call it a *side-effect*. In some cases, the side-effect can become the therapeutic effect and vice versa depending on circumstances. For example, the tricyclic antidepressant amitryptiline has a side-effect of sometimes causing retention of urine, yet it is sometimes given to 'treat' difficulty in controlling the bladder at night (nocturnal enuresis). One of the balancing acts to be achieved with antidepressant medication is that of preparing people for the side-effects which can appear *before* the therapeutic effect. Each of the above groups has particular side-effects. Comprehensive information on all of the drugs available cannot be provided here, so only pointers for good practice are suggested.

While it is not the role of most nurses to prescribe antidepressant medication it is often the role of the nurse to administer such medication and to monitor its effects. As such, it is important for nurses to be up to date with the medication that is in common usage in terms of:

- recommended dosages
- likely side-effects
- how long someone might need to take the drug before he or she can expect to experience any therapeutic effect

- any special precautions or contraindications (when the medication might be inappropriate or dangerous)
- the answers to any common questions that someone prescribed the medication might ask.

Information sources

This knowledge should be kept constantly under review. It is not sufficient, for example, to purchase a book on pharmacology for nurses during pre-registration training and consider that to be the end-word on medications. Drugs are constantly being developed. New drugs come onto the market, old ones fall out of favour or are removed from common usage. New precautions and instructions often appear after a drug has been in use for a while and nurses need to be up to date on these issues as well as aware of where to access information and where to point people who take the drugs for information.

A good point of reference for both nurses and people prescribed antidepressant medication is the Norfolk and Waveney Mental Health Partnership NHS Trust Pharmacy website: www.nmhct.nhs.uk/pharmacy. This provides information about drugs in common usage in mental health, in readily accessible language. The *British National Formulary* in the UK is also a useful reference manual when dispensing medication. More importantly, additional information can be accessed online, in a constantly updated form, at www.bnf.org/bnf/ once a free registration is completed.

Other physical approaches

Further physical methods of treating depression are electroconvulsive therapy (ECT) and transcranial magnetic stimulation (TMS). ECT is a well-known treatment for depression involving the administration of a controlled current of electricity across the skull of the person who has been anaesthetized and had a muscle relaxant administered. The aim of the treatment is to induce a seizure.

It is not clear how ECT works to improve symptoms for someone experiencing depression but many psychiatrists (and some people who have received ECT) do still consider it to be a useful weapon in the armamentarium against depression. The National Institute for Health and Clinical Excellence (NICE) recommends that ECT be used only after other treatment regimes have been used and found to be ineffective.[13]

ECT has been a contentious subject for many nurses, with some taking the view that they would not wish to be involved in the treatment. The ethics of ECT is beyond the remit of this chapter. As the law stands in the UK the only treatment from which a nurse may lawfully abstain is abortion, and so many nurses may find themselves working with people who are about to receive or have received ECT. In certain respects, the responsibilities of the nurse with a treatment such as ECT are similar to those with medication. The person's questions and fears should be addressed and information given regarding what the person might expect on waking after the procedure, e.g. headache and some memory loss.

TMS is a treatment that involves the application of controlled bursts of an electromagnetic field around the head of the person. This is thought to stimulate the activity of neurones and alleviate some of the problems of depression. Given the questions posed about the use of mobile phones and their ability to induce an electromagnetic field in the vicinity of the head and possible associated side-effects, it will be interesting to see how this form of treatment develops. At time of writing, NICE has entered consultation on the use of TMS but is yet to issue guidance.[14]

Psychological therapies

Psychological therapies to help people experiencing depression are based within the psychological theories discussed previously. Depending on availability, people may be offered one or more of psychodynamic, cognitive, interpersonal, behavioural and marital therapies. In the current system of psychiatry in the UK, it is rare for someone to be offered such therapies in the absence of medication. In spite of the public perception of the psychiatrist as a latter-day Freud using psychotherapeutic techniques in a purpose-built surgery, most psychiatrists operate within a biological mindset which recourses to medication as a first resort.[15]

Nevertheless, there are some tools developed in psychotherapy that nurses can use. An example would be the Beck Depression Inventory (BDI), which is a self-rating scale that covers 21 areas of a person's life and scores each of these between 0 and 3. The scores are totalled and scores over 16 in total are indicative of depression. Unfortunately, nurses often use this tool in such a way that does not do it justice. Often, it is merely used to obtain a score as a baseline on admission to hospital and then put away in the back of someone's notes and repeated after 3 weeks of antidepressant drug therapy to see whether the drugs have had any effect. The BDI is a useful tool for nurses to use because it enables them to focus on the particular areas that the person is experiencing as problematic. In other words, it enables the nurse to discuss things with the person in a focused way rather than just general conversation.

NURSING APPROACHES TO PEOPLE EXPERIENCING DEPRESSION

The nursing care of someone experiencing depression is a skilled activity that is neither medicine nor psychotherapy but might take from both of these disciplines and others in order to help people. On meeting the person for the first time it is worth considering the work of Peplau,[16] who considered roles in the relationship between nurses and people in care. She reminded us that the first role the nurse fulfils for the person is that of *stranger*. 'Trust me I'm a nurse' would probably not be a very successful opening for a conversation, yet there is an assumption that just because a person approaches someone wearing a badge saying 'Nurse' then that person must not only trust the nurse but also pour out his or her innermost feelings. When people do not do this, they may appear to be uncooperative.[17]

Curiosity skilled the nurse

It can often be difficult for people to remember that nurses are strangers to them because people assume that nurses *know* them. Whenever people enter the psychiatric system one of the first things that happens is that copious amounts of medical, nursing and other professionals' notes are generated about them. These then accompany the person throughout the journey made in the system and become, effectively, the person's biography. While notes are an obvious necessity for the purposes of communication between professionals there is always the danger that they can become *the* story about a person's life. This can have negative consequences.

- Because of the nature of the problem-solving approach employed by health professionals, people's lives can sometimes be seen in terms of their problems rather than their strengths.
- Professionals risk losing all curiosity about people because they know *the* story. Consider the 'man who throws refrigerators'. Dick had been resident in a large psychiatric hospital for many years and was known as the man who threw refrigerators. He was thus known because he had *once* thrown a refrigerator across the kitchen of the ward in 1973. His notes recorded, however, that 'when he gets angry he throws refrigerators'.

Reflection

Consider the stories told by different professionals about people in the mental health system.

- What stories might be told by the consultant psychiatrist, the nurse, the occupational therapist, the social worker and the psychologist?
- How might these stories differ from that of the person called patient?

Building relationships

One of the first principles of psychiatric–mental health nursing should be *curiosity*. Nurses should maintain an interest in people's stories. To allow people to tell their stories we need to create conditions in which this might happen. When a person is experiencing depression he or she often feels worthless and boring. Often, friends and relatives will have given up the arduous task of trying to 'cheer up' the person. The realization that a nurse might be willing to spend time with a person when other people find that person boring and difficult can be very reassuring. A nurse may need to sit with the person for a while *not* talking and *not* asking lots of questions but simply being there. This can be difficult. There is often a temptation to fill the silence or to talk to a more lively person or to find something else to do. At the same time a balance has to be achieved. Annie Altschul[18] described her feelings when she experienced depression as wishing both to feel safe in a ward environment and to have her own space.

People experiencing depression can develop a hostile way of relating to others as a way of maintaining their own ideas of worthlessness, i.e. 'people have no time for me because I'm worthless so I won't have any time for people'. In Joan's case, she had developed disdain for many health professionals because they had not helped her. Invariably, she would enter into what a professional thought was a 'therapeutic session' but Joan had no intention of allowing anything 'therapeutic' to happen. As a result, the professionals had quickly changed from what Watkins[19] describes as 'rescuer role' to the 'persecutor role'. Rescuers see people as in need of rescuing. There is a tendency among nurses to want to help people in distress and fix their problems. Once the problem will not be fixed the rescuer can turn into the persecutor and blame the person with the problem for not getting mended. When people may not 'mend' quickly we need to develop the skill of being neutral towards hostility and also not having expectations that the person can be fixed like some broken washing machine.

Nurses need to begin to build the relationship with the person slowly and carefully using the active listening skills and open questioning described in Chapter 11.

Here is a snippet of my early conversations with Joan.

Ian: Joan can you tell me a bit about how you feel just now?
Joan: I feel everything is hopeless, everything is just black.
Ian: Black?
Joan: I'm just going through the motions. I can't do anything and no one can help me.
Ian: You say no one can help you, can you say a bit more about that?
Joan: Yes well I've been to see psychologists, the last one I saw I ended up getting her to tell me all about her children [laugh] it was easier than talking about my problems.
Ian: So you have found that you could move the conversation away from discussing your problems. Does that help?
Joan: [Laugh] Well it makes me feel better in the short term but it doesn't get me anywhere.

By using simple questioning techniques I was able to listen to her and find out more about her feelings and experiences without putting words in her mouth. As our conversation developed it became clear that other professionals had begun their work with Joan assuming that she had to change. But they had not established where it was within Joan that this change should occur.

Ian: Can you tell me a bit more about what you see as the problem with therapy?

Joan: Well I've had loads of people sitting with me telling me that I've got to change to get better and there they are, every time I see them they wear the same clothes, they come to work at 9 o'clock and go home at 5 o'clock and do the same things every day. Where do they get off telling me I've got to change?

In spite of having seen a number of different therapists Joan felt that they were all too busy trying to 'cure' her to get to know her as a person. By adopting these simple techniques I was able to get to a point where, when I summarized what Joan had told me about herself and related it back to her, she responded by saying that no one had ever understood how she felt in a way that I had showed her that I did.

Despite being strangers, people do generally expect nurses to be doing something in clinical settings. People generally expect nurses to have a plan and also for that plan to be related to some of the problems that they are experiencing. Personal illustration 2 indicates how much people expect there to be a plan even in the face of contradictory evidence.

Personal illustration 20.2

Jeff was admitted to an acute psychiatric ward experiencing depression and found that he was placed in the day room of the ward while the nurses spent a lot of time in the office.

Three years after his discharge Jeff remained convinced that the nurses' plan must have been to check out his mental state by observing him from a distance and seeing how he behaved.

Negative statements

People experiencing depression may very often talk in very negative ways about their lives, their families and their futures. This can often be disconcerting for nurses because it can be very easy to get into confrontation with the person by taking the view typified by 'of course you are not worthless'. The nurse's advocacy merely confirms (paradoxically) that the nurse believes the person to be worthless. One way to address this is to use a cognitive technique known as the 'friend technique'.

Person experiencing depression: I'm a useless mother. I can't get anything right.

Nurse: If you had your best friend sat next to you and your best friend said 'I'm a useless mother, I can't get anything right!' What would you say to your friend?

Generally, the friend technique elicits one of three responses:

1 'I know just how you feel!'
2 'Pull yourself together, of course you're not useless!'
3 Some sort of helpful suggestion.

The first response – 'I know just how you feel' – seems, at first sight, to undermine the whole purpose of the friend technique, which is to try to elicit a more helpful way of thinking about the situation. If the person responds in this way it is worth exploring the feelings further: 'OK, so you know just how your friend feels, so what might you be able to say to your friend that might help her at the moment?'

If the person's response is something of the nature of 'pull yourself together!' the nurse might say 'OK, so has anyone ever said something like that to you?' 'Did it help you?' 'What else might you say to your friend?' On rare occasions the person may say something quite helpful straight away.

In each scenario notice that the response by the nurse is *not* to enter into argument but, simply, to try to elicit a more helpful response. The nurse aims to help the person to undermine the negative way of thinking. However, this will not happen by attacking the person's beliefs. Generally speaking, when our beliefs are directly attacked we hold on to them more strongly.

Discussing suicide

People who are experiencing depression often consider suicide. Nurses need to assess the risk that this poses to the person. We can do this only by talking *about* suicide. Joan had made several suicide attempts and it was important to assess the risk of another attempt. People expect nurses to be interested in their problems so it would be strange for someone who is feeling suicidal to find that no one wanted to talk about it. In Joan's case this is how the subject was discussed.

Ian: Anyone who had not met you before might say that, given you have tried to kill yourself on a number of occasions and you are still alive, you didn't really intend to die. What would you say to that?

Joan: Well the last time I took an overdose was very late at night in the middle of winter and I went up the mountain where I didn't think anyone would find me. You don't expect a group of soldiers to be out on exercise at that time. And you don't know that the cold slows down your metabolism so the tablets don't work so quickly do you? … But I'll remember next time!

Ian: OK so on a day-to-day basis what is it that stops you from killing yourself?

At no point did I say to Joan that I did not believe she was serious in her attempts at suicide. At the same time, however, I was able to ascertain the seriousness of her intentions. I could then move on to discussing with her the reasons why she may not have killed herself already. Viktor Frankl[3] took the view that the drive behind existence was our desire to find meaning in our lives. If a life has meaning then it will endure. In terms of working with someone who is feeling depressed this means that it is important to find out what positives there are in life. This can sometimes seem contrary to the way in which nurses are trained to think. After all nurses seek to assess people's problems and then plan care based on what those problems are deemed to be. If nurses simply concentrate on people's problems they get a very strange view of people's lives. Nurses define people in terms of problems and they see depression as a discreet entity that can be treated. Yet everyone has problems, but Frankl teaches us that people also have strengths. For example, they do not come into contact with services the moment they start to feel down; they adopt their own strategies for getting by. It is only when these strategies appear not to work that people seek help from others.

In Joan's case she often talked at length about her children and how the thought of them being without a mother prevented her from harming herself. One of the strategies that could therefore be developed was to discuss her children with her and to develop plans for how she might keep from harming herself. Barker and Buchanen-Barker[20] term this the 'personal security plan'. For Joan this included not drinking alcohol when she was alone in the house because this made her feel more depressed and for her to go round to her daughter's house when she felt particularly low.

Discussion that enables people to think in terms of taking some control of their situations creates the conditions for them to start to think about themselves in a more positive light and not simply to rely on the professional to always put things right. It also validates the person's own solutions as opposed to always having to rely on the received wisdom from the professional. In Joan's case, for example, she was able to move on to some extent after her dead child appeared to her in a dream and told her that she had experienced enough guilt and that she should get on with her life.

SUMMARY

- Nursing care of the person experiencing depression is not treatment in the sense of diagnosis and prescription of medication or physical treatment.

- Nurses do have a part to play in the administration of medication, and in monitoring of both the wanted and unwanted effects of that medication.
- Nursing care is not psychotherapy, although it shares the similarity of involving a discourse between the person experiencing depression and a professional and can usefully employ some psychotherapeutic techniques in the relationship with the person.
- Nursing involves a skilled relationship with the person experiencing depression to enable the person to develop ways of making sense of the experiences in his or her life.
- To do this, the nurse employs a variety of theoretical approaches to ensure that the relationship is purposeful and focused on the concerns of the person in care.

REFERENCES

1. Redfield Jamison K. *An unquiet mind: a memoir of moods and madness.* London, UK: Picador, 1995.

2. Gilbert P. *Counselling for depression.* London, UK: Sage, 1992.

3. Frankl V. *The doctor and the soul: from psychotherapy to logotherapy.* New York, NY: Vintage, 1986.

4. Barker P, Kerr B. *The process of psychotherapy: a journey of discovery.* Oxford, UK: Butterworth Heinemann, 2001.

5. Nelson-Jones R. *Six key approaches to counselling and therapy.* London, UK: Continuum, 2000.

6. Barker P. *Severe depression: the practitioner's guide.* London, UK: Chapman & Hall, 1992.

7. American Psychiatric Association. *Diagnostic and statistical manual of mental disorders, 4th edition, text revision.* Washington, DC: American Psychiatric Press, 2000 (DSM IV-TR).

8. World Health Organization, ICD-10. *The ICD-10 classification of mental and behavioural disorders: clinical descriptions and diagnostic guidelines.* London, UK: Gaskell/Royal College of Psychiatrists, 1992.

9. Wolpert L. *Malignant sadness: the anatomy of depression,* 2nd edn. London, UK: Faber & Faber, 2001.

10. Ackner B. *Handbook for psychiatric nurses,* 9th edn. London, UK: Baillière Tindall/Cassell, 1964.

11. Beeber L. The client who is depressed. In: Lego S (ed.). *Psychiatric nursing: a comprehensive reference,* 2nd edn. Philadelphia, PA: Lippincott, 1996: 201–7.

12. Brown G, Harris T. *The social origins of depression: a study of psychiatric disorder in women.* London, UK: Tavistock, 1978.

13. National Institute for Health and Clinical Excellence. *Depression: management of depression in primary and secondary care.* Clinical Guideline 23. London, UK: NICE, 2004.

14. National Institute for Health and Clinical Excellence. *Transcranial magnetic stimulation for severe depression (interventional procedures consultation).* Available from: www.nice.org.uk. Accessed 29 July 2007.

15. Barker P. Psychiatric Lara Crofts? Forget it. *Nursing Times* 2001; **97** (33): 31.

16. Peplau H. *Interpersonal relations in nursing*. Basingstoke, UK: Macmillan, 1988.

17. O'Hagan M. Two accounts of mental distress. In: Read J, Reynolds J (eds). *Speaking our minds: an anthology*. Basingstoke, UK: MacMillan, 1996: 44–50.

18. Altschul A. There won't be a next time. In: Rippere V, Williams R (eds). *Wounded healers: mental health workers'* *experiences of depression*. Chichester, UK: John Wiley & Sons, 1985: 167–75.

19. Watkins P. *Mental health nursing: the art of compassionate care*. Oxford, UK: Butterworth Heinemann, 2001.

20. Barker P, Buchanan-Barker P. *The tidal model: a guide for mental health professionals*. Hove, UK: Brunner Routledge, 2005.

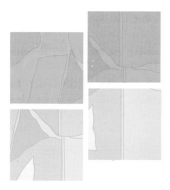

CHAPTER 21

The person who is suicidal

Elaine Santa Mina* and Ruth Gallop**

INTRODUCTION

Suicide is a major problem in all Western countries, most of which have specific targets aimed at reducing its prevalence. This chapter discusses the possible reasons why people commit suicide, and then focuses on the nursing role of assessment of suicidal risk and the development of specific care plans which might help reduce this risk. The importance of aftercare following suicide is also discussed.

A psychiatric–mental health nurse will inevitably care for persons who try to harm themselves or express feelings such as 'I wish I were dead' or 'there is nothing worth living for'. The act of self-harm is a *behaviour* – an expression of an internal feeling state. Being suicidal is not a disease – it is not a disorder. Although we are compelled to try to prevent people from killing themselves we will not always succeed. More importantly, we need to put most of our energy into *understanding* the internal state of the person and trying to help him or her deal with the feelings. Hopefully over time and with appropriate support the person will begin to feel that life is worth living.

Suicidal and self-harm behaviours can be found in clients who receive many different diagnoses. Suicidal behaviour is not restricted to patients diagnosed with depression. Patients with diagnoses of schizophrenia, bipolar affective disorder, personality disorder, eating disorders and post-traumatic stress disorders can all be at risk for self-harm and suicide. Everyone in the mental health system may be, at one time or another, at risk for self-harm and suicide. It is the responsibility of the nurse to be alert to the possibility of this behaviour, to have the knowledge to assess for suicide and to have the basic skills needed to support and care for the suicidal patient.

The term 'suicidal behaviour' is often used to cover many different behaviours:

- completed suicides
- non-fatal self-harm behaviours (including suicide attempts and self-harm without suicidal intent)
- suicide threats.

Sometimes self-harm reflects the wish to die, sometimes it does not, and often the wish to die overlaps with other intentions.[1] Trying to sort this out requires substantial knowledge and understanding plus clinical acumen. Here, we shall focus on the person who has the wish to be dead.

PREVALENCE OF SUICIDE

Death by suicide continues to be a serious problem in contemporary society. The most recent UK suicide rates

*Elaine Santa Mina is an Associate Professor at Ryerson University, Toronto, Canada. Her research focus is self-harm and suicidal behaviour, specifically in adults with histories of childhood trauma. Her clinical work is in acute care for mental health clients.

**Ruth Gallop is Professor Emeritus in the Faculty of Nursing and Department of Psychiatry, University of Toronto, Toronto, Canada. Her research, clinical work and writing focus on clients perceived as treatment and management challenges, who often receive diagnoses of borderline personality disorders, have histories of severe early trauma and have current self-harm behaviours.

are 17.5 males and six females per 100 000.[2] These statistics are similar to European and North American data.[3] More females than males attempt suicide (1.6:1), and more males than females complete suicide.[4] Approximately 4.6–6.6 per cent of the UK population have engaged in some type of self-harm behaviour.[5] There is a link between self-harm behaviour and suicide. Of those who complete suicide, 30–47 per cent have a history of self-harm behaviour. In the UK, 1 per cent of persons who engage in self-harm complete suicide within 1 year and 3–5 per cent complete suicide in 5–10 years.[6]

The current practice trends in mental health care focus on brief hospitalization for severely ill clients. Consequently, many clients in the community are experiencing acute and chronic states of depression and/or other mental illnesses. Therefore, the assessment of suicidal risk is an essential skill for mental health nurses regardless of their work setting.

THE NATURE OF SUICIDE

The novice clinician is often reluctant to ask about suicide. This may be because of a lack of understanding about the feelings and dynamics surrounding suicide. First, we shall list a few basic facts about suicide and then follow this with some of the theoretical and conceptual explanations that make suicidal behaviour understandable.

- *Asking about suicide does not make a person suicidal.* If you think a person is suicidal, then ask them! This is a *vital* question to ask, and should be part of all assessments (see below for assessment guidelines).
- *Most people who commit suicide have a previous history of self-harm.* Previous self-harm is always a cause for concern. Unfortunately, people who self-harm can be viewed as 'attention-seeking', or seen as a distraction from people in 'real need'. Research shows that many people who self-harm go on to complete suicide, so each incidence of self-harm needs careful assessment for risk.
- *Most people who are considering suicide have mixed feelings.* It is extremely important to understand the role of ambivalence in suicide. Patients who tell you that they want to die, or telephone you, saying that they are about to take an overdose, or leave a message that they have self-harmed may be indicating that they are not sure that they really want to die. She may *feel* like dying but some small part of her is unsure. However, communication about suicidal ideation or suicidal behaviour can be an expression of the ambivalence between the wish-to-live and the wish-to-die; and a means to reach out for help.[7] If the clinician recognizes this ambivalence, then they can capitalize on it as a way of helping the person to stay alive and to receive the needed help.

- *Many people who attempt or complete suicide give out warnings or clues.*[8] It is a misconception that people who talk about attempting suicide never do it. The opposite is actually true. Most people who have attempted or completed suicide have given warnings or clues of their intent. Although suicide may appear impulsive in many cases, as we shall discuss and illustrate below, it is not. People give out clues directly and indirectly:
  - personal items may be given away
  - a sense of calm may indicate that the final plan is in place
  - wills may be completed or letters sent
  - statements of a desire to die, of hopelessness, and of a will to kill themselves may be overtly expressed. All such warnings need to be received seriously.
- *Most people who commit suicide have a plan.* Suicide is often a carefully thought out plan. Many people 'feel' suicidal and experience suicidal thoughts or wishes to die but may not act on them. However, others move from thinking about suicide to creating and executing a plan. The plan or method of choice is often one which has a social context.[9] For example, more men than women use violent means such as firearms, and more women than men use overdoses. Many people do not change methods. If access to one method is removed, then the person may not choose another method. For example, if pills are removed from cupboards then the person may not choose a method other than overdose.

WHY PEOPLE COMMIT SUICIDE

Suicide occurs within a complex set of individual and social circumstances. Many different theories, developed by the respective disciplines, attempt to explain self-harm and suicidal motivations. A competent clinician will use the knowledge from different theories to understand the complexity of suicide. Multiple risk factors, occurring simultaneously, are indicative of a higher risk for suicidal behaviour.[10]

- *Social theories.* People who experience a lack of social support are more prone to suicide (e.g. divorced, separated or widowed people, or those who live alone); more men than women complete suicide (specifically men over 65 years of age); people who experience sudden losses, stressors, crises or unexpected change in economic circumstances (either wealth or poverty) are also at increased risk.
- *Biological theories.* It is suggested that some people may have a genetic predisposition towards chemical disturbances, such as depression or psychotic disorders, which make them more vulnerable to suicide. Studies have indicated that people with low levels of serotonin in the brain, as measured by the level of a main metabolite, 5-hydroxyindoleacetic acid (5-HIAA), are more

prone to depression and suicide.[11,12] Alteration of biochemical states through substance misuse such as alcohol or cocaine can also distort a person's perspectives, increasing a sense of hopelessness or distorting reality.

- *Psychodynamic or internal personal theories.* The loss of an important relationship or attachment (actual or perceived) is thought to precipitate tremendous psychological pain. Often, childhood experiences leave an individual vulnerable to the experience of loss. The person may experience overwhelming distress and despair. Life may seem hopeless and suicide the only option.
- *Learning theories.* Suicide is also seen as a mechanism by which people 'cope' with problems of living. As such, suicidal behaviour can become a part of a person's repertoire of coping skills.

Hopelessness

Psychological research indicates that a sense of hopelessness may be an important catalyst for the catastrophic event of suicide. Hopelessness is a manner of thinking and feeling which frames life with negative perceptions of the present and bleak expectations about the future.[13] Current and future situations, relationships and views about oneself are interpreted with pessimism. The person anticipates that life will never become better and that he or she is unable to effect any positive change.

People who experience hopelessness tend to think in a very narrow manner. This constriction in cognitive processes limits the range of understanding of situations and potential choices that may be available for problem resolution. When presented with a situational problem to solve, a person whose thoughts are hopeless and rigid may conclude that suicide is the only choice. Death is an escape from the pain of life.

Circumstances generating hopelessness and depression

Crisis

A suicide attempt is often preceded by some form of crisis. This may be an extreme life event – death of a partner or child, loss of a job or divorce – or it can be a less extreme life event that has significant meaning for the individual.

Personal illustration 21.1

Kim, a 15-year-old boy, jumped off a high bridge. Of Asian heritage, he was the only son of an immigrant family. The family had worked hard so that their son could get the best education. The boy had been caught and humiliated in a school prank. His parents were about to be informed. The shame was unbearable.

Loss and abandonment

Some people are exquisitely sensitive to loss and abandonment, whether real or imagined. When forming successful relationships is difficult for a person, disruption of an existing relationship can feel catastrophic. Sometimes, in the eyes of the observer, the relationship is seen as transient or not very substantial. However, for the individual the loss can re-evoke earlier feelings of being alone. It is not unusual for people with histories of childhood abuse or neglect to be highly sensitive to loss.

Personal illustration 21.2

Jane was hospitalized after taking an overdose. During her stay she formed a friendship with a male patient. After he was discharged she spent her time off the unit visiting him. After two meetings he told her he was too busy to see her and anyway had a girlfriend. Jane was angry and then upset. She left the unit and took a large overdose.

Social isolation

Humans are by nature interpersonal creatures. We all need connection with others. To be in the world without any others who know or care about us can be devastating. Having difficulty forming relationships can lead to isolation, as can certain illnesses, such as schizophrenia and depression. People may feel so unworthy that they isolate themselves from others.

Personal illustration 21.3

John had lived for years with his outgoing brother. After his brother died, John, who was naturally quite shy, gradually withdrew from activities and contacts. He rejected the visits of the community nurse. One night he turned on the gas and died.

Internal motivations

The reason for a suicide attempt is not always apparent. It may be driven by internal events – such as voices or other psychotic thoughts. Occasionally, the motivation is revenge or punishment of another – leaving a legacy of guilt in the survivor. For people with a history of severe abuse, the intense internal pain generated can lead to suicide.

Personal illustration 21.4

Mary experienced severe sexual abuse as a child and lived a chaotic life. When her father (the perpetrator) was nominated for a community award, she sent her diaries to the newspapers and then took an overdose.

Chronic depression, constricted thinking

Despite the best efforts of clinicians, depression can remain chronic and debilitating. Years of hopelessness, different medications without success and a feeling that this will never get better can lead to increased risk for suicide.

Reflection

How do the multiple theories about suicidal behaviour support the philosophy of holistic nursing care?

THE NURSING ROLE

The role of the nurse in caring for the suicidal person is grounded in the therapeutic relationship. All the principles outlined in earlier chapters on therapeutic practice are relevant. Treating each person with respect, dignity and empathy is essential for persons who often view the self as bad or worthless. However, working with a person who is suicidal requires additional knowledge. The nurse must be able to:

1 assess for *suicidal risk*
2 assess the *mental status*
3 promote *safety*
4 explore *precipitants*
5 promote *alternative* coping strategies.

Using a personal illustration, we shall demonstrate the application of this necessary knowledge.

Assess for suicidal risk

Rationale

A suicide attempt is very difficult to predict. However, assessment of a patient's risk for suicide will direct the provision of an appropriate level of protection and guide interventions. Risk for suicide is re-evaluated throughout the course of care to assess the patient's response to personal situational changes and clinical interventions. A suicide risk assessment is discussed with members of the healthcare team, incorporated into the care plan and documented in the clinical record. A careful review of the risk is critical for discharge planning.

The following outline reflects the broad areas to include in your assessment with examples of how questions might be posed. Remember, asking someone about his or her thoughts of suicide will not cause the person to attempt it.

Suicidal ideation

Nurse: Since you have been admitted to hospital do you continue to think about harming yourself or taking your life?

Fred: Well, maybe a little less so at the moment, but I still think everyone would be better off without me.

Nurse: Are you able to control these thoughts or do they occur spontaneously?

Fred: If I am distracted with other people around then the thoughts seem to go away, but when I am alone, I can only think about dying.

Suicidal plan

Nurse: If you were to make another attempt, how might you try it?

Fred: They took all my pills from me in the emergency department, but that's what I would do.

Nurse: Apart from this current overdose have you made other attempts in the past?

Fred: Once before, when my wife ended our marriage, I got drunk and took a handful of pain pills.

Nurse: During this current attempt, how did you arrive at the hospital?

Fred: I called my brother and told him what I had done. I wanted to say goodbye and ask him to keep an eye on my kids for me. He called the ambulance.

Nurse: Did you make any other preparations for your death such as writing a note or leave a will?

Fred: Yes, I wrote my sons.

Nurse: Fred, you have told me about your thoughts and plans to die. However, is there anything that would prevent you from taking your life?

Fred: I think about my sons. I remember how alone I felt when my father died and I worry that they might feel the same way.

Nurse: Do you think your concerns about them may be helpful in stopping you from carrying out your plan.

Fred: I don't know. They are my only reason for living but I still think they might be better off if I were gone.

Nurse: Might there be reasons, in addition to wanting to die, that prompted you to harm yourself?

Fred: I could not stand feeling so bad any more, I wanted to escape from all the emotions I am feeling.

You recognize that several risk factors exist for this patient. Although he says he thinks less about suicide you know that *ambivalence* between the wish to live and the wish to die is common in people who are suicidal. His intentions may also include a desire to escape the overwhelming affect. His thoughts can be distracted when in the presence of others. However, the suicidal thoughts are intrusive and relatively continuous when he is alone and continue to put him at risk.

Fred also has a plan to end his life and has used it in the past. You are aware that a history of previous attempts, especially within 1 year of the current attempt, is more likely to result in a completed attempt within the next year. In his previous attempt, he combined the pills with alcohol. His history of substance misuse creates a potential for impulsive and lethal choices.

The circumstances around his current attempt are of concern. He was alone at the time of his attempt and wrote a note to his sons. This indicates that he was anticipating life for others after his death. However, he reached out and called his brother. He was able to tell someone of his attempt, which initiated a rescue. His ability to reach out and notify someone of his feelings and his actions will also be important information to help him to protect himself in the future. He identifies reasons to live, his sons, but is unsure whether this reason would help him to stay alive. Fred also has a family history of completed suicide, which is an additional risk factor.

Recent stressors

Nurse: Have you experienced any recent problems or losses in your life?

Fred: I was fired from my job 2 months ago. They caught me drinking on the job again so I was let go. Now I can't afford my child support payments and my flat. I can't seem to do anything right. I'll never get out of this mess. My children don't want to see me. The only answer for everyone is for me to be dead.

Nurse: Things seem pretty hopeless to you now. When problems are overwhelming, it can be difficult to find ways to manage and work through them, one step at a time. Later on, we can explore options that you may want to consider trying.

Fred's recent losses and a lack of social support increase his risk for suicide. Each person's response to stress and loss is highly individual. Events that overwhelm one person do not necessarily overwhelm everyone. However, some people, such as Fred, feel desperate, alone and hopeless in the midst of surmounting problems. Acknowledging a state of hopelessness confirms for Fred that you accept his current feelings and do not try to falsely 'cheer him up'. However, you prepare him for future discussions about his coping strategies, and how you might support him to find alternative solutions to his problems. Validation of current and future supports, for example his brother, will be important to help the patient maintain and build on relationships which are protective and provide a sense of belonging.

Impulsivity and substance use

Nurse: You mentioned that you were fired for drinking. How much do you drink in a day on a regular basis?

Fred: I don't drink daily. I only drink when I'm worried or upset. Sometimes I'll go for weeks and not drink. Then a problem will come along and I drink until I fall asleep.

Fred is using alcohol as a means of coping. His use of chemicals adds to his suicide risk by impairment of judgement and perception and increasing lethality when mixed with medications. During another meeting with him you will explore this further. What recent problems triggered this episode of drinking, which resulted in his employment termination? Had he ever received treatment for alcohol use? In a similar manner to your assessment of alcohol misuse, you also understand that other street drugs will add to potential impulsivity and increase suicidality and, therefore, you assess for drug use.

Assess the mental status

Rationale

It is important for the nurse to assess the patient's mental status and level of suicidality *frequently* and *repeatedly* during an episode of care, to be sensitive to alterations in the person's current mental state. Assessment of the patient's mental status provides the nurse with clinical information about the patient's thoughts, feelings and behaviours beyond the aspect of suicide. This provides important clinical data to determine competency and an ability to engage with the treatment team. A suicidal patient's mental status can change in response to external events by internal biochemical changes. This may be indicative of mental and/or organic illness, or in response to medications or ingested chemicals. The severity of a depression can also be reflected in reduction or cessation of activities associated with daily living. Therefore, a mental status assessment needs to be frequently repeated. Also, a current assessment will ensure that the clinician alters the treatment approaches to be appropriate for the clinical status and requirements.

Personal illustration 21.7 (cont.)

After a few days of admission you have observed that Fred is spending almost all of his time in bed, sleeping. He is refusing to get up for meals. He is isolating himself and rarely interacts with other patients.

You meet with him to assess his mental status and revise his care according to his altered state and subsequent needs.

Assessment of affect

Nurse: Fred, you seem to be sleeping most of the day and I noticed that you were not up for meals. How have you been feeling today?

Fred: [He is slow to answer and keeps his face turned away from you.] I have nothing to get up for and I'm not hungry. Please go away and leave me alone.

Nurse: You seem very sad at the moment.

Fred: I have no life and I don't want your help.

You recognize the features of despair and hopelessness. He does not feel motivated even to eat.

Assessment of behaviour

Fred's non-verbal communication – his face and body turned away from you and no eye contact – is a further indication of the severity of his feelings of despair. He is unable to connect with others and participate in life-sustaining activities such as eating.

Assessment of cognition

Nurse: What are you thinking of while you lie there?

Fred: I try not to think. I try to block out these voices in my head.

Nurse: Sometimes when a person feels so awful, thoughts in the form of voices can occur. They sound very real and can be very disturbing. Is this sort of experience happening to you?

Fred: One voice in my head continually tells me to die, to kill myself, I am no good. If I don't eat, I'll die and that is what I should do.

Fred is hearing 'voices' which command him to take his life. You are aware that these voices can be very powerful and frightening and may indicate that the person is experiencing a distortion in reality. He is unable to consider other options for his life. His thoughts about himself are negative and intrusive with the presence of psychotic, self-destructive content that may put him at further risk for suicide. His refusal to eat has become a passive manner to end his life. His plan of care will need to incorporate a nutritional assessment and assistance with nutritional requirements, an increased frequency in observation and assistance with hygiene.

The components of this mental status assessment demonstrate that Fred is still severely depressed. He has a hopeless mood with rigid thinking and intrusive commands to end life. His behaviours are not life sustaining. Based on these observations you believe Fred is at risk for attempting suicide. You increase the level of observation for Fred and convey your concern to the clinical team.

Promote safety

Rationale

The balance between the maintenance of safety for a patient and the assurance of his or her integrity as a human being can be a challenge for nurses. Safety and integrity seem to be mutually enhancing ideals rather than conflicting values. However, in the care for someone who attempts to end his or her life the measures necessary to protect a patient from himself may inherently diminish individual choice and freedoms. Although individual suicides are difficult to predict, the clinician's responsibility is to assess foreseeable risk and to plan for safe measures.[14]

Patients who attempt suicide may resist protective efforts from clinicians and families. If the patient is either not competent to make treatment decisions or unable to develop an alliance with staff then the risk for suicide is higher and the need to ensure safety is enhanced in situations of uncertainty. One of the most meaningful interventions for someone in distress is the presence of a caring nurse. 'Being with' a client who is in despair and mutually engaging in activities of his or her interest fosters a therapeutic relationship, and promotes participation in living. Even the seemingly small and inconsequential activities can garner investment in life.

By its very nature, a hospital environment has numerous potential hazards. A psychiatric unit may have more than one suicidal client, with more than one preferred method. Therefore, most psychiatric environments consider the majority of suicide methods in the planning and development of the environmental structure. Mental health units frequently incorporate construction features to protect patients from suicide: all medications and patient belongings may be locked in cupboards which can be accessed only by nurses; all environmental finishes – which could be used as a means for suicide – may be constructed to counter self-destructive actions (e.g. collapsible curtain rods, weight-tested breakaway hardware, shatter-proof Plexiglas windows and mirrors; and locks that secure the environment yet enable rapid response from staff.[15]

Although immediate protection may be essential, it should neither be more extensive nor of greater duration than the patient clinically requires. The clinician must perform a careful balancing act – maintaining the dignity and self-responsibility of the person as much as possible while ensuring safety. Excessive containment or coercion may at the very least foster a maladaptive dependency. Worse, it can be punitive and an infringement of patient rights. If a patient feels punished and violated through excessive force, then any ambivalence that he or she may have about suicide may be eroded and the person may feel more determined to die. These negative outcomes counter the therapeutic goal to help the patient to a healthy life through the development of constructive adaptive skills and choices.

Although physical measures are important for safety, no measure is a replacement for being with the patient and providing human connection. Human interaction and responsiveness may itself convey a sense of belonging and hope. Also, frequent, direct observation and presence by a skilled clinician provides timely awareness of subtle and overt changes in a patient's mental status and associated behaviours. An observant nurse can respond to subtle patient cues and intervene at a time of increased distress. In the event of an actual attempt, the nurse can intervene immediately and provide emergency care to the patient who is frequently or constantly observed, and thereby diminish potential lethality. In a non-hospitalized scenario, the observation may be provided by a friend or family member who stays at home with the patient or by asking the patient to stay at a temporary residence in a crisis centre.

Example

You have increased your observation of Fred to every 15 minutes based upon your previous assessment. During one of your observations you notice someone visiting Fred and handing him a plastic bag of items. You introduce yourself to the visitor.

Nurse: I notice that your friend has brought you some items, Fred. It's very helpful to have a friend who cares about your needs. Our concern is also for your need for safety. Would you and your friend show me the articles that have been brought for you, then, if necessary, we can find safe places to store them for your future use?

Fred: I feel like a child if you check everything. The articles are mine and I don't want to give them over to anyone.

Friend: I would never do anything that would harm Fred. Why are you suggesting that I would?

Nurse: We know friends want to be helpful and caring, but sometimes items you may not recognize as risky are brought in. We can help to ensure your continued safety by identifying items that can pose a risk to you. This is something we can do together.

Among some toiletry items, there was a bottle of non-prescription pain pills for headache.

Fred: I need those pills for headaches. I want them at my bedside.

Nurse: If you are having headaches, it is important that we know; and how frequently you have them; and what medication you have found helpful. We will work with you to find safe ways to provide pain relief for you. These pain pills can either be sent home with your friend, or labelled and locked away for your security.

You recognize the need for choice in adult decision-making. Although Fred initially expresses a loss in adult integrity, you have provided him with choices that he can make which are congruent with ensuring his safety. You acknowledge the headaches are not viewed exclusively within the context of suicide.

Explore precipitants to suicidal thoughts and plans

Rationale

Suicide is an expression of feelings and thoughts. As a nurse it is useful to gain some understanding of what was going on in the person's life that precipitated suicidal intent or behaviour. Asking about suicide does not 'put the idea in the patient's head'. Honesty and trust are the core of the nature of the therapeutic relationship. Openness about the possibility of ending one's life facilitates discussion about the circumstances that can contribute to despair. When a person feels listened to, he or she may be able to tell the clinician if the distress has reached an intolerable point such that suicide feels imminent. Then a clinician can intervene. Careful listening can help the patient learn to identify the triggers behind the thoughts and behaviours. Being able to identify triggering events and feelings, associated with suicidal thoughts and behaviours, can lead to more adaptive problem-solving.

Example

Nurse: Fred you have been saying you have no future and you sound very hopeless about everything. I know it's very hard to talk about what has been going on in your life but it might be possible that, as we talk about what has been going on, together we can look at some ways to find some relief and move forward. For example, it might be helpful to talk about what was happening that led you to start drinking at work.

Promote alternative coping strategies

Rationale

Suicide is often seen as the only solution to a problem. It can be the permanent solution to a temporary problem. The overwhelming despair of a crisis can impede rational decision-making. Working with a patient to reframe situations more fully or realistically can be a challenge. However, gradual and continued assistance to consider alternative, meaningful coping strategies can be helpful.

Example

Nurse: You told me that when you are under stress you drink alcohol to excess and this adds to your problems. What other things have you done in the past to solve problems that have not created more difficulties for you?

At this point you are trying to build on the person's strengths and identify effective coping strategies. Problem-solving needs to be in *small* increments with positive reinforcement for each achievement. It is essential that clients are able to experience success as they try to modify behaviours or experiment with new coping skills. Even as you try to move forward you continue to monitor for risk and safety.

Nurse: You indicated that some of your reasons for self-harm may have included a wish to escape from all the bad feelings. There are measures to help you to decrease the intensity of the emotions you are feeling, other than alcohol or self-harm. We can explore the events that lead up to such emotions and help you to plan for alternative things to do that provide release and restore your feelings to a more manageable state. Would you like to talk more about this possibility?

Reflection

Suicidal thoughts and behaviours frequently persist and vacillate between chronic and acute states. How would you modify your assessments and plans of care in such a condition?

Aftercare in the community

Many clients return to the community still at risk for suicide. Although the patient's feelings of impulsivity may be reduced and he or she may no longer have a suicide plan, feelings of hopelessness may still be quite strong. The transition from the protective environment of the hospital to the community means that careful monitoring and assessment is still required. It is important that the link to community services happens rapidly after discharge, i.e. within the next 24 hours, or the emptiness of life, particularly if no partner or family support is in place, may be overwhelming. Transition therefore requires:

1 immediate aftercare
2 reduction of social isolation
3 bolstering of social support networks
4 meaningful opportunities for testing new coping strategies.

Aftercare for the nurse

A nurse may experience many feelings in the event of a patient's suicide attempt or completed suicide. A sense of helplessness, anger, sadness, a need to rescue, self-blame, frustration and rejection often leaves the nurse feeling 'manipulated' or 'victimized' by the patient. Clinicians have their own values regarding suicide, which are grounded in personal, social and cultural history. For example, a nurse who is a young mother may be bewildered and angry at a mother who tries to take her own life, risking leaving her children motherless. Or the nurse's religious beliefs may lead her to judge people who attempt suicide to be morally weak. The occurrence of suicide in a clinical setting can be very distressing for staff and patients. Both groups will need opportunities to talk about their feelings (see below). For patients, issues of safety may be foremost. Many clinicians will feel that somehow they did not do enough to save the patient. Despite our best vigilance and assessment, some people will be so determined to die that we cannot stop them. Responses to suicide have been compared to grief responses and post-traumatic stress with clinicians reporting flashbacks, hypervigilance, insomnia, fear and confusion. It is important for the nurse to be aware of and manage his or her own feelings and responses to the suicidal patient so that therapeutic care is not impeded by the nurse's own internal distress.

After a suicide: caring for the care-giver

Nurses, as individual clinicians and as members of a healthcare team, require attention to their responses to suicide. Critical stress-debriefing sessions are frequently offered to teams who have been affected by this type of trauma. These sessions provide confidential, non-judgemental opportunities for staff to explore their feelings about the event and scenarios leading up to it. Facilitated by a professional who is not a member of the team it provides a forum for sharing and support. Individual nurse supervision and counselling may also play an important role to help the nurse restore clinical confidence and prevent burnout.

SUMMARY

This chapter has focused on the role of nursing the person who is suicidal. The critical interventions outlined here emphasize the clinical knowledge required to keep the person alive and to start the process of recovery. These interventions are only a part of a longer journey directed at helping the person to develop a more positive sense of self or find ways to create meaning and relationships in his or her life.

- Suicidal thoughts and behaviours are to be taken seriously by the nurse and require assessment and intervention.
- Suicidal thoughts and behaviours have multifaceted aetiologies and usually require multiple intervention strategies to alleviate them.
- Safety of the suicidal client is always paramount.
- Care of the nurse's response to a patient's suicide is essential to prevent burnout and to prevent future intrusion of traumatic feelings in the nurse–patient relationship.

REFERENCES

1. Santa Mina EE, Gallop R, Links P *et al.* The self-injury questionnaire: evaluation of the psychometric properties in a clinical population. *Journal of Psychiatric and Mental Health Nursing* 2006; **13**: 221–7.

2. National Statistics UK. *Snapshot.* Available from www.statistics.gov.uk/cci/nugget. Accessed 25 June 2007.

3. Langlois S, Morrison P. Suicide deaths and suicide attempts. *Health Reports* 2002; **13** (2): 9–22.

4. Bland RC, Newman SC, Dyck RJ. The epidemiology of parasuicide in Edmonton. *Canadian Journal of Psychiatry* 1994; **39** (2): 391–6.

5. Meltzer H, Lader D, Corbin T *et al. Non-fatal suicidal behavior among adults aged 16–75 in Great Britain.* London, UK: The Stationery Office, 2002.

6. Hawton K, Arensman E, Townsend E *et al.* Deliberate self-harm: systematic review of efficacy of psycho-social and pharmacological treatments in preventing repetition. *British Medical Journal* 1998; **317**: 441–7.

7. Shneidman E. Classifications and approaches. In: *Definition of suicide.* New York, NY: Wiley, 1985: 23–40.

8. Linehan MM. A social–behavioral analysis of suicide and parasuicide: implications for clinical assessment and treatment. In: Clarkin JF, Glazer HI (eds). *Depression, behavioral and directive intervention strategies.* New York, NY: Garland STPM Press, 1981: 229–94.

9. Kral MJ. Suicide as social logic. *Suicide and Life-threatening Behavior* 1994; **24** (3): 245–55.

10. Fuse T. *Suicide, individual and society.* Toronto, Canada: Canadian Scholars Press, 1997.

11. Asberg M, Traskman L, Thoren P. 5-HIAA in the cerebrospinal fluid: a biochemical suicide predictor? *Archives of General Psychiatry* 1976; **33**: 1193–5.

12. Mann JJ. Psychobiological predictors of suicide. *Journal of Clinical Psychiatry* 1987; **48** (12): 39–43.

13. Beck RW, Morris JB, Beck AT. Cross-validation of the suicidal intent scale. *Psychological Reports* 1974; **34**: 445–6.

14. Jacobson G. The inpatient management of suicidality. In: Jacobs D (ed.). *The Harvard Medical School guide to suicide assessment and intervention.* San Francisco, CA: Jossey-Bass Publishers, 1999.

15. Sullivan AM, Barron CT, Bezmen J, *et al.* The safe treatment of the adult suicidal patient in an adult inpatient setting: a proactive preventive approach. *Psychiatric Quarterly*, 2005; **76**: 67–83.

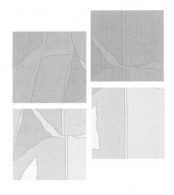

CHAPTER 22

The person who self-harms

Ruth Gallop* and Tracey Tully**

INTRODUCTION

Although self-harm is often confused with suicide attempts or suicidal gesturing, survivors cognitively distinguish these activities from attempts to kill themselves, and may in fact self-injure in order to avoid suicide.[1–4] Self-harm can take many forms ranging from intentional self-poisoning to severe body mutilation. This chapter will focus on self-harm that involves bodily self-injury. Bodily self-injury includes cutting, burning, abrading or hitting oneself, inserting sharp objects in the anus or vagina, pulling out body hair or other self-attacking behaviours that are idiosyncratic to the individual. In the general population, the prevalence of self-harm is in the range 0.75–4 per cent[5–8] and in clinical populations it is in the range 20–40 per cent.[4,5,9,10] In the UK, cutting is the second commonest form of self-harm after overdose.[11] The majority of people who injure their bodies in the ways considered here are women.[12]

Self-injury is often an attempt to communicate distress, relieve pain and maintain connection to oneself and others. Suicide attempts, on the other hand, are directed at discontinuing all connections and ending consciousness (see Chapter 21). However, it is important for nurses not to view self-injury as less serious than a suicide attempt and therefore respond to self-harm with less concern. A history of self-harm is a key predictor for repetition of self-harm and a subsequent completed suicide.[11]

Unfortunately, people who self-harm are often seen in a negative light by healthcare professionals, including nurses. These individuals may be viewed as attention-seeking, manipulative 'bad' patients undeserving of taking up time in an overburdened healthcare system. Caring for people who self-harm can be very stressful and difficult work. Because our role as mental health nurses is to help people grow and make sense of life events, it is often frightening and frustrating when people, in spite of our best efforts, continue to self-harm. The risk of working with these individuals is that we respond to our frustration and seeming lack of ability to help with anger and rejection.

To retain a balanced caring view of these patients and to engage in a therapeutic relationship, the nurse requires an understanding of the function of self-harm and the skill to engage in a relationship that is neither too caring nor too rejecting. Acquiring that knowledge and finding the balance that enables appropriate boundaries in the

*Ruth Gallop is Professor Emeritus in the Faculty of Nursing and Department of Psychiatry, University of Toronto, Toronto, Canada. Her research, clinical work and writing focus on clients perceived as treatment and management challenges. These clients often receive diagnoses of borderline personality disorders, have histories of severe early trauma and current self-harm behaviours.
**Tracey Tully is an Independent Consultant and was formerly a Clinical Nurse Specialist in the Women Recovering from Abuse Program (WRAP) at the Women's College Health Sciences Centre in Toronto, Canada.

nurse–patient relationship to be maintained will be the focus of this chapter.

EARLY TRAUMA AND SELF-INJURY

Recent studies indicate that the overwhelming majority of individuals who self-injure have a history of childhood trauma. Childhood trauma can include neglect, emotional, physical or sexual abuse, or experiences such as prolonged separation from parents for reasons such as serious illness or war. It is estimated that between 79 and 96 per cent of individuals who cut themselves were victims of childhood abuse or neglect.[4,5,13,14] Within the mental health system, research has shown that certain diagnoses are strongly associated with trauma and self-harm (see Chapters 28 and 61). These include *borderline personality disorder* and *dissociative identity disorder*. As research about self-injury remains in its early stages, the particular nature of the relationship between trauma and self-harm has not yet been fully determined. However, it is thought that one possible link between early trauma and self-injury lies in the set of fundamental beliefs about oneself and others that arise from a history of trauma. We do know that the earlier the age of abuse, the closer the relationship of the abuser and the longer the duration of abuse, the worse the self-harm.[15] What is clear is that people who self-harm have a negative view of themselves. They think they are bad, worthless and powerless. Feelings about their badness and awfulness are overwhelming and experienced as never-ending. Emotions are viewed as dangerous and potentially engulfing, and the individual does not trust his or her capacity to pass through intense emotions safely. Further, the self-injuring individual often lacks the words to name or describe the emotional experiences, thus adding to the distress. Action becomes the way to deal with overwhelming emotions and the body becomes the place for attack.

FUNCTIONS OF SELF-INJURY

Recently, several authors have proposed a number of psychological functions that self-injury may serve for an individual.[1,2,12,16,17] Self-injury may serve the purpose of re-enacting early trauma or abuse-related experiences and can render one powerless. Therefore, the act of inflicting harm on oneself may be a way to exert control, mastery, personal agency and autonomy in a life that seems otherwise chaotic and uncontrollable. One self-injuring woman commented:

> When I cut myself, I am the only one who has a say over how badly I am treated. I get to choose for myself how severely I hurt myself and when I want

to stop. I wish I could have said this about the abuse I got from my father.

The self-loathing that many traumatized women experience may generalize into thinking of both the self and the body as bad and ugly. In physical and sexual abuse, the body was violated and this abuse included both emotional and physical boundary violation. These boundary violations may lead to self-injury that temporarily helps define the body boundaries. Cutting the external body symbolically attacks the internal badness. Because of boundary confusion this represents (symbolically) an attack on the abuser.

Self-harm may also function to regain equilibrium, both emotionally and physiologically, when ability to self-soothe or sense of control is impaired. Self-harm is often a means to soothe oneself or create a sense of calm and equilibrium in overwhelming situations. In their early development, comforting experiences by nurturing care-givers have, generally, been absent in the lives of people who self-harm. As such, they did not acquire the internal ability to comfort themselves when in distress, and are unable to rely on more sophisticated means of coping in adulthood.[18] As one woman poignantly stated:

> When I'm feeling all alone, like nobody in the world cares about me, I have a very strong urge to cut myself. Some people are able to ask for a hug during a time like this. Other people can listen to a favourite piece of music, or eat comforting foods. I only know how to be calmed by cutting myself. My parents never showed me any love, only pain and suffering, so now I have no way of showing myself love.

Another woman said:

> Before I cut I feel like a volcano about to erupt. The feeling is so overwhelming that I literally feel like I will explode if I don't self-injure. As soon as I do it's like all that is built up inside is released.

Management and maintenance of dissociative processes may also be a function of self-injury. Dissociation is the compartmentalizing of experiences so they can be split off from consciousness. The act of harming oneself may move one into a dissociative state when escape from painful emotions or memories is needed. In this way, self-injury may provide needed distance and numbness. Conversely, self-harm may be a way to return one to a sense of reality, to remind oneself that one is alive after being stuck in a state of numbness. Another woman said:

> When I cut myself and see the blood flow out of me I know that I am alive. I spend so much of my life feeling nothing, feeling detached from the body I

live in. I desperately want to feel something, anything, other than nothingness.

Self-injury may also serve to express feelings, such as guilt, shame or rage, or to communicate needs. People who self-injure may not know the words, or trust the power of their words, to convey their pain. As a consequence, they may rely on their injuries as a way to speak for them, or as a means of having their needs met. As one person explained:

I don't know how to talk about what I'm feeling, I only know how to act on it. I realize this is a big problem because lots of people think I'm trying to get attention. Just because I got somebody's attention when I cut, it doesn't mean that I was trying to get their attention.

It is also important to consider when self-harm occurs. Cutting rarely occurs in the presence of others – whether family, friends or clinicians. It may occur minutes, hours or days *after* being in the presence of another. The benefit of being in the presence of another can drain away very quickly. Being alone invites the overwhelming pain and affect associated with the trauma and self-badness to start to be experienced.

Finally, as we consider the functions of self-harm it is apparent that self-harm is used to deal with intense, often overwhelming emotional states. In all of the quotations above, self-harm is experienced as an effective, reliable although problematic means by which to decrease the intensity of one's distress. The critical feature is that the feelings are intolerable and must be stopped and cutting serves a self-soothing capacity to relieve this distress.

Although an external activity, cutting shares some features with an internalized sense of soothing and object constancy, and can be relied upon to be available on demand to comfort and diminish pain. Cutting, unlike the childhood trauma, is within the control of the individual. Of course, the relief it brings is short-lived and often leads to shame and guilt at the activity and so the cycle of pain, relief and shame starts again.

SELF-INJURY IN OTHER POPULATIONS

Mental health nurses need to be aware of other populations in which self-harm may occur.

- *Psychotic populations.* While self-injury among individuals with a negative sense of self and/or trauma history generally follows a pattern of high frequency and low severity, psychotic individuals who self-harm may do so infrequently and sustain serious injuries. The most severe acts of self-injury are to be found in the psychotic population. Self-injury may take the form of limb amputation, autocastration or removal of eyes. These extreme acts are generally performed in response to disturbances in thoughts or perceptions such as persecutory or somatic delusions or command hallucinations.

- *Forensic populations.* As many as 50 per cent of incarcerated individuals exhibit self-injurious behaviours, although only about 10 per cent pose a serious threat to themselves. However, owing to the nature of the prison system, all attempts are treated as potentially life-threatening, which means that prisoners are transferred to the medical wing for treatment, an environment that is more tolerable than the general prison population. This has led some to suggest that self-injury among prisoners is motivated by secondary gain. Further research needs to be done in this area to gain knowledge of all possible functions of this behaviour. Given that many individuals in the forensic system have experienced violence, the functions of their self-injury may be similar to those seen in traumatized women. In addition, one must consider that self-injury among prisoners may be a form of stimulating oneself in a monotonous environment.

- *Developmentally or physiologically impaired populations.* Individuals who have Lesch–Nyhan syndrome, autism, de Lange's syndrome or Tourette's syndrome generally exhibit self-injurious behaviours. The type of self-injurious behaviour that may be observed in these individuals includes self-directed head banging, biting, hitting or slapping. The behaviour is generally repetitive and rhythmic in nature and occurs with much higher frequency, often for several hours daily, than in the population of traumatized women who self-injure. It is generally accepted that the behaviour provides sensory stimulation, or is consistent with obsessionality, impulsivity, compulsivity or motor tics.

- *Socially sanctioned self-injury.* The anthropology, theology and sociology literature offer several accounts of self-injury. Generally, these self-injurious acts are performed as rites of passage, or as a way of joining, remaining part of, or demonstrating one's commitment to a group.[19] Injuries may include self-flagellation, facial scarification, insertion of objects under the skin, or other self-mutilative acts that are consistent with cultural or religious practices.

Reflection

What is the attitude of your professional colleagues – nurses, doctors, therapists, etc. – towards people who self-harm?
In what way do these attitudes differ, across disciplines, and individuals?
How do you explain these differences in attitude?

THE NURSING ROLE

Personal illustration 22.1

Jane is a young woman with a long history of abuse perpetrated by various family members. Throughout most of her life she has told herself that she is a terrible, evil, dirty person for what happened to her. She believes that she deserves nothing good in her life and that she will achieve very little. Jane attempts to cope with her overwhelming sense of badness and worthlessness and her intense feelings of shame, fear and anger by cutting her forearms, thighs and breasts. She is requesting help at this time because her self-injury is worsening in both frequency and severity and is beginning to affect her work performance.

Establishing and maintaining clear and consistent boundaries

Rationale

Providing clear, reliable, consistent expectations of the relationship are essential. During your first meeting it is very important to establish a framework for working within the therapeutic relationship. This is important for work with all clients, but especially critical for trauma survivors who self-injure because their boundaries have been violated so severely. They have not known safe, reliable people and therefore have no expectations that someone will be safe and reliable.

Example

You first meet Jane when she arrives at an outpatient mental health clinic requesting to talk to someone about her self-injury. Near the end of the first session, Jane asks if she can have a hug from you.

You recognize this request could be potentially a boundary transgression, and should be considered carefully. Many survivors of childhood trauma have confusing reactions around physical touch. Touch may have been sexualized or associated with physical violence. As such, many mental health professionals develop a guideline around the use of touch so as not to re-play an earlier dynamic. This becomes your first opportunity to put into action the words you communicated about boundaries and conveys the importance of consistency in your message. It is critical that the discussion that follows her request does not have a punitive or rejecting tone, to which she will already be sensitive. Instead, ensure the discussion conveys your empathy and an openness to discuss her request. The following is one way that you *might* proceed with this request.

Nurse: Thank you for asking, Jane; however, a hug is something that I feel we need to talk about. As we are coming to the end of our time together today we can talk about this for a few minutes [adhering to the time frame is another way of maintaining consistent boundaries]. It seems that you have experienced some strong feelings today. Part of the work that we'll be doing together is putting into words what you feel inside of your body. Do you have an awareness of what you were feeling about me or about our time together today when you asked for a hug?

Jane: Nobody has ever listened to me like you did today. Most people think I'm crazy for what I do and they just tell me to stop or they won't see me any more. I felt that you cared about me. I wanted to see if that was really true because when people care for each other they hug.

Nurse: So is it fair to say that you were feeling close to me and you were curious about how I was feeling about you?

Jane: Yes.

Nurse: I also felt that we had a nice connection today and I would agree with you that many close relationships involve physical touch and intimacy. However, this relationship is unlike others that you may have in your life, therefore many of the social norms you are used to will be quite different in our relationship. Hugging is one of those areas that is different in this relationship. A hug can seem like a simple gesture to communicate caring, but I am more comfortable using my words to express how I'm feeling. This is also one of the goals that we will be working on — to help you move away from using actions to express feelings and towards using your words. I appreciate your courage for asking me for a hug. You may leave today and have some more feelings about this conversation. I encourage you to take note of what you may be thinking and feeling and I invite you to raise these thoughts and feelings with me when we meet next week.

Note how the nurse *supported* Jane and *confirmed* her connection to Jane. This will help to comfort and soothe her. Many nurses might feel the urge to hug Jane because her life has been so painful and to deny her could feel cruel and rejecting for a nurse. Further it can be very rewarding to know that a client experienced you as caring and you want to maintain that feeling. However, it is also important for the nurse to realize that Jane's emptiness cannot be filled in the short term by hugs or creating dependencies. Instead, she requires your help with developing the internal capacity to comfort herself so that she can begin to care for her own needs.

Boundary-related issues can take many forms with clients who self-harm. Below are three further examples of situations that require the nurse to be able to reflect on her own needs in the relationship. These situations can be the basis for further discussion of boundaries. After each we have given one of many possible explanations for conflict in the nurse as he or she responds. Nurses need to be aware of their own responses and seek help and supervision when confused about reactions and actions.

1 A client asks you if you self-injure or if you have a history of trauma; you may think that revealing your own history will make the client feel more understood.
2 A client asks you to place a brief call to her every day. You believe you really understand this person and by being available can effect real change.
3 A client asks if he can extend his appointments with you by 15 minutes. You do not have anything planned so this request feels reasonable.

Ensuring responsibility for change lies with the client

Rationale

Communicating the message that you believe a client is capable of keeping him/herself safe minimizes the potential for power struggles and offers an opportunity for the client to reflect on internal resources that can be called upon when making changes.

> ### Example
>
> Jane asks if you require her to sign a contract stating that she will not engage in self-injury.

Nurse: It is our belief that contracts aren't a useful way for you to learn how to keep yourself safe. Instead, we are going to work together to build your belief that you can cope with distress by not self-injuring.

As nurses, we cannot be anyone's constant protector. Rather, we need to work towards helping clients keep themselves safe. Clients may have difficulty maintaining a contract and then feel shameful that they have betrayed the contract.

One client said:

> I've signed lots of papers saying I won't cut, but when I really want to cut and I'm in that dark place I don't care that I signed my name to something. It's just a piece of paper that doesn't mean anything. I can find lots of places on my body where I can cut and nobody will know about it.

Asking a client to sign a 'no-harm contract' is probably serving the nurse's, rather than the client's, needs. It may help the nurse to feel less anxious and protected from litigation, but it does little to encourage responsibility and empowerment.

> ### Reflection
>
> In your view, what is the first responsibility of the nurse in caring for someone who self-harms?

Exploring the functions that self-injury serves for the individual

Rationale

Early in the therapeutic relationship it is important to explore the various ways in which self-injury has been helpful as well as the ways in which it has been unhelpful. Acknowledging the adaptive qualities of the behaviour communicates a message of non-judgement and non-blame. This serves to strengthen your alliance. In addition, it provides important clinical information for both of you.

> ### Example
>
> On Jane's second appointment with you she tells you that yesterday she overheard two women in a shop commenting on the scars to her forearms. One woman wondered if she had been in an accident. The other woman disagreed and stated, 'I heard about this from my friend who works in a hospital. These people are total freaks. They're absolutely nuts. They can't control themselves and need to be locked up in psych wards and even tied to the bed.'

Jane: I must be your craziest patient. I'm sure you tell all of your friends about the freak who hacks at herself. I almost didn't come back to see you because I'm afraid you'll have me locked away.

Nurse: This sounds as if this was a very powerful experience for you. It seems that you are wondering if I judge you in a similar way.

Jane: Yeah.

Nurse: I want to be clear that I do not believe that you are crazy. I think it's also important for you to know that hospitalization for self-injury is not a recommended form of treatment. I see you as doing your very best to cope with what life has thrown you [acknowledging the adaptive quality of self-injury]. From what you have already told me about your early life, it makes sense that you chose self-injury as a way of coping with distress. Self-harm can be a very effective, although ultimately destructive, way of dealing with pain. As with all ways of coping that are not beneficial in the long run, eventually they stop working as effectively, or they get in the way of living the life you want. Because you have come for help with your self-injury you have already acknowledged that your self-injury is no longer working for you in the way it once did. Perhaps we can use this as an opportunity to talk about the various ways that self-harm has helped you to get though life. We can also talk about the ways that it interferes with your life. This may give you some insights into the reaction that you had with the women in the shop.

At the end of this discussion, it may be useful to engage in a teaching piece around the functions of self-injury that have been previously identified. A reading list of books or articles can be very useful. This may serve to normalize her experience. Also encourage Jane to consider the ways in which her self-injury is no longer serving her well. What are the areas in her life that are affected by this way of coping? Examining the drawbacks of self-injury may assist with motivation for change.

Informing a client that inpatient admission is not ideal may also reassure her. After a careful assessment in Accident and Emergency where suicidality is ruled out, inpatient admission should be avoided, as it is often a hothouse for regression and re-enactment of previous conflictual relationships in this population.

Openness to engage in dialogue about self-injury

Rationale
Openness functions to decrease shame, stigma and secrecy of the act. It also communicates that you can tolerate all of who they are and not reject or abandon them. For those women whose self-injury occasionally functions to communicate an aspect of themselves, open dialogue and acceptance of the behaviour (not to be confused with condoning) encourages verbal forms of expression, rather than merely physical means. Finally, it can provide a means of gathering further information about her self-injury that is essential to consider when preparing for changing behaviour.

> ### Example
>
> Nurse: We have spent some time talking about the ways that self-injury serves you well. We have also talked about some of the drawbacks. Before we talk about how you might change your self-injury, we need to have more information about other aspects of your self-injury.

Let this be an opportunity to explore and gather information about the following areas:

- interpersonal stressors related to self-injury
- situational triggers to self-injury, both internal and external
- the thought process that accompanies self-injury, both before and after the episode
- the overwhelming affect that is associated with self-injury, both before and after the episode
- the confusing and threatening physiological responses that are experienced
- the role of flashbacks and dissociation.

Goal setting

Rationale
Although it is essential that we be empathic when working with individuals who self-injure, empathy alone is

not sufficient. We need to convey to people who self-harm that, if they want to, together we can work to change things. Goals need to be modest, attainable and mutually agreed upon.

Nurse: As a way to plan the remainder of the time, it is important that we focus on what you would like to achieve by the end of our time together. Have you thought about this?

Jane: Last time we met I thought a lot about all the parts of my self-injury that we talked about. I never thought much about my triggers, my feelings, my thoughts and the other aspects of my self-injury. I might like to work on decreasing the amount that I self-harm.

Nurse: That sounds like a goal that would be reasonable to work on in the time frame we have. You told me that you are cutting yourself weekly at present. When you say you want to decrease the frequency, do you have a sense of by how much you would like to decrease? [Ask Jane to get very specific and break down her goal into something measurable.]

Jane: I would feel a lot better if I cut down to once a month.

In addition to identifying her goal, there are also other areas to consider when working towards change. The following areas should also be explored with Jane.

- Why does she think this is an important goal to work on?
- Who does she need to have on her side to achieve this goal? What supports are essential?
- Who will not be helpful to have in her life when she is working towards this change?
- What might get in the way of achieving this goal and how will she manage this potential barrier?

Self-care of injuries

Rationale
A client you have a relationship with may come to you having self-injured. While you are concerned about the self-injury, your primary concern once you have established that urgent care is not needed is to focus on understanding triggers and developing alternative coping methods. Avoid turning excessive focus to the actual injury.

> ### Example
>
> Jane arrives for her appointment and she informs you that she cut her arm 2 hours ago. You can see through her shirt sleeve that the wound is bleeding.

It is important that you remain calm and do not respond as if the injury is a crisis. Remember that most cutting can be tended to with basic first aid. Ask Jane to reveal the injury. Assess the severity of the cut and establish the need for sutures. If you establish that she does not require medical intervention, encourage Jane to tend to her own wounds, i.e. direct her to the first aid kit at your clinic and invite her to use the washroom or an unoccupied private space. Since she has been self-injuring for many years, she is well aware of the appropriate intervention. If she is not, suggest that she apply pressure, irrigate the wound, dress the wound, keep it clean and monitor for infection.

Once Jane has returned from tending to her cut, invite her to talk about what triggered the self-injury, i.e. encourage her to put into words what she enacted on her body. At this time, it is important not to focus on the details of the act of injuring or the wound itself.

Use of distraction techniques

Rationale

The nature of the distraction activity may reduce its benefit. Maintaining a focus on immediate action to cope with overwhelming emotions reinforces a sense of urgency. Finding activities that reduce tension and reduce the urge rather than distract from the urge are more useful.

Example

Jane arrives for her appointment and tells you that she was surfing the Internet for self-harm websites. She tells you that several of the websites suggest using techniques such as rubbing ice on one's forearm, snapping elastic bands on wrists. She tells you that these techniques are apparently good because they distract from the urge to self-harm. She wants to know what you think about this.

While this is a relatively common technique that is suggested, we do not recommend this approach as it sends the message that one still needs to take immediate action when the urge to self-harm presents itself. If an individual responds to the urge to self-injure with another action (e.g. applying ice) he or she has already started to follow a similar pattern which may lead to self-injuring. Instead, we encourage working towards a place where action is not needed. That is, where she can sit with distressing thoughts, sensations and feelings without experiencing them as being intolerable. As one woman stated:

> In the last group I was in I learned a lot about distracting myself when I wanted to cut. This did not work for me at all. It was like a band-aid that covered up the real problem that was going on. They would tell me to use an ice cube or rubber band on my wrist when I want to cut. I thought this was a bunch of crap. It's like they don't get it that I want to stop doing destructive things to myself. Besides, by the time I get to the point of wanting to hurt myself, it's too late, the train is already going 100 mph and I can't stop it. I need to learn how to not let the train out of the station.

The development of alternative methods of comforting oneself, or dealing with affect is an important part of the work. This will happen over time. For example, you can work together to develop a list of activities that make a person feel less agitated, e.g. bathing, music, writing a diary.

Reflection

In your experience of nursing people who self-harm, what has been the biggest challenge you have faced?
How did you deal with that particular challenge?

SUMMARY

Working with a person who self-harms is demanding work. In addition to their responsibilities towards the people in care, nurses need to look after themselves, through maintaining supportive networks, engaging in pleasurable activities and finding a balance between personal and professional pursuits. Clinical supervision should be available to all psychiatric–mental health nurses. However, for nurses engaged in work with people who self-harm, supervision is essential. Like other areas of psychiatric–mental health nursing, this work is grounded in the therapeutic relationship. The specific knowledge about self-harm is layered upon this fundamental therapeutic use of self.

REFERENCES

1. Babiker G, Arnold L. *The language of injury: comprehending self-mutilation.* Leicester, UK: The British Psychological Press, 1997.

2. Connors R. Self-injury in trauma survivors. 1. Functions and meanings. *American Journal of Orthopsychiatry* 1996; **66**: 197–206.

3. Himber J. Blood rituals: self-cutting in female psychiatric inpatients. *Psychotherapy* 1994; **31**: 620–31.

4. van der Kolk B, Perry JC, Herman JL. Childhood origins of self-destructive behaviour. *American Journal of Psychiatry* 1991; **148**: 1665–71.

5. Briere J, Gil E. Self-mutilation in clinical and general population samples: prevalence, correlates, and functions. *American Journal of Orthopsychiatry* 1998; **68**: 609–20.

6. Favazza AR, Conterio K. The plight of chronic self-mutilators. *Community Mental Health Journal* 1988; **24**: 22–30.

7. Pattison EM, Kahan J. The deliberate self-harm syndrome. *American Journal of Psychiatry* 1983; **140**: 867–72.

8. Whitehead PC, Johnson FG, Ferrence R. Measuring the incidence of self-injury: some methodological and design considerations. *American Journal of Orthopsychiatry* 1973; **43**: 142–8.

9. Evans C, Lacey JH. Multiple self-damaging behaviour among alcoholic women: a prevalence study. *British Journal of Psychiatry* 1992; **161**: 643–7.

10. Zlotnick C, Mattia JL, Zimmerman M. Clinical correlates of self-mutilation in a sample of general psychiatric patients. *Journal of Nervous and Mental Diseases* 1999; **187**: 296–301.

11. NHS Centre for Reviews and Dissemination. Deliberate self-harm. *Effective Health Care* 1998; **4**: 1–12.

12. Conterio K, Lader W. *Bodily harm: the breakthrough healing program for self-injurers.* New York, NY: Hyperion, 1998.

13. Romans SE, Martin JL, Anderson JC, *et al.* Sexual abuse in childhood and deliberate self-harm. *American Journal of Psychiatry* 1995; **152**: 1336–42.

14. Zlotnick C, Shea MT, Pearlstein T *et al.* The relationship between dissociate symptoms, alexithymia, impulsivity, sexual abuse, and self-mutilation. *Comprehensive Psychiatry* 1996; **37**: 12–16.

15. Stone MH. Some thoughts on the dynamics and therapy of self-mutilating borderline patients. *Journal of Personality Disorders* 1987; **1**: 347–9.

16. Miller D. *Women who hurt themselves.* New York, NY: Basic Books, 1994.

17. Suyemoto KL. The functions of self-mutilation. *Clinical Psychology Review* 1998; **18**: 531–54.

18. Gallop R. The failure of the capacity for self-soothing in women who have a history of abuse and self-harm. *Journal of American Psychiatric Nurses Association* 2002; **8**: 20–6.

19. Favazza AR. *Bodies under siege: self-mutilation and body modification in culture and psychiatry.* Baltimore, MD: Johns Hopkins University Press, 1996.

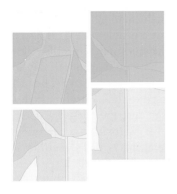

CHAPTER 23

The person who hears disturbing voices

Cheryl Forchuk* and Elsabeth Jensen**

1 Michael sat alone in the TV room on the inpatient psychiatric ward. 'NO, NO, NO! I will not do THAT! Now you leave me alone! Shut up! Get out of here!'

A student nurse, Donovan, stood in the doorway. Michael was his assigned patient for the day. How should he approach him?

2 Sally greeted the community nurse, Suchita, with a smile and a cup of tea. 'Sometimes, I think you and St Georgette are the only two true friends I have in the world.'

After a few minutes of conversation, Suchita enquired: 'So, how are you finding that new medication?'

'Terrible!' replied Sally. 'It was drowning St Georgette so I could barely hear her – so I had to stop taking it right away.'

3 'I'm really loving this "Women in History" course. It really has me thinking', Ngozi explained to her room-mate. 'But after today's class, one thing keeps coming back to me. If Joan of Arc were alive today – wouldn't we just say she was hallucinating and drug her up or lock her up?'

'Well', replied Nadine, 'how do we know she didn't have schizophrenia?'

VOICES AS AN EXAMPLE OF HALLUCINATIONS

Nurses will frequently encounter people who are hearing disturbing voices. 'Hearing voices' is frequently described as an auditory hallucination. Hallucinations can involve any sense. For example, in addition to auditory hallucinations there are visual hallucinations, olfactory hallucinations, taste hallucinations and tactile hallucinations. Something is generally described as a hallucination if others cannot perceive it.

Different kinds of situations may make different kinds of hallucinations more likely. For example, hearing voices or auditory hallucinations is quite common in people with a diagnosis of schizophrenia. It is therefore a phenomenon encountered quite regularly by psychiatric–mental health nurses. Visual hallucinations are more likely in a drug-induced situation, for example someone who has taken street drugs such as phencyclidine (PCP) or lysergic acid diethylamide (LSD), or someone taking opiates for pain control. Tactile hallucinations are common during drug withdrawal. For example, someone

*Cheryl Forchuk is a Professor in the School of Nursing and Department of Psychiatry at the University of Western Ontario, and an Assistant Director of the Lawson Health Research Institute. She has worked in a variety of mental health settings, including tertiary psychiatric care, acute care, community care and addictions. Her current research focuses on therapeutic relationships, models of discharge, peer support and housing.

**Elsabeth Jensen is an Assistant Professor in the School of Nursing, York University. She has worked in a wide variety of mental health settings and is specialized in working with survivors of childhood abuse. Her current research focuses on evaluation of discharge care models, knowledge translation, diversity, and the relationships between the determinants of health and mental health.

with alcoholism may complain it feels like 'bugs are crawling all over' during withdrawal. Taste hallucinations are more rare but, in our experience, have occasionally been noted with a drug-induced psychosis. All of these depictions are generalizations. For example, although people diagnosed with schizophrenia typically have auditory hallucinations (hearing voices), they can also sometimes report visual hallucinations (seeing things).

Another distinction sometimes made is that between a hallucination and an illusion. Both phenomena involve perceiving something that is not perceived by others. However, an illusion is based on the apparent misperception of something that can be seen by others. For example, a person may see something more sinister in a shadow – but others can, at least, see the shadow. Or, people may hear a ringing bell, but not that the bell is calling out a name.

As the scenario at the beginning of the chapter with Suchita and Sally illustrates, not all auditory hallucinations are disturbing. An early study[1] found that the relationship one had with the 'voice' was often an indicator of chronicity. People who had lived with their voices for a long time would sometimes develop a positive relationship with them. Miller et al.[2] found that the majority of patients who were hallucinating reported some positive effects of hallucinations. These attitudes did not change after treatment, but those people with more positive experiences of hallucinations were more likely to continue hallucinating after treatment.[3] Romme[4] compared 'patients' who heard voices with those who had not been identified as patients and found that non-patients were more likely to report a positive experience with the voices. They concluded that hearing voices lay on a continuum with normal functioning.

In a previous study, Forchuk[5] asked individuals with chronic mental illnesses about their social support. Almost all of the 124 clients in the study reported very small social networks (friends to whom they could turn for help). In two situations, the clients reported that their only supports were the community nurse and their 'voices'. In another two situations the only supports were the community nurse and a pet. When one has a very small social network, each individual in the network is very important. So, although the nurse or others may perceive the auditory hallucination as a *symptom*, the client may perceive it as a close friend. Obviously, these things need to be discussed and understood for nurses to be able to work with clients on their goals and not simply on their own assumptions of what constitutes a problem.

Interestingly, the idea that someone would have a relationship with a hallucination is not new to nursing. Nursing theorist Hildegard Peplau[6,7] adopted Harry Stacks Sullivan's[8] definition of interpersonal relationships. Interpersonal relationships are defined as any relationship involving two or more people. All but one of the people may be illusory.

Clearly, not all auditory hallucinations are disturbing. Does that mean they are not a problem? This is also a complex issue, and begs the question, a problem for whom? Consider a client who would spend all day in her room. It was difficult to encourage her to get her off her bed for meals or even to go to the bathroom. In discussing the issue with her, she described why she spent so much time in bed. She was listening to a centuries-old conversation among several angels, and sometimes if she was lucky she would hear God as well. They were discussing plans for the great flood. Details about the animals and the geography kept her fascinated for hours on end. How could she leave for lunch and miss the possibility of hearing God's input to the conversation? Were these voices a problem? She had lost contact with almost all her family and her level of functioning on a day-to-day basis was dramatically reduced by her constant focus on the voices. On the other hand, she saw herself as an important person, and involved in an important process. She felt that without her voices she would be 'nothing'. Not all auditory hallucinations interfere with functioning or the person's activities of daily living. These things need careful evaluation together with the client.

Some hallucinations are horrifically disturbing. Clients have described hearing screaming, tortured voices pleading with them for relief. Others have described taunting, insulting voices that can issue commands (called command hallucinations) such as to jump off a bridge or strangle a friend. Frequently, disturbing voices list every fault of the client before them and tell them that they are worthless or evil.

Clients have experienced multiple disturbing voices that make contact with another human being very difficult to even sort out among the other voices. Sometimes, in these situations, there are insulting voices and friendly voices all speaking at once, clamouring to be heard. The nurse trying to speak is simply one more voice competing for attention.

Reflection

What do you think about when you hear the term hallucinations?

WHY DO SOME PEOPLE HEAR VOICES?

Beyerstein[9] stated that 'Anything that prompts a move from word based thinking to imagistic or pictorial thinking predisposes a person to hallucinating.' He further states that things which bias 'the brain's representational system towards memory images at the expense of sensory information can also predispose to hallucinating'.

Voices as a symptom of psychosis

Hearing voices is most commonly considered a symptom of psychosis. Psychosis is a break with reality. Psychosis may accompany many different kinds of situations. People may experience psychosis as part of an illness experience (e.g. schizophrenia, a manic or depressive phase of a bipolar disorder, Wernicke's syndrome, high fever, or a brain tumour); it may be experienced with extremely stressful situations, e.g. intensive care unit psychosis, post-traumatic stress syndrome, massive losses, culture shock, a medication side-effect (e.g. disulfiram/Antabuse, opiates), illicit drug use (hallucinogens such as PCP, LSD), or a symptom of withdrawal from an addictive drug (e.g. alcohol, barbiturates). Delusions and disorganized thinking are other symptoms of psychosis.

Auditory hallucinations as a common symptom of schizophrenia

Although there are many causes of psychosis, mental health nurses will encounter this symptom most commonly among people who have been diagnosed with schizophrenia. Someone with schizophrenia is generally not psychotic all the time. They typically have periods of wellness between acute psychotic episodes. The pattern of psychosis and wellness varies considerably among individuals. For a few people, the symptoms of psychosis are chronic in nature and are unremitting, i.e. the symptoms do not fluctuate with acute periods followed by periods of wellness.

Hallucinations are considered to be a 'positive' symptom of schizophrenia. This means that they are present in schizophrenia, but not present in the 'normal' population. Other positive symptoms are delusions (unusual belief symptoms, described more fully in Chapter 24), and disorganized thinking. The 'negative' symptoms of schizophrenia are symptoms that reflect something is 'missing'. These include a lack of energy, a lack of motivation, emotional withdrawal, and difficulty in abstract thinking.[10] The experience of psychosis also varies considerably among individuals with schizophrenia. Some people may be more troubled by the positive symptoms, others by negative symptoms or a combination of both.

Men typically develop symptoms of schizophrenia in their late teens, whereas women typically develop the first symptoms in their early twenties. This means that men may be less likely to have completed vocational training or become independent from their family of orientation before developing the illness. Women are more likely to have completed their schooling and may have started families of their own, when the symptoms first strike. This difference in age of onset can create very different treatment and rehabilitation issues. For example, someone who has had the symptoms at a young age may need a lot of assistance to meet educational and vocational goals. Someone who developed the illness at a later age may have completed more developmental tasks and have additional strengths to draw on. On the other hand, there may be issues related to coping within the family of procreation. It must be understood that these are generalizations and the specific issues still need exploring with each individual.

Auditory hallucinations as a symptom of dissociative identity disorder

Disturbing voices are also experienced by people diagnosed with dissociative identity disorder (also known as multiple personality disorder).[11–13] This condition is usually a consequence of serious, life-threatening sexual abuse early in life. During periods when one personality is in charge, the voices of one or more other personalities are talking, sometimes to each other. These voices are experienced as being inside the head. Some voices can be frightening. The person may hear the voice(s) suggesting self-harm or suicide. The person hearing the voices will often believe that he or she is 'going crazy'. As a result, people are often reluctant to disclose that they hear voices for fear they will be locked away.

In cases of dissociative identity disorder, medication is usually ineffective. The intervention of choice is psychotherapy with a therapist sensitive to the issues of childhood sexual abuse, and skilled in working with people with personality disorders.

Biological reasons

The biology of actual perceptions and imagined perceptions appear to be the same.[9] This has been demonstrated with studies using electroencephalogram (EEG) recordings and positron emission tomography (PET) scans.[14–17] Beyerstein[9] states:

> Because functionally equivalent states of the central awareness system can arise from either memory or sensory sources, it is possible for dreams, perceptual memories, fantasies and hallucinations to become indistinguishable from real events. Hallucinations result whenever internal events trigger a pattern of brain activity equivalent to that normally generated when sense organs respond to a publicly observable event.

Spiritual and cultural reasons

There may also be spiritual/religious or cultural reasons for hearing voices. Within many traditions, it is considered normal to be able to communicate with the dead, including friends, relatives or even strangers. Similarly, many cultures would value communication with a spiritual power, spiritual guide, angel or higher being that may not have been previously alive on earth. Also, many people believe in a sixth sense that allows them to see or hear things that others do not. It is extremely important in these situations to be aware of cultural and family norms and not pathologize a spiritual situation. Often, involving other community members or family members can help to understand what kind of process is occurring. For example, in North America, many first nations (indigenous) people would be expected to communicate with a spirit guide. In the Northwest Territories of Canada the mental health legislation includes consultation with a First Nations or Aboriginal elder, to determine whether an involuntary admission status is appropriate if the potential patient is native. The assessment is complex and includes both a mental health specialist and a native elder since just because one has a spirit guide, it does not mean that one cannot suffer a psychosis or auditory hallucination.

Interpersonal reasons

Hildegard Peplau also described the potential interpersonal development of auditory hallucinations. She believed that hallucinations could develop to avoid anxiety and to mitigate loneliness. She describes this as developing through four stages.[7,18] These stages were further elaborated by Clack.[19]

The stages of hallucinations are as follows.

1 *Comforting*: The individual feels lonely and/or anxious and finds that focusing on comforting thoughts relieves the discomfort. At this stage the thoughts are clearly understood to be one's own.
2 *Condemning*: The person continues to court similar relief and increasing reliance on illusory figures to meet needs. The individuals gradually put themselves into a 'listening' mode and are unable to control their own awareness.
3 *Controlling*: There is a marked loss of ability to focus awareness, indicated by withdrawal from others in order to interact with the hallucination, the person gives up trying to combat the hallucination and may feel lonely when the voices leave.
4 *Conquering*: The voices become increasingly threatening, particularly when commands are not followed. There is a failure of strategies to conceal ongoing interactions with hallucinations. There is a continued loss of control over concentration and awareness.

Reflection

What are the responses of your colleagues to the term hallucinations?

INTERVENTIONS TO ASSIST WITH HEARING PROBLEMATIC VOICES

Assessing problematic voices

Before any intervention can be planned an assessment is needed. The nurse may simply ask the individual if he or she is hearing any unusual voices. It also needs to be ascertained as to whether or not the individual considers experiencing such voices to be a problem. Occasionally, a person who is experiencing problematic voices will deny this, or be unable to confirm this because of language or cognitive difficulties. Behaviours to note would include looking at a specific area where nothing is obviously present, talking to someone who others do not see, or giggling/laughing to oneself. Obviously, any of these behaviours can have other explanations, so one must be careful to observe and try to confirm but not to jump to conclusions.

Medical approaches

The primary medical approach to treat psychosis is with the use of anti-psychotic medications (also called neuroleptics or major tranquillizers). Nurses are involved in administering the medications, observing for the effectiveness of the medications, and monitoring for side-effects.

Anti-psychotic or neuroleptic medications are used mainly to treat schizophrenia but can also be used in manic states and delirium.[20] These medications are not curative and thus do not eliminate the underlying thought disorder. Rather, they may allow the patient to function in a supportive environment.[20]

Neuroleptic medications fall into two broad categories. The traditional agents (e.g. haloperidol, chlorpromazine) function by primarily blocking dopamine receptors. They are most effective in treating positive symptoms of schizophrenia such as delusions, hallucinations and thought disorders. The newer neuroleptics (e.g. clozapine, olanzapine) function by blocking serotonin receptors. They are most effective with patients resistant to traditional antipsychotics and are especially useful in treating the negative symptoms of schizophrenia such as withdrawal, blunted emotions and a reduced ability to relate to people.[20]

Side-effects from the use of neuroleptic drugs occur in almost all patients. These are significant in up to 80 per cent of patients.[20] The major side-effects of traditional neuroleptics are parkinsonian effects, tardive dyskinesia, dystonia/dyskinesia and akathisia. Parkinsonian effects are characterized by akinesia, rigidity, shuffling gait, drooling and tremors.[20]

Tardive dyskinesia can occur from long-term treatment. Symptoms include lateral jaw movements and 'fly-catching' motions of the tongue.[20] A prolonged holiday from neuroleptic treatments may diminish symptoms or cause them to disappear after 3 months. However, in many individuals, the effects are irreversible and continue even after medication is stopped.[20] Other side-effects include drowsiness (which usually occurs in the first 2 weeks of treatment), confusion, dry mouth, urinary retention, constipation and orthostatic hypotension. They can also result in the depression of the hypothalamus causing amenorrhoea, galactorrhoea, infertility and impotence.[20]

The newer antipsychotics also have potential side-effects. They have been associated with a higher risk of hyperglycaemia and type 2 diabetes mellitus.[21] The most serious side-effects are blood dyskrasias, including agranulocytosis, which are potentially fatal. Clients taking clozapine require regular blood monitoring of white blood cell counts to ensure the count is within normal limits. Such clients need to be taught to report symptoms such as lethargy, malaise and sore throat immediately. Other potential side-effects include central nervous system symptoms (e.g. seizures, drowsiness), orthostatic hypotension, cardiac abnormalities, gastrointestinal symptoms (e.g. constipation, diarrhoea), musculoskeletal effects (e.g. muscle weakness, pain) and respiratory (throat discomfort, nasal congestion).[22] Weight gain is a common complaint with these medications. Depending on the particular medication, one study reported that between 9.8 and 29.0 per cent of patients had a greater than 7 per cent increase in body weight.[23] In particular, clozapine and olanzapine were reported to produce a weight gain of between 4 and 4.5 kg after 10 weeks of standard dose treatment.[23] Weight gain can have serious clinical implications. It can have a negative effect on compliance and compound the stigma associated with mental illness, and it can increase the risk of physical diseases associated with obesity, such as diabetes and cardiovascular disease.[23,24]

The nurse's role is to monitor and document side-effects and therapeutic effects, to educate the client and family about the medication so as to promote compliance and minimize the impact of side-effects, and to provide support for clients experiencing adverse effects of the medication. In particular, nurses can play an important role in the early detection of tardive dyskinesia and in counselling clients and families so as to reduce the embarrassment associated with these symptoms.[22,25]

Cultural/spiritual approaches

Cultural and spiritual approaches begin with the recognition that a cultural or spiritual issue may be present. Family members or other members of the cultural/religious group will need to be consulted to understand the issue and to assist in identifying appropriate strategies. The nurse may facilitate referral to an appropriate healer/spiritual leader and assist in coordinating the traditional healing with the treatment plan.

Interpersonal approaches

The primary nursing role related to hallucinations relates to interpersonal approaches. The primary intervention is always to establish a therapeutic trusting relationship (see Chapter 36). To do this, it is essential to be patient and listen to what the individual is saying.

Peplau[7,18] suggests that nursing interventions reverse the process that occurred when the hallucinations developed.

To do this, it is first important to identify the phase of hallucination development. The nurse then helps the individual to identify and name the anxiety. The nurse provides regular opportunities to interact with real people to mitigate the loneliness the individual may be experiencing.

Clack,[19] in her classic paper on hallucinations, suggests several strategies to assist people with hallucinations.

1 The first step is always to establish a therapeutic relationship, show acceptance and listen.
2 Next, look and listen for cues or symptoms of the hallucination. Focus on the cue and elicit the individual's observation and description.
3 Then, identify whether the hallucination is emotionally or toxically based (e.g. street drugs). Clack suggests that, if asked, the nurse should acknowledge that he or she is not experiencing the hallucination.
4 Clack suggests that the nurse next follows the direction of the individual and help him or her to observe and describe the hallucination. Eliciting observations of current and past hallucinations is part of the process of establishing trust, as well as assisting in understanding what the person is experiencing. This helps the person in determining why the hallucinations are occurring. The individual is to be encouraged to observe and describe thoughts, feelings and actions. Clack suggests the person should observe or describe needs that may be underlying the hallucinations in order to see what needs it may be serving.
5 The nurse would then suggest and reinforce meeting needs through interpersonal relationships and explore other behaviour concerns.

Since Clack's paper was written we now have many more medications to assist the individual. This means a person may recover from the symptoms much more quickly than the early paper would suggest. Some nurses may even believe that their role can therefore be restricted to administering the appropriate medication. However, Clack's interventions are still useful. The importance of listening, accepting and being patient is still very important. Also, if the individual is obtaining a lot of secondary gains from the hallucinations, that person may be unwilling to continue the medication. Therefore, understanding whether additional needs are being met by the hallucination is as important today as it was in 1962.

Reflection

What do you think it would be like to experience hallucinations?

STRATEGIES TO ASSIST WITH COPING

People who continue to experience hearing problematic voices often develop specific coping strategies to deal with the problem. Finding out the pattern of when the voices occur may help in identifying appropriate coping strategies. For example, many people report that the voices are worse when they are alone. They may need to carefully structure their time to include ample opportunity for interacting with others. Some people have found that listening to something else helps to block out the voices. For this reason some people will use headphones and an MP3 player, portable CD player or radio to help block out problematic voices. It is useful to explore with each individual the pattern of when the voices are most problematic and when they seem to fade away. This can be used to strategize specific coping approaches.

Buccheri and co-workers[26] summarized several strategies that had been reported in the literature to manage auditory hallucinations. These include self-monitoring of the hallucinations; reading aloud and summarizing; talking with someone; watching and listening to television; saying 'stop' and naming objects; listening to music with headphones; listening to relaxation tapes with headphones; wearing a unilateral ear plug; and humming a single note. In testing whether these strategies were useful, they found all study participants found at least one strategy provided relief for the distress associated with auditory hallucinations. In a later study, Buccheri et al.[27] found that 82 per cent of the participants continued to use at least one strategy.

Frederick and Cotanch[28] asked research participants to report self-help techniques they had found useful for coping with auditory hallucinations. The responses were grouped into physiological approaches to reduce arousal (relax, lie down, sleep, calm music, alcohol, extra medication); physiological approaches to increase arousal (loud music, walk, pace, jog); cognitive approaches (acceptance of voices, reduced attention to voices); and behavioural changes (leisure or work activity, seek interaction, isolate self). The findings highlighted the variety of different techniques that different people find useful.

Consider again the people introduced at the beginning of the chapter.

---

1 Michael sat alone in the TV room on the inpatient psychiatric ward. 'NO, NO, NO! I will not do THAT! Now you leave me alone! Shut up! Get out of here!'

Donovan needs to remember that the first steps are always to listen and to work on establishing a therapeutic relationship. Since this is a new patient assignment, it would be unlikely that Michael would trust Donovan immediately. So patience is required. Donovan would need to introduce himself and let Michael know he is available.

'Michael, my name is Donovan. I am a student nurse and will be with you today … I heard you talking a moment ago and you sounded pretty upset. Perhaps you could tell me about that ….'

2 Sally greeted the community nurse, Suchita, with a smile and a cup of tea. 'Sometimes, I think you and St Georgette are the only two true friends I have in the world.'

After a few minutes of conversation, Suchita enquired: 'So, how are you finding that new medication?'

'Terrible!' replied Sally. 'It was drowning St Georgette so I could barely hear her – so I had to stop taking it right away.'

Suchita might explore with Sally the relationship with her auditory hallucination. Sally and Suchita could work together to explore ways to expand Sally's social network. For example, Sally may join a recreational programme or a consumer/survivor self-help group that facilitates making new friends. When Sally has more social supports she may be less reliant on St Georgette as her only friend.

3 'I'm really loving this "Women in History" course. It really has me thinking', Ngozi explained to her room-mate. 'But after today's class, one thing keeps coming back to me. If Joan of Arc were alive today – wouldn't we just say she was hallucinating and drug her up or lock her up?'

As nurses we need to be open-minded in our understanding of the experience of hearing voices. Such experiences may be considered part of a normal occurrence within various cultures and spiritual belief systems. Hearing voices may or may not be indicative of a mental illness such as schizophrenia. We need to consider whether or not the experience is creating any problems for the person. We need to listen carefully to people to work on their goals, rather than simply considering hearing voices as a symptom to be controlled.

REFERENCES

1. Benjamin L. Is chronicity a function of the relationship between the person and the auditory hallucination? *Schizophrenia Bulletin* 1989; **15**: 291–310.

2. Miller L, O'Connor E, DisPasquale T. Patients' attitudes towards hallucinations. *American Journal of Psychiatry* 1993; **150**: 584–8.

3. González JC, Aguilar EJ, Berenguer V et al. Persistent auditory hallucinations. *Psychopathology* 2006; **39**: 120–5.

4. Romme M. Listening to the voice hearers. *Journal of Psychosocial Nursing and Mental Health Services* 1998; **36**: 40–4.

5. Forchuk C. The orientation phase of the nurse–client relationship: testing Peplau's theory. *Journal of Advanced Nursing Practice* 1994; **20**: 532–7.

6. Peplau HE. *Interpersonal relations in nursing.* New York, NY: JP Putnam, 1952.

7. Peplau HE. Anxiety, self and hallucinations. In: O'Toole AW, Welt SR (eds). *Interpersonal theory in nursing practice: selected*

works of Hildegard E. Peplau. New York, NY: Springer, 1989: 270–326.

8. Sullivan HS. *The interpersonal theory of psychiatry.* New York, NY: WW Norton, 1952.

9. Beyerstein B. Believing is seeing: organic and psychological reasons for hallucinations and other anomalous psychiatric symptoms. *Medscape Mental Health* 1996; **1** (11): 1–10.

10. American Psychiatric Association. *Diagnostic and statistical manual of mental disorders, 4th edition, text revision.* Washington, DC: American Psychiatric Press, 2000 (DSM IV-TR).

11. van der Hart O, Nijenhuis ERS, Steele K. *The haunted self: structural dissociation and the treatment of chronic traumatization.* New York, NY: Norton, 2006.

12. Staford LL. Dissociation and multiple personality disorder: a challenge for psycho-social nurses. *Journal of Psychosocial Nursing and Mental Health Services* 1993; **31**: 15–20.

13. Stickley T, Nickeas D. Becoming one person: living with dissociative identity disorder. *Journal of Psychiatric and Mental Health Nursing,* 2006; **13**: 180–7.

14. Bentall RP. The illusion of reality: a review of psychological research on hallucinations. *Psychology Bulletin* 1990; **107**: 82–95.

15. Tiihonen J, Hari R, Naukkarinen H *et al.* Modified activity of the human auditory cortex during auditory hallucinations. *American Journal of Psychiatry* 1992; **149**: 255–7.

16. Cleghorn JM, Garnett ES, Nahmias C *et al.* Regional brain metabolism during auditory hallucinations in chronic schizophrenia. *British Journal of Psychiatry* 1990; **157**: 562–70.

17. Rockstroh B, Junghöfer M, Elbert T *et al.* Electromagnetic brain activity evoked by affective stimuli in schizophrenia. *Psychophysiology* 2006; **43** (5): 431–9.

18. Peplau HE. Interpersonal relations and the process of adaptation. *Nursing Science* 1963; **1** (4): 272–9.

19. Clack J. An interpersonal technique for handling hallucinations, in nursing care of the disoriented patient [Monograph 13]. *American Nurses Association Publication* 1962; 16–29.

20. Mycek M, Harvey RA, Champe PC *et al. Pharmacology,* 3rd edn. Philadelphia, PA: Lippincott-Raven, 2005.

21. Newcomer W, Haupt D, Fucetola R *et al.* Abnormalities in glucose regulation during antipsychotic treatment of schizophrenia. *Archives of General Psychiatry* 2002; **59** (4): 337–45.

22. Spratto G, Woods A. *2007 PDR Nurses' Drug Handbook.* Clifton Park, NY: Thomson Delmar Learning, 2007.

23. Allison DB, Casey DE. Antipsychotic-induced weight gain: a review of the literature. *Journal of Clinical Psychiatry* 2001; **62** (Suppl 7): 22–31.

24. Blin O, Micallef J. Antipsychotic-associated weight gain and clinical outcome parameters. *Journal of Clinical Psychiatry* 2001; **62**: 11–21.

25. Johnson BS. *Psychiatric nursing.* Philadelphia, PA: J.B. Lippincott, 1986: 251–3.

26. Buccheri R, Trystad L, Kanas N *et al.* Auditory hallucinations in schizophrenia: group experience in examining symptom management and behavioural strategies. *Journal of Psychosocial Nursing and Mental Health Services* 1996; **34**: 12–25.

27. Buccheri R, Trystad L, Kanas N, Dowling G. Symptom management of auditory hallucinations in schizophrenia: results of 1-year follow-up. *Journal of Psychosocial Nursing and Mental Health Services* 1997; **35**: 20–8.

28. Frederick JA, Cotanch P. Self-help techniques for auditory hallucinations in schizophrenia. *Issues in Mental Health Nursing* 1994; **16**: 213–24.

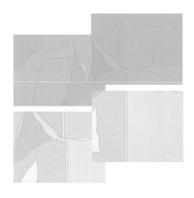

CHAPTER 24

The person who experiences disturbing beliefs

Elsabeth Jensen* and Cheryl Forchuk**

INTRODUCTION

Alcock[1] contracted a sore throat while in the Orient. He was offered an antibiotic and a Chinese herbal remedy based on snake bile. He accepted the antibiotic but declined the snake bile. Within a few days he was better, concluding that the antibiotic had worked. Later he learned his infection was viral, and that it had simply run its course. He struggled with the fact that he believed the antibiotic was responsible for his recovery. Like so many others, he had faith that the antibiotic would help, in spite of evidence to the contrary. Had he chosen the snake bile, he could as easily believe in its effectiveness, as the infection would have cleared in the same number of days.

Beliefs, simply defined, are convictions or opinions held as truths in the mind of the believer.[2] Many beliefs are supported by facts, many are held on faith. The common feature is that the believer holds his or her beliefs to be true. Even healthy people hold beliefs that may not hold up against facts and scientific evidence. Spiritual beliefs are based on faith and may be quite contrary to facts and evidence based on science. They are, however, considered valid and are known to contribute to good health.

History provides a long list of stories involving beliefs. When Columbus sailed west in 1492, he challenged the prevailing belief that the world was flat. However, despite his success, there are still people who believe the world is flat. Even in the presence of evidence, strong beliefs may not be given up easily. There are other, more ordinary, examples of beliefs that are held strongly in current times. How often have you heard someone say, 'I have no friends', 'I don't have a thing to wear', or 'I am so overweight', when the evidence is quite contrary? Superstitions provide another example of strongly held beliefs. Have you ever avoided walking under a ladder, or thrown salt over your shoulder after spilling it? Even educated people behave in ways that respect superstitions from time to time.

HOW DO BELIEFS DEVELOP?

Alcock[1] describes beliefs as our 'expectations about our world'. They derive from four sources: direct experience;

*Elsabeth Jensen is an Assistant Professor in the School of Nursing, York University. She has worked in a wide variety of mental health settings and is specialized in working with survivors of childhood abuse. Her current research focuses on evaluation of discharge care models, knowledge translation, diversity, and the relationships between the determinants of health and mental health.

**Cheryl Forchuk is a Professor in the School of Nursing and Department of Psychiatry at the University of Western Ontario, and an Assistant Director of the Lawson Health Research Institute. She has worked in a variety of mental health settings, including tertiary psychiatric care, acute care, community care and addictions. Her current research focuses on therapeutic relationships, models of discharge, peer support and housing.

observation; logical thought; and authority. Beliefs are developed out of direct experience. These are based on the patterns we observe in our world from the moment of birth. If two events occur together, they set up an association in the brain. The feeling of hunger is associated with unpleasantness. Mother providing milk leads to feeling satisfied. This leads to associating food with feeling good. Touching a hot stove causes pain, so stoves are associated with pain. Watching siblings cry from falling off the bicycle can lead to a fear of bicycles. Observing mother apply butter to the burn leads to believing that burns are helped by applying butter. Logical thought applied to reading about burn treatment later in life leads to the belief that it is best to apply cold water, and not butter, to the burn. Being taught by parents and teachers to wash hands after playing with something dirty leads to believing that one must always wash hands after touching anything that is dirty. Being told by parents that we are bright or stupid creates beliefs about self: 'I have the ability, I can do this' or 'I'm stupid, I'll never be any good'. We also learn about the world from authority figures. We are told, 'Don't trust strangers', 'This is how we do (don't do) it in our family'. These, and many other lessons, are combined to create our belief system about the world and how it works.

How do beliefs become disturbing?

Since many people hold false beliefs about themselves, their health and the world, why is this of interest to nurses? There are times when false, or groundless, beliefs can interfere with health and functioning. When a person's beliefs have the potential to cause them to do harm to themselves, or to another person, by commission or by omission, the beliefs come to be defined as disturbing. The beliefs may not disturb the person holding them, but they disturb other people. In such cases, the term 'delusions' is used. A delusion is a rigidly held, irrational belief that persists in spite of evidence that it is not true. Usually, people will have a cluster of beliefs that are groundless and extreme. This is referred to as a 'delusional system'.

Muse[3] observed, however, that 'The same type of delusion has caused certain persons to be canonized as saints in the early Christian period, persecuted as witches in the middle ages, and confined in an institution in the 20th century.' This observation is important as it alerts us to the social context of beliefs. What may be seen as a problem in one situation may not be seen the same way in another. In fact, culture can be a powerful influence on ideas and beliefs. Cultural ignorance in healthcare providers can result in misunderstandings and incorrect assessments. The following definition is helpful in understanding how to be clear that what is observed is a delusion and not something else.

The *Diagnostic and statistical manual of mental disorders*[4] provides the definition most often used in mental health care. According to this authority:

> A delusion is a false belief based on an incorrect inference about reality that is firmly held, despite the beliefs of almost everyone else, despite obvious proof or evidence to the contrary. The person holds a belief that is not ordinarily accepted by other members of the person's culture or subculture.

The belief is not an article of religious faith. A value judgement is considered to be a delusion only when the judgement is so extreme as to defy credibility. The person may talk about a delusion or it may be implied by his or her behaviour, e.g. eyeing other people with suspicion and mistrust. Delusions can occur on a continuum. Delusions can interfere with relationships, with work and with self-care. They are of particular concern when they jeopardize the person's safety, or the safety of others. When they do, the person will often come to the attention of the mental healthcare system.

Delusions can occur alone or in combination with other signs and symptoms of mental illness. They are a known feature of several psychiatric diagnostic categories including, but not limited to, schizophrenia, depression, psychotic depression, mania, schizo-affective disorder, anorexia nervosa, bulimia, delusional disorder, psychosomatic disorder, paranoid personality disorder, schizotypal personality disorder, and a variety of substance abuse disorders.[4] The experience of abuse in childhood is also a factor in the development of delusions in adults with mental illness.[5] In studying people with delusions, Read and Argyle[6] found that 50 per cent had a history of childhood sexual abuse or a history of childhood physical abuse, and an additional 29 per cent had experienced both forms of abuse. This means that 79 per cent of these people were abused as children.

Beliefs form in the brain, where they serve the purpose of reducing anxiety and increasing structure and consistency in the person's day-to-day dealings with the world. They result from the processing of information in both hemispheres. There is some evidence that false beliefs, or delusions, can result when the left hemisphere receives incomplete information from the right, or if the interpreter function of the left hemisphere is malfunctioning. Brain research provides some evidence that disturbing beliefs, or delusions, are at least modestly associated with impairment of the central nervous system.[6–8,9]

Delusions have been reported to be a feature of disorders of the central nervous system. Examples of this include Capgras' syndrome, and dementias resulting from substance abuse. Capgras' syndrome causes the person to believe that people close to him or her have been replaced by identical doubles or robots. This condition has been linked to diffuse or localized lesions, especially of the right hemisphere.[10,11]

Understanding delusions can be difficult for a beginning practitioner. They may or may not be a feature of many different mental health diagnoses. While delusions are a feature of these many conditions, not every person with that diagnosis will suffer from delusions. It is important to assess the person and to identify the presence or absence of delusions. If they are present, they are not all the same. Depending on their characteristics, they may require different interventions.

Reflection

What do you think about when you hear the term delusions?

NURSING THE PERSON WITH DISTURBING BELIEFS

The task of the nurse is to observe, from the perspective of a participant observer. Based on the nursing assessment, the nurse makes inferences through identifying themes and forming hypotheses. Finally, the nurse experiments with interventions in the nurse–client relationship that will effect changes favourable to the client.[12–14]

Peplau[12] defined delusions as one of several possible responses to repeated frustration. Fixed responses, such as delusions, occur after repeated frustrations that require reorganization of the personality in order to deal with the anxiety resulting from the frustration. The beliefs cannot be given up, as this would cause overwhelming insecurity in the person. In this sense, delusions are a defence against long-standing anxiety and insecurity. This view has support from others.[6]

It is easier to provide nursing care based on the type of delusion being suffered, rather than the psychiatric diagnosis. The different types of delusions cut across the different diagnostic categories. A person may suffer from more than one type of delusion. The client may also be suffering from more than disturbing beliefs. People with schizophrenia, for example, often experience both disturbing beliefs and disturbing voices, or other forms of hallucination. It is important to know that there is often a thread of truth at the core of most delusions, and that these often serve as a way of dealing with underlying anxiety.[14–16] This last fact is very important as delusions can be challenging for the beginning nurse. By their nature, delusions are bizarre and irrational. They challenge common sense. It is imperative, however, that one avoids challenging the belief. The nurse should, however, assess carefully.

When beliefs are suspected to be delusional, it is important to gather as much information from other sources as possible. This includes talking to family and friends. A colleague recently discovered, to her amazement, that the young man she had admitted *was* indeed a successful rock star, with a Porsche, a mansion and a large bank account, even though he was poorly dressed, penniless and dishevelled on admission. In this case, family members had been available to validate his story. Had they not been available, he might easily have found himself under treatment for delusions!

Three major types of delusions are encountered in nursing practice.[3,16] These are delusions of *persecution*, delusions of *grandeur* and *negative delusions*. Other categories may be encountered, including sexual delusions, somatic delusions and delusions that are difficult to understand. Case examples will be used to illustrate the major types.

Delusions of persecution

Delusions of persecution involve the belief that others are after the person, and that he or she is at risk of being harmed by these persecutors. These delusions can be dangerous. People may try to defend themselves from the danger that they believe is present. In the process, they can harm or even kill others. These occur more commonly in people who may have experienced danger from others at a point in their life and in abusers of some drugs, such as amphetamines.

Personal illustration 24.1

Mikel is a 25-year-old man admitted for assaulting the postman. He is under close observation as he is still potentially violent. As he speaks, his eyes move about, scanning his environment constantly. He sits forward on a chair in the dayroom, talking in a low voice.

Mikel: I don't know why I am here. I am not crazy. I don't like to be locked up.

Nurse: Can you tell me what happened just before you came here?

Mikel: A policeman came. He said he wasn't, but he had the uniform on. I know them. I tried to protect myself, then, others came. They took me here. What will happen to me?

Nurse: You say you 'know them'; have you had other experiences with the police?

Mikel: They came after me. The police, I don't trust them. They take people, and you never see them again. They beat me, left me for dead. I came to this country. I thought I would be safe here, but they are everywhere. Now they found me, and brought me here.

He continues to look anxiously about the room as they talk.

In Mikel's delusion, people wearing any kind of uniform are police, and they are the enemy. He sees his efforts to protect himself as legitimate. In his case, he had been a victim of the horrors of war. His beliefs about danger were formed in the past, but are out of place in the present. His belief that he needs to protect himself from the non-existent threat makes him dangerous to others. His beliefs are disturbing as they threaten the safety of other people, especially those wearing a uniform.

Delusions of grandeur

People with delusions of grandeur hold exaggerated beliefs about their abilities, status, worth or accomplishments. The content is boastful or egotistical. Others who know the individual do not substantiate the contents of the belief system. The behaviour resulting from the delusions is disturbing to others around the individual.

Personal illustration 24.2

Dr Fairchild is a 59-year-old physicist, admitted after his wife had taken him to the family doctor for an evaluation of strange behaviour. She discovered he had spent a large amount of money on laboratory equipment for the basement. When she asked him about this, he had told her that he had discovered time travel. She was told not to worry, as he had access to unlimited wealth through his discovery. On checking with his Dean, she confirmed that her husband had suffered a number of grant rejections, had been reported by a number of his students for bizarre grading of exam papers and, as a result, the University was considering suggesting early retirement. The Dean had spoken repeatedly with Dr Fairchild about these concerns.

Dr Fairchild carried his briefcase around on the ward. It was filled with papers with equations and strange symbols. 'My work will solve the great mysteries of the ages. I will be able to talk to the greatest scientists as they make their discoveries. The University is very fortunate to have my work based here. I can show you my work, but it is very complex and requires a genius to comprehend it. You should be grateful I am even sharing this information with you. Not everyone is worthy, you know.'

Dr Fairchild's beliefs are not disturbing to him. They are disturbing to his wife, who sees the family resources dwindling. They are also disturbing to his Dean, who is concerned about productivity and performance. He is at risk of squandering his resources and of damaging the relationships he has with his wife and his employer.

Negative delusions

Negative delusions usually occur in people who are depressed. They are mood congruent and involve themes of despair, inadequacy and hopelessness. These beliefs are disturbing as they can result in self-harm or suicide. The delusions also interfere with the person's ability to get on with his or her life tasks.

Personal illustration 24.3

Willow is a 15-year-old student, admitted for depression and delusions involving snakes. Her schoolwork has deteriorated over the past 6 months and she has gained weight. She looks downward, avoiding eye contact. Her clothes are plain and very baggy.

Willow: The snake is eating me. I am going to die.
Nurse: Can you tell me more about the snake?
Willow: It's inside me. It's eating everything. [Tears flow.] The monster put a snake in me because I was bad. He said it was my fault. He said the snake would eat me and I would die because I was bad. I'm not supposed to tell. But I'm scared, I don't want to die, but I'm bad. I have to die. The snake will kill me by eating me from the inside.
Nurse: You sound afraid.
Willow: I'm scared. I don't want to die. I wish I could get it out. [Her head is low. Her voice is barely audible.]

Willow is depressed and believes she is dying. Obviously, no snake could survive inside the human body, yet this is her belief. She is clearly troubled. By stating that she wishes she could get the snake out, Willow alerts the nurse to the possibility that she might do something that would result in self-harm. The content of the delusion should also alert the nurse to the possibility of sexual abuse. The nurse should not introduce the topic, but, should it arise, it will be important for her to be empathic and non-judgemental.

As with other delusions, it will take time for the individual to feel safe enough to begin to share the issues that are at the core of his or her beliefs. Although it may be tempting to simply point out the seemingly obvious, this action will only aggravate the individual and raise his or her anxiety even higher.

The two main approaches to helping people with disturbing beliefs are the interpersonal nurse–client relationship and appropriate medical evaluation and treatment.

Reflection

What are the responses of your colleagues to the term delusions?

INTERPERSONAL APPROACHES

The development of a therapeutic relationship with the client provides the necessary context for dealing with the underlying issues. Delusions are a way of coping with repeated frustrations and the anxiety they cause, and there is usually a core of truth, or fact, at the base of the delusions. As Donner[15] points out, the underlying core of the delusion must be decoded before the underlying need can be understood. Only when the underlying need is met in a healthier way can the delusion be given up. This can happen only in the context of a safe and trusting relationship. Donner cautions that the delusion should never be interpreted directly to the client. Neither should it be confronted, as this will only escalate the client's anxiety.

The *orientation phase* is the beginning of the therapeutic relationship. During this phase, the nurse and the client are getting to know each other, and are forming a contract about the focus of the therapeutic relationship. When the client is believed to be suffering from delusions, it is important to find out as much as possible from the client, family, friends, associates and any other source of information.

The nurse also needs to consider her or his comfort and confidence in working with people with delusions. Depending on the nature of the delusions, nurses have found that extended contact can lead to impatience and anger on the part of the nurse.[16] If the particular beliefs, or underlying issues, cause anxiety in the nurse, this must be examined. Peer consultation, or consultation with the multidisciplinary team, can be an important source of support for the nurse.

Given the nature of delusions, safety is always a concern. The clients may be on close or intensive observation for their safety or to protect others. The content of the delusion is an important consideration. For a person such as Mikel, who fears people in uniforms, it would be unwise to have a uniformed person provide close observation. In Willow's case, her 'monster' is a 'he'. She will experience less anxiety if observed by a woman. These suggestions may seem so obvious that the reader wonders why they are made explicit, yet there are many examples in the real world of problems arising from failure to consider the obvious.

Rosenthal and McGuinness[17] have clear recommendations for nursing the person with delusions. They caution against agreeing with delusions, suggesting the nurse tactfully avoid agreement. Agreement is as unhelpful as disagreement. At the same time, logic and debate are inappropriate, as this frustrates clients and escalates their anxiety, which is already overwhelming. That is why the client is suffering from delusions in the first place. Instead, it is recommended that nurses focus on the client's feelings as this validates the client's reality.[18]

To avoid agreeing *or* disagreeing with the delusional content and yet enter into a dialogue may seem to be a confusing set of guidelines to follow. One approach is to look for what is *true to the listener* about what is said, and then support or agree with that piece. For example, when Willow says she is frightened of the snake, the nurse can agree that she (Willow) is frightened. For example, 'It sounds like you are feeling very afraid of what is happening.' The nurse would not say 'It sounds like that snake in you is really frightening', because that would reinforce the delusion. Similarly, a statement like 'Don't you realise a snake would be killed by the acid in your stomach' would be seen as argumentative and would risk the establishment of trust in the nurse. At times, a patient will directly ask the nurse whether or not the nurse believes the client. Again, the nurse walks a tightrope to agree with the truth while neither reinforcing nor confronting the delusion. An example might be, 'I don't feel or see the snake, but I believe it is real to you.'

It can be tempting at times to try and use logic to talk someone out of a delusion. This tends to result in either the person not trusting the nurse's motivation or coming up with a more elaborate explanation to account for the logic presented by the nurse. An example from the clinical experience of one of the authors illustrates this problem.

Personal illustration 24.4

I had been providing clinical supervision, with the use of a one-way mirror, to a nurse who was pregnant while I was also pregnant. The patient appeared to be less and less willing to be open about his concerns as our pregnancies became more obvious. In discussing this with him the nurse discovered he was concerned that his 'crazy talk' might harm the unborn children. After further exploration he felt that if the unborn children were disturbed they would begin to kick and make the mothers uncomfortable. An agreement was made that he would discuss what was truly bothering him if we both agreed to let him know immediately if we experienced extreme kicking. This seemed to work well and he returned to his usual frankness in discussing his concerns during counselling sessions. Months later, on the first day I returned from maternity leave, this patient was waiting at the door of the hospital for my return, and demanding to know if the baby was alright. He wanted to see a baby picture 'for proof'. I told him the baby was fine, but did not share a picture. Every day for the next week this patient waited at the hospital door and again asked if the baby was alright. I thought his concern was related to the earlier issue of his 'crazy talk' potentially harming the baby. I decided to show him a picture to prove the baby was fine and allay his concern. Much to my surprise, he said, 'Just as I thought, that is my baby.' I asked him why he thought that and he replied 'See – the baby is bald just like me. That is my baby.' I foolishly argued the point by saying that there are many bald babies, to which he replied 'Yes, I have many children.'

When working with a client over a long period of time the nurse will observe periods of both wellness and difficulty. In these situations, it may be possible to discuss the delusional content while it is not being currently experienced. It is often helpful for clients to learn to recognize early signs of difficulty to prevent relapse. For example, a nurse case manager had been working with a particular client for 3 years. During this time, the client had several relapses. When this client was psychotic, he always had a delusion that his food was poisoned. He would eventually refuse all food and drink and be hospitalized for 4–6 weeks in order to recover both physically and mentally. The nurse case manager and client were able to establish that the early signs of trouble were finding that his food seemed to have a metallic taste. This client learned to alert the case manager to when this occurred, so he could have an early assessment and readjustment of medication. This strategy was successful in breaking the pattern of regular re-hospitalizations.

Reflection

What do you think it would be like to experience delusions?

MEDICAL APPROACHES

When strong beliefs are sufficiently disturbing, and interfere with health and functioning, they often result in admission to hospital. This allows the physician to evaluate the case, to test which medication will be of best benefit and to titrate the dosage. Hospitalization also provides intensive nursing care in support of the medical plan of care. As Nightingale[19] observed, 'I would go further, and state that to the experienced eye of a careful observing nurse, the daily, I had almost said hourly, changes which take place in patients, and which changes rarely come under the cognisance of the periodical medical visitor, afford a still more important class of data.'

Nurses are responsible for communicating their observations to the other members of the team. Nurses are also responsible for administering prescribed medications and reporting the person's responses to these. It is necessary for the nurse to have a good knowledge base of the classes of medications usually prescribed for persons with disturbing beliefs. It is only through careful observation that benefits and side-effects can be identified. Some side-effects are minor, while others may be transient. Still others can cause disability or even death. The nurse's role includes educating the person about the medication. The lessons should include information about the benefits of the medication, the importance of taking it as prescribed and the common side-effects. Knowledge of strategies for dealing with side-effects such as dry mouth and blurred vision can be very reassuring to the person.

One of the nurse's roles is that of teacher. Information about the medication is given as part of health teaching. It is important for the person to understand that the medications are intended to help them get better. Information should be given verbally and in written form, for the person to keep. Written materials should be in lay language for easy comprehension, and should be typed in size 14 or larger font. This is to compensate for the visual effects of the medication. The information should be succinct. Keeping it to one page per medication allows the person to post it in the medicine cabinet at home. The written material should always have contact information, should the client have any questions or concerns after discharge. More details about anti-psychotic medication are provided in Chapter 23.

Having a working-stage therapeutic relationship provides an easy vehicle for discussing the concerns or questions that the client may have. It will also allow that the nurse needs to be fully aware of how the medication is affecting the person. This information will be essential to the physician making decisions about the medical plan of care.

SUMMARY

We all hold some beliefs that others would disagree with. An extreme example of this would be a delusion. While some delusions may be innocuous, others may be very disturbing and can place the individual at risk. The nurse needs to help the person feel as comfortable as possible, to be honest about concerns, to listen carefully to what is being said, to assess for severity of problems and response to treatment, and to work with the client on mutually agreed goals. The particular challenge in communicating with the person with disturbing beliefs is to support and listen to the client without reinforcing or directly confronting the delusions.

REFERENCES

1. Alcock JE. Alternative medicine and the psychology of belief. *Medscape* 1999. Available from: www.quackwatch.com/01 QuackeryRelatedTopics/altpsych.html. Accessed April 2008.

2. *Webster's encyclopedic unabridged dictionary of the English language.* San Diego, CA: Thunder Bay Press, 2001.

3. Muse MB. *Psychology for nurses.* Philadelphia: WB Saunders, 1926.

4. American Psychiatric Association. *Diagnostic and statistical manual of mental disorders, 4th edition, text revision.* Washington, DC: American Psychiatric Press, 2000 (DSM IV-TR).

5. Hammerly P, Burston D, Read J. Learning to listen: childhood trauma and adult psychosis. *Mental Health Practice* 2004; **7** (6): 18–21.

6. Read J, Argyle N. Hallucinations, delusions, and thought disorder among adult psychiatric inpatients with a history of child abuse. *Psychiatric Services* 1999; **50** (11): 1467–72.

7. Butler RW, Braft DL. Delusions: a review and integration. *Schizophrenia Bulletin* 1991; **17** (4): 633–47.

8. Kunert HJ, Norra C, Hoff P. Theories of delusional disorders: an update and review. *Psychopathology* 2007; **40** (3): 191–203.

9. McKay R, Langdon R, Coltheart M. Models of misbelief: integrating motivational and deficit theories of delusions. *Conscious Cognition* 2007 [Epub ahead of print] Available from: http://homepage.mac.com/ryantmckay/Paper%20PDFs%20for%20Website/Models%20of%20Misbelief.pdf.

10. Buckwalter KC. Are you really my nurse, or are you a snake sheriff? *Journal of Psychosocial and Nursing Mental Health Services* 1993; **31**: 33–4.

11. Edelstyn N, Oyebode F, Barrett K. The delusions of Capgras and intermetamorphosis in a patient with right-hemisphere white-matter pathology. *Psychopathology* 2001; **34** (6): 299–304.

12. Peplau HE. Themes in nursing-safety. In: Mereness D (ed.). *Psychiatric nursing: developing psychiatric nursing skills*, 2nd edn. Dubuque, IA: WC Brown, 1971: 142–7.

13. Peplau HE. Peplau's theory of interpersonal relations. *Nursing Science Quarterly* 1997; **10** (4): 162–7.

14. Peplau HE. *Interpersonal relations in nursing*. New York, NY: GP Putnam, 1952.

15. Donner G. Treatment of a delusional patient. *American Journal of Nursing* 1969; **69**: 2642–4.

16. Jakes S, Rhodes J, Issa S. Are the themes of delusional beliefs related to the themes of life-problems and goals? *Journal of Mental Health*. 2004; **13** (6): 611–19.

17. Rosenthal TT, McGuinness TM. Dealing with delusional patients: discovering the distorted truth. *Journal of Mental Health Nursing* 1986; **8**: 143–54.

18. Brough C. Developing and maintaining a therapeutic relationship. Part 2. A case study. *Nursing Older People* 2004; **16** (9): 26–8.

19. Nightingale F. Notes on hospitals. In: Rosenberg CE (ed.). *Florence Nightingale on hospital reform*. London, UK: Garland Publishing, 1989 [original work published in 1863].

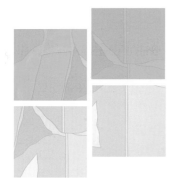

CHAPTER 25

The person with a diagnosis of schizophrenia

Tom Keen* and Phil Barker**

If I am mad I let you see
When I laugh I am looking at me
While I talk of hope you will understand
Why look at me I'm just another hand

My brain is like a big unpaid bill
What's the good when my fancies can't fulfil
Those who keep me I am keeping all them
How many points ponder this pen

From what I write if my righting is wrong
If you hark to its lilt you might make a song
Those who know me please treat me as not mad
That's good of you when you know you're not bad

You ask me where I put my pill
I digest it that's why I'm not ill
I put my thoughts before me and direct them after
Look there's a lot to learn from laughter

Limber[1]

DIAGNOSIS AND SYMPTOMATOLOGY

The diagnosis of schizophrenia refers to a complex and controversial[2] cluster of conditions occurring in roughly 1 per cent of people worldwide, and affecting about 250 000 individuals in the UK.[3] There are no diagnostic tests for the multifaceted condition, and aetiology remains uncertain, despite significant recent clarification of genetic and neurological factors.[4] Instead, the diagnosis is made on the evidence of a variety of subjective experiences (symptoms) and observable behaviours (signs) which commonly include:

- holding apparently false or incredible beliefs that seem at odds with one's cultural or educational background (*delusional thinking*);
- hearing sounds, thoughts-out-loud or voices (often making critical or abusive comments and threats) in the absence of any actual external stimuli or speakers (*auditory hallucinations, thought-echo*);
- experiencing one's thoughts, feelings, speech or bodily functions being controlled, interfered with or

*Tom Keen was a Lecturer in Mental Health at the University of Plymouth. He has had a long career as a nurse, therapist and manager in various situations, including acute admission wards, adolescent psychotherapy, therapeutic community and community mental health centres.
**Phil Barker is a psychotherapist and Honorary Professor at the University of Dundee, UK.

manipulated by some external force (*thought broadcasting, withdrawal or insertion; passivity phenomena; 'made' actions*);

- believing that neutral, outside events and people or insignificant objects have special meaning for or about oneself (*ideas of reference, delusional perception*);
- speaking (and therefore presumably thinking) idiosyncratically or unintelligibly, with unusual patterns of expression, disjointed sentences, repetitiveness or coining novel words and phrases (*thought disorder, loosened association, word salad, neologisms*);
- becoming unusually withdrawn, both socially and emotionally, or obsessively preoccupied with fantasy and esoteric ideas (*autism*);
- showing less interest, emotion or enthusiasm than usual (*impaired volition, anhedonia, blunt or flattened affect*);
- seeming to others to behave or feel differently from their normal expectations (*inappropriate behaviour, incongruous affect*).

All, some or none of these may persuade a psychiatrist to diagnose schizophrenia. Individuals also complain of anxiety, agitation, depression, moodiness, lack of concentration and memory problems. These are all common experiences not only as schizophrenia develops, but also during critical life-periods such as adolescence or mid-life, and make early psychiatric diagnosis difficult. Standardized diagnostic manuals recognize many other behavioural idiosyncrasies and experiential oddities as signs or symptoms of various schizophrenia subtypes and provide clear guidelines to psychiatrists, researchers or others needing to establish a diagnosis.[5,6]

Schizophrenia encompasses such a wide range of diverse presentations that evidence from countless incompatible clinical cases could contradict almost any generalized statement about the diagnosis. Schizophrenia has no typical course and no typical underlying gross pathology. Since its initial formulation, arguments about the validity of the diagnosis and its nature, causes and treatment have abounded and continue.[7] People unfamiliar with schizophrenia see nothing in common between the apparently spontaneous breakdown, dramatic imagery, persuasively surreal fears or frantically poetic outpourings of a 20-year-old student and the chronic torpor, expressionless features and superficially stagnant life of an unkempt middle-aged vagrant who seems to spend time and money on nothing but smoking. Schizophrenia disables people in innumerable ways, and almost anything that nurses do could be a valid intervention at some point in someone's diagnostic career. This chapter will of necessity miss out much that is important, and probably include much that is disputed, but presents a variety of perspectives on an intriguingly complex and continuingly controversial diagnosis.

Reflection

What do you think the various forms of schizophrenia have in common?
How well does this belief correlate with your experience?

Categories and classification

The core features of schizophrenia can be divided into three blurred categories.[8]

- *Positive symptoms* – so-called because they represent experiences that are qualitatively different from normal, or behavioural exaggerations of conventional social conduct. They include apparent exaggerations or distortions of thinking (delusional thought); perception (hallucinations); communication and language (incomprehensible speech, incongruous affect); and behaviour (catatonic posturing and impulsivity).
- *Negative symptoms* – which by contrast represent an apparent loss of normal function or a diminution from social norms. People diagnosed as schizophrenic sometimes seem unemotional or avoid intimate contact with others. They may become withdrawn and speak little, or seem inactive and apathetic with apparently little purpose or energy.
- *Schizophrenic thinking* – subtle changes in perceptual analysis and reasoning, which psychiatrists construe as 'formal thought disorder' and 'loosened associations'. These cognitive patterns may be analogous with, if not identical to, the kinds of thought patterns that cognitive psychologists call 'divergent thinking' and 'loosened constructs'.[9] Schizophrenic people often analyse reality from unusual perspectives and classify experiences or objects in innovative or surreal ways. Schizophrenic thinking seems sometimes unnecessarily complex, unconventionally abstract, or strangely literal and concrete.[10]

Although schizotypal thought patterns are sometimes subsumed within the category of 'positive symptoms', it is useful to consider them separately, not only because they are also found in 'ordinary', undiagnosed people (as are many of the negative and positive symptoms) but also because the three symptom clusters seem to respond differently to psychiatric treatments.

Positive symptoms tend to occur or predominate during acutely disturbed periods in patients' lives. Breakdowns tend to occur more frequently and with greater severity after stressful life events, such as accidents or illness, natural disasters, economic changes, celebrations, anniversaries, etc. Positive symptoms are especially likely to recur or intensify when a patient's socioemotional environment becomes tense or fraught with *communication deviance* – unclear or disguised meanings; denied or deviously articulated feelings; or high levels of *expressed emotion*.[11] Neuroleptic drugs, the mainstay of mainstream psychiatric treatment, target and often effectively suppress positive symptoms, but are less successful in banishing individuals' subjective unease or less florid symptoms.[3]

Negative symptoms are not so readily ameliorated by anti-psychotic medication. Indeed, sedation and other side-effects of injudiciously prescribed neuroleptic drugs may worsen them.[12] Apathy, withdrawal, self-neglect, uncommunicativeness, etc. may develop before the onset of, or continue in the absence of, more dramatic positive symptoms. These symptoms are not only compounded or mimicked by the effects of drugs (both psychiatric and recreational, e.g. cannabis) but are also worsened by impoverished economic, cultural or social circumstances.[7] Concerned others (e.g. relatives, friends, naïve professionals) often critically attribute negative symptoms to someone's personality and react by rejection, silent judgement, criticism or antagonism. Such responses by carers and staff have been shown to compromise patients' fragile personal integrity, aggravate their symptoms and increase pathological behaviour.[13,14]

The third category of schizophrenic phenomenology – the tendency to use heavily concrete, highly abstract or bafflingly divergent forms of thinking – tends to pre-date initial breakdowns and also persists as a stable part of patients' personalities, even after effective neuroleptic

suppression of p
commonly found
schizophrenics, as w
connection at all with
and schizotypal thinking
ophrenia, but occur thr
indolent and mildly to
superficially display the equ
Many creative people and soc
schizotypal thinking.[8,10] Recen
sively demonstrated that even
sional thought are much more ord
may appear the case to many profe
becoming blinkered by constant expo
pathologies encountered in clinical wor

Schizophrenia subtypes

The various characteristics used to diagnose s
tend to occur in loosely segregated clusters,
many different conditions nestle beneath the si.
nostic umbrella. Both official diagnostic manuals[5,]
schizophrenia into subtypes, whereas indepe
researchers have applied statistical factor analysis to sy
tom clusters and found three core syndromes that loos
conform to traditional diagnostic subtypes, and also
emerging neurological knowledge (Table 25.1).[18,19]

TABLE 25.1 Symptom clusters and diagnostic classification

Symptom cluster	DSM-IV	ICD-10
Reality distortion Hallucinations; delusions	*Paranoid* Preoccupation with delusions or frequent hallucinosis	*Paranoid* Delusions usually, with hallucinations predominately
Disorganized Incoherent speech; incongruous affect; thought disorder	*Disorganized* Disorganized speech or behaviour; flat or inappropriate affect	*Hebephrenic* Inappropriate mood; incoherent speech; negative symptoms
	Catatonic Motor immobility with waxy flexibility of limbs or stupor; excessive purposeless activity not externally influenced; extreme negativism – resistance to instructions, rigid stereotypical posturing, mutism; repetitive imitation of someone else's speech or movement	*Catatonic* Prominent psychomotor disturbances; catatonic excitement, stupor or posturing
Psychomotor poverty Lack of responsiveness; flat affect; poverty of speech; inactivity; anhedonia	*Residual* Absence of prominent delusions, hallucinations, disorganized speech and grossly disorganized behaviour; negative symptoms or continuing but attenuated positive symptoms, e.g. odd beliefs or unusual perceptions	

ists commonly attribute the various symptoms
al behaviour of diagnosed schizophrenics to the
ces of subtle defects in brain structure and func-
ch may respond to carefully targeted psychologi-
pharmacological treatments. Sharing this clinical
tive facilitates close cooperation among nurses, psy-
ts and the medical canon of diagnosis, treatment
re. It can reassure those who crave diagnostic cer-
and the potential security of professional harmony
t medical treatment. It also risks invalidating the per-
l hypotheses of other individuals, and constructing too
a knowledge-and-power imbalance between profes-
nals and some service users, leading to either unwar-
nted dependence or negativistic resistance. Some
sychiatrists have expressed concern about becoming too
dogmatically entrenched in biomedical explanations, and
propose more balanced approaches that acknowledge people's holistic integrity.[7,20] Clinical symptoms of schizophrenia can also (not necessarily *instead*) be thought of as
valid, if often miserable or misunderstood aspects of
people's experiences, thus enabling the establishment of
strong therapeutic alliances between patients and professional carers.[21] Problematic behaviour or psychotic experiences can be therapeutically construed as individuals'
attempted solutions to other more deeply lying, vaguely
troubling or intensely difficult problems. Withdrawal may
represent an individual's constructive response to unexpressed fear of others' judgement or opinion of himself; an
attempt to reduce the undifferentiated torrent of stimuli
pouring into his consciousness; or an admittedly lonely or
self-defeating solution to extreme shyness or feelings of
low worth. Shouting, talking to oneself or playing bad
music loudly may help an individual to express feelings,
avoid troubling conversations or sort out thinking, but it
may also silence the chattery background or frightening
foreground of hallucinosis. Hallucinations themselves may
be symbolic residues of past abuses; dramatically serving to
disguise pain, shift blame, maintain threat and shout a
warning; all in one elegant neuropsychological synthesis.[22]

To develop effective clinical relationships with people,
nurses should share their professional conceptual frameworks with patients. Once both parties are psychoeduca-
tionally initiated into each other's world views, a more
effective partnership can be established by pooling both
formal psychiatric nomenclature and subjective, personal
phenomenology. In such a shared enterprise, diagnoses,
symptoms and personal beliefs become equal partners in
a joint problem-solving approach. Symptom clusters
become potential frameworks for helping people to
clarify their experiences and collaborate with care planning. *Coping strategy enhancement* is the jargon term for
therapeutic strategies based on identifying what people
do that actually helps them, and working out ways of
doing that even more effectively or frequently.[23] If shouting helps silence voices, but attracts unwanted public
tion, how about singing or whistling?

The course and outcome of schizophrenic experience
varies widely. Some people only ever have one breakdown (22 per cent of diagnoses); others recover completely between recurrent attacks (35 per cent); whereas
about 40 per cent of diagnosed people either remain permanently affected or show progressive personal and
social deterioration.[4] Despite decades of research, psychiatrists have been unable to establish clear patterns of
biological, psychological or social causes,[12] although
expectations are increasingly expressed that rapidly
evolving brain-imaging technologies, advances in genetic
understanding and epidemiological studies will soon clarify the causes and underlying nature of schizophrenia.[24]

The lack of a consistent symptomatology, widely variant
prognoses and continuing difficulty to identify definite
aetiologies has led many people to condemn the diagnosis
as at best flawed[7] or at worst prejudicial and in itself
delusional.[25–27] However, mainstream psychiatry remains
unmoved by such criticisms. When tightly defined using
standardized diagnostic procedures, the incidence of
schizophrenia is found to be remarkably similar worldwide, however culturally and economically dissimilar the
populations studied.[11] This is an epidemiological rarity,
and suggests not only a profoundly widespread genetic
basis for the condition but also that the genetic differences
involved may be evolutionary in origin and derive from
complex human psychological and anthropological characteristics, such as language development and social group
diffusion rather than simple individual pathology.[8,10]
While people continue to suffer intensely from the distressing and socially disabling emotional, intellectual and
interpersonal experiences associated with schizophrenia,
mental health nurses will be needed to provide care, compassion and sensitive understanding, whatever the nature
of this complex diagnosis eventually proves to be.

SCHIZOPHRENIA: A MENU OF INTERVENTIONS

Clinicians and researchers have recently evolved a package of reasonably well-evidenced psychiatric interventions for the various forms of schizophrenia. Estimations
of the effectiveness of this treatment package vary, partly
according to whether outcome studies concentrate on
measuring formal reductions in clinical symptoms or
focus upon overall social recovery and subjective increase
in personal well-being.[28] Nevertheless, current policies
dictate that mental health services should be able to offer
the following menu:

1 community-based teams to ensure early intervention
in the course of the illness, prevent prolonged periods
of non-treatment and provide support during crises;
2 monitored anti-psychotic medication and flexible
compliance strategies;

3 applied cognitive–behavioural therapy;
4 therapeutic support for families;
5 social, occupational and vocational support and skills training;
6 targeted health promotion, and attention to patients' physical health.

COMMUNITY-BASED TEAMWORK

The UK Department of Health has published clear guidelines for the kinds of service structures needed for the effective integration of interventions.[29] As well as improved residential services such as acute admission wards[30] and hostel accommodation, local services should include a range of alternative provisions, as follows.

- *Early intervention services* are intended to help people when they first develop schizophrenic symptoms, and for the first few years of any subsequent illness. Because of the complexity of both adolescence and schizophrenia, services should focus on specific symptoms and preferred solutions, rather than strict diagnostic protocols. They need to be conscious of the risk of stigmatization and social censure, and focus on people's social integration and normal developmental process, not simply their pathology and clinical status. Staff must be family oriented yet also aware of the importance of separation and identity issues in people's lives. There should be seamless connections between children's, adolescents', families' and adults' mental health services, and firm partnerships with all other relevant agencies, including primary care, education, employment and social services.

- *Crisis resolution teams* provide 24-hour rapid response, with intensive but time-limited support to individuals, families or social networks early in the development of crises. Crisis resolution work stresses engagement with patients with schizophrenia and their carers, and strives for the active involvement of all protagonists within the situation. Interventions need to be pragmatic, and factually focused. Crisis resolution teams reduce immediate emotional heat by: effective containment of emotions and catastrophic fantasies; systemic engagement, empathic calmness and explorative clarity; and an emphasis on solution-focused problem-solving approaches, rather than custodial or medical interventions. They function as gatekeepers, referring people on as soon as the protagonists feel back in control of themselves or their situation.

- *Intensive home treatment* is linked to crisis intervention, and ensures the provision of close contact, active support and therapeutic interventions to individuals and families to prevent further crises. Interventions may include whatever is needed: sleeves rolled up practical help and instruction; liaison with other agencies; shared recreational or social activity; family management and therapeutic work; systemic or individual psychotherapy; medication management; etc.

- *Assertive outreach teams* establish and maintain contact with people who have complex needs and are difficult to engage, or who repeatedly withdraw from contact with services. Teams should communicate intensively with each other, users, social networks and agencies. They should be self-contained, well led and mutually supportive; oriented to long-term treatment and continuity of care; highly creative, flexible and imaginative in building, maintaining and repairing their relationships with users; and focused on risk management and physical health needs as well as psychosocial welfare.

- *Primary care liaison teams* epitomize the future integrated provision of mental health services based on the dissolution of rigid boundaries between agencies and artificial categories, such as *health* versus *social* needs. Primary care liaison teams should establish better partnership arrangements among social care agencies, mental health specialists and primary care staff; and enhanced mental health education and training for the latter. Teams can grow from pre-existing generic community mental health teams by professionals detaching from bases in specialist centres and moving fully into primary care situations or giving much more attention to inter-agency liaison.[31]

Such a comprehensive set of services reflects the logical implications of the 'stress–vulnerability' model of schizophrenia first propounded by Zubin and Spring.[32] Services should respond not only clinically to the individual who carries the diagnosis (i.e. to their *vulnerability*) but also preventatively by targeting resources and practical interventions at the very real social, economic and interpersonal *stressors* that can precipitate schizophrenic relapse in vulnerable individuals.

> **Reflection**
>
> How wide a range of care and treatment options are available within your area?
> How effective do you think these services are?

ANTI-PSYCHOTIC MEDICATION AND COMPLIANCE

Psychiatric treatment for people with schizophrenia almost always involves drug therapy to stabilize psychotic symptoms and reduce people's chances of relapse. Successful treatment should also improve people's ability to resume ordinary life and live independently; however, although current medication relieves some symptoms for many people, there remains a need for more effective, better-tolerated drugs. Some people avoid medication entirely, preferring their symptoms to side-effects; others try to manage their symptoms by flexible use of medication and other remedies, including dietary supplements.[12] Evidence of the prophylactic effectiveness of fish oil-based preparations is accumulating. These contain concentrated doses of two fatty acids that are essential for building and maintaining healthy brain tissue. Clinical trials of eicosapentaenoic and docosahexaenoic acids (EPA and DHA) are under way,[3] meanwhile many users are responding to anecdotal reports and adding the capsules to their shopping lists. Horrobin[10] provides a fascinating and full account of the significance of fatty acids in brain structure and function, and the evolution of schizophrenia.

Compliance – or informed choice?

The severe side-effects of anti-psychotic drugs discourage many individuals. Estimates of non-compliance vary, and professionals may often be quite mistaken in guessing how compliant people are;[33,34] surveys suggest up to 80 per cent of people fail to follow prescriptions.[35] Other reasons suggested for non-compliance include:[36]

- universal reluctance (detected by general physicians and others) for patients to adhere long term to medical prescriptions;
- poor therapeutic relationship; lack of trust, empathy, mutual respect, etc.;
- personal health beliefs that conflict with the illness models advanced by professionals;
- disagreements between patients and professionals about the predicted likelihood of relapse;
- recovered patients often recollect only slight or tolerable symptom severity and social handicap when unwell, whereas professionals dispute their evaluation.

Evidence suggests that people who avoid pharmaceutical treatment increase their risk of relapse; and subsequent hospitalization is extremely expensive relative to the cost of medication.[3] This has motivated professionals to develop effective systems of convincing people to take medication. Strategies vary, but generally emphasize:[37]

- the importance of maintaining good collaborative relationships;
- careful dosage titration and monitoring of medication;
- not trivializing people's reports of side-effects, and regular assessment of them, using tests such as Liverpool University Neuroleptic Side Effect Rating Scale (LUNSERS)[38];
- pragmatic, flexible, solution-focused approaches and compromise;
- shared exploration of health beliefs and resistances to treatment;

- objective evaluations of relapse risk and symptom severity;
- motivational interviewing techniques which help people to analyse the potential costs and benefits of specific decisions.

Depot preparations slowly release their active component over several days or weeks after intramuscular injection and represent another way of increasing compliance. People receiving such preparations require especial sensitivity and attention to their willing cooperation if they are not to relapse or become treatment drop-outs or service avoiders. The term 'compliance' has been challenged for perceived authoritarian connotations, and more collaborative language has been proposed:[39]

> Anyone faced with … serious mental health problems has … difficult decisions to make. Anyone in such a situation might value an ally who could help them … to come to decisions that are right for them … the person may then require assistance … to carry through their chosen course, and help to review their decision … in the light of events. But that is not *compliance*, rather *collaborative alliance*.
> **Perkins and Repper[40]**

Reflection

How much are the side-effects of anti-psychotic medication underestimated by clinicians?
How much are they overemphasized by patients?

Psychiatric medication for schizophrenia

The drugs used for schizophrenia are collectively described as *anti-psychotic* or *neuroleptic* and comprise a mixture of pharmacological subgroups, including the commonly distinguished *typical* and *atypical* anti-psychotics. This distinction is based upon the observation that many older drugs cause a *typical* range of side-effects, including especially movement disorders. In fact, the picture is more complicated. Although many newer drugs appear not to produce such severe side-effects, some older drugs were also *atypical*, and the newer drugs have their own emerging drawbacks. There is some equivocal evidence that the effects of standard anti-psychotic drugs may be enhanced by supplementing them with other medicines, particularly carbamazepine and beta-blockers.[3]

It is difficult to establish the truth about the relative merits and demerits of psychiatric drugs for various reasons. Experimental trials vary in their methodology and may use incompatible, bafflingly complex or obscure statistical analyses. They often feature patients, treatment outcomes or prescription schedules that match awkwardly with everyday clinical practice. Comparisons are not always made with realistic or relevant alternative treatment regimes. Most trials are funded by organizations that have specific financial or political interests in the outcome. Drop-out rates are often very high, making final results difficult to interpret. Publication and reporting biases may make less favourable or more critical findings difficult to access. Even relatively uncontroversial findings of effectiveness cannot guarantee that a specific medication will be efficacious for any one individual patient.[3]

Typical anti-psychotics

Haloperidol and chlorpromazine are among the most common classic anti-psychotics. They seem both more effective and more harmful than placebo in reducing positive symptoms, but not significantly different from each other in overall effect. Some, for example flupentixol, fluspirilene and haloperidol, are available as long-lasting 'depot' injections. Despite manufacturers' claims and counter-claims, there seems little convincing evidence that any one preparation is generally more efficacious than another.[3]

Sedation often occurs early in treatment, frequently accompanied by a vague, dream-like sense of oddness and anxiety. Dose reduction, drug switching or night-time single-dose administration may help people adjust to these effects.

Dry mouth, blurred vision, flushing, urinary retention, constipation, ejaculatory inhibition and impotence result from a specific neurochemical characteristic shared by many psycho-pharmacological agents. Dizziness and unsteadiness can result from lowered blood pressure. If people persist with the medicine, these effects often diminish and become more tolerable, but, for many others, the effects constitute the insufferable last straws that lead to non-compliance. Unfortunately, many professionals construe these as minor irritations that should be endured for the greater good of fewer psychotic symptoms.[41]

Movement disorders are perhaps the most distressing neuroleptic side-effects. Termed *extrapyramidal* effects, after the neuronal tract that generates them, these variously affect many patients and include:

- generalized muscle spasms and stiffness (*dyskinesia*, *dystonia*);
- muscle spasms in the head and neck that may be accompanied by rolling of the eyeballs (*torticollis, oculogyric crises*);
- a syndrome resembling Parkinson's disease – limb rigidity, tremor, expressionless face and shuffling gait (*parkinsonism*);
- restlessness and agitated movements, accompanied by an inner sense of unease and urgency – often misconstrued by professionals as symptomatic worsening requiring increased medication (*akathisia*).

Extrapyramidal effects are generally treated by anti-muscarinic drugs such as orphenadrine or procyclidine that can be given orally (or intramuscularly in emergencies), but these may cause an increase in dry mouth, etc. The anti-muscarinics are less effective against akathisia, which responds best to dose reduction or drug switching.

The most severe and distressing movement disorder is *tardive dyskinesia*. This consists of repetitive, involuntary movements of the face, tongue and neck muscles and sometimes of the arms and legs. People feel unable to control their lip smacking, tongue protrusion, chewing, blowing and sucking movements. They cross and uncross their legs, flap their hands or march on the spot. Tardive dyskinesia develops most commonly in people over 40 who have been on typical anti-psychotics for 3 months or more. It is usually irreversible, even when anti-psychotics are discontinued. Paradoxically, withdrawing established neuroleptics may even worsen the side-effect. Switching to one of the newer atypicals may be the only available pharmacological course of action.[3]

The movement abnormalities caused by extrapyramidal side-effects are difficult to endure. As well as being distressing, uncomfortable and often painful, they are also a source of stigma, being highly visible, and are commonly portrayed as an aspect of madness or a sign of disease, rather than a consequence of treatment. It is difficult for people to rehabilitate themselves after a breakdown and integrate successfully into work and community when they feel so uncomfortable and can readily convince themselves that they are as odd as they may look to others. Users' groups report that alternative self-help remedies to these problems include the recreational drug cannabis and dietary supplements such as vitamin E and vitamin B6. Evidence for these treatments remains both controversial and largely anecdotal.

Interference with metabolism of the hormone prolactin causes other distressing and embarrassing side-effects such as menstrual difficulties, breast enlargement and milk production in women, or impotence and breast enlargement in men. These effects generally respond to either dose reduction or neuroleptic discontinuation and replacement with another atypical preparation. Some anti-psychotics (especially chlorpromazine) also affect people's skins, causing sunburn and sensitivity to sunlight, pigment changes, rashes and granular deposits in the cornea. Patients should avoid sunbathing and use blocking lotions. Medication in liquid form should be handled carefully. Skin effects usually disappear after stopping treatment.

Blood disorders leading to loss of white cells (*agranulocytosis*) and susceptibility to serious infection are rare but important side-effects. Blood counts help to monitor this possibility, but nurses should be alert to signs of infection, such as sore throats and general discomfort. Body temperature is an unreliable indicator, as anti-psychotics can lower it. If serious infection is suspected, medication should be stopped. *Neuroleptic malignant syndrome* manifests by sudden onset of muscle stiffness and worsened extrapyramidal symptoms, accompanied by a fast pulse, high, low or variable blood pressure and a very high temperature. The individual may seem drowsy and be drooling or delirious, or may become very frightened and agitated. Medication should be stopped immediately and urgent medical aid summoned because the condition is potentially fatal (in 20 per cent of cases), owing to possible failure of the heart, kidney or respiratory functions. Rest and rehydration are the first priorities if there is any delay in admission to an emergency treatment facility. Thankfully, the condition is extremely rare.

Atypical anti-psychotics

Atypical anti-psychotics include clozapine, risperidone, olanzapine and quetiapine. Others are actively being produced but have either yet to complete laboratory and clinical trials (e.g. zotepine, aripiprazole) or have given grounds for concern after initially enthusiastic claims for their safety and effectiveness (e.g. sertindole, ziprasidone). Side-effects, especially extrapyramidal movement disorders, are supposedly much milder than typical antipsychotics, but these drugs are generally more expensive, leading to ambivalent prescribing policies.[3] The most commonly prescribed atypicals are clozapine, risperidone and olanzapine. Clozapine is particularly effective in people who have failed to respond to other neuroleptics, but because it can cause *agranulocytosis*, clozapine is often regarded as a last resort. Prescription must always be accompanied by stringent blood monitoring.

Many clinicians recommend that atypicals (except clozapine) should be given to people when first diagnosed, not only because of any increased efficacy but also because fewer, less severe side-effects would increase compliance. This would reduce the risks of relapse and subsequent expensive residential or intensive community treatment. Others disagree, claiming that atypical antipsychotics are not significantly different from conventional neuroleptics in either their efficacy or their side-effects. The most balanced view seems to be that atypicals represent a refinement of available treatments for schizophrenia, but not a revolution.[3] In the UK, prescribing guidelines from the National Institute for Health and Clinical Excellence should clarify this issue. Further research and development will continue, and the latest drug to be announced, aripiprazole, has a different more subtle mode of action than its predecessors, stimulating renewed excitement among both professionals and patients.

Atypical anti-psychotics seem less severe than the older neuroleptics, but are not entirely free of side-effects. Some, including clozapine, may lower the epileptic threshold, causing seizures in vulnerable individuals. People may prefer to take preventative anticonvulsants if continued anti-psychotic medication is advised. As clinical experience of these drugs grows, evidence of possible heart effects such as myocarditis is accumulating and causing concern. Diabetes is both a complicating factor (especially with olanzapine) and a possible side-effect. Weight gain is an obvious side-effect of atypicals as well as earlier neuroleptics. It may be due to metabolic changes, but it could also be secondary to either increased well-being and appetite, or decreased activity due to sedation and drug-induced lethargy. Either way, weight gain has knock-on psychological and physical health problems, including lower self-esteem, tiredness, cardiovascular disease and an increased risk of diabetes. In common with such effects as reduced sexual desire and breast enlargement, weight gain can be extremely upsetting and make people reluctant to continue with medication.

> ### Reflection
>
> How free should people be to refuse medication if they feel disabled by it?

PSYCHOSOCIAL INTERVENTIONS FOR SCHIZOPHRENIA

Psychiatric treatment has traditionally focused on the neurobiological nature of schizophrenia. Developmental, interpersonal and social facets have received relatively less attention in devising clinical responses, despite featuring strongly in research. Users, however, have repeatedly asserted the value of various psychosocial interventions, often from nurses, who spend large amounts of time in social contact with those who are diagnosed with schizophrenia, or from clinical psychologists, whose therapeutic orientation differs from medically trained psychiatrists.[42,43] Comprehensive care for schizophrenia comprises a holistic package which should include cognitive–behavioural therapy, family interventions, supportive education and life, social and vocational skills training.[44] Many of these interventions have been incorporated into the Thorn[45] and Psychosocial Interventions (PSI)[46] training courses, and should be integrated into basic mental health nurse education programmes.

Psychosocial help is usually offered in conjunction with medication, although some individuals prefer social support and psychological therapies as mainstay alternatives to drug treatment, either throughout their care or during their less disturbed periods.[12] Psychiatrists usually consider the clinical and social risks too high to base care upon non-pharmaceutical treatments, although some professionals believe they offer effective alternatives to drug-based treatment for many users. Therapeutic community, psychodynamic and other non-pharmaceutical approaches have reportedly helped people with their schizophrenic symptoms, but, although these approaches continue to develop,[47–50] psychiatrists generally consider them to be insufficiently evidenced and therefore unsound as sole foundations for clinical treatment.

APPLIED COGNITIVE–BEHAVIOURAL THERAPY

Cognitive–behavioural therapy (CBT), like some psychodynamic formulations, emphasizes the meanings that experiences have for individuals, and the consequences of their subsequent behavioural responses. CBT helps people become aware of connections made unconsciously between experiences, patterns of thinking and subsequent feelings and behaviour. Therapist and client collaborate to explore the meanings that individuals attribute to events. They examine the evidence for and against specific beliefs, meanings or attributions; devise challenges to habitual patterns of thinking and reacting; and employ logical reasoning and other, neglected, personal experiences to develop more rational and effective alternative responses. CBT is effective when expertly applied to symptoms of schizophrenia,[12,51] but could become more valuable if its principles could be absorbed, generalized and applied by nurses in everyday working situations. Individuals should benefit from working within CBT milieux, where supportive reality testing and modification of symptoms could occur early in someone's breakdown process, before pathology becomes deep rooted, chronic or confrontationally defended.[52]

For such therapeutic environments to become effective, staff should revise residual, traditional psychiatric thinking about psychotic symptoms. Delusions and hallucinations have traditionally been understood as simply abnormal phenomena, which are either present or absent and vary significantly in only one dimension – severity. Nurses intending to engage people in therapeutic conversation need to regard delusions and hallucinations as multidimensional. Delusions vary in intensity of conviction; degree of preoccupation; nature and depth of distress caused; and their motivational power.[53] They are not fixed, but alter with new experiences and collaborative analysis of evidence or logical basis. Hallucinations similarly vary in intensity, frequency, abusiveness and controllability.[54] The emotions of those with schizophrenia are not merely flattened; rather, their symptoms are often accompanied by significant emotion that can be empathically engaged. Hallucinatory and delusional content or themes can have both direct and metaphorical meaning derived from people's often long-neglected experiences. Nurses should not regard psychotic symptoms as simply meaningless pathologies, thereby running the risk of invalidating individuals' experiences and provoking

further alienation. Delusions and hallucinations can be meaningfully construed as complex psychological phenomena actively generated from the interaction of people's personalities with past and current experience.

Nurses working from this perspective can suggest normalizing rationales for psychotic symptoms, whereby people's pathological experiences and behaviours are interpreted as valid expressions of their vulnerability. Nurses have been enjoined to make more use of formal assessment measures[55] and many are now available.[45] Semi-structured interview formats [e.g. the Krawiecka, Goldberg and Vaughan (KGV) scale,[28] comprising detailed questions about every aspect of schizophrenia] enable closer, more attentive conversations about individual's personal experiences of illness. *Time–life diagrams* are simple parallel line diagrams that encourage people to reminisce about ordinary life events occurring along a narrative thread of well-being, often discarded in favour of preoccupation with illness events and a life story based upon treatment. Collaboratively devising time–life diagrams helps people to unpick the rich nonclinical threads of their experiences and re-stitch their narrative tapestry to incorporate less pathologically pessimistic possibilities. *Externalizing questions* explore the impact of illness as an outside intruder into personal life. They can help people to detach from preoccupation with internal defectiveness and devise coping strategies that deal more effectively with the intrusion of schizophrenia into their lives.[56]

Meta-representation

The clinical and academic discipline of cognitive neuropsychology attempts to integrate psychological and biological explanations of behaviour by developing insights into how electrochemical, hard-wired brain processes mediate mental phenomena such as thoughts and feelings, and how these intangible phenomena are behaviourally operationalized. One such explanation is that the failure of a neurocognitive function called *meta-representation* causes schizophrenic cognitive pathology.[57] Meta-representation underlies two other important cognitive functions: *theory of mind* and *self-monitoring*. Humans develop both faculties while wiring-up our plastic brains during the primary attachment phase of infancy.[58]

Theory of mind refers firstly to the realization that other people have minds too, but that they may well be different from our own. Secondly, it refers to our ability to form theories about other people's minds: to create accurate impressions of others' intentions or feelings; to make sense of their actions and communications; and to successfully predict or anticipate their behaviour. Effective communication and social activity require shared implicit understanding that others have thoughts, feelings and intentions similar or dissimilar to our own; that their behaviour is governed by discernible motives;

and that attentive interpersonal observation provides reliable clues to others' states of mind. Schizophrenics often report or display difficulty with these abilities.

Self-monitoring is an essential function for conscious intention and regulated action. The brain requires continuous feedback about thoughts or intentions in order to successfully maintain cognitive processes or actions until their purpose is accomplished. We need to remind ourselves whether the thought we are generating is a memory, wish, hope, plan or fantasy. Without such self-monitoring we would 'forget' that we are imagining, pretending, fearing or hoping that something is the case (e.g. 'I'm *pretending* that I'm rich' or 'I'm *afraid* he won't like me' or '*What if* the fire alarm is a bugging device?') and believe it to be so: 'I'm rich, he doesn't like me and the fire alarm is a bug!'

Meta-representation is the means by which the brain continuously checks the context for each representation of reality or intention. During cognition and action, meta-representation 'remembers' our purposes and intentions, our self-monitoring and our reading of others' minds. In its absence, we would not only fail to 'know our own minds' but we would also 'forget' that we are thinking about something that someone else said or thinks, and feel confused as to how we find ourselves thinking about such stuff at all. The hypothetical mechanism has been tentatively mapped onto known brain organization, and could help to construct intervention strategies for specific cognitive and communication anomalies.

> ## Reflection
>
> How confident do you feel about using everyday interactions to apply cognitive and psychosocial therapeutic interventions? Do you think nurses should perform this role? If not, why not?

WORKING FROM FAMILY PERSPECTIVES

The relationship between schizophrenia and family life has been contentiously debated for decades, and the various controversies are far too complex to be dealt with here. Two broadly different approaches to working with families exist – family therapy and family management – and, although both claim effectiveness, one (family management) dominates conventional psychiatric practice.[59] Family therapists, frequently from non-psychiatric backgrounds, base their interventions upon a theoretical proposition – that families function as complex organic social systems – and an assessed judgement – that some aspects of a family's organization are less than optimally effective and are disabling its functional capabilities. This dysfunction creates internal stress which has the largest effect on the most vulnerable individual or role within the family, and causes breakdown. Changes made to functional subsystems such as problem-solving, communication, family roles, affective responsiveness, affective involvement and behaviour control can enable the whole family to cope better with internal stress or external pressures and ease the strain on individuals.[60] Family management practitioners adopt similar rationales, but emphasize that schizophrenia is a serious organic disease which engenders a shared need for education and support to cope with the consequences of diagnosis. However, even family management interventions remain underused, despite evidence of their effectiveness.[44]

Professional interventions into the normally private environment of family life are usually justified in one of two interrelated ways:

- family members are stressed by burdens, e.g. caring for an unwell member, or economic distress and need support to manage responsibilities, resolve concerns or prevent further functional deterioration;
- the family system itself does not operate as effectively as it might, and consequently individual members are subjected to stressful interactive processes that can be eased by changes in family functions and relationships.

Families with a schizophrenic member experience considerable stress. There is often pain and puzzlement about their vulnerable relative's behaviour and obvious distress; grief over lost hopes and fear for future possibilities; anger and guilt about recrimination and self-blame. Equally, people with schizophrenia often experience aspects of family life as stressful, and relapse more often and more severely when there is an intense atmosphere of criticism, hostility or emotional overinvolvement. These behaviours can be measured to assess a family's quotient of *expressed emotion*, and it has been established that high expressed emotion environments constitute serious stress for individuals vulnerable to a range of physical and psychological disorders, including schizophrenia. Research suggests that reducing the intensity and frequency of high expressed emotion as a precipitating stressor helps, as also does limiting the time spent in overall interaction.[11]

The proposition that defective interpersonal family functioning prior to the onset of symptoms may precipitate initial conversion to active schizophrenia has been hotly disputed.[2] It remains a matter of contention[61] and has historically fuelled the development of some forms of family therapy.[59] Most family interventions for schizophrenia, however, are based upon relatives' needs for support with their caring responsibilities, or aim to reduce stressful interactions so that the diagnosed individual relapses less and the welfare of other family members is not so compromised.[62]

Potentially effective interventions derived from various schools of thought and practice include:

- education about schizophrenia: symptoms, vulnerability and stressors;

- facilitating discussions about each other's perspectives on specific problems and favoured solutions;
- validating and positively reframing family members' intentions and behaviours;
- support for family members' efforts to tolerate and appreciate individual differences and interpersonal boundaries;
- recognizing and finding ways of increasing the frequency of effective interpersonal behaviours;
- identifying and reducing the frequency and intensity of excessive emotional resonance, critical comments and hostile reactions;
- training and support in problem-solving strategies;
- reinforcing clear, direct communication and reducing less transparent, more evasive or ambivalent messages;
- clarifying expectations about roles, responsibilities and personal accountability;
- helping to adjust expectations of each other's behaviours to attainable standards;
- encouraging interaction between estranged or uncommunicative members;
- supportive collaboration with caring relatives, especially in acute crises;
- modified bereavement counselling for (especially parents') grief-like reactions to loss of idealized expectations for their child;
- planned respite and recuperative activity for all vulnerable members, both patient and carers;
- structuring activities and rationing time spent together.

Schizophrenia affects not only the individual but also family, friends, colleagues, neighbours and even wider social networks. Emotional reactions such as grief, anger, shame and fear are common, as are unhelpful responses such as rejection or infantilization. All may respond to supportive interventions, and family-based approaches are relevant to whatever social matrix is involved.[63]

Reflection

What communication difficulties have existed between you and your parents or children?

How did they arise?

How would you feel about your family relationships being investigated by outside professionals?

SOCIAL, VOCATIONAL AND LIFE SKILLS

Because of its impact on cognitive and communication processes, schizophrenia often disables people's abilities to conduct effective interpersonal relationships and to perform ordinary domestic or vocational tasks. Preoccupation with internal mental states; memory and attention difficulties; and the cumulative effect of negative symptoms and neuroleptic-induced deficits complicate everyday interactions. After several years of breakdown, withdrawal, treatment and relapse, people may lose technical skills and social abilities they once took for granted. If severely affected at adolescence, some individuals may never have acquired the social confidence and practical skills necessary to survive independently. Skills training programmes use a variety of techniques, including role play, video-recording and behaviour modification, and can be classified into three types.[44]

- *Life skills, or daily living programmes*, provide group or individual training in ordinary social survival and include teaching and supervised practice in financial management and budgeting; personal self-care; domestic skills such as cooking and cleaning; shopping and allied consumer skills such as complaining; civic skills such as voting.
- *Social skills training* aims to enhance people's abilities to perform well in social and interactive relationships. Training includes assessment of trainees' interpersonal skill deficits and excesses (i.e. not looking at people or staring too intently; speaking too loudly, quietly or monotonously); analysis of how well people pick up and cognitively process interpersonal cues; and graded practice of specific verbal and non-verbal communication skills.
- *Vocational skills* are needed to obtain and retain employment. Specific skills for particular jobs need to be learnt, but also people sometimes need help with their orientation towards work and fundamental issues such as time-keeping, rule-observance, taking orders, etc. Many services have developed their own supported employment programmes or industrial therapy units where sensitive support and training can be provided. Ultimately, the aim should be for people to be as fully integrated as possible into ordinary working life.

Skills training programmes offer nurses the opportunity to work closely not only with users but also with occupational therapists, whose professional preparation includes intensive experience of skills development techniques. However, skills training may be more effective when integrated into everyday life in supportive residential, outreach or daycare services. Benefits from formal training sessions alone may not endure long outside, or may generalize poorly into ordinary situations.[64]

PHYSICAL ILLNESS AND HEALTH PROMOTION

An unfortunate percentage of individuals go on to develop chronically relapsing or deteriorating forms of schizophrenia. Their needs for nursing care shift as negative symptoms dominate their clinical profile, and increasingly inactive or impoverished life-styles begin to take their toll. Mortality from all causes is higher in the psychiatric population than in the general public. Even when figures for suicide and accidents are excluded, the severely mentally ill population has an excessively high death rate. Long-term schizophrenia puts people in increased jeopardy from cardiovascular conditions, respiratory problems, infectious diseases and endocrine disorders.[65] Iatrogenic illness from cardiovascular, metabolic and endocrine side-effects of neuroleptics may explain some of these discrepancies. Life-style causes (which may also be secondary to neuroleptic-induced deficits) include increased tobacco use, reduced exercise and poor diet. People may also use street drugs or drink alcohol excessively. In addition, primary care and mental health professionals often fail to assess, recognize or treat physical illness in psychiatric patients. They may wrongly attribute reported symptoms to psychological causes, and interpret patients' physical problems as aspects of psychiatric illness. Some primary care professionals may be unfamiliar with, and feel uncomfortable dealing with, psychiatric patients. Patients may themselves not communicate their difficulties to professionals, through social skill deficiencies, fear of stigmatization, embarrassment or because of the effects of delusional beliefs, high anxiety, etc.

The UK Department of Health now requires primary care services to monitor the physical health of people with schizophrenia and provide effective health care. Patients should at least receive annual medical checks of blood pressure and urinalysis, be vaccinated against influenza and have help to reduce smoking.[66] Strategic interventions by mental health services include:

- liaison with accommodation, employment and benefit agencies
- regular meetings between primary health care and specialist mental health teams
- effective integration of health and social care agencies
- greater involvement of patients or their advocates in health and social care decisions.

Mental health nurses and social care staff in whatever setting should ensure that they collaborate with long-term patients and liaise with physicians to focus on physical health as well as on psychological and social welfare. Within therapeutic alliances, or as part of assertive outreach, nurses could help individuals to:

- enjoy more exercise and stimulating recreational life-styles
- maintain healthy accommodation and hygienic living standards
- limit the amount they smoke
- avoid excess alcohol and drug use
- eat well, as personal taste and finances allow
- monitor any damaging side-effects from medication.

Nurses' physical health promotion work should be characterized by the same empathic attitudes that prevent them becoming high-expressed emotion carers in relation to people's psychosocial needs. If nurses strive too zealously to manipulate, persuade or coerce people into pure, healthy life-styles, they run the risk of being experienced as health fascists. Individuals may feel misunderstood or threatened and label their supposed helpers as the enemy, as do-gooding types with little knowledge or understanding of alienation, isolation or poverty, or as uncaring, punitive strait-laced or interfering critics. People are more likely to value their own health and well-being if nurses validate them as adult personalities with the right to some peccadilloes and even venial sins. The keynotes should be harm limitation and a 'motivational interviewing' emphasis on the benefits of feeling more lively, being comfortable, eating well and having some spending money not earmarked for the next day's nicotine.

THERAPEUTIC RELATIONSHIPS WITH SCHIZOPHRENIC PEOPLE

Although treatment schedules and care plans consisting of various combinations of technical interventions are potentially clinically effective, they do not help nurses and patients to determine how best to establish and maintain trusting relationships, nor how to communicate positively with each other. One of the earlier accounts in the modern era of nursing people with schizophrenia contains some retrospectively interesting advice:

> We need careful re-thinking about our nursing methods; and about nurses' attitudes; and any tendency to institutionalised reactions; for such reactions are far more common than one would imagine, and inevitably the patient suffers. I can remember early on in my psychiatric training, I was playing a card game with a schizophrenic patient and endeavouring to make light conversation with her. She rarely spoke, but after an hour she put down her cards and said wonderingly 'You treat me as if I were normal.' I shall never forget the look on that patient's face as she said this. I believe it sums up what should be our attitude at all times to those suffering from schizophrenia.[67]

Nearly 30 years later, this quotation may seem quaintly platitudinous, but it also innocently throws into relief some recent criticisms of psychiatric services. The poem quoted at the beginning of this chapter expresses similar sentiments. One unintended consequence of nurses becoming increasingly associated with the psychiatric treatment of the biological bases of schizophrenia, rather than collaborative allies and advocates, is the risk of people feeling objectified or 'othered'.[68] 'Othering' attitudes can be benign, albeit infantilizing or dependence inducing, as well as malign, perverse or degenerate. An attitude of superior difference can be conveyed paralinguistically by tone of voice; by using technical, managerial or authoritarian language; by being purposely unclear and indirect in everyday or formal interactions; and by invalidating in various other ways, such as closed office doors, non-collaborative care, imposition of rules and strictures, thoughtlessly worded signs, casual unexplained use of psychiatric or legalistic jargon, and thinking, however unconsciously and however people may behave, that patients with schizophrenia are child-like, dull, dangerous or incomprehensible.

There are many ways in which staff can become unhelpful in their relationships with patients with schizophrenia. Patients can be puzzled, frustrated or dismayed by unclear, indirect, ambivalent, ambiguous or disguised communications. People who experience schizophrenic symptoms often speak and behave in apparently incomprehensible or simply unusual or challenging ways. When nurses or others respond in patronizing, dismissive, authoritarian or otherwise invalidating fashions, patients naturally feel even more confused, disturbed, distressed or angry.

The noxious effect of high expressed emotion within family life is replicated in studies of staff cultures. Criticism, hostility and emotional overinvolvement are just as potent precipitators of illness when portrayed by staff as they are when performed within the closer bounds of family life. Emotional overinvolvement in this context does not mean caring about, but rather uncontrolled emotional resonance – of whatever hue – in staffs' responses to patients' behaviours. If professionals are not to create a psychonoxious, non-therapeutic environment then individual therapeutic supervision and team support and sensitivity meetings are essential adjuncts to collaborative care planning.[14]

In reaction to the unhelpful impact of what they perceive as uncomprehending, uncaring or hostile attitudes within professional service organizations, patients and carers have recently developed self-help and user-led alternatives, such as crisis houses, drop-in centres and hearing voices groups. These less medically driven, non-prescriptive and more democratic resources are judged by many individuals to match their needs more sensitively and have led to many professionals adopting similar attitudes and strategies as traditional services are evaluated and improved to accommodate users' and carers' expressed wishes.[69]

Nurses should engage fully with the ordinariness (however unexceptional or extraordinary) of people diagnosed as schizophrenic, as well as be interested in or sympathetic to them as sufferers from clinical illness. Thus, care plans should take account of the importance of enjoying the company of persons diagnosed as schizophrenic; initiating and holding normal conversations; and sharing recreational, purposeful social activities. Nurses should be warm, empathic and positive. They should be fascinated companions, supportively encouraging people to clarify and make constructive sense of their experiences.

However, the diagnosis of schizophrenia often entails a fragile sense of self. People develop vulnerable identities, with weakness and potential erosion of normally secure personal boundaries.[70] Individuals are exposed to potential flooding by or fusion with their sociocultural environments. People, objects, events, ideas or emotions from outside can invasively pollute highly susceptible inner selves. In developing companionable relationships, nurses need to be aware of this heightened sensitivity. Feeling constantly under threat, many people with schizophrenia develop exquisitely delicate sensory antennae, and become subliminally aware of minute stimuli and implicit messages normally masked behind disguised verbal communication. This perception of an invasive, inexplicable and uncontrollable outside world leads not only to high anxiety and social withdrawal but also to mistrust of outside influences and uneasiness about social intercourse.[70] Thus, nurses' fascination and warmth should not only be genuine but it should also be carefully modulated. Watzlawick *et al.*[71,72] suggested 'the meaning of any communication is the response you get'. When in therapeutic interaction with people, nurses should carefully notice their companions' reactions, and engage no more closely than they seem ready to tolerate. There may be no intention to invade, invalidate or otherwise abuse. Nevertheless, because of differences in sensitivity and reliability of schizophrenic 'theory of mind' compared with most non-schizophrenic clinical staff, empathy will not be easily accurate. Basically, if people seem hurt by your communication, think of it as a hurtful communication; if they seem pleased, then score it as pleasant.

Because of anxiety and difficulties in controlling sensory input, people diagnosed as schizophrenic are potentially vulnerable to invasive intrusion from aspects of 'the outside world'. This vulnerability complicates their more ordinary needs for social communion and companionship. The conflict exposes patients to twin fears: of alternately being engulfed by overintimate outsiders, or disregarded and abandoned in isolation.[73] Nurses need to constantly monitor people's behavioural and emotional responses to maintain the most helpful, least threatening social distance. Interacting through shared activity may help to counteract relationship and communication difficulties. Incorporating a third point into the relationship, such as a physical activity, chore or creative project, helps triangulate or neutralize the struggle to achieve unthreatening empathy and engagement. Apart from the simple fact that people appreciate nurses' practical assistance and interested involvement,[74] painting and sculpture,[75] cooking, repairs, maintenance, gardening and other ordinary activities of everyday life offer unemotional absorption and neutral escape from interpersonal tension.[76,77]

What feelings do you have when trying to understand the inner worlds of people diagnosed as schizophrenic?

How easy or difficult is it for you to empathize with them, as distinct from feeling pity or sympathy?

CONTEMPORARY CONTROVERSIES AND DEVELOPMENTS

As noted at the outset, the concept of 'schizophrenia' is used, worldwide, to describe a complex and increasingly contested set of human problems. The British mental health nursing academic Liam Clarke[78] recently raised again some of the key issues regarding the validity of the diagnosis of schizophrenia, which Thomas Szasz[79] long ago described as the 'sacred symbol of psychiatry'. Addressing 'contemporary discussions' about 'schizophrenia' and other 'mental illnesses', Clarke discussed schizophrenia's 'capacity to induce cyclical psychological misery – at rates of 1 per cent in any population, worldwide'.[78]

Although it is correct to say that similar numbers of people, worldwide, are diagnosed for the first time with schizophrenia, not all of these people experience '*cyclical psychological misery*', with repeated 'breakdowns' and the need for psychiatric treatment. The study[80] carried out by the World Health Organization (WHO) of schizophrenia across 10 countries reported recovery rates of 63 per cent in 'developing countries' (i.e. *poor* and *disadvantaged*), compared with 39 per cent in the affluent Western nations. The WHO researchers concluded that living in a developed country was a 'strong predictor' that a patient with schizophrenia would *never* recover.[80] The most parsimonious explanation for this anomaly is that, in developing countries, less than 16 per cent of 'patients are maintained on neuroleptic drugs, compared with almost 60 per cent in the West'.[81] In short, there is more chance of recovering from 'schizophrenia' if one lives in a poor, underdeveloped country than if one lives in the USA or Europe, where the person has more chance of becoming a 'long term, chronic patient'.

It has long been believed that the introduction of antipsychotic drugs in the 1950s revolutionized the treatment of people with a diagnosis of schizophrenia. Indeed, much contemporary legislation is focused on ensuring that people take medication, even against their wishes. The 'need' to take medication in the long term is often found in advice written expressly for families, whose members are warned about the risk of 'loss of insight' where

they [the 'patient'] may also think that when their symptoms have been reduced or temporarily eliminated they won't need to take medication any more.
Mueser and Gingerich[82]

However, Hegarty[83] pointed out that the popular faith in medication was misplaced. Outcomes for people diagnosed with 'schizophrenia' are actually worse *now* than before neuroleptic drugs were introduced. The WHO study also corroborated the long-term follow-up carried out by Harding[84] of people discharged from hospital in the 1950s. Harding found that the group of people who recovered completely from schizophrenia had *all* weaned themselves off their neuroleptic medication, *not* kept on taking it. Harding[84] commented that this showed the popular notion that people with a diagnosis of schizophrenia needed to remain on medication *all of their lives* was a 'myth'.

These findings resonate with the WHO international study. In the absence of 'high-technology' and highly fraudulent medical explanations for their problems in living, people in poor countries probably get personal or social help to deal with their problems. In many instances, they remain embedded within the family unit or community. In affluent 'Western' countries, the 'patient' is invariably marginalized and ostracized, often forcibly injected with toxic chemicals, and 'taught' how to live a limited life, through some programme of 'psychoeducation'.[85]

Despite the growing influence of neuroscience in schizophrenia research, a competing body of evidence points to the possible influence of psychological factors on the development of the symptoms of schizophrenia. Morrison *et al.*[86] edited a series of papers that illuminated the *personal* and *social* factors, especially in early life, which appeared to be related to problems commonly diagnosed as 'psychosis'. They described at least two-thirds of people with a 'psychotic' diagnosis (such as 'schizophrenia') having experienced physical or sexual abuse. In a related book, Read *et al.*[87] brought together a range of international authors, who provided empirical evidence to show that, contrary to popular medical 'myth', hallucinations and delusions are understandable reactions to life events and circumstances, rather than symptoms of a supposed genetic predisposition or biological disturbance.

According to Morrison *et al.*,[86] the public also recognizes the importance of these 'psychosocial' factors. In almost every country where surveys have been conducted, the *public* believes the causes of psychosis are more likely to be adverse psychosocial events and circumstances (such as poverty, trauma and abuse) than biogenetic factors. Contrary to the view that schizophrenia 'originates' in brain pathology, the emerging evidence suggests that some people have such led such an awful life that they develop 'strange' ways of relating to themselves and others, as a means of coping with that life. For Morrison *et al.*,[86] the picture was clear: 'psychotic experiences are essentially normal phenomena'. These states may be 'strange', but they are not 'abnormal' and they certainly *cannot* be properly described as forms of illness.

However, some senior mental health nursing academics continue to value the 'disease concept (as) a useful

Personal illustration 25.1

Jim Limber was a middle-aged Irishman who was diagnosed as paranoid schizophrenic and formally detained in a psychiatric hospital after frequent attacks on strangers while he was working as a labourer. Jim claimed they were homosexuals who had stolen his ideas and money, and also intended to abuse him. Jim knew that he'd invented rocket propulsion, hovercraft and jet engines, among other things, but a conspiracy of homosexual men removed his brilliant ideas before he could patent them, and stored the profit in a docklands warehouse. Wandering around after a hard night's drinking, he'd seen the golden glow from his treasure gleaming through the pre-dawn mist.

One day a nurse suggested that Jim get involved in preparing the small garden being rehabilitated outside the ward. Once outside, Jim started furiously digging over a flowerbed. 'That'll be a well-prepared bit of soil! What would you like to plant there, Jim?' 'Pansies!' Jim grinned as he replied. 'Forgive and forget, eh Jim?' thought the nurse, and dared to share the joke. 'I wish I could.' Jim responded. 'Well, I suppose there's lots you'd like to forget,' replied the nurse, 'but then there's a lot we don't remember – like when we're small.' 'I remember Ireland, and the smoke of peat.'

For the rest of the morning, Jim told whimsical stories about childhood – poverty, drunkenness, abuse and a deep sense of nostalgia. 'It's strange, Jim. There's so much difference between life as it was, and the life you feel you should have been entitled to.' 'Strange to miss so much misery – there's no point getting nowhere I suppose,' Jim mused quietly, and there was no hint of madness in his conversation from then on, but there was a very well dug-over garden.

way of thinking about schizophrenia and its causation',[88] arguing that 'while it is true that the early promise of finding a single gene responsible for [schizophrenia and major affective disorders] will most likely never materialise, biological research, year on year, produces vast amounts of evidence to demonstrate biological underpinnings.'[89] Clearly, a huge gulf exists between the biological and 'psychosocial' theorists that seem unlikely ever to be bridged.

Biological research into the possible causes and treatment of schizophrenia is supported by massive government and pharmaceutical company funding, endowing this field of enquiry with considerable power and authority. Many families and people with a diagnosis of schizophrenia would be delighted to be told, *finally*, that this disorder, which has so upset their lives, is not only caused by some biological or genetic 'fault' but can also be remedied merely by taking some tablets.

The alternative perspective is that the 'symptoms of schizophrenia' are only the latest chapter in a complex life story, involving emotional and/or sexual abuse and damaged interpersonal and social relationships, with a resultant distorted way of 'being in the world'. This alternative perspective signals a call for action – on the part of both the individual 'sufferer' and the 'significant others' – to begin to 'do' something to make a change for the better. This perspective offers hope of recovery, but little comfort, since the route is likely to be complex and demanding.

It seems unlikely that it will ever be possible to 'prove' definitively which of these hypotheses on the 'cause' of schizophrenia is 'right' or 'best'. Time will tell, however, which of these perspectives is adopted most widely, and people – professionals, individual 'sufferers' and families – will give their own reasons for their choice.

REFERENCES

1. Limber J. One of many poems written by a man diagnosed with paranoid schizophrenia, who lived for several years on a 72-bedded locked ward.

2. Keen T. Schizophrenia: orthodoxy and heresies: a review of some alternative perspectives. *Journal of Psychiatric and Mental Health Nursing* 1999; **6** (6): 415–24.

3. NHS Centre for Reviews and Dissemination. Drug treatments for schizophrenia. *Effective Health Care* 1999; **5** (6): 1–12.

4. Frangou S, Murray RM. *Schizophrenia*, 2nd edn. London, UK: Martin Dunitz, 2000.

5. American Psychiatric Association. *Diagnostic and statistical manual of mental disorders, 4th edition, text revision.* Washington, DC: American Psychiatric Press, 2000 (DSM IV-TR).

6. World Health Organization (WHO). *ICD-10 classification of mental and behavioural disorders: clinical conditions and diagnostic guidelines.* Geneva, Switzerland: WHO, 1992.

7 Thomas P. *The dialectics of schizophrenia.* London, UK: Free Association Books, 1997.

8. Nettle D. *Strong imagination: madness, creativity and human nature.* Oxford, UK: Oxford University Press, 2001.

9. Bannister D, Fransella F. *Inquiring man*, 2nd edn. Harmondsworth, UK: Penguin, 1980.

10. Horrobin D. *The madness of Adam and Eve: how schizophrenia shaped humanity.* London, UK: Bantam Press, 2001.

11. Leff J. *The unbalanced mind.* London, UK: Weidenfeld & Nicolson, 2001.

12. Kinderman P, Cooke A (eds). *Recent advances in understanding mental illness and psychotic experiences.* Leicester, UK: British Psychological Society Division of Clinical Psychology, 2000.

13. Atkinson J, Coia DA. *Families coping with schizophrenia.* Chichester, UK: Wiley, 1995.

14. Kuipers E. Working with carers: interventions for relatives and staff carers of those who have psychosis. In: Wykes T, Tarrier N, Lewis S (eds). *Outcome and innovation in psychological treatment of schizophrenia.* Chichester, UK: John Wiley, 1998.

15. Leudar I, Thomas P. *Voices of reason, voices of insanity.* London, UK: Routledge, 2000.

16. Romme M, Escher S. *Accepting voices.* London, UK: MIND, 1993.

17. Jenner A, Monteiro ACD, Zagalo-Cardoso JA, Cunha-Oliveira JA. *Schizophrenia: a disease or some ways of being human.* Sheffield, UK: Sheffield Academic Press, 1993.

18. Liddle P. The symptoms of chronic schizophrenia: a re-examination of the positive-negative dichotomy. *British Journal of Psychiatry* 1987; **151**: 145–51.

19. Liddle P, Friston K, Frith C. Patterns of cerebral blood-flow in schizophrenia. *British Journal of Psychiatry* 1992; **160**: 179–86.

20. Clare A. Psychiatry's future: psychological medicine or biological psychiatry? *Journal of Mental Health* 1999; 8 (2): 109–11.

21. Repper J. Adjusting the focus of mental health nursing: incorporating service users' experience of recovery. *Journal of Mental Health* 2000; **9**: 575–87.

22. Coleman R, Smith M. *Working with voices: victim to victor.* Newton-le-Willows, UK: Handsell Publications, 1997.

23. Nelson H. *Cognitive behavioural therapy with schizophrenia: a practice manual.* Cheltenham, UK: Stanley Thornes, 1997.

24. Sharma T, Chitnis X. *Brain imaging in schizophrenia.* London, UK: Remedica Publishing, 2000.

25. Boyle M. *Schizophrenia: a scientific delusion?* London, UK: Routledge, 1990.

26. Johnstone L. *Users and abusers of psychiatry*, 2nd edn. London, UK: Routledge, 2000.

27. Bentall R. Why there will never be a convincing theory of schizophrenia. In: Rose S (ed.). *From brains to consciousness? Essays on the new sciences of the mind.* London, UK: Penguin, 1998.

28. Drake R, Haddock G, Hopkins R, Lewis S. The measurement of outcome in schizophrenia. In: Wykes T, Tarrier N, Lewis S (eds). *Outcome and innovation in psychological treatment of schizophrenia.* Chichester, UK: John Wiley, 1998.

29. Department of Health. *The mental health policy implementation guide.* London, UK: Department of Health, 2001.

30. Department of Health. *The mental health policy implementation guide: adult acute inpatient care provision.* London, UK: Department of Health, 2002.

31. Regel S, Roberts D. *Mental health liaison: a handbook for nurses and health professionals.* Edinburgh, UK: Baillière Tindall, 2002.

32. Zubin J, Spring B. Vulnerability: a new view of schizophrenia. *Journal of Abnormal Psychology* 1997; **86**: 260–6.

33. Hughes I, Hill B, Budd R. Compliance with antipsychotic medication: from theory to practice. *Journal of Mental Health* 1997; **6**: 473–89.

34. Smith JA, Hughes I, Budd R. Non-compliance with antipsychotic medication: users' views on advantages and disadvantages. *Journal of Mental Health* 1999; 8: 287–96.

35. Bebbington P. The content and context of compliance. *International Clinical Psychopharmacology* 1995; **9** (Suppl. 5): 41–50.

36. McPhillips M, Sensky T. Coercion, adherence or collaboration? Influences on compliance with medication. In: Wykes T, Tarrier N, Lewis S (eds). *Outcome and innovation in psychological treatment of schizophrenia.* Chichester, UK: John Wiley, 1998.

37. Kemp R, Hayward P, David A. *Compliance therapy manual.* London, UK: Bethlem & Maudsley NHS Trust, 1997.

38. Day J, Wood G, Dewer M, Bertall R. A self-rating scale for measuring neuroleptic side-effects. *British Journal of Psychiatry* 1995; **166**: 650–3.

39. Perkins R, Repper J. Compliance or informed choice? *Journal of Mental Health* 1999; 8 (2): 117–29.

40. Perkins R, Repper J. *Dilemmas in community mental health practice: choice or control?* Oxford, UK: Radcliffe Medical Press, 1998: 64.

41. Healy D. *Psychiatric drugs explained*, 2nd edn. London, UK: Mosby, 1997.

42. Rose D. *Users voices.* London, UK: Sainsbury Centre for Mental Health, 2001.

43. Rogers A, Pilgrim D, Lacey R. *Experiencing psychiatry: users views of services.* London, UK: Macmillan, 1993.

44. NHS Centre for Reviews and Dissemination. Psychosocial interventions for schizophrenia. *Effective Health Care* 2000; **6** (3): 1–8.

45. Gamble C, Brennan G. *Working with serious mental illness: a manual for clinical practice.* London, UK: Baillière Tindall, 2000.

46. Fahy K, Dudley M. An introduction to psychosocial interventions in services. In: Thompson T, Mathias P (eds). *Lyttle's mental health and disorder*, 3rd edn. Edinburgh, UK: Baillière Tindall, 2000.

47. Breggin P, Cohen D. *Your drug may be your problem: how and why to stop taking psychiatric medication.* New York, NY: Perseus Books, 2000.

48. Kuipers E. The management of difficult to treat patients with schizophrenia, using non-drug therapies. *British Journal of Psychiatry Supplement* 1996; **Dec** (31): 41–51.

49. Mosher L, Burti L. Is psychotropic drug dependence really necessary? In: Mosher L, Burti L (eds). *Community mental health: a practical guide.* New York, NY: Norton, 1994: Chapter 5.

50. Alanen YO. *Schizophrenia: its origins and need-adapted treatment.* London, UK: Karnac Books, 1997.

51. Tarrier N, Yusupoff L, Kinney C, *et al.* Randomised controlled trial of intensive cognitive behaviour therapy for patients with chronic schizophrenia. *British Medical Journal* 1998; **317**: 303–7.

52. Drury V. Recovery from acute psychosis. In: Birchwood M, Tarrier N (eds). *Psychological management of schizophrenia.* Chichester, UK: Wiley, 1994.

53. Garety P, Hemsley D. *Delusions: investigations into the psychology of delusional reasoning.* Hove, UK: Psychology Press, 1997.

54. Haddock G, Slade PD (eds.) *Cognitive-behavioural interventions with psychotic disorders.* London, UK: Routledge, 1996.

55. Standing Nursing & Midwifery Advisory Committee. *Addressing acute concerns.* London, UK: Department of Health, 1999.

56. White M, Epston D. *Narrative means to therapeutic ends.* New York, NY: W.W. Norton, 1990.

57. Frith CD. *The cognitive neuropsychology of schizophrenia.* Hove, UK: Lawrence Erlbaum, 1992.

58. Siegel DJ. *The developing mind: toward a neurobiology of interpersonal experience.* New York, NY: Guilford Press, 1999.

59. Burbach F. Family-based interventions in psychosis: an overview of, and comparison between, family therapy and family management approaches. *Journal of Mental Health* 1996; **5** (2): 111–34.

60. Epstein NB, Bishop D, Ryan C, *et al.* The McMaster model view of healthy family functioning. In: Walsh F (ed.). *Normal family processes.* New York, NY: The Guilford Press, 1993: 138–60.

61. Johnstone L. Do families cause schizophrenia? Revisiting a taboo subject. In: Newnes C, Holmes G, Dunn C (eds). *This is madness: a critical look at psychiatry and the future of mental health services.* Ross-on-Wye, UK: PCCS Books, 1999.

62. Kuipers L, Leff J, Lam D. *Family Work for Schizophrenia.* London, UK: Royal College of Psychiatrists/Gaskell, 1992.

63. Jones DW. *Myths, madness and the family: the impact of mental illness on families.* Brighton, UK: Palgrave Publishers, 2002.

64. Benton M, Schroeder H. Social skills training with schizophrenics: a meta-analytic evaluation. *Journal of Consulting and Clinical Psychology* 1990; **58**: 741–7.

65. Osborn DPJ. The poor physical health of mentally ill people. *Western Journal of Medicine* 2001; **175** (5): 329–34.

66. Cohen A, Hove M. *Physical health of the severe and enduring mentally ill.* London, UK: Sainsbury Centre for Mental Health, 2001.

67. Frost M. *Nursing care of the schizophrenic patient.* London, UK: Henry Kimpton, 1974: 8.

68. MacCallum EJ. Othering and psychiatric nursing. *Journal of Psychiatric and Mental Health Nursing* 2002; **9**: 87–94.

69. Newnes C, Holmes G, Dunn C (eds). *This is madness too: a further critical look at mental health services.* Ross-on-Wye, UK: PCCS Books, 2000.

70. Chadwick PK. *Schizophrenia: the positive perspective.* London, UK: Routledge, 1997.

71. Watzlawick P, Beavin J, Jackson D. *Pragmatics of human communication.* New York, NY: Norton, 1967.

72. Watzlawick P, Beavin J, Jackson D. Some tentative axioms of communication. In: Morse BW, Phelps LA (eds). *Interpersonal communication: a relational perspective.* Minneapolis, MN: Burgess Publishing Company, 1980: 32–42.

73. May R. *The courage to create.* New York, NY: Norton, 1994.

74. Perkins R, Repper J. *Working alongside people with long-term mental health problems.* Cheltenham, UK: Stanley Thornes, 1997.

75. Killick K, Shaverien J (eds). *Art, psychotherapy & psychosis.* London, UK: Routledge, 1997.

76. Wilson M. *Occupational therapy in short-term psychiatry.* London, UK: Churchill Livingstone, 1996.

77. Wilson M. *Occupational therapy in long-term psychiatry.* London, UK: Churchill Livingstone, 1996.

78. Clarke L. Sacred radical of psychiatry. *Journal of Psychiatric and Mental Health Nursing* 2007; **14**: 446–53.

79. Szasz TS. *Schizophrenia: the sacred symbol of psychiatry.* Syracuse, NY: Syracuse University Press, 1976.

80. Jablensky A. Schizophrenia: manifestations, incidence and course in different cultures, a World Health Organization ten-country study. *Psychological Medicine* 1999; **2** (Suppl. 20): 1–95.

81. Whitaker R. *Mad in America: bad science, bad medicine and the enduring mistreatment of the mentally ill.* Cambridge, UK: Perseus Books, 2002.

82. Mueser KT, Gingerich S. *The complete family guide to schizophrenia.* New York, UK: Guilford Press, 2006: 372.

83. Hegarty J. One hundred years of schizophrenia: a meta-analysis of the outcome literature. *American Journal of Psychiatry* 1994; **151**: 1409–16.

84. Harding C. Empirical correction of seven myths about schizophrenia with implications for treatment. *Acta Psychiatrica Scandinavica* 1994; **384** (Suppl.): 140–6.

85. Szasz TS. *Pharmacracy. Medicine and politics in America.* London, UK: Praeger, 2001.

86. Morrison A, Read J, Turkington D. Trauma and psychosis: theoretical and clinical implications. *Acta Psychiatrica Scandinavica* 2005; **112**: 327–9.

87. Read J, Mosher LR, Bentall RP. *Models of madness: psychological, social and biological approaches to schizophrenia.* London, UK: Routledge, 2004.

88. Clinton M. Biological psychiatry versus humanism: why taking meaning seriously in mental health practice In: Cutcliffe J, Ward M (eds). *Key debates in psychiatric/mental health nursing.* Edinburgh, UK: Churchill Livingstone, 2006.

89. Gournay K. Psychiatric/mental health nursing: biological perspectives. In: Cutcliffe J, Ward M (eds). *Key debates in psychiatric/mental health nursing.* Edinburgh, UK: Churchill Livingstone, 2006.

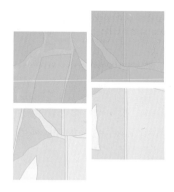

CHAPTER 26

The person who appears aggressive or violent

Eimear Muir-Cochrane*

INTRODUCTION

This chapter explores anger, aggression and violence in the workplace. Adopting a reflective practice, personal understandings of aggression are explored in the context of the challenges that face mental health professionals working in hospital settings. Nursing interventions that focus on prevention, de-escalation and management are discussed, using case studies and reflective exercises. The chapter aims to develop the reader's personal awareness of aggression and violence by:

- exploring personal understandings of anger and frustration;
- defining and differentiating between anger, aggression and violence;
- increasing knowledge of the dynamics of aggression;
- describing physical and physiological approaches to anger and aggression;
- identifying predisposing factors to the expression of anger and aggression;
- discussing different nursing interventions for clients exhibiting aggression;
- identifying ways of reducing the potential for aggression and violence in the workplace.

Definitions

- *Anger*: an emotion aroused because of a real or perceived threat to self, others or possessions.[1]
- *Aggression*: a disposition that may lead to constructive or destructive actions but that usually has long-term negative consequences.[2]
- *Violence*: the harmful and unlawful use of force or strength. The violent person is generally understood to refer to someone who attacks another.[2]

Violence and aggression in society and the workplace

Violence and aggression are universal phenomena and occur in all cultures, although some societies are perceived as more violent than others. The reporting of violence from around the world by means of television, the press, Internet and radio has dramatically increased over the last few decades, influencing how people perceive its prevalence. In the Western world, concerns for personal safety have generated the associated 'industry of protectionism'. This can be seen in the growth of sales of personal alarms, as well as home security systems. Sensationalist reporting is increasing, including images of

*Eimear Muir-Cochrane was Associate Professor at the University of South Australia, where she recently implemented a new postgraduate multidisciplinary mental health programme. In early 2008, she was appointed Professor and Chair of Mental Health Nursing at Flinders University, South Australia. Her research interests include the use of seclusion, absconding, the mental health needs of homeless young people and the involvement of consumers in postgraduate education.

mentally ill people as violent. Although there is little evidence to support such a view, the public often construe disorganized and agitated behaviour in people with mental illness as examples of antisocial conduct and hostility. Thus, the public, health professionals and psychiatric patients are often fearful of other psychiatric patients, believing them to be potentially aggressive and violent. It is generally assumed that aggressive and violent behaviour occurs more in psychiatric settings than in other healthcare settings, but this is not the case.[3] All healthcare settings have the potential for aggression since the experience of anger is a normal adaptive reaction. However, it is the intensity of the experience of anger, its duration and expression that causes people problems.[1]

The frequency of aggression towards nurses in healthcare settings is increasing and well documented, posing a major occupational health and safety hazard.[3,4] In mental health, between 64 and 80 per cent of staff are assaulted while at work.[3,5] Nurses now work in a diverse range of healthcare settings: home, hostels, health centres, police stations, as well as inpatient hospital units. The first week of hospitalization is recognized as a period in which the incidence of aggression or violence is higher than at any other time of inpatient care,[6] suggesting that the time around the admission of an individual ought to receive special attention by the mental healthcare team.

Merecz *et al.*[7] state that, out of all studied occupations, healthcare workers are particularly at risk of physical violence, with nurses four times more likely than other healthcare workers to be victims of violence at work. It is a sad reality that nurses need to prepare themselves with skill and knowledge to deal with aggression and violence in the workplace. The increasing risk of aggression and violence ranges from verbal abuse through to assault with violence.[1] It is vital that evidenced-based policies, procedures and training have a high profile in the management of aggression in all healthcare organizations. In 2001, the New South Wales (NSW) Nurses Association in Australia adopted a 'no tolerance' approach to violence in healthcare settings after an inpatient psychiatric patient bludgeoned an elderly resident to death.[8] Unfortunately, the necessity of anger management practices for patients (particularly in those healthcare settings where patients reside for long periods) received little attention. Instead, the commitment of the NSW government to increase the number of security guards in healthcare settings[8] suggests a containment focus rather than a therapeutic approach to the problem of workplace aggression and violence.

Notably, many aggressive incidents go unreported, perhaps because nurses see aggression as a frequent but unfortunate reality; perhaps because they become accustomed to such experiences; or perhaps because of the paperwork required to report incidents.[3] Although aggression cannot be avoided altogether, its incidence can be reduced through prediction measures and prevention strategies.[1] While it would seem reasonable to suggest that the characteristics of the human environment have a powerful effect in mitigating or precipitating aggression and violence, research cannot yet demonstrate this. There is some evidence that training and experience in aggression management help reduce injuries to staff, but it has not yet been proven that this leads to a reduction in the overall incidence of violence.[9]

Anger

Anger is an energy – a normal and powerful human emotion that people may experience several times a week. It is an under-researched emotion and a satisfactory definition of anger is difficult to achieve. Although on an individual basis, we can all understand what it is to be angry, it is more difficult to define what anger means for other people.

Mental health nurses recognize that making judgements about those in our care is unhelpful for the patient.[1] Yet, if someone is angry and we do not make a judgement about the appropriateness of their anger, how are we to help them? Thus, it is not always inappropriate or unhelpful to make a judgement about someone's anger to assist in the resolution of the situation.[1] However, making generalizations about people (e.g. people who are angry have no self-control) is to be avoided.

The difference between anger and aggression

Anger and aggression differ. Anger can be understood to be an immediate emotional arousal whereas aggression is an enduring negative attitude.[2] We can be angry without becoming aggressive, and we can be aggressive without being angry (e.g. during war).[2] It is generally accepted that anger can be conceptualized as having three core components.[10]

1 *Physiological arousal* occurs as a result of the stimulation of the cardiovascular and endocrine systems and results in physical tension and irritability.
2 *Cognitive arousal* shows in antagonistic thought patterns and in suspicious and negative thinking.
3 *Behavioural arousal* is manifested by verbal aggression and impulsive reactions.

This model proposes that exposure to stressors in the environment can cause irritability and tension, which over time can result in distorted and angry thinking patterns and ultimately aggressive behaviour. Generally speaking, this kind of aggression is interpreted as a maladaptive coping strategy and frequently causes problems for the person in daily living and interacting with others.[11]

For newly qualified health professionals, working with people who are potentially violent may be their biggest fear. There is conflicting evidence concerning the sex of staff in association with risk of assault in the workplace.[3,12] However, women and gay or lesbian people often perceive themselves to be in a vulnerable position and at most risk of becoming victims of violence. It is vital that such perceptions are recognized and dealt with appropriately so that staff can feel confident and empowered in the workplace.

Reflection

How do you feel when a patient becomes agitated or angry? Think about how you regulate your emotions.

Theories of violence

Common themes in the study of theories of violence include fear, frustration, manipulation, intimidation and pain or altered state of consciousness.[1] The various assumptions underpinning theories of aggression include whether or not aggression was learned; whether processes were cognitive or affective; and whether determinants were internal or external.[13]

Trait anger is attributed to individual differences in personality, whereas *state* anger refers to the temporary emotional state that arises from stress frustration or irritation. Each act of aggression depends on the person's values, personality and attitude. There are many evolutionary theories that stem from the perspective that aggression is a universal instinct. From a psychoanalytic perspective, Freud saw aggression as a response to frustration and/or pain. Aggression is conceptualized as an instinct, balanced by Thanatos (the death instinct) and Eros (the representation of love and self-preservation).

Other behavioural and cognitive perspectives focus on the tenet that aggression is learned. Neurophysiological research has indicated that damage to the amygdaloid nucleus in the brain may be associated with violence.[1] There is some evidence to suggest that temporal lobe epilepsy has been associated with episodic aggression and violence.[4] Other implications for the manifestation of aggression and violence are trauma to the brain that has resulted in cerebral changes and diseases such as encephalitis and tumours in the brain, particularly the limbic system and the temporal lobes.[1] Medical conditions such as chronic obstructive pulmonary disease, stroke, dementia, polypharmacy and urinary tract infection have roles to play in the increase of anxiety and aggression they cause, owing to frustration and cognitive confusion.

Biochemical factors such as hormonal dysfunction (e.g. Cushing's disease or hyperthyroidism) may contribute to the expression of aggression. There is anecdotal evidence, but no proven correlation, between the experience of premenstrual syndrome and violence. Research continues to attempt to identify which neurotransmitters (e.g. dopamine, serotonin, epinephrine, norepinephrine and acetylcholine) may be linked with the manifestation of aggressive and violent behaviour.[1]

Socioeconomic and environmental factors

As noted, violence and the expression of aggression in all Western societies is increasing. Explanations for the increase include the lack of infrastructure in the community for health, housing and education; increasing casual employment; the experience of alienation in individuals due to family break-up; race, sexual and religious discrimination; and poverty. Alcohol, street drugs and firearm use are all associated with the incidence of violent behaviour. Physical overcrowding in housing or institutions such as prisons and lack of recreational facilities to expend energy and natural aggression also contribute to an increased potential for violence in the community and have been recognized as proximal factors.[14]

Measuring aggression

The assessment of risk of aggression is notoriously difficult. Nevertheless, several tools may assist in the detection and rating of aggression, for example the Nurses' Observation Scale for Inpatient Evaluations (NOSIE) and the Modified Overt Aggression Scale (MOAS). Self-rating scales are of limited use as their utility depends on the person having insight, self-understanding and good communication skills. Other scales involve the nurse or other health professional completing them during an observation period of the patient. Most scales involve the rating of aggressive behaviour as verbal, physical, aggression against property or self-harm, with items within these categories on a five-point ordinal scale. Other behavioural and affective components may be included.[1]

The experience of the nurse in working with potential aggression and violence

Without education, skills training and clinical supervision, nurses tend to respond to inappropriate or aggressive behaviours as they would outside the work environment. Because of the powerful nature of anger as an emotion, people exposed to anger may feel fearful and intimidated. It is generally accepted that nurses will avoid patients if they are fearful of them. Patients experiencing paranoia are often neglected by nurses in this way and the avoidant behaviour reinforces their suspicious thinking and may increase the potential for aggression. Clearly, this is not therapeutic for either the nurse or the patient. A number of other common, but unhelpful, responses have also been identified, which might explain why nurses avoid patients.[11] Wishing to punish or humiliate the patient is a response that counters the patient's threat. This is a *reaction*, not a considered response, and is inappropriate when working with people who are aggressive regardless of their diagnosis.

Condoning or approving of violence, either among patients or between nurse and patient, is serious and destructive. Many such practices have existed up until recently in mental health institutions and have reportedly included the sexual assault of female patients[13] by health professionals. Such behaviour contravenes codes of ethics and professional conduct. Another negative response involves the adoption of a passive attitude or the use of professional verbal clichés in response to the aggressive behaviour by patients.

Imagine that you discovered that a friend had disclosed confidential information about you to someone you did not know very well. How would you feel when, on confronting your friend in an angry and upset manner, he or she replied 'I understand that you are very angry right now' or 'I know how you feel'. You are likely to feel enraged and certainly not appeased by such responses!

Genuinely helpful responses by nurses involve reflection of issues such as 'What was the aggressive patient thinking at the time?' and 'What is the context of their anger?' These can serve to work through the situation in a therapeutic way. Self-management of our own anger and frustration is necessary to develop effective skills in working with aggressive patients.[1]

Individual responses by staff to aggression and violence in the workplace will be influenced by childhood experiences, and the adults who were our role models. Working with aggressive patients can evoke feelings of frustration, exasperation, irritation and distress. Nurses need to recognize the need for clinical supervision to process feelings and reflect on their practice.

> ### Reflection
>
> Consider a situation in which you observed the demonstration of anger either by a patient or by a relative.
>
> - Write a list of what you think indicated that the person was angry.
> - Compare your list with Box 26.1.

These defining characteristics are signals for nursing staff to continue close assessment and observation of the patient and to plan care that might maintain emotional and physical safety for all in the immediate environs.

Patients with mental health problems may exhibit behaviours that may lead to an aggressive or violent incident, and being alert to these behaviours and early interventions can assist in the prevention of escalation of angry behaviour. Patients who are sarcastic in conversation, who express ideas of self-harm or harm to others, who are experiencing paranoid thoughts or general suspiciousness, or who have difficulty concentrating because of disturbances of thought or perception may also be at risk of becoming aggressive.

> ### Box 26.1: Observable characteristics of anger[1,p.642]
>
> - Intense distress
> - Pacing
> - Gritting or grinding teeth
> - Increased energy
> - Agitation
> - Change in tone of voice (raised or lowered)
> - Raised or lowered eyebrows
> - Flushed face
> - Withdrawal
> - Staring
> - Fatigue
> - Clenched fists

Indicators of biologically based aggression are useful in identifying the possibility of an organic basis to aggressive or violent behaviour. If the aggressive incident is unprovoked, if the episode involves a sudden shift in emotion to aggression from calm, if the episode is out of character for the individual, or if the person shows no remorse, nurses ought to be alerted to the possibility of pathophysiological causation and advise the multidisciplinary team of the need for further investigation.

KEY CONCEPTS IN AGGRESSION MANAGEMENT

Prevention

In most areas of practice aggressive behaviour can be expected. Staff must be adequately prepared to identify types and levels of aggression, to communicate problems among themselves simply and clearly, and to confront aggression directly. Appropriate training will decrease fear and hostility and will also help staff maintain a therapeutic environment. The prevention and management of aggression and violence is an interdisciplinary function, facilitating a multifaceted approach involving individualized interventions to minimize aggressive episodes. Aggression management has cognitive, behavioural and social components. Management should begin with those measures that have the least possibility of causing harm. Behavioural and environmental strategies are fundamental in maintaining a therapeutic atmosphere and are used as preventive measures with the careful use of medication as required in consultation with the multidisciplinary team (Box 26.2). Decision-making with regard to restraint and seclusion lie with the most senior staff. This involves a balance between the individual's personal freedom and their physical safety, and that of other patients and staff.

Limiting choices may be useful when cognitive impairment is a factor. For example, ask whether the person would like to go for a walk or watch television, rather than asking an open-ended question such as 'What would you like to do?' For patients who have difficulties thinking, concentrating and carrying out activities independently, an increased level of structure to their day can reduce anxiety and thus the potential for frustrated or agitated behaviour. For patients who are medicated and experiencing side-effects of neuroleptic drugs, or lethargy, a rest time after lunch can help maintain a sense of calm in both staff and patients. Identification of trigger events (meal times, before and after visiting time, weekends) that may contribute to patient's outbursts, and careful assessment at these times, can reduce the opportunity for the escalation of aggression.

Nursing management of aggression and violence

In aggressive situations the aggressor is often agitated, may be sweating, talking quickly or shouting and pacing around. Nursing interventions that can 'slow down' and ease the overstimulated individual can be extremely useful in preventing aggression from turning into actual violence.

While senior nursing staff manage the situation, continuous assessment, observation and documentation by other team members is important. Monitor how other patients are reacting to the situation. Witnessing aggression is potentially stressful and distressing.

Remaining calm when dealing with an angry person may sound simple but is a learned skill. Setting verbal limits and clearly distinguishing between acceptable and unacceptable behaviour while negotiating with the distressed relative can prevent further escalation. As a rule of thumb avoid touching patients and relatives when they are aroused. Although comments made to nurses by patients and relatives may be derogatory, personal and hurtful, they are merely words and the best course of action is to ignore them. Do not argue with the person as this is most likely to make matters worse. Approximately 3 per cent of the general population use alcohol harmfully but, as a socially endorsed activity in society, alcohol is readily available to people in times of distress. Close assessment of signs of drug or alcohol intoxication or withdrawal can prevent associated aggressive events.

Restraint and seclusion

In some cases it may be necessary to physically restrain an individual when preventive and de-escalation measures have failed to calm the patient. For some nursing interventions – such as the giving of intramuscular tranquillizing medication – it may be necessary to physically restrain the patient, if he or she is unwilling to take the medication. In the past, formalized staff development and training in self-defence and physical restraint was uncommon in health organizations. However, current standards of practice require staff to have mandatory preparation in the general principles of physical restraint. The English National Board (for example) recommended that all pre-registration courses for nurses and midwives contain material on aggression and violence.[15] For staff working in areas of potential aggression and violence, two basic rules apply:

1 never attempt to restrain someone on your own, unless life is in immediate danger
2 call for help if you cannot reach alarm systems.

Each organization should have its own policies and procedures regarding types of physical restraint and self-defence strategies, including breakaway techniques.

As noted, decision-making with regard to the use of restraint lies with the most senior staff and involves a delicate balance of an individual's personal freedom and the safety of others. The use of reasonable force and the patient's removal of freedom can be justified to take control *for* the patient, for the time they are 'out of control'. In some cases patients may be physically restrained so that they can be placed in seclusion. Seclusion involves the confinement of an individual in a secured room, from which individuals cannot leave of their own volition.[16] Seclusion is a last resort, used when other nursing interventions have failed or are unavailable. The literature suggests that patients often associate seclusion with punishment,[1] emphasizing the importance of open communication between staff and patients, when someone is secluded, to reduce anxiety and fears associated with confinement. Seclusion can offer physical and emotional safety for both patients and staff and the opportunity for counselling interventions.

Open and ongoing communication between all members of the multidisciplinary team is necessary to alert staff to changes in the individual's mental state and to plan care accordingly. This is not to say that all violent incidents can be foreseen or even prevented, but that safety concerns for staff and patients can be minimized. Debriefing of all incidents of aggression and violence for staff as well as patients is an important component of aggression management. Individuals need opportunities to work through their own feelings and to evaluate the efficacy of nursing interventions, to reduce burn-out and enhance personal and professional growth.

Personal illustration 26.3

A social worker is approached and verbally threatened by a female patient after a one-to-one session discussing social security benefits. Nursing staff intervene, and the patient eventually calms down. In the debriefing session that follows, the social worker explains that the patient had been expressing paranoid thoughts about the staff, thinking that they were conspiring to steal her money and possessions.

Reflection

What can you do in debriefing sessions to help yourself and your colleagues get the most out of them?

TEACHING MANAGEMENT OF AGGRESSION

On a one-to-one basis, nurses have an important role in assisting patients to manage their anger and aggression. Keeping a diary and recording negative feelings on a daily basis can identify personal triggers for anger and frustration. Exploring alternative ways of coping with stress such as physical outlets (exercise) and seeking out staff when feeling angry or agitated can also reduce the potential for aggression and help patients feel more in control of their emotions. Activities that include mental and physical stimulation (regular exercise and relaxation strategies) can offer routine and structure to a patient's daily activities. Token economies are contractual agreements that identify target behaviours and reward patients with tokens for good conduct. Rules ought to be predetermined, and these programmes require expert psychology assistance in their establishment within a prescribed care plan. Non-aggressive behaviour can be successfully rewarded through verbal reinforcement, although a consistent staff response is required for this to be effective. Assertiveness training helps patients express their needs and wishes and helps them get the attention they need. This kind of training in one-to-one and group settings can also help patients deal with the frustration of activities of daily living in the community such as standing in queues and being on hold on the telephone for periods of time.

Common mistakes

In stressful situations it is not uncommon for individuals to react in a way that at the time appears to be of use but that is ultimately counterproductive.

- Disagreeing or raising your voice (unless it is to be heard) with people who are angry is of no value and will cause the situation to escalate.
- In a similar way demonstrating emotions such as frustration, distress or anger yourself is likely to increase the tension of the situation.
- Never approach an angry person without back-up. Continuous assessment of safety is important as the situation may deteriorate quickly.
- Do not attempt to use humour or sarcasm or to touch the patient.
- Above all, learn by observing those who have successfully managed such situations, learn by your mistakes and the insights gained from debriefing critical incidents.

Reflection

- Think of a time when you have witnessed violence or aggression but were not directly involved. How did you feel? What were your thoughts about what was happening?
- Think of a time when you have spoken to someone who was angry about something. What conclusions did you draw about the strength of their feelings? How would you define anger in your own words?
- Think of a time when you have been aggressive, perhaps when you were very young or an adolescent. Try and remember what you were feeling and thinking and how you behaved. Such recollections can cause feelings of discomfort, fear, shame and regret as we acknowledge that we may have lost control over a situation. Hold onto this feeling of discomfort as this may be exactly how patients feel when they become aggressive or violent.

SUMMARY

Working with patients who are angry and frustrated arouses a range of emotions in those who care for them. Aggression and violence are not symptomatic of mental illness, but reflect the general expression of these emotions and behaviours in mainstream society as well as the powerlessness and frustration that patients often experience when they are within the healthcare system. Nurses need special personal attributes, skills, education and training to manage difficult situations safely and therapeutically. This chapter has explored personal and professional strategies for exploring the experience of anger and aggression in the workplace. Ongoing reflection and critique of personal and team practices are significant elements in maintaining therapeutic environments for patients under duress.

REFERENCES

1. Hamolia C. Preventing and managing aggressive behavior. In: Stuart G, Laraia M (eds). *Principles and practice of psychiatric nursing*, 7th edn. St Louis, MO: Mosby, 2001:635–57.

2. Rippon TJ. Aggression and violence in health care professions. *Journal of Advanced Nursing* 2000; **31** (2): 452–60.

3. Farrell GA, Bobrowski C, Bobrowski P. Scoping workplace aggression in nursing: findings from an Australian study. *Journal of Advanced Nursing* 2006; **55** (6): 778–87.

4. Ferns T. Violence, aggression and physical assault in health-care settings. *Nursing Standard* 2006; **21** (13): 42–6.

5. Royal College of Nursing. *One third of service users 'experience inpatient violence'*. London, UK: RCN, 2005: 26 May.

6. El-Badri SM, Mellsop G, Aggressive behaviour in an acute general adult psychiatric unit. *Psychiatric Bulletin* 2006; **30**: 166–8.

7. Merecz D, Rymaszewska J, Moscicka A. Violence at the workplace: a questionnaire survey of nurses. *European Psychiatry* 2006; **21** (7): 442–50.

8. NSW Nurses' Association. Violence against nurses still a significant problem. In: *NSW hospitals and nursing media release*. NSW, Australia: NSW Nurses' Association, 2006.

9. Deane DP. A critical review of the prevalence and effectiveness of workplace violence prevention programs. Dissertation Abstracts International: Section B. *The Sciences and Engineering* 2007; **67**: 7-B.

10. Glancy G, Saini MA. An evidenced-based review of psychological treatments of anger and aggression. *Brief Treatment and Crisis Intervention* 2005; **5** (2): 229–48.

11. Horsfall J, Stuhmiller C, Champ S. *Interpersonal nursing for mental health*. New York, NY: Springer, 2001.

12. Daffern M, Mayer, M, Martin T. Staff gender ratio and aggression in a forensic psychiatric hospital. *International Journal of Mental Health Nursing* 2006; **15**: 93–9.

13. Cutting P, Henderson C. Women's experiences of hospital admission. *Journal of Psychiatric and Mental Health Nursing* 2002; **9**: 705–12.

14. Meehan T, McIntosh W, Bergen H. Aggressive behaviour in the high-secure forensic setting: the perceptions of patients. *Journal of Psychiatric and Mental Health Nursing* 2006; **13**: 19–25.

15. Beech B. Sign of the times or the shape of things to come? A 3 day unit of instruction on 'aggression and violence in health settings for all students during pre-registration nurse training'. *Accident and Emergency Nursing* 2001; **9**: 204–11.

16. Muir-Cochrane EC, Holmes CA. Legal and ethical aspects of seclusion: an Australian perspective. *Journal of Psychiatric and Mental Health Nursing* 2001; **8**: 501–6.

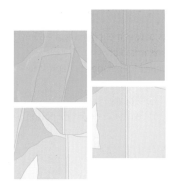

CHAPTER 27

The person with a diagnosis of bipolar disorder

Ian Beech*

INTRODUCTION

Bipolar disorder is usually ranked, along with schizophrenia, as a serious mental illness.[1] Although nurses' primary responsibility is neither to diagnose nor prescribe treatment, they do have a role in the delivery of treatment regimes and need to understand the diagnosis and medical responses to bipolar disorder.

This chapter focuses on the care of the *person* who is experiencing bipolar disorder and the alliance that nurses need to build in order to enable the person to recognize and take control of mood swings.

DIAGNOSTIC CRITERIA

Although long known as manic depression, both the *World Health Organization*[2] and the *American Psychiatric Association*[3] now use the term *bipolar disorder* to indicate the fluctuation of the person's mood between the two poles of depression and mania. The American Psychiatric Association divides bipolar disorder into two types. *Type I* is characterized by the person having experienced one or more manic episodes, whereas *type II* is characterized by the person having experienced one hypomanic episode and one major depressive episode. The difference between mania and hypomania is considered to be the length of the episode, with mania lasting for 1 week or longer, and hypomania lasting for 4 days.

THE EXPERIENCE OF MANIA

The experience of mania or hypomania is not simply being overexcited. There is an important qualitative difference between being happy, or 'full of the joys of spring', and experiencing mania. A manic episode involves the person showing some or all of the characteristic changes in *emotion, cognition, behaviour and physicality* listed in Table 27.1.

Table 27.1 indicates the possible signs and symptoms of mania but does not help us understand what the *experience* might be like for the person. Let us consider the case of Jane (see the Personal illustration over the page).

Jane believes that her bipolar disorder was the result of a combination of the stress of coping with living away from home for the first time, the work at university and her excessive partying. She has heard that both her grandfather and her uncle 'suffered with their nerves' and wonders whether her condition may be genetic. This view of the 'cause' of bipolar disorder is not unusual as it is sometimes seen to 'run in families'. Genetic research has indicated that there may be a risk factor for bipolar disorder.[5] Individuals also often describe a stressful event or events in their lives to which they believe they can trace back the onset of their

*Ian Beech is Head of the Mental Health Division at the University of Glamorgan, Pontypridd, UK, and is researching a history of Cardiff City Mental Hospital.

Personal illustration 27.1

Jane is in her forties and is a self-employed financial advisor. When at university she started to go to overnight parties and to drink and dabble with cannabis. Initially, she could still study, but then found that she was having difficulty concentrating and also that she could get by on less and less sleep. She eventually had to take a break from university because of poor results.

She has experienced mood swings for the past 25 years. When she has experienced 'highs' she has spent money on clothes and luxuries that she cannot really afford. She has also gone to nightclubs and pubs and had numerous sexual partners. Her mood can swing very quickly into depression when she is consumed with feelings of guilt over her actions while high, and she ruminates on thoughts that she has acquired a sexually transmitted disease. She lives alone and says that the main reason for this is that she has never been able to sustain a long-term relationship because partners have found her behaviour too difficult to live with.

Since being diagnosed in the 1980s Jane has been treated with a variety of drugs and found that, although they have helped for periods of time, nothing has stabilized her mood for longer than about a year.

About 5 years ago Jane attended a self-management training course run by the Manic Depression Fellowship. On the course, she says she learned to adapt her lifestyle and to take ownership of her problems by developing an advanced agreement with mental health services.

Although she still experiences mood swings she feels more confident about the future and feels more able to exercise some control over her life.

TABLE 27.1 Symptoms of manic/hypomanic episode[4]

Emotional changes	Mood swings between euphoria and elation to anger and irritability
	Switches of affect from happy to depressed and hostile
	Uncritical self-confidence
	Wish to be gratified in whatever the person does
Cognitive changes	Racing thoughts
	Distractible
	Rapid and loud speech that is difficult to interrupt
	Flight of ideas
	Impaired judgement
	Ideas of reference, delusions and hallucinations
Behavioural changes	Dramatic mannerisms, flamboyant dress and make-up
	Increase in goal-directed activity
	Intrusive, demanding, domineering and sometimes aggressive
	Resists efforts to treat
	Dislikes having wishes thwarted
	Impulsive
	Acts in sexual ways that are unusual for the person, e.g. hypersexual
Physical changes	Full of energy, does not easily tire
	Extreme motor activity leading to exhaustion
	Insomnia with decreased need for sleep
	Change in appetite
	Lack of attention to personal hygiene, appearance and general health

problems. The well-known comedian and writer Spike Milligan,[6] for example, traced his problems back to having been caught in a shell blast in the Second World War. However, his father was someone who was prone to mood swings. On an ordinary day, it may be that meteorologists can identify what causes rainfall, but for most people their main concern is whether or not they need to put on a raincoat or carry an umbrella; in other words, people's concerns are how to deal with problems on an everyday basis, and this is the same with bipolar disorder.

Kay Redfield Jamison[7] described her experiences thus:

When I am high I couldn't worry about money if I tried. So I don't. The money will come from somewhere; I am entitled; God will provide. Credit cards are disastrous, personal checks worse. Unfortunately, for manics anyway, mania is a natural extension of the economy. What with credit cards and bank accounts there is little beyond reach. So I bought twelve snakebite kits, with a sense of urgency and importance. I bought precious stones, elegant and unnecessary furniture, three watches within an hour of one another (in the Rolex rather than Timex class: champagne tastes bubble to the surface, are the surface, in mania), and totally inappropriate siren-like clothes. During one spree in London I spent several hundred pounds on books having titles or covers that somehow caught my fancy: books on the natural history of the mole, twenty sundry Penguin books because I thought it could be nice if penguins could form a colony.

At first sight it may seem that to feel so full of energy, with no worries about finances, and being sexually active must be a wonderful feeling to which many people might aspire. However, this is not the case. People often find that they feel great as a manic episode commences but soon the fall-out both for themselves physically and mentally and for their relationships is immense. Mary Ellen Copeland,[8] for example, described her experience as one in which:

I feel unable to stay physically still or to quiet my brain. My body hurts all over. Every cell says I want to rest, but the body and mind cannot and will not co-operate.

It is important, therefore, for nurses to be aware that what the person is experiencing is not merely exuberance but moving beyond this to being 'out of control' and likely to perform actions that the person would not usually wish to perform.

NURSING APPROACH

The nursing approach to someone diagnosed with bipolar disorder has three dimensions.

1 When a person is in the acute manic phase, the main considerations are to address the physical, psychological and social consequences of behaviour while manic.
2 Ensure that, if a mood-stabilizing drug is prescribed, the person experiences no major problems with the drug and can maintain a therapeutic level in the body.
3 When the manic phase has abated, try to develop the person's awareness of possible trigger factors so that self-management strategies may be developed.

The manic phase

An often underestimated complication of an acute phase of mania is that the person does not rest and is on the move continually, resulting in a very rapid use of calories. This can be coupled with an excitability that prevents the person concentrating on mundane matters like eating and drinking. It is easy, therefore, for the person to become physically exhausted and dehydrated. With this in mind, the nurse should consider ways of providing food and drink that do not require the person to sit for prolonged mealtimes. It is unprofitable to get into an argument with the person about mealtimes. This will result only in the creation of tension between the nurse and the person, so undermining the relationship.

Mania is often characterized by excitability and distractibility and consequently the person often reacts quickly and excitably to environmental stimuli. Therefore, it is a helpful nursing approach to try to aim to promote a quiet and relaxed environment for the person. This is not always possible in an inpatient environment because of distractions provided by the other people present. Given that some people in mania can often be amusing and entertaining, there is a risk that nurses and other patients might provide an 'audience' for the person (wittingly or unwittingly) as a means of providing light relief from the everyday humdrum of the ward. Wherever possible, nurses should be relaxed and quiet in their approach and avoid getting into protracted arguments and conflict with people as this provides distraction and further, unhelpful, stimulation.

People in manic phases are often given high dosages of medication in an attempt to lower the mood and control behaviour. If this is the case there are a number of considerations that have to be taken into account. Anybody subjected to high dosages of drugs such as haloperidol and Acuphase (clopixol) may experience drowsiness, extrapyramidal side-effects and blurred vision. Therefore, it is important for nurses to be aware of a possible lack of

coordination and the risk of tripping and/or falling and of spilling hot drinks. National Institute for Health and Clinical Excellence (NICE) guidelines recognize these problems and recommend that haloperidol should not be the drug of choice and that olanzapine and lorazepam are preferable because of their having fewer severe side-effects.[9]

People in mania can sometimes be argumentative and apparently difficult to take issue with. Discussions about such things as personal hygiene and self-care are seen as mundane interruptions to the great scheme on which the person is embarked. In such situations, the nurse should maintain a calm, relaxed approach and avoid entering into protracted arguments with the person, which will merely provide further stimulation, generating more frustration and argument. Instead, a gentle calm encouragement in which the issue does not become a battleground is more likely to bear fruit.

Another common feature of mania is hypersexuality (heightened sexual activity), often coupled with lowered inhibition. This can be very difficult for both the partners of people with bipolar disorder and for nurses charged with caring for them. For partners there is the emotional rollercoaster of living with someone who is apparently seeking other sexual partners. The difficulty revolves around whether or not the behaviour being exhibited is a result of the bipolar disorder or the person exercising free will in following his or her own desires. For nurses, it is often difficult to strike a balance between not wishing to interfere in the private matters of people in care and being reluctant to abdicate responsibility under the duty to care for people. Ron Coleman[10] distinguished between nurses caring *for* people and caring *about* them. He considers that when nurses care *for* people they try to wrap them in cotton wool and not allow any personal freedom, whereas when nurses care *about* people they are prepared to take risks and allow personal autonomy. Each case must be considered on its own merits and sexual behaviour, like any other behaviour, should be assessed within the context of the whole person. It should always be borne in mind, however, that if a person's mood were to swing into depression following a manic episode there could be overwhelming feelings of guilt and self-disgust associated with any actions that the person carried out during a manic episode.

Mood-stabilizing medication

People diagnosed with bipolar disorder are often prescribed two types of mood-stabilizing medication: lithium compounds and anticonvulsant medication (the same drugs used to treat epilepsy). Neither medication works for everybody, but both have been found to have some beneficial effects in mood stabilization for many people.

In either case the nurse should remember that it is paramount that people receive comprehensive and detailed information about drugs they are prescribed. Very often, people taking mood-stabilizing drugs are expected to take them for prolonged periods during their lives, often for years. To expect anyone to comply with a long-term prescription of any medication without first ensuring that the person has access to full information is simply laying the foundations for conflict. Nevertheless, it is remarkable how many nurses will willingly condemn people for not complying with prescriptions of psychiatric medication while, when asked, openly admit to never completing a prescribed course of antibiotics. It is not unheard of for people who were prescribed lithium carbonate in the past to have been told that it was not a proper medication at all; it was a salt (technically true for a student of chemistry, since a salt is a compound of a metal and lithium is a metallic element). The result was that some people were under the misapprehension that lithium tablets were neither more hazardous nor more effective than the condiment they put on their fish and chips.

People need to be given full information about what they might expect from medication in terms of both therapeutic effects and side-effects and special precautions they should take, especially in terms of eating and drinking. People should also be informed about the blood tests that will be necessary at regular intervals while they are taking lithium.

There are many useful sources of information about medication. One of the most accessible in terms of language and explanation is the Norfolk and Waveney Mental Health Trust pharmacy website (www.nmhct.nhs.uk/pharmacy).[11] There are, however, a number of points that need to be considered.

Lithium products

Lithium is produced pharmaceutically in two forms – lithium carbonate and lithium citrate. The exact way lithium acts on the body to produce its mood-stabilizing effect is unknown.[12] It has a very narrow therapeutic blood level range of between 0.4 and 1.2 mmol per litre of blood, although the usual effective range is even narrower at 0.6–1.0 mmol per litre.[11] Outside this range, at the lower end lithium is *ineffective* and at the higher end it is *toxic*. Consequently, people prescribed lithium need to have regular blood tests to monitor levels and also to monitor the function of the thyroid gland, which can be adversely affected by lithium.

Because of the fairly narrow therapeutic range, and because of the relative ease with which people can slip into toxicity, nurses need to be aware of both the signs and likely causes of toxicity, and also to inform people of this risk. People should be informed that, should they begin to experience blurred vision, unsteadiness in walking and standing, diarrhoea and vomiting, slurred speech, a bad hand tremor, clumsiness, increased thirst or passing urine and/or drowsiness/confusion, they should seek medical advice.

There can be a number of causes of toxicity, but common factors can be anything that might lead to dehydration, as this increases lithium concentration in the blood (e.g. drinking large amounts of tea, coffee or cola drinks as these contain caffeine, which is a diuretic), sweating in hot weather, drinking alcohol (another diuretic), vomiting and diarrhoea, and taking aerobic exercise.

Problems might also develop if a person chews lithium tablets rather than swallows them whole. Lithium is designed to be absorbed slowly over a few hours. Chewing the tablet increases the rate of absorption and so increases the concentration in the body.

It may seem that giving people all of this information when they may never experience adverse effects is playing hostage to fortune. Might it not simply reinforce anyone's reluctance to take their medication? However, lithium has the potential to be a dangerous drug if taken without taking its problems into account. Nurses must address the issue of toxicity in order to provide safe care for people. Furthermore, the potential damage to the therapeutic relationship should someone experience adverse effects after a nurse had given reassurance would be irreparable.

Personal illustration 27.2

Bob has had a number of manic episodes over the last few years and, during these, he has sometimes become agitated and had nocturnal enuresis.

When he was admitted to a new unit for the first time, Bob wet the bed on his first night. Following this, it was decided by the nursing staff to limit Bob's fluid intake, particularly in the evenings to try to stop him from wetting the bed at night.

Unfortunately, Bob was prescribed lithium carbonate and began to have toxic symptoms as a result of dehydration.

Physical care

It is important to give holistic care for people who are diagnosed as having bipolar disorder and blood tests alone are insufficient. NICE[9] recommends that people with bipolar disorder should also receive a comprehensive annual physical health check, which should include:

- lipid levels, including cholesterol in all people over 40
- plasma glucose level
- weight
- smoking status and alcohol use
- blood pressure.

Anticonvulsant medication used to control mood

Carbemazepine, sodium valproate and lamotrigine are all used as mood stabilizers either alone or in conjunction with lithium products. These products have various side-effects and interactions with other drugs which require attention by nurses. Carbemazepine, for example, reduces the effectiveness of oral contraceptives whereas sodium valproate has a potentially adverse effect on fetal development. Therefore, great care should be taken to offer detailed contraceptive advice if a woman of child-bearing age is prescribed carbemazepine. NICE recommends that sodium valproate should be given to women of child-bearing age only in exceptional circumstances, along with detailed contraceptive advice.[9] It is fundamentally important that such issues are discussed with people and that they are given the information required to make an informed choice about their life-style.

Other medication

People with a diagnosis of bipolar disorder may sometimes be prescribed major tranquilizers and/or antidepressants.

Given the nurses' responsibility for the safe administration of medication, they need to be fully conversant with appropriate dosages, effects and side-effects, etc. and also the need to engage in a collaborative approach with the person in care in order to ensure that full information is given.

Reflection

What are your responsibilities in administering medication? What resources are available to you to help you fulfil your responsibilities?

SELF-MANAGEMENT

It is only through ownership of problems of living and ways of coping that people are enabled to embark on the road to recovery. Mary Ellen Copeland[8] encouraged people with bipolar disorder to develop a personalized chart that might help them to build up a profile of the nature of any mood swings to which they might be subject. From this, people can develop awareness of the things in their lives that might trigger swings into mania and/or depression. Nurses can play an important role in this process by providing with information about ways of monitoring moods, providing people with contacts with organizations such as the Manic Depression Fellowship, which runs courses on self-management. Nurses are also in a position to provide encouragement that recovery is possible. Barker[13] has shown that people who are susceptible to manic phases may feel themselves to be powerless in the face of what they feel are inevitable, uncontrollable mood swings. By beginning to address likely precursors to mood changes, not only do people begin to identify triggers but they also gain a sense of ownership of the problem. Rather than passively waiting for the latest wonder drug from professionals, people enter into a collaborative approach to finding a way of living their lives that does not result in their lives

being constantly defined and then redefined in terms of problems rather in terms of their strengths.[14]

In order to take control and ownership of their own lives, people need to feel that they might have influence over what professionals term symptoms. Copeland[8] suggested that people should try to identify early warning signs of *depression* (e.g. lethargy, sleep patterns, negative thought patterns) and early warning signs of *mania* (e.g. thrill seeking, increased sexual activity, being argumentative), alongside a series of things to do every day (e.g. eat well, take moderate exercise). In so doing and by reviewing their mood charts regularly people can establish patterns in their lives of what causes them problems and what they find helpful. In this process it is important that nurses do *not* suggest what they should be charting. To be effective, such a chart should be personal and, potentially, meaningful as an educational vehicle for self-management.

Personal illustration 27.3

Mary was diagnosed with manic depression over 30 years ago and has had a number of compulsory admissions to hospital under both the 1959 and 1983 Mental Health Acts.

In recent years, Mary has learned to build close alliances with professionals with whom she feels that she can work effectively.

Mary trusted Jack, a nurse on her ward, when she was admitted a few years ago. Her trust was grounded in the nurse having faith in her. Whereas she felt other professionals often dismissed how she felt and what she was saying as symptoms of her illness, often reaching for medication when they felt it was required, Jack used to sit with her and listen to what she was saying while she told him about how she felt, how she had slept and what had helped her get through the day.

After Mary's discharge from hospital Jack would make himself available to her when she called or visited. If he was busy he would make her a cup of tea and return as soon as he had 'cleared the decks'. He would then answer her questions honestly or help her to reaffirm her ways of coping.

Even though it is now many years later, Mary is still subject to swings in mood but she has accurately identified, with Jack's help, what helps and what makes things worse. Jack was the first person in what has become, for Mary, a network of relationships with professionals whom she feels she can trust. She has also identified those professionals with whom she cannot develop trust and who are best avoided.

Nurses should be careful *not* to allow knowledge about a person's diagnosis to lull them into explaining everything that happens in the person's life in terms of that diagnosis (see Chapter 15). For example, Mary, a woman with a 30-year diagnosis of bipolar disorder, was very active in the voluntary sector. She went to a meeting with a senior nurse about a project she wished to set up in the community. She had worked on the project for some months and was very keen to see it succeed. Many years after the meeting, Mary had access to her medical notes and in them found a letter from the nurse to her consultant, dated the same day as her meeting, saying that, at the meeting, Mary had been enthusiastic, expressed strong opinions and was forceful. Perhaps, the nurse suggested, Mary was going high and should have her medication reviewed.

Reflection

Remember that people are neither manic depressive nor bipolar: they have a diagnosis of manic depression or bipolar disorder.

Be careful not to assign everything that happens in the person's life to the diagnosis that he or she has been given.

Advanced directives

Being able to take control of your life when you are not showing symptoms of bipolar disorder is one way of feeling that you have ownership. However, when a person is showing psychotic symptoms such a sense of ownership might be more difficult to achieve. One important way of addressing this is to work with people to develop advanced directives.[15] These are documents within which people have considered the possibility of their having mood swings in the future and have set down in clear terms the issues that are important to them with the view that, should decisions have to be made about care at some future date, the advanced directive might inform the process and allow the person's own wishes to be an integral part of the decision-making of the clinical team even if, at the time, the person is deemed to be incapable of making decisions.

The advanced directive has no legal status currently in the UK, but it is recommended by the NICE guidelines[9] for bipolar disorder as being best practice. In New Zealand, the Mental Health Commission has recognized advanced directives as being a vital component of care for people who are diagnosed as manic depressive.[16] In Australia, the National Mental Health Plan[17] puts forward the concept of people's rights and involvement even though there is no legal status to advanced directives there, or in the majority of states in the USA. Nevertheless, in each of these there is an increasing moral force gathering behind the practice.[18] Minnesota in the USA authorized advanced directives in 1991 and has been followed by Alaska, Hawaii, Idaho, Illinois, Maine, North Carolina, Oklahoma, Oregon, South Dakota, Texas and Utah.[18] It seems, therefore, that in countries such as the UK, Australia, New Zealand and the USA there is a groundswell of opinion in favour of adopting more consensual approaches to care planning and treatment,

giving advanced directives a widespread moral if not legal force. As Ron Coleman[10] says:

> We do not want you to work on us any more. We want you to work with us and that means on our terms not your terms. And we don't want you to perceive our needs because that is what professionals do, they are wonderful at it: 'This person needs this, this, this and this.' You never ask us what we need.

Advanced directives may be as simple or as detailed as the person wishes. For example, the person may simply state a preference for a certain type of medication over another type based on his or her experience of side-effects and therapeutic benefit. Or there might be a statement that the person would rather not receive electroconvulsive therapy (ECT). On the other hand, the person might go into a level of detail about who might have power over credit cards, car keys, post and money or who might care for the dog and the goldfish. As previously stated, the current state of law is that if a person is detained under Section 3 of the Mental Health Act 1983, and subject to a second opinion, ECT can be given legally against the person's will even if that person has expressed a preference not to receive ECT (and this is not likely to change under the Mental Health Act 2007). But professionals have to consider that they will need to work with the person for a number of years and anything that undermines the trusting relationship will mean years of trying to rebuild bridges.

Reflection

Think back to people who you have worked with who have been diagnosed with bipolar disorder.

How might you help these people to develop an advanced statement of their needs?

Providing information

In learning to take control of their changes in mood, people usually find that the support of significant others is of paramount importance. This support is more likely to be forthcoming and lasting if it is predicated on sound up-to-date information about the diagnosis and prognosis.

There now exists a wealth of information about bipolar disorder, in the publications of organizations such as the Manic Depression Fellowship, in libraries and on the Internet. However, firstly, people often expect nurses to be knowledgeable about their diagnosis and treatment – the source of all knowledge.[19] Secondly, nurses attempt to engender trust in people for whom they care. This is extremely difficult if all the information to which the person has access comes from sources other than the nurse. Thirdly, people often worry about whether or not their children might develop bipolar disorder in the future. Nurses need to be able to address these issues while neither overstating nor diminishing them.

- The person diagnosed with bipolar disorder presents in different ways to the nurse.
- When the person is in the manic state the nurse needs to address this in a calm, rational way to promote a calm environment and avoidance of harm.
- If the person has become depressed, the nurse needs to address this (see Chapter 20).
- When the person is prescribed mood-stabilizing medication, the nurse should be sufficiently knowledgeable to avoid complications and help to negotiate a medical approach with which the person can live.
- When the person feels that his or her mood is stable, the nurse and that person together need to develop ways of the person taking control and ownership and feeling empowered.
- The nurse's role involves a complex set of skills and knowledge – from physical considerations such as hydration to complex interpersonal processes involving negotiation and facilitating empowerment.

REFERENCES

1. Gamble C, Brennan G (ed.). *Working with serious mental illness: a manual for clinical practice*, 2nd edn. Edinburgh, UK: Elsevier, 2006.

2. World Health Organization. *ICD-10: The ICD-10 classification of mental and behavioural disorders: clinical descriptions and diagnostic guidelines*. London, UK: Gaskell/Royal College of Psychiatrists, 1992.

3. American Psychiatric Association. *Diagnostic and statistical manual of mental disorders, 4th edition, text revision*. Washington, DC: American Psychiatric Press, 2000 (DSM IV-TR).

4. Lego S. The client who is diagnosed bipolar. In: Lego S (ed.). *Psychiatric nursing: a comprehensive reference*, 2nd edn. Philadelphia, PA: Lippincott, 1996: 213–17.

5. BBC News. *Scientists make bipolar find*. Available from: http://news.bbc.co.uk/1/hi/wales/6728133.stm. Accessed 14 July 2007.

6. Milligan S, Clare A. *Depression and how to survive it*. London, UK: Arrow, 1994.

7. Redfield Jamison K. *The unquiet mind: a memoir of moods and madness*. London, UK: Picador, 1995.

8. Copeland M. *The depression workbook: a guide for living with depression and manic depression*, 2nd edn. Oakland, CA: New Harbinger, 2001.

9. National Institute for Health and Clinical Excellence. *Bipolar disorder: the management of bipolar disorder in adults, children and adolescents, in primary and secondary care*. Clinical Guideline 38. London, UK: NICE, 2006.

10. Coleman R. The politics of the illness. In: Barker P, Stevenson C (eds). *The construction of power and authority in psychiatry*. London, UK: Butterworth Heinemann, 2000: 59–66.

11. Norfolk and Waveney Mental Health Partnership NHS Trust Pharmacy. Available from: www.nmhct.nhs.uk/Pharmacy. Accessed 11 July 2007.

12. Healy D. *The creation of psychopharmacology*. Cambridge, MA: Harvard University Press, 2002.

13. Barker P. Locus of control in women with a diagnosis of manic-depressive psychosis. *Journal of Psychiatric and Mental Health Nursing* 1994; **1**: 9–14.

14. Watkins P. *Mental health nursing: the art of compassionate care*. Oxford, UK: Butterworth Heinemann, 2001.

15. Manic Depression Fellowship. *Planning ahead for people with manic depression*. London, UK: MDF, 2001.

16. Mental Health Commission. *Advanced directives in mental health care and treatment*. Available from: www.mhc.govt.nz/publications/2003/MentalHealth_HDC_Broch.pdf. Accessed 14 July 2007.

17. Australian Government. *Department of Health national mental health plan 2003–2008*. Available from: www.dh.sa.gov.au/mental-health-unit. Accessed 14 July 2007.

18. Honberg RS. *Advanced directives*. Available from: www.nami.org/Content/ContentGroups/Legal/Advance_Directives.htm. Accessed 12 July 2007.

19. Jackson S, Stevenson C. What do people need psychiatric and mental health nurses for? *Journal of Advanced Nursing* 2000; **31**: 378–88.

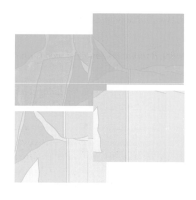

CHAPTER 28

The person with a diagnosis of personality disorder

Marie Crowe* and Dave Carlyle**

INTRODUCTION

Personality disorder (PD) has become an overused diagnosis, often applied to people who present themselves in a difficult or challenging manner. However, clearly there is a group of people who are distressed greatly by their personal experience and who, for whatever reason, are unable to contain this, resulting in a variety of socially disturbing forms of behaviour. This chapter critically examines the diagnostic features of what is constructed in psychiatric discourse as PD and suggests possible alternatives for understanding these behaviours that may result in more effective mental health nursing care.

Reflection

What type of behaviours do you think about when you hear the term 'personality disorder'?

What are the responses of your colleagues when they hear the term?

HISTORICAL OVERVIEW

There are two classificatory systems for PD. The *International classification of diseases* (ICD), which incorporates mental disorders into a broader classification of medical conditions, is primarily used in Europe and was developed by the World Health Organization (WHO). The *Diagnostic and statistical manual* (DSM), which is specifically focused on psychiatric disorders, is primarily used in the USA and to a large extent Australia and New Zealand, and was developed by the American Psychiatric Association (APA).

In describing the history of PDs in the context of the DSM, Millon and Davis[1] outline how the first clinical interest in personality arose when psychiatrists at the end of the eighteenth century were drawn into the age-old arguments concerning free will, and whether certain moral transgressors are capable of understanding the consequences of their acts. The first psychiatrist to organize personality into categories was Kraeplin, who, in 1913, proposed two premorbid personality types to dementia

*Marie Crowe is an Associate Professor in the Department of Psychological Medicine and Centre for Postgraduate Studies at University of Otago, Christchurch, New Zealand. She also works as a clinical nurse specialist in adolescent mental health. Her current research is related to the use of psychotherapies for depression and bipolar disorder.
**Dave Carlyle is a Lecturer in the Department of Psychological Medicine, University of Otago, Christchurch, New Zealand, and a community mental health nurse with adults. His research interests include Lacanian discourse analysis and the role of the mental health nurse. His current research projects include a study of how mental health nurses make moral decisions and the effects of psychotherapy.

praecox and maniacal–depressive insanity – the *cyclothymic disposition* and the *autistic temperament*. However, many theorists began proposing different classificatory systems until attempts to reign in the confusion was a driving force behind the DSM-I (1952).[2] This text outlined five subclasses of PDs – personality pattern disturbances, personality trait disturbances, sociopathic personality disturbance, special symptom reactions and transient situational PDs. The text was revised in 1968 (DSM-II) as attempts were made to align the classification with the ICD-8. New personality syndromes were added and all but the sociopathic personality disorder removed. The DSM-III (1980)[3] was explicit in its aim to expunge theoretical biases and to establish a separate axis. Attempts were made to maintain compatibility with the ICD-9 and the PDs were grouped into three clusters: the first characterized by odd or eccentric behaviour; the second by dramatic, emotional or erratic behaviours; and the third by the notable presence of anxiety or fear. A significant refinement of the diagnostic criteria for each PD was made in the DSM-IV (1994),[4] and the next revision of this text is due for publication in 2010.

Reflection

How did you develop your understandings about 'personality disorder'?

DEFINITIONS

Both ICD-10[5] and the DSM-IV[4] define PD similarly: a PD is a type of condition consisting of *deeply ingrained* and *enduring* behaviour patterns manifesting themselves as *inflexible responses* to a broad range of *personal* and *social* situations. They represent either extreme or significant deviations from the way the average individual in a given culture perceives, thinks, feels and particularly relates to others. Such behaviour patterns tend to be stable and encompass multiple domains of behaviour and psychological functioning. They are frequently, but not always, associated with various degrees of subjective distress and problems of social performance (World Health Organization). However, there are some differences in how the different types of disorders are defined (Table 28.1).

TABLE 28.1 ICD-10 and DSM-IV personality disorders

Description	ICD-10	DSM-IV
Characterized by being suspicious, believes that other people will treat you wrongly, insists on own rights	Paranoid PD	Paranoid PD
Characterized by social detachment and restricted emotional expressions, indifferent to the emotional expressions of others and not interested in social relationships	Schizoid PD	Schizoid PD
Characterized by social and interpersonal deficits marked by acute discomfort with, and reduced capacity for, close relationships		Schizotypal PD
Characterized by callous unconcern for others, disregard for social norms, lack of remorse and tendency to frustration and aggression	Dissocial PD	Antisocial PD
Characterized by affective instability, impulsivity, fear of abandonment, unstable relationships, explosiveness and chronic feelings of emptiness	Emotionally unstable PD – Explosive type – Borderline type – Aggressive type	Borderline PD
Characterized by a need to always be the centre of attention, shallow and labile affectivity, theatricality and easily influenced by others	Histrionic PD	Histrionic PD
Characterized by preoccupation with details and rules, perfectionism, rigidity and excessive pedantry and adherence to social conventions	Anankastistic PD	Obsessive–compulsive PD
Characterized by a fear of being judged, social discomfort, fear of criticism or rejection and views self as socially inept and inferior	Anxious (avoidant) PD	Avoidant PD
Characterized by desperate need to be in a relationship, needs others to assume responsibility, avoids conflict, subordinates own needs to others and uncomfortable when alone	Dependent PD	Dependent PD
Characterized by grandiose sense of self-importance, a tendency to take advantage of others to meet own needs, and a strong sense of entitlement and need for admiration	Narcissistic PD	Narcissistic PD
Characterized by a pervasive pattern of negative attitudes and passive, usually disavowed resistance in interpersonal or occupational situations	Passive–aggressive PD	

PD, personality disorder.

Besides these two mainstream classificatory systems, another psychological model takes a dimensional approach to classifying personalities, referred to as the Big Five Factor Model.[6] This is concerned with the degree to which particular traits are evident in a person's personality: neuroticism, extraversion, agreeableness, conscientiousness, and openness to experience. It considers personality style to be on a continuum as opposed to the categorical approach of the other classifications, which take either a disordered or not approach.

Reflection

In your practice, how do nursing interventions differ for axis I and axis II disorders?

SOME PROBLEMS WITH THE DIAGNOSTIC CRITERIA

There are a number of problems with the way in which PDs are constructed by the two main psychiatric classificatory systems, DSM and ICD:

- the lack of diagnostic validity
- the lack of conceptual credibility
- the lack of scientific or theoretical rigour
- gender bias.

The lack of diagnostic validity

The PD categories raise the issue of diagnostic validity – the ability of a standard to measure what it claims to measure. The diagnostic criteria are highly subjective and judgemental and are based on an assumption about 'normal' personality when no such knowledge is available. There is also a lack of reliability in distinguishing one PD from another and a PD from other disorders, e.g. it is not clear where the boundaries of obsessive–compulsive personality disorder lie in relation to obsessive–compulsive disorder; paranoid personality disorder or schizotypal personality disorder and psychotic disorder; avoidant personality disorder and social phobia.

The lack of validity in the diagnostic categories has been noted by a number of authors (e.g. Kutchins and Kirk,[7] Pilgrim[8] and Tyrer[9]). The manuals have no consistent requirement that the everyday behaviours used as diagnostic criteria are actually the result of mental disorder and not the result of other life experiences.[7] The text generally evades the question of validity by its utilization of the construct of 'co-morbidity' – the simultaneous existence of more than one set of diagnostic criteria.

Tyrer[9] has noted that the degree of overlap between and among the different PDs is far too great and the specious use of the term 'co-morbidity' hides diagnostic

confusion. Moreover, there is insufficient emphasis on the concept that 'personality disorder' refers to long-term functioning, and too much reliance is placed on self-report. He concludes that these diagnostic categories still lack validity in clinical practice.

The two manuals also have different thresholds for diagnosis. The prevalence estimates in the ICD-10 are lower than those in the DSM-IV, which is possibly due to the higher threshold for disorder in the ICD-10 (a greater proportion of criteria must be present for the diagnosis to be made). This suggests that behaviour in one cultural context, for example the USA, is more likely to be considered disordered than if it were displayed in a European context.

The lack of conceptual credibility

The major concepts used in constructing PD in both the ICD and DSM are:

1. an enduring pattern of inner experience and behaviour
2. leads to distress or impairment, and
3. deviations from the expectations of the individual's culture.

A number of studies have found that there is a lack of endurance or stability in what is supposed to represent an 'enduring pattern'. One example is Zanarini et al.,[10] whose 6-year prospective follow-up of the phenomenology of borderline personality disorder found that remissions in symptoms were common over the 6 years: 75 per cent of the participants had full remission of symptoms over 6 years and within 2 years there was a 30–40 per cent remission rate. This suggests that when a diagnosis is given at a particular point in time it is based on what is observed during that time period with little concern for evidence of whether these symptoms are enduring.

It is also debateable whether a substantial amount of the criteria provided as evidence of PD represent clinically significant distress or impairment in functioning. The following are some examples of when it is difficult to understand how the behaviour is either distressing or impairing to the point of requiring psychiatric intervention:

- schizoid PD[4,p.568] – 'appears indifferent to the praise or criticism of others'
- schizotypal PD[4,p.645] – 'behaviour or appearance that is odd, eccentric or peculiar'
- histrionic PD[4,p.568] – 'consistently uses physical appearance to draw attention to self'
- narcissistic PD[4,p.661] – 'is interpersonally exploitative i.e. takes advantage of others to achieve his or her own needs'.

The classificatory systems pathologize a range of behaviours that are not necessarily distressing or impairing to the individual.

There is no scientific evidence that proves biological aetiology conclusively, which suggests that what is considered to be a PD can also be regarded as a cultural construction. As Hirshbein[11] has noted, what gets called scientific truth is very contingent on social, cultural and professional factors. Some authors have argued that PDs reflect social trends in Western culture, including a growing sense of social isolation and the dissolution of social structures that lent coherence to self-identity.[12]

Lack of scientific or theoretical rigour

The criteria for PDs lack scientific evidence and yet actively eschew theoretical rigour. The current constructions of PD are described as 'atheoretical' but assume biological or neurological aetiology, despite a continuing lack of evidence for this supposition. This is based on an observational approach that assumes that 'patterns of inner experience' are observable by clinicians.

Despite its reliance on scientific objectivity as the basis for practice, psychiatry has come with little scientific evidence to support its assertions. The assumption that mental disorder is biological and observable through scientific methods is contradicted in the DSM-IV with its statements that 'no laboratory findings have been identified that are diagnostic of schizophrenia'[4,p.28] (or major depressive episode or bipolar disorder or any of the PDs). It goes on to state that 'perhaps the most common associated physical findings are motor abnormalities. Most of these are likely to be related to side effects from treatment with antipsychotic medication'![4,p.280]

Gender bias

There is considerable research into the gender bias inherent in the different personality disorders, and the DSM-IV has identified that three of the PDs are diagnosed more often in females (dependent, histrionic and borderline) and six of the PDs are more commonly diagnosed in males (paranoid, schizoid, schizotypal, antisocial, narcissistic and compulsive). Hartig and Widiger[13] found the following gender ratios with each disorder:

Paranoid	Male > female
Schizotypal	Male > female
Borderline	Three females:one male
Narcissistic	One to three males:one female
Dependent	Female > male
Schizoid	Male > female
Antisocial	Male > female
Histrionic	Female > male
Avoidant	Male = female
Compulsive	Two males:one female

Many authors have identified the gender bias inherent in the diagnostic criteria and have suggested that many of the criteria reflect excessive displays of stereotypical gendered behaviour.

Reflection

What difficulties have you encountered nursing someone who has a diagnosis of 'personality disorder'? How have you managed these difficulties?

THE CLINICAL SETTING

The use of the term 'personality disorder' is frequently, and sometimes capriciously, used in clinical settings, but is based on some flawed assumptions. However, the behaviours of individuals who are labelled in this way are often challenging and distressing for mental health nurses. The 'personality disorders' that are considered to require the most ongoing clinical intervention are those constructed as 'borderline' or 'antisocial'.

Some authors have called for the reform of borderline personality disorder as a psychiatric diagnosis[14,15] because of its clear relationship to past trauma, its lack of stability as a diagnosis and its similarity to the post-traumatic stress disorder. McLean et al.[15] have identified high rates of sexual abuse in borderline personality disorder and complex post-traumatic stress disorder. Virtually all the women with a history of childhood sexual abuse met diagnostic criteria for both borderline personality disorder and complex post-traumatic stress disorder. They suggest that these findings support the proposal that such symptoms be subsumed as complex post-traumatic stress disorder. One could reasonably expect that if these people were given this diagnosis the way in which clinicians perceive and respond to them would alter.

It is curious that antisocial (dissocial) personality disorder is regarded as a mental disorder when there is little if any subjective distress associated with it. Any distress is possibly only as a result of contact with justice systems. By including people who exhibit primarily criminal (or unempathic behaviours) it could be argued that psychiatry is attempting to extend its domain into 'bad' rather than 'mad' behaviours. It is not clear why this should be the case. One study in Britain found that 48.7 per cent of all prisoners met criteria for antisocial personality disorder[16] and psychiatry is unable to offer any successful treatments or interventions that diminish such behaviours.

Other 'personality disorders' most commonly appear in the clinical setting as co-morbid to a more significant mental disorder. Dependent, avoidant and obsessive–compulsive personality disorders appear to be diagnosed as co-morbid with major depression, and most of these symptoms no longer persist past an improvement in mood. The way in which nurses construct behaviours that are challenging or difficult as personality disorders or symptomatic of overwhelming distress effectively forms the basis to the way in which they respond. If the nurse regards the behaviours as personality disorders then the consequent response is to employ a medical model approach. If the nurse constructs the behaviours as responses to overwhelming distress then his or her course of action and mode of response become more client centred.

Reflection

What interventions have been used in your clinical area to treat someone with a diagnosis of 'personality disorder'? Were they successful or not?

MENTAL HEALTH NURSING CARE

The use of psychiatric discourse limits the practice of mental health nursing to medication dispensers and agents of social control in relation to those people whose behaviour is so challenging and disturbing. We are proposing here what we call a discursive approach to providing mental health nursing care for someone experiencing overwhelming distress:

- recognizing the nature of the distress
- making connections between how the person has learned to cope with their fears and her or his current distress
- situating the fear and distress in its sociocultural context
- promoting acceptance of difference
- exploring alternative subject positions for managing distress.

The aim of this approach is to assist the person experiencing overwhelming distress to develop alternative subject positions that demonstrate an awareness of the sociocultural context of the development and expression of that distress, and represent a self-image that is more emotionally aware and can engage in interactions with others as an equal participant. The focus of these interventions is to encourage awareness of how the person positions him- or herself in relation to others, and the patterns of interaction that perpetuate the feelings of distress.

Recognizing the nature of distress

The recognition of the nature of the person's distress can begin by seeking information about the person's feelings and relationships with others, particularly incidents in which the distress is triggered. This recognition is part of a psychotherapeutic process of recognizing the person and accepting his or her differences while helping that person to recognize and accept him- or herself and

develop alternative, more fulfilling subject positions. If an individual's behaviour is recognized as symptomatic of a personality disorder which suggests a lack of hope this may intensify the person's distressing feelings.

Establishing connections

The nurse can then help the person to make connections between the sources of distress and the effects of this on his or her life. This involves helping the person to put into words something that is often very painful and requires a trusting relationship with the nurse. This relationship includes a trust in the nurse's skills and the nurse's ability to contain strong outpourings of feelings. The establishment of connections also involves enabling the person to see how patterns from the past shape and give meaning to the present. This involves exploring how apparently disconnected present day experiences, behaviours and feelings may be connected to past fears and anxieties.

Situating the distress in its sociocultural context

The nurse can assist individuals to explore their experiences of distress within the sociocultural context in which they occurred. This is a sociocultural context in which some subject positions are apportioned more value than others. Such positions reflect the Western cultural norms of unitariness, rationality, productivity and moderation.[17] Feelings of distress may be reinforced by considering the problem as faulty individual functioning without taking into account the person's sociocultural context.

The nurse can begin this by raising questions about the values and beliefs that underpin the person's perspective of distressing events to enable the person to begin his or her own questioning. This questioning can be used to explore how these culturally imposed values and beliefs may be contributing to or maintaining feelings of distress.

Promoting the acceptance of difference

The nurse could help individuals accept differences in the way they may experience a sense of self and the attributions they make about others. An initial step in this process is to help individuals to identify and name these feelings. The nurse can encourage the individuals to explore the expectations that they have of others and begin to hypothesize about what others may expect of them. The emphasis is on helping people to develop the capacity to reflect on their own and others' behaviour and interactions. An important aspect of this process involves helping people to manage ambiguity and contradictions in their relations with others.

Exploring alternative subject positions

This nursing approach can also provide the person with the opportunity to engage with different subject positions in his or her interactions with others. These subject positions can be regarded as those modes of being that constitute a sense of self. People have a range of subject positions from which they can respond to others. The performance of particular subject positions can be regarded as particular intersections of culture, gender, class and race. A sense of self is constituted by the repeated performance of particular subject positions, and meaning is determined by the subject positions to which people have access. The meanings that can be attributed to subject positions are developed through relations with others and the experiences of acceptance or rejection. The experimentation with alternative subject positions within the support of the nurse–patient relationship allows for this creation of meaning.

CLINICAL SCENARIO

The case of Jane A

Jane is a 22-year-old woman who had a very unstable childhood, having been abandoned by her birth mother at age 6 months after she was admitted to an alcohol treatment centre. She has not met her father and has no knowledge of him or his whereabouts. She was made a ward of the state and during her childhood she lived in a series of foster homes and generally described her experience in these homes as unhappy. She performed poorly at school and was often expelled because of disruptive behaviour. In three of her foster homes, beginning at the age of 6 years, she was sexually abused by adult and teenage males from these family homes.

Jane describes her upbringing as 'crappy' and states she never felt cared for. She gave an example of having hurt herself while playing outside one day and being told by her foster mother to go to her room and 'get over it'. Subsequently, it was discovered she had a bone fracture in her forearm.

Jane uses alcohol and other illicit drugs on a daily basis. She says that she could quit these at any time, but chooses not to as these help her 'get through the day and the night'. Without these she says she has too many nightmares and would not be able to sleep.

She has lived independently since the age of 16 years, in boarding houses and flats. She came under the care of the mental health services at the age of 18 years after presenting to emergency services having taken an overdose of over-the-counter medications. At that time, Jane stated that she had wanted to die as she had been raped 2 weeks before by a fellow resident of her boarding house. Following this presentation, and subsequent admission to an acute inpatient psychiatric ward she was diagnosed as having a borderline personality disorder.

Since that time, Jane has presented to community services or after hours emergency services many times having taken non-lethal overdoses. One year ago, Jane presented having made a deep laceration in her inner forearm. Presentations with lacerations that have required medical intervention to close these wounds have continued. Often, Jane will present to her community nurse in distress, spend time with her and become more settled. Sometimes following this, she may present again within a short period of time again in a distressed state.

The current view of the community team is that Jane has a severe borderline personality disorder. Jane has been referred for alcohol and drug counselling, but has failed to comply with attendance at appointments. She has not responded significantly to treatment with antidepressants and anti-psychotic medications, although she remains on these. She is also prescribed sleeping medications and benzodiazepines. Jane is described by the outpatient team as a 'difficult, demanding and challenging' patient who requires a lot of staff time. The current aim of the treatment plan that the team has developed is to limit the amount of time available to Jane and to avoid hospital admissions as it is believed that all this 'will only make her worse'.

The team does acknowledge that admission is necessary at times though to 'keep her safe' when she is highly suicidal. When Jane is admitted to a psychiatric hospital this is to the intensive care unit and often results in conflict, further episodes of self-harm and, at times, Jane needs to be physically restrained by nursing staff. Staff there describe Jane as attention-seeking, manipulative, overinvolved with other patients and disruptive on the ward.

Jane's story

Jane says she has never had a mother. She says she feels abandoned, uncared for, unloved and unlovable. She has not felt anyone has ever kept her safe and protected her from harm. Jane says she was sexually abused by men all her life and still is. She has felt angry about this and when she was a teenager often was unable to control her anger. This often led to her getting into physical fights with others and becoming hurt or injured. She feels she was often told it was her fault when this happened.

Now Jane says she just feels empty. 'There is nothing left inside. I have done so many bad things I might as well die, I can't go on.' She says she no longer feels angry at others as 'it's not their fault, its mine'.

Jane says though that she is scared of dying, and would rather just go to sleep and never wake up. Jane tends to use alcohol and other drugs to dull her feelings of distress and to 'make myself unconscious'. She says that she cuts herself not to die but that she often 'feels good' for a short time afterwards. 'It doesn't make the bad feelings go away, but I can feel different.' Leading up to cutting, sometimes 'I think about it for days before I do it. I can think of nothing else and that's kind of good.'

Jane says she does not like going to hospital as none of the nurses there like her and just want her discharged. She says she feels they do not care about her and they 'always tell me to go to my room when I'm upset or crying'. She says that being in the 'nut house' makes her feel worse and can make her angry again, particularly when she sees other patients being treated 'badly' and she feels compelled to involve herself in the care of these patients.

Often when she sees her community nurse, who she describes as 'really caring', she is able to talk and can feel better afterwards, but when she gets home to her flat she looks around and nothing has changed. She just feels bad and empty again, a brittle shell with nothing inside.

Recognizing the nature of distress

In the Jane A scenario, the perception of Jane's experience is only partially complete, substituting her experience for clinicians' observations, e.g. observing that she is 'non-compliant' with attending to treatment for her alcohol and drug use. Filling in around these observations to complete the picture are transferential experiences of the clinicians themselves, e.g. when she is described as 'difficult, demanding and challenging'. These are in fact experiences the clinicians have had and are not attributes of Jane herself. The assignment of invalid behavioural labels will intensify Jane's feelings of distress. By adopting an alternative approach that recognizes Jane's own experience of her world can be validating for her and be confirming that her experiences have been real and are being understood as such. Without this validation of her then it will be difficult for Jane to safely explore other potential ways of being.

Establishing connections

With acknowledgement and acceptance of her experiences and her distress as real the nurse is able to offer the opportunity for a real human connection. This is not an easy situation for the nurse, who may be required to engage with Jane in very emotionally charged narratives. Jane's experience has been to be told she should contain her strong emotions and 'get over it'. The underlying message in that is that other people are unable to deal with her feelings and the nurse here with her now may be the same. Jane will undertake some degree of testing in order to confirm her assumption of others who are there ostensibly to care for her, but do not. Without some testing then, for Jane, trust in the nurse's strength, skills and abilities cannot be verified and therefore it limits Jane's potential for engaging in a more open relationship. Without this confidence in the nurse, a move

from a position of self-defence against invalidation will not be achieved and exploration of other ways of being in the world will not be possible.

Situating the fear and distress in its sociocultural context

Here, in assigning Jane a dysfunctional personality and the invalidation of her life experience that led her to this point will confirm her assumption that it is her responsibility for what has happened to her. This will close off her ability to consider other potential ways of conceiving of herself and of her position and way of being in the world.

Promoting the acceptance of difference

By the nurse demonstrating an acceptance of Jane as a valid person with real experiences the relationship between them can be nurtured into areas of therapeutic development. With a relationship established then areas of ambiguity and contradiction in their relationship can begin to be explored. The nurse can then more effectively and more ably extrapolate these into other relationships that Jane has and will have with others.

Exploring alternative subject positions

Jane has developed a view of herself as 'bad' and 'unlovable' over a long period of time. She has been told repeatedly that the bad things that have happened to her have been her fault. Her place in the world and her relationship with others has been confined to a narrow and distressing role. With patience the nurse can support Jane to explore alternative ways of interacting with others that may lead to more meaningful and fulfilling experiences for Jane.

Reflection

Could this approach be used in your practice?
What might be some of the problems with the approach?
How could your practice focus more on the person's story than on their diagnosis?

SUMMARY

By adopting a position of being interested in the person and the story of their experiences, while being aware of one's own assumptions with regard to the person sitting in front of you, it is possible to engage with that person in a way that could offer an effective avenue for change to occur (see Chapter 2). Latent potential for change can become lost to opportunity when the nurse becomes

bound to preconceived notions of outcomes associated with particular diagnostic labels. By attending to and altering the inner aspects of our own selves it may just be possible to alter the outer aspects of the lives of others.

The diagnosis of personality disorder is often fraught with problems and is not particularly useful in directing the approach to mental health nursing care. However, this is not to deny that people who receive such diagnoses are not experiencing significant distress. It has been proposed that working the person's narrative and engaging in a manner that allows the person to explore less distressing subject positions may be a more effective approach to mental health nursing care.

REFERENCES

1. Millon T, Davis R. Conceptions of personality disorders: historical perspectives, the DSMs and future directions. In: Livesley WJ (ed.). *The DSM-IV personality disorders*. New York, NY: Guilford Press, 1995: 3–28.

2. American Psychiatric Association. *Diagnostic and statistical manual of mental disorders*, 1st edn. Washington, DC: American Psychiatric Association, 1952.

3. American Psychiatric Association. *Diagnostic and statistical manual of mental disorders*, 3rd edn. Washington, DC: American Psychiatric Association, 1980.

4. American Psychiatric Association. *Diagnostic and Statistical Manual of Mental Disorders*. Washington, DC: American Psychiatric Association, 1994.

5. World Health Organization. *The ICD-10 classification of mental and behavioural disorders: clinical descriptions and diagnostic guidelines*. Geneva, Switzerland: World Health Organization, 1992.

6. Goldberg LR. The structure of phenotypic personality traits. *American Psychologist* 1993; **48**: 26–34.

7. Kutchins H, Kirk S. *Making us crazy*. New York, NY: Free Press, 1997.

8. Pilgrim D. Disordered personalities and disordered concepts. *Journal of Mental Health* 2001; **10**: 253–65.

9. Tyrer P. Are personality disorders well classified in DSM-IV? In: Livesley WJ (ed.). *The DSM-IV personality disorders*. New York, NY: The Guilford Press, 1995: 29–42.

10. Zanarini MC, Frankenburg FR, Hennen J, Silk KR. The longitudinal course of borderline psychopathology: 6-year prospective follow-up of the phenomenology of borderline personality disorder. *American Journal of Psychiatry* 2003; **160**: 274–83.

11. Hirshbein LD. Science, gender, and the emergence of depression in American psychiatry, 1952–1980. *Journal of the History of Medicine & Allied Sciences* 2006; **61**: 187–216.

12. Millon T. Sociocultural conceptions of the borderline personality. *Psychiatric Clinics of North America* 2000; **23**: 123–36.

13. Hartig C, Widiger T. Gender differences in the diagnosis of mental disorders: conclusions and controversies of the DSM-IV. *Psychological Bulletin* 1998; **123**: 260–78.

14. Tyrer P. Borderline personality disorder: a motley diagnosis in need of reform. *Lancet* 1999; **354**: 2095–6.

15. McLean LM, Gallop R, Zanarini MC. Implications of childhood sexual abuse for adult borderline personality disorder and complex posttraumatic stress disorder. *American Journal of Psychiatry* 2003; **160**: 369–71.

16. Yang M, Ullrich S, Roberts A, Coid J. Childhood institutional care and personality disorder traits in adulthood: findings from the British national surveys of psychiatric morbidity. *American Journal of Orthopsychiatry* 2007; **77**: 67–75.

17. Crowe M. Constructing normality: a discourse analysis of the DSM-IV. *Journal of Psychiatric and Mental Health Nursing* 2000; **7**: 69–77.

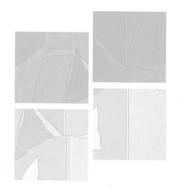

CHAPTER 29

The person who experiences mental health and substance use problems

Philip D. Cooper*

... services for people with 'dual diagnosis' – mental health and substance misuse – the most challenging clinical problem we face.

Department of Health[1]

INTRODUCTION

This chapter highlights the key issues for the person experiencing co-existing mental health and substance use problems. Here, we explore some of the reasons why people experiencing mental health problems use substances and identify the processes involved when a person attempts to make changes to their substance use. Understanding the motivations for using substances, the nature of change and recognizing the long-term nature of work with individuals with co-existing problems reduces the likelihood of professionals becoming frustrated in their interactions with clients. This increases the likelihood of worker and client remaining positively engaged in therapeutic relationships.

WHAT IS 'DUAL DIAGNOSIS'?

The term 'dual diagnosis' is commonly applied to individuals who experience a co-existing mental health and substance use problem(s) (drugs and/or alcohol). Ryrie and McGowan[2] indicate 'dual diagnosis' encompasses a diverse group of individuals with differing types of mental disorder, with varying degrees of severity, who may be using one or more psychoactive substances in varying frequencies and in varying amounts.[2] This deliberately broad and inclusive definition reflects the wide range of co-existing problems seen by clinicians on a daily basis.

*Philip D. Cooper is a Practice Educator at Suffolk Mental Health Partnership NHS Trust. He has a background in assertive outreach, community mental health and acute admissions wards. Phil is also the editor of *Mental Health and Substance Use: Dual Diagnosis* (www.informaworld.com/mhsu).

The term has been criticized as a restrictive and unhelpful label. It encourages a focus on two distinct problems, which may lead to inaccurate case formulations and inappropriate interventions or no intervention at all. 'Dual diagnosis' is more than simply 'two problems' or 'diagnoses'. Individuals often experience a multitude of problems. Compared with those with a mental health problem alone, individuals with a dual diagnosis are likely to experience:

- more severe mental health problems
- homelessness/unstable housing
- increased risk of being violent
- increased risk of victimization
- more contact with the criminal justice system
- family problems
- history of childhood abuse (sexual/physical).
  They are also:
- more likely to slip through the gap between services
- less likely to be compliant with treatment.[3,4]

The needs of individuals with co-existing problems are complex and the relationship between their mental health and substance use is often one of mutual dependence. The effect of one will undoubtedly affect the other. Attempting to separate and address mental health and substance use as individual problems can be fraught with difficulty. Adopting a holistic approach, which recognizes and respects the relationship between an individual's mental health and his or her substance use is therefore essential. In recognition of these complex issues, this chapter avoids the term 'dual diagnosis' in favour of *co-existing problems*, to emphasize that mental health and substance use problems exist together and should be addressed as one.

PREVALENCE OF CO-EXISTING PROBLEMS

Substance use is seen as usual, rather than exceptional, among the mental health population.[5] The high level of co-existing problems in mental health service users has become increasingly recognized over the past 20 years. This may be linked to the rising levels of substance use across the general population and/or due to an increased awareness and identification of co-existing problems by professionals.[3]

Approximately one-third of the UK mental health population has a substance use problem and half of the individuals seen by substance use services have some form of mental health problem.[3] Substance use is implicated in up to 50 per cent of psychiatric admissions.[6] This figure rises to 73 per cent when patients have a diagnosis of schizophrenia.[7] The resulting hospital admissions are estimated to be 1.8 times as long as for those with a mental health problem alone.[8]

WHY DO PEOPLE WITH A MENTAL HEALTH PROBLEM USE SUBSTANCES?

Alcohol, tobacco and cannabis are the most commonly used substances among individuals with a mental health problem, as they are in the general population. This is closely followed by stimulants and heroin. The physical, psychological and social effects of these substances are widely documented and are not covered in this chapter. However, it is important that professionals have an understanding of these substances, and their effects. Therefore, readers are directed to *KFX: Learning of Substance* website (www.ixion.demon.co.uk) for further information.

There are several theories why people with a mental health problem use substances.

- *For the same reasons as others in the community.*[9,10] People with mental health problems generally use substances for the same reasons as everyone else, e.g. to socialize, celebrate, reduce anxiety or simply to relax.
- *As an attempt to alleviate the symptoms of a mental health problem.*[11] The symptoms of many mental health problems lead to people feeling unmotivated, socially withdrawn and anxious. The use of alcohol and/or drugs can induce feelings of motivation and confidence and reduce anxiety in certain situations. In addition, individuals with a mental health problem may find it more socially acceptable to be part of a drug subculture, as opposed to a mental health subculture.
- *To reduce the side-effects of medication.*[9] Psychotropic medication can lead to feelings of apathy, poor motivation and depersonalization. The effects of certain substances may assist people in overcoming the unpleasant side-effects of medication. For example, some studies have shown cannabis to have an anticholinergic effect, reducing tremors and muscle stiffness commonly found in Parkinson's disease, or as the result of side-effects of anti-psychotic medication.[12]
- *Substance use as a coping strategy.* Individuals may have learnt and believe that the use of a substance aids their ability to cope with the stresses of daily life or certain situations.

Understanding why a person uses substances is essential. For some, the use of alcohol and/or drugs can be a pleasurable experience that does not result in harm. For others, the use of substances assists them in managing life and/or physical and/or mental health problems. The perceived benefits of substance use in managing problems are short lived and the risk of harm is increased with repeated use. Therefore, it is important to explore a person's reasons for using substances and provide interventions based on their beliefs and understanding of substance use.

APPROACHES TO TREATMENT

While concern for this group has increased in recent years, current service provision remains unable to adequately meet their needs.[1,8] Traditionally, the NHS has provided two service models of care:

1 *serial*: individuals are treated for one condition before progressing to treatment for the second, or
2 *parallel*: individuals are treated for both conditions simultaneously but by different services.

These models of treatment promote a culture in which health problems are treated as separate entities. Service users are often passed between services, with neither service feeling it can meet the needs of the individual. Service users frequently fall between this gap in services and their needs remain unmet. Serial and parallel approaches are viewed as inadequate for individuals with co-existing problems. The Department of Health (DoH)[5] highlights that individuals with co-existing problems have the right to high-quality, patient-focused and integrated care, and call for an *integrated service model*, in which service users' needs are addressed by one service. Mental health services have been identified to take lead responsibility in providing care for this group, referred to as *mainstreaming*.[5] The DoH,[5] Care Services Improvement Partnership (CSIP),[13] and Turning Point[4] suggest a multiagency approach is essential and highlight the importance of shared care as an effective intervention for this group.

The four-stage model

Osher and Kofoed[14] identify four stages of treatment for individuals with co-existing problems. The model aids clinicians in acknowledging the long-term nature of the work and in identifying and offering appropriate and timely interventions.

1 *Engagement*: the development and maintenance of a therapeutic clinician–client relationship that is empathic, non-judgemental and non-confrontational.
2 *Motivation (persuasion)*: a non-confrontational approach which draws on the principles of motivational interviewing by exploring ambivalence and motivation to change.
3 *Active treatment*: can take place only if goals are realistic and set by the client. Unrealistic goals will reinforce feelings of failure and self-worthlessness if the client is unable to achieve them.
4 *Relapse prevention*: educating clients about their early warning signs, anxiety management and coping skills training.

SCREENING AND ASSESSMENT

Competent assessment is viewed as the first step in a 'stepped care' approach to co-existing problems.[13]

In addition to being concerned with gathering information, the assessment can assist in establishing and enhancing the engagement process.[15] Four objectives are identified when carrying out an assessment, which can be applied to both a mental health and a substance use assessment.[16]

1 *Measurement*: nature, duration and frequency of the problem.
2 *Clarification*: how, where and when the problem occurs.
3 *Explanation*: the impact of the problem on the individual and others.
4 *Variation*: possible changes in the pattern of the problem.

Assessing co-existing problems requires drawing together a mental health and substance use assessment. Both assessments possess a number of core features, including history of the presenting problem, personal history and current social situation. However, each requires elaboration on the specific areas it assesses and may potentially be a lengthy process.

Problems may arise when the person being assessed finds it difficult to communicate needs, or when memory and concentration are poor.[3] It is unlikely that a full understanding of an individual's presenting problems and the relationship between them will be achieved in one session. A comprehensive assessment is likely to take a number of sessions, weeks or even months, using a number of methods. This highlights the need for assessment to be an ongoing process. Active feedback of assessment outcomes, presented in a non-confrontational, empathic and user-friendly manner, can be regarded as a minimal intervention[17] and should routinely occur.

The 'primary' diagnosis

Professionals may become preoccupied with diagnosis during the assessment of individuals with co-existing problems and attempt to define the 'primary' problem. This can prove a difficult task because of the nature and complexity of the individuals presenting problems.[3] Co-existing problems do not typically fall neatly into 'primary' and 'secondary' categories and the relationship between the two often changes over time.[18]

Attempts to identify which problem came 'first' are seen as unhelpful in the treatment of this client group. Assessments should instead attempt to determine the relative importance of each problem and how they interact with, and affect, one another. The relationship between them is most often one of mutual influence.[19] Identifying a *primary diagnosis* can often be seen as an attempt to redirect service users to other services, and the use of assessment for punitive reasons, such as refusal of care, should be avoided.[20]

A *primary* focus may also lead to the signs of a mental health or substance use problem being overlooked. The symptoms of mental health problems and signs of substance use can overlap and both share common features. For example, a younger person who regularly uses cannabis may experience social withdrawal, flattening of affect, paranoid ideation and vague auditory hallucinations. This may be attributed to cannabis use and individuals could be advised to stop using cannabis, add structure to their day and be redirected to voluntary services. However, it is possible the individual is experiencing the prodromal phase of a first psychotic episode. Therefore, it is essential to ensure that screening and assessment of an individual's mental health and substance use is thorough and undertaken routinely for all clients in contact with mental health services. Early interventions are essential in improving the long-term outcomes and functioning of individuals with co-existing problems.

Screening tools

A range of screening tools are available to assist clinicians in detecting mental health and substance use problems. However, specific and effective screening tools for identifying co-existing problems are unavailable at present.

Considering the high prevalence of substance use among mental health service users, routine substance use screening for all individuals in contact with services is advocated. However, screening does not replace a full and comprehensive assessment but should form part of an initial assessment. When screening identifies problematic substance use, the clinician proceeds to complete a full assessment of the individual's substance use. The Alcohol, Smoking and Substance Involvement Screening Test[21] (ASSIST) identifies hazardous, harmful and dependent use of a range of substances, including cannabis and stimulants, and is an extremely valuable tool. Croton[22] provides a useful review to screening and assessment tools for mental health and substance use problems, which is available online.

ENGAGEMENT

Engagement is described as the development and maintenance of a therapeutic clinician–client relationship that is empathic, non-judgemental and non-confrontational.[14] The aim of engagement is to understand individuals' view of their problems and respond to their needs accordingly.[23] Acceptance of the client's substance use is important at this stage and care should focus on the individual's immediate needs, as opposed to the cessation of substances.[2] Assisting in areas such as housing, finances, daily living and leisure activities are essential elements of the engagement process.[24]

Professionals should be flexible and adaptive in their response to meeting clients' needs.[25] A collaborative

approach between the client and professional is crucial. Clients must be central to all decisions made, thereby increasing their level of control and improving self-efficacy. The value of the engagement process in building a foundation of trust and mutual respect between the client and care coordinator cannot be overemphasized. Without a process of effective engagement, subsequent interventions may not be successful in their aim.

Three main barriers to effective engagement are identified.[26]

1 *Services*: separate systems of care (mental health and substance use); exclusion, rather than inclusion criteria; clash of treatment philosophies (abstinence versus harm minimization); lack of resources.
2 *Staff*: lack of training; poor communication; negative attitudes; focus on primary diagnosis; treatment not matched to need; policing not treating; lack of time.
3 *Service users*: services do not meet needs; not ready to change; past negative experiences of services; not being listened to/heard; fear of disclosing substance use; fear of losing peers/symptom control/side-effect management.

Professionals' values, attitudes and beliefs can affect the quality of care provided and the process of engagement will undoubtedly be affected by negative attitudes. Negative attitudes toward substance users are commonly held by professionals and arise from a lack of understanding and inadequate preparation in pre-/post-registration training. Individuals who use substances are often viewed as unmotivated, manipulative and self-destructive,[3] and professionals may find it difficult to work with someone perceived as demanding. Many professionals feel ill-equipped to address the substance use needs of individuals with mental health problems. Clinicians may feel unable or reluctant to engage with this client group for a number of reasons.[27]

- *Role adequacy*: a perceived lack of knowledge and skill in identifying and responding to substance-using clients.
- *Role legitimacy*: uncertainty as to whether, or how far, harmful substance use falls within their role as a mental health professional.
- *Role support*: insufficient access or support from specialist services/clinicians should they identify a harmful substance user.

When clinicians feel uncertain in either or all of these areas, negative attitudes are high. However, the provision of training and ongoing support has been shown to increase clinicians' confidence in role adequacy, legitimacy and support and improve their attitudes and response to substance-using clients.[27] This highlights the need for comprehensive training packages to be available to all staff working with individuals at risk of co-existing problems.

BEHAVIOUR CHANGE AND THE CYCLE OF CHANGE

Professionals often find it frustrating working with individuals who appear unmotivated and unwilling to change, or who are unable to maintain changes in behaviour. It is not unusual for staff to become dismissive and unsupportive of clients during repeated attempts at change. However, changing behaviour is difficult both to achieve and to maintain. It is uncommon to achieve a change in behaviour on the first occasion and it may take a number of serious attempts before the chosen goal is reached.

Often, many other factors are involved, apart from motivation and willpower, that affect an individual's ability to maintain a behaviour change. Relationships, social and financial pressures, and fluctuations in mental state may all impede change attempts. Changes achieved during admission to hospital, for example, may not be maintained at discharge, when the client faces the same stressors that led to admission. External pressures and influences are often not acknowledged by professionals, who then become disillusioned with repeated patterns of admission involving substance use. Dismissive and unsupportive attitudes can arise and beliefs that 'a leopard never changes its spots' may be present. This wisdom is true; leopards cannot change their spots. However, people can change their behaviour.

The cycle of change[28] (Figure 29.1) assists clinicians in understanding the process of change, identifying an individual's readiness to change, and matching subsequent interventions to reflect this. Equally, the model is useful for clients in aiding understanding of their own experience of change. Moreover, it assists in viewing relapse as part of a natural process and *not* as a failure. Each time a person moves round the cycle of change, they develop existing and learn new coping strategies. This enhances their ability to manage subsequent change attempts and increases the likelihood of maintaining new behaviours. The model comprises four stages.

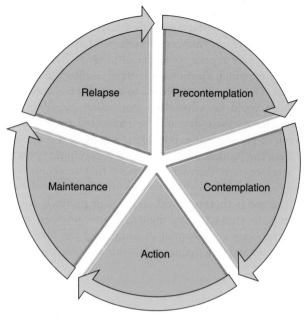

Figure 29.1 **Cycle of change**

1 *Pre-contemplation.* At this stage, the individual is not aware of a problem. This could be because of ambivalence, denial or selective exposure to information. As the individual becomes aware of the problem, progression to the next phase is made possible.
2 *Contemplation.* At this point, the individual identifies that something is wrong and begins to think seriously about behaviour change. Ambivalence is common during this phase. This stage may last for a few weeks to many years, and some individuals never progress beyond this point.
3 *Action.* Here, the individual makes a commitment to alter the problematic behaviour. This is a brief stage; when the decision has been made, the individual progresses to the next stage.
4 *Maintenance.* At this point, the new behaviour is strengthened and develops into self-efficacy; the individual's feeling of being in control is maximized. At this stage, an individual may exit the cycle of change.

At the maintenance stage, the individual may temporarily lapse as a result of the extreme effort required to maintain the change in behaviour. Occasionally, this extends to relapse, in which case the individual often goes back to the contemplation stage of the cycle. On average, a typical self-changer makes three revolutions of the change cycle before exiting into a relatively dependency-free life.[29] However, some individuals do become arrested at one particular stage and change may not be achievable.

Appropriate interventions to assist people in changing behaviour need to be offered at the right time, by the right person and in the right way. It is essential that the individual and professional are in agreement as to which stage of change is relevant at a given time. Any resistance to therapeutic interventions often comes as a direct result of the clinician and client working at different stages. Interventions not matched to an individual's stage of change are unlikely to result in positive outcomes. This can have negative consequences for the individual, who may perceive themselves as a failure, thus further reducing self-esteem.

Reflection

Despite the difficulties in changing our own behaviour, we often place unrealistic expectations on clients to maintain change at the first attempt. Recognizing our own difficulties in negotiating change can help us to become more therapeutically engaged in supporting clients on a long-term basis.

- Think of a time when you attempted to change your behaviour – perhaps stop smoking or lose weight.
- How long did you think about changing your behaviour before attempting it? Days, weeks, months, years? Are you still thinking about it?
- How did you feel when you first made this change? Happy, sad, irritable, relaxed?
- When did you find it most difficult to maintain the changes?
- What stressors led to your lapse back into old habits?
- How did you feel about yourself when you were unable to maintain your change?
- What did you learn about yourself and how you cope with stressful situations?
- How many times did you attempt to change before succeeding?
- Think about a client you worked with who has attempted to change his or her behaviour on a number of occasions. Do you think the client experienced similar thoughts and feelings?

INTERVENTIONS AND TREATMENT

Many interventions share common themes and have been proven beneficial in their respective fields (mental health or substance use). However, evidence for their efficacy in the treatment of co-existing problems is limited, although early studies appear to indicate that they are as effective for this client group.

The importance of supportive and collaborative partnerships with clients cannot be underestimated in achieving positive treatment outcomes. Clients must be central to all decisions, and goals should be identified by the individual and not clinician or service led. Interventions do not have to be abstinence. For some, this goal may be unachievable and even undesirable. Assisting individuals to use substances in a safer manner and/or at a reduced level is equally important in the management of substance use problems.

Brief intervention

Brief intervention (BI) is an approach that is typically less intensive in terms of time than traditional treatment methods. BI may range from 5–10 minutes of giving information to three to five individual or group sessions. BI is usually opportunistic and aimed at non-dependent substance users whose use is harmful but who are not experiencing consequential major health problems. BI is motivational in nature and should encourage the individual to conclude that a reduction in use, or less harmful use, is beneficial. Information, written and verbal, should be provided regarding the health risks associated with the particular substance use and any advice given should be tailored to individual needs. BI is particularly beneficial for individuals at the contemplation stage of change.

Bein et al.[30] identified six elements shown to be effective in brief intervention, described as the **FRAMES** model:

1 Feedback – assessment and evaluation of the problem.
2 Responsibility – emphasizing personal choice.
3 Advice – explicit advice on changing behaviour.
4 Menu – aiding the development of alternative goals and strategies.
5 Empathic interviewing – a non-confrontational reflective approach.
6 Self-efficacy – instilling optimism that chosen goals can be achieved.

All professionals should be capable of offering this intervention (Box 29.1). BI is effective in the delivery of

---

Box 29.1: Information offered during a brief intervention

- *Practical advice and information*, tailored to meet the needs of the individual.
- *Offering information on the consequences of substance use* should be considered, paying attention to the harms associated with intoxication, binge drinking and/or excessive substance use.
- If alcohol is the person's substance of choice, information on weekly and daily drinking is provided, in addition to how to calculate units.
- The individual is aided to consider the *positive and negative consequences of substance use* in relation to social, physical, psychological and spiritual needs.
- *Practical advice can be given on how to reduce substance use.*
- *Written material* to complement and build on, if necessary, the information provided during an intervention should be offered.
- Appropriate *contact details of local drug and/or alcohol services* should be provided when necessary. If referral to a specialist agency is required and the individual agrees, the healthcare worker may make contact to arrange a full assessment or provide written details.

a wide range of health education activities. The FRAMES model can be used for interventions related to smoking cessation, healthy eating and exercise, or for specific mental health problems/symptom management. Its use is not confined to substance use-related interventions. The World Health Organization[31] offers an excellent manual to guide clinicians in delivering BI for alcohol and other drugs, which is available to download online.

Useful tools in a brief intervention

Substance use diaries (Figure 29.2) are useful in identifying the amount of a substance used, possible patterns and triggers to use and in highlighting the associated cost implications. Clinicians may assist clients in completing the diary or review their diary with them. These interactions can provide a valuable platform for discussion on patterns and triggers to substance use and enable the professional to understand this from the individual's perspective. In addition, diaries can be a useful means for providing health education, especially in relation to alcohol 'units' for which individuals can be educated on what a 'unit' is and be encouraged to calculate their daily/weekly use.

Retrospective diaries are completed for a *normal* week, e.g. completing a diary for a week spent in hospital would probably not reflect the individual's usual patterns or levels of use. Contemporaneous diaries can be useful in assisting individuals to monitor substance use over a period of time, especially if they are attempting to reduce the amount they use.

Decisional balance sheets (DBSs; Figure 29.3) are a useful way of encouraging individuals to consider the pros (benefits) and cons (costs) of either maintaining a current behaviour or changing that behaviour. DBSs are beneficial as they acknowledge that substance use does have some positive aspects for the individual. DBSs are usually completed with the client and provide a platform for further discussion on the points listed. The pros of using substances are usually completed first, followed by the cons. For individuals at the contemplation stage of change, the list of cons is likely to be longer than the pros. This observation can be useful to highlight and may assist in encouraging individuals to conclude for themselves that change is beneficial. For those at the pre-contemplation stage, the benefits are likely to outweigh the costs. In this way, DBSs can be useful in identifying appropriate interventions depending on the individual's stage of change.

Day	Time started and finished using?	Type of substance used?	Amount used?	Where?	Who with?	Cost?	How were you feeling before using?
Monday							
Tuesday							
Wednesday							
Thursday							
Friday							
Saturday							
Sunday							

Figure 29.2 Sample substance use diary

What I enjoy about using alcohol/drugs What are the advantages/benefits?	What I don't enjoy about using alcohol/drugs What are the disadvantages/costs?

Figure 29.3 Decisional balance sheet

Motivational interviewing

Motivational interviewing (MI) is a style of counselling that is particularly beneficial for individuals in the early stages of the cycle of change,[3] predominantly contemplation. MI adopts an empathic, person-centred and collaborative approach that incorporates skilful reflective listening and aims to understand the client's perspective. MI aims to raise individuals' awareness of the impact their behaviour has on their biopsychosocial health and to increase motivation for positive change.

The clinician does not propose changes in behaviour but creates and amplifies discrepancies arising from ambivalence between the individual's current behaviour and his or her broader values or future goals/aspirations. Although MI is non-confrontational, it is directive, moving the client towards change by inducing the individual's inherent motivation and resources for change.[32] In essence, MI encourages individuals to conclude for themselves that change is necessary.

MI has been shown to increase the likelihood of behaviour change, improve engagement in treatment and enhance an individual's ability to maintain changes.[33] MI with clients experiencing co-existing problems has been shown to increase engagement with services and treatment and reduce substance use and related problems.[34]

Cognitive–behavioural therapy

Cognitive–behavioural therapy (CBT) adopts a flexible, client-centred approach that develops from an understanding and acceptance of the client's experience. CBT is based on the cognitive model, which assumes that thoughts, feelings and behaviour are interrelated. How people perceive the world around them and interpret events affects these areas. It is not the actual event that affects mood but the individual's interpretation of that event, based on core beliefs.[35] CBT is seen to be effective in a range of mental health problems, including depression and psychosis.[36,37] There is increasing evidence to suggest that this approach may be useful for individuals with co-existing problems, not only in addressing mental health issues but also in encouraging the identification and evaluation of thoughts that result in substance use.[38]

Relapse prevention

Relapse prevention applies to both mental health and substance use. It involves identifying triggers that may result in a relapse of either mental health symptoms or substance use. Triggers may include exposure to certain stressful situations or contact with certain people. Once triggers have been identified, a plan of how to cope with the situation and, if necessary, who to contact can be developed by the service user and professional. The use of distraction techniques, relaxation, exercise and music therapy can be extremely beneficial coping strategies during high-risk periods. Assisting individuals to identify the early warning signs (EWSs) of a mental health relapse is a key feature of relapse prevention. EWSs are subtle changes in a person's mood, thoughts and behaviour that, typically, present before more overt psychotic symptoms. Each person has his or her own unique EWS, which may change during each relapse. Guiding clients in recognizing their EWSs and accessing services earlier during relapse reduces the risk of more severe episodes.

Harm reduction

Harm reduction recognizes that abstinence in substance use is often an unachievable goal for many people, and those wishing to continue using should be enabled to do so in a safer manner. The underlying philosophy is that, although it may be impossible to eradicate the illegal use of substances, it is nonetheless beneficial for individuals and society to make existing substance use as safe as possible. Harm reduction involves providing users with advice on the safer use of substances; clean needles, syringes and containers for disposal to reduce the risk of blood-borne viruses through sharing equipment; health promotion on substance use and safe sex and free condoms.

Medication management

The reasons for individuals either continuing or discontinuing medication are complex and can be determined by personal beliefs and social issues.[39] Unwanted side-effects, negative beliefs about medication and complex treatment regimens may all influence a person's decision to discontinue medication.[40] 'Compliance therapy'[41] incorporates a combination of cognitive–behavioural approaches with psychoeducation and MI. Compliance therapy recognizes an individual's readiness to change and allows discussion on past experiences of treatment. It enables individuals to explore ambivalence regarding medication, considers the positive and negative aspects of such and modifies false beliefs while assisting individuals in making a connection between effective medication management, reduced symptomatology and relapse. Medication management is best viewed as an ongoing process of collaboration and exploration that adjusts attitudes, reinforces positive behaviours and increases knowledge and understanding, rather than a single intervention at the beginning of treatment.

SUMMARY

This chapter has highlighted some of the issues and concerns associated with the treatment and management of the person experiencing co-existing mental health and substance use problems. Emphasis has been placed on the importance of effective assessment and engagement. If problems are not identified through thorough assessments and clients are not adequately engaged in therapeutic relationships with professionals and services, subsequent interventions will not be successful in their aim.

Working with clients with co-existing problems can be challenging. Their needs are complex and multifaceted and assisting individuals in the process of recovery takes time and dedication. It is essential that professionals are mindful of their own values, attitudes and beliefs regarding substance use and the difficulties that clients experience when attempting to change behaviour. Awareness of these issues and how they affect relationships with clients enables professionals to become emotionally available and therapeutically engaged with individuals experiencing co-existing problems. The importance of ongoing training and effective clinical supervision cannot be underestimated in assisting professionals to address therapeutic impasses and improve client outcomes.

The key points of this chapter are:

- 'Dual diagnosis' is more than two distinct problems.
- It is more important to understand the relationship between a person's mental health and substance use problems than it is to attempt to define which problem came 'first'.
- Assisting with housing, benefits and social activities is often more important in the early stages of treatment than directly addressing mental health and substance use needs.
- Effective assessment and engagement are essential if subsequent interventions are to be successful.
- If a person is unable to achieve a change in his or her behaviour on the first occasion, this does not mean that all future attempts will be unsuccessful. Take time to reflect on your own past attempts to change.

REFERENCES

1. Department of Health. *The National Health Service framework for mental health – 5 years on*. London, UK: Department of Health, 2004.

2. Ryrie I, McGowan J. Staff perceptions of substance use among acute psychiatric inpatients. *Journal of Mental Health Nursing* 1998; **5**: 137–42.

3. Banerjee J, Clancy C, Crome I. *Co-existing problems of mental disorder and substance misuse (dual diagnosis): an information manual 2002*. London, UK: The Royal College of Psychiatrists Research Unit, 2002.

4. Turning Point. *Dual diagnosis: good practice handbook; helping practitioners to plan, organise, and deliver services for people with co-existing mental health and substance use needs*. London, UK: Turning Point, 2007.

5. Department of Health. *Mental health policy implementation guide: dual diagnosis good practice guide*. London, UK: Department of Health, 2002.

6. Department of Health. *Dual diagnosis in mental health inpatient and day hospital settings: guidance on the assessment and management of patients in mental health inpatient and day hospital settings who have mental ill-health and substance use problems*. London, UK: Department of Health, 2006.

7. Smith J, Frazer S, Bower H. Dual diagnosis in patients. *Hospital and Community Psychiatry* 1994; **45** (3): 280–1.

8. Menzes P. Drug and alcohol problems among individuals with severe mental illness in south London. *British Journal of Psychiatry* 1996; **168**: 612–19.

9. McDermott E, Pyett P. *Not welcome anywhere*. Melbourne, Australia: Victorian Community-Managed Mental Health Services, 1993.

10. Mueser KT, Drake RE, Wallach MA. Dual diagnosis: a review of etiological theories. *Addictive Behaviours* 1998; **23**: 717–34.

11. Noordsy DL. Subjective experience related to alcohol use among schizophrenics. *Journal of Nervous and Mental Disorders* 1991; **179**: 410–14.

12. Mathre ML. Cannabis series – the whole story. Part 2. Current research findings on cannabis and cannibinoid therapies. *The Drug and Alcohol Professional* 2001; **1** (2): 4–11.

13. Care Services Improvement Partnership. *Changing habits. North West dual diagnosis intelligence report: informing commissioning, management and provision of integrated service provision for dual diagnosis treatment populations*. Hyde, UK: CSIP North West Development Centre, 2007.

14. Osher FC, Kofoed LL. Treatment of patients with psychiatric and psychoactive substance abuse disorders. *Hospital and Community Psychiatry* 1989; **4** (10): 1025–30.

15. Jeynes P, Minett R. Engagement in people with mental health problems: a case study. *British Journal of Therapy and Rehabilitation* 1999; **6** (10): 487–91.

16. Barker P. *Assessment in psychiatric and mental health nursing: in search of the whole person*. Cheltenham, UK: Stanley Thornes, 1997.

17. Baker A, Velleman R. *Clinical handbook of co-existing mental health and drug and alcohol problems*. London, UK: Routledge, 2007.

18. Kavanagh D, Mueser KT, Baker A. Management of co-morbidity. In: Teeson M, Proudfoot H (eds). *Co-morbid mental disorders and substance use disorders: epidemiology, prevention and treatment*. Canberra, Australia: Commonwealth of Australia, 2003.

19. Mueser KT, Kavanagh D. Treating comorbidity of alcohol problems and psychiatric disorder. In: Heather N, Stockwell T (eds). *The essential handbook of treatment and prevention of alcohol problems*. Chichester, UK: John Wiley & Sons, 2004.

20. Gafoor M, Rassool GH. The co-existence of psychiatric disorders and substance misuse: working with dual diagnosis. *Journal of Advanced Nursing* 1998; **27**: 497–502.

21. Henry-Edwards S, Humeniuk R, Ali R *et al. The alcohol, smoking and substance involvement screening test (ASSIST): guidelines for use in Primary Care*. Draft Version 1.1 for Field Testing. Geneva, Switzerland: World Health Organization, 2003. Available from: www.who.int/substance_abuse/activities/en/Draft_The_ASSIST _Guidelines.pdf.

22. Croton G. *Screening for and assessment of co-occurring substance use and mental health disorders by alcohol and other drug*

and mental health services. Victoria, Australia: Victorian Dual Diagnosis Initiative Advisory Group, 2007. Available from: www.dualdiagnosis.org.au/

23. Rassool G. Substance misuse and mental health: an overview. *Nursing Standard* 2002; **16** (50): 46–52.

24. The Sainsbury Centre for Mental Health. *Keys to engagement: review of care for people with severe mental illness who are hard to engage with services.* London, UK: The Sainsbury Centre for Mental Health, 1998.

25. Heraghty M, Anipa F, Bryant A, Tallon C. *The Friday group; engaging and empowering service users with a dual diagnosis.* First interim report. Innovation and Creative Practice Awards 2004. London, UK: The Queen's Nursing Institute, 2004. Available from: www.alcoholconcern.org.uk/docs/889

26. Heraghty M. The 'Friday Group': engaging and empowering service users with a dual diagnosis. In: *Good thinking: supporting the mental health and alcohol fields.* Mental Health and Alcohol Misuse Project Newsletter 9, Winter 2005. London, UK: Alcohol Concern, 2005.

27. Shaw S, Cartwright A, Spratley T, Harwin J. *Responding to drinking problems.* London, UK: Croom Helm, 1978.

28. Prochaska JO, Di Clemente CC. Towards a comprehensive model of change. In: Miller WR, Heather N (eds). *Treating addictive behaviours: processes of change.* London, UK: Plenum, 1986.

29. Prochaska JO, Di Clemente CC. Stages and process of self-change of smoking: towards an integrative model of change. *Journal of Consulting and Clinical Psychology* 1983; **51** (3): 390–5.

30. Bein T, Miller W, Tonigan S. Brief interventions for alcohol problems: a review. *Addiction* 1993; **88**: 315–36.

31. Henry-Edwards S, Humeniuk R, Ali R *et al. Brief intervention for substance use: a manual for use in primary care.* Draft Version 1.1 for Field Testing. Geneva, Switzerland: World Health Organization, 2003. Available from: www.who.int/substance_abuse/activities/en/Draft_Brief_Intervention_for_Substance_Use.pdf.

32. Miller MR, Rollnick S (eds). *Motivational interviewing: preparing people for change,* 2nd edn. New York, NY: Guilford Press, 2002.

33. Noonan WC, Moyers TB. Motivational interviewing. *Journal of Substance Misuse* 1997; **2**: 8–16.

34. Kavenagh DJ, Young R, White A *et al.* A brief motivational intervention for substance use in recent onset psychosis. *Drug and Alcohol Review* 2004; **23**: 151–5.

35. Beck JS. *Cognitive therapy: beyond the basics.* London, UK: The Guildford Press, 1995.

36. National Institute for Health and Clinical Excellence. *Schizophrenia: core interventions in the treatment and management of schizophrenia in primary and secondary care.* Clinical Guideline 1. London, UK: National Institute for Health and Clinical Excellence, 2002.

37. National Institute for Health and Clinical Excellence. *Depression: management of depression in primary and secondary care.* Clinical Guideline 23. London, UK: National Institute for Health and Clinical Excellence, 2004.

38. Mueser KT, Noordsy DL, Drake RE, Fox L. *Cognitive behavioural counselling. Integrated treatment for dual disorders: a guide to effective practice.* New York, NY: The Guildford Press, 2003.

39. Gray R, Robson D, Bressington D. Medication management for people with a diagnosis of schizophrenia. *Nursing Times* 2002; **98** (47): 38–40.

40. Gray R, Brewin E, Bressington D. Psychopharmacology and medication management. In: Hannigan B, Coffey M (eds). *The handbook of mental health nursing.* London, UK: Routledge, 2003.

41. Kemp R, Hayward P, Applewhaite G *et al.* Compliance therapy in psychotic patients: randomised controlled trial. *British Medical Journal* 1996; **312**: 345–9.

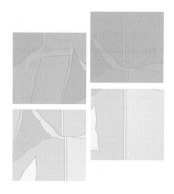

CHAPTER 30

The person who appears paranoid or suspicious

Denis Ryan*

INTRODUCTION

The term paranoia has a long history. The term has Greek origins and roughly translated means that the mind is 'beside itself'. The early Greeks used it to refer to almost any form of mental disturbance or bizarre thinking. Over time, the term has changed in meaning but remains synonymous with the concept of insanity.[1] More recently, paranoia has acquired a shared professional and lay meaning. The popularity of the term in lay circles has led to a situation in which the term is widely used and simultaneously poorly understood.

Within health care accuracy of definition is obviously important. Having a shared language, through the use of diagnostic classification, has many potential benefits for both clinical and administrative practice. Three general purposes which classification serves have been noted.[2] These relate to the standardization of language across disciplines; the study of the natural history of particular disorders and development of effective treatments; and finally to the development of an understanding of the causes of various mental disorders.

Language and precise terminology also have implications in relation to the broader social contexts for the individuals to whom such classifications are applied. For example, diagnoses have long-term implications for people who have to live with their social as well as medical consequences, especially labelling and stigmatization. This situation clearly includes those who demonstrate paranoid and/or suspicious thinking or behaviour.

Reflection

Consider the social implications of a diagnosis of a paranoid disorder.

DEFINITIONAL ISSUES

The changing nature of the diagnosis of paranoid conditions has been an issue of considerable debate within the literature and has persisted since the time of Kraepelin and Bleuler, when many of the debates on classification began.[3] Differences have existed in relation to symptomatology and presentation and have revolved around the issue of whether or not paranoia could be considered a distinct diagnostic entity.

Some have argued that paranoid conditions became subsumed into the concept of schizophrenia because of

*Denis Ryan is Senior Lecturer at the University of Limerick, Ireland.

the dominance of the Bleulerian concept of schizophrenia, which was extremely loose.[4] Others argue that there is a clear distinction to be drawn between *paranoid personality* and the various manifestations of schizophrenic disorder. There is also a move to consider any form of psychotic-type disorder within a 'symptom-based' rather than diagnostic category approach,[5] which influences how paranoia might be understood.

While the origins of the term paranoia seemed to date from at least the early 1800s, when the terms 'paranoia' and 'madness' effectively had a shared meaning,[1] the identification and acceptance of paranoia as either a distinct entity or an element of a broader clinical categorization has changed over time. Some argue that paranoia presents in both non-clinical and clinical populations.[6] In his original categorization of mental disorders, Kraepelin drew a clear distinction between paranoia and dementia praecox, and, although Bleuler subsequently disagreed with Kraepelin in terms of specific diagnostic criteria, he agreed that paranoid disorders should, in fact, be seen as a separate entity. Kraepelin originally described individuals with paranoid disorders as those who would present with systematized delusions, but would not present with hallucinations. He proposed that paranoid disorders were characterized by their prolonged course without recovery but not at the same time leading to mental deterioration.[7] By contrast, Bleuler believed that hallucinations could be a feature in some patients.[8]

In the 1960s it was acknowledged that there were 'no reliable statistics concerning the incidence of paranoia and paranoid reactions'.[9] While both major international classification systems [the *Diagnostic and statistical manual* (DSM)[10] and the *International classification of diseases* (ICD)[11]] have established diagnostic criteria with ongoing refinements over time, there remain inconsistencies between them which do not inspire confidence in the validity or reliability of the term paranoia. In more recent editions of the DSM and ICD, a distinct classification of paranoid conditions within schizophrenic disorders has continued, but paranoid reactions have been largely subsumed within the broader categorization of delusional disorder. Some authors argue that the accuracy of diagnosis is complicated by the fact that many people who have the condition either present with differing complaints or have co-morbid conditions and will not necessarily present to mental health services.[12]

Paranoia is frequently associated with schizophrenia or delusional disorder. What distinguishes the nature of the delusions arising in schizophrenia from paranoid delusions is that in paranoia they tend to be clear, logical and systematic, the personality remains intact and social functioning remains high. Paranoia is also associated with other conditions such as substance abuse and mood disorder. Several authors have reported that paranoia is associated with cocaine abuse,[13] although this appears to be a transient feature, mainly evident when individuals in a cocaine intoxicated state are 'hypervigilant' relating to potential environmental threats.[14,15] However, paranoia is most associated with three categories of disorder:

1 paranoid personality disorder
2 delusional (paranoid) disorder
3 paranoid schizophrenia.

This explains the trend towards understanding and dealing with such manifestations from a 'symptom-based' rather than a 'syndrome-based' perspective.[5]

> ### Reflection
>
> Consider the implications of understanding 'paranoia' as either a 'symptom' or a 'syndrome' from the perspective of the individual and society.

PARANOID IDEAS AND THEIR PRESENTATION

The word paranoia is generally understood to describe exaggerated suspiciousness or mistrust, or unwarranted suspiciousness. One of the key misunderstandings is the relationship of paranoia to suspicion. Suspiciousness, in its own right, does not necessarily constitute paranoia, and can be justifiable based on past experience or earlier learning. In a professional sense, suspiciousness can be seen as a desirable attribute and professionally mandated.[16] All healthcare and social care practitioners are trained to look 'at' or 'underneath' or 'beyond' that which is not initially obvious. Indeed, such approaches to enquiry can be seen as a fundamental aspect of thorough assessment practice and are a highly valued skill or attribute among such practitioners. In such instances, suspiciousness is nurtured on the basis that it is positive, necessary and justifiable.

The most obvious feature which distinguishes suspiciousness and paranoia is that the level of mistrust is either out of keeping with the past experience or wholly unjustified. Paranoid ideas are also usually persistent in nature, such persistence distinguishing paranoid ideas from normal suspicion. There is also a tendency for individuals with paranoid conditions or symptoms to persistently seek out supportive evidence to confirm their beliefs while ignoring objective or contradictory evidence. Also, the level of severity and impact on functioning may vary to such an extent that some individuals function relatively well in society whereas others become severely incapacitated.

Paranoia usually presents with cognitive or behavioural manifestations or both. Paranoid ideation is increasingly understood as a manifestation of a health condition or a 'symptom'. However, when it occurs as part of a disease process, perhaps the most frequent conditions with which paranoia is associated are when those who have it manifest delusions of importance or persecution.[1] While ideas of exaggerated importance or prosecution may present as a feature of a range of conditions or disorders, the issue that clearly distinguishes paranoid disorders relates to the delusional nature of the ideas.

A complicating factor is that paranoid delusions often co-exist with other disorders, or indeed individuals may present with conditions such as depression or anxiety while denying the existence of delusional ideation.[17] The importance of distinguishing the delusional nature of paranoid ideas was highlighted in a recent study of risk factors for depressive episodes that identified subclinical suspiciousness as a risk factor of new episodes of depression.[18] This highlights the necessity of clearly distinguishing suspiciousness and paranoia.

A distinction is required between the so-called *'poor me'* and *'bad me'* presentations.[19] In the first case, individuals believe that they are innocent victims of persecution and their energies are focused on blaming or condemning those who they believe are responsible for their persecution. The second group believe that they are wholly deserving of persecution and are more like people with depressive conditions or low self-esteem who link this persecution to previous behaviour or past aspects of their lives.[20]

To assist with appropriate identification of paranoia, mental health nurses need to be aware that there exists a range of 'at risk' people. While not exclusively the case, paranoia is more likely to manifest itself in middle or later life and is more prevalent among women than men.[8] It would also seem that those who present are more likely to be either currently or formerly partnered. Although variable rates of presentation among married, separated, widowed and divorced persons are reported, it would seem that partnered people have higher rates than unattached persons.[8]

CARING FOR PEOPLE WITH PARANOID CONDITIONS

Nurses help individuals or groups to care for themselves when they are unable to do so alone.[21] However, there is also a common understanding that there needs to be a clear and identified *need* or legitimate basis for nursing intervention. The International Council of Nurses[22] defines nursing as an occupation which

> encompasses autonomous and collaborative care of individuals of all ages, families, groups and communities, sick or well and in all settings. Nursing includes the promotion of health, prevention of illness and the care of ill, disabled and dying people. Advocacy, promotion of a safe environment, research, participation in shaping health policy and in-patient and health systems management, and education are also key nursing roles.

There still exists, however, a range of difficulties in arriving at an adequate definition of the primary function of the mental health nurse.[23] Although there are clear arguments that the core function of nursing deals with the manifestations of illness, psychiatric–mental health nursing has distinctive features and at least part of the role of the mental health nurse is to work collaboratively with other professions – especially psychiatrists.[24] Historically, little attention has been paid to the role of nursing in health promotion, illness prevention or roles with families and the wider community. In that regard, while there are clear roles for mental health nursing in relation to the promotion of health and the prevention of illness, the thrust of the remaining sections of this chapter will focus on the role of the nurse with those who manifest paranoid thoughts or ideas.

Reflection

Given that paranoia presents in non-clinical as well as clinical populations, consider the role of the mental health nurse in health promotion, illness prevention and disorder management.

ASSESSMENT AND DIAGNOSTIC ISSUES

Individuals who present for treatment or diagnosis are likely to have concerns and fears. Frequently, these may be misinterpreted as suspiciousness, irritability or negativity. It is also important to remember that paranoid ideas, as suggested earlier, may present in a range of disorders or in none. Indeed, it has been noted that many with paranoid conditions continue to function at a high level, many never seek clinical intervention and many have no obvious identifying characteristics.[25]

This highlights the importance of adequate assessment and screening to identify pathological elements or to distinguish between *paranoid ideation* and *paranoid delusions*, which, in turn, may lead to a distinction between psychotic and non-psychotic disorders. As previously acknowledged, collaborative care is increasingly the norm in mental healthcare practice, and in that regard rigorous attention to appropriate distinction of symptomatology may also help in the collaborative process of arriving at an accurate diagnosis of the particular condition of which paranoia is a feature.

Although paranoid delusions may occasionally present as an isolated feature on their own, more frequently they will present in association with features such as different kinds of delusions, hallucinations, changes in speech content or form, alterations in affect, level of orientation, agitation or aggressive behaviour.[26] In addition, paranoid ideation or delusions should also be considered in the context of an individual's physical health status and use of substances of abuse. The levels of impairment and the range of areas of impairment also need consideration. These types of considerations point to the necessity for accurate, integrated and comprehensive assessment. While it may be relatively easy to identify severe forms of paranoia,[1] it is quite a challenging issue for assessors to distinguish between clinical paranoid states and understandable levels of suspicion.

Probably the most profound complicating factor in both the assessment and indeed the treatment process with people who present with paranoia is the fact that much of the assessment must rely on interview methods with both the individual and the family or concerned others. In that regard, it is likely that the interview process itself will be complicated by the nature of the paranoid ideas or delusions if present.

In arriving at an accurate diagnosis, it is vital that an adequate history of a range of areas is obtained. This will include such issues as psychiatric, psychological, social and medical histories. This relates to the fact that paranoia may present alone or in association with a wide range of conditions which are associated with paranoia. These might include neurological disorders; metabolic and endocrine disorders; vitamin deficiencies; sex chromosome disorders; infections; alcohol and drug abuse disorders; toxic disorders; pharmacological disorders; delusional (paranoid) disorder; mood disorders; schizophrenia; schizo-affective disorder; schizophreniform disorder; paranoid personality disorder; brief reactive psychosis; induced psychotic disorder; primary degenerative dementia (Alzheimer's type); and organic personality disorder.[26]

Co-morbid conditions, of which paranoia may be a feature, must be adequately diagnosed. The distinctions between the different manifestations of paranoia may be important to distinguish the associated condition. For example, the DSM-IV[10] suggests that paranoid schizophrenia will be characterized by a preoccupation with one or more delusions, but is also frequently associated with auditory hallucinations, unfocused anger, anxiety, argumentativeness or violence. In addition, interpersonal interactions tend to be very stilted and quite formal or extremely intense. The presentation of paranoia in delusional disorders differs from that in schizophrenic disorders, insofar as that the delusions described are systematized, encapsulated and non-bizarre in nature.[8] Essentially, the nature of the delusions in delusional disorders are such that they are characterized by connectedness and being part of an overall theme.[1] The fact that they tend to be non-bizarre in nature means that it is not implausible that the situations which are the subject of the delusions could potentially occur in real life situations, such as being followed by another person,[8] and the condition is not generally associated with significant impairment in most areas of living.

The characteristics most associated with paranoia tend to include self-consciousness, hypersensitivity, mistrust and fear.[15] However, *paranoid personality disorder* needs to be distinguished as a distinctive disorder in terms of its level of persistence, pervasiveness and inappropriateness. Individuals with paranoid personality disorder tend to manifest levels of suspiciousness of the motivation of other individuals that are ongoing, pervasive and inappropriate. People with paranoid personality disorder are likely to present as tense, guarded, hypervigilant and frequently question (without objective reason or justification) the motives, trustworthiness or loyalty of people around them – commonly friends or family. They have a tendency to be solitary and frequently invest significant energy and time in interpreting ordinary events or interactions as 'evidence' of malevolent intent. In addition, they frequently misinterpret completely benign events or actions as those which are intended to be, or have the effect of being, demeaning or threatening to them personally. The DSM-IV[10] distinguishes paranoid personality disorder from other disorders such as paranoid schizophrenia and delusional disorder in that delusions or other perceptual distortions and eccentric behaviour are not dominant features of the disorder.

> ### Reflection
>
> Consider the role of the mental health nurse in the diagnosis of conditions in which paranoia and suspiciousness are dominant features.

TREATMENT ISSUES AND THE ROLE OF MENTAL HEALTH NURSING

Given the obvious difficulties in accurately defining paranoia, it is hardly surprising that these difficulties also feature in any discussion of the role of the mental health nurse in the treatment and management of people with paranoid and suspicious manifestations. Practitioners should be aware that manifestations of paranoia can range from normal caution and vigilance, through transitory beliefs and/or expressions of pathological suspiciousness to psychotic conditions in the absence of any objective threat or potential harm, including paranoid reactions to delusional and schizophrenic disorders or personality disorder.[1]

Irrespective of the point on this continuum when paranoia occurs, the central feature relates to the issue of *mistrust*. Another key feature is that of being misunderstood. While paranoia is associated with a sense of victimhood, it is equally important to be aware that individuals with paranoid conditions may actually be the victims of mistreatment, or have been wronged. Specifically in relation to paranoid personality disorder, some core beliefs have been identified which such individuals are likely to hold, and consequently these beliefs are likely to influence how individuals perceive themselves and behave.[27] These beliefs include a persistent sense of foreboding; belief that the world is full of enemies; that accidents are doubtful and that negative events are initiated by others with hostile intent; that all events relate to the person themselves; they are never to blame and that guilt is not attributable to them but to others; a belief that they are in some way different from the rest of humanity; and often they have the belief that they have unique awareness or insight which is not shared by others.

Consistent with these core beliefs, individuals who are paranoid are likely to believe others either exploit or deceive them. They are likely to demonstrate a strong sense of hurt and express beliefs that they have been deeply and irreversibly injured, despite objective evidence to the contrary. In the initial period of contact with healthcare professionals – including nurses – interaction with the paranoid patient is likely to be characterized by difficulty in forming and/or maintaining a therapeutic relationship. The therapeutic engagement must, of course, be understood in the context of the core beliefs and characteristics of mistrust and suspiciousness. It is most likely that there will be considerable difficulty in obtaining accurate histories through direct interview processes with clients themselves. Paranoid individuals will most likely be reluctant to share information, and may withhold personal information for what they understand are reasons of self-protection.[10]

This tendency should be understood within the context of paranoia itself. In the case of paranoid delusions, individuals are more likely to jump to conclusions on the basis of less information[28] than those without paranoia. It is also likely that paranoid patients will attribute negative events to external sources or causes, and will do the exact opposite in relation to positive events, i.e. attribute the source of positive events to some internal cause related directly to themselves.[29,30]

With regard to interpersonal relationships, which have been identified as the primary medium through which mental health nurses practice,[24] the DSM-IV[10] notes that paranoid individuals have consistent difficulties in interpersonal behaviour. Mistrust and suspiciousness may manifest through hostility argumentativeness, guarded behaviour, secretiveness, aloofness or deviousness. In addition, paranoid individuals may be quick to take offence, reluctant to forgive but ever willing to counterattack.[31] This type of behaviour is understandable because paranoid people believe themselves to be vulnerable to shame and humiliation at the hands of others – especially those in authority.[32] In addition to seeing themselves as victims, paranoid individuals are also likely to see themselves as

blameless in conflict situations, and are likely to explain, legitimize and understand aggression on their part as a justified counterattack.[27] Understanding why interpersonal difficulties arise will not automatically decrease the types of difficulties that arise between paranoid patients and others. However, awareness of such difficulties may help in the overall management of the individual.

It is ironic that the symptomatology of paranoid conditions is the very issue that is likely to impede treatment. The suspiciousness and mistrust that are central to paranoid conditions mean that it is less likely that people with paranoia will present for treatment, especially on a voluntary basis. The reluctant nature of the engagement with treatment services is likely to be interpreted as evidence (either new or confirmatory) of persecution or harm – directed at the person themselves. The imagined source of that harm or further persecution may be family or concerned others, or the healthcare professionals or agency involved in the provision of care.

Full consideration must be given, therefore, to the nature and level of suspiciousness, fear, sense of threat or persecution in terms of the overall approach to such patients. It is, of course, most likely that care will be provided in a multi- or interdisciplinary manner and that a collaborative approach will be taken. One of the greatest challenges when dealing with paranoid patients is persuading them of the necessity both to access and accept treatment and to comply with the requirements of the treatment approach. It is most likely that the initial phase of treatment will concentrate on the establishment and development of a trusting and therapeutic relationship between service provider and user. Above all other types of patient, it is extremely important to emphasize the issue of confidentiality. Simultaneously, one needs to be conscious that guarantees of confidentiality, although a central feature of the therapeutic relationship, are likely to be tested on an ongoing and sometimes unreasonable basis.

Many individuals who present with paranoid conditions may never fully reject the delusional system or ideas which they hold, despite achieving improvements in their level of functioning.[33] This has implications for the level and type of support necessary or the nature of intervention that the mental health nurse is likely to engage in. Although medication has been a consistent feature in the overall management of paranoid conditions, there is a lack of consensus regarding its usefulness or efficacy. The orthodox view is that anti-psychotic medication has a role to play in the management of individuals with paranoid personality disorder, whereas others caution that medication will have limited (if any) use in patients whose paranoia is non-delusional in nature.[26] Likewise, there is some argument that the use of anti-psychotic medication has never been properly evaluated in relation to delusional disorder.[8] When medication forms a part of the overall treatment approach, the mental health nurse will have a vital role as part of the multidisciplinary team in helping to ensure compliance with medication regimes. This may involve the direct administration of medication and psychoeducational approaches to explaining issues around usage, management and unwanted side-effects of medication to both the individuals and their families. It may also involve teaching self-medication management techniques as well as monitoring compliance.

While medication and pharmacological methods of treatment have perhaps been a very significant element in the overall approach to the management of paranoia, there has been an increasing reliance on the use of psychological and psychosocial interventions such as cognitive–behavioural therapy. Promising results have been achieved with these interventions in individuals with schizophrenia,[34] and in the case of individuals with paranoia promising short-term results have been reported.[35] Reference has already been made to the difficulties relating to the issue of late access to treatment and non-compliance. These issues either in isolation or combined are likely to make treatment of any nature more complicated. A further complication in this instance also relates to the fact that it is highly likely that individuals who present with paranoid conditions or manifestations will do so in the context of having a complex presentation[26] or in the presence of co-morbid conditions.[32]

However, the key challenge for mental health nurses relates to helping individuals to manage the manifestations of their illness. This will involve the forging of an alliance with clients, within the limits of their paranoid ideation. This will, of necessity, involve an ongoing process of evaluation on the nurse's part to ascertain the level of 'investment' the person has in their own paranoid experience or ideas.[33] It will also mean combining the apparently conflicting, though in fact complementary, roles of building trust – through acceptance of the individual – while not being drawn into or validating individuals' particular world view. It is likely to involve a process of challenging falsely held assumptions, as well as re-structuring the thoughts or re-framing their meaning. It will mean in many instances bridging the gap between individuals and significant others in their lives, such as spouse, family members or other people who are seen as the source of persecution or threat.

Although the core unfounded paranoid belief or idea may never go away completely, there is some evidence that irrational ideas of delusional proportions may in fact be capable of alteration in terms of the intensity with which they are held. In that sense, they may not, in all cases, be 'fixed' in the traditional understanding of delusions.[36] In addition, the significant others as well as the clients need to arrive at an understanding of the condition and perhaps ultimately an accommodation with and between each other in order to best manage their lives.

A belief that the role of the nurse in the care and management of people who present with paranoia is central and vital[1] draws on the work of early nursing theorists such as Travelbee[37] and Peplau.[38] These arguments suggest, with some validity, that the central role of nursing in the care of such people lies in the practice of 'active' listening and therapeutic engagement. In fact, Barker[1] argues that Travelbee's proposals[37] in relation to such techniques or processes of active listening and effective deconstruction of the validity of irrational beliefs over time are historical forerunners of cognitive approaches that are in extensive use currently. The work of early nurse theorists are, therefore, reflected in more recent definitions of psychiatric–mental health nursing, which understand therapeutic engagement as relying heavily on the personal and professional characteristics of the nurse. This understanding of the interpersonal process of the therapeutic relationships among nurse, patient, family and indeed the broader community is particularly important when dealing with complex presentations such as paranoia.

REFERENCES

1. Barker P. Persecution complex: the enigma of paranoid disorders. *Nursing Times* 1997; **93** (2): 30–2.

2. Williams JBW. Psychiatric classification. In: Hales RE, Yudofsky SC (eds). *Synopsis of neuropsychiatry*. Washington, DC: The American Psychiatric Press, 1996.

3. Adityanjee AYA, Theodoridis D, Vieweg VR. Dementia praecox to schizophrenia: the first 100 years. *Psychiatry and Clinical Neuroscience* 1999; **53** (4): 437–48.

4. Fear CF, McMonagle T, Healy D. Delusional disorders: boundaries of a concept. *European Psychiatry* 1998; **13**: 210–18.

5. Combs DR, Michael CO, Penn D. Paranoia and emotion perception across the continuum. *British Journal of Clinical Psychology* 2006; **45**: 19–31.

6. Gracie A, Freeman D, Green S *et al*. The association between traumatic experience, paranoia and hallucinations: a test of the predictions of psychological models. *Acta Psychiatrica Scandinavica* 2007; **116** (4): 280–9.

7. Kendler KS. Kraepelin and the diagnostic concept of paranoia. *Comprehensive Psychiatry* 1988; **29** (4): 4–11.

8. Black DW, Andreasen NC. Schizophrenia, schizophreniform disorder, and delusional (paranoid) disorder. In: Talbott J, Hales R, Yudofsky S (eds). *Textbook of psychiatry*, 2nd edn. Washington, DC: American Psychiatric Press, 1994.

9. Cameron N. Paranoid reaction. In: Freedman AM, Kaplan HI, Sadock BJ (eds). *Comprehensive textbook of psychiatry*. Baltimore, MD: Williams & Wilkins, 1967: 666–7.

10. American Psychiatric Association. *Diagnostic and statistical manual of mental disorders*, 4th edn. Washington, DC: American Psychiatric Association, 1994.

11. World Health Organization. *ICD-10. The ICD-10 classification of mental and behavioral disorders: clinical description and diagnostic guidelines*. Geneva, Switzerland: World Health Organization, 1992.

12. Hsiao MC, Liu CY, Yang YY, Yeh EK. Delusional disorder: retrospective analysis of 86 Chinese outpatients. *Psychiatry and Clinical Neuroscience* 1999; **53** (6): 673–6.

13. Rosse RB, Fay-McCarthy M, Collins Jr JP *et al.* The relationship between cocaine-induced paranoia and compulsive foraging: a preliminary report. *Addiction* 1994; **89** (9): 1097–104.

14. Satel SL, Southwick SM, Gawin FH. Clinical features of cocaine-induced paranoia. *American Journal of Psychiatry* 1991; **148** (4): 495–8.

15. Brady KT, Lydiard RB, Malcolm R, Ballenger JC. Cocaine-induced psychosis. *Journal of Clinical Psychiatry* 1991; **52** (12): 509–12.

16. Winfrey ME, Smith AR. The suspiciousness factor: critical care nursing and forensics. *Critical Care Nursing Quarterly* 1999; **22**: 1–7.

17. Kendler KS. The nosologic validity of paranoia (simple delusional disorder). A review. *Archives of General Psychiatry* 1980; **37**: 699–706.

18. Messias E, Kirkpatrick B. Subclinical suspiciousness as a risk factor for depressive episodes. *Acta Psychiatrica Scandinavica* 2001; **103** (4): 262–6.

19. Trower P, Chadwick P. Pathways to defence of the self: a theory of two types of paranoia. *Clinical Psychology: Science and Practice* 1995; **2**: 263–77.

20. Fornells-Ambrojo M, Garety PA. Bad me paranoia in early psychosis: a relatively rare phenomenon. *British Journal of Clinical Psychology* 2005; **44** (Pt 4): 521–8.

21. Orem D. *Nursing concepts of practice*, 6th edn. St Louis, MO: Mosby, 2001.

22. International Council of Nurses. *The ICN definition of nursing*. Geneva, Switzerland: International Council of Nurses, 2002.

23. Hamblet C. Obstacles to defining the role of the mental health nurse. *Nursing Standard* 2000; **14** (51): 34–7.

24. Peplau HE. Psychiatric nursing: challenge and change. *Journal of Psychiatric and Mental Health Nursing* 1994; **1**: 3.

25. Grover S, Parthasarathy B, Ajit A. The relationship between childhood abuse and adult personality disorder symptoms. *Psychiatry and Clinical Neurosciences* 2007; **61** (5): 462–70.

26. Bloch B, Pristach CA. Diagnosis and management of the paranoid patient. *American Family Physician* 1992; **45** (6): 2634–41.

27. Kantor M. *Diagnosis and treatment of the personality disorders*. Tokyo, Japan: Ishiyaku EuroAmerica, 1992.

28. Bentall RP, Corcoran R, Howard R *et al.* Persecutory delusions: a review and theoretical integration. *Clinical Psychology Review* 2001; **21** (8): 1143–92.

29. Bentall RP, Kaney S. Content specific information processing and persecutory delusions: an investigation using the emotional Stroop test. *British Journal of Medical Psychology* 1989; **62** (Pt 4): 355–64.

30. Bentall RP, Haddock G, Slade PD. Cognitive behaviour therapy for persistent auditory hallucinations: from theory to therapy. *Behavioral Psychotherapy* 1994; **25**: 51–6.

31. Fenigstein A. The paranoid personality. In: Costello CG (ed.). *Personality characteristics of the personality disordered*. New York, NY: Wiley, 1996: 242–75.

32. Maina G, Badá AA, Bogetto F. Occurrence and clinical correlates of psychiatric co-morbidity in delusional disorder. *European Psychiatry* 2001; **16**: 222–8.

33. Botman JA. Paranoid patients benefit from alliance with therapist. *Behavioural Health Treatment* 1997; **2** (10): 8.

34. Cormac I, Jones C, Campbell C. Cognitive behaviour therapy for schizophrenia. *Cochrane Database of Systematic Reviews* 2002; **1**: CD000524.

35. Sullivan J. Cognitive behavioural nursing therapy in paranoid psychosis. *Nursing Times* 1997; **93** (2): 28–30.

36. Garety PA, Hemsley DR, Wessely S. Reasoning in deluded schizophrenic and paranoid patients: biases in performance on a probabilistic inference task. *Journal of Nervous and Mental Disease* 1991; **179**: 194–201.

37. Travelbee J. *Interpersonal aspects of nursing*, 2nd edn. Philadelphia, PA: FA Davis, 1971.

38. Peplau HE. *Interpersonal relations in nursing*. New York, NY: Putnam, 1952.

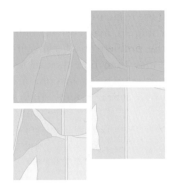

CHAPTER 31

The person with experience of sexual abuse

Mike Smith*

INTRODUCTION

This chapter deals with working with adult survivors of childhood abuse. The principles used in dealing with abuse in younger people are similar; however, the legal framework is quite different.

I receive referrals from other nurses because they do not feel confident or competent to work with sexual abuse. Indeed, some professionals are afraid to work with people's stories and narratives when they include sexual abuse. My understanding of sexual abuse is based on both personal and professional experience. My knowledge is, therefore, the result of an exploration of those twin experiences and their results on the person as an adult. I believe in a very simple approach to people with an experience of sexual abuse. All that you need to help most people is a warm, interested and caring human approach. If people can explore their experiences, help them to own them and then to make decisions in their life about how they wish to move on and thrive (see the *THRIVE* manual[1]).

The process of recovery and thriving is natural. Clients have the necessary knowledge to work out their road to recovery once they have hope. Help from you, the practitioner, is an added bonus. It is the *technician* who is important, not the technique, when it comes to helping people come to terms with their abuse; the underlying philosophy of helping is far more important than the particular techniques you may wish to use to help you on your way. Many therapies to help the abused person are touted and some undoubtedly may contribute something to helping the abused person. However, people's experience of their survival and recovery tells us that it is the therapist rather than the therapy that is most important in these days of evidence-based practice.[2]

This chapter outlines the nature and scope of the problem and its effects upon the person, along with some ways of helping people who have been abused to move on in their lives.

SEXUAL ABUSE: A DEFINITION

Sexual abuse is the sexual molestation of a child by an older or more powerful person seen as a figure of trust or authority such as parents, relatives, family friends, youth leader and teachers.

Sexual abuse may be any sexual act with a child/young person, performed by an adult or an older child. Such acts include fondling the child's genitals, getting the

*Mike Smith was overall winner of the RCN Nurse of the Year in 1997 and is known for his campaigning approach to change beliefs about the nature of psychotic experiences and the 'treatments' offered. Mike has written many practical books about working with psychotic experiences and now works freelance at www.crazydiamond.org.uk.

child to fondle an adult's genitals, mouth to genital contact, rubbing an adult's genitals on the child, or actually penetrating the child's vagina or anus. There are other, often overlooked, forms of abuse. These include an adult showing his or her genitals to a child, showing the child obscene pictures or videotapes, or using the child to make obscene materials. The definition and interpretation of *molestation* is probably the most debated concept, i.e. what constitutes molestation. If people believe that they have been abused then they have. However, this is not a legal definition and some cases of abuse, when explored by the victim, have little recourse to legal satisfaction.

The term *sexual abuse* in psychiatric practice most commonly refers to the involvement of a young person below the age of 16 in sexual activity with a significantly older and/or powerful person. It is referred to as *abuse* since it is assumed in Western society that the older person must, by definition, be taking advantage of the younger one, since a person under 16 cannot give informed consent (in law) to sexual activity. As with many things, this legal framework for what is and is not abuse differs from country to country, and may be radically different from continent to continent.

Usually, the victim of the abuse cannot understand fully the implications of what is happening at the time. Therefore, although he or she may appear to consent to the activity, the consent is not truly *informed* in the legal sense. Although the abuser may also be young, there is usually a significant age and status difference between the parties, which puts the abuser in a position of power. This power difference means that, even when there is apparent acquiescence, this is usually based on fear of the consequences of refusal and so is not true consent.

Sexual abuse can be an isolated or a recurrent event and may be disclosed or hidden. There are, however, vast differences not just in the physical way in which a person is abused but also in the social and emotional circumstances in which the abuse takes place.

Abuse can range from inappropriate or unwanted touching to sexual penetration. It may be perpetrated with 'love' or with violence. The abuse can be disguised as play or it may be a more overt assault. The abuser may be a relative, an acquaintance or a stranger. Abuse can be limited in its occurrence, happening only a few times to the person, or it may be a part of everyday life for the person. Some abused people may only realize that they have been abused much later on in life when they talk with other adolescents or adults and find that their experiences were 'different'. For some people, abuse may be related to one specific person. Others may be abused on a number of occasions by different adults. This further reinforces their feelings that it was their fault or destiny. A small proportion of people may be victims of organized circles of sexual abuse for the gratification of paedophiles.

The way people experience abuse, and its subjective meaning to the abused person, is critical to how they respond as adults. Some of these responses, be they coping strategies or survival techniques, may even become pathologized and seen as the problem itself, e.g. self-injury or self-harm. People may then find themselves diagnosed with a mental disorder such as schizophrenia or borderline personality disorder (BPD). Some studies of people in general psychiatric populations have found that a large number of people with a variety of diagnostic labels attribute the origin of their psychotic experiences to life events,[3,4] especially those with histories of abuse.

Commonly, those who are currently experiencing abuse are referred to as *victims* of sexual abuse; those whose experience of abuse is in the past are referred to as *adult survivors* of sexual abuse.

How abuse may be perpetrated: some examples

Some examples of how abuse may be perpetrated are shown in Box 31.1.

Box 31.1: How abuse may be perpetrated

- A girl was sexually abused by her father until her teens. She eventually reported what was happening to the authorities as an adult, and her father was tried and imprisoned.
- A girl was involved in the making of pornographic material by her stepfather until her teens, when she eventually reported what was happening. She was removed, along with her younger sister, from the family home and was brought up by the state as a 'looked after' child.
- A 9-year-old boy was touched by a teacher while showering after physical education, under the pretence that he was helping him wash. He thought he was alone in this experience until a number of boys reported similar abuse several years later.
- An altar boy was touched during prayer by a priest and was told that he was an evil, filthy heathen who needed the priest's help to prevent him from going to hell.
- A teenager living in care was befriended by a policeman and his family, treated as a member of the family and then sexually assaulted. She did not wish to lose the affection of the family so tolerated the sexual molestation, eventually blaming herself when it was discovered because she had enjoyed and indeed encouraged the abuse.
- A young girl's teenage stepbrother used to play games with her at an early age that she later realized (at puberty) had been sexually abusive.
- A boy was often sent to stay with his aunt and uncle, and was regularly abused by the aunt with the knowledge of the uncle. This abuse took place over several years, during which time he was unable to say why he did not wish to visit these relatives.
- A young girl was recruited to work as a prostitute from the age of 13 by a much older man whom she says she loved.

Gaining an overall view of who gets to say 'yes' and 'no' in sexual relationships is an important starting point to understanding our constructions of sexual abuse (see *Understanding child sexual abuse*,[5] chapter 2).

The scale and scope of the problem

Figures on sexual abuse are often contentious and vary according to reporting techniques, definitions of abuse, etc. However, abuse is common in the general population, and far more common among people treated for mental health problems as adults. It is reasonable to assume, therefore, that sexual abuse is a major contributor to mental distress among adults and those in the psychiatric population.

Sexual abuse is not as infrequent as society likes to think, and some have referred to society as complicit in the abuse of children, especially for further blaming and pathologizing the victims later in their life. General population statistics have shown that between one in three and one in four girls will be victims during childhood and between one in five and one in six boys.

The experience of abuse is not restricted to one gender and abusers are not always male. Most recent estimates in Britain suggest that at least 10 per cent of children suffer sexual abuse at some time, with two-thirds of the victims being girls. In over 90 per cent of the cases, the perpetrator of the abuse is male. However, it is not exclusively men who abuse. Because of the small numbers of those abused by women, the victims have a further specific reason to blame themselves for the abuse. This is explored by Warner (see *Understanding child sexual abuse*,[5] chapter 3). A large percentage of abusers are known to their victims and/or families, and one in five of those who abuse are close relatives.

In the psychiatric population, however, the incidence of sexual abuse is much higher than in the general population. Prevalence studies of sexual abuse in the life histories of psychiatric and other populations have remarked upon the significance of sexual abuse among those who hear voices[4] and those who self-injure.[6,7] Diclemente's[7] research with adolescents in a psychiatric service who reported sexual abuse in their life history showed that 83 per cent cut themselves.

Estimates of abuse vary within psychiatric populations – from around 30 per cent (three times greater than the general population) to 83 per cent among specific populations.

Often, the trauma, guilt and self-blame caused by childhood sexual abuse affects a person for life and, in a very pervasive way, affects relationships, learning and maturation and can lead to suicide. The UK has the highest suicide rate in Europe with 5000 deaths per year, and is the foremost cause of death for young men aged 18–25.

Research by the UK Home Office published in February 2000 suggests that the 6000 rapes and 18 000 indecent assaults reported to the police in 1996 (plus the one-third of sex assaults reported to the police that are not recorded by them as crimes) represent probably only one-tenth of the actual number of sex attacks. This suggests that the true figure for UK sex crimes may be between 118 000 and 295 000 per year. However, most sexual abuse is never reported as a sex crime.

TYPES OF ABUSE

Sexual abuse varies not just in its effects upon the person but, more significantly, in:

- the way in which it is perpetrated
- the degree to which the victim is groomed to be abused
- the degree to which the victim is made to feel responsible for the abuse
- the accompanying physical and psychological abuse
- the degree and nature of repetition of the sexual abuse
- the number of ways, times and by whom a victim is abused
- whether the victim is abused serially by different abusers and in different ways.

All these factors can form the substance of a person's exploration of their own abuse. A common question asked by the person is 'why has it affected me so much when 10 per cent of the population have been abused?' The way abuse is socially and emotionally constructed varies greatly from case to case. Consequently, this question reflects the 'unfair punishment' victims and survivors inflict upon themselves, so continuing the damage of their abuse.

GENERAL EFFECTS OF ABUSE ON THE PERSON

Diagnosis

Many different diagnoses or sets of symptoms may loosely explain the *consequences* of sexual abuse upon the person.

Therefore, both professionals and clients have questioned the validity of any relationship between a mental disorder and an underlying pathology. Diagnosis of many mental disorders implies a pathology that has little scientific validity[8] and is currently the subject of a campaign to eradicate the label of schizophrenia[9] as it says nothing of the origins or causes nor does it say anything about coping with the experiences that arise. At its simplest, people who have been abused may argue that their problem is that, as children, they were locked in a cycle of abuse. This, they say, is their *real* problem. This is what they have to overcome, not a pathology or a disease caused by some biological vulnerability. Victims point to emerging and often ignored evidence that it is the *nature* of the abuse that is significant in the development of a mental disorder, not any biological difference.

These problems are vital because if the mental health worker is unaware of them, or does not acknowledge them, they can be a barrier between the worker and client.

What is most important, however, is not just the *way* in which a person was abused but also the *social circumstances* in which it occurred:

- whether it was disclosed
- how that was dealt with
- how the abuse affected the way in which the person interacts with other people
- the person's learning from the point of abuse
- the degree to which the person 'dissociated', and other survival methods used by the person at the point of abuse and thereafter.

Some effects of abuse in later life may, more appropriately, become pathologized when they occur to such an extent that they begin to define the person, rather than represent a part of the person, or interfere with the person's life to such a degree that he or she has problems and seeks help.

Escape

Dissociation is probably the most significant effect upon individuals who are abused in circumstances from which they cannot *physically* escape. There are many different ways and levels in which a person may dissociate, and it is often missed as a symptom by many clinicians. There is a validated tool available – the Dissociative Experience Scale (DES) – which has been used in several psychiatric populations (including chronic schizophrenia) and shows that many people have clinically significant problems with dissociative experiences and may be misdiagnosed.

In research studies participants have recalled their responses, as children, to sexual abuse. A wide variety of attempts to escape from abuse are common. These include both physical action and mental processes. Those who could escape physically did so when possible, either by running away, keeping busy or dressing protectively. Others who could not physically escape engaged in mental processes ranging from pretending the sexual abuse was not happening, to day-dreaming, to isolation of affect and dissociation, to partial or complete repression of memory of the abuse. These responses are conceptualized along a continuum from conscious and voluntary to unconscious and involuntary escape mechanisms. Despite this complex array of escape attempts, most people in a wide range of research studies continued to blame themselves for the abuse.

Denial

Denying – not just to others but also to yourself – that the abuse happened is a common response. Many people with chronic patterns of depression, mood disorders or other psychiatric labels eventually disclose, sometimes in an offhand way, that they were abused as children. When one reflects on their experiences of abuse, often it is not difficult to understand why they behaved or felt that way. Denial of course is associated with shame and the way in which the abuse was constructed. By exploring these aspects of the abuse with victims, we can help them to recover their lives.

Memories may resurface, however, when the person is settled in a safe environment, or may be triggered by specific events such as beginning a sexual relationship, falling in love, being in a further abusive relationship or becoming a parent.

Denial for some people is often unconscious, as we know from narrative work. However, it is doubtful that we can usefully infer abuse. Indeed, repressed memories and 'false memories' are often discussed as major problems in the literature. I have worked with some people who tell me that they cannot recall being abused in childhood but feel sure that they must have been, given their present experiences. I have found that the only way forward is to *agree to assume* that, if they cannot recall it, it may not have happened and we should put those ideas to one side while they look for alternative explanations. Alternatively, we can agree that the origins of the experiences – if they are unclear at this time – are not as important as how people now live, and cope, with such experiences. The nurse may therefore agree to shelve the dilemma of 'why' for the present, until the person's recollections, if ever, become clearer.

The intermediary language of abuse

Sharon Lefevre[10] and Sam Warner[5] have both written about sexual abuse resulting in an 'intermediary language' for the victim.

The person's psychological pain cannot be expressed verbally and therefore other forms of language (an intermediary language) emerge. Lefevre says that it is the language between the abused and non-abused. The commonest forms of these intermediary languages are self-harm and dissociative identity problems (or personality disorders as psychiatry labels them). However, survivors of sexual abuse have described many other forms of mental disorder as manifestations of an intermediary language.

Splitting

Splitting is a complex psychological phenomenon, often reported as a direct consequence of traumatic experiences in early life, especially abuse in its many forms. It is most commonly associated with the diagnosis of BPD; however, other authors have suggested it is a *logical* consequence of abuse, rather than a symptom of a disorder. Splitting occurs when the person appears to swing between idealizing and devaluing people in relationships. The person pits people against one another, making allies of one group and enemies of the other. When people engage in 'splitting', they perceive a person is either good or bad and they are unable to accept that there is both good and bad within a person. Such 'categorization' is extremely changeable, shifting from day to day. One day the person is good and bad the next. Splitting presents the survivor of abuse with particular difficulties in forming and maintaining long-term relationships, especially therapeutic relationships.

OTHER PRACTICAL CONSEQUENCES

- *Intense feelings*. Memories of abuse and surrounding events can bring intense feelings and other experiences, which can be very intrusive to the extent of becoming flashbacks.
- *Flashbacks and nightmares*. Recollections of the abusive experience may intrude into the person's waking thoughts, or may recur in dreams. These are often triggered by subtle events that the person can begin to recognize over time. With support the person can learn to live with these disturbing experiences, by anticipating them or avoiding the situations that 'trigger' them.
- *Shame and guilt*. Survivors frequently blame themselves, suffer from low self-esteem or feel deeply embarrassed about seeking help. They may become depressed, harm themselves and have thoughts of suicide. Mental health workers are very positive and well intentioned when they tell the person that they are not to blame. However, victims who have disclosed abuse accept that this is what everyone else thinks, but they still *know* that they are to blame. This is one result of how the abuser made the person feel at the time of the abuse, and when he or she was groomed for the abuse. Consequently, people find it hard to come to terms with their shame and guilt.

- *Intense anger*. This may be directed at the abuser, and may be linked with a wish to confront or to completely avoid them. It may also be directed at others who seem to have colluded with the abuse or may be directed at people in general. Often, people find it hard to understand their anger and this further reinforces their view that they are a bad person.
- *Self-harm and self-injury*. People who have been sexually abused are far more likely to demonstrate self-destructive activity.[6] This may be because of anger, internalization of shame, or may be a symbolic way of cutting out the filth, dissociating and reintegrating. The literature contains many examples of 'why' a person who has been abused may go on to self-harm. A workbook has been developed for people who self-harm, to explore how their life experiences resulted in them self-harming and how they might cope with their feelings and so reclaim their lives.[11]
- *Internalized feelings of shame*. Harrison[12] wrote about how female survivors of sexual abuse internalized their shame and anger, resulting in self-harm, self-loathing, poor self-esteem and alternative ways of displaying distress.
- *Disrupted relational patterns*. Some survivors avoid intimate relationships and are distrustful of others' motives. Other survivors may find that they tend to form very intense intimate relationships, which can be emotionally draining. These are also features of BPD, a label often attached to abused people who find themselves in the psychiatric system. This raises the question of whether BPD is a biological entity caused by some genetic vulnerability or whether it is a description of some people's coping strategies for dealing with abusive experiences. If the latter is true then pathologizing people's distress and coping, by attributing pathological diagnoses, further reinforces their distress by increasing their shame and sense of self-blame.
- *Coping and adjustment*. Sigmon et al.[13] found that coping and adjustment were seriously affected among both male and female survivors. In response to sexual abuse experienced during childhood, avoidance coping emerged as the most frequently used strategy by both sexes. Although there were no gender differences in current use of problem-focused and avoidance strategies, men described greater use of acceptance whereas women utilized more emotion-focused coping. In general, women reported significantly greater trauma-related distress than men, including higher levels of anxiety, depression, and post-trauma symptoms.
- *Using substances to assist in coping*. Men who have suffered sexual abuse are more likely to suffer from psychological problems than the general population, including alcohol misuse and self-harm.
- *Sexual identity, emotional and sexual relationships*. In their study of 10 adult male survivors, Gill and Tutty[14] found that the men described the abuse as having

significantly affected their sexual identity, as well as their emotional and sexual relationships as adults.

- *Sexual difficulty or dysfunction.* People often report difficulties in enjoying normal sexual activities, which further increases their feelings of abnormality and shame, and reinforces, for them, the experience of grooming by their abuser.
- *Fear of the consequences of the abuse.* Survivors may wonder whether they will ever be able to form normal relationships or whether they might become abusers themselves. This can lead to people ruminating to a degree that is further damaging to them. For some, this fear can have dissociative consequences. Some men and women hear voices telling them that they will abuse children or become a paedophile or a rapist as a direct consequence of their own childhood abuse. In a lesser, but equally damaging, way these fears can also take the form of intrusive thoughts when not dissociative, resulting in a diagnosis of obsessive–compulsive disorder, or identifying the person as a 'high risk' because of these intrusive thoughts.
- *Isolation and stigmatization.* Survivors may feel that they are totally alone with their experience. They can feel that they have been marked out and that somehow others know of their history, even without being told, and so treat them differently.

As with any human response to trauma, the degree of the person's reaction can vary widely between individuals. Some people apparently come to terms with very severe abuse comparatively easily; others find the abuse has a lasting effect on them.

THE VICTIM'S EXPERIENCE

Victims often report feeling very alone with the experience of abuse. Often, they are afraid of telling others, because of the fear of retribution or the consequences for their family.

Victims frequently feel that they will not be believed or taken seriously if they tell others what has happened. Often, this fear is confirmed when they do try to raise the matter. The social conditions in which people are abused, and how disclosure is mitigated against, are important when people reflect on their experiences, as they seek greater understanding of their abuse.

Victims frequently feel guilty. The abuser may suggest that they are to blame for the abuse or they may take responsibility upon themselves. Children naturally tend to assume responsibility for events that are not of their making, and this is particularly true in the case of abuse. I have seen this phenomenon extended into a 'delusional disorder' in which a person comes to believe that he or she is responsible for all the evil in the world.

The guilt and shame is increased if the child has found any aspect of the abuse gratifying. In this context, it is

important to note that the sexual response of many people, at the time of abuse, is normal.

Victims commonly report feeling extremely scared and confused by the abusive experience. They are often alone, or groomed into feeling alone, by the abuser. For some people fear is used to prevent disclosure.

Abusers often control their victims with threats that may be real or psychological. Living for long periods in fear can affect people's development. A number of victims have told me that all they can remember about their childhood is being scared.

Perhaps the most personally damaging effect, at the time of abuse and later, is when the victim feels responsible for the abuse of others – friends or siblings or their other parent. Many abused people have been prepared to take the abuse to spare a brother or sister. Some young children are encouraged to bring other friends into the circle of abuse. Later, this is something they find very difficult to live with and often is more difficult to manage than their own experience of abuse.

Reflection

Do you think that society is complicit in the continuing abuse of people abused as children, for instance by blaming them for the abuse or by labelling behaviour as attention seeking, personality as disordered or coping strategies as maladaptive? Can you think of other ways in which people may feel blamed as adults for their childhood experiences and how this may also affect them today?

HELPING THE ABUSED PERSON

Some general principles underpin the help that might be offered to survivors of sexual abuse. *Talking* about abuse, *being believed* and being helped to come to his or her own conclusions are all intrinsically helpful for the abused person.

Here the structure is described that I use to work with sexually abused people. This is based on my own research, which focused on 'how' people managed their recovery. This is not a panacea for sexual abuse, but merely describes the mental processes that many people follow in reclaiming their experiences, so that they might move on from the mad times of their life.

In general, people describe reaching a:

- *Turning point* in their lives, in which they experience a resolve to move on from their current situation, and to reclaim their life, so that they might move beyond that to enjoy their life again. *People do this by:*
- *Identifying* what they are recovering *from*, i.e. their life experiences to date and the practical manifestations of their abuse in their current life – relationships, feelings

Reflection

Think of something you have survived or recovered from –
perhaps as simple as a cold or a fall or perhaps an emotional
loss. Explore the process of recovery, write about it or discuss
it with a friend.

* What was important, who was important, what did you
  and they do, who did you tell?
* Ask yourself whether it is any different for emotional problems, or is recovery and thriving a relatively common process?
* How can you use this knowledge to help clients?

of shame and blame, and being clear about *how* they
were abused, groomed and its effects on their early
life. *People then need to*:

* *Explore* in depth, the meaning, symbolism, metaphor
  and consequences of these experiences, how they
  were perpetrated, how they felt about them then, and
  how they feel about them now. *Then they begin to*:

* *Understand* their abuse, its links to their life, some of
  the more subtle consequences of the abuse, how they
  cope with their feelings, their beliefs about their abuse
  and their abuser and what they want to do about that.
  For some people, this leads to:
* *Accepting* and resolving to move on with their life, and
  growing again. This may include acknowledging their
  experience of abuse but doing nothing overtly about it,
  or developing less harmful ways of coping. Exploring
  their experiences, in greater depth with someone the
  person trusts, is perhaps the final step towards reclaiming their life.

This approach is a structure for helping people to
address their experience of abuse and perhaps reclaim
their lives through the recovery process. This structure
leads the person and the helper to ask a great number of
questions of each other, and provides a framework within which to ask the questions that might help. I believe
this is a natural process that most people eventually
arrive at in their lives, even if left alone. If recovery is a

Personal illustration 31.1: Paul's story of recovery

Paul was a 30-year-old man with a diagnosis of schizophrenia. He
had been treated with traditional and atypical neuroleptics and
was now thought to be suffering from a personality disorder of
the borderline type (BPD). Paul had been in an intensive care unit
for 13 months and was compulsorily detained. I was informed
that, after reasonable periods of stability, Paul had sabotaged
attempts to help him leave hospital by burning himself or attacking staff. Paul told me he was desperate to leave hospital. He had
no contact with any friends or relatives (i.e. having no social network outside the mental health arena was an obvious hurdle to
reclaiming his life). However, he had one strong relationship with
a nursing assistant, Ricky. This relationship was questioned as
some staff felt that Paul 'manipulated' the staff and was using
Ricky to get what he wanted. Ricky felt that they had a common
interest in the same football team, were a similar age and he
understood him (it later transpired that Ricky also had similar life
experiences to Paul).

At first, we met on an ad hoc basis over 3 weeks, as Paul and
Ricky began to trust me a little more and I focused on telling them
that I was not a therapist but a resource for them to use to bounce
some ideas off about why Paul harmed himself. As a first step, Paul
agreed to write his life history over a 2-week period with Ricky's
support in typing it up in the evenings and at night (Ricky was
working nights at the time).

Paul told a disturbing account that had been unknown to the
people supporting him. He recalled a number of incidents in his
life that he felt had influenced him as an adult.

* His father had killed himself when Paul was 6. He had argued
  with his mother and hung himself from the shower above the
  bath. Paul found his father and had vivid flashbacks of his

father hanging and himself and his mother trying to lift him and
also his baby sister crying in the background.

* Paul's mother began a new relationship when he was 8 and
  married again when he was 9. This stepfather occasionally sexually assaulted Paul, but more frequently physically punished
  him. This included severe beatings and locking him in a cupboard for long periods. Paul's sister was sexually abused far
  more often by this person and he twice recalls his mother being
  beaten by this man with vivid memories of her crying.

* Paul began to be absent from school at about 11 and became
  involved in sniffing solvents and petty crime. He also ran away
  from home after being locked up for 3 days by his stepfather. He
  received more frequent beatings and ran away from home more
  often, only to be returned. He left the family home aged 14 and
  entered the care system as a 'looked after child' as his mother
  and stepfather felt he was uncontrollable after he had set fire to
  the family home when he was locked in a room.

* Paul's sister committed suicide by overdose when he was 17;
  she was aged 13.

* Paul went to prison for a long catalogue of crimes – mostly violent assaults, including racially motivated assaults – until the
  age of about 25, when he entered psychiatric hospital for the
  first time. He did not return to prison, neither was he prosecuted for a crime after that point.

Paul wrote a 25-page life history, which he felt was therapeutic
and gave people a picture of him as he believed he was. We then
began to explore two specific things: the voices that he heard and
his self-harm behaviour. Paul heard several voices. Six of these
predominated, but two were significant. He was terrified of a
man's voice, which reminded him of his dead father. He also
heard a supportive voice of a friend he met in prison, called Leroy.

His stepfather's voice commanded him to 'do it', which he believed meant to kill himself. However, he didn't want to kill himself. He found in prison that harming himself helped him in a number of ways:

- He felt clean.
- He felt that he had bargained with the voice.
- He was left alone by the voice when in pain.
- He could see his hurt in the burns and showed it to others. 'They respond to that', he said, 'and not the pain inside'.

We decided to do two things: to agree a plan with his team that would help him return to his flat. This relied on working closely and honestly together. This was almost spoiled, Paul told me later, when unreliable staff (not regular staff) tried to make him fail. Secondly, we agreed that he wanted to explore his feelings about the death of his sister, the beating of his mother and finally his own physical and sexual abuse with someone independent of his care (at that time, this was myself).

We followed a loose framework, which allowed us to explore what his life experiences meant to him now; how he felt to blame for the death of his sister and the pain of his mother; and how he had always felt that he was a bad person who had to be punished. Paul eventually decided that he was continuing his own abuse by punishing himself and that he had to do something about it by resolving to move on.

To help him to do this I taught him some coping strategies to deal with his voices and the desire to self-harm.[15] He set limits, structured the time spent with his voices, learned to say 'no' to his voices and reduced the influence of his powerful voice by renaming it the 'coward' and the 'pervert'. He also focused upon the voice of Leroy and chatted with him when he felt down. Leroy was a powerful man in real life, and he asked Leroy's voice to protect him from the coward, which it mostly did. When he thought about harming himself he used a variety of techniques to interrupt his thoughts and would have a range of things to do that he liked, such as having a hot bath, watching football and running continuously around a set track.

Paul eventually left the hospital after 3 months, moving back into his flat. Ricky spent 2 days working closely with him, transferring his care to a person introduced some weeks earlier from an assertive community team. Ricky continued to see Paul as a friend. Paul has not been back to hospital, although once he set fire to his legs with lighter fuel 'as a bargain', after 2 days spent listening to his voices. Paul felt he was relapsing and was terrified of going mad. His voices reinforced this. I visited him once then and explained that he was in control, was not going mad and that sometimes we all just have bad patches. He was, however, afraid of his voice, so again we explored what had already been agreed: that the voice (of itself) was not the problem but rather it was its identity, and its meaning in his life, which gave it the power.

Paul's fear of this voice was the issue that he needed, again, to surmount – not the idea that he had 'relapsed'. We explored again the reasons why his voice had appeared again, so powerfully. Paul had experienced a series of flashbacks after seeing (although not meeting) his abuser in a supermarket. Having clarified what was the real problem this then enabled Paul to regain control in his life.

---

journey, however, then there must be some short cuts or a route map. Nurses can be guides along this journey, and can offer expert advice on the most appropriate way to reach a destination. The person sets the destination, but the nurse can advise the person, from their experience, as to what might be the best way to get there.

It is important to remember, however, that for some people looking back at their life is not practical, or possible, or perhaps something they want to do. What a nurse can do is to adopt Florence Nightingale's approach – placing the person in the best position for nature to take its course.

In other words, if the person does not want to do all the above things, this is acceptable. It is not compulsory. The nurse needs to help the person to be in a position where they are not disadvantaged or stopped from recovering, when they feel the time is right. Generally, I do this by dealing with practical problems, teaching ways of coping with distressing consequences of the abuse – such as the feelings of shame – and letting the person know that it's all right not to do anything about the abuse. This is handled far better when the person feels ready.[15]

There are further underpinning principles in the process of recovery that can be used as a structure to help people on their recovery journey. These principles and detailed exercises are explained in the *THRIVE* manual[1] that aims to help the client and the nurse to understand and have a framework for approaching the deeply personal and dynamic process that constitutes recovery and thriving.

REFERENCES

1. Aslan M, Smith M. *THRIVE, the thrive approach to mental wellness.* Warrington, UK: Crazy Diamond, 2007.

2. Talking Cure. *What works in therapy.* Available from: www.talkingcure.com/docs/What_Works.doc. Accessed August 2007.

3. Romme M, Escher S. *Accepting voices.* London, UK: Mind Publications, 1993.

4. Ensink B. Trauma: a study of childhood abuse and hallucinations. In: Romme M, Escher S (eds). *Accepting voices.* London, UK: Mind Publications, 1993.

5. Warner S. *Understanding child sexual abuse: making the tactics visible.* Gloucester, UK: Handsell, 2000.

6. Shapiro S. Self mutilation and self blame in incest victims. *American Journal of Psychotherapy* 1987; **61**: 1.

7. Diclemente R, Ponton L, Hartley D. Prevalence and correlates of cutting behaviour. *Journal of the American Academy of Child and Adolescent Psychiatry* 1991; **30**: 735–9.

8. Boyle M. *Schizophrenia: a scientific delusion?* London, UK: Routledge, 2001.

9. CASL. *The campaign against the schizophrenia label*. Asylum Publications. Available from: www.asylumonline.net. Accessed August 2007.

10. Lefevre S. *Killing me softly. Self-harm, survival not suicide.* Gloucester, UK: Handsell, 1996.

11. Smith M. *Working with self-harm: a workbook*. Gloucester, UK: Handsell, 1998.

12. Harrison D. *Vicious circles. An exploration of women and self harm in society*. London, UK: Good Practices in Mental Health, 1994.

13. Sigmon M, Green R, Nicholls K. Coping and adjustment in male and female survivors of childhood sexual abuse. *Journal of Child Sexual Abuse* 1996; **6**: 57–75.

14. Gill M, Tutty L. Male survivors of childhood sexual abuse: qualitative study and issues for clinical consideration. *Journal of Child Sexual Abuse* 1996; **6**: 19–33.

15. Smith M (ed.). *Psychiatric first aid in psychosis*. Gloucester, UK: Handsell, 2002.

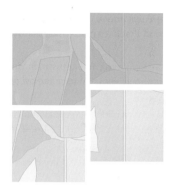

CHAPTER 32

The person with an eating disorder

Rachel A. Keaschuk* and Amanda S. Newton**

An eating disorder is not usually a phase, and it is not necessarily indicative of madness. It is quite maddening, granted, not only for the loved ones of the eating disordered person, but also for the person. It is, at the most basic level, a bundle of contradictions: a desire for power that strips you of all power. A gesture of strength that divests you of strength. A wish to prove that you need nothing, that you have no human hungers, which turns on itself and becomes a searing need for the hunger itself. It is an attempt to find an identity, but ultimately it strips you of any sense of yourself …

Hornbacher[1]

INTRODUCTION

The quote from Marya Hornbacher's personal memoir, *Wasted*, reflects the complicated psychological world experienced by the person with an eating disorder. Collectively, eating disorders are part of a spectrum of eating pathology that extends from severe self-starvation to the severe overconsumption of food. What makes eating disorders illnesses are not just the severe disturbances in eating behaviours but also the acute cognitive distress associated with the behaviours. This chapter provides an overview of the eating disorders and discusses in detail appropriate forms of therapeutic support for this clinical population.

DEFINING EATING DISORDERS

There are four recognized eating disorders, each differentiated by their unique behavioural disturbances and accompanying psychological sequelae. Anorexia nervosa (AN) and bulimia nervosa (BN) are the two eating disorders most extensively documented in popular media, and, diagnostically speaking, have been classified the longest. In the 1970s, AN became the first eating disorder to be classified with medical diagnostic criteria, followed by BN in 1979. In the 1980s, atypical eating disorders, or disorders that were not readily classified under the criteria for AN and BN, were recognized as eating disorders not otherwise specified (ED NOS).[2] More recently, binge eating disorder (BED) has begun to receive recognition as another form of eating pathology, but is not yet diagnosable as a syndrome in its own right.[3]

Anorexia nervosa

The cardinal psychological feature of AN is a pervasive fear of weight gain and unrealistic evaluation of physical

*Rachel A. Keaschuk is a clinician and researcher in the Pediatric Centre for Weight and Health at the Stollery Children's Hospital in Edmonton, Alberta, Canada. Her interests include the development of eating disorders, gender differences in eating and body image pathology, and psychological correlates of paediatric obesity.

**Amanda S. Newton is an Assistant Professor and Clinician Scientist at the University of Alberta in Edmonton, Alberta, Canada. She has worked extensively in mental health nursing as a cognitive–behavioural clinician and currently leads a research programme focused on addressing paediatric mental health emergencies in Canadian emergency departments.

shape, despite a starved appearance. Refusal to maintain body weight above minimum recommendations generally translates to being 15 per cent below recommended weight for age and height. Because of the extreme weight loss in this disorder, amenorrhoea (loss of menstruation for at least 3 consecutive months) is experienced in women and included as a diagnostic criterion for this gender. Self-employed strategies to achieve weight loss include lengthy periods of food restriction/starvation (classified as the restricting subtype of AN) and/or food restriction/starvation coupled with excessive exercise and purging behaviours such as the use of laxatives or self-induced vomiting (classified as the binge/purge subtype of AN).[4]

Bulimia nervosa

BN is similar to AN in that size and shape are unrealistically valued, but this disorder is marked by recurrent episodes of binge eating (considered the eating of an unusually large amount of food in a discrete period of time). What makes this eating experience unique for an individual with BN, and unlike a large meal eaten by someone with an unusually large appetite, is that the binge is accompanied by feeling out of control and by recurrent behaviours to undo or compensate for the binge episode. This includes self-induced vomiting and laxative/diuretic misuse (classified as the purging subtype of BN) and excessive exercise or periods of fasting (classified as the non-purging subtype of BN).[4] The weight of an individual with BN is dependent on caloric intake during binges as well as the extent to which they engage in purging behaviours. However, weight can be within normal (recommended) guidelines when bingeing behaviours exceed purging behaviours. Many individuals demonstrate a combination of both anorexic and bulimic behaviours; 50–64 per cent of individuals with AN develop bulimic symptoms, and individuals with BN can go on to be diagnosed with AN.[4]

Eating disorder not otherwise specified and binge eating disorder

Individuals with eating disorders that meet some of the diagnostic criteria for either AN or BN, but not all, are diagnosed with ED NOS. This is a diagnosis given to more than 50 per cent of individuals with eating disorders. While individuals diagnosed with ED NOS may not present with all of the symptoms of other eating disorders, their cognitions regarding weight, shape and body are significantly distorted. Like BN, weight for individuals with ED NOS can be within recommended guidelines. BED is identified as a form of ED NOS in individuals who engage in binge eating, but do not engage in compensatory behaviours (such as those observed in BN) to counter the binge.[3,4] The weight of individuals diagnosed with BED is typically well above recommended guidelines (e.g. obese) as caloric intake from bingeing for exceeds energy-expending activities.

Reflection

Compare and contrast the possible clinical features of anorexia nervosa, bulimia nervosa, eating disorder not otherwise specified and binge eating disorder.

THE PREVALENCE AND COMPLEXITY OF EATING DISORDERS

In modern societies, the prevalence of AN is estimated at 0.5–1 per cent and that for BN is 1–4 per cent.[5] This prevalence increases fivefold when accounting for ED NOS.[4] BED has a broad prevalence range, occurring in approximately 2 per cent of the community population and in 1–30 per cent of individuals seeking obesity treatment. For AN, BN and ED NOS, the male–female prevalence ratio ranges from 1:6 to 1:10, whereas for BED the male–female prevalence ratio is approximately 3:10.[4,5] The increasing prevalence of eating disorders in men has become well documented. Woodside et al.[6] suggest that eating disorders are underdiagnosed/under-recognized in men and that prevalence rates for partial symptom eating disorders are approaching equivalence between the genders for AN (male–female = 1:1.5) and BN (male–female = 1:1.8).

Evidence to date highlights complex interactions in the disorder's development and persistence, which includes the influence of personal (i.e. developmental and psychological make-up), socioenvironmental (i.e. sociocultural and peer norms, familial environment) and behavioural (i.e. eating, weight management and coping) features.[7,8] From this perspective, eating disorders alter physiological functioning, cognitions (i.e. thinking patterns), self-concept and relationships. Although these alterations vary on an individual basis in terms of degree of severity and the number of manifestations, they are particularly important when considering appropriate forms of therapeutic support for this clinical population.

EATING DISORDERS IN TREATMENT

The course of treatment for individuals with an eating disorder will depend on the severity of their disorder, and can span from outpatient treatment to inpatient care. For patients requiring inpatient care, there is evidence to suggest that specialized inpatient treatment offers better clinical outcomes than general inpatient settings in which healthcare professionals have limited training and experience specific to working with individuals with eating disorders.[9] Patients with eating disorders require the expertise and input of a core multidisciplinary team of healthcare professionals including psychiatrists, nurses, psychologists, dietitians, social workers and specialized therapists (i.e. cognitive–behavioural, occupational and/or art therapists). The specific role of each professional will vary depending on the organizational structure of the programme and the professionals' specialized training.[4] Other medical specialists may be consulted for management of acute and ongoing complications, and in the treatment of children and adolescents, school teachers, counsellors and sports coaches may be asked to collaborate.

Assessing eating disorders

All patients with an eating disorder should initially receive a full medical assessment and should receive interim assessments during treatment. An important contribution from nurses in the medical management of eating disorders is their conduction of assessments alongside other health professionals that profile the patient's eating disorder symptoms and behaviours.[10] Formal assessment measures, including self-report questionnaires and semi-structured interviews, can be employed by the nurse, and will assist in identifying target symptoms and behaviours that should be addressed in the treatment plan. Examples are listed in Table 32.1.

The physical impact of eating disorders and its management

The physical impact of eating disorders varies. Some individuals may have minimal medical concerns, despite the severity of their illness, whereas other individuals may experience multiple complications. Major body systems can be affected by eating disorders, including the cardiovascular, endocrine, gastrointestinal, reproductive, dermatological and haematological systems.[18] Physical symptoms commonly result from self-starvation and compensatory behaviours (e.g. self-induced vomiting, laxative misuse). Extreme weight loss from self-starvation is known to be related to cardiac arrhythmia (abnormal heart rate), bradycardia (slow heart contractions) and amenorrhoea, while self-induced vomiting can lead to glandular inflammation (the parotid glands), oesophageal erosions (from stomach acid exposure) and electrolyte abnormalities.[4,18] Physiological and medical management of eating disorders primarily targets nutritional restoration and maintenance along with the treatment of associated physical complications.[4] The role of the nurse in this management is supportive to the medical team and involves monitoring physical signs and symptoms experienced by the patient.

Reflection

What physical complications are associated with eating disorders?

Psychological treatment of eating disorders

The quote at the beginning of this chapter illustrates the paradoxical and complicated psychic and physical relationship that individuals with an eating disorder have with themselves. Several treatment models acknowledge this complexity and offer interpretations of how this self-relationship develops, what it represents, and how to treat the eating disorder based on the specific model's interpretation.

TABLE 32.1 Eating disorder assessment tools

Tool	Description
Bulimia Test – Revised (BULIT-R)[11]	A self-report tool that assesses eating behaviours and attitudes related to BN
Eating Attitudes Test (EAT)[12]	A self-report tool that screens for symptoms and concerns characteristics of eating disorders
Eating Disorder Examination (EDE)[13]	A tool administered by healthcare professionals that measures the presence and severity of eating disorder cognitions and behaviours and provides diagnostic interpretations
Eating Disorder Examination Questionnaire (EDE-Q)[14]	A self-report version of the EDE, designed for clinical situations when an interview cannot be used
Eating Disorders Inventory 2 (EDI-2)[15]	A self-report tool that measures psychological traits and symptom clusters for eating disorders
Eating Disorders Questionnaire (EDQ)[16]	A self-report tool that assesses eating disorder symptoms, time course and treatment
Yale–Brown–Cornell Eating Disorder Scale (YBC-EDS)[17]	A tool administered by healthcare professionals that assesses eating disorder symptoms

A psychodynamic approach

In general, psychodynamic theorists believe that eating disorders are symptomatic expressions of unresolved psychological conflicts.[19] Psychodynamic understandings of eating disorders emphasize the impact of early experiences on the development of the self, emotional regulation and coping skills. Early experiences form the basis for how we come to understand ourselves, others and the world around us. These experiences help us to learn to regulate drives for physiological needs and for relationships. When there are conflicts in early relationships, individuals may form distorted views of themselves and others, or may be unable to regulate their emotions and responses. For an individual with an eating disorder, conflicts in early relationships can lead to self-reliance for pleasure, reward and security/comfort. Eating disordered behaviours become a simultaneous way to avoid interpersonal needs and conflicts, and to self-regulate distressing emotions.

Underlying all psychodynamic treatments is an understanding that treating the symptoms will not result in disorder remission. In fact, from this perspective it is necessary to treat the underlying conflict or cause before the symptoms will begin to change. Many psychodynamic theorists believe that treating the symptom through therapy without treating the cause will only cause the symptom to change how it is expressed, and will not lead to remission of the disorder.[2,4]

An interpersonal approach

Interpersonal psychotherapy (IPT) is a short-term therapy initially developed for treating individuals with depression; however, it has been applied in the interpretation and treatment of eating disorders, primarily BN.[20] IPT views the symptoms of the eating disorder as being intertwined with the individual's interpersonal relationships. Similar to psychodynamic theories, IPT does not treat the symptoms of an eating disorder directly; however, IPT does differ from psychodynamic theories in that the focus of treatment is on *current* interpersonal problems, rather than historical conflicts. The goals of treatment are to decrease symptoms and improve ways of relating to and experiencing interpersonal relationships. There are four categories of interpersonal problems that may be the focus of IPT: grief (e.g. loss of important relationships), interpersonal role disputes (e.g. conflict in a significant relationship), difficulties with role transitions (e.g. leaving home, marriage, beginning a new job) and interpersonal deficits (e.g. few satisfying relationships, social isolation).[21]

A cognitive–behavioural approach

Cognitive–behavioural conceptualizations of eating disorders focus on the interplay between the individual's thoughts (cognitions), feelings (affect) and behaviours. Thoughts, feelings and behaviours all influence each other, and often a single thought, feeling or behaviour will affect a chain of thinking, feeling and/or actions.

According to cognitive–behavioural theorists, there are significant cognitive disturbances that characterize eating disorders and these are central to the development of eating disordered behaviours. A fundamental cognitive disturbance is the tendency to primarily judge self-worth on the basis of weight, eating and appearance, rather than assessing performance in multiple domains (e.g. interpersonal, academic, work). Cognitive distortions related to this disturbance may include low self-esteem (excessively negative self-evaluation), perfectionism and rigid rules regarding eating and exercise.[22] Eating disordered behaviours can also occur in relation to negative affects. For example, bingeing or restricting when feeling sad are common affect–behaviour pairings. In general, cognitive–behavioural theorists hold that disturbed cognitions and negative affects may precede eating disordered behaviour. However, eating disordered behaviours can also contribute to the maintenance of disturbed cognitions (e.g. restricting leads to weight loss, which provides the individual with positive feedback) and the resolution of negative affects (e.g. an adrenaline rush after bingeing or purging). In this sense, eating disordered behaviours perpetuate the cycle of thoughts, feelings and behaviours that maintain the disorder.

Of the psychological approaches presented thus far, the cognitive–behavioural approach is the only one with therapeutic techniques that directly treat the eating disordered behaviours. Unlike psychodynamic therapy or IPT, cognitive–behavioural therapy (CBT) does not necessarily address factors that may have contributed to the development of eating disorders; rather, it focuses on the factors within the individual that are maintaining the disorder.[22]

> ### Reflection
>
> What are the strengths and limitations of the different psychological approaches for treating eating disorders?

THERAPEUTIC RELATIONSHIPS WITH INDIVIDUALS WITH AN EATING DISORDER

Working with an individual with an eating disorder necessitates the appreciation of the patient's self-relationship and how to approach the therapeutic relationship based on this appreciation. This section will present basic roles that nurses may adopt, irrespective of the clinical setting they are working in, along with essential principles to consider during the development of the nurse–patient therapeutic relationship.

In a recent analysis of UK nurses' experiences of working with patients with eating disorders, there were three principles that were felt to be related to this type of nursing,[23] two of which were related to relationship building. The first of these was providing *empathic support*, which involved conveying positive regard and warmth. The second was nursing as *discipline and surveillance*, which involved setting consistent, firm boundaries with respect to expectations and behaviours. In building relationships with patients the key is to be able to combine both roles: to be warm and empathic while still setting strong boundaries.[23]

Nurses as empathic professionals

A therapeutic relationship built on empathy is foundational and essential, as it will serve as the basis for ongoing exploration and treatment of the problems associated with the patient's eating disorder. Empathy involves the patient feeling understood and heard by the nurse he or she is working with. This involves interactions between the nurse and patient that convey trust, respect and openness to the patient's experience. Empathy in theory is easy to appreciate, but empathy *in action* can often be difficult. Working with patients does not always involve them wanting to receive treatment (e.g. 'I'm not doing this. You can't make me.'), and they may convey a lack of respect for the nurse they work with (e.g. 'I hate you! You don't even know what you're doing.'). Recognizing these behaviours as disorder-related phenomena can be a challenge, but reacting to these behaviours at face value can create barriers to fostering empathy. It is important for patients to feel valued as people and not as behaviours. In this way, nurses provide an opportunity to support the development of a patient's identity outside their eating disorder. Help-resistant patients are trapped in mistrust; this may be based on past interpersonal experiences or current ones in treatment. Trust grows through empathy. Nurses who listen to their patient's concerns, convey respect for these concerns, and shape these concerns for the patient to better understand their origin (i.e. the concern's relationship to the patient's eating disorder) will build trust. Personal illustration 32.1 provides an example of how nurses can convey empathy with their patient.

Nurses as consistent professionals

Receiving treatment for an eating disorder requires the eventual replacement of eating disordered behaviours and disturbed cognitions with healthier behaviours and thoughts. For many patients with eating disorders, the only consistency they have had in their lives is their eating disorder, and replacing their eating disordered experience can be stressful given that the eating disorder has provided comfort and a sense of control over difficult situations. Along with adopting an empathic approach, a consistent approach can help to mitigate the patient's fear and concerns.

Consistency in the therapeutic relationship relates to providing consistency in the care, messages and responsibilities carried by the patient. Consistency in the therapeutic relationship will help patients to understand their treatment experience and know what to expect in certain circumstances. Consistency is reinforced with validation to ensure that both the nurse and the patient understand what is being communicated and what is expected in the therapeutic relationship. In this sense, consistency involves being clear and concise. Clear expectations are easier for patients to understand, especially when they are stressed.[24]

When working in a multidisciplinary treatment setting, consistency can be a challenge as it will involve all healthcare professionals working together to provide complementary messages from their specific disciplines. For treatment to be effective, all professionals must work closely together and maintain open communication in order to reduce the potential of providing the patient with confusing and inconsistent treatment messages. Consistency also encourages the patient to work with the team as a whole versus working with or valuing the input of certain providers and not others.

Nurses as therapeutic communicators

Therapeutic communication is one of the most important skills nurses can develop. This skill not only underpins both empathy and consistency, but also enables the nurse to respond to patients when they are ready to talk, are in crisis, or are coping with change. Therapeutic communication involves listening to what patients are saying and allowing them to finish their thoughts. This can be a challenge when patients are communicating distorted perceptions related to their eating disorder, but in order to foster empathy and trust it is important to allow patients to express their experiences. Underpinning this approach to listening is adopting a non-judgemental stance. This involves the nurse refraining from judging the experience the patient is sharing, or providing suggestions and

---

Personal illustration 32.1

Patient: You can't make me go! I'm not putting up with that crap today! You're just being horrible to me!

Nurse: You're right. I can't make you do anything. [pause] You seem really upset right now.

Patient: Of course I'm upset, you're making me go and join everyone in the group.

Nurse: You're feeling forced to do things you don't want to do.

Patient: Everything here feels like something I don't want to do …

Nurse: Sounds like you are feeling pretty helpless right now.

Patient: I can't make any of my own decisions and I'm afraid of doing the things I need to do.

Nurse: It's pretty scary to feel like you don't have any control over what you do, but you know that you need to do certain things to be healthy again. That's a tough spot to be in.

solutions to 'solve' the experience. From a therapeutic standpoint, a more effective approach is for the nurse to encourage patients to explore the emotions behind what they are experiencing, to validate their feelings and experiences, and to help guide them towards making their own healthy decisions based on those feelings and experiences. When patients feel judged or dismissed, or feel that they are instructed to do something a certain way, they may become more resistant to making a change. On the other hand, when patients feel that they have formulated their own plan of action through guidance with their healthcare professional, and have been treated in a respectful way, they are more likely to follow through with the treatment plans that are made.

Therapeutic listening is communicated through both verbal and non-verbal behaviours. Verbal communication that demonstrates listening includes reflecting, summarizing and encouraging patients to share their experience. This type of communication allows nurses to fully understand the patient's experience and to gather information that may be helpful in the therapeutic relationship. Non-verbal communication that demonstrates listening includes providing patients with undivided attention during contact, making eye contact and nodding encouragement. Patients may be initially reluctant to share their experiences and will benefit from verbal and non-verbal therapeutic communication to encourage self-exploration. Further, during the course of their treatment they may be reluctant to look beyond immediate symptoms to explore their relationship with themselves (intrapersonal) and with others (interpersonal). Conversely, some patients may be hesitant to discuss eating disorder thoughts and behaviours in favour of focusing on 'core personal issues'

as a way to avoid addressing their eating disorder. Using therapeutic communication strategies to explore patients' approaches to treatment can help reframe their experiences and allow them to progress towards wellness.

Patients will also communicate using verbal and non-verbal means, and it can be difficult to discern which of these modes to respond to. Often, time focusing on the overt verbal messages will be less productive than focusing on the non-verbal messages. For example, a nurse discussing food with a patient who is refusing to eat is unlikely to enable the patient to make healthy changes. However, the nurse's observation that the patient appears agitated and therefore focuses the discussion around this observation may be a more productive therapeutic dialogue. From this approach it is possible that a new solution, other than restricting food, can be found to manage the patient's distress and agitation. Personal illustration 32.2 presents a nurse–patient dialogue focused on this type of interaction.

Nurses engaging in self-care

Working with patients with eating disorders involves maintaining consistent boundaries to promote a healthy therapeutic relationship. In order to accomplish these tasks nurses need to engage in self-care. Self-care refers to the actions that healthcare providers engage in to nurture and care for themselves. Caring for individuals with eating disorders can affect issues for the healthcare provider, and it is important for providers to be able to separate themselves from their jobs. Separating oneself as an individual from professionally being a nurse can be a difficult task. It involves taking responsibility for nursing care but also expecting patients to take responsibility for their care as well. Nurses can feel personally responsible when patients do not take the steps towards recovery that are expected. In the case of eating disorders, it is important to acknowledge that the nature of the disorder makes change difficult. It is also impossible to change another person's disordered eating: he or she must make the decision to act towards change. Nurses must also be aware of their own personal beliefs about eating disorders and individuals with eating disorders. These beliefs and biases can affect the type of care that is given. In this sense, it is important for nurses to engage in self-exploration and reflection to better understand how they interact with their patients. A series of questions to encourage self-reflection is outlined in Box 32.1.

Personal illustration 32.2

Patient: I'm not finishing my lunch, and I'm not drinking that Ensure either. Can't you see how fat I am?

Nurse: You seem really bothered right now, what's going on for you?

Patient: Can't you see I'm upset by this lunch?

Nurse: You're feeling too fat to eat lunch, and you've had a pretty intense morning with your parents being in the unit.

Patient: They're really frustrating, but I can't tell them that because it will hurt them too much.

Nurse: You didn't get a chance to tell your parents that you feel frustrated because you're afraid that it will hurt them. Now you are really upset because you feel like you didn't say what you needed to.

Patient: Exactly. I can't seem to stop replaying the conversation or worrying about what will happen if I don't say something.

Nurse: What do you think we can do to help you manage your anxiety right now?

Reflection

Which aspect of the nurse–patient therapeutic relationship do you personally consider the foundation of your clinical care? Reflect on which aspects you feel comfortable with and which aspects you need to develop as a healthcare professional.

SUMMARY

Eating pathology has increasingly become the most prevalent of psychiatric issues in women and female youth, and is an increasing psychiatric issue in males. Eating disorders can be identified by their disturbances in eating behaviours coupled with acute distress during eating periods, as well as distress over body shape and weight. The key features of eating disorders are the coupling of cognitive distortions with disordered behaviours. Given this, their impact is far-reaching; they alter physiologic functioning, thinking patterns, self-concept and interpersonal relationships. Understanding these sequelae is crucial because they will guide decision-making for appropriate therapeutic support. For nurses, it is important to consider the nature of the patient's disorder when building a therapeutic relationship. Empathy, firm and consistent boundaries, and the use of therapeutic communication can foster a healthy, therapeutic relationship. The health of this relationship is important for the recovery of the patient and the professional well-being of the nurse who is providing care.

The key points of this chapter are as follows:

- Eating disorders are characterized by disturbances in eating behaviours coupled with cognitive distortions related to weight and appearance.
- Eating disorders can have a systemic impact on an individual's physical and mental health as well as their interpersonal relationships.
- The nurse's understanding of how eating disorders affect cognitions and behaviours is essential to building a therapeutic relationship with an individual who has an eating disorder.
- The nurse's use of empathy, boundaries and therapeutic communication are cornerstones to fostering and maintaining a therapeutic relationship with an individual who has an eating disorder.

REFERENCES

1. Hornbacher M. *Wasted*. New York, NY: Harper Collins Publishers, 1998.

2. Fairburn CG, Brownell KD (eds). *Eating disorders and obesity: a comprehensive handbook*, 2nd edn. New York, NY: The Guilford Press, 2002.

3. Devlin MJ, Goldfein JA, Dobrow I. What is this thing called BED? Current status of binge eating disorder nosology. *International Journal of Eating Disorders* 2003; **34**: S2–S18.

4. American Psychiatric Association. Practice guidelines for the treatment of patients with eating disorders (revision). *American Journal of Psychiatry* 2000; **157**: 1–39.

5. Hoek HW, van Hoeken D. Review of the prevalence and incidence of eating disorders. *International Journal of Eating Disorders* 2003; **34**: 383–96.

6. Woodside DB, Garfinkel PE, Lin E *et al*. Comparisons of men with full or partial eating disorders, men without eating disorders, and women with eating disorders in the community. *American Journal of Psychiatry* 2001; **158**: 570–4.

7. Rosen DS, Neumark-Sztainer D. Reviews for options for primary prevention of eating disturbances among adolescents. *Journal of Adolescent Health* 1998; **23**: 354–63.

8. Stice E. Risk and maintenance factors for eating pathology: a meta-analytic review. *Psychological Bulletin* 2002; **128**: 825–48.

9. Palmer RL, Treasure J. Providing specialised services for anorexia nervosa. *British Journal of Psychiatry* 1999; **175**: 306–9.

10. Kaplan AS. Medical and nutritional assessment. In: Kaplan AS, Garfinkel PE (eds). *Medical issues and the eating disorders: the interface*. New York, NY: Brunner/Mazel, 1993: 1–16.

11. Thelen MH, Mintz LB, Vander Wal JS. The Bulimia Test, revised: validation with DSM-IV criteria for bulimia nervosa. *Psychological Assessment* 1996; **8**: 219–21.

12. Garner DM, Olmsted MP, Bohr Y, Garfinkel PE. The Eating Attitudes Test: psychometric features and clinical correlates. *Psychological Medicine* 1982; **12**: 871–8.

13. Fairburn CG, Cooper Z. The Eating Disorder Examination. In: Fairburn CG, Wilson GT (eds). *Binge eating: nature, assessment and treatment*, 12th edn. New York, NY: The Guilford Press, 1993: 317–60.

14. Fairburn CG, Beglin SJ. Assessment of eating disorders: interview or self-report questionnaire? *International Journal of Eating Disorders* 1994; **16**: 363–70.

15. Garner DM. The Eating Disorders Inventory-2 (EDI-2). In: Sederer LI, Dicky B (eds). *Outcomes assessments in clinical practice*. Baltimore, MD: Williams & Wilkins, 1996: 92–6.

16. Mitchell JE, Hatsukami D, Eckert E, Pyle RL. The Eating Disorders Questionnaire. *Psychopharmacological Bulletin* 1985; **21**: 1025–43.

17. Sunday SR, Halmi KA, Einhorn A. The Yale–Brown–Cornell Eating Disorder scale: a new scale to assess eating disorder symptomatology. *International Journal of Eating Disorders* 1995; **18**: 237–45.

18. Pomeroy C, Mitchell JE. Medical complications of anorexia nervosa and bulimia nervosa. In: Fairburn CG, Brownell KD (eds). *Eating disorders and obesity: a comprehensive handbook*, 2nd edn. New York, NY: The Guilford Press, 2002: 287–5.

19. Goodsit A. Eating disorders: a self-psychological perspective. In: Garner DM, Garfinkel PE (eds). *Handbook of treatment for eating disorders*, 2nd edn. New York, NY: The Guilford Press, 1997: 205–28.

20. Fairburn CG, Jones R, Peveler RC, *et al.* Three psychological treatments for bulimia nervosa: a comparative trial. *Archives of General Psychiatry* 1991; **48**: 463–9.

21. Weissman MM, Markowitz JC, Klerman GL. *Comprehensive guide to interpersonal psychotherapy*. New York, NY: Basic Books, 2000.

22. Fairburn CG. Cognitive behavioral therapy for bulimia nervosa. In: Fairburn CG, Brownell KD (eds). *Eating disorders and obesity: a comprehensive handbook*, 2nd edn. New York, NY: The Guilford Press, 2002: 302–7.

23. Ryan V, Malson H, Clarke S *et al.* Discursive constructions of 'eating disorders nursing': an analysis of nurses' accounts of nursing eating disorder patients. *European Eating Disorders Review* 2006; **14**: 125–35.

24. George L. The psychological characteristics of patients suffering from anorexia nervosa and the nurse's role in creating a therapeutic relationship. *Journal of Advanced Nursing* 1997; **26**: 899–908.

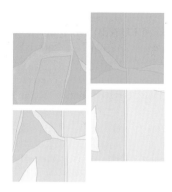

CHAPTER 33

The person who is homeless

Paul Veitch*

INTRODUCTION

This chapter offers the reader an introduction to the problems facing homeless people and to the practice implications for psychiatric–mental health nurses (PMHNs). We will explore who the homeless are and then consider the special challenges faced by different health and social care practitioners in trying to meet their needs. Most of the issues and related nursing approaches outlined here will have a UK focus, but will be applicable to the many other mental health service users who are insecurely housed, living in poverty and facing restricted access to health care in other countries.

Homeless people provide a graphic illustration of both the enmeshed nature of social and health problems and the structural deficiencies of the services attempting to address them. The range and intensity of health and social problems faced by homeless people are often daunting to professionals; however, we consider that the PMHN has a valuable set of skills to offer and is well placed to address the multiple needs of homeless people. To be helpful to homeless people, we need to address issues of poverty, stigma and social exclusion. This calls for a varied knowledge base, encompassing mental illness, drug and alcohol use, physical health, housing, social security systems and an awareness of the agencies addressing them, as well as the underlying ethical dilemmas

produced.[1] The 'inverse care law' is evident here, in which homelessness is an extreme form of social exclusion with huge health problems yet homeless people have great difficulty accessing and negotiating their way to utilizing health care.

For specialist practitioners who work in homelessness teams in particular, this work demands an ability to work outside the familiar clinically orientated multidisciplinary setting and in partnership with a network of providers, some of whom may be philosophically at odds with traditional mental health services. It is these PMHNs who are often evolving new and innovative practices with homeless people and who set the benchmark of good practice in this area. However, such services are often viable only in urban settings with big populations and PMHNs working without recourse to specialist advice should not consider the difficulties of homeless people as beyond the remit of their everyday practice.

WHAT IS HOMELESSNESS?

Absolutes and universal truths relating to homelessness and homeless people do not exist.[2] There has never been a consensus about what homelessness means or who homeless people are, and the PMHN should exercise caution when confronted by generalizations about the

*Paul Veitch has worked as a psychiatric nurse in the north-east of England for 25 years. He has a Masters degree in Psychiatric Nursing and has specialized for 7 years in working with people who are homeless. Presently, he works as a manager and practitioner in an Early Intervention in Psychosis Team.

needs of 'the homeless' in the literature and media. What is true of one subgroup of homeless people may be the opposite for another. Attempts at quantification usually reflect the professional and political interests of those framing them and are additionally problematic as even people generally agreed to be homeless at a given point in time are notoriously hard to count and easy to discount. Definitions are particularly critical, however, because they determine the moral agenda and the shape and extent of the services available.[3]

In the UK, homelessness has been defined in legislation as having no accommodation which one might 'reasonably' occupy. This includes those who are:

- 'sleeping rough' (rooflessness)
- living in direct access hostels and shelters aimed at homeless people
- using temporary accommodation (including families), such as hostels or bed and breakfast hotels, or occupying empty buildings
- in prison, hospital or care, without access to 'move-on' housing
- staying with family and friends (often called the 'hidden homeless').

The demographic and health profiles of the subgroups of homeless people moving between those forms of non-tenure vary considerably. Homeless people include asylum seekers and refugees, young people, older people, children, families, people from ethnic minorities, single people and couples. The focus here will be on the subgroup known as 'single homeless people' because they experience considerably poorer physical and mental health than any other section of society and arguably of any other homeless subgroup. They are the most likely to experience physical and mental health problems as a direct result of their lack of tenure. The single homeless are adults who usually sleep rough or in institutional settings (prisons, hostels, shelters and squats), and no statutory authority has accepted a responsibility to re-house them.[4]

Personal illustration 33.1

Simon, a 50-year-old man who had been successful in business, was made homeless following a series of disastrous losses. Depression and alcohol use had contributed to his downfall and he came to live in a hostel. He had to ask permission to leave the building, was unable to find a satisfactory degree of privacy and felt humiliated by his lack of financial independence. Although not seeking psychiatric help, Simon spoke to the PMHN who visited the hostel. The PMHN was able to convey an understanding of Simon's frustration, which enabled Simon to decide to find a less restrictive hostel.

More holistic conceptions of homelessness attempt to encompass processes that people experience in losing access to housing – perhaps the single most important component of health. Brandt's[5] definition attempts a synthesis between housing status (the quality and tenure of accommodation) and features of structural and personal social relationship:

> A person is homeless when he or she does not have a place to live that can be considered to be stable, permanent and of a reasonable housing standard. At the same time, this person is not able to make use of society's relations and institutions (understood in the broadest sense, such as family networks and private and public institutions of all kinds) due to either apparent or hidden causes relating to the individual or to the way in which society functions.

Belonging to the 'homeless family' and the social support it provides can be central to why many remain homeless or do not succeed in what from the outside appears to be a suitable abode. Qualitative research allows us some insights into this world.[6,7] An illustration from practice is a homeless man who had been admitted to a psychiatric facility and then discharged to a flat of his own. This man had been found what most would describe as 'suitable' accommodation. It was warm, safe and secure, offered a variety of support systems and was well integrated with the healthcare and social systems the man otherwise utilized. However, what it did not provide was the camaraderie and sense of place that he had found over a number of years living in street locations. To experience this, he regularly slept rough with groups of drinkers in a disused cemetery while maintaining the tenancy and remaining well.

In the UK, approximately 90 per cent of the single homeless are men aged between 25 and 50 years, although there is a recognized recent increase in youth homelessness. It is problematic to determine the degree to which ethnicity is a factor, but black people are over-represented in overall homelessness figures, while being less so in hostels and shelters. Particularly in the London boroughs, Irish people are over-represented, with London having about half the single homeless people in the UK. Military backgrounds are over-represented as are young people leaving the care of statutory social services. The single homeless are generally estranged from their birth and extended family with high divorce rates.

Personal illustration 33.2

Alan was, for the first time, willing to share time with the PMHN over a cup of tea at the day centre. However, he was tearful and unable to concentrate on the simple conversation. He soon left the building, but tolerated the company of the nurse on a walk. When crossing the bridge he talked of feeling compelled to jump but was agreeable to a formal interview in the emergency room where his active suicidal intent led to a hospital admission.

Some experiences such as a history of childhood parental abuse and unemployment appear to make people vulnerable to homelessness. Specific crisis points often precede an episode of homelessness (such as prison discharge or relationship breakdown). In the UK, discharge from long-stay psychiatric hospital does not appear to have been a major cause of homelessness so much as the closure of large-scale hostels and lodging houses in the 1980s and 1990s.

Reflection

Think about the homeless people you have worked with or passed on the street.

- How do you think these people became homeless?

THE HEALTH IMPACT OF HOMELESSNESS

A strong body of evidence points to markedly higher rates of psychiatric problems in populations of homeless adults than among the securely domiciled.[8–10] Most studies support the finding that unusually high rates of psychosis and substance misuse are a common feature of homeless populations. That mental health problems exist for young homeless people,[11] homeless children and families,[12] homeless mothers,[13] and homeless people from ethnic minorities[14] have also been reported. A relationship between homelessness and offending behaviour is identified in the literature.[15] The difficulties of addressing combined substance misuse and mental illness, which exists in this group, has long been acknowledged.[16] However, consistent criticism has been directed at health research on homeless people because of methodological flaws.

The physical health of homeless people has also been investigated. Those at the most extreme end of the homeless continuum (the roofless) are more at risk from poor physical health with high rates of trauma, skin conditions, respiratory conditions and venereal infections. Chronic problems with hypertension, obstructive pulmonary disease, diabetes and dental problems are also a feature. There is a likelihood that previously non-existent disorders will develop with a prolonged period of homelessness.[17] Primary preventative strategies could be aimed at homeless children. Many of the behavioural consequences of substance misuse may appear superficially to be presentations of mental illness, and sometimes substance misuse (either acute or long term) can cause mental illness. Being able to distinguish between presentations of intoxication, overdose, delirium and withdrawal are important as all can have serious medical psychiatric consequences requiring careful assessment and sometimes hospitalization.

Personal illustration 33.3

Police arrested Alf because of threatening behaviour towards a man walking his dog in the park where Alf had been sleeping rough. This led to a compulsory psychiatric admission to hospital, where Alf was considered to be mentally unwell. At the first opportunity Alf absconded from the ward and has never been seen since. Opportunities to engage with Alf prior to this episode may have led to an improved outcome.

As well as combinations of substance misuse and mental illness, homeless people may also have physical illnesses that require treatment and that may have an impact on psychiatric management, e.g. epilepsy. Trauma is frequently encountered, but often secondary to substance misuse, injecting injuries/infections and falls during drinking sessions. Cognitive impairment can hinder people utilizing some psychotherapeutic interventions and rehabilitation interventions. Because of the above, we recommend that PMHNs give the assessment of the physical state a high priority when working with people who are homeless.

High rates of alcohol and street drug use are also found in single homeless populations and companionship (within a group of fellow drug users) is recognized as a factor in sustaining drug use. Mental disorder plays a role for some in becoming homeless, although these individuals tend to have a pre-existing heavy loading of poverty and familial instability. For those who become homeless following an episode of mental ill health, alcohol and substance misuse are often a major factor.[18]

Personal illustration 33.4

Eddie was living in some woods 12 miles from the primary care centre. The PMHN was unable to engage him in formal assessment despite concerns expressed about his obvious distress. The PMHN was very concerned with attending to Eddie's personal hygiene and finding him dry clothes. Following a team discussion, the PMHN was able to obtain a good local supply of the necessary items as well as some emergency cash for Eddie. Following the assessment, in which Eddie now participated, a suitable hostel was found and Eddie accepted treatment and support for a depressive illness.

SPECIAL ISSUES FOR SERVICES

Because people who are homeless are more likely to utilize 'ordinary' services than specialist homeless mental health teams, this section considers the special issues which will be apparent in the following clinical settings. Although based on experience in the UK many developed countries will have similar service organizations.

Joint working with homeless agencies

Jointly managing a case with homelessness agency staff is a pragmatic and enabling extension of the nursing function. People who are homeless frequently present with crises, hostile behaviour or safety needs. This demands careful negotiation and a thorough mastery of the communication systems in the homelessness agency.[19,20] Roles may be shared, or separately delineated. There are opportunities for mutual role modelling and learning, and the PMHN may also offer clinical supervision and advice. The PMHN's role can be central in organizing other mental health resources for the care of an individual.

The person who is homeless in the primary care setting

The difficulties faced by homeless people in accessing primary health care are well documented. Often, consultations in primary care will be problematic for both the practitioner and the individual seeking help as the availability of comprehensive notes about the patient will be compromised. The modernization of primary care records into electronic systems that are available nationwide may see homeless people as unforeseen beneficiaries. A homeless person may be presenting with multiple problems, all needing careful evaluation. Mental health assessment in a primary care setting should ensure that a screening includes a substance misuse profile and a specific awareness of the present housing problems as these are significant stressors. Simple interventions such as considering the need for immunization and whether the homeless person has been unable to keep up with routine outpatient appointments can be supportive and promote good engagement.

The person who is homeless and in crisis services

Crisis teams in mental health are asked to give opinions about very many individuals and are well placed to consider the needs of the homeless person who presents in a crisis, e.g. in the emergency room. When seeing so many people over short periods of crisis, clinicians need to guard against stereotyping homeless people and making judgements based on such notions. Additionally, clinicians should be aware of local homeless resources (hostels and day centres typically), which are usually adept at offering large amounts of personal support during crisis periods. A primary therapeutic role of the PMHN is to plan for and manage crisis collaboratively. Many homeless agencies provide, or are aware of, daycare support, which is often more widespread than mental health-orientated facilities. The advanced practitioner in this field should also develop additional expertise, particularly in substance dependency work.

The person who is homeless in the care of the assertive outreach team

Specialist teams offering active case work to people with serious and enduring mental health problems will almost inevitably encounter homelessness, which can act as a chronic stressor that destabilizes pre-existing severe mental health problems. Such services have at their heart the active follow-up of people who often have had very negative experiences of mental health service provision and also of institutional authority in other forms. This assertive stance is often ideally suited to homeless people, and these teams are potentially a suitable base for the specialist PMHN in homelessness.

Young homeless people in early intervention in psychosis teams

Intervention in early psychosis is aimed not only at prompt symptom resolution but also at helping young people to address their developmental needs. Psychosis often affects young people during the individuation process, and incipient psychosis development with a long prodrome or period of unrecognized and untreated psychosis is particularly harmful. Case management in such services should be 'assertive', and only when the PMHN is satisfied that the appropriate management plan has been developed should the young person involved be supported to utilize less intensively resourced teams or the primary care team. The PMHN in the early intervention team is unlikely to be effective without an ability to tolerate and intervene when substance misuse is a focus for attention.

The homeless person in an acute psychiatric hospital

To be nursed in an acute psychiatric facility would be disorienting and disconcerting to most of us. For a person who is a hostel dweller or has been street homeless a psychiatric ward may feel more secure than other circumstances that they have recently known. When homeless people are inpatients of psychiatric units there is rarely a day-to-day critical audience (someone with an awareness of their powerlessness) to challenge clinical decision-making. The first task of the PMHN working with a homeless patient, particularly in the inpatient setting, is to understand the structural powerlessness of the person and to address this with concrete strategies. A reliance on experience with securely domiciled populations can lead to false assumptions about the appropriateness of behavioural or nursing interventions.

- *Talk to the patient about the services they use in the community.* For example, hostels vary hugely in terms of philosophy, staffing levels and ability to manage challenging behaviour. Some hostels allow for alcohol use on the premises whereas others do not. If the person agrees, initiate contact – the hostel staff may be an important resource when planning leave and discharge.

- *Recognize that homeless people have 'carers' and offer them a role in the clinical process.* These may include peers, partners, staff of voluntary organizations, housing workers, outreach workers or advocates. A hospital admission may provide an opportunity for family reconciliation. The families of homeless people may be excluded from local initiatives to meet the needs of families and carers in the locality (such families are stigmatized too).
- *If the patient has no access to temporary accommodation, get him or her some housing advice quickly.* Many homeless people are referred unnecessarily to high care mental health hostels because alternatives have not been considered. Statutory authorities usually have an obligation to assess the needs of homeless people.
- *Homeless people need advocates more than any other section of society.* You may have to explain what advocates are and take extra steps to engage the patient with them. Workers (who may have been trying to manage difficult behaviour for some time) sometimes have an interest in extended hospital stays for their clients. Homeless people need *independent* advocates when these are available.
- *Ensuring linkage with community mental health services.* Specialist homeless services themselves may not be ideal and can carry a stigma of their own. Linkage into 'ordinary' local mental health and primary care services (which may be more comprehensive than the specialist homeless team) is important and needs careful negotiation. This is often more than simply referral and involves ensuring that people can utilize such resources, thus preventing a breakdown in continuity. A period of 'shared care' is often necessary with support for those workers who might have limited experience of working with homeless people.
- *Discharge arrangements.* For people who are homeless, these should involve enhanced aftercare packages.

The homeless person in a substance misuse setting

This chapter has already stressed the importance of substance misuse capability in the PMHN dealing with a person who is homeless. Substance misuse workers are regularly asked to help homeless people with substance misuse problems and often have an intimate awareness of the local homeless resources in their area. However, although many such workers are by background also mental health workers, the impact of psychiatric difficulties in addition to substance misuse and homelessness can create a sense of being overwhelmed – 'Where do I start?' – and good liaison/case discussions with staff who

already know the homeless person and creation of a mini- 'care team' is often productive.

Refugees

Many refugees have had traumatic experiences and faced very significant adversity. Refugee children can sometimes arrive in countries unattended by adults. Such individuals and families pose major challenges to the health and social care structures of their host countries and refugees can become reliant upon homeless resources such as day centres for many basic needs because they offer a social 'safety net'. The PMHN can be well placed to identify individual refugees at risk for psychiatric disorder, and utilizing appropriate interpreting help is always advised when necessary. However, the multiple needs of this grossly marginalized group will usually be best met by seeking advice from specialist teams if these are available, or by offering psychiatric–mental health nursing skills if they are not available within such multiagency teams. Often, refugees will seek reports regarding their health in order to support their legal status (see Chapter 59).

Psychotherapy

Family interventions are problematic as single homeless people are invariably estranged from their family. Case work aimed at helping such individuals reintegrate with family members, especially young people, can be an intervention with long lasting benefit. Consulting with colleagues who are advanced practitioners in family therapy would support such an intervention. Local authorities in the UK have a responsibility to ensure homeless families are given the appropriate help and support to live as a unit. The PMHN will often have some experience of engaging with families, and promoting such work by involving other support staff offers insights into functioning as well as creating therapeutic possibilities. Individual psychotherapy might be deemed unsuitable when there is an unsecure domicile, but this should not be a reason for exclusion per se. Often, people are resident in homeless hostels that offer semipermanent shelter.

Reflection

- What special skills do you think staff working with homeless people should possess?
- What particular values do you think would be important in working with this group of people?

THE ASSESSMENT OF RISK

Personal safety

Settings that the PMHN may need to access such as day centres may not have the safe interviewing facilities many PMHNs are accustomed to, and homeless people are sometimes interviewed without the kind of information usually available from referrers such as primary care staff. Owing to the complexities of need and the variety of agencies attempting to help, fragmentation can occur and clinical notes are often unavailable.

Seeing homeless people accompanied by other staff members or in a joint assessment has the potential to compromise an assessment because of inhibiting the patient. A balance needs to be found whereby the advantages of a multidisciplinary assessment are acknowledged and may outweigh such disadvantages. Some facilities search people for weapons (especially in the USA), but a more subtle approach may be to have a high index of suspicion that any person may be potentially carrying an offensive weapon (usually for personal protection). If people report a previous use of weapons, it is important to ascertain whether they are currently armed. Patients may be intoxicated with drugs or alcohol leading to an increased possibility of impulsive violence.

If people are visited in a domiciliary setting, for example a squat or shared house, then the possibility of individual patients being accompanied by an unknown person makes precautions necessary. The PMHN should consider the use of joint visits (including police accompaniment) and reserve the right not to visit the temporary domicile when this is justifiable.

Suicidality and homelessness

The homeless are a group that is often unpopular with workers because of the perception or expectation that such persons will present with multiple needs, causing difficulty in assessment and clinical management. An inquiry into suicide and homicide by people suffering from mental illness[20] makes special mention of homelessness, with 3 per cent of suicides in England and Wales, 2 per cent in Scotland and 1 per cent in Northern Ireland being those of homeless individuals. Some 71 per cent of these suicides in England and Wales occurred when homeless people were psychiatric inpatients or had been discharged from hospital within the previous 3 months. Half of these individuals were being formally followed up; yet, two-thirds were out of contact with care providers at the time of death.

These findings led the inquiry team to recommend that all homeless patients who had received inpatient care should receive the most enhanced aftercare packages. Reliable evidence about rates of self-harm and attempted suicide in homeless populations is subject to even more complex epidemiological difficulties than diagnosable mental disorder. However, research with young people in the north-west of England that was concerned with service utilization found 43 per cent of the sample reported previous suicidal intent. The most important protective factors identified (social support of

family or partners) are often absent in the case of many single homeless people.[21] This focus on suicide and self-harm belies the fact that many homeless people are themselves at risk of violence from others.

Exploitation and victimization of the homeless mentally ill

The homeless mentally ill are particularly at risk of exploitation from others. Such persons can potentially have relatively high incomes compared with their peers (from social security) and are more likely to carry cash and possessions with them at all times. They can be 'obvious' victims because of their appearance and the places they frequent. Hiday and colleagues[22] found a substantial rate of violent criminal victimization among a homeless mentally ill sample, with the combination of substance misuse and homelessness being more likely to put an individual at risk. Careful assessment of interpersonal relations is necessary as what from the outside appears to be an exploitative relationship may provide a person with companionship and protection. Providing a third party payee who takes charge of an individual's finances has not been shown to benefit such people and may be perceived as an unwanted intrusion.[23] Helping people to find an address where they can receive mail or store possessions is a helpful and less intrusive strategy.

The sharing of confidential data concerning an individual's welfare is necessarily done within disciplinary expectations concerning professional practice, as well as with regard to human rights legislation. Information made available to agencies providing care can also be used to an individual's detriment if such information is misunderstood, e.g. some psychiatric diagnoses are treated pejoratively and can prejudice an individual's chances of housing or another benefit.

Reflection

Imagine that you became homeless.

- What would be your first priority?
- What kind of help would you hope to receive?
- What would 'keep you going'?

SUMMARY

People who experience mental health problems and are homeless remain some of the most socially excluded and vulnerable persons in contemporary societies. PMHNs have the potential to fulfil a role as the champions of these people as they have the right blend of skills and flexibility of role (across clinical and social domains) to meet the multiple needs of people who are homeless. The need is to develop and adapt nursing practices and to be aware of the services which homeless people utilize.

REFERENCES

1. Timms P, Borrell T. Doing the right thing: ethical and practical dilemmas in working with homeless mentally ill people. *Journal of Mental Health* 2001; **10** (4): 419–26.

2. Neale J. Homelessness and theory reconsidered. *Housing Studies* 1997; **12**: 47–61.

3. Scott J. Homelessness and mental illness. *British Journal of Psychiatry* 1993; **162**: 314–24.

4. Pleace N, Burrows R, Quilgars D. Homelessness in contemporary Britain: conceptualisation and measurement. In: Burrows R, Pleace N, Quilgars D (eds). *Homelessness and social policy*. London, UK: Routledge, 1997.

5. Brandt P. Reflections on homelessness as seen from an institution for the homeless in Copenhagen. In: Avramov D (ed.). *Coping with homelessness: issues to be tackled and best practices in Europe*. Aldershot, UK: Ashgate, 1999: 529.

6. Payne J. An action research project in a night shelter for rough sleepers. *Journal of Psychiatric and Mental Health Nursing* 2002; **9**: 95–101.

7. Baumann SL. The meaning of being homeless. *Scholarly Inquiry for Nursing Practice: An International Journal* 1993; **7**: 59–73.

8. Dennis DL, Buckner JC, Lipton FR, Levin IS. A decade of research and services for homeless mentally ill persons: where do we stand? *American Psychologist* 1991: **46**: 1129–38.

9. Munoz M, Vasquez C, Koegel P *et al*. Differential patterns of mental disorders among the homeless in Madrid (Spain) and Los Angeles (USA). *Social Psychiatry and Psychiatric Epidemiology* 1998; **33**: 514–20.

10. McAuley A, McKenna HP. Mental disorder among a homeless population in Belfast: an exploratory survey. *Journal of Psychiatric and Mental Health Nursing* 1995; **2**: 335–42.

11. Sleegers J, Spijker J, van Limbeck J, van Engeland H. Mental health problems among homeless adolescents. *Acta Psychiatrica Scandinavica* 1998: **97**: 253–9.

12. Herth K. Hope as seen through the eyes of homeless children. *Journal of Advanced Nursing* 1998; **25** (5): 1053–62.

13. Zima BT, Wells KB, Benjamin B, Duan N. Mental health problems among homeless mothers. *Archives of General Psychiatry* 1996; **53**: 332–8.

14. Leda C, Rosenheck R. Race in the treatment of homeless mentally ill veterans. *Journal of Nervous and Mental Disease* 1995; **183** (8): 529–37.

15. Gelberg L, Linn S, Leake BD. Mental health, alcohol and drug use, and criminal history among homeless adults. *American Journal of Psychiatry* 1988; **145** (2): 191–6.

16. Drake R, Osher F, Wallach M. Homelessness and the dual diagnosis. *American Psychologist* 1991: **46**: 1149–58.

17. Gerlberg L, Linn LS. Assessing the physical health of homeless adults. *Journal of the American Medical Association* 1989; **262** (14): 1973–9.

18. Sullivan G, Burnham A, Koegal P. Pathways to homelessness among the mentally ill. *Social Psychiatry and Psychiatric Epidemiology* 2000; **35**: 444–50.

19. Timms P. Management aspects of care for the homeless mentally ill. *Advances in Psychiatric Treatment* 1996; **2** (4): 158–65.

20. Department of Health. *Safety first: five-year report of the national confidential inquiry into suicide and homicide by people with mental illness*. London, UK: DoH, 2001.

21. Reid P, Klee H. Young homeless people and service provision. *Health and Social Care in the Community* 1999; **7**: 17–24.

22. Hiday VA, Swartz MS, Swanson JW, *et al*. Criminal victimisation of persons with severe mental illness. *Psychiatric Services* 1999; **50**: 62–8.

23. Rosenheck R, Lam J, Randolph F. Impact of representative payees on substance use by homeless persons with serious mental illness. *Psychiatric Services* 1997; **48** (6): 800–6.

RECOMMENDED READING

Bhugra D (ed.). *Homelessness and mental health: studies in social and community psychiatry*. Cambridge, UK: Cambridge University Press, 1998.

Health Advisory Service. *People who are homeless: mental health services. Commissioning and providing mental health services for people who are homeless*. London, UK: HMSO, 1995.

Orwell G. Down and out in Paris and London. In: Davison P (ed.). *The complete works of George Orwell*. London, UK: Secker and Warburg, 1933.

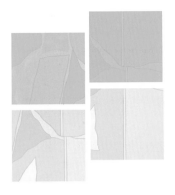

CHAPTER 34

The person with dementia

Trevor Adams*

INTRODUCTION

The past 20 years has witnessed a growth of interest in mental health nursing of people with dementia, partly because of the increasing number of older people in Western society and their greater likelihood of developing dementia. Butterworth[1] noted that people with dementia have often been a marginal concern within mental health nursing and have frequently been seen as an undesirable area of clinical practice. Dementia care has now become a dynamic, progressive and exciting area of mental health nursing. However, in many places, standards of care remain poor and there is no room for complacency.

Until recently, people with dementia were often placed in mental hospitals and, like other patients, found themselves under the control of mental health nurses through a regimen of nursing tasks such as feeding and dressing. This shared many features typically found in institutional settings in which preference is given to the needs of the staff rather than the needs of the people with dementia. The culture of institutionalization in mental hospitals had a harmful effect on people with dementia *and* their nurses and was identified in numerous reports on mental hospitals in the 1960s and 1970s, notably *Sans everything*,[2] which dealt specifically with older people. In

Sans everything, an acting chief male nurse reported that[2,p.13]

> [A]fter six months in certain hospitals, there are ways in which mental health nurses are no longer like ordinary people. Their attitude to mental illness changes – as it does to old age, to cruelty, to people's needs, and to dying. It is as if they become numbed to these things.

In this way, people with dementia often found themselves in difficult and sometimes humiliating situations – devalued, disempowered and marginalized by mental health nurses.

More recently, newer discourses relating to personhood and hearing the voice of people with dementia have entered mental health nursing and have reconstructed people with dementia and their care. In many dementia care units these discourses exist alongside traditional medical–custodial discourses that identify people with dementia as having a brain pathology that prevents them from making worthwhile choices about their own care. This latter way of constructing people with dementia is often convenient to mental health nurses and other care staff as it positions them as having no obligation to ask people with dementia what they actually want. The

*Trevor Adams lectures in mental health nursing at the University of Surrey, Guildford, UK. He has specialized in dementia care nursing for 25 years within practice, education and research. He has written over 50 chapters and papers and edited three books.

newer discourses, however, represent people with dementia as people who, like everyone else, are able to make sense of the world, experience selfhood, and display identity. The emergence of these alternative discourses has done much to challenge and deconstruct discriminatory and oppressive practices towards people with dementia. Indeed, their availability has raised the possibility that a new culture of dementia care may be possible. However, in many places, the old culture of dementia still exists and there is frequently a constant conflict between discursive practices that construct patients with dementia as people and those that construct them as 'demented'.

This chapter draws on these newer discourses to construct a sensitive and politically aware approach to mental health nursing with people who have dementia. Common threads running through the chapter are that mental health nursing of people with dementia should be underpinned by discursive practices that, firstly, construct people with dementia as people, rather than just a diagnosis; secondly, construct the nature and quality of the 'relationship' between people with dementia and others within the provision of care; and, thirdly, set the provision of care within a whole systems approach. These approaches support contemporary developments in health and social policy.

THE EXPERIENCE OF PEOPLE WITH DEMENTIA AND THEIR FAMILIES

People can develop dementia at any age, although its likelihood increases with age. Various studies have described the subjective experience of people with dementia as they come to realize that they are becoming forgetful.[3,4] Keady and Gilliard[5] describe eight stages that people pass through as they develop dementia (Box 34.1). Their work provides worthwhile insights into the subjective experience of people in the early stages of dementia.

However, it is not just the person who is diagnosed that suffers from dementia. In a very real way their relatives, friends and work colleagues all experience the effects of dementia. For various reasons, such as denial and a lack of knowledge about dementia, close family members and friends may take some time to realize the full implications of their relative's or friend's behaviour. Eventually though, often as the result of a crisis, one or more family members will come to realize that their relative has a serious, though at this stage undiagnosed, mental disorder. Then, family members often seek help from a local medical practitioner. The amount of help and support they receive will depend partly on the doctor's view of the situation, the doctor's sensitivity and willingness to involve the family, and the doctor's decision about whether to refer the case to a specialist agency. The person with dementia should receive from the medical practitioner a physical examination and an assessment of his

> ### Box 34.1: The development of dementia
>
> - *Slipping*. The person gradually becomes aware of trivial slips and lapses in memory and/or behaviour.
> - *Suspecting*. Increased number of slips, which the person cannot 'explain away'. The person begins to suspect that there may be something seriously wrong. By 'covering up' the person makes a deliberate effort to compensate for these slips and hides them from other people.
> - *Revealing*. The person reveals to close friends and relatives that he or she is having problems.
> - *Confirming*. The person openly acknowledges that he or she has a problem.
> - *Maximizing*. The person uses strategies to adjust to the dementia.
> - *Disorganization*. Cognitive and behavioural difficulties increasingly dominate the person with dementia.
> - *Decline*. Semblance of normality and reciprocal relationships with other people is gradually lost. Meeting the person's bodily needs becomes the prominent feature.
> - *Death*. Finally, the person with dementia dies.

or her mental state and should have investigations that clarify the diagnosis and exclude other possible causes.

The medical assessment should include an interview with someone who knows the person with dementia well, such as a close family member who can give an account of what has happened. It should be recognized that this account may be very different from that of the person with dementia. Of course, the account of the person with dementia should not be dismissed in preference to that of a family member or healthcare professional, but rather listened to and understood as contributing to the information available to the nursing assessment. Moreover, many medical practitioners do not share the diagnosis with people who have dementia and thus prevent them making decisions about their own care.

Medical practitioners may then refer people with dementia and their primary informal carers to various specialist health and social care agencies. In the UK, the *National service framework for older people*[6] has outlined the pathway along which people with dementia pass following consultation with a general practitioner.

Medical practitioners may then refer people with dementia along with their primary informal carers to community-based mental health teams specializing in people with dementia. Mental health nurses often work alongside people with dementia, and their families, throughout the various stages of dementia, including the later stages when palliative care is required.[7] Mental health nursing care occurs in a variety of settings, including the home, the memory clinic, the day hospital and the long-stay ward. Complexity does not just lie in cases of end-stage dementia, but rather complexity may arise throughout the duration of the dementia and each of these clinical settings may be seen as complex.

HEALTH AND SOCIAL CARE OUTCOMES FOR PEOPLE WITH DEMENTIA AND THEIR FAMILIES

Until recently, people with dementia were never asked about the sort of care they wanted. Various writers such as Goldsmith,[8] Barnett[9] and Allen[10] have argued that many people with dementia are quite able to contribute to decision-making about their own care. In the UK, the importance of older people, including people with dementia, making decisions about their own services is recognized in Standard Two of the *National service framework for older people*.[6,p.23]

It is important that policy and practice in mental health nursing sees meeting the needs of the person with dementia as the most important, though not exclusive, concern. Every effort should be made to seek the opinions and preferences of people with dementia.

NURSING PEOPLE WITH DEMENTIA

Mental health nurses can make a distinctive contribution to people's mental health. Barker *et al.*[11] have outlined four premises upon which mental health nursing is based. These premises assert the following.

1 Mental health nursing is an interactive, developmental human activity that is more concerned with the future development of the person than the origins or cause of their present distress.
2 The experience of mental distress associated with mental health disorder is represented through public behavioural disturbance or reports of private events that are known only to the person concerned.
3 Mental health nurses and the people in care are engaged in a relationship based on mutual influence.
4 The experience of mental health disorder is translated into problems of everyday living in which the mental health nurse is concerned with addressing human responses to mental health distress, not the disorder.

These premises are just as applicable to mental health nursing of people with dementia as they are to other specialties within the profession.

Important ideas in the mental health nursing of people with dementia

Among the other ideas important to mental health nursing of people with dementia and their families, are the following.

Well-being

Well-being has been defined as 'The subjective state of being healthy, happy, contented, comfortable and satisfied with one's quality of life. It includes physical, material, social, emotional ("happiness"), and development and activity dimensions.'[12,p.99] We would include within this understanding of 'well-being' psychological, social and physical dimensions of aspects and would recognize the contribution of purposeful activity to the maintenance of people's well-being. We would take a broader approach that views well-being as something that should be possessed not only by people with dementia, but also by their families and nurses.

Reflection

Jasper[13] defines 'reflective practice' as the means by which 'we learn by thinking about things that have happened to us and seeing them in a different way, which enables us to take some kind of action'.[13,p.2] In this way, reflection is a way of gaining new knowledge in and about dementia care settings. We would want to adopt a more critical and systemic view of reflection and say that, first, nurses should reflect upon the distribution of power in dementia care settings and consider who occupies positions of power and how power is used. We would suggest that often people with dementia can find themselves powerless, and that nurses need to identify and challenge these situations. Different family members and health and social care workers will have their own agenda which may undermine the choices and opinions of the person with dementia.

Body

People with dementia, family members and nurses all have bodies, and the idea of 'the body' needs to be incorporated into any understanding of dementia care nursing. As Kontos[14,p.565] urges, 'We must develop a new paradigm that respects individuals with Alzheimer's disease as embodied beings deserving dignity and worth.'

The body is important in dementia care nursing because it is through changes in the brain and other bodily organs that people experience dementia. Moreover, when a person with dementia is wet or in pain, it is through their body that it is experienced. As one man with dementia notes, 'When I trip over something, I get mad. I do believe that Alzheimer's does include what your feet do and what your hands do, as well as what your brain does.'[15,p.8] In addition, it is through the body that nurses come into contact with people who have dementia and through which they assess and implement nursing care.

The body also has a semiotic role and constitutes a collection of signs that are displayed by the person with dementia and read by family members and nurses. 'Reading the body' is an important part of dementia care nursing, as many people with dementia find it difficult to communicate through talk and can make themselves understood only through their bodies.[16] But, also, the way nurses and carers use their bodies when working alongside people with dementia has a significant impact upon the promotion of well-being.

Voice

People with dementia have views and opinions, and nurses have a moral obligation to listen to what people with dementia are saying as they make their views and choices known. The idea of 'voice' used here has a more political connotation than is generally used in everyday speech. It is the voice of the less able and marginalized person, in this case the person with dementia, and is closely associated with not having power. Often, people with dementia find that their views, interests and agendas have been passed over in favour of those of other people, and that family members, medical practitioners, nurses and informal carers are given priority. Sometimes, stories shared within dementia care situations represent people with dementia as not having the ability to say anything worthwhile so that their voices are never heard and sometimes never sought. Thus, people with dementia often have no opportunity to make their views known and no opportunity to take part in decision-making processes. There is a close relationship between voice and well-being as people who are able to express their voice are more likely to find themselves included within decision-making and ensure their well-being.

Story

Stories that arise and are shared between people with dementia, family members and nurses are particularly important, as they enable people to understand their own experience of having dementia or giving care and allows them to construct a view of what has, what will and what may happen.[17] Stories told by people with dementia and their carers have two purposes in dementia care situations. First, they allow people with dementia and their carers to explore and articulate their own experiences and set them within a broader personal narrative that offers a coherent and storied understanding of events. Second, stories contribute to the organization of clinical settings by identifying different participants as having various identities, responsibilities and obligations. One story may, at a particular point in the interaction, identify a person with dementia or a carer as attention-seeking, whereas another story may identify them as needing care. The story told within case may give these participants a different set of identities. Each story may be used at various points during meetings with clients and multidisciplinary team meetings to achieve different things, such as raising the concern of the nurse or perhaps gaining admission to much sought-after respite care.

Within this context, we would suggest that stories that are available and used in clinical settings may contribute to the well-being of the person with dementia and his or her family. It is important, however, to note whose stories are being told, who is telling them and who benefits from them. In this respect, people with dementia

and, to a lesser extent, their relatives are often at a disadvantage as their stories are not usually as universally recognized as those of professionals, and people with dementia and their relatives may lack the ability to share the stories convincingly because of their impaired cognitive ability or lack of professional training.

Implicit in this view of 'story' is that there is often not just one dominant story that may be applied to a particular dementia care setting such as the story of a particular family member or the expert story of the doctor but rather that various stories may be mapped onto clinical settings, each giving a particular view of events.

Evidence

Alongside the growing recognition of the importance of voice and story, there has been an increased recognition of the need to guide and direct practice though the use of evidence.[18] This evidence is usually seen to emerge from research, the most authoritative being randomized controlled trials (RCTs).[19] We would suggest that the elevation of one sort of research over another is problematic as it devalues evidence gained from other research methods such as surveys and different types of qualitative methodologies. In addition, it assumes that practitioners only use or should only use RCTs within clinical decision-making (see Chapter 4). We would, however, take a broader and more inclusive view and argue that the evidence that mental health nurses use when working with people who have dementia comes not just from one source but rather arises from:

- past experience – professionals seeing what works best with particular clients and/or personal experience taken from everyday experience of life situations;
- theoretical approaches – such as Kitwood's person-centred care;[3]
- views and opinions of people with dementia, family members and other health and social care workers;
- role models and experts;
- policy directives.

Thus, we see evidence in dementia care nursing as not merely contained in expert bodies of knowledge that are detached and separate from the clinical setting but rather as also including evidence that arises in clinical settings.

Reflection

What other ideas do you think should underpin mental health nursing of people with dementia?

Theoretical basis for practice

We would suggest mental health nursing of people with dementia is underpinned by a whole systems approach that captures the ongoing interrelationship between biological and social systems within dementia care nursing.

As Rolland[20,p.17] argues, 'The heart of all systems-orientated biopsychosocial inquiry is the focus on interaction.'

The approach we adopt identifies the following systems.

- *Biological system*: within the person with dementia, their family members and paid-for carer(s).
- *Psychological system*: within the person with dementia, their family members and paid-for carer(s).
- *Family system*: concerned with roles, rules, boundary and the construction of family life.
- *Health and social care system*: includes all aspects of health and social care provision and the design of accommodation for older people with dementia, along with the financial aspects of the provision and organization of accommodation.
- *Cultural system*: values, religious beliefs and customs possessed by different people involved with the provision of care for those with dementia.
- *Sociopolitical system*: administration of health and social care for people with dementia and their carers.

In this approach, the care of people with dementia is seen in terms of the interdependency among the person with dementia, the family and other agencies. Carpenter and Treacher[21,p.4] note that 'The family as a system should always be considered in terms of its interaction with other systems.' Systemic approaches have been developed by a long line of theorists (see Dallos and Draper[22]). Herr and Weakland,[23] Hargreave and Hanna[24] and Curtis and Dixon[25] have applied systemic approaches to older people; Benbow *et al.*,[26] Fisher and Lieberman,[27] Garwick *et al.*[28] and Szinovacz[29] have applied them to people with dementia; and Friedman *et al.*[30] and Wright and Leahey[31] have applied them to nursing.

Systemic theory recognizes that each family is unique and that family membership is affected by different systems, such as those relating to biological, legal, affectional, geographical and historical ties.[32] These ideas are underpinned by the General Systems Theory[33] and offer a way of understanding bio-psycho-medical phenomena, such as those that nurses encounter when working with people who have dementia. Underpinning systemic approaches are a number of ideas that include:

- the importance of boundaries between different systems;
- the organization of subsystems, e.g. the person with dementia and his or her primary family carer is a subsystem of the family;
- the semipermeability of boundaries, i.e. one system will affect another; for example, whatever is happening in the family system will affect what is happening in the system that constitutes the person with dementia, such as when a carer is tired and irritated with a relative with dementia it will affect what the person with dementia does and feels;
- the importance of patterns of interactions: what happens in one system will affect what happens in another;

- the acknowledgement that behaviour in systems is governed by rules.

Systemic thinking has been applied to people with dementia, their family members and the wider community and is supported by the work of numerous academics, researchers and practitioners.[34]

Within this whole systems approach, we would draw on ideas that are contained in various approaches that have emerged in dementia care. The first is person-centred care, which was initially developed by Kitwood,[3] who saw care in terms of ensuring that the person (with dementia) comes first, and more recently by Brooker[35] in the equation:

$$\text{Person-centred care} = V + I + P + S$$

in which V is a value base that asserts the absolute value of all human lives regardless of age or cognitive ability, I is an individualized approach, recognizing uniqueness, P is understanding the world from the perspective of the service users, and S is providing a social environment that supports psychological needs.

Person-centred care is important in mental health nursing as it challenges traditional institutional approaches towards people with dementia that meet the needs of the organization but do not allow people with dementia to exercise choice about the services they want to receive.

An additional idea developed by Kitwood[3] highlights the 'dialectical' nature of the dementia process. Although Kitwood's later work seems to highlight interpersonal aspects of dementia care, Downs *et al.*[36] reaffirms Kitwood's earlier ideas that outline the contribution of physical/neurological impairment *and* social/psychological phenomena to the dementia process. This reaffirmation is important because of the growing importance of diagnosis within dementia care, the development of new pharmacological treatments[37] and discoveries relating to genetics.[38] The dialectical approach prevents undue polarization towards either a medical or a psychosocial representation of dementia care and recognizes that dementia arises out of pathological changes to the body.

These ideas correspond with a third idea – that of the 'embodied selfhood' of people with dementia –which is described in the work of Phinney and Chesla,[39] who state that bodily and somatic phenomena are commonly experienced by people with dementia. Kontos[14] argues that the body is an active and communicative agent that is imbued with its own wisdom, intentionality and purposefulness, and is separate and distinct from cognition. 'Embodied selfhood' is a new and important idea that not only offers nurses a fuller understanding of people's lived experience of dementia but also allows people with dementia to be seen as able to express themselves through their body. This idea is supported by Activity Theory,[40] which argues that optimal mental health occurs when older people undertake purposeful activity, and by the work of Archer,[40] who supports the primacy of practice in the development of selfhood.

We would also highlight the importance of relationships within dementia care. This idea is implicit though limited in the work of Kitwood, who seems to see the formal or informal care as the person who initiates but fails to 'capture the interdependencies and reciprocities that underpin caring relationships.'[41,p.203] We therefore draw on relationship-centred care as a contributing theoretical basis to mental health nursing of people with dementia and highlight the importance of mutual relationships.

Legal and ethical framework

Mental health nurses working with people who have dementia should be aware of, and able to articulate, the ethical and legal framework upon which their practice is based.[42] The ethical implications of working with people who have dementia has been examined by such writers as Brannelly.[43] This framework is dependent upon codes of conduct such as those that have been made available by the International Council of Nurses[44] and also national laws that have relevance to the care of people with dementia and their informal carers.

In addition, mental health nurses have an important role to play in maintaining a positive and humanitarian attitude towards people with dementia within contemporary society. One has only to think of the Holocaust in the 1930s and 1940s to see the extent to which a society can construct cognitively mentally impaired people as worthless. Ethical frameworks that mental health nurses use to underpin their practice must assert the essential value of people with dementia. Owing to the relocation of mental health nursing education into higher education, mental health nurses are now in a better position to make and articulate an ethical basis towards their practice.

Reflection

Do you think that the recent highlighting of the voice of the person with dementia and the carer has led to less attention being given to what mental health nurses have to offer?

ASSESSMENT

To ensure the validity of the assessment, a number of features should be displayed.

- First, assessments should not be based solely upon one 'assessment meeting' but rather information should be gathered over the course of a number of visits.
- Assessments should take place in a setting in which the person with dementia feels most comfortable.
- Mental health nurses should do their best to help people with dementia and their carer(s) to relax by facilitating an informal and sociable relationship.
- Mental health nurses should do everything they can to help people with dementia talk about their views and preferences.
- The assessment should be based on what the person with dementia and his or her relatives can do, rather than, as is often the case, what they cannot do.
- Mental health nurses should collect additional and supplementary data from people such as family members and friends, and other members of the multidisciplinary team.
- Case notes should be written as soon as possible after the assessment meeting so that as little as possible is forgotten or misremembered. It is easy to put off writing up an assessment especially after a long day!
- Finally, the assessment should be written up on appropriately designed documentation. The written assessment should be available to any member of the multiprofessional team as well as to informal carers and the person with dementia.

The primary focus of the assessment should be the person with dementia. The mental health nurse must make sure that family members do not take over and speak on behalf of, or perhaps instead of, the person with dementia. This denies people with dementia the right to talk about what they want and prevents them feeling that they have a sense of ownership about the decisions they make. It is essential that information is not taken from only one informal carer but from the whole family. Mental health nurses can use a variety of assessment schedules when assessing the person with dementia, such as the Mini-Mental State Examination.[45] The assessment, and for that matter the intervention, should be sensitive to the cultural background and social context of the person with dementia. Most of all, the assessment should not disable and should be directed at identifying the strengths that the person with dementia possesses and not his or her shortcomings.

INTERVENTION

Mental health nurses working with people who have dementia need a range of skills similar to those used by nurses in other areas of mental health care. Good communication skills are essential to ensuring that people with dementia have a sense of personhood and are treated with respect and dignity. A range of specialist approaches are available to nurses working with dementia, such as reality orientation, validation therapy, reminiscence therapy and various art-based approaches, e.g. art therapy, music therapy and Snoozlem. Various approaches have been developed to promote well-being in family carers. All approaches should accept people's ethnic, religious and sexual orientation and develop care plans that take them into account.

TABLE 34.1 Whole systems approach

Overall skill	Constituent skills
1. Promote settings and cultures that value and respect the diversity of people with dementia and their families	Work with people to create an inclusive culture that respects and values the dignity of people with dementia and their families through transparent decision-making Demonstrate an ability to work with a range of stakeholders to promote capacity for the inclusion of people with dementia Encourage the active participation of people with dementia and their carer(s) to participate in care on the basis of informed choice Represent positive views of people with dementia and their informal provision of care by valuing their stories and life experiences
2. Improving outcomes for service users	Use a range of communication skills to establish, maintain and manage relationships between people who have dementia, their families and key people involved with their care Be approachable, spend time with people who have dementia, understand and support their interests, needs and concerns Demonstrate safe and effective use of interpersonal and basic counselling skills Give feedback to others about clinical situations that is constructive and facilitates positive change
3. Promote physical health and well-being for people with dementia and their families	Identify and assess the physical needs of people with dementia Assess the capacity of people with dementia to maintain activities of daily living Communicate with people who have dementia and groups and communities about promoting their health and well-being Promote sexual well-being that is relevant and appropriate to the person with dementia and others Undertake physiological measurements of people with dementia and encourage their family members to fully participate in the assessment, planning, implementation, monitoring and assessment of therapeutic interventions
4. Work with people with dementia, their families and colleagues to maintain health, safety and well-being	Demonstrate the application of appropriate legal and ethical frameworks to support practice Ensure all records are kept in line with local policy and procedures and stored according to the legal and regulatory requirements of data protection Take immediate action to reduce risk when there is a danger to an individual's health, safety and well-being Demonstrate under supervision the safe, correct, effective and appropriate use of physical intervention techniques in the presence of challenging behaviour
5. Work with people with dementia, their families and colleagues to maintain health, safety and well-being	Demonstrate the application of appropriate legal and ethical frameworks to support practice Support the health and safety of nurses, people with dementia, their families and society Demonstrate the ability to work in partnership with people with dementia and their carers to promote privacy, dignity, health, safety and well-being Work in partnership with people who have dementia to enable them to communicate their fears and knowledge of potential and actual danger, harm and abuse, particularly if their autonomy or learning ability is impaired Promote, monitor and maintain health, safety and security in the clinical setting Ensure all records are kept in line with local policy and procedures and stored according to the legal and regulatory requirements of data protection Discuss implications and contraindications of all procedures with people who have dementia and their families Obtain valid informed consent for all procedures, with attention to the special and exceptional needs of people with dementia Recognition of signs and circumstances associated with aggression and violence Demonstrate an awareness of prevention and risk-reduction strategies for aggression Assess the level of risk and consider how the risks can be controlled to minimize harm Contribute to the prevention and management of abusive and aggressive behaviour Use, under supervision, methods from the National Institute for Health and Clinical Excellence guidelines on effective methods of working with people whose behaviour is harmful to self or others Contribute, as a member of the therapeutic team, to the safe and effective assessment, management and reduction of any identified risks

(Continued)

TABLE 34.1 (Continued)

Overall skill	Constituent skills
	The ability to work as a member of the therapeutic team in making a safe and effective contribution to the de-escalation and management of anger and violence
	Take immediate action to reduce risk when there is a danger to an individual's health, safety and well-being
	Demonstrate under supervision the safe, correct, effective and appropriate use of physical intervention techniques in the presence of challenging behaviour
	Provide frameworks to help individuals to manage challenging behaviour
	Act in accordance with relevant practice guidelines from the National Institute for Health and Clinical Excellence to reduce risks to an individual's health, safety or well-being
	Assess older people's risk of falls and implement evidence-based interventions
	Develop and agree individualized care plans with older people at risk of falls
	Maintain a safe, clean and welcoming environment
	Follow universal precautions for infection control
	Take immediate action when you find aspects of the environment are unsafe, unclean and unwelcoming
	Observe and monitor the general cleanliness of the environment and report to the appropriate person when there is concern over the level of cleanliness
	Check whether equipment is fully operational and free of defects before use
	Demonstrate the safe use of equipment in emergency situations, e.g. automatic defibrillators
	Use of correct personal protective clothing for your role and the procedure you are undertaking in line with organizational policy
	Take correct precautions for the safe handling of blood, body fluids, specimens and toxic or corrosive substances in line with control of substances hazardous to health risk assessments
	Identify hazards which could result in serious harm to people at work or other persons
	Take relevant and timely corrective action to manage incidents or risks to health, safety and security
	Respond appropriately to environmental emergencies
6. Work collaboratively with other disciplines and agencies to support people with dementia and their families to develop and maintain social networks and good relationships	Work effectively and assertively in a team, contributing to the decision-making process and taking responsibility for delegated action associated with the assessment, planning, implementation and evaluation of care
	Clarify and confirm your role in the overall care programme and single-assessment process with people who have dementia and family carers
	Coordinate the integration of care for people with dementia, working with team members and other agencies who affect directly, or indirectly, the health and social care of the person with dementia
7. Demonstrate a commitment for continuing professional development and personal supervision activities, in order to enhance the knowledge, skills, values and attitudes needed to implement safe and effective nursing of people with dementia and their families	Using the clinical supervision and support systems available within and outside your organization
	Taking responsibility for your own personal and professional development, seeking and accessing developmental opportunities to enhance your provision of dementia care nursing
	Use reflective practice, supervision and support to facilitate ongoing insights into your emotional state and its impact on your work with people with dementia, their families and colleagues
	Set professional goals that are realistic and achievable
	Clarify the expected learning outcomes to be achieved when teaching others and how success is to be measured
	Give constructive and timely feedback to others on ideas and options being explored
	Demonstrate key skills, including literacy, numeracy and use of information technology
	A working knowledge of the support needs of others
	Enable other workers to reflect on their own values, priorities, interests and effectiveness
	Delegate nursing care or associated tasks safely and appropriately
	Engage actively in peer supervision

Various writers have outlined a range of skills and competencies that nurses working with people should possess. However, these skills and competencies usually do not emerge out of a theory base and are atheoretical. We, therefore, suggest that mental health nursing of people with dementia should display skills and competencies that arise out of a theoretical approach. This may be achieved using the whole systems approach accordingly (Table 34.1).

Reflection

How should theory, research and practice in mental health nursing of people with dementia develop in the immediate future?

SUMMARY

Until recently mental health nursing of people with dementia has typically been constructed by biomedical discourses. This chapter has reconstructed the specialty using newer discourses, which construct people with dementia and their care within a psychosocial and sociopolitical framework. By constructing dementia care in this way, mental health nurses will not only focus on the biomedical features of people with dementia that give rise to their being seen and treated as objects, but will also emphasize their status as people, with preferences and rights like anyone else. Under the biomedical discourse, mental health nursing was largely oblivious to the ethical and political consequences of its practice. However, psychosocial and sociopolitical discourses have enabled mental health nursing to emphasize the subjective and interpersonal context of caring for people with dementia.

REFERENCES

1. Butterworth T. Breaking the boundaries. *Nursing Times* 1988; **34**: 36–9.

2. Robb B. *Sans everything: a case to answer.* London, UK: Nelson, 1967.

3. Kitwood T. *Dementia reconsidered: the person comes first.* Buckingham, UK: Open University Press, 1997.

4. Sabat SR. *The experience of Alzheimer's disease: like through a tangled veil.* Oxford, UK: Blackwell Publishers, 2001.

5. Keady J, Gilliard J. The early experience of Alzheimer's disease: implications for partnership and practice. In: Adams T, Clarke C (eds). *Dementia care: developing partnerships in practice.* London, UK: Baillière Tindall, 1999: 227–56.

6. National Health Service. *National service framework for older people.* London, UK: NHS, 2001.

7. Kovach CR. *Late-stage dementia care.* Washington, DC: Taylor & Francis, 1997.

8. Goldsmith M. *Hearing the voice of people with dementia.* London, UK: Jessica Kingsley, 1996.

9. Barnett E. *Including the person with dementia in designing and delivering care.* London, UK: Jessica Kingsley, 2000.

10. Allen K. *Communication and consultation; exploring ways for staff to involve people with dementia in developing services.* Bristol, UK: Policy Press, 2001.

11. Barker PJ, Reynolds W, Stevenson C. The human science basis of mental health nursing: theory and practice. *Journal of Advanced Nursing* 1997; **25**: 660–7.

12. Department of Health. *Commissioning framework for health and well-being.* London, UK: HMSO, 2001.

13. Jasper M. *Beginning reflective practice.* Cheltenham, UK: Nelson Thornes. 2003.

14. Kontos PC. Embodied selfhood in Alzheimer's: re-thinking person-centred care. *Dementia: The International Journal of Social Research and Practice* 2005; **4**: 553–70.

15. Henderson CS. *Partial view: Alzheimer's journal.* Dallas, TX: Southern Methodist University Press, 1998.

16. Hubbard G, Cook A, Tester S, Downs M. Beyond words: older people with dementia using and interpreting nonverbal behaviour. *Journal of Aging Studies* 2002; **16**: 155–67.

17. Adams T. Developing partnership in dementia care: a discursive model of practice. In: Adams T, Clarke C (eds). *Dementia care: developing partnerships in practice.* London, UK: Baillière Tindall, 1999: 37–56.

18. Rolfe G. Evidence-based practice. In: Jasper M (ed.). *Professional development, reflection and decision-making.* Oxford, UK: Blackwell Publishing, 2006: 135–53.

19. Sackett D, Rosenberg W, Gray J *et al.* Evidence-based medicine: what is it and what it isn't. *British Journal of Medicine* 1996; **312**: 71–2.

20. Rolland JS. A conceptual model of chronic and life-threatening illness and its impact. In: Chilman S, Nunnally EW, Cox F (eds). *Chronic illness and disability. The trouble with families*, vol. 2. Beverly Hills, CA: Sage Publications, 1988.

21. Carpenter J, Treacher A. Introduction: using family therapy. In: Treacher A, Carpenter J (eds). *Using family therapy.* Oxford, UK: Basil Blackwell, 1984.

22. Dallos R, Draper R. *An introduction to family therapy: systemic theory and practice*, 2nd edn. Maidenhead, UK: Open University Press, 2005.

23. Herr JJ, Weakland JH. *Counselling elders and their families: practical techniques for applied gerontology.* New York, NY: Springer, 1979.

24. Hargrave TD, Hanna SM (eds). *The aging family: new visions in theory, practice and reality.* New York, NY: Brunner/Mazel, 1997.

25. Curtis EA, Dixon MS. Family therapy and systemic practice with older people: where are we now? *Journal of Family Therapy* 2005; **27**: 43–64.

26. Benbow SM, Marriott A, Morley M, Walsh S. Family therapy and dementia: review and clinical experience. *International Journal of Geriatric Psychiatry* 1993; **8**: 717–25.

27. Fisher L, Lieberman MA. Alzheimer's disease: the impact of the family on spouses, offspring, and inlaws. *Family Process* 1994; **33**: 305–25.

28. Garwick AW, Detzner D, Boss P. Family perceptions of living with Alzheimer's disease. *Family Process* 1994; **33**: 327–40.

29. Szinovacz ME. Caring for a demented relative at home: effects on parent–adolescent relationships and family dynamics. *Journal of Aging Studies* 2003; **17**: 445–72.

30. Friedman M, Bowden VR, Jones E. *Family nursing: research, theory and practice*, 5th edn. Upper Saddle River, NJ: Prentice Hall, 2003.

31. Wright LM, Leahey M. *Nurses and families: a guide to family assessment and intervention*, 4th edn. Philadelphia, PA: F.A. Davis, 2005.

32. Carr A. *Family therapy: concepts, processes and practice.* Wiley, UK: Chichester, 2000.

33. Bertalanffy L. *General systems theory.* New York, NY: Brazilier, 1968.

34. Richardson CA, Gilleard CJ, Lieberman S, Peelerg R. Working with older adults and their families: a review. *Journal of Family Therapy* 1994; **16**: 225–40.

35. Brooker D. *Person centred care.* London, UK: Jessica Kingsley, 2006.

36. Downs M, Clare L, Mackenzie J. Understandings of dementia: explanatory models and their implications for the person with dementia and therapeutic effort. In: Hughes JC, Louw SJ, Sabat SR (eds). *Dementia: mind, meaning, and the person.* Oxford, UK: Oxford University Press, 2006: 235–58.

37. Page S. Dementia care and cholinesterase inhibitors. *Professional Nurse* 2001; **16**: 1421–4.

38. Schutte DL, Holston EC. Chronic dementing conditions, genomics, and new opportunities for nursing interventions. *Journal of Nursing Studies* 2006; **38**: 328–34.

39. Phinney A, Chesla CA. The lived body in dementia. *Journal of Aging Studies* 2003; **17**: 285–99.

40. Archer M. *Being human: the problem of agency.* Cambridge, UK: Cambridge University Press, 2000.

41. Nolan M, Ryan T, Enderby P, Reid D. Towards a more inclusive vision of dementia care practice. *Dementia: The International Journal of Social Research and Practice* 2002; **1** (2): 193–211.

42. Hughes J, Baldwin C. *Ethical issues in dementia.* London, UK: Jessica Kingsley Publications, 2007.

43. Brannelly T. Developing an ethical basis for relationship-centred and inclusive approaches towards dementia care nursing. In: Adams T (ed.). *Dementia care nursing.* Basingstoke, UK: Palgrave Macmillan, 2008.

44. International Council of Nurses. *Code for nurses.* Geneva, Switzerland: International Council of Nurses, 1973.

45. Folstein MF, Folstein SE, McHugh P. Mini-mental state: a practical method for grading the cognitive state of patients for the clinician. *Journal of Mental Health Research* 1975; **12**: 189–98.

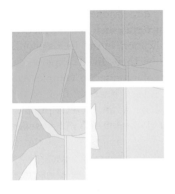

CHAPTER 35

The person with a diagnosis of autism

Andrew Cashin*

INTRODUCTION

Although autism emerged from Kanner's[1] seminal paper in 1943, recently there has been a sharp increase in its prevalence.[2] This chapter offers a definition of autism, discusses its relevance to psychiatric–mental health nursing, and explores how nurses might help people with a diagnosis of autism deal with their problems of living.

WHAT IS AUTISM AND WHY SHOULD PSYCHIATRIC NURSES CARE?

History

Phenomena do not exist as separate entities 'out there' waiting to be identified and studied.[3] Autism was not a concrete thing, waiting to be picked up, identified and given a label.[4] Autism is a *construct* derived from the observation of a set of commonly experienced ways of being first articulated in 1943 when Leo Kanner, a Baltimore psychiatrist, explored the cluster of 'fascinating peculiarities' that he saw in clinical practice. From his attempts to describe this group of children the modern construct of autism was born. At the same time, Hans Asperger, a Viennese paediatrician, was exploring similar phenomena, which he called *autistic psychopathy*.[2,5] Both of these phenomena were based upon behavioural observation and, like all psychiatric conditions, autism remains a behavioural diagnosis.[6]

All knowledge development is context dependent, and Asperger and Kanner had no opportunity to share their observations or work together because of the outbreak of the Second World War. Kanner's work in the West progressed whereas Asperger's was not translated into English until the 1980s. Both had identified groups of young people with common impairments in three areas: *communication*, *social skills* and *behavioural flexibility*.[7] In Kanner's early observations, he noted that people with this impairment triad tended to be aloof and closed off from the world. The diagnosis, phenomena of autism, sat squarely within the province of child psychiatry. Once any phenomenon is observed and its structures articulated, the next question is *why*? The earliest answers came from the psychogenic theories of the day.[8] In 1967, Bruno Bettleheim[9] coined the term 'refrigerator mother'. Bettleheim made the observation that children with autism looked like people in concentration camps who had lost the will to live. In his view, this was the result of the cold uncaring interpersonal style of the camp guards, so he leapt to the conclusion that autism was the result of the mother's cold and unloving parenting style, a theory

*Andrew Cashin occupies a clinical chair as Associate Professor in Justice Health Nursing in the faculty of Nursing, Midwifery and Health at the University of Technology Sydney. Andrew is an authorized mental health nurse practitioner with a private practice on the central coast of New South Wales.

consistent with Freudian psychoanalysis.[9] Bettleheim was honoured by being made a Professor of Education Emeritus and Professor Emeritus of both psychiatry and psychology at the University of Chicago.

The backlash to the refrigerator mother theory began with the more rigorous investigations led in America by Bernard Rimland, a psychologist and parent of a child with autism. Parent groups were formed in the USA and the UK that challenged the psychoanalytic view, proposing, instead, that autism be seen as a neurobiological developmental disorder.[2,5] Until the 1980s, although Kanner's sample group was seen as largely intelligent,[1] autism was recognized only in people with a co-existing intellectual delay. Professionals interested in developmental disability were largely the only ones interested in autism. Autism had shifted from being a *psychiatric disorder* to a *developmental disability*, yet still clarity regarding the causation was absent. Autism remained a behavioural diagnosis.

Although it makes sense that a disorder recognized in children and labelled as a life-long disability would be present in adults, most research focused on children and adolescents. For nurses, autism fell squarely within the realms of intellectual disability services. In the 1980s clinicians began to recognize that people with average or above intelligence showed the same 'autistic' cluster of impaired communication, social skills and repetitive and restricted ways of being in the world. However, the diagnostic practice of the time would allow recognition of only those with severe intellectual disability or non-remittent behavioural disturbance, which prevented their participation in school or family life. Lorna Wing, an English psychiatrist, then published the first account of Asperger's work in English.[10] This provided the platform for a professional dialogue concerning the construct of autism. Asperger's description of autism had included Kanner's triad, but had also considered those with the triad who were *not* shut off, cold and aloof. His sample included the active but odd group of individuals who sought social interaction, but who were clumsy about it. Although Asperger included such observations, physical clumsiness was soon dropped as an essential criterion for the modern version of what became known as *Asperger's disorder*.

The new construct of Asperger's disorder became a distinct subtype of autistic disorder, and entered the fourth edition of the *Diagnostic and statistical manual* (DSM-IV) in 1994, opening the way for consideration by a range of clinicians.[11] It was recognized that autism *could* co-exist with intellectual disability, but the majority of new diagnoses of autism now are people of average intelligence or above. Autism was recognized as a *spectrum disorder:* existing at the macro- and micro-level. The degree of impairment was variable both *within* the diagnostic group but also *across* each of the elements of the triad of impairments. As autism is a behavioural diagnosis, impairment fluctuates dependent on the external demands imposed on the person. Impairment is dimensional as opposed to categorical,[12,13] and qualifying terms, such as mild, moderate or severe, offer little clarification. In the 1990s people with autism began to describe their 'lived' experience, providing an important source of information, complementary to professional observation and research. One of the most famous writers is Temple Grandin.[14] Description of the experience of autism led to insights into the presence of sensory sensitivities, crippling anxiety and, at times, depression that are part of the lived experience.[14,15]

In keeping with its spectrum nature, three constructs are represented in autism.

1 The original *autistic disorder* (sometimes referred to as Kanner's autism).
2 *Asperger's disorder*.
3 A subthreshold category of *pervasive development disorders not otherwise specified* (PDDnos or *atypical autism*). PDDnos are used to denote people who have the requisite triad of impairment at a level less than that required for a diagnosis of Asperger's disorder or autistic disorder, or for people who showed no signs of the triad of impairment until after the age of 3 years.

Interestingly, although it allowed the broadening vision of clinicians, Asperger's disorder has now collapsed into redundancy. At first, the need to have average or above intelligence, as measured by a standardized tool, would appear to be a useful separation from the diagnostic category of autistic disorder. However, the classification of autistic disorder makes no reference to intelligence. Further, the diagnostic criteria for Asperger's disorder state that if an individual meets the criteria for autistic disorder then this is the diagnosis to be given.[16] *No one* can be given a diagnosis of Asperger's disorder based on our current classification system.[11,17]

Reflection

The language we use structures how we think about things. What language is being used in your service related to the diagnosis of autism?

Much energy has been expended on testing the hypothesis of difference; however, all attempts have required changes in diagnostic criteria.[18,19] These result in circularity, as lower functioning individuals are placed in the autistic disorder cohort. This is good evidence of our habit as professionals of holding the attitude that:[20,p.37]

where the phenomenon refuses to conform to the categorical Procrustean bed, it is the phenomenon that must be altered to fit. Reality is reformed in the image of assumptions which must be reiterated again and again.

Even with the broadening of the diagnostic vision, autism remained in the realm of developmental disability. For those practitioners for whom this was not their area of expertise the triad of impairment was often seen to satisfy other diagnostic criteria. Missed diagnosis and confusion with personality disorder, mood disorder, obsessive–compulsive disorder and disorders of language, attention and conduct are not uncommon.[2,13,21]

Epidemiology

The prevalence of autism has continued to rise in keeping with the historical developments outlined above. The expansion of the clinician's vision to include those with average or above intelligence and the apparent validation of these efforts through inclusion of Asperger's disorder as a recognized classification in the mid-1990s sowed the seeds of the recently well-publicized 'epidemic'. As the vision enlarged, those at the centre of the phenomena increased, and those accepted to be on the periphery were far removed from those identified within the vision inspired by Kanner. The increased prevalence is largely attributed to wider recognition of autism and precision with diagnosis.[2] Epidemiological studies are difficult to interpret because of variance in diagnostic constructs across time (PDDnos entered DSM-III and Asperger's disorder entered DSM-IV) and methodological differences including the process of case identification.[22] Logically, epidemiological studies that could draw on samples of screened child populations had higher prevalence than studies that relied on case identification based on previous diagnosis from health and school systems.[2] Whether there is something beyond better recognition contributing to increased numbers in a subgroup of those with autism we will not know until causality is established.

CAUSE: THE BIG WHY?

There is no known causative factor for autism,[23,24] which poses great difficulty. In *Smiling at shadows*, Junee Waites[15] describes her response to her son Dane's diagnosis.

> My first reaction to Dane's official diagnosis was relief. I felt grateful that my son's problems weren't the result of poor mothering skills, or inadequate diet or allergies or heaven knows what else. Then the shock hit me. Why, God? Why Dane? What caused this? Was it those dreadful forceps at his birth? Was it genetic, or my diet.

Like many other psychiatric 'disorders', the focus in autism research has now turned to genetics, environmental pathogens and diet, but as yet the answer has not been found. Although genetic findings, such as specific changes on chromosome 7, have been heralded with much excitement,[25] this fades when it is considered that at some point small changes have been found on every chromosome excepting 14 and 20 in some people with autism.[24] It is also important to remember that often small genetic effects on a phenotype account for only a small degree of variance in the phenotype.[26] Nothing has been identified that could account for the pervasive pattern of impairment in communication, social skills and behavioural flexibility. Heritability points to the presence of a genetic link and through twin studies it has been determined that autism is highly heritable.[26,27] Like many conditions involving thought, it is likely that genes are involved, but science has not evolved sufficiently to deliver the answers.

Reflection

When engaged in psychoeducation, how often do you field the question of why?

Environmentally, the most intense focus was placed on the mercury-based preservative Thimersol, used in the triple antigen vaccine for measles, mumps and rubella. After much scrutiny, no causal link was determined.[2] Dietary theories of immune-mediated responses and the circulation of partially digested gluten and casein were considered, as endogenous opioids burst onto the autism scene. It was proposed that, for the presumed genetic vulnerability to be expressed, a complex interaction with environmental factors was needed. It was felt that such an interaction could be mediated by a *dysregulated immune system*.[28] No research has established diet to be a causal factor. It of course makes sense for those with autism and dietary sensitivity/allergies to avoid certain foods, but no studies have established a causal link with autism. In terms of the circulation of endogenous opioids (the leaky gut theory),[13] the offending opioids molecules are too large to cross the semipermeable blood–brain barrier.

Anatomical variance

Autism remains a *behavioural diagnosis* based upon the triad of impairment of impaired communication, impaired social skills and reduced behavioural flexibility, varying in intensity across a spectrum for which causality has not been established. Much attention has been paid to determining whether there are any physically distinct properties or *pathology* in those with autism, involving imaging and theorizing from knowledge of people with injured or diseased brains and the effects of medication.

Statements such as 'Autism is a complex, behaviourally defined, static disorder of the immature brain that is of great concern to the practicing pediatrician' suggest that there has been an established understanding of brain changes.[29,p.472] However, there remains *no* universally accepted structural change or imbalance in neurotransmitters. As with the non-specific and non-universal genetic profile, changes in brain cells and structure have been observed, but none are *specific to autism* or could account for the behavioural expression of autism.[24,30] (For details of contemporary 'biological' research, see references 31–33.)

If the psychiatric–mental health nursing role is to conduct psychotherapy with people with a behavioural diagnosis, then autism fits squarely within that realm. 'Psychotherapy involves the psychological treatment of the problems of living, by a trained person, within the context of a professional relationship, involving either removing, reducing or modifying specific emotional, cognitive or behavioural problems; and/or promoting social adaptation, personality development and/or personal growth'.[34,p.8] Discussion of the triad of impairment provides further justification for a broadly 'psychotherapeutic' approach.

THE TRIAD OF IMPAIRMENT

Around 500–550 BC Pythagoreans believed and taught that the earth was round and revolved around a central fire in the universe. Two centuries later, Aristotle revised this, stating that the earth was indeed round yet it

---

Personal illustration 35.1: Nathan's story

Nathan, who is 15 and in ninth grade, was referred to the child and adolescent mental health team for assessment following expression of suicidal ideation. His medical history began when he was 4 and his parents took him to the paediatrician because, unlike his two brothers, he seemed 'difficult to manage', displaying tantrums if his routine was changed, even slightly. Everything needed to be on Nathan's terms.

The paediatrician saw Nathan's behaviour as 'attention deficit' and prescribed a stimulant. Nathan returned the following year on the insistence of his preschool staff, who thought that he did not follow verbal instructions and, if things were not going his way, Nathan would tantrum. They also thought he lacked empathy, was selfish and a bully. The only pupils Nathan related to were two 6-year-old girls who 'mothered' him. The paediatrician added 'oppositional defiant disorder' to his diagnosis and prescribed a *selective serotonin reuptake inhibitor* (SSRI) to accompany the stimulant.

Nathan entered school when he was 6, and appeared to fit in for the first two terms. In his last year at preschool Nathan had stopped 'spinning and flapping' and had become intensely interested in *Thomas the Tank Engine*. In the transition to school Nathan included Thomas in every sentence and developed some vigorous motor tics of blinking and head shaking. At the end of term as two distinct peer groups began to form, the teacher noted that Nathan was often left out, and spent time in the playground alone. The exception to this was when a small group of relatively mature girls would include him in their games. In years 1 and 2 Nathan did well in counting and maths, but was poor at stories and writing in general. There was a big difference between his academic strengths and relative deficits.

In year 3 Nathan did not cope with the increased responsibility, and had several outbursts in class. He was suspended one day after throwing a chair at a relief teacher who had given the class complex verbal instructions about how their day would be restructured for adventure. The school counsellor wondered why Nathan often did just not 'get it'. An IQ test showed he was of average intelligence, but when he next saw the paediatrician he was diagnosed with Asperger's disorder. The paediatrician replaced the SSRI with an atypical antipsychotic. This medication change had a 'miraculous' effect for 6 months. Nathan became less obsessional and more flexible in his behaviour, and had fewer motor tics as his anxiety dropped. After 6 months the original anxiety returned. The atypical antipsychotic appeared effective if the dose was adjusted (sometimes up and sometimes down) every 6 months. It worked even better when the paediatrician stopped the stimulant. Nathan's parents had been worried about ceasing the stimulant, fearing what would happen if his behaviour became worse.

The transition to high school was a challenge as Nathan struggled to negotiate the new routines and peer pressures developed, as in his first year of school. Nathan was 'different' and ripe for persecution. The same group of girls were there to pick up the pieces, including Nathan in their activities. Towards the end of year 9, things went badly for Nathan as pubertal social relations became more intense and complex. The girls who had supported Nathan since primary school abandoned him, as the implications of talking to a boy and the consequent teasing were too much. Nathan often stumbled over social conventions and was the focus of jokes, becoming confused, anxious and alone.

Nathan slept little as he could not quieten his mind. His parents often heard him, late at night, going over conversations word for word, to the point that it sounded as though other people were in the room. His diet had always been restricted to favourite foods that had to be served in a particular fashion, but his appetite now declined and he was losing weight. Nathan had always had difficulty talking about his feelings, so his parents had given up asking how he felt. The night before the referral, Nathan's parents tried to encourage him to join the family in the living room. He yelled out, 'I want to die', describing an elaborate plan to jump under a train.

Because of poor social skills and lack of adaptability, Nathan had great difficulty fitting into the social world of school. Although he wanted to do well, he struggled to keep up with lessons. He was often criticized by teachers as being wilfully obstructive and neglectful. He wanted to do better but did not know how and became hopeless. In the playground, Nathan worked at being invisible and was alone and anxious. Nathan was overtaken by the very human problems of pervasive sadness and anxiety. The journey to this point was through struggles to adapt, the very stuff mental health teams are geared up to work on.

remained stationary at the centre of the universe, an idea which remained current until the Copernican revolution in the seventeenth century.[35,36] These philosophical/scientific 'arguments' are relevant to today, in which we still argue about the extent to which medicine is central to health. Autism represents a different way of thinking and hence of *being in the world*. Understanding the triad of impairment allows the clinician to develop an understanding of where the 'shoe pinches', where the issue hurts both the person and those with whom he or she relates.[37] This understanding equips the nurse to move beyond being a mere agent of surveillance, who categorizes behaviours within the dominant medical paradigm. Instead, the nurse might develop a new horizon from which to project into a relationship with a 'person' in autism, developing a meaningful therapeutic engagement.

Darwin provided an excellent example of the failure to 'recognize' something, simply because it had not been *previously* witnessed. 'The Fuegians, whom Charles Darwin visited from the Beagle, were excited by the sight of the small boat which took the landing party ashore, but failed to notice the ship itself, lying at anchor in front of them.'[38,p.19] The Fuegians could 'recognize' small boats (since they had similar ones of their own), but could not see the previously 'unseen' large ship.

By exploring the triad of impairment, we might 'recognize' the ship that is *autism*: something beyond our experience. It is useful to discuss each point of the triad individually, but, to recognize the impairment fully, we need to appreciate how the three elements interrelate alongside the underpinning cognitive processing style. The accepted triad of impairment in autism is represented by the three behavioural elements: impaired communication, impaired social skills and restrictive and repetitive behaviour. This triad is underpinned, in turn, by a triad of *cognitive processing differences*, of visual as opposed to linguistic processing, impaired abstraction ability and lack of theory of mind.

Cognitive processing style in autism

Listing behaviours that characterize the triad is less important than attempting to grasp the underlying cognitive processing style that appears to characterize autism. As with all people the array of possible behavioural variants is unlimited in autism, but what remains consistent is a unique way of *being*, based on a unique cognitive processing style. This is not 'normal' or 'abnormal' but rather a feature of autism, perhaps best described as not neurotypical.[39] In terms of our rudimentary understanding of how people think it would appear that, broadly speaking, there are only two main processing styles: those with autism and those without autism.

Of course, there is variance within both groups in terms of relative balance between visual and auditory processing for instance, and preference for attending to visual, auditory or tactile stimuli. However, this variance occurs within two main processing styles. People often ask: 'What about intellectual disability?' The answer is simply that if the intellectual disability is not co-existing with autism then the person has a typical processing style, but the amount of information that can be processed or speed of processing may be limited. The person may be able to process less and at a slower rate than the typical person. Others ask about people who have schizophrenia and, in general, the answer is that psychosis is episodic, and although the individual interpretation of information fluctuates the person's processing style remains neurotypical.

Neurotypical processing and autism

Take the case of the Honourable Henry Cavendish FRS (1731–1810), whose introversion went beyond a social phobia. He was so reclusive he forbade his bankers to speak to him about his money or his housekeepers to speak to him at all. He was painfully shy, and could not bear to be interrupted about trivial matters. To ensure his privacy, he developed an elaborate ritualized system of letter boxes and double doors within his house. After meeting a maid on the staircase by accident, he had a second stairway built to spare himself any further close encounters. His contemporary, Lord Brougham, recalled Cavendish's nervous quirks at scientific meetings – the shrill cry he uttered as he shuffled from room to room. He probably spoke fewer words in his seventy-eight years than any septuagenarian in history, not at all excepting monks of the Trappist order. Yet Cavendish was a brilliant scientist, the first to realize that water was not a single element, but composed of hydrogen and oxygen. He also discovered, but neglected to publish, two fundamental principles of electricity – Coulomb's Law and Ohm's Law – years before they dawned on Charles Coulomb or George Ohm.

Weeks and Ward[36,p.21–22]

The behaviours seen in autism that characterize the triad of impaired communication, social skills and behavioural flexibility are underpinned by a unique cognitive processing style. People with autism are *visual* as opposed to *linguistic* processors of information. The neurotypical/ordinary platform of processing is one of linguistics; thought is based on a form of personal language or *mentalese*.[40] People with autism favour the visual processing of information.[41,42] People with an ordinary cognitive processing style are blessed with what Aristotle described as the great gift of abstraction.[43] People with autism did not receive this gift and have a marked deficit in this area.[5] Abstraction is the gift that allows ordinary beings to linguistically categorize their interpretations, which constitute their information about the world in an ordered fashion based on like and similar concepts. This unified base of knowledge of the world has been likened to a personal 'in-head' filing cabinet.[12] People with an ordinary cognitive processing style are self-referential; to make sense of incoming stimuli they pull information in and relate it to what is in their filing cabinet, their interpretations about the world.[33] This unified base of knowledge is critical in recognizing the world.

There is a strong central coherence in the way information is processed that is dependent on context and individual interpretations of the world. People with autism have poor *abstraction abilities* and hence have great difficulty forming a unified base of knowledge about the world. Information is stored on the basis of visual, as opposed to linguistic, code and stored in chunks in the order received without being unified with past experience based upon the quality of being like or similar.[5] People with autism are not constructionists in terms of thought and have weak central coherence. Another great gift of which people with autism were deprived is that of *theory of mind*, which can be described as the basis of empathy. The innate knowledge that other people possess a mind (like our own) is used to make a guess about what other people are thinking and feeling. This is an intentional category; something we can attend to or take notice of.[44] Theory of mind ability allows neurotypical beings to regulate communication and social contact. The combination of an ever-expanding unified base of knowledge about the world and theory of mind allows people with an ordinary cognitive processing style to adapt in an ever-changing social world. Of course, to adapt requires flexibility of thought and behaviour. The ordinary individual when confronted with novel stimuli can reach into their unified base of knowledge and bring forth the successful behaviour from the closest or most like circumstance. The ordinary individual then has behaviour to try and for a short while anxiety subsides. If the behaviour is successful, adaptation has occurred and more worldly knowledge is added to the personal database. If the behaviour is not immediately successful, anxiety may rise but the behaviour can be modified until successful. The database is added to in such a case by not only a new context but also a new behaviour.

Although the expression is used in popular parlance, it is rare for an ordinary person to 'not have a clue', even though the first behaviour tried may be a long way off the mark. For people with autism, who store information visually, when confronted with a novel situation they may in fact have no behaviour to try out: they may, literally, 'not have a clue'. Anxiety rises and the only way to control it is to engage in a flight or fight response.

Autism does not affect what might be called temperament or personality, so some people with autism lean predominantly towards internalizing and others towards externalizing. *Externalizing* in autism often means behaviour related to taking control. This may be tantrums or application of rigid ritualistic ways of doing things to avoid any novel stimuli or situation. *Internalizing* may

well be to engage in obsessional pursuits or thought. It is of interest that an element of personality disorder is often the rigid pattern in which people continue to trial non-successful behaviours as a way of coping, without adaptation. Neurosis has been described as a form of shut-up-ness, a case of rigid and non-responsive ways of being.[37] The neuroprocessing style of autism in a world dominated and structured by ordinary processors clearly predisposes people with autism to anxiety and the need for assistance to adapt and cope.

THERAPY

If nurses can appreciate the cognitive processing style of the person with autism, they might be able to help 'translate the world' for the person with autism and 'translate the person with autism' for the world.[45] Although each person with autism is an individual, understanding the structures of autism gives some potential insight into the elements sitting behind a person's experience of the world. Nurses can be aware of the possibilities and incorporate them into their interpretation with patients where relevant.

The question remains: how might we adapt psychotherapy for use with people with autism, given that it is devised to work with neurotypical/ordinary constructionist thinkers? One potentially useful area lies in the realms of narrative therapy, which explores the individual construction of meaning by working on the stories a person or family tells themselves *about their world*.[46] This is the discussed ordinary trait of the linguistic coding of information that leads to an individual construction of meaning. This constructed meaning or world interpretation is built on grouping of similar ideas in engrams or concepts.[47] However, the lack of abstraction ability that characterizes autism is well catered for by the externalization techniques employed in narrative therapy. Further to this, the notion of dealing with small concrete chunks works well, as opposed to hopelessness inducing problem-saturated narratives: problems that are too big and complex to begin working on. The origin of narrative therapy was Epston and White's work[46] with children and adolescents in which person centredness was taken for granted. Engaging the participant as co-conspirator or co-therapist is an often used strategy that is clinically potent.

The creative approach can be bent to obsessive interests of spying, in spying on one's own behaviour or experimentation with data collection. A combination of such techniques with a cognitive–behavioural approach and social stories shows great promise. The cognitive–behavioural approach of engaging the person as an apprentice in problem-solving through the systematic trial of solving a problem and examining the associated cognitions is fruitful.[48] Social stories are an approach that involves creating complete chunks of social information around a particular event or behaviour that can be applied by the person in the particular situation. The story includes information on the effect of the person's behaviour on others. This approach, devised by Carol Gray,[49] caters for the chunk style learning and theory of mind deficit.

By appreciating the distinct cognitive processing style of the person with autism, we can use narrative therapy techniques to engage the person and begin to define 'the problem', moving on to use a cognitive–behavioural model for planning, trialling and modifying behaviour. This behaviour them forms the basis of the social story. *Engaging* the person with autism is vital. In the book, *Smiling at shadows*,[15] Dane, a person with autism, described how if he wrote a story, he had an obsessional need to follow it and apply it to his behaviour, even if he did not want to. The structures and support derived through such a process can assist with the boundary-expanding work of chaos therapy.[50]

SUMMARY

Autism is a clinical construct that has been refined and expanded since its inception in 1943. Responsibility for working with people with autism on their problems of living in nursing has migrated from psychiatric nursing to developmental disability nursing, and now back to a shared domain of care in which the stake for psychiatric nurses is both clear and significant. The exciting implication for psychiatric nurses from this rewarding area of endeavour is that the role can be articulated beyond the trap of diffuse collaborator and therapeutic engager. Understanding the underlying cognitive processing style of autism allows nurses to articulate clear nursing therapies in an area that is not dominated by the current medical paradigm.

Reflection

How do impaired communication, social skills and behavioural flexibility render the person with autism particularly vulnerable to depression and anxiety, associated with problems of living in a social world?

Can you think of a particular example from your practice of working with people with autism?

REFERENCES

1. Kanner L. Autistic disturbances of affective contact. *Nervous Child* 1943; **2**: 217–50.

2. Wing L, Potter D. The epidemiology of autistic spectrum disorders: is the prevalence rising? *Mental Retardation and Developmental Disabilities Research Reviews* 2002; **8**: 151–61.

3. Schutz A. *The phenomenology of the social world*. Evanston, IL: Northwestern University Press, 1932/1967.

4. Heidegger M. Understanding and interpretation. In: Mueller-Vollmer K (ed.). *The hermeneutics reader*. Oxford, UK: Basil Blackwell, 1927/1985: 215–27.

5. Scott J, Clark C, Brody M. *Students with autism characteristics and instruction programming*. San Diego, CA: Singular Publishing, 2000.

6. Szatmari P, Volkmar F, Walter S. Evaluation of diagnostic criteria for autism using latent class models. *Journal of the American Academy of Child and Adolescent Psychiatry* 1995; **34**: 216–22.

7. Gillberg C. Asperger syndrome and high functioning autism. *British Journal of Psychiatry* 1998; **172** (3): 200–9.

8. Nash M. The secrets of autism. *Time* 2002; 6 May: 50–60.

9. Bettleheim B. *Recollections and reflections*. London, UK: Thames and Hudson, 1990.

10. Wing L. Asperger's syndrome: a clinical account. *Psychological Medicine* 1981; **11**: 115–30.

11. Cashin A. Two terms – one meaning: the conundrum of contemporary nomenclature in autism. *Journal of Child and Adolescent Psychiatric Nursing* 2006; **19** (3): 137–44.

12. Cashin A. Autism: understanding conceptual processing deficits. *Journal of Psychosocial Nursing and Mental Health Services* 2005; **43** (4): 22–30.

13. Berney T. Autism: an evolving concept. *The British Journal of Psychiatry* 2000; **176**: 20–5.

14. Grandin T, Scariano M. *Emergence labelled autistic*. New York, NY: Warner Books, 1996.

15. Waites J, Swinbourne H. *Smiling at shadows*. Sydney, Australia: Harper Collins, 2001.

16. American Psychiatric Association. *Diagnostic and statistical manual of mental disorders, 4th edition, text revision*. Washington, DC: American Psychiatric Press, 2000 (DSM IV-TR).

17. Macintosh K, Dissanayake C. Annotation. The similarities and differences between autistic disorder and Asperger's disorder: a review of the empirical evidence. *Journal of Child Psychology and Psychiatry* 2004; **45** (3): 421–34.

18. Szatmari P, Bryson S, Streiner D et al. Two-year outcome of preschool children with autism or Asperger's syndrome. *American Journal of Psychiatry* 2000; **157**: 1980–7.

19. Szatmari P, Archer L, Fisman S et al. Asperger's syndrome and autism: differences in behaviour, cognition, and adaptive functioning. *Journal of the American Academy of Child and Adolescent Psychiatry* 1995; **34**: 1662–71.

20. Adam B. *The survival of domination. Inferiorization and everyday life*. New York, NY: Elsevier North Holland, 1978.

21. Bejerot S. An autistic dimension. A proposed subtype of obsessive–compulsive disorder. *Autism* 2007; **11** (2): 101–10.

22. Fombonne E. Epidemiology of autistic disorder and other pervasive developmental disorders. *Journal of Clinical Psychiatry* 2005; **66** (10): 3–8.

23. Edwards D, Bristol M. Autism: early identification and management in family practice. *American Family Physician* 1991; **44**: 1755–64.

24. Committee on Children with Disabilities. Technical report. The pediatrician's role in the diagnosis and management of autistic spectrum disorder in children. *Pediatrics* 2001; **107** (5): e85.

25. Buitelaar J, Willemsen-Swinkels S. Autism: current theories regarding its pathogenesis and implications for rational pharmacotherapy. *Paediatric Drugs* 2000; **2**: 67.

26. Viding E, Blakemore S. Endophenotype approach to developmental psychopathology: implications for autism research. *Behaviour Genetics* 2007; **37**: 51–60.

27. Bailey A, Le Couteur A, Gottesman I *et al.* Autism as a strongly genetic disorder: evidence from a British twin study. *Psychological Medicine* 1995; **25**: 63–78.

28. Goldberg M. *Autistic syndrome: a medical problem.* Tarzana, CA: Avalar Medical Group, 1997.

29. Muhle R, Trentacoste S, Rapin I. The genetics of autism. *Pediatrics* 2004; **113** (5): 472–86.

30. Wing L. *The autistic spectrum: a guide for parents and professionals.* London, UK: Constable, 1996.

31. Zilbovicius M, Garreau B, Samson Y *et al.* Delayed maturation of the frontal cortex in childhood autism. *American Journal of Psychiatry* 1995; **152** (2): 248–52.

32. Ferstl E, Cramon D. What does the frontomedian cortex contribute to language processing: coherence or theory of mind? *Neuroimage* 2002; **17**: 1599–612.

33. Burnette C, Mundy P, Meyer J *et al.* Weak central coherence and its relations to theory of mind and anxiety in autism. *Journal of Autism and Developmental Disorders* 2005; **35**: 63–73.

34. Barker P. The healing of the mind: meaning and method. In: Barker P (ed.). *Talking cures: a guide to the psychotherapies for health care professionals.* London, UK: Nursing Times Books, 1999: 7–22.

35. Williams J. *Pooh and the philosophers.* London, UK: Methuen, 1995.

36. Weeks D, Ward K. *Eccentrics. The scientific investigation.* Glasgow, UK: Stirling University Press, 1988.

37. May R. *Psychology and the human dilemma.* New York, NY: D. Van Nostrand, 1967.

38. Polyanyi M. *The logic of liberty.* London, UK: Routledge and Kegan Paul, 1951.

39. Gray C, Attwood T. The discovery of Aspie criteria by Attwood and Gray. *The Morning News* 1999; **11** (3).

40. Pinker S. *How the mind works.* New York, NY: W.W. Norton and Company, 1997.

41. Grandin T. *Thinking in pictures.* New York, NY: Doubleday, 1995.

42. Grandin T. An anthropologist on Mars. Georget A (director). New York, NY: Gloria Films, 2000.

43. Gadamer H. Man and language. In: Linge D (ed.). *Philosophical hermeneutics.* Berkeley, CA: University of California Press, 1966/1976: 59–69.

44. Lauer Q. The other explained intentionally. In: Kockelmans J (ed.). *Phenomenology.* New York, CA: Doubleday and Co, 1967.

45. Cashin A. Letters to the editor: reply from the author. *Journal of Child and Adolescent Psychiatric Nursing* 2006; **19** (4): 168–9.

46. Epston D, White M. Termination as a rite of passage: questioning strategies for a therapy of inclusion. In: Neimeyer R, Mahoney M (eds). *Constructivism in psychotherapy.* Washington, DC: American Psychological Association, 1995: 339–54.

47. Ogden C, Richards I. *The meaning of meaning,* 10th edn. London, UK: Routledge and Kegan Paul, 1952.

48. Fishman K. *Behind the one-way mirror. Psychotherapy and children.* New York, NY: Bantam Books, 1995.

49. Gray C, Garand J. Social stories: improving responses of students with autism with accurate social information. *Focus on Autistic Behaviour* 1993; **8**: 1–10.

50. Cashin A, Waters C. The under-valued role of over-regulation in autism: Chaos Theory as a metaphor and beyond. *Journal of Child and Adolescent Psychiatric Nursing* 2006; **19** (4): 224–230.

Preface to Section 5

Success in psychotherapy – that is, the ability to change oneself in a direction in which one wants to change – requires courage rather than insight

Thomas Szasz

Increasingly, we explain ourselves and our actions by invoking one school of psychological thought, or another. In the words of the sociologist Frank Furedi, we live in a 'therapy culture' where much of the language and only a little of the original ideas about 'psychotherapy' have leaked into our everyday conversation, coming to dominate our thinking.

This can be seen as a 'dumbing-down' of important ideas about human helping; ideas, which have emerged over millennia, but have been scripted specifically over the past 100 years. Many of these ideas about human nature, human conduct and human development now inform nursing practice. Over the past 50 years a wide range of models has been developed, which serve as templates for the development of ways of relating to people in care and their families and friends. Increasingly, nurses are involved in researching and sometimes actively developing some of these core constructs of human helping.

In Section 5 we review some of the more important uses of 'therapeutic conversation' as they apply to mental health nursing. Since nursing practice is invariably an intimate relationship, often located in the most ordinary of social surroundings, we open with a detailed consideration of the therapeutic one-to-one relationship and the development of empathy. If nurses are to get close to the people in their care they need to understand *how* this might be achieved, and they need also to know how to make the person aware that they appreciate the story, which is unfolding.

Most nursing practice is predicated on storytelling, either as an individual encounter or in a small social group. Working with children and adolescents presents special challenges, which illustrate that working with adults, individually or in groups, is different yet often remarkably similar. The next three chapters emphasize the psychodynamic basis of the relationship between nurses and individuals or groups, of whatever age. These chapters all illustrate the key 'facts' of human helping: the relationship is always *mutual* and that much of its power is dormant or *invisible*.

The next four chapters illustrate models of counselling and therapy that either feature a distinct theoretical perspective or are related to specific situational contexts.

Finally, we introduce a consideration of mindfulness – one of the most ancient forms of 'self-knowledge' – which is gaining a wider audience within a therapy setting, and a reflection on the history of 'therapeutic communities', where people find support by actively 'being with', and 'living with', others in need of support and succour.

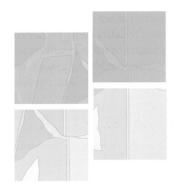

CHAPTER 36

Developing therapeutic one-to-one relationships

Bill Reynolds*

INTRODUCTION

The therapeutic nurse–patient relationship is not a nebulous, kind-hearted, well-intentioned relationship. The purpose of the nurse–patient relationship also differs from the purpose of the doctor–nurse relationship and social relationships with friends and chums. The nurse more than the physician must relate positively to the reaction of patients to illness, including the psychological and social changes that illness forces upon the patient. The nurse spends more time with the patient than does the physician, and therefore has more opportunity not only to observe but also to talk with and come to know the patient. Thus the nurse has an opportunity to help the patient to become aware of and to make sense of, reactions to illness, particularly in terms of long-term personal consequences.

All nurse–patient contacts provide opportunities to implement the purpose of nursing to come to know the patients as *human beings in difficulty*, and to help them stretch their capabilities to achieve more favourable health outcomes. For the patient, illness can be a source of new learning that can be applied in subsequent life situations. In order to provide this kind of meaningful relationship, the

nurse must be a sensitive observer and have a range of theories within which to interpret and extend observations, and on which to base the interpersonal actions of the nurse.

In this chapter the concept of the one-to-one therapeutic relationship in nursing is introduced. Operational definitions of a therapeutic relationship are examined and the aims or purposes of the therapeutic relationship are discussed. It is argued that the therapeutic relationship is the crux of clinical nursing. Practical examples (cases) of the therapeutic relationship in action are provided and evidence supporting the importance of one-to-one relationships to healthcare outcomes is reviewed.

OPERATIONAL DEFINITIONS OF THE THERAPEUTIC RELATIONSHIP

Therapeutic relationships are the cornerstone of nursing practice with people who are experiencing threats to their health, including, but not restricted to, those people with mental illness. The concept of the therapeutic nurse–patient relationship evolved from the work of Hildegard Peplau in the 1950s.[1] Peplau introduced an interpersonal relations

*Bill Reynolds is a mental health nurse from Scotland who now lives and works in Finland. His research and teaching interests are the development and measurement of empathy in nursing and the promotion of discharge models that enable patients to adjust to community living.

paradigm for the study and practice of nursing that was grounded in the clinical experiences of herself and her graduate students.[2] The paradigm held that nurse and patient participate in and contribute to the relationship and, further, that the relationship could be therapeutic. The view was that while relationships may contribute to dysfunctional behaviour, people can also heal within relationships.[2] Theorists studying the focus of psychiatric nursing[3] have also acknowledged the importance of the input of the patient in a two-way relationship. They stated that:

> The proper focus of psychiatric nursing is located in the careful (i.e., methodological) examination of the whole lived experience of people in care. This examination demands an active collaborative role between nurse and patient.

These writers also claimed that the focus of nursing involved a study of human responses to threats to the patients' health that could be observed during nurses' relationships with their patients. The idea that the one-to-one relationship has the potential to influence positive health outcomes for patients (i.e. is a form of treatment) has been stated in the nursing literature for several decades. Reynolds cites Kalkman, who (in the 1960s) referred to the nurse–patient relationship as relationship therapy.[4] The following description illustrates that view:

> Relationship therapy refers to a prolonged relationship between a nurse-therapist and a patient, during which the patient can feel accepted as a person of worth, feels free to express himself/herself without fear of rejection or censure, and enables him/her to learn more satisfactory and productive patterns of behaviour.

The view that the therapeutic nurse–patient relationship should be used to establish an interpersonal climate for nursing assessment and ultimately enable patients to learn more satisfactory and productive patterns of behaviour has prevailed until the present time. For example, it has been suggested that using therapeutic communication, the nurse can begin to assess the individual in crisis,[5] and it has been shown how a non-defensive relationship with nurses relieved embarrassment and anxiety in incontinent patients.[6] This is an important finding since it has been pointed out in the literature that severe anxiety can result in impaired problem-solving ability.[7]

In a similar vein Peplau informs us that anything not talked about, merely acted out, is less likely to be understood and addressed by the nurse or the patient.[8] Her theory of interpersonal relations provides an explanation for why people do the things that they do in respect of concepts such as anxiety, negative self-views and hallucinations. However, the opportunity to assist patients to struggle towards full development of their potential for productive living is dependent upon nurses' ability to understand and apply such concepts within the context of a therapeutic nurse–patient relationship. Evidence supporting the efficacy of the nurse–patient relationship in clinical nursing is considered later in this chapter.

Reflection

What attitudes and behaviours, on the part of the nurse and the patient indicate that a relationship is therapeutic?

THE AIMS OR PURPOSES OF THE THERAPEUTIC RELATIONSHIP

The therapeutic nurse–patient relationship is an important goal for working with individuals in most situations. In spite of the fact that psychiatric or mental health nurses have used Peplau's theory most frequently, the literature shows that it transcends all clinical nursing specialties. This is particularly true of the therapeutic relationship, since a great deal of clinical nursing is based on the interpersonal process and relationship that develops between nurse and patient. This point was emphasized by an Australian nurse academic[9] who stated that:

> Regardless of the apparently different clinical knowledge and skills required to function effectively in different clinical specialities, there is one reliable constant across all nursing settings, and that is the nurse–patient relationship.

Irrespective of the context of the therapeutic relationship, it has the same aims and purposes.[10] These include:

1 Initiating supportive interpersonal communication in order to understand the perceptions and needs of the other person.
2 Empowering the other person to learn, or cope more effectively with their environment.
3 The reduction or resolution of the problems of another person.

The achievement of these aims requires nursing strategies that orientate the patient to the purpose of the relationship, and aid the patient to resolve obstacles that stand in the way of full development and health. Obstacles are primarily of two kinds: (i) disturbances in thought, feelings and action, which might be called pathological use of one's potential; and (ii) lacks and gaps in the development of intellectual and interpersonal competencies that are essential for healthy social interaction and positive health.[11] The nursing strategies needed to address such matters will facilitate the therapeutic nurse–patient relationship from the beginning to end and require that the nurse attends to the interpersonal processes that occur between nurse and patient.

PHASES OF THE THERAPEUTIC RELATIONSHIP

The work of theorists referred to in this chapter, identifies the nurse–patient relationship as the crux of nursing.[12–14] The early studies of the therapeutic relationship revealed that it evolves through identifiable overlapping phases. The phases include orientation, working and resolution. The relationship form developed by Forchuk and others[15] provides an overview of the nurse and patient behaviours at each phase (see Appendix 36.1).

Orientation phase

The initial phase of the relationship is the orientation phase, during which the nurse and patient come to know each other as persons and the patient begins to trust the nurse. This phase is sometimes referred to as the strangers phase, because the nurse and the patient are strangers to each other. The time in orientation phase can vary from a few minutes of an initial meeting to weeks or months of regular contact. During this phase, the nurse is often confronted with interferences or blocks that hinder progression to the working phase of the relationship.

Common interferences are that the patient is unaware of the purpose of the relationship and has not learned to trust the nurse. Patients' confusion about the purpose of the nurse–patient relationship is illustrated by the following patient statements to my students during their clinical work: 'what do you want to talk about nurse?' and, 'I'm not very interesting nurse'. This indicates that the role expectations of the patient are unclear. What goes on between nurses and patients seems to be related to the expectations that each hold of the sick role and the nurse role. At the beginning of a new relationship, the patient needs to be provided with an explanation for one-to-one contacts. Since the role of the nurse is more diverse and unlike the role of other professionals (who may only provide formal counselling or psychotherapy), patients are often unclear why nurses are talking to them. Since the eventual outcome of the nurse–patient relationship is unknown during the orientation phase, it is sufficient to provide a simple explanation that does not produce unrealistic expectations that might not be met. For example:

> I would like you to talk a bit about yourself as a person. This will help me to understand your needs as you see them and to understand what I can do as a nurse to help.

The dialogue arising from providing simple explanations provides the nurse and the patient with an opportunity to assess the 'boundaries' of the relationship, i.e. the purpose and limitations of the relationship.[16] It is also worth remembering that at this stage the patient needs time to learn that the nurse can be trusted. This can be particularly problematic when patients have extensive experience as an inpatient, since it has been revealed that the number and length of hospitalization is significantly related to movement through orientation phase.[17] During the orientation phase the patient is closely watching the nurse. Trust will be established if nurses carry out their stated intentions over a period of time.

Sometimes patients will test out nurses in order to see whether stressors such as hostility and avoidance force the nurse to reject them. The following account from one of my student's diaries describes testing out behaviour.

Personal illustration 36.1

I invited my patient to meet with me for half an hour each day in a semi-private part of the ward. The explanation that I gave was that it was his time to talk about was important to him. He agreed to talk but on the first day he didn't turn up. My supervisor told me to stay in the arranged meeting place for the arranged time. On the second day he didn't turn up, but staff noticed that he was checking to see whether I was there. Between scheduled one-to-one meetings I approached him and said: 'I'm sorry that you were unable to come and talk to me today but I will be there each day in case there is anything important to you that you would like to discuss.' Eventually he came, but at first he rarely stayed for the entire half hour. I always told him that I would stay just in case he felt the need to return. Eventually he always turned up on time and talked for the scheduled period of time. I felt that he now trusted me and understood the purpose of our relationship.

This personal illustration shows how being consistent can help the patient to trust you. Acceptance of the patient's difficulties and the physical presence of the nurse, within identified time limits, demonstrate that the nurse is consistent and will deliver what has been promised.

Working phase

The second phase of the relationship, the working phase, is subdivided into identification and exploitation subphases. In the identification subphase the patient begins to identify problems to be worked on within the relationship. The nature of the problems identified can be as diverse as the scope of nursing practice. Examples include loneliness, anxiety and unresolved relationship difficulties. The exploitation subphase occurs as the patient makes use of the services of the nurse to work through identified problems. The nurse does not usually 'solve' the patient's problems but rather gives the patient an opportunity to explore options and possibilities within the context of the relationship with the nurse. The following clinical data from nurse–patient verbal interaction illustrate some of the clinical work that needs to be done during the working phase.

Patient: I felt confused, uncertain what to do when my daughter left home. I try to keep the peace, but the thing is, her father doesn't realize how upset she is by his interference.

Nurse: Sounds as if you were really upset at that time; what did you feel?

This is an example of a nurse working with her patient during the identification subphase of the relationship. It is a good example of an investigative response that does not challenge the relief behaviour or symptoms of the behaviour. It resulted in the patient confirming that she felt anxious. For example:

Patient: I avoided confronting him because I knew that would make things worse for me. I felt 'in a million pieces', didn't know where to turn, I felt anxious I suppose.

Nurse: What were you doing to avoid being anxious?

Essentially, the clinical work of the nurse during the working phase of the nurse–patient relationship should be investigative. Nurses should assist patients to investigate their experience of threats to their health, the efficacy of their human responses, and to meet needs in a manner that reflects their preferences. Nurses should always view patients as autonomous and free persons. The language of the nurse is intended to provide prompters that stimulate the work that the patient needs to do for his/her own therapeutic benefit. Patients often use vague generalizations rather than description, for example 'I had a lousy day in town today'. Unless this statement is investigated neither the nurse nor the patient will learn anything. The nurse should say something like, 'I have 20 minutes, talk about that experience'. If the patient does not begin, the nurse could say, 'What happened at that time?' Only by listening and hearing a full description from the patient, can the nurse understand the meaning of the patient's experience.

Reflection

Since inpatient care is generally of a brief duration, unplanned (abrupt) termination of therapeutic relationships may result in the patient returning to earlier, less adaptive behaviour. How would you prepare your patient for termination of the nurse–patient relationship?

Resolution phase

The resolution phase of the relationship is the final phase that is sometimes referred to as the termination phase. Resolution is usually a gradual weaning off process where dependence is relinquished and the patient resumes independence. Ideally, resolution should be carried out by mutual agreement when the patient has demonstrated a greater level of functioning. In practice, it more often occurs with patients in an unplanned manner. This can be a problem since it has been reported that abrupt termination of nurse–patient relationships because of a change in staff resulted in patients returning to behaviour exhibited during the orientation phase of the relationship.[17] As a consequence nurses should anticipate and prepare the patient for resolution at a very early stage.

Assuming that resolution can be planned there is no single criterion sufficient to demonstrate readiness to terminate a relationship. However, the following criteria are useful indicators.

1 An improved sense of autonomy, i.e. ability to 'stand on your own feet'.
2 A reduced need to be defensive.
3 The ability to use new-found insights to adaptively alter day-to-day functioning.

The resolution phase of the relationship can be viewed as a separation of what was unique to the nurse and to the patient, and temporarily shared in a one-to-one relationship. It replicates some of the feelings of disconnectedness that follow bereavement. Termination of a relationship can engender feelings of discomfort, pain and anger. The difficulties confronting the nurse may be similar to those confronting the patient. Nurses too need to overcome an unwillingness to separate and to give up exalted roles the patient has assigned to them. Although the therapeutic relationship ends with an expanded appreciation of the stories and convictions that motivate the patient, it can also end on the same conflictional note on which it began, with expressions of ambivalence and a recounting of successes and failures. The nurse may have to endorse sadness, the patient's disappointment in them and their disappointments in themselves.

The following example highlights some of the problems that emerge during the resolution phase of the therapeutic relationship. This example has been selected from the author's work while supervising nursing students' clinical work in the USA.

Personal illustration 36.2

A young student nurse, providing a final counselling service to a young man, scheduled a final counselling session on the final day of his clinical placement. Previously his patient had regularly turned up for appointments and, on the surface, appeared to be enjoying interaction with his nurse.

The patient failed to appear for his final counselling session and the student spent a frustrating hour waiting for him in the appointed place. He felt very confused and angry.

Later on seeking an explanation from his patient, the student was told: 'You are leaving to get on with better things, while I am stuck in this dump'. This response indicates regression on the patient's part that he has returned to a more dependent state. It also reveals that the relationship has reverted back to the orientation phase.

The student had failed to prepare the patient for termination; in fact, it had never been spoken about. Following consultation with his supervisor the student identified his failure to prepare his patient for termination and immediately scheduled a further meeting with his patient to discuss termination. During that session the patient was assisted to identify ways of coping with termination. The remainder of the day was spent introducing the patient to other patients and a new nurse therapist. The friendship relationships and the new nurse–patient relationship would act as interpersonal support networks when the student left the clinical area.

In conclusion, the nurse must be alert to the surfacing of any behaviour during the resolution phase of a relationship that indicates that the relationship has moved back to an earlier phase. Behaviours to be concerned about include regression, repression, anger, denial and sadness. The nurse may respond by repeatedly observing that the patient is not addressing issues of impending separation, and may move to explore this avoidance. The patient who reverts to a previously abandoned life pattern with the message, 'I can't make it without you', demonstrates regression. When the patients are regressing they give no evidence of an emotional response.

The following therapeutic interventions offer a humanistic approach to the resolution phase of a relationship.

1 Identify the circumstances under which the relationship may be terminated.
2 Assist the patient to discover new interests, such as hobbies, friendship relationships and personal achievement.
3 Encourage transference of dependence to other support systems such as spouse, relative, employer, neighbour, friend or new therapist, for emotional support.
4 As the patient's independence from you grows, allow time and space for interactions with significant people in his/her life.
5 As the time for termination nears, increasingly focus on future-orientated material.
6 Assist the patient to work through feelings associated with the resolution phase.

The course of termination is influenced by the work that precedes it. The more that patient and nurse discuss their successes and failure, their gratitude and disappointments, the more the patient will have benefited from the therapeutic relationship.

Reflection

What favourable health outcomes can be achieved by the patient during a therapeutic relationship with the nurse?

THE CLINICAL SIGNIFICANCE OF THE THERAPEUTIC NURSE–PATIENT RELATIONSHIP

A considerable amount of evidence exists in the literature to support the view that the therapeutic nurse–patient relationship is a significant variable in health care and that it can enable people to cope more effectively with threats to their health. The evidence varies from the theoretical to research evidence accumulated from different types of research designs. The cumulative evidence is encouraging and some of it is reviewed in the next section of this chapter.

Some of the evidence relating to the clinical significance of the nurse–patient relationship has been elicited from the recipients of health care, the patients themselves. A review of the literature reveals that patients are in a position to advise professionals about how to offer a therapeutic relationship. A paper reporting the findings from two qualitative studies conducted on opposite sides of the Atlantic[18] showed that the type of relationship that psychiatric patients wanted from their nurses in Canada and Scotland is similar. This indicates that the concepts of the therapeutic relationship, which has its origins in the USA, can cross some national boundaries. Since cultural sensitivity can facilitate open, non-defensive relationships, that is an important finding. In both studies patients identified the relationship with the nurse as important to their overall recovery. Listening, availability and a friendly approach were identified as critical in the nurse–patient interactions in the Canadian study. Participants wanted to see that action was taken on issues that were identified.

In the Scottish study, similar themes were identified. Patients wanted nurses to listen, be sensitive to feelings, seek clarification of confused messages, help them to 'anchor' accounts of problems in the personal time and setting of the problem, help them to focus on solutions to problems, and to sound warm and genuine. Canadian patients valued help to see things more clearly. Scottish patients valued nurses' attempts to help them gain more detail about the emotional experience. The clinical significance of these data is indicated by the consensus in the literature[19] that the consumer of health care is an important, active collaborator in treatment and outcome goals.

Patients' perceptions of the nurse–patient relationship have been a focus for studies in various clinical contexts. For example, the findings of a pilot study into nursing observation from the perspective of the patient showed that the experience was predominately negative for the majority of patients. A key variable in positive experience was a therapeutic relationship with the observing nurse and the provision of information about the observation process.[20] In a different type of clinical environment[21] chemotherapy patients and their families placed a high value on a warm reciprocated personal relationship with a nurse. They claimed that it could create a supportive atmosphere in what might otherwise be a threatening environment for patients. Data from these studies indicate that the nurse–patient relationship can humanize care and reduce stress levels. The reduction of stress in chemotherapy patients would seem particularly important since stress can lower the efficiency of the autoimmune system.

Several other studies show that there is now widespread belief in the therapeutic relationship as a means of generating favourable outcomes for patients. In a Hong Kong study,[22] 10 registered nurses were interviewed on their perceptions of caring behaviours in their clinical setting. Findings showed that respondents valued the importance of interpersonal relationships in providing holistic care. In a Japanese study,[23] experienced psychiatric public health nurses revealed that they used an empowering relationship with families, neighbours, educators and employers in order to enable their patients' healthy living in the community. Finally, a German study[24] used clinical vignettes and observed that nurses used their relationship with psychotic patients to understand psychotic functional behaviour and that this enabled patients to return to the non-psychotic world.

The efficacy of the nurse–patient relationship is further supported by a Canadian study that revealed that overlapping hospital and community services enabled the therapeutic nurse–patient relationship to be maintained after discharge from hospital. Findings revealed improved quality of life for discharged patients, reduced re-admissions, and a saving to the tax payers in Western Ontario of $500 000 in the initial year.[25] Subsequently a major randomized controlled study in Western Ontario has revealed that the continuation of the therapeutic nurse–patient relationship in the community for a short period after discharge has reduced time in hospital and reduced re-admission rates by 50 per cent.[26]

The Canadian study was replicated in the Highland Region of Scotland. The intervention, which was called a Transitional Discharge Model, was viewed as a solution to a very high relapse/re-admission rate to acute psychiatric wards in that region due to the inability of many individuals to adjust to community living.[26] The supportive relationship with hospital staff is generally lost during discharge, and often terminated in an unplanned manner. This is a problem because it can take several weeks to form a new working relationship with community staff; thus individuals are often left with minimal support at a time when they need to mediate the stress of adjustment to community living. The transitional discharge model included (1) overlap of inpatient and community staff in which inpatient staff continue to work with the discharged patient until a working relationship is established with a community care provider; and (2) peer support, which is assistance from former patients who provide friendship, understanding and encouragement. A comparison was made between patients' discharge with a transitional discharge model and a control group of patients discharged under the usual discharge arrangements. The findings showed that the usual treatment subjects in the control group were more than twice as likely to be re-admitted to hospital.[26]

Discharge programmes that involve bridging therapeutic relationships from hospital to community build on the work of Forchuk in Canada and Reynolds in Scotland.[27] The conclusions drawn from this work are that the quality of interpersonal relationships will promote less need for expensive intervention in mental health, such as hospitalization.[27]

SUMMARY

The literature indicates that psychiatry is focusing on a biomedical approach to mental health. The work of the psychiatrist incorporates ongoing brain research and pharmaceutical research, and utilizes sophisticated equipment for forms of laboratory measurement and the study of within-body phenomena of psychiatric patients. It would therefore seem urgent that mental health nurses develop their own area of interest, the human responses of psychiatric patients. Examples of human responses observed by nurses during their relationships with psychiatric patients include anxiety, self-esteem problems, loneliness, grief and hallucinations. Mental health nurses need to study such problems, make themselves experts in a humanistic alternative approach to such problems of psychiatric patients and to speak out on the prevention of such problems. Such human responses of patients can only be studied effectively in a therapeutic (investigative) relationship that enables a person to examine life experiences.[28] This implies that the patient should have an active role in the treatment of disease and the recovery of health. Additionally, research into molecular biology, including notions of neuroplasty, the effect of life events on the brain and behaviour, and the interaction of genes and the environment, indicate that environment can result in the same effect on the brain as medication. This indicates that therapeutic relationships can enable nurses to influence the human condition positively.[29]

REFERENCES

1. Forchuk C, Reynolds W. Interpersonal theory in nursing practice: the Peplau legacy [guest editorial]. *Journal of Psychiatric and Mental Health Nursing* 1998; **5** (3): 165–6.

2. Peplau H. *Interpersonal relations in nursing*. London, UK: Macmillan Education, 1988.

3. Barker P, Reynolds W. The proper focus of psychiatric nursing: a critique of Watson's caring ideology. *Journal of Psychosocial Nursing* 1994; **22**: 17–23.

4. Reynolds W, Scott B. Do nurses and other professional helpers normally display much empathy? *Journal of Advanced Nursing* 2000; **31** (1): 226–34.

5. Smith D. Flight to Los Angeles: crisis at 30,000 feet. *Journal of Psychosocial Nursing* 2000; **38** (10): 38–45.

6. Shaw C, Williams K. Patients' views of a new nurse led continence service. *Journal of Clinical Nursing* 2000; **9**: 574–82.

7. Barry F. *Psychosocial nursing care of physically ill patients and their families*. Baltimore, MD: Lippincott, 1996.

8. Peplau H. Interpersonal relations model: theoretical constructs principles and general applications. In: Reynolds W, Cormack D (eds). *Psychiatric and mental health nursing: theory and practice*. London, UK: Chapman and Hall, 1990.

9. Martin T. Something special: forensic psychiatric nursing. *Journal of Psychiatric and Mental Health Nursing* 2001; **8** (1): 25–32.

10. Reynolds W. *The measurement and development of empathy in nursing*. Aldershot, UK: Ashgate, 2000.

11. Reynolds W. Peplau's theory in practice. *Nursing Sciences Quarterly* 1997; **10** (4): 168–70.

12. Peplau H. Interpersonal techniques: the crux of psychiatric nursing. *American Journal of Nursing* 1962; **62**: 50–4.

13. Forchuk C. *Hildegard E. Peplau: interpersonal nursing theory*. London, UK: Sage Publications, 1993.

14. Reynolds W, Scott A, Austin W. Nursing, empathy and perceptions of the moral. *Journal of Advanced Nursing* 2000; **32** (1): 235–42.

15. Forchuk C, Brown B. Establishing a nurse–client relationship. *Journal of Psychosocial Nursing* 1989; **27** (2): 30–34.

16. Lego S. *Psychiatric nursing: a comprehensive reference*. Baltimore, MD: Lippincott, 1996.

17. Forchuk C. The orientation phase: how long does it take? *Perspectives in Psychiatric Care* 1992; **28** (4): 7–10.

18. Forchuk P, Reynolds W. Clients' reflections on relationships with nurses: comparisons from Canada and Scotland. *Journal of Psychiatric and Mental Health Nursing* 2001; **8** (1): 45–51.

19. The Scottish Office. *Designed to care: renewing the National Health Service in Scotland*. London, UK: The Stationary Office, 1997.

20. Jones J, Lowe T, Ward M. Inpatients' experiences of nursing observations on an acute psychiatric unit: a pilot study. *Journal of Mental Health Care and Learning Disabilities* 2000; **4** (4): 125–9.

21. Walker A, Wilkes L, White K. How do patients perceive support from nurses? *Professional Nurse* 2000; **16**: 902–4.

22. Yam Brassier J. Caring in nursing perceptions of Hong Kong nurses. *Journal of Clinical Nursing* 2000; **9** (2): 293–302.

23. Kayama M, Zerwekh J, Murashima S. Japanese expert public health nurses empower clients with schizophrenia living in the community. *Journal of Psychosocial Nursing* 2000; **39** (2): 40–7.

24. Teising M. 'Sister, I am going crazy, help me': psychodynamic-orientated care in psychotic patients in inpatient treatment. *Journal of Psychiatric and Mental Health Nursing* 2000; **7**: 449–54.

25. Forchuk C, Martin ML, Chan Y, Jensen E. Therapeutic relationships from psychiatric hospital to community. *Journal of Psychiatric and Mental Health Nursing* 2005; **12**: 556–64.

26. Reynolds W, Lauder W, Sharkey S *et al.* The effects of a transitional discharge model for psychiatric patients. *Journal of Psychiatric and Mental Health Nursing* 2004; **11**: 82–8.

27. Forchuk P, Reynolds W, Sharkey S *et al.* Transitional discharge based on therapeutic relationships: state of the art. *Archives of Psychiatric Nursing* 2007; **21** (2): 80–6.

28. Peplau H. Investigative counseling. In: O'Toole A, Rouslin S (eds). *Hildegard Peplau: selected works*, Chapter 16. London, UK: Macmillan, 1994.

29. Gallop P, Reynolds W. Putting it all together: dealing with complexity in understanding of the human condition. *Journal of Psychiatric and Mental Health Nursing* 2004; **11**: 357–64.

Appendix 36.1

	Non-therapeutic Relationships		Therapeutic Relationships		
	Mutual withdrawal	**Grappling**	**Orientation** Start	**Working phase** Identification	**Resolution phase** Exploitation
Client:	Forgets appointment/planned times Cannot recall who nurse/service provider is Unaware if nurse/service provider is available Content kept superficial Actively avoids nurse/service provider	Frequent changes of topics and approach Increasing frustration Sense of lack of connection Begins to dread meetings	Seeks assistance Conveys educative needs Asks questions Tests parameters Shares preconceptions and expectations due to past experience	Identifies problems Aware of time Responds to help Identifies with nurse Recognizes nurse as person Explores feelings Fluctuates dependence, independence and interdependence in therapeutic relationship Increases focal attention Changes appearance (for better or worse) Understands purpose of meeting Maintains continuity between sessions (process and content) Testing manoeuvres decrease Increases focal attentive	Makes full use of services Identifies new goals Rapid shifts in behaviour; dependent–independent Exploitative behaviour Realistic exploitation Self-directing Develops skills in interpersonal relationships and problem-solving Displays changes in manner of communication (more open, flexible) Abandons old needs Aspires to new goals Becomes independent of helping person Applies new problem-solving skills Maintains changes in style of communication and interaction Positive changes in view of self Integrates illness Exhibits ability to stand alone
Service provider:	No time for client meetings Client meetings very short if they occur at all Focus on instrumental tasks Decision that client is atypical of usual relationship Avoids client contact	Frequent changes of therapeutic approach Sense of lack of connection Increasing frustration Length of meetings vary Place of meetings vary	Respond to emergency Give parameters of meetings Explain roles Gather data Help client identify problem Help client plan use of community resources and services Reduce anxiety and tension Practise non-directive listening Focus client's energies Clarify preconceptions and expectations	Maintain separate identity Unconditional acceptance Help express needs, feelings Assess and adjust to needs Provide information Provide experiences that diminish feelings of helplessness Do not allow anxiety to overwhelm client Help focus on cues Help client develop responses to cues Use word stimuli	Continue assessment Meet needs as they emerge Understand reason for shifts in behaviour Initiate rehabilitative plans Reduce anxiety Identify positive factors Help plan for total needs Facilitate forward movement of personality Deal with therapeutic impasse Sustain relationship as long as patient feels necessary Promote family interaction Assist with goal setting Teach preventive measures Utilize community agencies Teach self-care Terminate relationship

Note: Phases are overlapping

MW	GR	O	WP	RP

Please mark on the following scale where the check marks are concentrated within the above table. Check lists designed to assist in evaluating phase.

Completed by: _____ **Date:** _____

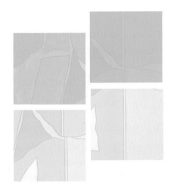

CHAPTER 37

Developing empathy

Bill Reynolds*

INTRODUCTION

Empathy is crucial to all forms of helping relationships. Although there is a considerable debate about whether empathy is a personality dimension, an experienced emotion, or an observable skill, empathy needs to involve the patient's actual awareness of the helper's communication in order that patients know whether they are being understood. Accurate empathy is a form of interaction, involving communication of the helper's attitudes and communication of the helper understanding of the patient's world. It is an essential component of the therapeutic, one-to-one nurse–patient relationship discussed in Chapter 36, since without empathy, there is no basis for helping. The cumulative research evidence supports this view in spite of attempts by some contributors to the literature to argue that empathy may not always be useful.

Here the historical and theoretical background to empathy will be discussed. Different definitions of empathy will be considered and a construct of empathy that is relevant to clinical nursing will be described. The author's own research-based empathy scale is used to illustrate the dimensions of empathic relating, which occurs within the therapeutic relationship, and can be measured. Clients' views of their relationships with nurses and other research evidence will be presented to illustrate that empathy is crucial to the goals of clinical nursing.

EMPATHY: HISTORICAL AND THEORETICAL BACKGROUND

Essentially the concept of empathy originated from the German word *Einfulung* as used by Lipps,[1] which literally means feeling within. This contribution led to empathy being viewed for many years as a perceptual rather than a communicating skill. For several decades references to empathy as a trait or human quality indicate that a necessary condition of empathy is that the observer understands in some sense the affective state of the other person. The tendency to conceptualize empathy as a kind of attitude or way of perceiving, which therapists assume, and not something that they say or do, is illustrated by the following quote from the early 1960s.[2]

> In order to help, one has to know the patient emotionally. One cannot grasp subtle and complicated feelings of people, except by this emotional knowing, the experiencing of another's feeling that is meant by the term empathy. It is a very special mode of perceiving.

The work of many individuals in the helping and healthcare disciplines, over several decades, has helped us to recognize that empathy has many more components than was originally recognized. This work has clarified the meaning of empathy and helped professionals to know when they are offering empathy. In spite of this

*Bill Reynolds is a mental health nurse from Scotland who now lives and works in Finland. His research and teaching interests are the development and measurement of empathy in nursing and the promotion of discharge models that enable patients to adjust to community living.

work, some contributors to the nursing literature continue to misrepresent the meaning and value of empathy. This problem will be discussed in the next section.

The client-centred paradigm

The development of the construct of empathy was stimulated by the work of Carl Rogers and others from clinical psychology in the 1950s and 1960s. Rogers[3] developed an approach to counselling that was at first called non-directive, but is now called client-centred. At first, this approach was applied only in one-to-one relationships but in later years Rogers became involved in the group movement and extended his theory to encounter groups and other treatment modalities such as play therapy. He also became interested in the application of his theory to education, and extended it to interpersonal relations in general.

Like all theories, the client-centred approach is built on several inter-related concepts. One concept is that people are basically rational, socialized, forward moving and realistic. Furthermore, the client-centred point of view sees people as being basically cooperative, constructive and trustworthy when they are free of defensiveness. As individuals we possess the capacity to experience, and to be aware of, the reality of our psychological maladjustment, and to have the capacity and the tendency to move from a state of maladjustment towards a state of psychological adjustment. These capacities and this tendency will be released in a relationship that has the characteristics of a helping (non-threatening) relationship.

Rogers' view that the relationship should be non-defensive chimes with the suggestion in Chapter 36 that the therapeutic relationship should enable patients to experience freedom to express themselves without fear of censure or rejection. The questions that we need to ask ourselves are: how does a non-defensive relationship occur, or, what are the helping attitudes and behaviours, which create a relationship that enables patients to study the effectiveness of their coping strategies? Rogers postulated that three core (facilitative) conditions were necessary and sufficient to achieve a non-defensive relationship and to enable the patient to learn more satisfactory and productive patterns of behaviour.[3] The facilitative conditions were described as warmth, genuineness and empathy.

Despite his tendency to refer to empathy as an attitude, Rogers' descriptions of the facilitative conditions emphasize the communicative aspect of empathy, and the complexity of empathy.[4] He suggests that the facilitative conditions operative in all effective relationships relate to the helper's attitude, cognition and behaviour. Rogers argues that the patient learns to change when the helper communicates commitment (warmth) and non-defensiveness (genuineness), and is successful in communicating understanding of the patient's current feelings (empathic). He expressed the view that the attitudes and cognitive ability of the helping person are communicated to the patient through the communication of the helper. This suggests that when attitudes and understanding are shown to the patient, empathy is a skilled interpersonal behaviour.

Many theorists recognize that the core facilitative conditions in therapeutic relationships, postulated by Rogers, are inter-related and that the three conditions have an interlocking nature.[5] By this is meant that they interact in such a way as to increase and complement each other. For instance, the communication of empathy (the ability to see things from another person's point of view) can be hollow or threatening if the empathizing individual is defensive, and is not genuine. This suggests that warmth and genuineness are part of an empathic response to the patient and are of equal importance to therapeutic outcome. It appears that empathy cannot exist in the absence of the other two conditions.

This seems logical since it is difficult to understand the feelings behind the patient's words (empathic), if external stressors such as dissatisfaction or anger prevented the nurse from showing commitment (warmth), by seeking clarification when the patient's message is unclear. Putting it another way, a barrier to the exploration of the meaning of the patient's experiences, is a very natural tendency to judge, evaluate or disapprove, when the patient's personal communication is threatening. When this happens the helping person may become defensive, often transmitting this to the patient through unwanted advice or unfriendly voice tone. Unless the helper can work on achieving genuineness, the helper's moment-by-moment empathic grasp of the meaning and significance of the patient's world will be impeded.

Despite extensive research and literature supporting the clinical usefulness of empathy, some writers have suggested that empathy might not always be useful during nurse–patient relationships. In some instances these challenges have revealed a lack of understanding about how empathy works. For example, it has been suggested that empathy might not always be necessary because sometimes it might be more therapeutic to allow the patient to use denial as a coping strategy.[6] The problem with that idea is that it misrepresents what empathy is about. Empathy is not about pushing a patient into revealing what he or she is not ready to discuss, since this can be harmful. It might result in the intensification of anxiety which might exist as a consequence of health problem(s), or maladaptive living. If this happens it will be a problem because severe anxiety can result in loss of control and impaired problem-solving ability.[7] Judging when to ask questions about the patient's health or coping patterns is a strategic therapeutic decision. Timing is dependent upon an empathized awareness of the patient's state of readiness to talk. Therefore, a high empathy nurse is more likely to be sensitive towards a patient's need to use denial than a low empathy nurse. That is what is meant by a client-centred approach.

An alternative challenge to empathy is based upon an assumption that it has no value in certain clinical contexts. For example it has been suggested that therapeutic empathy, comprising primarily cognitive and behavioural components that are used to convey understanding of the patient's reality, is particularly unsuited in clinical settings such as surgical wards.[8,9] The basis of this criticism is that the concept of empathy was based on a counselling model developed by clinical psychology, and that nurses working in non-psychiatric contexts do not have sufficient time to offer accurate empathy. In response, it could be argued that the literature reviewed in later sections of this chapter indicates that just because barriers to empathy exist, this does not mean that empathy is not necessary. Additionally, a measure of empathy now exists which has its antecedents in patients' views about the type of relationship that they would like to have with nurses.[10] The items on the Reynolds Empathy Scale (RES) are discussed later in this chapter.

Reflection

What type of attitudes and behaviours do you think about when you hear the term empathy?

THE MEANING AND COMPONENTS OF EMPATHY

For several decades the literature has illustrated that there is disagreement about what empathy means and that there is a need to find a common definition of empathy. The reason for this debate is that while empathy is a complex multidimensional construct involving cognition, behaviour, attitudes, emotions and personality, many writers have viewed it narrowly as a unitary construct.

The components of empathy that are most frequently referred to are cognitive (the helper's intellectual ability to identify another person's feelings and perspectives from an objective stance) and behavioural (a communicative response to investigate and then convey understanding of another's perspective). A possible explanation is that professionals tend to look for definitions that reflect the aims of the therapeutic relationship. Clinicians, such as nurses should communicate understanding of the patient's experience (i.e. offer cognitive–behavioural empathy) in order that this can be validated by the patient.[10]

The clinical significance of moral/trait empathy (an internal altruistic force that motivates the practice of empathy), and emotional empathy (the ability to subjectively experience and share in another's psychological state or intrinsic feeling) has not been determined.[10] While it is logical to believe that a predisposition to offer empathy is essential, at the present time, there is little evidence that personality traits are significantly correlated with an actual ability to offer empathy. In other words, the desire to help does not always manifest itself in supportive behaviours. It is reasonable to suggest that emotions can enrich a relationship. Emotion may even play a fundamental role in perceiving the moral dimensions of clinical practice. This has been suggested in the literature.[10] However, the amount of emotion necessary to respect the perspective of the patient is unknown. Emotional empathy has sometimes been viewed as a synonym for sympathy. Sympathy (an innate biological tendency to react emotionally to the emotions of another) may even block cognitive–behavioural empathy since emotions, such as anxiety, can cause inattention to detail. It has also been reported that high levels of emotional empathy can cause individuals to be sensitive to rejection and to engage in behaviours related to approval-seeking tendencies. For those reasons it has been argued that there needs to be fixed (minimum) levels of emotion necessary in a helping relationship.

The relationship of the many components of empathy to each other is poorly understood. Clearly, a great deal of work needs to be done in order to understand how all of the variables in the empathic process interact with each other. What is currently understood is that empathy involves several concepts or stages. Several writers have offered the following explanation about the sequence of the stages and how each of these stages affect the next stage.[10] First, the helper must be receptive to another's communication (the moral component). Second, the helper must understand the communication by putting himself in the other's place (the cognitive component). Third, the helper must communicate that understanding to the patient (the behavioural or communicative component). Finally, the patient needs to validate the helper's perception of the patient's world. The final stage has been referred to as the relational component of empathy, the patient's awareness of how well they are being understood.

The final stage of empathy (the relational component) is important since it offers the patient an opportunity to comment on the accuracy of the helper's perceptions and to experience being understood. The patient's actual awareness of the helper's communication allows him/her to say, 'Yes that is how I see things' or 'No that is not what I mean'. This assumption is consistent with the Barrett-Lennard multidimensional model of empathy, which he described as the empathy cycle. He described it in the following manner:

Phase 1: The inner process of empathic listening to another who is being personally expressive in some way, reasoning and understanding.

Phase 2: An attempt to convey empathic understanding of the other person's experiences.

Phase 3: The patient's actual reception/awareness of the helper's communication.

When the process continues, phase 1 is again the core phase and 2 and 3 follow in cyclical mode. The total interactive sequence in which these phases occur begins with one person being self-expressive in the presence of an empathically attending helper and this characteristically leads to further self-expression and feedback to the empathizing helper.

The clients' perception of empathy

An interesting finding from the literature is that most measures of empathy tend to reflect professionals' views rather than patients' views of empathy. Since empathy is closely associated with the client-centred paradigm, the failure to consider patients' views seems paradoxical. If patients are able to observe the amount and nature of empathy existing in a helping relationship, they are in a position to advise professionals about how to offer empathy. Patients are likely to be better judges of the degree of empathy than professionals and their perceptions of helping relationships can contribute to our understanding of empathy.

In the late 1990s an empathy scale was developed that had some of its antecedents in patients' perceptions of their relationships with nurses.[11] The research responsible for the development of that scale revealed that patients knew a great deal about the degree of empathy existing in a relationship. Findings also suggested that patients' experience of the nurse–patient relationship is a fertile source of information about the phases of the empathic relationship, and how it is best brought about. The issues identified from patients' reports, when matched with views in the professional literature formed the basis for an item pool for the Reynolds Empathy Scale.[11]

Twelve items were developed for the empathy scale that was considered to reflect patients' descriptions of helpful and unhelpful interpersonal behaviours. Since the item pool reflected patients' perceptions of their relationships with nurses, the instrument was considered to measure a construct of empathy that was relevant to clinical nursing.

THE REYNOLDS EMPATHY SCALE AND PATIENTS' VIEWS ABOUT HELPING

The relationship of items on the new empathy scale to patients' views about helping is illustrated by the following patient comments selected from interviews carried out in acute psychiatric admission wards in Scotland.[11] The discussion that follows reveals a relationship between patients' views about effective and ineffective interpersonal behaviour and variables critical to empathy. Positive scale items (effective behaviours) are discussed first.

High-empathy items

Item 1 on the empathy scale (Attempts to explore and clarify feelings) is an example of the extent to which the nurse is attempting to listen actively. Patients' descriptions of the early phase of their relationships with nurses indicated that sensitive understanding or accurate understanding on the part of the nurse was not happening at that point. However, patients revealed that nurses' attempts to listen determined whether accurate understanding was going to happen at some later point in the relationship. Patient statements supporting this conclusion included:

> It is very hard for her to understand me but she is trying very hard.

And

> We haven't discussed my problems yet but she is listening and we are getting there.

Item 3 on the scale (Responds to feelings) reflects patients' needs for nurses to be sensitive to their feelings. For example:

> I don't know her very well but she is very thoughtful. She doesn't object to my feelings and tries to understand my feelings.

And

> He tries very hard to understand my feelings. That must be very hard for him because I talk too much.

Responding to feelings enabled nurses to demonstrate that they were willing to journey alongside the patient in an attempt to 'get inside their shoes'. Patients indicated that this was critical during the early stages of a new relationship.

Item 5 (Explores personal meaning of feelings) relates to the need for nurses to help patients to clarify their often confused messages by providing more detail about their emotional experiences. Essentially patients were stating that they found it helpful when nurses sought to investigate feelings that they had been approaching hazily and hesitantly. This is emphasized by the following statements:

> It's not like getting your brains picked. She helps me to let it flow out.

And

> It's like speaking to myself or looking into a mirror. She helps me to explain the reasons for my distress.

Item 7 (Responds to feelings and meanings) relates to patients' need for nurses to help them to 'anchor' accounts of problems in the personal time and setting of the problem. When that help was provided patients indicated that they were able to move from the general to the particular, from the past to the present. The following comments illustrate this point:

> He helps me to get to the point and helps me to look at the current situation.

And

> She helps me to move from the past to the present. She is interested in what I am like today.

Item 9 (Provides the patient with direction) reflects patients' needs for nurses to help them to focus on solutions to problems. Essentially patients want nurses to assist them to find solutions to personal problems in a manner that reflects their preferences. Patient statements supporting that view included:

> She worked with me on my problem. She helped me to identify how I would like to change my response to family crisis, and to discover what I want to achieve.

And

> We talked about what I would like to happen and how I was going to bring that about.

Item 11 (Appropriate voice tone) relates to patients' views that nurses ought to sound committed (warm) and open (genuine). Patients suggested that the communication of these attitudes can promote an interpersonal climate of respect, neutrality and trust. Item 11 is a reminder of the fact that the way that a person perceives another is often based on the non-verbal, rather than the verbal communications. The following patient statements illustrate how influential voice tone can be:

> He sounds as if he would rather be in the pub having a pint, rather than listening to my rubbish.

And

> She sounds genuinely interested. This gives you a lot of confidence in yourself.

These statements indicate that item 11 is crucial to determining the extent to which verbal inputs are judged to be warm. Patient statements have also revealed that the empathy cycle, described earlier in this chapter, can be stalled at any stage. The origin of negative items on the Reynolds Empathy Scale (ineffective interpersonal behaviours) stemmed from patients' descriptions of threatening behaviours.

Low-empathy items

Item 2 on the scale (Leads, directs and diverts) is an example of manipulative communication that is not patient-centred. This is illustrated by the following statement.

> She is very clever. I don't want to talk about myself, but she judges what I say and somehow I find that we are talking about me. This is not comfortable.

Item 4 (Ignores verbal and non-verbal communication) refers to the nurse's inability to listen. Patients suggested that when nurses failed to hear their communicated message, they felt that they did not care. For example:

> She failed to understand what I was trying to explain to her. I felt that she couldn't have cared less.

Item 6 (Judgemental and opinionated) measures the extent to which a nurse is judgemental or neutral. Patients suggested that when the nurse was judgemental, this damaged the emotional quality of the relationship. This is illustrated by the following statement:

> If someone criticizes me, or doesn't respect me, I just clam up.

Item 8 (Interrupts and seems in a hurry) reflects patients' dislike of being interrupted. For example:

> She didn't give me time to explain: it felt as if I didn't matter.

Item 10 (Fails to focus on solutions) reflects a lack of acceptance. Patients suggested that this conveyed an impression that the nurse was not taking them seriously. For example:

> We haven't got around to discussing solutions to my problems yet. I'm not sure if she believes what I am saying.

Item 12 (Inappropriate voice tone) reflects patients' dislike of an unfriendly nurse. The following patient statement illustrates this point:

> I felt defensive because she sounded so hostile.

Patients indicated that nurses needed to select interventions that are appropriate to the phase of the helping relationship and the needs of the individual receiving help. Under some circumstances it might be appropriate to investigate feelings, coping strategies and health goals. The following statement illustrates this point:

> She can be trusted. You can talk to her about things you would be reluctant to talk to other people about.

However, patients have indicated that at a certain phase of the relationship, in-depth probing might threaten them. For example:

> When I don't want to talk about something she recognizes this mood and asks me about it. She won't persist if I am reluctant.

These statements reveal that nurses need to have an empathized awareness of patients' readiness to talk. If a patient signals a reluctance to discuss feelings, the nurse might not find exploration of the personal meaning of feelings (item 5 on Reynolds Empathy Scale) very productive. An alternative approach would be to say, 'Talk about what is comfortable for you at the moment'. That is an example of helping the patient to clarify the meaning of their communication by providing more detail about their emotional experience (item 1 on the empathy scale). It differs qualitatively from item 5 because it allows patients to continue to feel accepted, but able to make choices.

The findings from the study reported here are similar to research conducted in Canada. The Canadian study[12] reported that patients wanted nurses to respect them, to listen to their (often confused) stories, and to help them to see things more clearly. Interest in the findings has also been expressed by Spanish nurses working in non-psychiatric areas such as digestive pathology.[13] The Empathy Scale has been translated into Spanish and Chinese, indicating that the construct of empathy being measured may have practical utility across several cultural boundaries.

Reflection

What favourable health outcomes for patients might empathy achieve? Alternatively, what unfavourable experiences might the patient have with a nurse exhibiting low empathy?

It is likely that the ability to offer the construct of empathy described in this chapter will enhance ethical care and cultural sensitivity. It enables nurses to identify the problems of patients that need to be addressed by the skills of the nurse. A concern is the use of labels to convey complex concepts and the consequent compartmentalization of a person's problems into standardized terminology that fails to recognize and understand the feelings and needs of an individual, as perceived by them. Accurate empathy can avoid such problems since it involves an empathized sensitivity to the uniqueness of a patient in terms of their human responses to health threats. The next section illustrates the application of empathy in different nursing contexts

APPLICATION OF EMPATHY IN DIFFERENT NURSING SETTINGS

The cumulative evidence in the research and professional literature provides strong support for the hypothesized relationship of empathy to therapeutic relationships. The papers referred to in this section are only a sample of the available evidence. They have been selected in order to illustrate the clinical usefulness of empathy across a wide range of inpatient and community contexts.

Psychiatric and mental health contexts

The practical utility of empathy to psychiatric and mental health contexts would seem self-evident. In these contexts nurses need to gain understanding of complex behaviours such as withdrawal, anxiety and dysfunctional family systems. They need to understand the purpose of dysfunctional behaviour and what prevents people from giving up patterns of behaviour that reduce satisfaction with living. Nurses who work in psychosocial areas have opportunities to help move the patient in a direction favouring productive social living, and to learn about the purpose of dysfunctional behaviour. The focus should be on the experience of the patient, an outcome that is dependent on empathy. The following papers illustrate this assumption.

Reynolds and Scott[14] summarized several studies carried out between 1970 and 1990. Empathy was shown to be a more important facilitator of a helping relationship than the helper's ideological orientation. For example, one study found that behavioural therapists who scored highly in empathy were more potent reinforcers of adaptive behaviour than therapists who were low empathizers. Empathy was shown to be a significant variable influencing improvement among children with learning disability in both verbal and behavioural spheres. Similarly, empathy was found to be central to clinicians' effectiveness when working with hyperactive and uncontrollable children. With respect to confrontation of unpleasant or maladaptive behaviour, it has been shown that high-empathy helpers used approaches which focused on the here-and-now and emphasized the patient's resources. On the other hand, low-empathy helpers were found to be more likely to confront patients with pathology rather than with their resources.[14]

In more recent times it has been shown how empathy enables nurses to investigate and understand the individual experience of persons experiencing a state of chaos as a consequence of psychiatric disorder.[14] It has also been shown that there is a strong positive relationship between empathy, reduction in aggression and higher rates of behaviour compliance among abused group home youth. Additionally it has been demonstrated that empathy enabled partners of men with AIDS to provide increasingly sensitive care as the clinical course of the disease developed. Finally, it has been reported that teaching parents how to nurture empathy in their children can help to prevent family violence.[15] The last two studies illustrate that mental health is not restricted to psychiatric diagnosis per se, and that all forms of interpersonal experiences (from lay persons and professionals) can be therapeutic.

Non-psychiatric and mental health contexts

The closeness of nurses to the medical (disease) model may have led some nurses to believe that empathy has no relevance to non-psychiatric clinical areas. It has been argued that empathy is not possible in acute medical/surgical settings because workload does not usually allow a nurse to listen to a patient for 30 minutes or more. However, the development of psychiatric liaison nurses is now starting to reveal that patients in general hospitals have an extensive list of psychosocial needs that are likely to remain unrecognized unless nurses are able to offer empathy to their patients.[16] Furthermore, there is extensive evidence that empathy is an important facilitator of constructive interpersonal relationships across a diverse range of clinical environments. The evidence suggests that patients often experience health needs that have their origin in the medical problem. These health needs are frequently psychosocial in nature, but they are not part of the disease diagnosed and treated by medical doctors. Concerns about body image, sexuality or death are human responses to actual and potential health problems that arise in day-to-day nurse–patient relationships and which call for responsible, helpful nursing actions. This section examines evidence for this assumption across a variety of non-psychiatric clinical areas.[17]

Several studies have emphasized the importance of the nurse understanding the patient's experience of illness and the healthcare system.[18] For example, it has been shown that women were more likely to experience a depressive breakdown following a severe life event, such as mastectomy, if they lacked an opportunity to confide regularly to someone who understood them. In relationship to breast cancer victims, several studies indicate the importance of nurses meeting patients' information needs regarding chemotherapy and breast reconstruction. Evidence exists to support the view that such information is beneficial to the patient's postoperative progress. This suggests that there is a need for nurses to anticipate the information needs of their patients. Apart from the need to use empathy to humanize care, studies have shown that empathy has a positive correlation with relief from pain, improved pulse and respiratory rates, protection of the autoimmune system and patients' reports of reduced worry and anxiety.

Furthermore, studies have demonstrated[19] that patients with hypertension attributed greater importance to discussing with their care provider their responses to health care, compared with personal problems and life-style matters. Since these patients expressed a need to discuss their responses to health care, nurses need to demonstrate commitment to listening to them. Otherwise, an opportunity for patients to have an active role in problem-solving will be lost and nurses will fail to appreciate patients' individuality.

A study of the effect of nurses' empathy on the anxiety, depression, hostility and satisfaction with care of patients with cancer is encouraging. Less anxiety, depression and hostility was found in patients being cared for by nurses exhibiting high empathy. Alternative groups who are at risk emotionally are the terminally ill. Terminally

ill patients have reported that nurses' empathized awareness of the patient's need to talk about death and dying was very highly valued.[20]

Recently, evidence has steadily accumulated in support of the clinical utility of empathy. The following papers illustrate the clinical significance of empathy across a broad spectrum of contexts and clinical issues. For example, a study investigating the psychological distress experienced by patients receiving bone marrow transplants found that psychological distress and life satisfaction could be positively influenced by empathy.[21] Another study[22] illustrated the relevance of empathy to ethical care. This study showed that nurses' ability to make ethical decisions related to the termination of pregnancy requires empathy, respect for human rights and unconditional acceptance of a person. Empathy has also been shown to be a crucial component of care provided during pregnancy.[23] It enables midwives to differentiate between ordinary emotional turbulence, which inevitably accompanied child-bearing and rearing, and experiences of unbearable distress or massive denial requiring psychotherapeutic help. Finally, it has been shown that all chronic and progressive problems, including ageing, have emotional and spiritual aspects that demand attention. Grief or shame at growing older and denial of these feelings must be recognized; otherwise, patients will ignore or resist direction on life-style or medications. A study[24] has identified patients with type 2 diabetes as being individuals falling into this category. It was concluded that empathy with these patients' distress can individualize care and strongly influence positive health outcomes for patients.

Reflection

Despite the frequent claims that empathy is crucial to all helping relationships, a low level of empathy has been reported in clinical nursing. Why do you believe that low empathy exists and how may the problem be resolved?

SUMMARY

Empathy is essential in order to create an interpersonal climate that is free of defensiveness. This enables individuals to talk about their perception of need. This is important since it is unlikely that patients will trust nurses if they do not view them as being helpful and appreciative of their individuality. This may result in a failure to establish patients' needs as seen by them, and, as a consequence, a failure to address. When nurses assist patients to find solutions to personal problems, in a manner that reflects their preferences, favourable health outcomes will occur. Numerous studies have established a correlation between high empathy and improved health.

For those reasons it is regrettable that the literature consistently reports a low level of empathy in nursing and other professional helpers. Whether this is due to the cultural norms of the workplace or ineffectual education is an interesting question. What is known is that education can help nurses to offer higher levels of empathy to patients. One experimental study,[25] using the Reynolds Empathy Scale to measure outcomes reported that an experimental group of registered nurses (RNs) significantly outperformed a control group of RNs post-education and 6 months after education. The frequent reports of low-empathy nurses challenge nurse educators to review their practices.

Implications for health services

The relevance of empathic relationships to the goals of health services are suggested by the increasing focus on patient-centred care and the growth of consumerism. The client-centred focus is illustrated in Scotland by the NHS (Scotland) Patients' Charter, which emphasizes the clinicians need to collaborate with users of health services in the prioritizing of clinical needs and the setting of treatment goals. The following standards have been set for clinical care. Patients should

- share in the responsibility for their own health
- tell professionals what they want
- be entitled to be treated as a person, not a case.

Although the aims of the Patient's Charter seem desirable, it is difficult to understand how this might be achieved unless professionals are able to offer an empathized awareness of the patients' expectations and needs. This possibility is emphasized by Hogg[26] who pointed out that users, such as women with HIV, or those with the experience of living in pain, have different expectations and needs of the health service from professionals. Empathy can be learned but nurses need to be taught how to offer it to patients. Additionally, nurses need uninterrupted clinical time in order to listen to their patients and hear what they want to happen. Otherwise, the aims of the Patient's Charter are likely to remain unfulfilled rhetoric.

REFERENCES

1. Lipps T. Einfuhlung Innere Nachahmung and Organempfinungen. *Archives of Gestalt Psychology* 1903; **20**: 135–204.

2. Greenson R. Empathy and its vicissitudes. *International Journal of Psychoanalysis* 1960; **41**: 418–24.

3. Rogers C. The necessary and sufficient conditions of therapeutic personality change. *Journal of Consulting Psychology* 1957; **21**: 95–103.

4. Rogers C. Empathic: an unappreciated way of being. *The Counseling Psychologist* 1975, **5**: 2–10.

5. Reynolds W. Roger's client-centred model: principles and general applications. In: Reynolds W, Cormack D (eds). *Psychiatric and mental health nursing: theory and practice.* London, UK: Chapman and Hall, 1990.

6. Reynolds W. The concept of empathy. In: Cutcliffe J, McKenna H (eds). *The essential concepts in nursing.* Edinburgh, UK: Elsevier Churchill Livingstone, 2005: 93–108.

7. Reynolds W, Scott B. Do nurses and other professional helpers normally display much empathy? *Journal of Advanced Nursing* 2000; **31**: 226–34.

8. Morse J, Anderson G, Botter J *et al.* Exploring empathy: a conceptual fit for nursing practice? Image. *Journal of Nursing Scholarship* 1992; **24**: 273–80.

9. Reynolds W. Barriers to empathy does not mean that empathy is not needed. A response to Morse et al. (1992) Beyond empathy. Expanding expressions of caring. *Journal of Advanced Nursing* 2006, **53**: 88–9.

10. Reynolds W (ed.). *The measurement and development of empathy* in nursing Aldershot, UK: Ashgate, 2000.

11. Reynolds W. Developing empathy. In: Barker P (ed.). *Psychiatric and mental health nursing: the craft of caring.* London, UK: Arnold, 2003: 147–54.

12. Forchuk C, Reynolds W. Clients' reflections on relationships with nurses: comparisons from Canada and Scotland. *Journal of Psychiatric and Mental Health Nursing* 2001; **8**: 45–51.

13. Gisbert A, Reynolds W, Vivas C *et al.* La importancia de una buena traduccion: Adaptation Al Espanol De La Encuestia De Empatia De Reynolds, W. *Revista de enformeria Rol* 2004; **27**: 65–70.

14. Reynolds W, Scott B. Empathy a crucial component of the helping relationship *Journal of Psychiatric and Mental Health Nursing* 1999; **6** (5): 363–70.

15. Swick K. Preventing violence through empathy development in families. *Early Childhood Education Journal* 2005; **33** (1): 53–59.

16. Roberts, D. Liaison mental health nursing: origins, definitions and prospects. *Journal of Advanced Nursing* 1997; **25**: 101–8.

17. Reynolds W, Cormack D (eds). *Psychiatric and mental health nursing: theory and practice.* London, UK: Chapman & Hall, 1990: 11–17.

18. Tait A. Interpersonal skill issues from mastectomy nursing contexts. In: Kagan C (ed.). *Interpersonal skills in nursing: research and applications.* London, UK: Croom Helm, 1985.

19. Dawson C. Hypertension, perceived clinician empathy and patient self-disclosure. *Research in Nursing and Health* 1985; **8**: 191–8.

20. Friehofer P, Felton G. Nursing behaviours in bereavement: an exploratory study. *Nursing Research* 1976; **25**: 332–7.

21. Murdaugh C, Parsons M, Gryb-Wysocki T, Palmer J, Glasby C, Bonner J, Tavakoli A. Implementing a quality of care model in a restructured hospital environment. National Academies of Practice Forum. *Issues in Interdisciplinary Care* 1999; **1** (3): 219–26.

22. Bates A. Critical thinking by nurses on ethical issues like termination of pregnancies. Curationis. *South African Journal of Nursing* 2000; **23** (3): 26.

23. Raphael-Leff J. Professional issues: psychodynamic understanding and its use and abuse in midwifery. *British Journal of Midwifery* 2000; **8**: 686–7.

24. Rappaport W, Cohen R, Riddle M. Diabetes through the life span: psychological ramifications for patients and professionals. *Diabetes Spectrum* 2000, **13** (4): 201–8.

25. Reynolds. A study of the effects of an educational programme on registered nurses' empathy. PhD Thesis, Open University, 1998.

26. Hogg A. *Working with users: beyond the Patients Charter*. London, UK: Health Rights, 1994.

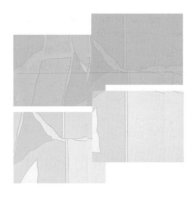

CHAPTER 38

Groupwork with children and adolescents

Sue Croom*

INTRODUCTION

There is compelling evidence that responding effectively to child and adolescent mental health (CAMH) issues represents a critical area for mental health nurses.

- One in five children and adolescents suffer from moderate to severe mental health problems.[1]
- Links have been established between mental health problems in children and adolescents and issues of public concern such as juvenile crime, alcohol and drug misuse, self-harm and eating disorders.[2]
- A significant number of severe problems in childhood, if not adequately treated, can lead to lifelong mental illness in adulthood.[3]
- Emotional and behavioural problems in the young not only carry an increased probability of adult mental illness, but may also indicate an increased risk of delinquency as the child grows up and continuing anti-social behaviour in adulthood.[4]
- Children with a parent with mental illness are known to be at higher risk of developing a mental health difficulty of their own.[5]
- The rate of mental health problems is higher in young offenders, particularly persistent offenders.[6]
- Difficult behaviour is the most common reason for children to be excluded from schools and the risk of further mental health problems is high.[7]
- Children who do not do well at school are at increased risk of mental health problems. The low self-esteem, and sense of 'in-competence' that this creates, can have an impact on job prospects and relationships leading to a risk of social isolation and difficulties with parenting, which may then affect the next generation.[8]

*Sue Croom is Lead Nurse for Northumberland and North Tyneside Mental Health Trust. Over her 25 years' experience in CAMH she has combined clinical work with university teaching and research in order to develop clinically relevant degree/masters programmes and participative action research focused on improving partnership with young people and carers. She had received two international fellowships and has lectured widely including in Canada and Russia.

Key factors, which appear to protect young people from child and adolescent mental health problems include the development of self-esteem, sociability and autonomy and engagement in social systems, which encourage personal effort and coping.[9] These protective factors can all be promoted through groupwork. For adolescents, such groupwork can improve social and communication skills through role-modelling feedback and practice.

Groups can be differentiated according to the developmental tasks, which children and young people need to achieve to meet their individual, social, emotional and developmental goals. Younger children can learn *turn taking*, *sharing* and participating in *cooperative play*; middle age range children can use activities and discussion to explore a sense of *who they are*, their *strengths* and *vulnerabilities*, and how to achieve a positive place in their *peer group* and to reflect on their *wider role in society*.

Research supports the efficacy of group therapy and groupwork for children and adolescents. A critical success factor appears to be the relationship of the children to the group therapist. Children who seem to get on better with adults, who can develop a warm positive rapport with them, are outgoing, and have a sense of humour.[10]

THERAPEUTIC PRINCIPLES OF GROUPWORK WITH CHILDREN AND ADOLESCENTS

The following principles, essential to successful groups, have been adapted from the work of Yalom[11] and Kolvin et al.[10]

1 *Promoting and conveying optimism*: It is crucial that the children and adolescents are helped to see how they have moved on, e.g. 'That's such a good way of looking at things – I don't think you could have done that the last time we met – it's great to see how much you're progressing'. This allows children and young people to see themselves and their peers improve in different ways.

2 *Developing shared experiences and a sense of connection*: All children and adolescents need to feel a sense of belonging. This can help them to appreciate that others can feel or react in similar ways to them – e.g. 'Has anybody else ever felt like that?'

3 *Helping children/young people to develop their self-awareness and a sense of who they are*: Supporting children/young people in exploring how they think and feel; developing an awareness of their values, e.g. through activities such as art work, discussion and games.

4 *Developing a sense of giving and empathy*: Through adult modelling, and the promotion of supportive, respectful, empathic interactions, children and young people learn to support each other, and thus feel

needed and useful. Comforting and supporting a peer can be a mutually rewarding experience.

5 *Recreating a nurturing and supportive group experience*: Through experiencing the sense of nurture, safety and caring in the group, children/young people can experience alternative patterns to the maladaptive ones they may have experienced in their families.

6 *Developing social skills*: Learning skills which promote successful social interactions can increase the likelihood that the young people will be able to experience positive interactions in the group and to transfer these to their everyday lives.

7 *Role modelling by either peers or adults*: Children and young people have the opportunity to observe alternative ways of responding constructively to frustration or embarrassment.

8 *Developing psychosocial learning in the here and now*: Using the group experiences to explore how the group members relate to each other and the meaning and consequences of these experiences.

9 *Learning how to discharge distressing feelings or impulses in socially acceptable ways*: For example, when upset with a peer, attempting to discuss the situation or, if angry, to hit a drum instead of hitting out at a peer or adult.

10 *Exploring how to cope with the challenges and experiences of everyday life*: Groups can help children and young people to acknowledge and share some common life experiences, e.g. for younger children sharing situations which may not seem to be fair and for adolescents, recognizing that individuals must take responsibility for the way they live their lives.

GROUPWORK WITH YOUNGER CHILDREN

Groups for young children with emotional or behavioural problems can recreate the experience of a normally developing child from infancy onwards. This can be achieved through the routine and predictability of the group's structure, which is underpinned by a strong nurturing philosophy.[12] Children can build on this safety net of security and trust to meet their developmental tasks, such as the ability to trust, explore, acquire a sense of achievement and begin to develop a sense of internal control.[13] Recreating the nurture of infancy can be achieved through meeting basic needs, e.g. for food. Meal and break time can be informal, enjoyable and very powerful opportunities to express nurture. Meeting emotional needs can be facilitated through studying the child, 'tuning in' to their feelings and needs, e.g. through maintaining proximity to the child, giving eye contact, encouraging activities. The nurses in such groups can model how adults can demonstrate confident, polite and supportive behaviour while engaging in the everyday tasks of living with the children. The nurses thus have the opportunity to use each event in the group as a therapeutic learning experience. As young children cannot be seen in isolation from their family systems, any groupwork needs to be complemented with parallel work and liaison with parents.

Personal illustration 38.1

Tommy, aged 3, has difficulties trusting adults to meet his needs. This tends to manifest itself through aggressive behaviour with adults and peers. His single parent mother, Tracey, is just beginning to get over depression, which started when he was born. This has meant that Tracey has had difficulties tuning in to Tommy's cues, and he has learned that hitting an adult is effective, if he wants their attention.

In the group, a nurse, who is allocated to stay close to him, supports him with activities. During the session, he becomes engrossed with building a high tower with a set of wooden bricks, but he finds that it always falls down before he has completed it. Although the nurse is beside him, attempting to engage with him, he ignores her until he fails for the third time, when he charges at her, aiming to hit her. She takes him to one side until he calms down and then suggests they go and build the tower together. She attends closely to Tommy's activity and provides positive encouragement about his progress in order to show her interest and to reinforce his capabilities. She notices that once he starts to find the task difficult, he does not ask for help, but hits his head hard with the brick. She achieves eye contact with Tommy and comments that they appear to have got to a difficult stage of building. She wonders aloud if the tower needs straightening and when Tommy agrees, she asks if she can help him with it.

She continues to subtly support Tommy each time he seems to be getting frustrated until he finally succeeds and she verbalizes her delight at Tommy's achievement. Tommy learns in this session that playing with an adult can be enjoyable if they encourage him, but don't take over his activity. The nurses share this with his mother, who admits she has been worried about Tommy hitting himself for what she perceived was no reason. The nurse and mother both agree to try to proactively respond to Tommy's ineffectual ways of asking for help. At the next session, Tommy is much more trusting of the nurse and seeks her help through eye contact instead of hitting her. Once she feels Tommy is confident, the nurse introduces another little boy, Andrew, whom Tommy seeks to like, to the activity. Andrew is able to verbally ask her for help and Tommy learns how effective this can be, from observing the consequences.

Eventually, the nurse moves the boys on from building their own towers to building one together and helps them to take turns. The nurse shares the successful strategies with Tommy's mother, so that there can be generalization of his learning to the home setting. Over time, Tommy and his mother develop a much more trusting and rewarding relationship and Tommy builds on his confidence to begin to interact more spontaneously with other peers in his group.

GROUPWORK WITH CHILDREN AGED 7–11

The developmental task for younger children (7–11) is to build on the sense of trust and initiative[13] they have learned from previous stages of development. This helps them acquire a sense of themselves as competent individuals. Group sessions that focus on play and activities can be used to develop a sense of achievement and skills with social interactions and peer relationships.[14] Children can be helped to explore relationships and the expression of feelings through the use of play materials, fantasy and conversation. Although the sessions enable children to express themselves, there are clear limits and boundaries that guide children to behave in socially and developmentally acceptable ways.

Activity groups involving games and exercises can help children to meet their developmental goal of achieving a sense of competence and to explore a range of solutions to cope with issues such as peer relationships and life, even changes such as separation and loss. Structured activities can be particularly useful for children with behaviour problems or impulsivity who find unstructured time difficult to cope with. The activities can thus facilitate:

- the development of *positive group dynamics* such as feeling a sense of cohesion and belonging;
- the child to work through *conflicts, hostilities* and *frustration* through games, which can develop and promote their *social adjustment, peer relationships and leaderships skills.*

Negative behaviours such as aggression usually elicit a negative response and can set up a cycle of negative feelings – rejection, anger and frustration. Children who have experienced this need time to develop their trust in the group before they can be helped to give up their well-established defence of rejecting others, as a way of avoiding rejection themselves.

Personal illustration 38.2

During an activity where the children have been making lemonade, Tim accidentally spills some juice onto Annie, who becomes very angry and tries to throw some juice back at him. The nurse uses a calm tone of voice to convey to the children that she is in control of the situation. (Children need to have the opportunity to observe how adults resolve situations when they are annoyed or frustrated, so that the child can learn to trust adults to be able to contain difficult feelings. This helps them to internalize alternative ways of successfully managing frustration in everyday life.) The nurse calmly and supportively cleans Annie up, giving eye contact to Tim to reassure him that this can be worked out. Annie is convinced Tim did it on purpose, because her 'world belief' is that 'everyone is out to get me'. The nurse attempts to soothe Annie's distress by empathizing with how upset she must feel in getting wet and in thinking that Tim did it on purpose. At the same time, she reiterates the group rules that throwing things at each other is not allowed. Acknowledging distress while setting limits can be helpful for other children in the group who may also have experienced similar situations. Once Annie's body posture and voice tone suggest that she is calm enough to be able to listen, the nurse appeals to the rest of the group to think of the possible reasons why Tim may have spilled the juice and how he could handle this.

Using the peer group to generate alternative explanations is helpful in encouraging Annie to consider other interpretations for Tim's behaviour and a range of solutions. The nurse helps the group to develop a solution of Tim apologizing to Annie. She praises Tim when he does this, commenting on his body posture, tone of voice and eye contact. When Annie accepts his apology, she also praises Annie and asks the group to explore how they feel the situation has been managed and how they may use this learning in the future. The situation may only take minutes to deal with, but provides a powerful way of modelling alternative behaviours for children within a group setting.

GROUPWORK WITH ADOLESCENTS

Groups are important for adolescents, whose developmental tasks include developing a positive identity, a confident place among their peers, gradually developing more intimate relationships and finding their role in society.[13] As individuals are born into, live and work in groups throughout their lives, they formulate their identities and learn behaviours associated with their ascribed roles, through dynamic, interactive processes, which often occur in groups. Group therapy can maximize this group interactive process to explore interpersonal fears, fantasies, conflicts and feelings.[15] Adolescents can use the group process to improve their interactive skills, gain acceptance and peer support and give and receive corrective feedback. The group experience can enhance the young person's positive sense of self/identity and their capacity to perform in expected and selected roles. Modelling and role-play can also be used to develop the young person's social skills, coping skills, insight into their problems and strengths and ways of coping through rehearsal, feedback and social reinforcement. Developing these skills can significantly increase the likelihood of eliciting positive responses from significant others such as teachers, parents and peers.

Personal illustration 38.3

Peter is a 14-year-old boy who has a history of somatic complaints. This has led to long absences from school, strained relationships at home and withdrawal from his peer group. He has had intensive investigations, but no physical cause has been found to account for his symptoms. He speaks in a barely audible voice with his head lowered and rarely initiates any interaction.

He is initially very reluctant to join the group. The group facilitator strategically organizes the session so that Peter sits next to a 15 year old, Gary, who is verbal and well liked by peers because of the kindness and consideration that he often shows them. Gary has a problem with impulsivity and aggression towards adults in the classroom or at home and resents what he perceives as their hostile interference in his life. The facilitator noticed in the first session that Peter appeared able to respond to Gary. She is thus trying to capitalize on the capacity of youths to connect to each other in the groups. After a couple of weeks, Peter seems to be enjoying the group activities, the humour and the support of the group. He is able to engage in a role-play where he has to practise asking his parents if he can stay out 1 hour later than usual because of a special event. The facilitators have previously modelled the use of eye contact, body posture, tone of voice and negotiation skills. Peter receives positive feedback from his peers and the facilitators. He is amazed at how good he feels about doing this and reflects that usually he wouldn't bother trying this with his parents, because it never works. He is encouraged by the group to explore how he feels when he gives up and whether it may be worthwhile giving the skills that have been modelled a try and to reflect on what some of the benefits may be.

Gary also engages in this role-play and reflects that although in real situations he would feel irritated at having to ask, he admits there may be benefits to using these skills. Both young people are able to identify how angry they feel with adults, but the different ways in which they express this. Over time, Peter becomes much more assertive and his reliance on physical symptoms to express his feelings reduce. His parents have needed support to relate to their son, who now has the confidence to express himself and whom they initially perceived as a demanding 'stroppy teenager'. Gary finds that he can use his innate sense of empathy to begin to explore how adults feel and how to respond assertively rather than aggressively and this has reduced the conflict in his life.

Reflection

Consider a family you are working with, where children or adolescents are vulnerable to mental health problems:

* What do you feel would be opportunities and challenges in providing group work for the child/young person?
* How could you ensure that the group is provided in a developmentally appropriate way?

GROUPWORK WITH YOUNG PEOPLE WITH SERIOUS MENTAL HEALTH PROBLEMS

Groupwork can provide an integral component of a holistic treatment programme for young people with serious mental health problems, such as thought disorders. It is essential to identify the exact nature of the thought disorder and the ways it impacts on the young person's experience in order to clarify how to help the young person interpret social and environmental cues. There must therefore be a constant reassessment of the capacity of the young person to interact with their environment in order to judge their suitability for groups. After a period of stabilization, group treatment may be beneficial. It is crucial, however, to assess the other group members' level of functioning and the group dynamics relative to the young person with a thought disorder. The group members may scapegoat the young person because of their bizarre behaviour or use it to avoid exploring their own issues. As the young person with thought disorder may find psychotherapeutic exploration too anxiety provoking or overstimulating, they may need to be present initially for only a part of the time. They will initially be able to tolerate more structured activities and may find that focusing on group activities will help them to orientate themselves to reality, whereas the intensity of dealing with past issues and feelings may be too anxiety provoking.

Returning to school or college may be a specific issue for many young people who are experiencing psychosis. Groups that can focus on cognitive strategies such as developing effective study strategies, improving attention and concentration, increasing the use of memory and learning strategies and improving academic performance and coping with social interaction can be critical in helping the young person to achieve their potential.

Groupwork can also be effective for adolescents with eating problems. The emotional support, reality testing and the hope engendered from seeing others improve are important elements of the group experience. The power of peer groups can be particularly useful in challenging dysfunctional cognitive schema and in motivating individuals, e.g. those with bulimia to abstain from vomiting. A number of major issues can be explored. Social skills are important for young people with eating disorders, who often have difficulties establishing close friendships. Assertiveness skills can also be useful for young people with anorexia who often play a very compliant role, and for young people with bulimia who often play a passive role. Their difficulties in acknowledging and expressing anger may underlie their problems.

NEED FOR SUPERVISION AND SUPPORT FOR GROUP FACILITATORS

For nurses to maintain their consistent demonstration of nurture, stimulation, limit setting and facilitation of personal growth, good supervision and support is needed. Nurses may experience the child's transference of the feelings of hate and anger, which they may wish to communicate to their caregiver. Furthermore, children may feel a need to severely test out the nurse to see if he/she

will reject him/her as other adults have done. Without support from the rest of the team and the development of insight, the nurse could develop unhealthy countertransference towards the child, feeling, for example, that this child 'is deliberately trying to wind me up'.

PLANNING A GROUP

Planning the group is an essential component of the overall group process. Group facilitators need to explore the type of group they wish to run, e.g. for vulnerable young people who are referred to CAMH services or a group that is universally available to all, e.g. a social skills programme for a particular school year group. The advantage of the former is that it can be focused on the presenting problems. Universal groups have the advantage of being non-stigmatized and are therefore useful in promotion of CAMH and prevention of CAMH problems. Facilitators also need to decide if the group will be 'open' throughout the course of the group or closed once members have been selected in order to build up a group identity.

The venue of the group needs to be carefully considered to ensure it can convey a sense of comfort, safety and confidentiality. The size and organization of the room is important. For discussion groups, sitting too closely together or being in a large open space can be threatening. However, for young children, and children or young people who tend to act out their feelings, there needs to be enough room to carry out activities and engage in exercises, which can draw away pent up emotions. The length of the groups, their frequency and the time at which they are scheduled, needs to be negotiated with parents, schools and with other relevant organizations. It may be helpful to run a group for children alongside a group for parents in order to maximize the effects.[14]

The mix of the groups for targeted and clinical populations of children or young people also requires careful thought. Much has been written about the contagion effects of acting out children in groups.[15] It can therefore be more productive to have a mixture of acting out children alongside more socially withdrawn young people. There is also a need to balance gender and cultural needs within groups.[15]

GAINING ORGANIZATIONAL SUPPORT FOR RUNNING A GROUP

It is crucial to think how a group fits into an overall CAMH strategy to ensure maximum support for the group's sustainability. For children and young people, developing a sense of trust and consistency is critical to their being able to engage in work, which can help them meet their developmental tasks. Thus, it is important that group facilitators attend each session unless there is an unforeseen circumstance. This provides a powerful message that the group is valued. Contingency arrangements need to be planned in case one of the facilitators is ill to ensure the group goes ahead. The minimum number of facilitators is two, but more may be required depending upon the age of the participants, the group mix and the severity of the problems.

MAINTAINING ATTENDANCE

Children/young people who have low self-esteem and difficulty with developing trusting relationships may need particular encouragement to attend the group and to maintain attendance. Outreach work involving contacting any young person who did not attend is essential to give the message that they are valued, that their presence was missed by the group and to try to solve any problems related to the following week's attendance.

MANAGING THE GROUP

Children and young people with conduct or behaviour problems can be difficult to work with in a group setting. It is therefore critical to establish ground rules right at the beginning, which the group can refer back to, e.g. only one person speaks at a time, name calling and hitting is not allowed, no criticizing without coming up with a positive solution.

Routines in the group are important in developing a sense of predictability, continuity, consistency, security and group identity, e.g. always starting with an ice-breaker and establishing a set time for a break. Food and drinks are essential to convey a sense of nurture and of being valued. It is essential to negotiate the provision of these in advance. At the beginning of the group or with very young children, the group leaders will be in charge of snacks, but as the group develops, members can take more responsibility for the planning of snacks and so reflect the dynamic development of the group and the growing autonomy of the participants.

In the initial *exploration phase*, the members need time to build up a sense of trust and ownership. The group may initially be highly dependent on group workers and so compliant to their wishes. As the group progresses, they will probably re-enact their early care-giving relationships and so will need to feel that the group workers can contain their feelings and behaviours while providing a consistent flow of nurture and support. This may mean that the children/adolescents engage in varying degrees of 'testing out' to see whether the group worker's limit-setting and the group's ground rules can be manipulated, and whether the group worker can still like and value them despite being presented with difficult behaviour. Children/young people may be reluctant to reveal very much about themselves because of fear of rejection and an unwillingness to trust the group because of situations in the past where they feel they have been let down. The group leaders need to be in tune with the degree of vulnerability felt by the young people, so that they are not overexposed to stress before the supportive bonds of the group have emerged. Warm-up sessions can be helpful, such as passing around a bowl of sweets and inviting each participant to take as many as they want and then asking them to share information related to the colour. At first the colours may be related to trivia to help the group to relax, e.g. if you have a red sweet, tell the group your favourite pop star. As the group becomes more confident, the colours can represent more exploratory issues, such as blue means 'share the best thing that happened in the past week' or orange means 'share with the group what you like about yourself'. Such group exercises also ensure that everyone has the opportunity to participate and learn about each other, and so it is useful for developing group cohesion. This early phase provides an opportunity to develop group trust and the group identity/norms, e.g. it's OK not to get it right!

In the *middle phase*, members can learn alternative ways of coping with difficult situations or distressing feelings. Here they can develop a greater rapport with each other and can use the group to discuss/try out ideas rather than constantly needing to check back to the group leaders. This is the most productive stage of the group. Group leaders need to listen actively, checking out and summarizing points, e.g. 'So what I'm hearing is that it can be difficult to negotiate with adults – is that right/'. They also need to help the group develop solutions, e.g. 'I wonder how that could be handled?' Positive feedback is crucial for all age ranges. This may take the form of positive comments on activities, positively reinforcing an interesting discussion point or an innovative solution to a problem or pointing out a situation, when one peer has been kind or supportive to another.

In the last stage, there is a need to work through the feelings of loss when the group comes to an end. Group facilitators can liaise with community groups to try to help the children/young people access other groups when they have completed the therapeutic group, e.g. cubs, youth clubs, football or dance classes. In this way, the young people can continue to use and apply the skills they have learned in other settings.

MANAGING CONFLICT AND SCAPEGOATING

If a young person is allowed to monopolize the group, other members may respond with hostility and ridicule. This increases the potential of scapegoating the young person when the group members project all of their negative feelings on to them. This may also occur towards the most vulnerable members. The response of the group facilitators in modelling a sense of fair play and justice is crucial while simultaneously exploring with the group what they feel is happening and how it can be resolved. In this way, the young people can develop the skills to cope and problem solve in social situations.

HELPING YOUNG PEOPLE TO UNDERSTAND AND COPE WITH SILENCES IN THE GROUP SESSIONS

Many children and adolescents can find silence threatening and difficult to cope with. The group facilitators need to be able to sensitively explore with the group what is underlying the silence, e.g. being bored, wanting to avoid the current topic of discussion or simply needing the time to think things through. In this way, the silence can be used productively within the group. Any quiet or withdrawn members may need support to speak in non-threatening ways, e.g. 'You made a very interesting point about this a couple of weeks ago' or 'I guess from your expression that you find this interesting – is there anything you would like to add?'

Personal illustration 38.4

Marilyn stands out in her adolescent group because of her slightly awkward manner and clumsiness. At first, the group are tolerant towards each other but as they get to know each other, a range of difficult emotional and interpersonal issues arise, and Marilyn appears to become their scapegoat. Just before break, she drops the papers she has just collected in following a group exercise. The group get angry, saying that she always makes them late for their snack. The group leader reflects back to the group that they seem to be irritated this morning and suggests that it may not be about Marilyn, but about how they are feeling about other things. Through a discussion on how it is possible to project our feelings on to others and an exploration of group experiences related to this, she manages to appeal to the group sense of fair play to explore the impact of their behaviour on Marilyn. Through this, they acknowledge that each person in the group deserves the support of the group. This kind of discussion can help develop a sense of group norms and values, provides an opportunity for the group to explore alternative ways of coping with difficult feelings other than getting angry with someone else and gives them insight into why they may blame others or get the blame themselves and how to deal with this.

FAMILY SUPPORT GROUPS

Family members are critical to the care and emotional well-being of young children. In partnership with other key systems in the community with which the children and young people interact, e.g. schools, youth clubs, recreation, families are also central to the promotion and well-being of older children and adolescents. With support, the family can play a pivotal role to the support and recovery of young people with mental health problems and disorders. A range of evidence-based groups programmes is most effective when combined with group interventions for the children and young people.[2,14]

Family support groups can be designed for parents, partners, children, siblings, extended family, close friends, and anyone who carries out a care-giving function in the young person's life. Joining a support group can encourages families to talk openly and freely in an understanding environment, learn from others who are in similar situations, learn how to ask for assistance and to access services, develop friendships to overcome any sense of isolation, and receive emotional support. They can also be very reassuring to new families or carers who can have their questions answered by people who have had first-hand experience of providing support to a young person with a mental health problem or illness.

EVALUATION

It is crucial to write up the group sessions afterwards in order to:

1 reflect on the group content;
2 debrief emotionally laden situations which may arise, e.g. from transference or the group splitting the facilitators into the 'good' leader and 'bad' leader;
3 document each participant's progress, e.g. their interaction/involvement in the group and their verbal and non-verbal communication;
4 write notes on the functioning of the group as a whole: interactions, mood, body posture, alliance, pairing, power hierarchies, group problem-solving.

The group can thus be evaluated using an analysis of such reports, allowing staff to explore how effective the group has been in helping the members achieve their developmental goals, develop their sense of self-esteem and competence, and gain skills in problem-solving and social interaction. The group can also be evaluated using standard questionnaires, such as Goodman's Strengths and Difficulties[16] Questionnaire. This offers an insight into changes in the profile of the child/young person's strengths and needs, before and after participation in the group.

Reflection

Imagine you are asked to set up a CAMH group:

- What are the critical factors for planning, implementing and evaluating groups with children, young people and their families?
- How could you deal with: a child/adolescent, who is being scapegoated in the group; or who easily loses control in a group; or when hostility and negativity is projected onto you as a group facilitator?
- How would you ensure that the group was accessible and acceptable to the young people and their families?
- Consider a child/adolescent/family who would benefit from a group. How might this reduce their needs and promote their strengths?

SUMMARY

Groupwork holds great potential for responding to the needs of younger people of different ages, in CAMH services. Factors crucial to the success of the group include the ability of the facilitators to convey warmth, a sense of humour, and ensuring that the safety and integrity of group members is preserved, and having a good understanding of social, cultural and developmental issues. Groups held in combination with groups for parents, carers and family members can be particularly effective. Planning the group in terms of the aims, venue, recruitment and mix of the group, together with evaluation and supervision, can help to guide the group to be a supportive, learning experience for the young people and an effective component of the overall strategy to reduce the individual, social and community distress arising from child and adolescent mental health problems.

REFERENCES

1. Green H, McGinnity A, Meltzer H *et al. Mental health of children and young people in Great Britain*. London, UK: Office National Statistics, 2004.

2. Swenson CC, Henggeler SW, Taylor IS, Addison OW. *Multisystemic therapy and neighbourhood partnerships: reducing adolescent violence and substance abuse*. New York, NY: Guildford Press, 2005.

3. Target M, Fonagy P. *What works for whom? A critical review of psychotherapy research*. New York, NY: Guildford Press, 2002.

4. Barker P. *Basic child psychiatry*, 7th edn. London, UK: Blackwell, 2004.

5. Place M, Reynolds J, Cousins A. Developing a resilience package for vulnerable children. *Child and Adolescent Mental Health Review* 2002; **7** (4): 162–7.

6. Tiffin P, Kaplan C. Assessment and management of risk. *Child and Adolescent Mental Health Review*. 2004; **9** (2): 55–64.

7. Appelton P, Hammond-Rowley S. Addressing the population burden of child and adolescent mental health problems: a primary care model. *Child Psychology and Psychiatry Review* 2000; **5** (1): 9–16.

8. Mental Health Foundation. *Bright futures: promoting children and young people's mental health*. London, UK: Mental Health Foundation, 1999.

9. Peters R DeV. A community-based approach to promoting resilience in young children, their families, and their neighbourhoods. In: Peters R DeV, Leadbeater B, McMahon RJ (eds). *Resilience in children, families and communities: linking context to practice and policy*. New York, NY: Springer, 2005: 157–76.

10. Kolvin I, Garside RG, Nicol AR *et al. Help starts here: the maladjusted child in the ordinary school*. London, UK: Tavistock, 1981.

11. Yalom ID. *The theory and practice of group psychotherapy*. New York, NY: Basic Books, 1975.

12. Bennathan M, Boxall M. *Effective interventions in primary schools: nurture groups*. London, UK: David Fulton Publishers, 1996.

13. Erikson EH. *Identify and the life cycle*. New York, NY: Norton, 1980.

14. Richardson J, Joughin J. *Parent-training programmes for the management of young children with conduct disorder*. London, UK: PCP/Gaskell, 2002.

15. Dwivedi K. *Groupwork with children and adolescents: a handbook*. London, UK: Jessica Kingsley, 2003.

16. Goodman R, Meltzer H, Bailey V. The strength and difficulties questionnaire: a pilot study on the validation of the self-report version. *European Child and Adolescent Psychiatry* 1998; **7**: 125–30.

CHAPTER 39

Psychodynamic approaches with individuals

Brendan Murphy*

Upon my word, I think the truth is the hardest missile one can be pelted with.

George Eliot
Middlemarch

INTRODUCTION

Models of the mind

Over the past 100 years, the nature of mental health and illness has been widely debated, investigated and disputed. This discussion of the nature of mental health and distress has drawn on a number of influential psychological models of the mind. These include the *behaviourist*, *cognitive* and *psychodynamic* models.

All these models offer explanations for the development and maintenance of mental distress and propose psychological techniques or psychotherapies that, it is claimed, will ease or remove mental distress.

The *psychodynamic* model draws upon the insights of Freud and other significant theorists. This approach takes account of unconscious as well as conscious elements of the personality and seeks to resolve unconscious conflicts

with the aim of enhancing the overall development of the personality. The psychodynamic approach has developed over a long period, at least 100 years, and it is composed of a number of theories and concepts that can be applied to any therapeutic relationship. It is central to the understanding of psychoanalysis, psychotherapy and counselling. It is perhaps the oldest and most influential approach used in modern talking therapies.

This chapter addresses the psychodynamic approach with individuals, outlining its development, key concepts and values.

Derivation of psychodynamic

A look at the derivation of the word 'psychodynamic' helps to explain some of its meaning. It is composed of two Ancient Greek words, *psyche* meaning 'mind' and *dynamic* meaning 'moving force'.[1] The term 'mind' is used here to refer to the sum total of the thoughts, feelings, emotions, impulses and memories that may occur in an individual, both conscious and unconscious. Mind and 'moving forces' implies that the mind is not a static entity; it is in motion, active and has the ability to transform.

*Brendan Murphy is Clinical Nurse Specialist Psychotherapy with the Derbyshire Mental Health Trust, England. Previously, he was Charge Nurse at University of Sheffield Department of Psychiatry and Charge Nurse at the Norfolk Park Community Mental Health Project and Deputy Co-ordinator, Leeds City Council Crisis Centre.

Freud[2] took the concept psychodynamic from the then recently invented device, the dynamo. In a dynamo, mechanical energy, pedalling a bicycle for example, is transformed into an electric current through a coil rotating in a magnetic field. If the properties of the magnetic field or the mechanical force varies then the electric current will vary, and perhaps will not flow at all. So we have a variety of elements (coil, mechanical force, magnetic field) and a result that is entirely different – electricity. The result can be seen as a product of the interaction of two or more ingredients. Clearly, the analogy between the human mind and an electromechanical system like the dynamo is of limited value. The mind is a much more complicated and subtle system. However, paradoxically, this analogy helps to capture something of the intricate nature of the mind and its constituents.

THE DEVELOPMENT OF THE PSYCHODYNAMIC APPROACH

It is generally agreed[2,pp.5–12] that psychodynamic theories and interventions evolved from the work of Freud and several of his close colleagues, who developed the theories and practice of psychoanalysis at the beginning of the twentieth century in Vienna. It is interesting to note that at about the same time as Freud was producing his psychoanalytic theories in Central Europe, behaviourist theory was developing in the USA.

Ellenberger[3] has shown that many of the key ideas and concepts in psychodynamic thought have a history dating back long before the work of Freud. For example the 'unconscious', elements of the human mind of which we are unaware, is often thought to be Freud's most important discovery. However, the philosopher Leibenitz had discussed this many centuries before Freud.[3] According to Brown and Pedder,[2] at the time that Freud was developing his own theories of the mind 'a work on Aristotle's concept of catharsis was being much talked of in Vienna in the 1880s and may have influenced Freud and his collaborator Breuer'.

Freud and his disciples

Freud was born in 1856, the year that Charles Darwin finally published the *Origin of species*. Like Darwin's theory of evolution by natural selection, Freud's psychoanalytical theories had a profound impact on the way that people understood themselves and their place in the world, at least in the Western world. It is difficult today to understand the impact his new views of humanity had when first produced, because they are such familiar ways of thinking today. For example Masson[4] claimed that Freud revised his original trauma theory of the origins of neurosis,[5] because its thesis – that neurosis was often the direct result of the sexual abuse of children by adults – was so unacceptable to his medical colleagues that it threatened his career.

Freud's achievement was to develop a systematic approach to the investigation of the mind. Freud took the insights of earlier philosophers and writers and combined them with his own careful observations as a trained scientist. He used his insight and understanding to synthesize a new account of the human psyche and developed a technique for treating individuals, which he called *psychoanalysis*. This model has been very influential in many areas of medical, cultural and social thought throughout the twentieth century.[2] Two of Freud's most influential colleagues, Adler and Jung, had fundamental disagreements with Freud's psychoanalytic theory and went on to develop their own schools of therapy, individual psychology and analytical psychology, respectively.[2]

Post-Freudian developments

Since Freud's death in 1939, his work – and subsequently that of the other pioneer theorists – has undergone much development and revision. Today there are a very large number of important theorists who can be described as *psychodynamic*. They include Anna Freud, Reich, Klein, Fairbairn, Horney, Fromm, Erikson, Winnicott, Bowlby, Sullivan and Kohut. In turn, other workers have developed and modified these ideas and techniques so that today many therapists, counsellors and nurses who do not practise psychoanalysis or analytical psychology would acknowledge the pioneering work of Freud and his co-workers. They would argue that they are working in the psychodynamic tradition initiated by Freud. Today, there is a wide variety of psychodynamic practice and theory. There is no single set of theories, accepted by all therapists and mental health workers using the approach. Having said that, although there is no unchallenged theoretical position in the psychodynamic approach, there are some key psychodynamic principles that are widely discussed and used across the field.[2]

Reflection

In what way is your work influenced by Freudian ideas of the 'mind'?

Which theorists have most influenced your approach to helping people deal with mental distress?

KEY PSYCHODYNAMIC CONCEPTS

This brief, and very selective, account of some of the most important concepts that make up the psychodynamic approach, draws on the works of Freud[6] and Malan.[7]

Hughes describes three important ideas derived from Freud's main theories, which have been influential in the development of the psychodynamic approach.

* That our behaviour is influenced by unconscious thoughts and feelings, and that symptoms may arise because of conflict between conscious thoughts and wishes and unconscious thoughts and wishes. This was part of Freud's topographical theory.[8]
* That we are born with innate instincts, which affect our behaviour. This was part of Freud's structural theory.[8]
* That early development has an important influence on adult behaviour. This was part of Freud's developmental theory.

These areas of psychodynamic theory will now be discussed in turn.

The dynamic unconscious

The unconscious is defined[9] as 'an area of mental experience not available to normal awareness'. This is a part of the mind that is as active as the conscious but of which we have no knowledge. The term may be used to refer to different levels of awareness, from something of which we are 'totally unaware' to that which we do not 'wish to acknowledge'. Freud believed that the conscious and the unconscious opposed each other; so that only through some sort of exploratory effort or work could we succeed in making conscious that which is unconscious. However, the deeper inaccessible regions of the unconscious, that of which we have no knowledge, could find expression by influencing the more accessible regions of the unconscious, that which we do not *wish* to acknowledge. These more accessible regions of the unconscious are called the *preconscious*.

Mental conflict

We are all familiar with the experience of conflicting wishes, which are an inevitable part of all our lives.
Consider the following example:

Mr E is offered a new job with more money. He then develops a series of physical symptoms, particularly pains in his chest near his heart. Mr E describes it as 'heartache', and he feels he is unable take up the job. Concern for his health leads Mr E to turn the job offer down, after which the pains disappear. When he visits his doctor, there does not appear to be any physical cause for the pains in his chest. He is very healthy.

This is a conflict of which Mr E is aware. Other conflicts may be unconscious. Conflict can be extremely painful and anxiety provoking. Our ability to solve such conscious conflict is often based upon our feeling of personal security and integrity. Those people who have a poor sense of personal security, low self-esteem, may find the conflict intolerably painful. Conflicts that we meet in adult life may resonate with earlier conflicts that we encountered as a child and these may become active again if they are still unresolved.

Mr E wants a better job with more money yet knows that this entails giving up a home and friends that he loves and moving to another part of the country. Mr E wants more money and a better job and wants to keep the home and friends that he loves. In this case he cannot have both.

Here only one side of the conflict is obvious. The wish for the new job is conscious. We could suggest that the other side of the conflict is unconscious, but finds some means of expression through the chest pains.

Human motivation and instincts

Any psychological model needs to explain human motivation: why we do the things that we do. More simply, what is it that makes us get up in the mornings? Freud thought that humans had a particular sort of nature, much like that of other animals, and that most of our behaviour is driven by very basic innate instincts or drives, such as the drive to reproduce and survive. These drives are represented in our minds in the forms of wishes or desires and become associated, from an early age, with the key figures in our life, for example our mothers and fathers.[9]

The drives are tendencies towards or away from certain types of experiences such as pleasure or pain. They are however very mobile and can be affected by the ways in which the outside world reacts to our needs or desires. This is especially important in our early life when the nature of our mind is open and very impressionable. This means that they can become strengthened, blocked, diverted or modified.

In his early theories, Freud thought that there were only sexual and aggressive drives. Later modifications to his theory produced two very basic principles or drives, those of life and death. Thus there are the drives associated with life such as the sexual and nurturing aspects of human nature and those associated with death such as the aggressive and destructive aspects of human life.[10]

Reflection

Have you ever had a problem in your life – work, relationships etc – that showed itself by a particular feeling in a part of your body – headache, stomach upset, etc?
To what extent were you aware of what was 'going on'?

THE STRUCTURAL MODEL

In 1923 Freud[9] introduced his structural model, suggesting that the mind was made up of three regions the *Ego*, the *Id* and the *Super Ego*. The Ego, the rational thinking part of the mind, is conscious and can be modified through experiences with the outside world. The Id is the instinctual, largely unconscious area of the mind, and is the seat of the basic drives such as sex and aggression. The Super Ego is often described as corresponding to the Conscience, that is, the self-critical aspect of the mind. There are both conscious and unconscious aspects of the Super Ego.

Although the three regions of the mind are clearly separated and easily distinguishable, Freud thought that the division was more like that of the political region known as the Balkans, a complex mix of different races, creeds and languages, often in complex conflicts where borders shift and alliances change.[9]

Later theorists[2] criticized aspects of Freud's structural theory of the mind and pointed out that he had missed out some very important aspects of human nature. A more comprehensive list of the basic drives would include:

* relatedness
* aggression
* sexuality
* hunger
* curiosity.

Human development

According to the psychodynamic model the individual develops physically and psychologically from childhood, through adolescence and into adulthood. The development of the mind and the body are inextricably linked. There are definite stages of growth and development, which are registered in body and mind. For example, consider the difference in the body and mind of a young infant and an adolescent.

In psychodynamic theory, early childhood relationships mould the individual's mind. The patterns of early relationships, especially with mother or other early carer, are held in the mind. They become a major influence in determining the nature of future relationships. An understanding of the individual's development in the *past* is important for understanding the individual *now*.

Most of us will have suffered shocks, frustrations, rejections and disappointments in the past, especially in our relationships with other people. Many different psychodynamic descriptions have been devised to try to capture the way in which the mind responds to the frustrations inevitable in relationships. All the descriptions agree that past experiences affect the development of personality and exert their influence in the present by contributing to the way we negotiate current relationships.[8]

UNDERSTANDING INDIVIDUAL DISTRESS

According to Malan, the psychodynamic model approaches human distress in a specific way.

> As human beings we adopt various defensive mechanisms in order to avoid mental pain or conflict or to control unavoidable impulses. These defences vary from being almost wholly conscious to being completely unconscious. The end product of these mechanisms is often a form of maladaptive behaviour or a neurotic symptom.[7]

Malan offers a basic psychodynamic view of how distress and disturbance are created and maintained by individuals. This can be represented by the *Triangle of conflict*[7] (Figure 39.1).

The *Triangle of conflict* refers to the relationship between the *defence*, the *anxiety* and the *hidden feeling*, wish or impulse. It is represented by a triangle that stands on its apex with the defence and anxiety above the hidden feeling. This denotes the idea that the hidden feeling involves the more unconscious of the elements of the triangle.

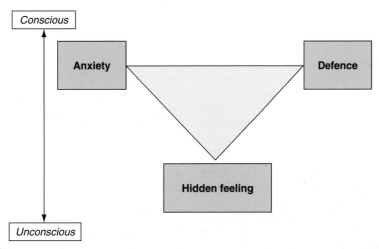

Figure 39.1 Triangle of conflict

From surface to depth

In psychodynamic theory it is thought that it is best to work from those elements near the surface and then to gradually reveal more depth or unconscious material. The defences are gradually explored together, with the anxiety and the hidden feeling or impulse usually being the last element that is approached. This means that as defences are modified, and anxieties are understood and acknowledged, the hidden feeling may safely come into awareness and be expressed.[7]

Let us consider the three elements of the triangle in more detail starting with its most *unconscious* aspect – the 'hidden feeling'.

Hidden feeling

The psychodynamic model starts from the observation that we suffer mental conflicts, usually conflicting feelings, impulses, 'wishes' or 'desires'. This conflict causes pain, distress and disturbances within us and we look for ways of removing or escaping from the pain and distress that is caused. Unacceptable impulses, ideas or feelings are rejected and forced into the unconscious area of the mind. This process of making something unconscious is termed *repression*.

Anxiety or mental anguish

The repressed material is active and seeks expression, yet is forcefully kept out of awareness. If there is a danger that the material repressed become conscious, this is experienced as anxiety. Anxiety occurs because the threat of loss, or some other distressing wish or impulse, causes the disturbing aspects of mental life.

Defence mechanisms

Think how common it is when we lose somebody close to us, either in death or through loss of a relationship. We deny what has happened. Denial is the means by which we, albeit temporarily or partially, are able to forget what has happened to us in reality. It can be thought of as a 'defence mechanism'. The defence mechanism removes from our conscious awareness the conflicting impulse, wish or desire, thus rendering it unconscious.

A hierarchy of defences

The psychodynamic approach thinks of *defence mechanisms* as being the normal human reaction to difficult and impossible situations. There is a view that some defences are more debilitating and constricting to individual development than others.[8] For example, *denial* may be very important at some periods of our life, following the bereavement of a loved one, for example. However if denial becomes a habitual way of dealing

---

> ### Personal illustration 39.1: a common defence
>
> Jack, who is a community mental health nurse, attends an early morning referral meeting. At the end of the meeting, while discussing the best referral for a patient whom Jack thinks needs to be seen urgently, his ideas are contradicted and rudely rejected by his manager. The patient is referred to another service with a long waiting list. Jack leaves the meeting feeling angry.
>
> At home, Jack's partner playfully contradicts him. He becomes furious, tells his partner that she does not know what she is talking about and startles himself with the intensity of his reaction.
>
> We might be as puzzled as Jack about his reaction, until we consider that he may be 'displacing' the anger he feels towards his manager onto his partner. Jack's partner is a safer and more understanding person, with whom Jack can become angry without fear of retaliation.
>
> In this example we can see that the defence is a displacement of anger from one person to another.

with problems, there is a real possibility that this will grossly distort our relationships with other people. Think for instance of the way in which people who drink alcohol, to the extent that it is destroying their relationships with partners, children and friends, may deny that they have any problems or difficulties associated with drinking alcohol. We all use defences, to some degree, to deal with the inevitable pains and frustrations of life.

The psychodynamic approach involves examining *habitual* defence strategies that have developed unconsciously, encouraging the relinquishing of old defences that are no longer necessary, or their substitution by more useful strategies some of which may be thought of as defences.

DEVELOPING THERAPEUTIC RELATIONSHIPS

Although it might appear obvious, all mental health work assumes that we are involved in some type of relationship with our patients (Box 39.1).

Introspection

Introspection involves looking into oneself, or encouraging another person to tune into memories, thoughts, ideas, motives and feelings. In the psychodynamic approach introspection is thought to be a means of discovering useful information. With the implication that developing the ability to understand and find out about oneself is beneficial. The method of working in the psychodynamic approach is to create the conditions, through a relationship with the patient that allows the patient to talk freely about what is currently on their mind; this is known as *free association*.[2]

Repetitive patterns of relationship

As was stated earlier the psychodynamic approach asserts that early childhood experiences influence the way in which we subsequently relate to others. We internalize a particular set of relationships and these patterns are stored in our mind. Freud observed that people had a tendency to repeat patterns of relating and behaviour, sometimes at great cost to themselves. Freud termed this the 'compulsion to repeat'.[2,p.115] There is an important implication in this pattern of repeating relationships for any caring relationship, in that the person seeking help is likely to repeat in the relationship with the nurse or helper, important aspects of their habitual relationships.

Transference

Hughes[8] defines *transference* as, 'the transfer of feelings, which belong to a relationship from the past into a present relationship'. These attributions are inappropriate to the present relationship and this process is unconscious. In a general sense we respond to any new situation in terms of our past experience. At times we may respond to people as though they were specific people from our past. This is particularly likely to happen if we are distressed, when regression is more common. Freud saw that transference could be used as a therapeutic agent of change.

Counter-transference

Hughes[8] describes *counter-transference* as 'the feeling or feelings elicited in the therapist by the patients behaviour and communication'.

It may be understood as a way in which the particular aspects or qualities of the relationship that the patient forges may be experienced by the helper. This will give valuable information about the model of relationship that the patients have internalized.

Carol's transference

Helping relationships often brings to light the particular patterns of relating of the patient through the feelings that the person transfers onto the nurse or therapist. In the example above we can see that Carole has transferred her feelings of anger onto Nurse Zeta, who is trying to help her. Carole has been offered help by Zeta. At first this was acceptable and helpful. After a time, however, Carole appears to have become convinced that the help being offered was not sincere. Zeta could not possibly want to listen to her without having some other motive. Carole is showing us something about her understanding and expectation of relationships.

Nurse Zeta's counter-transference

Nurse Zeta is left feeling unwanted and rejected. These are similar to the feelings that Carole often talks about in her relationships. This may be important information for Nurse Zeta, if she can reflect on the situation rather than angrily retaliate and reject Carole. This impulse to retaliate might be another important piece of *counter-transference*.

Nurse Zeta's wish to help Carole, is in conflict with her wish to reject her and her feeling of anger. There is, therefore, a danger of repeating Carole's particular pattern of relationship and confirming her belief that she will always be rejected.

Now Nurse Zeta's experience of relating to Carole means that she may be able to avoid the danger of repeating the pattern of rejecting Carole. This could allow Carole to gain a valuable insight into how and why she relates as she does. The therapeutic relationship becomes a means of helping Carole to understand and change her pattern of relationship. Carole and Zeta may be able to construct a different relationship, by using aspects of the knowledge and experience of the way in which Carole relates to her helper.

Personal illustration 39.3

In supervision with a colleague, Zeta is able to express her own feelings of rejection and anger. Her supervisor, while understanding her wish to forget about Carole, urges her to try and use her understanding of the relationship to help her.

They consider that Carole's feeling may, in some ways, be similar to the feelings of rejection and anger experienced by Zeta. They conclude that if Zeta is able to convey this understanding to Carole, it may help to develop the therapeutic relationship and allow Carole to begin to express her feelings of loss.

Zeta asks to meet with Carole again the following day and is surprised when she agrees. After a short silence:

Carole: I am surprised that you want to see me again. Usually people just leave me alone after I have told them that I think like that.

Zeta: Perhaps Carole you are afraid of me getting close to you and then leaving you alone again, as other people have done this in the past. Your anger is a way of protecting yourself when you are afraid that this is happening.

At this, Carole began to talk about a friend who had spent time with her, and then had abruptly disappeared, taking with her some of Carole's property. Carole spoke about how lonely she felt and how she missed her partner who had left recently and then began to cry.

ANXIETY, DEFENCE AND HIDDEN FEELINGS

Using Malan's *Triangle of conflict* we might form a hypothesis. Carole fears (*anxiety*) rejection, so she angrily rejects the help offered to her and withdraws (*defence*).

It is not yet possible to understand fully what the *hidden feeling* or impulse may be. We could make another hypothesis, that Carole has a lot of unexpressed feelings about the loss of her relationship, and the rejections that she has experienced in the past.

Reflection

Consider your own experience of clinical supervision. How easy do you find it to express feelings about patients? What kinds of feelings do you find yourself discussing most in supervision?

THE VALUE OF THE PSYCHODYNAMIC APPROACH

Here, the development and key concepts of psychodynamic theory have been outlined. The value of the psychodynamic approach is that it offers a way of thinking about any human relationship, based upon a coherent and flexible understanding of the human mind. The psychodynamic model of mind is based upon direct observations of the development of the human infant, as well as numerous clinical observations of patients suffering emotional distress. These clinical observations have been continuously developed for over 100 years. In turn the observation of infants and adult patients has led to innovations and developments in theory and practice. This approach can offer the nurse or therapist a wealth of understanding of the development of human relationships and how these relationships are maintained.

The psychodynamic approach offers an understanding of the development of mental distress, and how by developing a therapeutic relationship, the patient may be helped to develop new and more fulfilling ways of relating.

REFERENCES

1. *The new Oxford English dictionary*. Oxford, UK: Oxford University Press, 2001.

2. Brown D, Pedder J. *Introduction to psychotherapy*, 2nd edn. London, UK: Routledge, 1991.

3. Ellenberger HF. *The discovery of the unconscious*. London, UK: Allen Lane, 1970.

4. Masson JM. *The assault on truth: Freud's suppression of the seduction theory*. New York, NY: Farrar, Straus and Giroux, 1984.

5. Freud S. The neuro-psychoses of defence. In: *The complete psychological works of Sigmund Freud*, Vol. 3, standard edn. London, UK: Hogarth Press, 1894.

6. Freud S. *Inhibitions, symptoms and anxiety*, Vol. 20, standard edn. London, UK: Hogarth Press, 1926.

7. Malan DH. *Individual psychotherapy and the science of psychodynamics*. London, UK: Butterworth, 1979.

8. Hughes P. *Dynamic psychotherapy explained*. Oxford, UK: Radcliffe Medical Press, 1999.

9. Freud S. *The Ego and the Id*, Vol. 19, standard edn. London, UK: Hogarth Press, 1923.

10. Freud S. *New introductory lectures*, Vol. 22, standard edn. London: Hogarth Press, 1933.

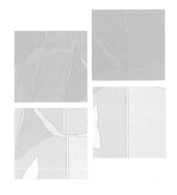

CHAPTER 40

Psychodynamic approaches to working in groups

Phil Luffman*

INTRODUCTION

The psychodynamic approach to group work utilizes and explores the experiences group members have in relationship to one another, to their significant past relationship experiences and their current situation. The aim is to enable the individual to overcome psychological problems and associated symptoms. By harnessing the experiential learning component that is present in the group, members can find support, receive important feedback about themselves and make changes that endure and advance their lives creatively.

The most essential components are the participants themselves, including the groupworker who facilitates the group. The nurse practitioner is a groupworker, in a dynamic sense, when they view the group as the main instrument of change. The structure of the group may vary, as can the setting, and may include more than one groupworker. However, the *purpose* of the group – to understand better the problems the individual faces within a group context, via interpersonal group relations – remains the same.

The patient/member as auxiliary therapist is one of the most powerful therapeutic factors in making the group an effective medium for change. Giving and receiving of feedback – both supportive and confrontational – and the interventions and interpretations that seek to clarify meaning, are all functions that promote the self-help culture of the group.

Within the psychodynamic approach theory and practice are woven together at the point of application, focused on the relationships developing in the *here and now* of the group. The experiences each group member brings to the attention of others is the operational basis for further exploration and elucidation, involving all participants. This joint venture can be difficult and uncomfortable as thoughts, emotions and hidden wishes surface from the unconscious at any time, and may be projected into the group. What can be disclosed and shared depends on the group's level of support and cohesion. The lasting benefits go beyond increased self-understanding to a greater sense of intimacy and belonging based on empathy and respect.

The processes and content – what is said, what preoccupies the group – are similarly inter-related. Even when a

* Phil Luffman RMN, Dip group analytic pschotherapy, works part-time for Hywel Dda NHS Trust in West Wales in a psychotherapy centre where a number of models of care may be integrated. He is a counsellor for a local school and has a small private practice. A lengthy involvement in Buddhism has contributed greatly to his work as a psychotherapist. He lives in Powys, Wales with his wife and two children.

group is short-lived or when someone participates in only a few sessions, processes and outcomes are still evident, as are some of the therapeutic benefits. A helpful outcome in the early stages of the group is being able to recognize similarities between one's own and others' problems.

The group analytic method utilizes concepts derived from a number of theoretical sources, especially classical psychoanalysis and object relations theory. The concept of transference phenomena, discussed later, helps explain how the patient's past is reactivated and remembered in the current relationships between group members.

Freud's hypothesis that our lives and aspects of our behaviour are influenced or determined by unconscious processes, underpins the psychodynamic approach.[1] Freud described defence mechanisms operating within a structural model of Id, Ego and Superego, where the individual unconsciously seeks mastery over primitive impulses and wishes that are in conflict with the higher order aspects of the personality. According to Freud's model this comes under the censorship of the Superego. Object relations theory moved away from instinct and drive/conflict theory, to a model that saw humans as essentially *relationship seeking* from birth. Winnicott[2] saw the mother–infant relationship as critical in terms of helping the baby differentiate itself from others.

Here, I shall also consider groups *outside* the treatment setting, especially naturally occurring social groups, such as friends or colleagues, which Foulkes[3] called 'life groups'. For the family or primary group, Foulkes gave the name 'root group'. I describe group psychotherapy in terms of its broadest therapeutic factors, which are observable in many group treatment methods. However, they become the focus for exploring at the conscious and unconscious level in the analytic group. Therapeutic factors occur in everyday 'life groups'. For example, reducing one's isolation could be achieved by joining a club that meets regularly. By careful planning and preparation of the group, the safe boundary provides the conditions whereby therapeutic factors can be realized and exploited as they occur. It is rarely the case, however, that the individual experiences benefits without 'working through' difficulties and conflicts. Similarly when an isolated person joins a club they may initially experience an increased sense of isolation if they cannot fit in.

I also consider, briefly, two aspects of the evolving nurse–patient relationship: the *transference relationship* – an unconsciously derived symbolic relationship – and the personal qualities and attributes of the *professional relationship*. What one wishes to establish in the two-person relationship – especially in the assessment and selection of group members – is a degree of trust and working alliance, which needs to carry over to the group situation.

Some patients may need specific instruction to help them acquire a less critical view of themselves, their feelings and of their world. Group treatments designed for those with complex personality problems, where self-harming, impulsivity and lack of trust may feature, must take account of both benefits and limitations to the reflective methods of analysis, and the more directed or taught method of CBT (cognitive–behavioural therapy). Elsewhere, the method can be used in programmes incorporating large group dynamics such as therapeutic communities, staff groups, or within clinical supervision.[4–6]

Reflection

How do you feel when you are in a group?
If invited to *lead* a group, how do you feel?

WHAT IS A PSYCHODYNAMIC APPROACH?

A psychodynamic approach to groupwork covers several well-defined experiential treatment methods in a variety of settings. The small outpatient 'stranger group', of between seven to eight members meeting once or twice weekly, is one well-defined, well-documented example. It has served as a valuable blueprint by which other applications can be developed, compared and contrasted. As Rutan[7] points out there is no single form of 'psychodynamic group psychotherapy'. Core concepts, however, do exist – such as the influence of unconscious processes. These provide both a framework and orientation and remain fairly constant for all treatment methods within the psychodynamic approach. The analytic framework also helps us understand our own experiences and unconscious processes when interacting with others.

The diversity of group psychodynamic treatment methods rests more on the emphasis given to the *group structure*, than to the content process and outcome. For example:

- *psychodrama* emphasizes action methods whereby the group, with the directors help, set the stage for the protagonist's internalized drama to be re-enacted; the *audience* – far from passive – fulfils the function of auxiliary egos;
- the *group analytic* method emphasizes the experience of self and others via dialogue and language, to bring into conscious awareness interpersonal conflicts, resistances and possible solutions; this group is *not* directed, but allowed or encouraged to discover its own meaning and possibilities through communication;
- the *therapeutic community*, although usually incorporating small group therapies, places more emphasis on *large group dynamics* within the context of a living, learning environment; engaging in purposeful community tasks focused on daily living brings to the surface traumas and conflicts from past relationships that become the communities concern. Hinshelwood refers to these as *unconscious dramatizations* occurring between people attempting to fulfil their roles and responsibilities within the community.[8]

Although these methods differ structurally, the common thread is experiential learning of 'self and others' within a group setting.

Groups are also structured differently to meet the developmental needs of the patient group to whom they are applied. In the group treatment of young people, for example, a psychodynamic orientation requires certain modifications to make the group environment both safe and comprehensible to its members. Young people have a shorter concentration span, so therapy time needs to be shorter than for an adult or late-adolescent group. Refreshment breaks may be built in midway. 'Acting out' may require more input on the conductor's part, to protect the boundary. Dwivedi[9] talks of the 'indigenous peer culture', which the facilitator must join before therapeutic peer culture can be established.

The psychodynamic approach refers to communication, conscious and unconscious, verbal and non-verbal, between people. In a group perspective we enter what Foulkes[3] described as 'a hypothetical web of communication', where the individual comes with their internal world of past and present relationships. For the experience to be therapeutically meaningful, and effective, members must feel safe and contained enough to work with their personal and often distressing material.[10]

Therapeutic factors refer to desirable change outcomes, both immediate and in the longer term. For example, being able to talk about an embarrassing or painful feeling or memory is a *process*. Having the experience that one's feelings are acceptable to others is an *outcome*. Group psychotherapy is the method used to explore all communications on a number of different levels, their latent and manifest content, making sense of this for the benefit of both the individual and the group as a whole. The group conductor, and in turn the group members, become engaged with *translating* and *interpreting* those resistances that block communication, and therefore impede the development of the group.

People find it difficult to *disclose* – for fear of an angry or rejecting response – or find it difficult to *hear* – because the truth is painful. How can this be resolved and better understood through further exchange by the group? Much will depend on a safe and protected environment, where anxiety can more easily be tolerated. This is a crucial part of the conductor or facilitator's role and is fundamental to the dynamic administration of the group.

GROUP RELATIONS IN A SOCIAL CONTEXT

Groups play a significant part in the structure of all societies or communities. Governments, councils, work groups, schools and teams are *formal* groups with a specific interest or *purpose*. We gather in groups on special occasions like weddings, birthdays and funerals. By so doing we share in both the joy and the sorrow of these events. Through these *interpersonal associations* – where closer relationships are also formed – people learn about themselves in relationship to others. This will have important implications for self-reliance, self-identity and social well-being. We must add to this the experience and influence of the past, and how this can be reactivated in current relationships. How we manage and convey emotion in our interactions with others is also a significant feature for group and social relatedness.

A group may also reflect an important developmental stage in an individual's life and in meeting the needs appropriate to this stage. A nursery or preschool group represents the need for the young to play and socialize. For the very young, this offers an opportunity to re-enact, through play, ongoing conflicts at home, such as sibling rivalry. A traumatized child exposed over time to conflict and/or emotional neglect could find the cooperative, sharing aspects of play difficult or impossible to manage.

Adolescents are particularly concerned with peer-group identification. Being able to share with others in these newly formed allegiances is a step away from dependence on the family group, where the turmoil of adolescence can be seen more clearly. These are mainly groupings around home, school and social life, each requiring an adaptation to a different set of norms and expectations.

We need look no further than the family, the *primary group*, to understand the fundamental nature of our need to belong, relate to and be identified with others. The long incubation of the infant/child transition from complete dependency to ever increasing self-reliance allows ample time and exposure to a network of interpersonal relationships. Many types and levels of experience, positive and negative, are imprinted on the young within their primary relationships and may determine how conflict is tolerated in adult life, how attachments are formed or affection shown.

In group therapy we are working with the adversities the patient brings from their current situation. However, it is also relevant to consider the person's background – the shared common ground, from which relationships, and what has disturbed them, originate.

> ### Reflection
>
> If you have brothers and sisters, what effect has this had on you as a person?
>
> If you are an only child, what was it like growing up without brothers and sisters?

THERAPEUTIC FACTORS

Group psychotherapy is a way of helping people understand problems and conflicts together. Being able to express and share difficulties in a group can help reduce isolation. Many find it a great relief that their suffering does not have to be borne alone. The group can impart new learning on its members via the diverse feedback available. Yalom[11] extensively researched the therapeutic basis of the group, identifying 12 therapeutic factors from patients' self-statements following group treatment. These included, *group cohesiveness, universality, catharsis* and *family re-enactment*. By Yalom's own account the high level of subjectivity in the design could not produce hard evidence. However, the results have demonstrated the effectiveness of interactive group psychotherapy.

A further factor, *interpersonal learning*, occurs because the person's assumptions, attitudes and beliefs, can be 'reality tested' by the many points of view available in the group. New learning or insight can be disturbing. However, it can also be enlightening, as can learning from experience. The image we like to have of ourselves is often challenged. For example, a male group member who shows much care and concern for others in the group says that he sees his own problems as trivial compared to those of others, whom he tries to support. A fellow member suggests that perhaps he must work hard supporting others, to justify his place in the group as one with only minor problems. He now takes up the subject of his 'triviality', talking more openly about how his needs are trivialized by their family group. In this way he begins to accept the group's support, for what he now realizes is a profoundly distressing problem. A pattern of relating to others outside the group is re-enacted and repeated within it. His disclosure, having resonated with other members, brings about sharing of similar experiences.

Our *protagonist* in this example provides a reflective space in which others can make contact with their own experiences. This process has been likened by Foulkes to a 'hall of mirrors': seeing oneself in the experience of another. Such exchanges would typically engage others not only because of similarity but also because of difference. Being able to express how we *differ* from each other is as important to group cohesion as the experiences we have in common. This factor brings contrast and often tension into the group and prevents it becoming too cosy.

These therapeutic factors are linked with how the group develops over time. Reduced isolation *and universality* – knowing that we are not alone with our problems – are apparent in exchanges in the early sessions of the group, often called the *orientation phase*. Nitsun[12] makes a comparison with our earliest experiences of infancy, linking this with the first few months of life, when the infant's developmental task is integration with others, in new and unfamiliar surroundings. Like the infant, members of a new group, often strangers to each other, face considerable anxiety if they do not feel that the environment is sufficiently safe and containing. Cohesiveness and catharsis is unlikely, or would be less apparent, unless the group has worked through the orientation phase. This is distinguished by the members' dependency on the conductor to provide answers and solutions to the difficulties the group faces. Taking the patient's point of view, we might ask 'is it not reasonable to expect the conductor to have expert knowledge, and therefore answers and solutions?' The conductor, although not rejecting these appeals to their expertise, cannot gratify them. This can cause frustration as group members are thrown back on their own resources. However, the conductor never avoids any issue that is important for group development. The conductor manages and contains the anxiety of the group members by repeatedly drawing attention to what may be happening in the group – whether painful or simply confusing – by interpreting the mood of the group, and sometimes by engaging the group member who has, so far, remained silent.

Mirroring is not exclusive to the group treatment setting, and may be an important aspect of empathy. For example, when listening to a friend describe a recent loss we *recognize* something of our own feelings concerning a similar loss. In group treatment, mirroring is different, because what passes for familiar (what Foulkes called the 'foundation matrix'[3] – our common cultural shared experience) is amplified and condensed within the framework that contains all group experience and communication.

TWO ASPECTS OF THE NURSE–PATIENT RELATIONSHIP

Nurses aim to develop therapeutic relationships with patients, which is central to groupwork. The nurse brings relationship qualities, which are encompassed within the humanistic tradition of therapy, in particular Rogers'[13] client-centred approach. Genuineness, unconditional positive regard, warmth, empathy and understanding are attributes we value in all human relationships. Within the clinical setting this composite of professional skills and personal attributes represents an investment the nurse makes to engage patients in their own recovery.

Although the nurse maintains professional boundaries and neutrality the relationship will always have a number of qualities resembling a personal relationship, especially when the therapeutic work becomes deeper in meaning and resonance. When the patient begins to see the relationship as a resource for change, then we describe this as a *working alliance*. Cognitive and emotional resources are mobilized for learning at this stage. It is important to emphasize that learning from experience, the basis of a psychodynamic approach, requires the nurse to be as interested and curious in their *own* thoughts and feelings as they are in their patients. Derlega *et al.*[14] offer a well-researched account of *personal relationship theory*. Personal disclosure can be painful and distressing but brings much needed emotional relief (*catharsis*). For some patients this may prove to be unique if they have only experience of traumatic or otherwise uncaring relationships. The positive attributes of a non-judgemental, uncritical supporting relationship, limited as it must be by professional constraints, may put the patient in touch with anxieties concerning closeness and rejection. If the nurse can stay with what is most uncomfortable for them and their patient then the disturbance becomes more manageable.

The nurse–patient relationship, in whatever setting, will inevitably end. This reality needs to be brought out into open discussion, and its meaning for the patient explored. To some extent it is part of natural loss and mourning that we all face at some point in our lives.

By extension we can now broaden our focus on the individual by locating our attention on what happens between people. We move from the *intrapersonal* to the *interpersonal*. We do not lose sight of the individual, but see them more in the context of their relationships, particularly in groups.

The nurse is also an important transference figure for the patient. This means that feelings towards a significant figure from the past, often parental, are transferred onto the nurse and this can provide valuable material for understanding conflicts in the patient's current relationships, including the nurse–patient relationship, as well as making greater sense of what past relationships meant.

GROUP-SPECIFIC FACTORS: THE ANALYTIC METHOD

The group analytic method is essentially a Foulkesian means of group psychotherapy.[15] Foulkes' own training in psychiatry and psychoanalysis enabled him to create a new paradigm for treating individuals within a shared-group context. The standard analytic attitude and reflective stance, whereby unconscious processes are brought into conscious awareness by free association and interpretation was something he believed could be facilitated by each group member. Foulkes called this 'analysis *in* the group, *by* the group, including the conductor'.

The following factors can be found in many group situations, both clinical and non-clinical. Other central concepts important in group therapy, but not specific to groups and not detailed here, are *counter-transference*, *resistance* and *acting out*.[6]

The nurse is often ideally placed to observe interactions between patients and the interpersonal dynamics of both the staff and patient subgroups. Where these can be made sense of for the benefit of the patient a psychodynamic culture will emerge, and the nurse will function as a 'nurse therapist'.

Mirroring

Mirroring is probably the most important factor in the process of the experiential group, promoting sharing and deepening of the group's commitment and shared sense of purpose. The mirror provides an accurate reflection of what is placed before it. Our thoughts and feelings, our self-image, how we see ourselves, or would like to see ourselves, is not always what is reflected back to us. The individual is confronted with different aspects of their reflection by other group members. Pines[16] describes human mirrors in the group that 'offer us multiple perspectives on ourselves, on how we are seen by others and let us see the many facets of human development, our conflicts and attempts to solve them'.

Through inner assessment, individuals gain a more accurate and realistic understanding of themselves and their problems. Foulkes called this 'ego training in action'. In the example of the man who saw his problems as trivial, the view given back to him – the reflection – was accepted as a more accurate or complete interpretation.

Although difficult to convey in words, mirroring involves the multiplicity of cause and effect. One person's disclosure, even a relatively minor comment, can bring about a chain of associations for others that promote further disclosure and in turn further reflecting back of different points of view. It would be misleading to describe mirroring as only of value in verbal exchange, when for example two people reflect upon each other's experience. The remainder of the group, although silent, will invariably see and hear what there is in this exchange that reflects upon their *own* experience.

Group illustration

In the fifth session of a new outpatient group, meeting weekly, six members are present. A seventh left abruptly after announcing in the previous group his intention to take a job offered in another part of the country. The themes predominating in previous sessions tended towards trying to manage symptoms and how medication is a mixed blessing. This group is in the *orientation* phase.

A group member (A) is telling others how doubtful she feels that the antidepressants she takes are having any effect.

A: I'm not sure, though, if I can do without them. I don't want to become dependent on this treatment because – well this is a sign of weakness.

Another member offers an *interpretation*.

B: Perhaps this is about depending on the group, which like the medication is an evening treatment. Feeling that you are weak if you come to depend on the group?

A: I don't know that I agree. The group and medication are two quite different treatments, and anyway the group is new and I don't think I've got that dependent on it.

Patient A seems uncertain, then says:

A: I suppose I don't know whether either are going to work.

Other members pick up the theme of 'two treatments'. Views become polarized as members weigh up having one or more treatments to depend on.

C: I rely on my medication. I don't have any problem with it. I know what I've been like without it.

There is ongoing heated discussion on symptom relief as though the members expect this group to be like a medication whose action they do not know.

D: I do think we spend a lot of time discussing medication in this group. It's not what I'm here for. I've had a lousy week and maybe others have too, but we are staying with this and not sharing other experiences.

An awkward silence ensues. The conductor is prepared to wait. Allowing this silence to continue promotes reflection and greater tolerance to anxiety. This has been an important challenge to the rest of the group who seem to be seeking comfortable unity around a subject they have in common. This challenge is far more significant coming from a fellow patient who usually takes a risk by opposing a majority consensus. We will see, by what happens next, that patient D is making another important challenge. The conductor notices that patient D looks tense and uncomfortable and asks if he can say what he is feeling and whether it's to do with the lousy week he's had.

D: Well I've had my father and sister staying and they are so wrapped up in their own interests I just think they don't want to know what has been going on for me. I could never tell them I'm coming here. Since my mother left him, no one wants to look at this loss.

Conductor: I wonder if you are angry with the group as well for not noticing how upset you are?

D: Well it seemed like everyone here was busily discussing things that had nothing to do with me.

Conductor: And you felt shut out?

D: Yes I did, I also feel angry with you because I wanted you to come in and do something to get us away from this preoccupation with medication. During that silence I was thinking about my father who never explained anything to me, and I suppose because you don't explain what's happening here to us I get into all this negative stuff about him.

The conductor explores further the significance of the transference to him by patient D, then addressing the group as a whole.

Conductor: I think the group is also struggling to know whether others can be depended upon, perhaps like a medicine when we don't know the effects.

Other members contribute at this more personal level having been cast to some extent as the siblings who have the father/conductor to themselves. In the second half of the session, members are more at work on the difficulties that underlie symptoms, rather than the symptoms themselves. A further deepening of the intimacy in the group occurs when a member links the departure of patient D's mother to the recently departed patient in the previous session. Issues of loss, particularly of this valued group member, and the real disruption to the group are acknowledged in a way that did not seem possible in the first half of the session.

Mirroring was more apparent in the second half of the session when the more personal disclosures of patient D were mirrored in the experiences others had concerning lack of emotional contact with a parent, unresolved rivalry with siblings, repressed feelings and experiences of loss due to bereavement, divorce and mental illness. Mirroring is an important phenomenon in the group, leading to greater cohesiveness because it promotes the sharing of experiences as a benefit to all rather than a benefit only to the individual. Foulkes said, 'the patient sees himself, or part of himself, in particular a repressed part of himself in the other members. He can observe from the outside another member reacting in the way he himself reacts, and can see how conflicts and problems are translated into neurotic behaviour'.

Reflection

If you had been a member of the group described, what would you have said to A?

What would you have said in response to the conductor's input?

The transference group

Within the dynamic matrix of the group, multiples of people significant in the individuals' past are transferred onto *one* or *more* members of the group, including the conductor. For patient D, feelings of jealousy towards his sisters were transferred on to those in the group whose interests excluded him. Similarly, the conductor was experienced as the distant father who disappointed him and frustrated his need to engage. By exploring his past relationship, in the light of displaced and projected feelings onto another in the current relationship, D made greater sense of his experiences.

Figure–ground relationship

The conductor always sees the individual against the *background* of the group. Depending on what is happening in the group this view may be reversed. The group as a whole is now *foreground* and the conductor will intervene, addressing the group as a single entity. The conductor needs to shift his point of view, the location between what's happening for the individual and the collective meaning in the group. This does not discount the individual's disclosure but relocates it within a shared context.

Family re-enactment

The group come to represent at different times, for different individuals, a reconstituted family of origin. This can be applied to many group structures and it may be apparent at the conscious level. Problems that had no solutions in the past, and are therefore likely to have been forgotten or denied, can be reworked. For example, patient D expressed anger with those in the group who were avoiding an important task. This may not ever have been possible in the past. This is important as a rehearsal for future relationships, and can loosen up defences so that further material can be remembered.

Socialization

The group is a social entity representing a sample of social convention. The less socially skilled can be 'brought on', and more dominant 'impatient' characters can be held back. A therapeutic benefit of the structure of the treatment group is the deepening social relatedness and the reduction of isolation. Making valuable connections in the group can inspire similar social behaviour outside the group.

Interpretation/translation

The great value of psychodynamic group treatment is the frequency in which the group develops its own therapeutic agency. The conductor only interprets when analysis fails. We saw how patient B made an interpretation suggesting an unconscious link between dependency on drug treatment and dependency on the group. The conductor participates less when the group works in this way, following rather than leading the group. Interpretation is not an exact science applied by the conductor. Even when it is certain that an interpretation will be accurate, it is better to wait and see what group members do before intervening. However, *translation* is somewhat different. Its purpose is to bring into language form unconscious processes of communication whose meaning would remain lost without this translation. In the awkward silence following patient D's challenge, the group has suddenly become a difficult place. The conductor will judge when best to intervene to help translate the mood of the group in the light of other factors preceding the silence. In practical terms, this may simply mean seeking clarification about what one person says and its impact on others. As with the example of figure–ground configuration, the conductor locates their attention at one moment with the individual and at another with the group.

For example, the fear of dependency on treatment may arise as an issue for one member but it is also an issue for others. The process of translation can help the silent member of the group to participate. This is important for a newly formed group or when a member joins an established group.

Scapegoat phenomenon

The *scapegoat* in biblical history carried away the sins of the community from which it was cast out. Similarly, one group member, or a pair, may embody all that is disturbing for others to face in themselves. Though not made explicit in the example given above, there were occasions when one or more members wondered if it were something unbearable about their problems that had 'driven out' the member in the previous session. Issues concerning rejection, and when this becomes acted out, were taken up during subsequent sessions. A patient who sees their experience as highly singular, or unique, may feel 'outside' the more common experiences of others, and may act out in a way that provokes the very responses they fear. This is a type of self-induced scapegoat phenomenon. Much effort is needed to help contain the individual who always feels at odds with the group, and it is quite possible they will drop out in the early sessions of the group.

Pairing and subgroups

Pairing in the group is common and can be easily overlooked. When two people find they can share an experience, they become a *pair*. This occurs when individuals are the only men in the group, or have experience of an emotionally distant father, which was the case for patient D and A. Sometimes opposite poles attract. Having very contrasting experiences can bring about pair bonding. Often, we are attracted to people for many different reasons. In the therapy group, members share thoughts and feelings towards one another. They sometimes express hitherto forbidden wishes, expressing things that they could not be so open about outside the group. This is an important aspect of developing intimacy, which is held and contained within the boundary of the group. Pairing is not generally problematic, as different associations bring different combinations of people together. Occasionally there is tension in the group if the pair are experienced at excluding the others. Usually this is temporary. When it is not, it can be understood as a form of acting-in and the couple will need help to see the value of integration within a whole-group perspective. As mentioned earlier the conductor need only intervene when what happens in the group impedes its development.

Subgroups may arise for equally valid reasons. People who have children form a subgroup as do those without children. A medication subgroup and a non-medication subgroup can at times work hard at not looking at what they have in common. This was the case in the group I have described. The conductor's role here is to draw to the group's attention the value of the pair or subgroup relationship when it is used defensively to avoid a common problem.

The dynamic matrix

Communication at the current conscious level in Foulkes' model is seen as of equal importance to communication at unconscious projective and transference levels. All processes and therapeutic factors belong to this *dynamic matrix*. Ahlin[17] provides an elegant definition: 'A group matrix is truly a group work creation and its aims and shape bear witness not only to the individual in it but to their ancestors, histories, cultures'.

The conductor's role

How and *when* we use a psychodynamic approach will depend on the setting and resources within which we work. The degree to which we feel able to work in a psychodynamic way is usually related to where we find ourselves during our professional lives. The opportunities available to start working in groups may depend on having like-minded colleagues with whom to share ideas and make plans. Here, I consider our role as groupworkers from two opposite ends of the spectrum of group facilitation.

The first focuses on the assessment, selection and preparation of patients for group psychotherapy and our involvement as *boundary keepers* and therapists within such groups. These groups are generally longer term, requiring considerable commitment of time and resources. The less experienced nurse can gain many useful group skills as co-therapist, working alongside a more experienced conductor. A supportive infrastructure is, however, necessary for this to succeed. The hard work that goes into preparation is never wasted.

The second focus is to consider where less formalized groups are already in place. A daily community meeting on an acute admissions ward, for example, might benefit from a psychodynamic approach, becoming more centred on experiential learning rather than on tasks.

In the assessment and selection of patients for group psychotherapy, I usually employ the following procedure.

Having welcomed the patients and explained the purpose and structure of the meeting, I invite them to describe their problems and also to give a *personal history*, starting as far back as possible. The order in which a person brings information into this meeting is not so important. What really matters is the *way* in which the story is told. Weighing up the different selection criteria – for example, psychological mindedness, motivation, curiosity about one's past and how this may link with present difficulties – are at the forefront of the assessment. The patient's capacity, or ego strength, needs to be sufficient

to manage the emotional upheaval that the dynamically orientated group process is likely to bring about.

Exclusion criteria

It is easier to consider who would *not* benefit from the group experience and who *should not*, in their own interests, be referred. Although there are many types of groups for many types of problems/disorders, the group I have described would not be suitable for people who are addicted to drugs or alcohol, or are paranoid, psychotic or sociopathic. Patients with borderline personalities can be very difficult to hold within a group. Most group therapists agree that the severely depressed patient would be too retarded to use the group, and patients who are actively suicidal are too threatening and disruptive. Also unsuitable would be those people in the midst of an acute illness or major crisis. Group psychotherapy is not recommended for people about to embark on major events such as childbirth, marriage or divorce. Their motivation is always worth noting, however, and they could be encouraged to return at a later date. People who have had no experience of at least one stable and satisfying relationship in their life will find the group too threatening and would be better directed toward individual therapy/counselling in the first instance.

Inclusion criteria

The most important inclusion criteria is motivation. Patients rarely do well in groups if they have been 'sent'. Uncertainty about the group process can be dealt with along with normal anxieties in pre-group assessment but the patient ultimately must decide that they want to enter the group for themselves. Yalom[11] said that

> an important criterion for inclusion is whether a patient has obvious problems in the interpersonal domain: loneliness, shyness and social withdrawal, inability to be intimate or to love, excessive competitiveness, aggressivity, abrasiveness, or argumentativeness, suspiciousness, problems with authority, narcissism, including an inability to share, to empathise, or to accept criticism and a continuous need for admiration, feelings of unlovability, fears of assertiveness, fears of depending.

He adds that 'patients must be willing to take responsibility for those problems or, at the very least acknowledge them and entertain a desire for change'.

PREPARATION OF THE PATIENT

People suitable for groups need basic information. This helps to dispel some anticipatory anxiety and conveys some of the therapist's beliefs in the process itself.

Practical arrangements may need to be discussed in the light of making an important commitment to treatment. Personal resources are often important, as therapy is an investment in time and often money (travel costs, etc.). Support of the family or partner may be important and the possible 'postponement' of travel arrangements, moving house, etc., may be necessary. These preoccupations, prior to therapy beginning, are important considerations for all and referring agencies in particular can do much in the preparation process.

At the other end of our spectrum are settings where brief group interventions are applied. The aims and service objectives of the departments within which we work determine how a psychodynamic approach can be used, particularly if time is a decisive factor. We have considered in this chapter a broad range of therapeutic factors and processes that can develop over time, especially in longer term group treatments. How can we now adapt this model to much shorter group interventions while maintaining a psychodynamic perspective? A personal experience may provide at least one possible answer. It represents a point on a learning curve to do with being creative with what you have got!

Many years ago I was on a placement in an acute admission department and wanted to provide a time-limited closed psychotherapy group. There was little interest. I took this to my supervisor who invited me to look at what existed in the prevailing culture of the department and to join whatever I could that involved group relations, and to observe the dynamic processes, which included me. By starting from this point of view I was able to see my own short-sightedness. A psychotherapy group of the kind I had in mind would take 6 months to put together! Instead, I joined a social worker who conducted a 'leavers group' and this proved to be a very worthwhile experience. The leavers group had two important focuses. It allowed time to look at external issues about going home such as finance, accommodation and work, but it also provided a valuable experiential forum for more interpersonal dynamics to unfold. Patients could share their anxiety about facing the outside world, returning to pick up the pieces of their lives. They could share what the hospital admission had meant to them and much more. The group successfully bridged the often difficult gulf of combining tasks and dynamics. Within these types of groups we begin to see how psychodynamic processes take shape and are incorporated alongside the more obvious theme or occupation of the group which in this example is to do with leaving hospital.

One of the conductor's key functions is in ensuring a safe and protected environment. This is about *boundary maintenance*. It is closely linked to confidentiality and containment and is ongoing throughout the life of both brief and longer term groups. Securing an undisturbed space, arranging chairs so that all participants can see each other, minimizing unnecessary distractions, precise time-keeping are all aspects that help the group focus on the task in hand.

Many groups do not focus on the dynamic interpersonal relationships as they develop in the group. It may not be of primary importance. For example, group treatments may be themed around a particular problem like addiction, or eating disorders. In an anxiety management group, the facilitator is likely to determine objectives for the group from tried and tested procedures. The therapist's role would be to educate and then direct members, much like a teacher, towards achieving these objectives, and so better manage their anxieties. However, it is unlikely that when we are involved in such groups we will fail to notice the dynamics between individuals at the interpersonal level. One only has to experience one's own counter-transference feelings of anger towards a silent or vulnerable looking individual, to appreciate this.

> ### Reflection
>
> How will this chapter influence the next group in which you participate?
> What, in particular, will you be thinking about, when you sit in the group?

WIDER APPLICATIONS

The *therapeutic community* employs a combination of group approaches and modifications of the therapeutic community model may be possible in day and inpatient settings. The key purpose is to involve the patient as much as possible in the routine administration of the unit. This returns to the patient a sense of responsibility and empowerment that the more medicalized treatments take away. Large-group dynamics often evoke anxiety and this is increased without tasks and recreational activities to offset them. The therapeutic community frequently manages to combine in a balanced way the more intense 'therapy' groups with the task group. A living and learning environment promotes equal status and valued roles. Even though distinctions must be made between the carers and the cared for and the specific responsibilities each participant carries out, the democratization principle places all members of staff and patients within the same culture of enquiry.

Training and supervision

To process what happens in psychodynamic groups, personal experience of group treatment is invaluable. This is built into many dynamically focused training courses and is mandatory as the personal component on all qualifying courses. This need not discourage the nurse who finds groupwork rewarding, challenging and at times enjoyable, and who may already possess a range of interactive and reflective skills. You will begin to appreciate that it is a lived experience, a personal reality and cannot simply be taught.

A psychodynamic approach to *group supervision* is another application that has value for those nurses, and of course other disciplines, interested in extending or developing their thinking about the nurse–patient relationship. In my experience working with community nurses, these small groups provide a forum for examining the transference and counter-transference issues that arise in their ongoing work with patients. Like the treatment group a reflective space helps each to share and make sense of their work via a psychodynamic perspective. This is not 'therapy' for staff however. The task is work focused but takes what can be learnt from group dynamics that is common to all.

REFERENCES

1. Freud S. *An outline of psycho-analysis.* London, UK: The Hogarth Press, 1979.

2. Winnicott DW. The beginning of the individual. In: *Babies and their mothers.* London, UK: Free Association Books, 1998: 51–8.

3. Foulkes SH. Outline and development of group analysis. In: *Therapeutic group analysis.* London, UK: Maresfield Reprints, 1984 [1964]: 66–82.

4. Wright H. The structure of the supervision seminar. In: *Groupwork: perspectives and practice.* London, UK: Scutari, 1989.

5. Faugier J, Butterworth CA. *Clinical supervision: a position paper.* Manchester, UK: University of Manchester, School of Nursing Studies, 1993.

6. Lego S. Psychodynamic group psychotherapy. In: *Psychiatric nursing: a comprehensive reference,* 2nd edn. New York, NY: Lippincott, 1996.

7. Rutan JS. Psychodynamic group psychotherapy. *International Journal of Group Psychotherapy* 1992; **42** (1): 19–35.

8. Hinshelwood RD. Resources for unconscious dramatization. In: *What happens in groups.* London, UK: Free Association Books, 1987: 38–45.

9. Dwivedi KN. Conceptual framework. In: *Group work with children and adolescents.* London, UK: Jessica Kingsley, 1993: 28–45.

10. Peplau HE. The history of milieu as a treatment modality. In: O'Toole AW, Welt SR (eds). *Hildegard E Peplau: selected works – interpersonal theory in nursing.* London, UK: Macmillan, 1989.

11. Yalom ID. The therapeutic factors. In: *The theory and practice of group psychotherapy.* New York, NY: Basic Books, 1985: 70–101.

12. Nitsun M. Early development. In: *Linking the individual and the group. Group Analysis.* London, UK: Sage, 1989; **22**: 249–60.

13. Rogers C. The characteristics of a helping relationship. In: *On becoming a person. The therapist's view of psychotherapy.* London, UK: Constable, 1979: 39–58.

14. Derlega VJ, Hendrick SS, Winstead BA, Berg JH. A social exchange analysis. In: *Psychotherapy as a personal relationship.* New York, NY: The Guilford Press, 1991: 42–74.

15. Roberts J, Pines M. Group analytic psychotherapy. *International Journal of Group Psychotherapy* 1992; **42** (4): 469–94.

16. Pines M. Reflections on mirroring. Sixth SH Foulkes annual lecture of the Group Analytic Society, 10 May, 1982. *Group Analysis* 1982; **15** (Suppl): 3–26.

17. Ahlin G. On thinking about the group matrix. *Group Analysis* 1985; **18** (2): 111–19.

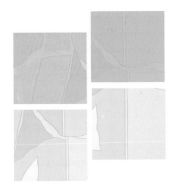

CHAPTER 41

Using counselling approaches

Philip Burnard*

INTRODUCTION

The research jury cannot make up its mind about counselling. It is neither easy to define nor easy to research. This chapter considers some of the things that mental health and psychiatric nurses may want to consider before doing counselling. It considers the research evidence and it offers a practical framework for offering counselling to those in emotional distress. Finally, it addresses some cultural issues that need to be considered and closes with some thoughts about integrating these sections.

What is counselling?

In recent years, a range of questions about *what* counselling is, *who* should do it and whether or not it *works* have been asked, both in the literature and in the national newspapers. As consumers become more aware of their rights and more discerning about the nature of the treatments that they are offered, they are – appropriately – asking questions about whether or not counselling is a 'good thing'. The answer to the question remains unanswered, convincingly, at the time of writing this book. All we can surmise is that talking about things seems to help a lot of people. Whether or not 'formal counselling'

makes a long-term difference has yet to be clarified. In the meantime, a useful distinction, for nurses, can be made between *counselling* and *using counselling skills*. It is argued that the *latter* are of particular use to the nurse.

There are many published, formal definitions of counselling. Just one is offered here, by Nelson-Jones,[1] a prolific and respected writer in the counselling field:

> Essential counselling and therapy skills are communication skills, accompanied by appropriate mental processes, offered by counsellors and therapists in order to develop collaborative working relationships with clients, identify problems, clarify and expand understanding of these problems and, where appropriate, to assist clients to develop and implement strategies for changing how they think, communicate/act and feel so that they can attain more of their human potential.

As with all definitions of this type of activity, it is only *a* definition and not *the* definition. Although Nelson-Jones' definition is wide-ranging and inclusive, we might ask questions about what he means by the abstraction 'attain more of their human potential'. Any definition necessarily reflects the author's own belief and value systems and this one is no exception. There are, of course, numerous others in the literature on the topic.[2]

*Philip Burnard is Professor of Nursing at Cardiff University, Wales. He has published widely in the fields of counselling, ethics, research and stress. He is currently Visiting Professor at the Royal Thai Army Nursing College in Bangkok, Thailand and lectures internationally. His current research is into stress in community mental health nursing and also into culture and its effects on communication.

COUNSELLING AND COUNSELLING SKILLS

What, then, are the differences between the two concepts? Counselling, it might be argued, is something that is carried out by people whose job it is to counsel. Such people will be known by the job title 'counsellor' and it seems likely that they will pursue this job on a full-time basis. Counselling skills are part of the things that they use to pursue that job. Such skills, however, are also transferable to other jobs and, in particular, to nursing. Nurses, without being 'counsellors' in the strict sense of the word, can use a range of counselling skills to help their patients talk through problems, express feelings and make decisions. Such nurses do not practice as counsellors but use the skills that are available appropriately and carefully.

Is counselling effective?

The question often arises whether or not counselling 'works'. A similar but perhaps clearer question is often asked: 'Is counselling effective?' This section offers a short review of some of the current thinking in this area. It is based on the NHS Centre for Reviews and Dissemination, The University of York publication, vol. 5, issue 2, August 2001, *Counselling in primary care*.

The primary interest of those collating evidence for clinical effectiveness, through systematic reviews of the research literature, is the randomized controlled trial or RCT. The use of RCTs to evaluate counselling and other psychological therapy treatments is contentious.[3–6] However, a number of RCTs of counselling in primary care have been conducted.

Rowland *et al.*[7] published a systematic review of counselling in primary care. The latest update of the review includes seven RCTs of counsellors trained to the standard recommended by the British Association for Counselling and Psychotherapy. The review focused on counsellors meeting these standards as they are increasingly recognized as a useful benchmark in primary care. The counsellors in these trials treated patients with mild to moderate mental health problems (such as anxiety and depression) referred by GPs. In six of the trials, the comparison group was 'usual GP care', including support from the GP within normal consultations, medication and referral to mental health services.

One RCT used a comparison group of 'GP antidepressant treatment' and was considered separately. The results of six RCTs (with 772 patients) indicated that counselled patients demonstrated a significantly greater reduction in psychological symptoms such as anxiety and depression than patients receiving usual GP care when followed up in the short term (up to 6 months). Psychological symptoms were measured using validated questionnaires such as the Beck Depression Inventory and General Health Questionnaire. These psychological benefits were modest: the average counselled patient was better off than approximately 60% of patients in usual GP care (if counselling and usual care were equally effective, the proportion would be 50%). There were no significant differences between counselling and usual care in the four RCTs (with 475 patients) reporting long-term outcomes (8–12 months).

Generally, the RCTs reported high levels of patient satisfaction with counselling and that patients were more satisfied with counselling than with usual GP care. However, this comparison of GPs and counsellors is difficult to interpret because of the differences in time each has available to spend with patients.

Two RCTs have compared counselling with other mental health treatments routinely provided in primary care.[8–11] The first compared counselling with cognitive–behaviour therapy provided by qualified psychologists. There were no differences between the two therapies in their overall effectiveness at short- or long-term follow-up. Both therapies were superior to usual GP care in the short term, but provided no significant advantage in the long term.

The second RCT compared counselling with antidepressant treatment provided by GPs who were given specific guidelines on antidepressant use. However, the study was designed to reflect antidepressant prescribing as provided routinely by GPs, and the prescription of medication was not standardized. There were no differences in outcomes between patients receiving counselling and medication at 8 weeks or 12 months of follow-up.

> ### Reflection
>
> What does 'counselling' mean to you?
> What would you expect a 'counsellor' to do for you?

HOW DO YOU CHOOSE AN APPROACH TO COUNSELLING?

There are lots of different ways of doing counselling, based on different sorts of philosophical views of people. In this section, I want to explore, in a general way, how our beliefs about people will affect the approach we use in counselling or, indeed, whether we do counselling at all.

One point seems more important than all the others when we consider views of the person. It is simply this: to what degree, if at all, do we feel that people can *change* and to what degree, if at all, can individuals *choose* that change? Presumably, if we do counselling, we must believe that people can change and that they can decide on that change. If we believe that people cannot change then we are unlikely to believe that counselling will be effective. In the paragraphs that follow, I explore the various philosophical points that relate to this idea.

Free will

Philosophically, there are at least three different views we can have about the human condition: free will, determinism and fatalism.[12] Free will involves the idea that we can choose our mental states and, to a greater or lesser degree, our futures. If I consider what choices I have as I write this, I may be led to thinking that all I can do is sit and finish my writing. However, if I think for a bit longer, I will realize that I can choose a huge range of options. Here are just some of them. I can choose to finish this writing task. I can choose not to finish it and to delete everything I have written so far. I can tell the editor that I refuse to write the chapter. I can write complete nonsense and submit it as a chapter. And so on. The point, by extension, is that, arguably, at any point in my life, I can *choose* a considerable range of things to do and not to do. In doing this and in choosing what I do, I am exercising free will. The most extreme statement of this comes in the branch of philosophy known as *existentialism*.[13,14]

The existentialists argue that, because we have consciousness and because we can reflect on our situation, we are free, psychologically, to choose our lives. This is a mental freedom. We cannot choose to change our physical status in any profound way. I cannot, for instance, choose to wake up tomorrow with blue eyes. But, according to existential theory, I do choose my psychological state. I am, according to existentialism, free to choose at any moment in my life – once I have reached an age where I am aware of being able to choose. Furthermore, I must choose. And in doing so, I become the author of myself. In choosing, I create who I am as a person.

So what is the point of this sort of freedom? Well, simply, perhaps, that many of us deny it. We prefer, instead, to believe that we are controlled either by our pasts or by other people. We sometimes feel *safer* believing that what we do is beyond our control. In that way, we can simply 'give in' to life and accept our lot. Also, in doing this, we do not have to take *responsibility* for who we are. Instead, we can blame our parents, or a 'bad marriage' or any number of other factors for our being in the situation we are in. The evangelizing aspect of existentialism is to convince people of the reality of their freedom to choose and also of their subsequent responsibility. For we cannot be free and not responsible. If I say, for instance, that I am free to do anything but that I must first check with my wife, I am clearly not free. However, if I *do* exercise my freedom, then I *have* to take responsibility for my actions. For, in choosing, I alone decide what I will do and I must face the consequences of my actions.

All of this fits very well with the notion of counselling as an activity – particularly with the client-centred approaches to counselling in which the counsellor refrains from offering the client advice or ideas or suggestions about how to live but, instead, helps them to make their own decisions about their life. This is completely compatible with the notion of personal free will and with the belief in our ability to choose our lives.

Determinism

An alternative way of thinking about people is to see their mental states as being *determined*. What might this mean? In the physical world – the world that surrounds us – the laws of *causality* are always and everywhere at play. If I consider the computer that I am using to help me write this, I will realize that before this computer existed, it was made up of plastic, metal and some other ingredients. These, in turn, existed in another state (the metal, as ore, for example) before they were used in making the computer. These are facts about the way computers come into being. Any object in the world was, previously, something else. We can always trace, for example, iron, back to its source as ore. This process of things becoming other things is known as a *causal chain*. It is never going to be possible to point to a computer and say 'this never existed as other chemicals and minerals before, it simply came into being in this room!'

Similarly, the argument goes, people's thoughts and actions do not simply spring into being. Instead, they can be traced back to previous events and thoughts. An argument for why I have the personality I have today is that it was in some way *caused* by previous life events. Sigmund Freud, the creator of the psychotherapy known as psychoanalysis, referred to all this as *psychic determinism*. He argued that our minds are situated in physical bodies, which themselves, are subject to causal law. Similarly, he argued, our minds are *determined* by previous life events, actions and thoughts. We do not, according to Freud, simply *choose* at any given point but, instead, there is a certain *inevitability* about how we turn out as people. Our thoughts, feelings and actions are not really *chosen* but, instead, *determined* by what has happened to us. This, then, is the counterposition to the argument for free will.

Psychoanalysis and determinism

Psychoanalysis, itself, seems to take an interesting line on determinism. Although it acknowledges that we are shaped and influenced by our past to the degree that it is our past that makes us who we are, it also argues that understanding these links between past and present can free us to make life choices. This seems something of a contradiction. It seems that our lives are determined up to a point and then, through the process known as psychoanalysis, we are somehow freed to choose our lives. Again, anyone coming to counselling needs to consider their own position on the free will–determinism axis. Suffice to say, at this point, that there is a middle, compromise position in all of this. It is possible to see people in terms of relative determinism. That is to say that at any given time, we have a wide but not limitless array of choices from which we choose. Whereas the existentialist would say that I can choose anything and the determinist would say that freedom of choice is a myth, the relative determinist would talk of a limited range of choices, but would also acknowledge that such choices are possible.

Fatalism

For completeness, it is interesting to note a third (or perhaps fourth) position that we might adopt in thinking about the nature of people. Another view is that of *fatalism*. Fatalism is the idea that our lives are, in some way, laid out for us. All we have to do is to *live* our lives, as those lives are already *chosen* for us. There is little we can do to change the ways in which our lives 'work', since a blueprint for them already exists somewhere. This position is usually seen in followers of the sects of certain world religions. However, it can also be found in everyday folk culture. It is not rare to hear people say 'well, if it is meant to be, then it will happen', suggesting that someone, somewhere, has already planned everything. This can, of course, be either a good thing or a bad thing. In cultures where fatalism is pervasive, it is usual to see a quiet acceptance of things as they are and a lack of determination to try to change things.

However, in certain settings, such a position leads to despair and what might be called a loss of the locus of control. In certain depressive states, for example, it is not unusual to find a person believing that nothing they can do will ever change their condition. Sometimes, then, the counsellor's role might be to help a nominally 'fatalistic' person to appreciate that it is the *person* who controls his or her life,[15] or is it? Debating and answering this sort of question is at the heart of deciding on an approach to counselling and also in deciding whether or not to counsel at all.

Reflection

How does 'counselling' differ from psychotherapy?

COUNSELLING INTERVENTIONS

All those who take up counselling will have to consider their basic beliefs about the nature of people, as outlined above. After this, it is necessary to consider the degree to which we feel people can make their own decisions, unaided. In counselling terms, there are a range of ways of thinking about this. At one end of the spectrum lies the *client-centred approach* to counselling.[16] This approach involves the view that people can and must choose their own lives and that counsellors should never offer advice or suggestions how clients lives might be

changed. At the other end of the spectrum is what might be called the *didactic* approach to counselling. This involves the view that it is always worth helping people to *question* their views of the world and to suggest alternative ways of doing things. Thus a cognitive–behavioural approach to counselling would be very different to the client-centred approach in that it would involve the counsellor in being confronting and very assertive in relation to what the client says.[17] For the cognitive–behavioural counsellor, it is not sufficient merely to agree with the client's view of his or her world. Instead, it is the counsellor's job to challenge that view and help to change it with concrete suggestions and instructions. It is also the counsellor's role to help spot faulty and illogical thinking on the part of the client. There is, again, a huge literature on the different approaches to counselling. One useful guide to these is published by the British Association for Counselling.[18]

To enable us to choose the sorts of interventions we make, ranging from client-centred to cognitive–behavioural methods of counselling, it is useful to have a *general framework* that covers all possible effective counselling interventions. Such a general purpose framework is now offered here in the form of Heron's Six Category Intervention Analysis.[19,20]

This conceptual framework was developed by Heron out of the work of Blake and Mouton.[21] It was offered as a conceptual model for understanding interpersonal relationships, and as an assessment tool for identifying a range of possible therapeutic interactions between two people.

The six categories in Heron's analysis are prescriptive (offering advice), informative (offering information), confronting (challenging), cathartic (enabling the expression of pent-up emotions), catalytic ('drawing out') and supportive (confirming or encouraging). The word 'intervention' is used to describe any statement that the practitioner may use. The word 'category' is used to denote a range of related interventions.

Heron calls the first three categories of intervention (prescriptive, informative and confronting) 'authoritative' and suggests that in using these categories the practitioner retains control over the relationship. He calls the second three categories of intervention (cathartic, catalytic and supportive) 'facilitative' and suggests that these enable the client to retain control over the relationship. In other words, the first three are 'practitioner-centred' and the second three are 'client-centred'. Another way of describing the difference between the first and second sets of three categories is that the first three are 'I tell you' interventions and the second three are 'You tell me' interventions.

What, then, is the value of such an analysis of therapeutic interventions? First, it identifies the *range* of possible interventions available to the nurse/counsellor. Very often, in day-to-day interactions with others, we stick to repetitive forms of conversation and response, simply because we are not aware that other options are available to us. This analysis identifies an exhaustive range of types of human interventions. Second, by identifying the sorts of interventions we can use, we can act more precisely and with a greater sense of intention. The nurse–patient relationship thus becomes more particular and less haphazard. Since we know *what* we are saying and also *how* we are saying it, we have greater interpersonal choice.

Third, the analysis offers an instrument for training. Once the categories have been identified, they can be used for students and others to identify their weaknesses and strengths across the interpersonal spectrum. Nurses can, in this way, develop a wide range and comprehensive range of interpersonal skills.

It is worth repeating that the skills identified in this chapter as counselling skills are exactly similar to the basic human skills used in day-to-day nursing interactions. Thus an understanding of the full range of the six categories can enhance and enrich the quality of the nurse's approach to care. It should be noted, too, that the analysis does not offer a mechanical approach to interpersonal skills training. This is an important issue. The analysis indicates a *type* of response. The choice of words, the tone of voice, the non-verbal aspects of a particular response must develop out of the individual's belief and value system and out of their life experience. Those aspects of the response are also dependent upon the situation at the time and upon the people involved. All human relationships occur within a particular context. It is impossible to identify what will necessarily be the right thing to do in *this* situation at *this* time. A mechanical, learning-by-heart approach to counselling or interpersonal skills would, therefore, be inappropriate.

One of the great strengths of Heron's analysis is that it allows the mental health and psychiatric nurse to consider *all* types of counselling intervention. Often, in the literature, it is possible to find a description of the client-centred approach *or* the cognitive–behavioural approach. Heron's analysis allows the nurse to consider the full range of possible interventions as they relate to helping the patient or client.

Although cultural issues are discussed in the next section, it is important to note the cultural limitations of Heron's analysis. In many Asian countries and cultures, the framework would not be particularly appropriate. In such cultures, it is often considered inappropriate to express strong emotion, thus the cathartic category of intervention would be inappropriate. Similarly, in such cultures, a person may often go to a more senior person for *advice* and would consider it strange to be 'drawn out' or encouraged to make their own decisions on certain issues. For example, in Muslim cultures, it would be normal to go to a 'religious advisor' for a Koranic solution to problems. It would certainly not be usual to find one's own solution through careful consideration of one's life circumstances. Finally, in various Asian cultures, 'face' or self-respect and dignity is very important. It may be considered a potential risk to 'face' if a counsellor was confronting in any way.

The point of the analysis, in this chapter, is to allow nurses to consider what counselling interventions may be appropriate for use with their patients. There is no room, in a chapter of this sort, to offer a detailed account of all aspects of counselling practice and the reader is referred to other chapters in this book about psychotherapy, psychoanalysis and other therapies for further details about what effective interventions may be used with different client groups. More details of this analysis and research undertaken by the present author into it are described elsewhere.[22]

> ## Reflection
>
> What are the human skills needed to practice counselling? How could you improve or enhance these skills?

CULTURAL AWARENESS

Although counselling is widely recognized as a reasonable practice in so-called Western countries, it is certainly not the only approach to personal problem-solving. In particular, the client-centred approach to counselling, in which the person receiving counselling is encouraged to identify his or her own problems and also their solutions, is acceptable only in cultures that value individualism and the primacy of the individual. Anyone working in multicultural settings (and that must surely include most nurses) must remain sensitive to cultural differences among client groups. Although it is beyond the scope of this book to highlight particular cultural issues involved in counselling, it is valuable to note the following points, adapted from McLaren's[23] guidelines for multicultural counselling practice.

- There is no single concept of 'normality' that applies across all people, situations and cultures. Mainstream concepts of mental health and illness must be expanded to incorporate religious and spiritual elements. It is important to take a flexible and respectful approach to other therapeutic values, beliefs and traditions: we must each of us assume that our own view is culturally biased.
- Individualism is not the only way to view human behaviour, and must be supplemented by collectivism in some situations. Dependency is not a bad characteristic in many cultures.
- It is essential to acknowledge the reality of racism and discrimination in the lives of people, and in the therapy process. Power imbalances between therapists and clients may reflect the imbalance of power between the cultural communities in which they belong.

- Language use is important: abstract 'middle-class' psychotherapeutic discourse may not be understood by people coming from other cultures. Linear thinking/storytelling is not universal.
- It is important to take account of the structures within the client's community that serve to strengthen and support the client: natural supporting methods are important to the individual. For some clients, traditional healing methods may be more effective than Western forms of counselling.
- It is necessary to take history into account when making sense of current experience. The way that someone feels may not only be a response to what is happening now, but in part a response to loss or trauma that occurred in earlier generations.
- In some cultures, talking about your problems, to a stranger, is not usually an option. The tendency to disclose, in Western cultures is not universal. It may be possible to talk to family members and very close friends but even this is not always the way in which problems are managed. In some cultures, the role of a 'helper' is simply to cheer the other person up and try to distract them from their problems rather than to examine and explore them.
- Be willing to talk about cultural and racial issues and differences in counselling sessions.

Almost all of the above points can be adapted to communication in everyday nursing practice. It is easy, perhaps, for all of us to be ethnocentric – to believe that the way *we* do things is in some way the 'right' way. Only by studying cultures and by listening closely to what clients, patients and colleagues are telling us about other cultures will we begin to avoid this trap.

SUMMARY

Thus, we have come full circle. This chapter started by considering fundamental views we might have of human nature. It outlined the possibilities of *free will, determinism* and *fatalism*. It then explored a *general framework* for considering what we might do as counsellors. Finally, given that we almost all work in culturally mixed settings, it considered the cultural aspects of counselling. Any nurse hoping to help patients and clients through counselling might usefully consider, first, their own beliefs about the nature of people, followed by their views of the cultural contexts of different people. It should be noted, too, that different cultures place different emphases on the issue of free will and determinism. Although, as a general rule, many American and Northern European people will value free will, many people in Asian and other cultures will not. The idea that our particular belief system is in some way superior is only one more trap that the would-be counsellor can become ensnared in. We share the world with lots of different sorts of people. It is likely that

some will be helped by counselling and others will not. Counselling is usually a fairly non-invasive and inexpensive form of therapy, but it is by no means universally applicable. It should be the aim of every mental health and psychiatric nurse to be able to help select the most helpful therapy for *this* particular patient or client at *this* time. If it is decided that counselling might help, then the framework offered by Heron, in this chapter, can help to shape the counselling experience.

REFERENCES

1. Nelson-Jones R. *Essential counselling and therapy skills.* London, UK: Sage, 2002.

2. Burnard P. *Counselling skills for health professionals,* 3rd edn. Gloucester, UK: Stanley Thornes, 1999.

3. Hazzard A. Measuring outcome in counselling: a brief exploration of the issues. *British Journal of General Practice* 1995; **45**: 118–19.

4. Bower P, Byford S, Sibbald B *et al.* Randomised controlled trials of non-directive counselling, cognitive-behavioural therapy and usual GP care for patients with depression. II. Cost effectiveness. *British Medical Journal* 2000; **231**: 1389–92.

5. Roth A, Fonagy P. *What works for whom? A critical reader of psychotherapy research.* London, UK: Guilford Press, 1996.

6. Seligman M. The effectiveness of psychotherapy: the consumer reports study. *American Psychologist* 1995; **50**: 965–74.

7. Rowland N, Bower P, Mellor-Clark J *et al.* Counselling for depression in primary care (Cochrane review). *Cochrane Database of Systematic Reviews* 2001; Issue 1, Art No: CD001025.

8. Ward E, King M, Lloyd M *et al.* Randomised controlled trial of non-directive counselling, cognitive behaviour therapy and usual GP care for patients with depression. 1. Clinical effectiveness. *British Medical Journal* 2000; **321**: 1383–8.

9. Sibbald B, Ward E, King M. Randomised controlled trial of non-directive counselling, cognitive behaviour therapy and usual general practitioner care in the management of depression as well as mixed anxiety and depression in primary care. *Health Technology Assessment* 2000; **4**: 19.

10. Bedi N, Chilvers C, Churchill R *et al.* Assessing effectiveness of treatment of depression in primary care: partially randomised preference trial. *British Journal of Psychiatry* 2000; **177**: 312–18.

11. Chilvers C, Dewey M, Fielding K *et al.* Anti-depressant drugs and generic counselling for treatment of major depression in primary care: randomised trial with patient preference arms. *British Medical Journal* 2001; **322**: 775.

12. Stevenson L. *Seven theories of human nature.* Oxford, UK: Oxford University Press, 1987.

13. Sartre JP. *Being and nothingness.* New York, NY: Philosophical Library, 1956.

14. Sartre JP. *Humanism and existentialism.* London, UK: Methuen, 1973.

15. Van Deurzen-Smith E. *Existential counselling in practice.* London, UK: Sage, 1988.

16. Nelson-Jones R. *Essential counselling and therapy skills*. London, UK: Sage, 2002.

17. Hawton K, Salkovskis PM, Kirk J, Clark DM (eds). *Cognitive behaviour therapy for psychiatric problems – a practical guide*. Oxford, UK: Oxford Medical Publications, 1989.

18. Palmer S, Dainow S, Milner P (eds). *Counselling: The BAC counselling reader*. Rugby, UK: Sage Publications in association with the British Association for Counselling, 1996.

19. Heron J. *Six category intervention analysis*, 3rd edn. Guildford, UK: Human Potential Resource Group, University of Surrey, 1989.

20. Heron J. *A handbook of facilitator style*. London, UK: Kogan Page, 1989.

21. Blake RR, Mouton JS. *Consultation*. New York, NY: Addison Wesley, 1976.

22. Burnard P. *Learning human skills: an experiential and reflective guide for nurses and health care professionals*, 4th edn. Oxford, UK: Butterworth Heinemann, 2002.

23. McClaren MC. *Interpreting cultural differences: the challenge of intercultural communication*. Dereham, UK: Peter Francis, 1998.

CHAPTER 42

Bereavement and grief counselling

Clare Hopkins*

INTRODUCTION

Bereavement involves loss: of a person, object or state. *Grief* is the human emotion of that loss – 'a reaction of intense pining or yearnings for the object lost'.[1] *Mourning* is the behaviour that expresses grief over the loss. Loss is part of every human life, although the meanings and responses are unique. Each person's feelings of grief, and their expressions of mourning, will be influenced by the culture and society within which they live.[2]

The terms 'bereavement', 'grief' and 'mourning' are most usually connected with loss through death. However, bereavement can be experienced through any kind of loss: relationships ending; people losing their jobs; families breaking up; pets dying; miscarriage, stillbirth and infertility depriving us of the family we hoped for. When we cannot fulfil our life plans because of economic circumstances, unemployment, lack of choice, abuse or deprivation, physical or mental distress or disability, we may be bereaved of our *expectations*, and may grieve these losses. Receiving a diagnosis of illness – physical or mental – may bring pain and loss and this may cause the person (and their family) to grieve. Although this chapter focuses on loss and grief through death, its content applies equally to these other losses.

GRIEF AND LOSS

Perhaps the experiences of loss and grief are common because people, in general, have positive expectations about life. Anyone who can allow themselves to love is also open to the possibility of loss. As Parkes[1,p.1] writes:

> It is the very transience of life that enhances love. The greater the risk, the stronger grows the attachment. For most of us, the fact that one day we shall lose the ones we love, and they us, draws us closer to them but remains a silent bell that wakes us in the night.

How we are able to form bonds of affection that may predict our reaction to the loss of those bonds. Bowlby[3]

*Clare Hopkins is a Primary Care Mental Health Worker with Newcastle Primary Care Trust. She works with adults of working age suffering from common mental health problems. Her interests are in family therapy, crisis work and suicide/self-harm.

wrote extensively about attachment – the formation of these bonds and the importance of the quality of the early relationship between infants and their parents or carers for later psychological functioning.

He identified that these attachment bonds could be secure or insecure. The formation of secure attachment provides the child with a 'secure base'[4] from which to explore the world. Parkes[1,5] later expanded on this work by exploring the complicated interaction between early attachment styles, adult attachment and reactions to loss and bereavement. Bowlby[3] identified two categories of insecure attachment and this was later expanded (for a comprehensive review see Parkes[1]). Parkes[1] points out that all attachment styles may also be adaptive to situations, may have been essentially protective of the individual during their childhood and may be mediated in adulthood by the formation of a secure adult attachment.

Grief is an emotion expressed in every culture. We all react to loss but the meanings we give to loss will, to some extent, be dictated by the culture in which we live and this will influence the way in which we mourn. Grief can be seen as socially constructed, in terms of which losses are viewed as bereavement and processes of mourning are seen as acceptable. In this way, our culture, in the form of our regional, national, ethnic and religious affiliations will determine how we feel, perceive ourselves and act when faced with losses.[1,6]

We are all affected by our society's understandings of what represents loss and who is, by consequence, entitled to grieve and take part in public mourning and who is denied that right. For example, in Western cultures, which value the sanctity of marriage and the family, the widow's right to show publicly her distress at her husband's funeral will be seen as legitimate. A similar expression of grief from his extramarital lover might be heard with horror and, by consequence, invalidated. Society would expect her to grieve but that her expressions of grief should be muted and private.

Widespread expressions of grief over the death of well-known public figures (such as Diana, Princess of Wales) challenge personal understandings about grief. The mass media play a key role in both reporting and encouraging these expressions of public grief but then raise questions about their legitimacy.[7] Mass grief of this kind may represent an opportunity for individuals to safely express their own previously unmourned losses[8] but may also be symbolic of contemporary national concerns.[9]

NURSING AND LOSS

As nurses we will encounter people who have experienced losses of many kinds. Twenty-first-century families may be more often fragmented and geographically distant. Prior to the middle of the twentieth century, families were more likely to support their members at times of loss and this process was made clear through defined religious, funeral and mourning rituals.[10–12] This allowed for expressions of grief by the bereaved and also indicated the kind of support they could expect from others. In the twenty-first century, grief is often viewed as a medical responsibility.

THEORIES OF BEREAVEMENT AND GRIEF

Many twentieth-century writers have studied bereavement and developed theories that relate to the process of grief and mourning and the prevention of mental illness.

Elisabeth Kübler Ross[13] described the process of accepting the diagnosis of terminal illness. She identified a series of *stages* through which the dying person may pass. Rarely are these stages sequential, but often occur randomly and occasionally simultaneously.

- *Denial and isolation*. A necessary, though usually temporary, stage. Denial acts as a form of protection against overwhelming feelings of powerlessness and loss. Occasionally it may continue until death.
- *Anger*. Expressions of anger ('why me?') that they are facing death.
- *Bargaining*. Often described as an 'attempt to postpone' – bargaining may be with the person's conception of a Higher Being or with the staff who are treating them.
- *Depression*. A sense of loss and sadness, but perhaps also guilt, regret and helplessness.
- *Acceptance*. A stage 'almost devoid of feelings' but perhaps characterized by peace and acceptance.
- *Hope*. A complex state that can encompass hope of cure (a miracle) or hope for a pain-free death or hopefulness gained through a sense of acceptance of death.

Colin Murray Parkes[5] identified common factors in the grieving process found among young widows. He stressed that these are not clear-cut and there may be considerable oscillation between phases, and that it is never possible to predict a time-scale.

- *Searching*. Closely related to 'pangs' of grief that may be experienced spontaneously in the immediate post-bereavement stage and later in response to reminders. The bereaved may have a sense of the lost person being with them or may 'see' them.
- *Mitigation*. Ways in which the bereaved comfort themselves. This may include a sense of the 'presence' of the dead person, a sense of disbelief, avoidance of reminders, a sense of numbness or unreality. The dead person may be 'idealized'.
- *Anger and guilt*. Feelings of anger and irritability addressed either to the deceased or to others are

common. The loss may be perceived as a personal insult and blame apportioned to others or themselves.

- *Depression.* Sometimes expressed as apathy and despair.
- *Gaining a new identity.* Taking on roles previously carried out by their dead spouse in practical matters, personal mannerisms, characteristics and interests.

Studying partner loss, Wolfgang Stroebe and Margaret Stroebe[14] identified four possible phases:

- numbness
- yearning and protest
- despair
- recovery and restitution.

All these theories see grief following bereavement taking a broadly similar route, moving from shock and disbelief, through seeking and yearning for the lost person or object, to a state of abjection and depression. If the grieving process is uncomplicated, the person will gradually regain a sense of stability and will be able to carry on with their lives without the object of their loss.

However, these accepted theories of loss and grief have been challenged.[1,15,16] There is a growing understanding that culture influences grief as well as mourning, and there is no longer an acceptance that grief is complete once the bereaved person has 'moved on' from their loss and made new links with life. Newer theories suggest that, through conversation with other people who knew the lost person, the bereaved are able to integrate and experience an 'inner representation' of the deceased as part of the grieving process. There is also an increased acceptance that mourners may not 'get over it' or 'move on', but instead reach a sense of 'accommodation'. Accommodation is not a static phenomenon but 'is a continual activity, related both to others and to shifting self-perceptions as the physical and social environment changes and as individual, family and community developmental processes unfold'.[16]

PHYSICAL RESPONSES TO BEREAVEMENT

The bereaved person may also be at risk of health problems.[5,14] Loss and grief often result in changes in behaviour: for example, increased smoking or alcohol consumption, changes in eating patterns and self-neglect. The grieving person may also experience stress, which is related to increased rates of infection, cancer, coronary heart disease and gastrointestinal disorders such as ulcerative colitis and peptic ulcers.[14] There may also be an exacerbation of an existing condition.[5] Following the death of a loved one, the bereaved person may develop symptoms that mimic those of the person they are mourning,[17] or may experience greatly heightened feelings of anxiety or panic which may result in physical symptoms – tense muscles, racing heart, sweating, breathlessness, sleeplessness.

Personal illustration 42.1

Jeannie is 33, a solicitor who currently lives alone. Throughout her life she has experienced a series of traumatic losses, which culminated in a serious episode of depression 2 years ago. She was born the eldest of her parents' three children and remembers a secure childhood until she was 14, when her mother was diagnosed with cancer. Since then, everything changed and she, her sister and brother were often left to their own devices. Her mother's illness was never fully explained to the children – at the ages of 14, 12 and 6, they became watchful children picking up information about what was happening through half-understood overheard conversations and by the number of visitors to their home. Jeannie had just started her law degree when her mother died suddenly. Her father was grief-stricken and seemed unable to consider how his children were grieving. When she became pregnant at the age of 25 she was ambivalent about becoming a mother and was aware that her partner was not committed to the relationship. When she suffered a spontaneous miscarriage at 10 weeks she was surprised by the depth of her emotion, but she and her partner did not discuss what had happened; they split up soon afterwards.

When her younger brother Sam became depressed, she did everything she could to support him as she had when her mother died, but often felt less than equal to the task. When he went missing and was later found dead in his car, although distraught and overwhelmed by grief, she felt that it was best to 'get over it' and returned to work within 2 weeks.

Reflection

Think about the losses you have experienced: the death of a significant person in your life; when you failed to achieve your aims and grieved this loss. How did you feel? What did or did not help you to feel better?

WORKING WITH THE BEREAVED

There are many ways of working with people experiencing grief because of bereavement. The most generally accepted is the person-centred approach,[18] although other forms of grief work include a cognitive–behavioural approach to address complicated grief[19] and family-focused grief therapy.[20]

Central to person-centred counselling is the use of the 'core conditions' within the therapeutic relationship: warmth, empathy, genuineness and unconditional positive regard.[21] The person will need a safe environment in which to complete the 'work' of grieving. Family-focused grief work aims to reduce the negative effects of loss within the family by working with the family while the member who is approaching death is alive and continuing this work following their death.

Grief responses are highly individual. There is no right or wrong way to grieve and a wide spectrum of experiences are 'normal'. However, in the majority of cases the person who is grieving will need to be heard. At each stage of the grief process they will need to speak their thoughts aloud to try to make sense of them. As Parkes[1,p.258] says:

> while they are explaining themselves to us they are explaining themselves to themselves and this, it seems, is a therapeutic experience.

Describing events to a sensitive, empathic, non-judgemental listener will help the person, who is in the stage of numbness and disbelief, come to a gradual realization of their situation and its implications. It is vital to gain an understanding of the bereaved person's beliefs about what happens beyond death as this may affect their response to the loss.

If the person becomes agitated, angry, blaming or guilty, it is important that they are able to express these feelings in safety, without the need to fear that they will either overwhelm their listener or that their listener will reject them because they are expressing strong feelings.[22] By accepting and tolerating the person's strong feelings, the nurse can help the grieving person feel less overwhelmed, and to experience a sense of 'containment'. By being empathic to the content and the emotional expression of what the person is saying, and by being genuine in their responses to the person, the nurse can help the person to feel valued, when they may be experiencing threats to their sense of security and life aims.

People who are grieving may be vulnerable to suggestion. Being with someone who is grieving can be stressful. For this reason, family and friends – who may also be grieving or who may be exhausted from the business of supporting the grief-stricken individual – may tend to be directive and prescriptive. Comments such as 'time is a great healer', 'you'll get over it' or 'what you need is … !' will not only have no meaning for the person but may be perceived as insensitive and dismissive. The well-meaning phrase 'I know how you feel' is always inaccurate. Even if the person using the phrase has experienced a similar loss, it will never be the same loss.

> Jeannie was referred for help by her GP. Dr Smith knew of Jeannie's life story and wondered if her many losses might be affecting her mood. However, Jeannie did not think that this was the case and said that she 'just wanted to get on with my life'.

> At her first appointment with the nurse, Jeannie said quite firmly that she had 'got over' the traumatic death of her brother. Her body language too gave very clear messages to the nurse to stay away from any difficult subject. It appeared that she was 'frozen' and unable to talk about any of her feelings and she seemed simultaneously sad, angry and preoccupied with a sense that her world was out of control.

In 1982 Worden[23] published his work on grief counselling and grief therapy which highlighted the 'four tasks of mourning':

- to accept the reality of the loss
- to experience the pain of grief
- to adjust to an environment in which the deceased is missing
- to withdraw emotional energy and reinvest it in another relationship.

These 'four tasks' provide a framework for remaining flexible, receptive and reactive to the person's shifting and changing needs. It is vital to accept that 'people do not necessarily pass through the stages smoothly; indeed they may go through all the stages in the space of a few minutes'.[24] Change is an important feature of loss and bereavement – changes in roles, relationships, view of self and ways of coping.[25] Following the loss of a loved person, the world has changed for ever and nothing can reverse it. Adjustment to these changes is central to the grieving process, whether the person is accepting their loss and forming new relationships or developing a strong internalized representation of their loved one.

ACCOMPANYING THE GRIEVING PERSON

Hearing the story

People who have experienced loss need to tell their story and express their feelings to someone who can comprehend the significance. They may be hurt, angry, despairing, puzzled, uncomprehending but they will all need to talk, possibly going over the same story many times. Only those who are at the stage of incomprehension and disbelief may find difficulty in testing reality by talking to others. On these occasions the nurse has an important role in finding ways which are sensitive to help the person who is 'stuck' to talk about their loss.

Allowing Jeannie time and space to talk about her experience of life without suggesting that she concentrate specifically upon loss, gave her the opportunity to 'explain herself to herself'. She talked about what it had meant when her mother became unwell, how she had felt when her mother died and how her father's response to grief had cast her into the role of being responsible for everyone. It seems that the only way she could do this was by holding tightly to her distress and keeping it under control, a control which had begun to slip when she suffered the miscarriage and to shatter completely when her brother committed suicide.

When Jeannie began to express her feelings she also seemed to feel that the control she was striving for was moving further out of her grasp and she responded by becoming even more depressed and by herself having suicidal thoughts.

Solace can be gained by talking about the person with others who knew them, framing an enduring biography for the deceased, creating their ongoing presence in the lives of the living. At such times, the role of the listener is that of a helpful 'editor'. Walter[15] suggests that for this reason funeral rights are important. The British reticence in mentioning the dead, for fear of upsetting the person most intimately connected to them, prevents this healing process. There exists a similar reluctance to use the word 'dying' and to discuss what facing death might mean to all concerned.[26] Walter[15] suggests that bereavement is part of the process of each person's autobiography and that bereavement behaviour – grieving and mourning – are connected to the need to make sense of our own stories of who we are and who we have been.

Supporting

People who have experienced loss may value practical help in the aftermath of that loss. Often, they need to take on new roles and confront new experiences when their personal resources are low. They need help to gain information or encouragement when struggling to complete new tasks, solve problems and test reality. This is a subtle process and should not be confused with acting *for* or *giving advice* to the person. Rather it involves giving support in the process of regaining individual power and agency.

Part of the supportive role involves literally 'being beside' the person while they accomplish a painful healing task or ritual.

Nursing hope

Following loss, hope may be absent for a time. Life may seem pointless and the person's behaviour may reflect these feelings. Loss of hope may also lead to thoughts about suicide. The person may fantasize about the possibility of being 'reunited' with the lost person, leading them to ruminate about killing themselves.[5,27] This can become chronic. For some, such thoughts are profoundly shocking. They may perceive themselves as 'going mad' and feel distressed and ashamed.[28] Exploring these fantasies and establishing the level of risk is important. This delicate process requires us to ask about the thoughts the person finds most frightening and shameful, while reassuring them that such experiences are not unique and may be part of the grieving process. There is need for special vigilance when the loss has been traumatic and the process of mourning has become derailed, especially when suicide has occurred in a first-degree family member and symptoms of severe depression are present.[29]

Jeannie's experience of suicide within her family made her extremely vulnerable to having thoughts of wishing to die. The nurse enquired not only about her thoughts, plan and intent to carry these through but also sought to know the meaning of the thoughts for Jeannie. Her sense of intense grief was accompanied by feelings of the pointlessness of her existence. The belief that she had lost control of her life had caused her to think about taking the step that she felt would prove that she did in fact have the ultimate control.

Hope needs to be 'grounded in reality'.[30] Discussion of the 'hard facts' of a situation may need to be in 'bite size chunks' that can be easily digested.[28,30] Hope may reappear gradually and will need to be fostered slowly.[27,31,32] In its emerging state, hope may be different from that which existed before the loss. It may be fragile and subject to many reversals during the process of its reconstitution and needs to develop at its own pace. Having one's individual worth affirmed is hope-inspiring.[27] Cutcliffe's[33] work on the inspiration of hope in bereavement counselling suggests that the counsellor's ability to maintain hopefulness and to incorporate this implicitly into their work with the bereaved is essential. It seems that hope is something that we 'do together'.[34]

If the person is to regain hope then they must be able to imagine other possibilities, learn new roles and gain new skills.[30] People who have experienced loss may find that they experience guilt when hopefulness returns. They may feel – or others may imply – that there is something shameful in once more experiencing pleasure in life.[33] Asking what the deceased person would have wanted of them in such situations may help to challenge this sense of guilt and give them 'permission' to regain hope.

Many people do not wish to 'forget' or 'move on' from the person who is lost to them. Continuing to grieve may retain the dead person's presence in their life when letting go may feel frightening or disloyal.[35] This may be especially true for older people.[36] Mourners may be given the message that talking of their loss is only permissible for a defined period of time. If they also experience a sense that their loved one is 'still there' because they sense a 'presence' or some other physical experience, they may feel confused and alone until reassured that there is nothing abnormal about these experiences. Costello[37] described an elderly widow who, 4 months after her husband's death, experienced the bed 'sag' as if her husband was getting into it. When asked how this felt she said, 'Oh once I knew it was him I felt fine, in fact, it felt rather nice.'

> ## Reflection
>
> Think about ways in which you might nurture hope in someone who is grieving and also in the obstacles to inspiring hope under these circumstances.

NORMAL OR UNCOMPLICATED GRIEVING

Similarities exist between coming to terms with the prospect of loss of one's *own* life and the prospect of life without a *loved person* or a *lost dream*. Grief is necessarily a disorganized and painful process. However, 'normal' grieving will inevitably move towards being able to remember the deceased without discomfort or even with equanimity or pleasure. Estimates for the time it takes for an 'uncomplicated' grief to reach resolution vary considerably from months to years.

COMPLICATED GRIEF

Any form of grieving that does not lead to resolution of the symptoms of grief and the ability of the person to get on with their lives can be termed 'complicated' grief. The person may resolutely inhibit all signs of their grief or may experience a grief that fails to lessen and is not amenable to consolation over a long period of time. Specific circumstances are implicated.

The nature of the relationship with the deceased

- The loss of a partner or child is recognized as being especially significant.
- If a relationship was ambivalent or unresolved at the time of death, if the bereaved person was highly dependent upon the deceased or if they viewed them as an extension of themselves this may bring complications in mourning.

Where the loss is sudden, unexpected or untimely

- Although all deaths are 'untimely' to the mourners, with increasing age and infirmity friends and relatives often expect loss before it occurs.
- When the loss is through suicide, accident or sudden illness of a previously healthy person, or where a child dies, if the prospect of our own happy and fulfilling

life is snatched away without warning, the shock can be intense and the mourning process complex.
- Accidental deaths where there is no body to serve as the focus for grief, can present special complications.

Where many bereavements have occurred together or in quick succession

- If accident or illness claims several members of a family, the severity and enormity of the loss will be difficult to comprehend and to mourn.

How the losses occurred

- The dramatic nature of some deaths can complicate the grieving which follows. The sudden and often unpredictable nature of suicide, homicide or death in war/terrorist attacks may also bring unanswerable questions and a strong sense of 'unfinished business'. Guilt and anger, which are common in bereavement, may be felt strongly by the survivors of suicide. There may also be strong feelings of rejection and stigma, or even a sense of relief.[38,39] After a disaster, survivors may suffer a strong sense of 'survivor guilt'.[40]

When a loss re-evokes an insufficiently mourned previous loss

- Grief can often appear to others to be 'out of proportion' to the loss experienced. When this happens it is crucial to explore with the person what previous losses they have suffered as well as the meaning of those losses.
- Occasionally, people put their own mourning 'on hold' because they are dealing with the grief of others, until forced to mourn by new losses.

Personal vulnerability of the survivor

- This may include previous experience of mental illness, existing high levels of anxiety, or having a grief-prone personality, perhaps related to other bereavements or incomplete grieving of a previous loss.[5]
- Where there is no family or social support network to provide a buffer to grief.

> It took Jeannie a long time to allow herself to become connected to the sense of grief and loss, which she had carefully locked away. It was a painful journey and she shed many tears. The symptoms of depression and anxiety persisted over 6 months during which time she was unable to work. From time to time the suicidal thoughts returned, which she found very frightening. Nevertheless, she eventually began to share with friends and family the meaning of her loss and began to pick up the threads of her life. When she returned to work, she was convinced that she would not be able to cope and was very surprised to find she could. She is still very often sad, especially on significant days and anniversaries. However, now she can share fun with friends and enjoy activities.

BEREAVED CHILDREN

When children experience loss, they need a prompt, mindful and carefully articulated response. It is important to consider both their chronological and developmental age: research suggests that children do not begin to develop an understanding of death until they have achieved concrete operational thought, usually between 7 and 12 years.[41] To understand what has happened they need to comprehend that death is universal and irreversible. The language used about the death should be clear and unambiguous; terms such as 'passed away' or 'gone to heaven' may create confusion. The child should be encouraged to ask questions, even when the same question is asked repeatedly. Taking part in funerals and other bereavement rituals can help them to appreciate the finality of death. They will also need to be reassured that there will be someone there for all their needs even if they do not ask about this.

The child bereaved by suicide may be deeply traumatized, especially if present at the event or its aftermath. This may prevent them accessing happier, softer memories of the person who died.[42] Guilt is common following a suicide and if a child is at an early stage of ego development they may feel responsible. Therefore, it is important to ask the child why they think the death happened, offering an opportunity to talk about their fears.

ANTICIPATORY GRIEF

Forewarning of loss may allow for adjustment to loss. However, the bereavement experienced, for example, over a lengthy terminal illness may reduce in emotional intensity as death approaches, but may also lead to premature withdrawal from the dying person.[37]

THE LINK BETWEEN GRIEF AND MENTAL ILLNESS

Just as mental illness may be associated with many losses, grief may result in mental illness. Grieving people often feel as if they are 'going mad.'[5] They may 'see' the lost person or experience their 'presence'. This can be comforting or distressing. As we have already heard, grief can bring suicidal fantasies – feeling that they want to 'be with' the person they have lost; or the feeling of loss, loneliness and misery is so profound that they feel that they cannot carry on alone.[26]

It is common for the grieving person to experience extreme anxiety or episodes of panic. This is understandable. The loss may have robbed the person of the sense of certainty about life that we all take for granted, both their own and that of others. The physical experiences of the early stage of grieving – sighing, a sense of hollowness in the abdomen, restlessness, the need to swallow, are clearly linked to anxiety. The author C. S. Lewis described his experience of his wife's death:

> No one ever told me that grief felt so like fear. I am not afraid, but the sensation is like being afraid.[43]

Where death or loss has been traumatic – homicide, suicide or sudden death to which the person has been witness – there should be careful monitoring for the symptoms of post-traumatic stress disorder. This can be a complicated process as many of the symptoms are also present in 'ordinary' grieving. Maintaining this awareness and carefully monitoring will allow referral for specific trauma work should this become necessary.[44]

Sometimes bereavement will bring to light a mental illness that has existed for some time but has been masked. The lost person or object may have been a crucial element in helping the person in managing the symptoms; the stress of loss may disrupt a fragile coping strategy or the experience of grief may open up the possibility of 'legitimately' requesting help with the problem.

Reflection

Think about people you have met who have any form of mental illness. What losses may be part of having this kind of diagnosis? What kind of losses might precipitate mental illness? Can you identify any factors that might have been helpful and hope-inspiring for each individual in dealing with their losses?

SUMMARY

Bereavement, loss, grief and mourning are part of all our lives, although how we experience and act on them will be influenced by our own early experiences – our style of attachment – and the culture in which we live. As nurses we will encounter bereavement loss and grief in many, diverse forms. This offers a unique opportunity to listen when grief is expressed by the people whom we nurse, to support them in their grieving journey and to help them in regaining hope.

The main points of this chapter are summarized below.

- Bereavement is a universal experience. Grief and mourning are culturally mediated responses to loss of loved objects or expectations.
- Our individual style of attachment will influence our response to loss.
- 'Uncomplicated' grief will resolve over time, allowing the bereaved to remember the lost person without pain.
- Grief reactions may become 'complicated' and fail to resolve because of the nature of the relationship with the person who has died: if the bereavement has been traumatic, if a series of losses have remained unmourned or the bereaved person is vulnerable for some other reason.

- If grief fails to remit or is linked to traumatic loss, then it is important to monitor for post-traumatic symptoms, acute anxiety and depression.

REFERENCES

1. Parkes CM. *Love and loss. The roots of grief and its complications.* Hove, UK: Routledge, 2006.

2. Walter T. *On bereavement. The culture of grief.* Buckingham, UK: Open University Press, 1999.

3. Bowlby J. *Loss, sadness and depression. Attachment and loss,* vol. 3. London, UK: Penguin, 1980.

4. Holmes J. *The search for the secure base. Attachment theory and psychotherapy.* Hove, UK: Brunner-Routledge, 2001.

5. Parkes CM. *Bereavement. Studies of grief in adult life,* 3rd edn. Harmondsworth, UK: Penguin, 1996.

6. Reimers E. Bereavement – a social phenomenon? *European Journal of Palliative Care* 2001; **8** (6): 242–4.

7. Walter T, Littlewood J, Pickering M. Death in the news – the public invigilation of private emotion. In: Dickenson D, Johnson M, Samson Katz J (eds). *Death, dying and bereavement,* 2nd edn. London, UK: Open University/Sage, 2000: 14–27.

8. Durston D. Community rites and the process of grieving. In: Martin R, Anderson TY (eds). *Loss and bereavement. Managing change.* Oxford, UK: Blackwell Science, 1998: 213–31.

9. Merrin W. Crash, bang wallop! What a picture! The death of Diana and the media. *Mortality* 1998; **4**: 41–62.

10. Clark D. Death in Staithes. In: Dickenson D, Johnson M (eds). *Death, dying and bereavement.* London, UK: Sage, 2000: 4–11.

11. Firth S. Cross-cultural perspectives on bereavement. In: Dickenson D, Johnson M (eds). *Death, dying and bereavement.* London, UK: Sage, 2000: 254–62.

12. O'Gorman S. Death and dying in contemporary society: an evaluation of current attitudes and the rituals associated with death and dying and their relevance to recent understandings of health and healing. *Journal of Advanced Nursing* 1998; **27** (6): 1127–35.

13. Kübler Ross E. *On death and dying.* London, UK: Routledge, 1970.

14. Stroebe W, Stroebe MS. *Bereavement and health. The psychological and physical consequences of partner loss.* Cambridge, UK: Cambridge University Press, 1987.

15. Walter T. A new model of grief: bereavement and biography. *Mortality* 1996; **1** (1): 7–25.

16. Silvermann PR, Klass D. What's the problem? In: Klass D, Silverman PR, Nickman SL (eds). *Continuing bonds. New understandings of grief.* London, UK: Taylor and Francis, 1996: 3–27.

17. Martocchio BC. Grief and bereavement: healing through hurt. *Nursing Clinics of North America* 1985; **20**: 327–41.

18. Rogers C. *Client centred therapy.* Boston MA: Houghton Mifflin, 1965.

19. deGroot M, Keijser J, Neeleman J *et al.* Cognitive behavioural therapy to prevent complicated grief among relatives and spouses bereaved by suicide: cluster randomized controlled trial. *British Medical Journal* **334**: 994–1000.

20. Kissane D, Bloch S. *Family focused grief therapy.* Buckingham, UK: Open University Press, 2002.

21. Means D, Thorne B. *Person-centred counselling in action.* London, UK: Sage, 1988.

22. Clark A. Working with grieving adults. *Advances in Psychiatric Treatment* 2004, **10**: 164–70.

23. Worden JW. *Grief counselling and grief therapy.* London, UK: Tavistock Publications, 1983.

24. Tschudin V. *Counselling skills for nurses,* 4th edn. London, UK: Baillière Tindall, 1995.

25. Duke S. An exploration of anticipatory grief: the lived experience of people during their spouses' terminal illness and bereavement. *Journal of Advanced Nursing* 1998; **28** (4): 829–39.

26. Flaming D. Improve care and comfort: use the label 'dying'. *Journal of Palliative Care* 2000 **16**, 2, 30–6.

27. Cutcliffe J. Hope, counselling and complicated bereavement reactions. *Journal of Advanced Nursing* 1998; **28** (4): 754–61.

28. Parkes CM. Coping with loss: consequences and implications for care. *International Journal of Palliative Nursing* 1999; **5** (5): 250–4.

29. Stroebe M, Stroebe W, Abakoumkin G. The broken heart: suicidal ideation in bereavement. *American Journal of Psychiatry* 2005, **162**: 2178–80.

30. Hegarty M. The dynamic of hope: hoping in the face of death. *Progress in Palliative Care* 2001; **9** (2): 42–6.

31. Snyder CR. To hope, to lose, and to hope again. *Journal of Personal and Interpersonal Loss* 1996; **1**: 1–16.

32. Gamlin R, Kinghorn S. Using hope to cope with loss and grief. *Nursing Standard* 1995; **9** (48): 33–5.

33. Cutcliffe J. *The inspiration of hope in bereavement counselling.* London, UK: Jessica Kingsley, 2004.

34. Weingarten K. Witnessing, wonder and hope. *Family Process* **39** (4): 389–402.

35. Paul C. Guilt and blame in the grieving process. *Bereavement Care* **25** (3): 50–2.

36. Costello J. Grief and older people: the making and breaking of emotional bonds following partner loss in later life. *Journal of Advanced Nursing* 2000; **32** (6): 1374–82.

37. Costello J. Anticipatory grief: coping with the impending death of a partner. *International Journal of Palliative Nursing* 1999, **5** (5): 223–31.

38. Wertheimer A. *A special scar. The experiences of people bereaved by suicide,* 2nd edn. London, UK: Routledge, 2001.

39. Parkes CM. After a terrorist attack. Supporting the bereaved families. *Bereavement Care* 2001; **20** (3): 35–6.

40. Hodgkinson P, Stewart, M. *Coping with catastrophe.* London, UK: Routledge, 1991.

41. Mitchell A, Wesner S, Brownson L *et al.* Effective communication with bereaved child survivors of suicide. *Journal of Child and Adolescent Psychiatric Nursing* **19** (3): 730–6.

42. Trickey D. Young people bereaved by suicide: what hinders and what helps. *Bereavement Care,* **24** (1): 11–14.

43. Lewis CS. *A grief observed.* London, UK: Faber, 1961.

44. Turnbull G, Gibson M. The aftermath of traumatic incidents. *Bereavement Care* 2001; **20** (1): 3–5.

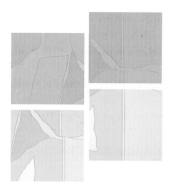

CHAPTER 43

Cognitive–behavioural therapy

Paul French*

INTRODUCTION

Despite the fact that cognitive–behavioural therapy (CBT) has been around for some time, the last few years have seen a growing interest in this form of psychological intervention. Training courses have developed to capitalize on this current interest; however, not all deliver the same high degree of skill acquisition. Some people believe that attending short courses can equip them with the necessary skills to deliver CBT, which is clearly not the case. Recognized courses, which provide up-to-date knowledge of developments in cognitive theory and provide clinical supervision by experienced therapists, may be costly but worthwhile. If individuals are adequately trained and have access to regular clinical supervision within a CBT framework, there is no reason why clinicians from any background cannot provide CBT. Many nurse therapists now practise CBT at the highest level. Recent developments in the UK in the provision of access to psychological therapy have further extended this interest.

This chapter will explain the framework of CBT and highlight the application of this approach with a personal illustration, using the approach to CBT developed by Aaron T. Beck, in which the author has most experience.

RATIONALE

CBT has evolved over a number of years, predominantly through the work of Beck[1] and Ellis.[2] This form of therapy has been widely adopted, originally as a specific treatment for depression, and now as a treatment option for a diverse range of problems.

Over 20 years ago a treatment manual was developed, which allowed CBT for depression to be taught, replicated, standardized and researched.[3] Since then several research trials have tested the efficacy of CBT in treating depression and the evidence clearly identifies CBT as a useful treatment option.[4–7] CBT was found to be *as effective* as medication in terms of treating the depressive episode but, significantly, also helped to protect the person against future relapse.[8] This is clearly important in terms of long-term management strategies, not only for the client and family, but also offsetting cost issues associated with the treatment. CBT aims to teach the person new skills in managing their depressive symptoms, whereas medication merely reinforces the medical model of the illness and the need for further intervention should symptoms occur in the future. Therefore, this skill acquisition is associated with reduced chance of relapse.

*Paul French is Associate Director of the Early Intervention Services based at Bolton, Salford and Trafford Mental Health Trust, UK. He has worked in mental health since 1986 with a particular interest in services for people with psychosis.

Cognitive therapy is often represented as a cold, clinical and technique-driven form of therapy. How would you sell it to a client?

These factors have led to the popularity of CBT as a treatment option. The initial treatment manual for depression has been applied to other psychological disorders, such as panic disorder,[9] obsessional disorders[10,11] and more recently psychotic disorders.[12] Despite their diversity each have models that allow a cognitive conceptualization of the problem, identifying specific treatment interventions that apply to it.

Cognitive theory of psychopathology is constructed around information processing[13] that is considered to be faulty, maintaining the psychological disorder. This is accessible in the conscious state through *negative automatic thoughts*, which emerge from the schemas that have a dysfunctional element to them. Automatic thoughts can be a stream of thoughts that just seem to enter our minds. For some people these thoughts can be in the form of mental images. The purpose of the therapy is to assist the client to recognize these thoughts and teach methods to challenge them, usually through the dysfunctional thought record (dtr),[3] which has since been further developed.[14]

Negative automatic thoughts are, by definition, negative in content and pop into our mind spontaneously, hence with no control over them. They frequently happen at times of uncertainty or stress. Hence when a person is in the midst of a depressive or anxious state then their occurrence is generally more frequent. These thoughts trigger certain emotions and subsequently certain patterns of behaviour, which frequently maintain them. This can be in seen Figure 43.1.

In Figure 43.1 we can see that the event itself does not necessarily *result* in depression or sadness, rather it is the *interpretation of the event* that determines or mediates the subsequent mood. Following from this the mood can determine the behavioural response to the original triggering event and this behaviour can maintain the original belief. What this indicates is that it is not necessarily the events themselves which lead to distress, rather it is how we make sense of these events. Enabling an individual to recognize patterns of thoughts, which may have become distorted, is a vital component of CBT. Developing skills to challenge these distorted patterns of thinking in a structured manner, by examining all available evidence, is the next step in assisting the individual to overcome these difficulties.

At this point critics of CBT may point out that an individual may have good reason to feel distress regarding an event, or their belief about an event may be an accurate evaluation. This can be the case in many situations and it is not the aim of CBT to encourage people to think in a positive manner contrary to popular belief. The aim of CBT is to enable people to *understand* how they think about situations, and enhance their ability to evaluate their thoughts based on available evidence, as opposed to a gut reaction based on intuition. If people are evaluating events accurately and they feel upset about these things, they should be encouraged to undertake alternative strategies to manage their distress such as develop problem-solving skills.

WHAT ARE THE COMPONENTS OF CBT?

CBT is a short-term, structured approach to therapy. A problem list is developed with the individual and these problems are systematically targeted throughout the therapy process with cognitive formulations developed to understand these problems.

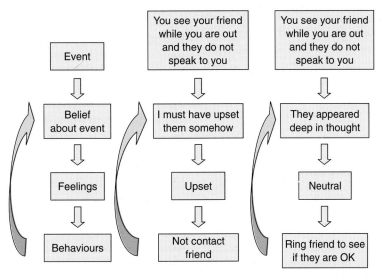

Figure 43.1 Maintenance formulations indicating the different emotional and behavioural responses elicited through appraising a single event in multiple ways

Structure

CBT is associated with a structured approach to therapy, which can be off-putting at first. However, this structured approach allows a means of maximizing the time spent in therapy and ensures that the individual has their problems prioritized and dealt with in a collaborative manner. This means that there is a set pattern associated with a CBT session, which can be seen below.

Brief review

This allows the individual to summarize what has been happening to them since the last therapy session without getting bogged down in details that may have little part to play in the problems.

Agenda setting

This involves developing a collaborative agenda of topics to be covered during the session, which is prioritized and time is allocated to each item on the agenda. Factors influencing agenda items will include the stage in therapy; joint prioritization of problems; items put on the agenda from previous sessions; and finally any hidden agendas.[2] Setting the agenda allows the session to proceed in a structured manner and without it discussion can often drift with no specific purpose; it can be seen as the first step in socializing the patient to the model.

Feedback

This allows a process of checking out what was or was not useful regarding the previous session. It also ensures that any potential miscommunication is clarified straight away. Feedback should also be utilized throughout the therapy session and each agenda item summarized to ensure understanding.

Homework review

Homework is set following a therapy session in order to test out or monitor items that have been discussed within session. This is an important part of therapy, allowing in-session skills to be transferred and tested in a real world setting. If someone is going to the trouble to undertake homework then there should be a point in the session that is dedicated to wanting to know the results of this. If the therapist does not ask about results of homework then the individual may feel what is the point of it.

Main agenda Item

This entails focusing on the main concerns the individual has raised, discussing them in greater detail, developing a cognitive formulation of the problem and collaboratively discussing strategies to overcome these problems.

Set homework

The process of setting homework to be undertaken between therapy sessions can be quite difficult. This important aspect of therapy should have sufficient time allocated in order to consider what task could be undertaken, and a useful strategy is to ask the individual what they think they should do for homework.

Feedback

This involves checking the content of the session to ensure that client and therapist felt understood in the things they were discussing.

Reflection

Do you think that too much structure can inhibit a session?

Structure is vital to the delivery of CBT, providing a framework for its delivery. There are a number of other skills that need to be integrated into this framework. Many people assume that the structure of therapy indicates a cold and sterile approach. However, this is not the case and the usual therapeutic skills of warmth, trust and honesty are valued as highly as the other elements of CBT and, indeed, are felt to be a prerequisite to providing therapy.

The cognitive therapy scale (CTS)[15] provides a check that the structure is being adhered to but also provides a means of measuring the other skills associated with CBT. This scale defines the 13 core components of cognitive therapy and rates each item between 0 and 6, which can be marked accordingly as the therapist develops in competency. The CTS has been seen to be reliable and valid when measuring therapist competency[16] and is used to rate videotape, audiotape or live observation rather than the therapist's perception of what took place during therapy. It is this ability to rate a therapist's performance that has enabled this type of psychological therapy to be used within research settings, because it is possible to state whether a therapist is doing CBT or not.

A major component of CBT is that it should be undertaken in a questioning style, which is termed *guided discovery*. This means that instead of the therapist providing ready-made solutions to problems, they work with the individual in an attempt to allow them to come to conclusions themselves. This can be particularly challenging for a therapist to undertake, especially if they have been brought up in a culture where it is assumed that they have specialist knowledge and know best. However, providing ready-made solutions does not allow the individual the opportunity to learn how to overcome the problems. The process of guided discovery attempts to guide the individual towards an understanding of their difficulties, how they came about and how they are maintained.

These processes are drawn up in a formulation describing the individual's problems. Next, potential strategies can be discussed and subsequently tested, to see whether they work. This process of guiding the individual towards coming up with their own solutions means that the person holds this information with a great deal more passion than they would if provided with a 'ready-made' solution. Through guided discovery, the individual is encouraged to develop a thorough understanding of their problems themselves in order to become their own therapist in the future, which could then impact on future episodes of illness.

Case formulation

A formulation relating to the development and maintenance of problems is a vital aspect of the therapy. Without a clear formulation interventions can be seen as a haphazard application of techniques without any rationale for their use. A formulation should be developed early in therapy generally within sessions one and two, although the formulation should be added to throughout the therapy process and in light of any data generated by experiments. Therapists should be aware of the variety of formulations for individual disorders and utilise these models and the indicated intervention strategies allied to them.

Personal illustration 43.1

Jane was seen following a referral by her GP because of concerns about a postnatal depressive illness. Jane had a 5-week-old baby daughter called Karen. Jane had been in hospital for 4 days following the birth of Karen, during which she felt quite well; however, as soon as she returned home she started to experience overwhelming feelings that Karen would die. Jane was extremely tearful and depressed and had little or no appetite and was extremely reluctant to let her child out of her sight because of fears over her safety. Jane was unable to leave Karen alone with anyone, feeling that she was the only person able to look after her properly. This included her mother and the baby's father, Joe. At times Jane feels that Karen gets so upset that she will die. Jane has developed a strict routine and is unable to vary from this, e.g. Karen must be woken up at certain times in order to be fed, if this does not happen she feels the baby may not have the energy to wake up and may die.

CHALLENGING NEGATIVE AUTOMATIC THOUGHTS

A clear focus of therapy was to access negative automatic thoughts and work scientifically and collaboratively to examine these thoughts. Jane's fears had a definite pattern in that she believed her baby was going to die. This could be because it got upset, which she could not really explain just that if the baby got so upset it might die. Or, because of a feeling that someone might harm the baby. An example of this was when Jane attended the local baby clinic. The doctor gave Karen an injection and physical examination causing the baby to cry. This led to Jane thinking that the doctor deliberately wanted to harm her

and Jane held this belief with a conviction of 10/10. This belief was challenged utilizing the technique of 'evidence for and against', with a result that the conviction level was reduced to 3/10. There was also a shift in emotion with fear being initially 10/10 and reduced to 4/10. Further sessions focused upon challenging negative automatic thoughts, and in one session Jane explained that when she went to the doctors the doctor measured Karen's head twice and this indicated that there was something wrong with Karen. Jane believed this with a conviction of 9/10 and an emotion of fear 8/10. This was understood and formulated as previously discussed (Figure 43.2).

Again the technique of evidence for and against was utilized as this seemed the most appropriate and Jane's conviction decreased to 4/10 in her original belief, and fear to 5/10 associated with the situation. An alternative thought about the situation was then generated based on the evidence, which was that perhaps the doctor had become distracted by one of the other babies crying and forgot the original measurement or perhaps just wanted to check it.

Jane would frequently utilize checking behaviours in order to prove to herself that Karen was not ill. A major checking behaviour that prevented disconfirmation was to check Karen's temperature frequently throughout the day. Jane would have the thought that something was wrong with Karen and become frightened and need to check her temperature; if she did not do this then Karen might die. An experiment was set up to help with this behaviour.

During the initial phase we focused upon the thought that Karen could die. The behaviour, which prevented disconfirmation, was the checking behaviour related to temperature. In order to challenge this behaviour we set up the experiment, which consisted of Jane not checking the temperature unless there was significant evidence to warrant this.

We thoroughly explored the occasions and reason behind temperature checking, going to great lengths to emphasize what the experiment was about. Jane should check her temperature if there was evidence for this; however, if there was no evidence for checking this may suggest there was no need for doing this. We generated a list of things that might indicate the need to check Karen's temperature, and if none of these things were present then Jane would not check. However, if there were any conditions on her list then Jane was quite correct to check her temperature. Jane felt that she usually checked the temperature when Karen was upset, so these were identified as high-risk times.

Jane understood the rationale behind this experiment and recognized that her checking behaviours had become a problem. She was now secretly checking the temperature and the frequency had increased to around eight or nine times per day.

Jane was exposed to the situation as a homework task to be carried out each day until we next met, which would be 4 days, and during that time she was going to

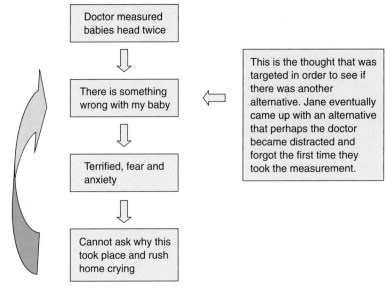

Figure 43.2 Individualized maintenance formulation

TABLE 43.1 Number of behavioural responses following problematic cognitions

Days	Number of times had the thought to check temperature	Number of times actually checked the temperature
Day 1	8	0
Day 2	9	0
Day 3	8	0
Day 4	7	0
Total	32	0

try to check the temperature only if any of the conditions on her list were present.

At our next session Jane was incredibly enthusiastic to recount the details of this experiment and the results are shown in Table 43.1.

Despite having this thought that she must check Karen's temperature 32 times over the 4 days, she did not check it once and actually reported that Karen appeared much more settled in her behaviour. There was also an observation by Jane that she tended to have the checking thought more when Karen was asleep, which she had not expected. This does, however, fit with Karen being more settled in that she was not being woken up several times a day to have her temperature monitored; this was a conclusion Jane arrived at and the experiment appeared to have a strong element of guided discovery about it. Her thoughts about temperature checking reduced over the next few weeks.

The next session focused upon another of the vicious cycles highlighted in the formulation. This was to do with Jane believing that if Karen got herself upset and tearful then she could die. This led to Jane feeling that she had to

be with her all the time to prevent her from getting upset. Guided discovery was utilized to ascertain the reasoning behind this train of thoughts. It transpired that Jane became extremely anxious, soon after she left hospital with Karen and experienced what sounded like a panic attack with the usual associated catastrophic misinterpretations. Subsequently she attributed her feelings to the baby and felt that if Karen becomes upset then she might die.

In order to tackle this we utilized some educational material about panic and anxiety and their associated symptoms. This equipped Jane to understand the physiological symptoms she was experiencing. We also arranged to go out of the house for a short walk to simulate a trigger situation for her anxiety symptoms. This again was negotiated with collaboration being a key factor. Jane was actually quite anxious about trying it but went through with the experiment as we had planned. Her partner was going to look after Karen while we were out of the house. Jane explained that she started to get anxious as soon as we left the house complaining of physiological symptoms, initially concerned with her breathing. The strategy employed was to allow disconfirmation of her catastrophic misinterpretation of this event. As we walked Jane realized that she was not going to stop breathing and began to relax a little more. The main purpose of the exercise was to demonstrate to Jane that becoming anxious and subsequently upset would not lead to death. This is what she envisaged would happen to Karen. On return from the walk, Jane was able to recognize that her interpretation of bodily sensations was not what she initially expected.

The final vicious cycle was to do with her belief that if she thought something then it would happen. It transpired that she frequently experiences what she describes as bad thoughts and then these become stronger and stronger in her mind till she cannot get rid of the thought and believes that it will happen. This becomes worst if she speaks her thoughts out loud because this adds further weight to her belief. Her strategy for dealing with this was through the use of thought suppression, although this appeared ineffective. Her compulsive thoughts followed a typical ego dystonic pattern in that she thought about her baby dying. In order to plan a strategy to overcome this problem Jane was introduced to the analogy of trying not to think of a green rabbit for a full half minute. This enabled her to recognize the difficulties inherent in attempting thought suppression and the fact that things can become worst. She was also introduced to some normalizing data and encouraged to undertake a polling experiment whereby she asked five other mothers whom she considered to be good parents if they had experienced thoughts that their children might die. Alongside this we planned a further experiment feeling flushed by success from the previous ones. (This had actually given Jane an incredible belief in the model and she readily accepted the fact that things could change and undertook homework assignments with great vigour.) The results from her polling experiment were that 5/5 parents had experienced thoughts that their children might die.

We decided to use the previous exercise of going for a walk but focusing upon alternative cognitions. Previously, when Jane had tried to go out of the house leaving Karen behind, she had gone with a close family member. That person had encouraged her to utilize suppression (unknowingly), telling Jane not to think about Karen. Unfortunately this led to strong thoughts of Karen and that she was screaming, and this activated strong visual imagery that Karen was becoming extremely upset and could die. We planned to go out of the house and Jane was going to be allowed to talk about her feelings and thoughts and not attempt to suppress them in an attempt at habituation training.

As soon as we left the house Jane started to experience thoughts that Karen was becoming upset. We explored these thoughts and discussed them in detail as we walked along. Jane felt that her anxiety levels changed from 3/10 before we left the house to 9/10 when we got out of the house and subsequently reduced to 4/10 after we had been walking for a period of time. This gave Jane the confidence she required to practise this method and stop the avoidance and suppression, which had not been working.

Jane continued to improve and a blueprint of what had taken place in therapy was devised. This consisted of the formulations and how we had arrived at them, the experiments we had undertaken and the results we had achieved and techniques we had utilized to challenge some of her cognitions. In short, it is a summary of therapy, and this is provided as a prompt for the client if such problems should arise again in the future. It can provide a guide in terms of self-help material with the aim of preventing future relapse by encouraging early intervention with problems.

Reflection

How might you describe CBT to a client new to this form of therapy?

SUMMARY

CBT is very much in vogue at present, with many people wanting to develop skills in this form of therapy. The reasons for the success of CBT lie in the results it has achieved through research trials, thereby meeting the criteria of evidence-based practice. At times critics challenge CBT therapists, regarding their philosophy and approach and expect an almost fanatical defence of CBT; however, most CBT therapists have a fanatical belief in what works for their clients. So if an alternative therapy comes along with greater evidence to suggest its ability to impact upon our clients' problems, most would happily adopt this type of intervention. However, at the present time, CBT appears to provide the most useful form of psychological therapy that can impact upon a wide variety of problems experienced by our clients.

For many years I worked as a community psychiatric nurse with people with serious mental health problems, predominantly schizophrenia. During that time I felt that I worked hard to develop relationships with people and understand their problems. However, almost without exception when someone I was working with started to express some concern that things were getting worse, such as increased voices or distress regarding their delusions, my intervention was to become a taxi. We would jump in the car and go and see a psychiatrist to get their medication reviewed. I always felt that this was not a particularly good nursing intervention.

Since I developed skills in CBT, I now feel as though I have an armoury of tools at my disposal that can be used *before* becoming a taxi. These frequently have a positive effect and it has enabled me and the individual to feel empowered to tackle problems without constantly settling for the taxi option. I believe that my nursing background has given me a unique opportunity to deliver these interventions to people in extremely difficult situations and believe that nurses are ideally placed to deliver these interventions.

REFERENCES

1. Beck AT. *Depression: clinical, experimental and theoretical aspects.* New York, NY: Harper & Row, 1967.

2. Ellis A. *Reason and emotion in psychotherapy.* New York, NY: Lyle Stuart, 1962.

3. Beck AT, Rush AJ, Shaw BF, Emery G. *Cognitive therapy of depression*. New York, NY: John Wiley & Sons, 1979.

4. Rush AJ, Beck AT, Kovacs M, Hollon SD. Comparative efficacy of cognitive therapy and pharmacotherapy in the treatment of depressed outpatients. *Cognitive Therapy and Research* 1979; **1**: 17–37.

5. Blackburn IM, Bishop S, Glen AIM *et al.* The efficacy of cognitive therapy in depression: a treatment trial using cognitive therapy and pharmacotherapy, each alone and in combination. *British Journal of Psychiatry* 1981; **139**: 181–9.

6. Simons AD, Murphy GE, Levine JE, Wetzel RD. Cognitive therapy and pharmacotherapy for depression: sustained improvement over one year. *Archives of General Psychiatry* 1986; **43**: 43–9.

7. Hollon SD, Shelton RC, Loosen PT. Cognitive therapy and pharmacotherapy for depression. *Journal of Consulting and Clinical Psychology* 1991; **59**: 88–99.

8. Blackburn IM, Eunson KM, Bishop S. A two year naturalistic follow up of depressed patients treated with cognitive therapy, pharmacotherapy and a combination of both. *Journal of Affective Disorders* 1986; 10: 67–75.

9. Clark DM. A cognitive model of panic. *Behaviour Research and Therapy* 1986; **24**: 462–70.

10. Salkovskis PM. Obsessional compulsive problems: a cognitive behavioural analysis. *Behaviour Research and Therapy* 1985; 23: 571–83.

11. Wells A. *Cognitive therapy of anxiety disorders: a practice manual and conceptual guide*. Chichester, UK: John Wiley & Sons, 1997.

12. Morrison AP. The interpretation of intrusions in psychosis: an integrative cognitive approach to hallucinations and delusions. *Behavioural and Cognitive Psychotherapy* 2001; **29**: 257–76.

13. Beck AT. Cognitive models of depression. *Journal of Cognitive Psychotherapy* 1987; **1**: 5–37.

14. Greenberger D, Padesky CA. *Mind over mood: change how you feel by changing the way you think*. New York, NY: Guilford Press, 1995.

15. Young J, Beck AT. Cognitive therapy scale: rating manual. Unpublished manuscript, University of Pennsylvania, Philadelphia, 1980.

16. Dobson K, Shaw B, Vallis T. Reliability of a measure of cognitive therapy. *British Journal of Clinical Psychology* 1985; **24**, 295–300.

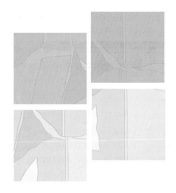

CHAPTER 44

Using solution-focused approaches

Denise Webster*

INTRODUCTION

As the name implies, solution-focused therapy (SFT) focuses on solutions and, some would say, does not even have to define the 'presenting problem' in any detail to be effective. At its inception, SFT was seen as a brief therapy, and the emphasis was on rapid resolution of a circumscribed problem. Although this is still a valid focus for the therapy, SFT has since been used successfully with people who may require ongoing support or with multiple problems.

SFT is an approach to working with clients that can be extremely challenging for counsellors who are comfortable with being simply a caring, reflective listener and/or focusing on clients' problems. Although many of the necessary skills are shared by other schools of therapy, the underlying assumptions about how to help people may be diametrically opposed to other forms of therapy.

As in *cognitive–behavioural therapy*, there is an expectation that the therapist is active, focusing on what is occurring in the present, recognizing that clients need resources to manage their situation. However, solution-focused therapists do not use programme-based, psychoeducational interventions for specific problems. Nor do they believe that noticing more about the problem is likely to be helpful. They also believe that clients already have most of the resources they need to effectively manage their situation. Both these resources and the way the client views the situation are likely to be unique.

Furthermore, a focus on a specified preferred future is central to a solution-focused approach. The explicit central belief in cognitive–behavioural theory – that faulty thinking is responsible for ineffective coping *and* must be challenged – is contrary to a solution-focused philosophy, which accepts clients' realities as valid *for them*. Unlike psychodynamic approaches, there is no attempt to determine the *source* of the situation (not automatically called a 'problem'), either in the client's personal and family history, or in the identification of *motives* (conscious or unconscious) or defence mechanisms. Although there is an explicit attempt to develop a strong relationship as a client advocate, there is no attempt to discuss the therapeutic relationship itself or to offer theory-based interpretations of material the client presents. The concept of 'resistance' is seen by solution-focused therapists as a problem the therapist has *with hearing the client*, rather than a client's problem in accepting the therapist's interpretations.

Evolving from the therapy approaches modelled by Milton Erickson[1] SFT has been called:

- a form of *hypnotic therapy*, to the degree that it utilizes a hypothetical preferred future (a form of hypnotic 'crystal-ball gazing');

*Denise (Denny) Webster is Professor Emerita from the University of Colorado at Denver and Health Sciences Center. She has taught, practised and written about solution-focused therapy for nearly 20 years. She currently enjoys family, fibre art and retirement in Georgia.

- a form of *strategic therapy*, (paradoxical interventions);
- a pattern intervention as well as a 'radical constructivist' therapy[2] because it supports the concept of multiple realities, all of which are dependent on how an individual 'constructs' both problems and solutions to problems.

The last view situates SFT as a *language-based* or *narrative therapy* that helps clients retell their 'stories' in ways that uncover positive interpretations and possibilities for change.

Reflection

Think of a 'problem' you have experienced.

- How did you begin to solve it?
- What aspect of yourself, or your life experience, played a part in moving through or beyond this problem?

CORE PRINCIPLES

Assumptions

SFT is not based on explicit theories of personality, psychopathology, aetiology or pathology. A successful solution-focused therapist has a positive philosophy about human potential, the human condition and the inevitability of change in the lives of humans, as in all life cycles. As a health-oriented, strength-based approach to helping people, the therapist seeks evidence of competency, rather than failure or weakness. Because the psychiatric language tends to be pathologizing, diagnosis or other forms of labelling is avoided. Identifying a client's 'defence mechanisms', whether or not these are interpreted to clients, would be seen as both pathologizing and distorting the client's story, whereas learning about clients' unique ways of *coping* would be honouring differences that can be developed to facilitate solutions. Clients' world views, values and language provide the framework for identifying relevant solutions and ways to achieve them. Realistically, many clients enter therapy with a well-developed language of problems and the therapist has the challenge of using the client's language and helping them shift their language to how they would describe the absence of the problem. For example, clients may label themselves as 'depressed'. In developing a 'picture' of what it's like *not* to be depressed, one person may describe an ability to be in a meaningful relationship, whereas others may describe having the energy to return to mountain climbing or finding everyday activities less stressful and more rewarding.

Both the acceptance of clients' realities and language and the search for the language of solutions are grounded in an acceptance of multiple realities or multiple, equally plausible, interpretations of any situation. People have a *unique* definition of their situation and what would be a 'solution' to any problem. This precludes the use of most problem-based programmes, which rely on the shared dimensions of human experience and generic theories about problem intervention.

The relationship

The development and maintenance of the therapeutic relationship is paramount in SFT. The therapist must be active and develop a collaborative, egalitarian relationship with the client. The therapist may define him or herself as an expert at helping people discover solutions. Clients are, however, the *most important experts*: they know most about their situation, circumstances, resources, and what they think is most likely to be helpful. The therapist practises '*radical acceptance*', respecting the client's expertise, all the time trying to frame questions that will communicate understanding of the client's view and support for their efforts.

Solution-focused counsellors are aware that clients can become overly dependent on the counsellor when the therapy process is prolonged. Therefore, conscious efforts are made to identify important relationships outside therapy (family, friends, community resources), encouraging clients to develop these 'natural' connections, which will be enduring after the immediate need for counselling has been met.

Role of change

'Change' in SFT is seen as inevitable, since nothing stays the same, people change in response to changes in circumstance, development, life experience and their perspectives. 'Readiness to change', then, is less about the client's motivation than about having found a goal and approach to a solution that is important to the client. deShazer's[1] early description of SFT identified client's 'relationship to the problem' (and by implication to the therapist) to help counsellors match homework assignments to the client's relationship to the problem and how much clients believe they can influence the situation. For example, if a client is sent for therapy, by a court, to address a problem they believe was not their fault, they would not be motivated to work on remedying that problem. This is not dissimilar from the problem of parents bringing in a child who thinks the parents are unreasonable and don't understand the situation. In both examples, however, the 'identified client' might be motivated to avoid further problems with the law or parents and/or to get them to 'stop picking on' him or her. If the 'client' does not describe having any relationship to the problem, they would be considered a 'visitor' and would be thanked for their time and openness to providing information about their unique perspective. If clients recognize that there is a problem that is affecting them, but feel they have no real role in changing the situation, they would be considered a 'complainant' and would be given homework assignments to help them gather information about the situation (specifically when it does *not* occur, as described below). Clients who believe they can have some influence in changing the situation would be considered 'customers' and would be given homework tasks that would build on their predisposition to 'do' something active, the specifics of which would very likely be unique to the client and situation.

Solution-focused questions

Defining and refining the focus of therapy and unique client solutions is dependent on the questions posed by the therapist. Questions are generally directed towards real world, present and future-oriented phenomena in the context of real relationships, i.e. those occurring outside the therapy session, in everyday circumstances. If time limitations are part of the reality, then these will be built into the questions. For example, if only eight visits are allowed, goals and solutions will be based on what can be realistically addressed within that time, and specific ways to generalize what is being learned to times and situations beyond that period will be explored. The client's past is explored by the therapist, only for the purpose of identifying forgotten resources and coping strategies, or to draw parallels between other times that once felt difficult and were successfully managed or are now seen more positively than they initially were seen.

- *Presuppositional questions* utilize 'presuppositional' language – i.e. they *imply* that a future experience is likely to be successful by using '*when*', rather than '*if*' when exploring the possible consequences of various solutions.
- *Pre-session change questions* build on observations that 'doing something', such as making an appointment, is already the *beginning* of a positive momentum. For example, 'we have noticed that sometimes/often between the time someone makes an appointment [or has sought other help] some things are already better. What have you *noticed* since [you made the appointment]?
- *Exceptions questions* focus on 'when the problem is *not* occurring'. Avoiding 'problem talk' can be difficult unless alternatives to the problem are identified. There are several approaches (locating, identifying, unearthing, naming) to exceptions. For example, after learning what brought the client to therapy, the therapist might ask: 'Can you tell me about the time when [name for the problem] has either not been present when it might have been', or 'was not as big a problem' or 'was not so distressing?' 'What was different about those times'? Another way is to begin the first session with the question, 'when you no longer feel the need to [seek therapy *or* come here] what will be different in your life?'
- The '*Miracle question*' also identifies possible *exceptions*, by projecting a possible future in which the problem no longer exists. When possible, the language used should reflect some awareness of the client's background or beliefs. For example, 'I'd like you to pretend for a moment that when you go to sleep tonight, during the night, a miracle happens, and the problems that brought you here today are gone. Since you were asleep you would not know a miracle had happened – but you would notice because things would be different. What is the *first thing you notice*, after the miracle occurs?'

  Although initial responses may be fanciful, clients usually describe in concrete terms the differences they would observe. For example, someone who has been depressed may say 'I would notice that I woke up without a sense of dread', to which the therapist would reply 'If you did not feel dread – what would you feel?' The latter step is important for generating positive language and providing increasing amounts of detail to the anticipated solution. The personal illustration that follows provides a sample conversation building on exceptions.

- *Amplifying differences questions* derives from Gregory Bateson,[3] who took the view that 'difference' in and of itself was not important unless it 'made a difference'. In addition to amplifying the exceptions identified by any of the questions posed, it is important to ask, '*and what difference will that make* (e.g. when you have the energy to "organize things around the house?")' [using the client's example]. '*And what difference will it make for you when* [the children notice that things seem in better order'?] etc. '*When the children are less critical, what difference will that make?*' '*What specific things do you think it would be important to do first?*' '*What difference will it make when you can get* [e.g. that one small thing] *completed?*'

- *Normalizing.* In contrast to identifying differences, clients may find it helpful to learn that their experiences and responses are 'normal' and *not* evidence of inherent pathology. Counsellors can normalize by indicating they have had similar experiences or would respond similarly. In other cases, looking at problems as normal within a developmental perspective or as part of known trajectory can have a normalizing effect.

- *Scaling questions* help people notice that change is a critical part of building *hopefulness*, reinforcing the client's appreciation of the small steps that lead to greater change. Scaling can be done at any point for different purposes. Among the many possibilities, scaling can be done to determine progress toward solutions, commitment to working towards identified solutions, or confidence that progress will be maintained.

Generally, scaling involves seeking information about what the scaling represents to the client. For example, if an identified solution is 'taking better care of myself by getting enough exercise' one might ask, 'On a scale of 0 to 10 where would you rate the exercise you are getting now?' 'If "10" is getting enough exercise, what would you be doing to rate a 10? If you are at [a "2"] now, what would you need to be doing to get a 2.5?'

- *Coping questions* acknowledge and build on strengths that are not always apparent to the client. Among these are: 'How have you prevented things from getting worse?' 'How did you manage to get yourself up this morning?' 'What keeps you going?'

Other important processes

- *Compliments*: In contrast to many therapies, active encouragement and enthusiasm for successes (based on progress towards the client's goals) is provided whenever the client seems open to hearing positive feedback. Statements such as *'that's terrific – how did you do that?'* not only support but can be the 'next question' for clarifying how best to continue progress toward desired solutions.
- *Reframing*: Reframing focuses on what *can* be controlled, i.e. our *interpretations*. Since multiple truths are seen as likely, the therapist explores the acceptability of different plausible content frames, based on a consideration of the positive meaning the behaviour might hold. Context frames can also be the basis for reframes, e.g. is there a place where this behaviour might have positive value? Negotiation of assumptions must be done cautiously, using questions, rather than statements, if the therapist is to avoid taking the role of the expert and distorting the client's views.
- *Homework*: Most solution-focused therapists will take a break (often leaving the room) after getting a picture of the solution and exceptions and prior to assigning 'homework', explaining the need to think for a moment about what has been learned and what might be most helpful. Such assignments are based on the client's own information about what has been working (i.e. sustaining exceptions) and based on the client's relationship to the problem, as described above.

Clients then receive feedback that incorporates compliments about coping, a 'bridging statement' linking the proposed homework to what the client has described, and an assignment to be carried out, with the client's approval, before the next meeting. Often clients come to therapy as 'complainants' and will benefit from actively seeking exceptions. If so, they are often given the assignment of 'noticing when the problem does not occur' and what seems to be different about those times. For clients who have already become aware of ways to create exceptions, homework will usually be directed toward continuing that

behaviour and *noticing what difference* it makes to them and others.

- *Modelling openness to change*: When clients try a new behaviour that does not work, or repeat old solutions that no longer work, it's time to try 'something different'. Some therapists discuss clients' ideas during the therapy session for doing something different before the next meeting. In other cases, therapists suggest that clients 'do something different' and report what it was and how it worked at the next meeting. Often clients come up with highly original ideas when they are not asked to specify a proposed action during the session.
- *Format for solution-focused interviews*: We often start initial sessions asking 'how can I help' and sometimes 'why now' in exploring the client's perspective on the situation. The majority of the session is spent identifying client goals, identifying exceptions and client strengths and steps toward goals. Follow up interviews usually start by asking 'what is better?' and seeking details about any improvement, specifically asking 'how did you do that' and complimenting clients on any progress. Next steps are identified, often using scaling and specifying what difference it makes when the new behaviour is enacted and what difference they think it will make when they continue that behaviour over time.
- *Solution-focused nursing process*: For those who find it helpful to translate practice in a nursing process Table 44.1 shows how the elements of the nursing process can be mapped onto the process of SFT.

TABLE 44.1 The solution-focused nursing process

Subjective	(Solution)
Objective	(Solution-relationship)
Assessment	(Goal and scaling)
Planning	(Next steps)
Implementation	(Homework)
Evaluation	(Scaling/differences)

Reflection

Postmodern therapies[4] are often described as avoiding taking ethical positions in the service of accepting clients' views and supporting multicultural perspectives.

- Can a therapist respect client's world views *and* maintain personal integrity?

APPLICATIONS

SFT has wide application in mental health and psychiatric care, in both inpatient and outpatient/community settings.[5] It can be incorporated into crisis work with

Personal illustration 44.1

The following is an abbreviated example of seeking solutions when Greg came to therapy at the urging of his sister, who was worried about his being more withdrawn.

Counsellor: Hello, Greg. I'm glad you could make it here today. How can I be helpful?

Greg: I'm not really sure you can be. I'm not even sure there is a problem, but my sister insists I talk with someone.

Counsellor: Do you have any idea why she wants you to talk with someone?'

Greg: She thinks I'm depressed.

Counsellor: Why would she think that?

Greg: I think I'm just going through a kind of 'down' time – I just finished school and don't have a job so I don't really have to be anywhere or do anything – I think it bothers her that I'm not 'going anywhere'. She's kind of a worrier.

Counsellor: Is it important to you that your sister is not worried about you?

Greg: It's more important to me that she lets me be who I am – but she worries how we'll pay the bills if I'm not working.

Counsellor: So when your sister lets you be who you are, what will you be doing?

Greg: I know what I won't be doing – I won't get a job in an office just to pay the bills.

Counsellor: What will you be doing instead?

Greg: I'm not sure … I guess that's really the problem.

Counsellor: Can you remember a time when you felt you really were able to be who you are and your sister was not so worried?

Greg: Yeah, when I was in school, before our dad died, I was taking classes in drama and working at a restaurant as a waiter.

Counsellor: What was different about then and now?

Greg: Well, my sister wasn't so worried about money and she knew how important it was to me to do something creative.

Counsellor: What else was different?

Greg: I really liked what I was studying and the job was as a 'singing waiter' so I got to entertain people while I got paid for waiting tables.

Counsellor: How else was that different from having a job in an office just to pay the bills?

Greg: Well, for one thing I could move around – I have trouble staying still for long – that was always a problem in school until I got into drama. My sister wants me to get a 'respectable job' in an office and have a regular income.

Counsellor: If you'd humour me for a moment, I'd like you to imagine that when you go to bed tonight, while you are asleep, a miracle happens and the script of your life story gets rewritten so that you are able to be who you are and your sister isn't so worried. Since you were asleep when this happened, the only way you will know is what you will notice when you awaken. What do you think will be the first thing you will notice?

Greg: Well, for starters, it would be later in the day when I woke up. I've never been a morning person, which is why I liked working in the restaurant at night and doing late rehearsals sometimes.

Counsellor: What else will you notice?

Greg: Well, my sister would not have made breakfast for me; she'd trust that I could fix my own meals – it always makes me feel guilty when she hovers over me.

Counsellor: What else might you notice?

Greg: I would be looking forward to the day – I'd have some plans to meet people and I would have the money to go out.

Counsellor: What difference would that make for you?

Greg: I wouldn't feel like such a loser – I'd be around people who can understand what's important to me.

Counsellor: What difference will it make for your relationship with your sister when you are able to spend more time with people who understand you and you have enough money to be able to go out sometimes?

Greg: Well, realistically, I'd have to be making enough to help pay the bills and go out. I know that would make her less worried and then she might stop complaining about me so much.

Counsellor: So how do you think you might be able to help pay the bills and still have enough money to go out with your friends, so your sister will not complain so much?

Greg: I'm not going to get a job in an office – but maybe I could look for some kind of job that I can move around in, and be around people like me … .

After some time spent specifying the requirements he would have for any job he would consider, the counsellor takes a break and returns with a homework assignment:

Counsellor: Greg, I'm really impressed that you came here today and that you have some ideas about how you can be who you are and how to help your sister be less worried about you. Between now and next time I see you I'd like you to notice a few things that may help you get a clearer picture of how you would like to proceed. First, I'd like you to think about people you know that you think are like you and understand you. Then I'd like you to notice how they spend their time and the ways they are still able to be who they are. Are you OK with that?

Greg: I guess so – I'll have to think about it a bit, but I think I can do that.

Counsellor: Great – and we can discuss what you have noticed the next time I see you.

In this example, the client and counsellor defined a relationship (one dependent on working within the client's perspective) and developed a direction for future work that is based on the client's preferred future and past successes.

individuals, couples and families and has been successfully used in family-based services, including child protection, and in school settings with children and adolescents. Solution-focused treatment has also been described for sexual abuse, eating disorders, relationship problems and depression, as well as problems associated with serious mental illness.

Use of SFT also has been described in primary care, helping individuals manage habit problems (such as tobacco cessation, alcohol/drug use) and to facilitate treatment adherence that is consistent with client goals and values. More recently there are examples of working with clients with chronic pain and chronic illness from a solution-focused perspective.[6] Programmes using a group format for clients dealing with similar conditions or problems, can effectively utilize solution-focused principles, often in combination with psychoeducational approaches, as long as the emphasis remains on the centrality of client strengths and goals and is respectful toward clients' idiosyncratic methods of coping and viewing their situation.

Many SFT therapists have developed unique ways to work with younger clients, e.g. encouraging them to draw pictures or act out with dolls what they wish there were more of in their lives. Because there are no requirements that all clients express emotions, develop insight or comply with predetermined goals, SFT provides a flexible approach for working with clients from different sociocultural and ethnic groups and across the age continuum. When working with clients from different cultural backgrounds it may be important to ascertain what types of questions are considered appropriate and to whom they may be properly addressed. Older clients and those experiencing grief can also benefit from attention to the practices and beliefs that are most important to them in their healing from multiple losses and changing circumstances. Solution-focused reminiscence therapy can help clients recall times and places and people who helped them grow and change in the ways they personally most value. The respect for the individual's world view can be particularly empowering to women and to clients who may distrust that the 'system' has any concerns about the clients' situation or ability to make decisions on their own behalf.

OUTCOMES

One challenge for SFT outcome measurement is that clients with similar problems (or in medical settings, similar diagnoses) may have quite disparate goals as well as many different ways to attain those goals. Outcome assessment of SFT can be challenging if therapists or agencies have predefined goals, critical paths, or specify how problems must be resolved. It is possible to measure change in symptom complaints across individuals if reduction of symptoms is a goal shared by clients (and is possible). For example, it may be possible to measure increased ability to function in specified life arenas if a group of clients share the same goal (e.g. regular work attendance among people with substance abuse). For clients who have some debilitating or fluctuating conditions, however, it may be challenging to attribute changes to any specific therapeutic intervention. On the other hand, it may be possible to determine if clients feel they are managing a situation more effectively (if this is a goal clients share).

Client satisfaction is another potentially shared outcome that can be measured; however, it's likely that what leads to client satisfaction may be radically different from one client to another. For example, if two depressed women both want to be able to function effectively in their relationships, the ability to identify and express emotions might be the preferred and most effective way for one client to reach her goals, while the ability to act, despite emotional distress, might be the preferred approach for another client with the same goal. Depending on the purpose for assessing outcomes, and the methods used, aggregate results may be differentially useful to counsellors and agencies.

Many agencies have shifted to a more solution-focused philosophy for the purpose of increasing efficiency and improving the economic health of the agency. Unless this type of transition is done with great care and respect for what counsellors believe they do that is helpful, it can lead to counsellor resentment and conscious or unconscious sabotage of the therapeutic approach. The rush to be brief can also be difficult for therapists who derive much of their professional reward from the opportunity to work with clients over time and help them grow and change. Ideally, the same sensitivity to clients' views about 'what works'[7] should be extended to therapists (as long they do not impose those beliefs on unwilling clients). In my experience, counsellors who may be initially unenthusiastic about the approach often become energized by seeing clients rally more quickly than anticipated and find satisfaction in hearing clients' reports of successful 'experiments' using strategies that had been forgotten or trying something 'different'. Realistically, some clients do best with longer term, often intermittent, therapy for problems that may be continuing and for which a range of changing or different 'solutions' may be appropriate over time. A *consultation model of care* may be most appropriate for these situations, permitting clients to seek support when they need it without being obligated to spend time and money during times when they are managing effectively.

LIMITATIONS

In addition to the difficulty comparing outcomes, there are some populations for whom any verbal therapy may have a limited role. Clients who are acutely psychotic, severely regressed, or have serious cognitive impairments may be unable to benefit from an approach that depends on active client participation in defining goals, strengths, options and progress.

Risk assessment may appear counter to solution-focused principles and must be carefully planned to protect the client without undermining the focus on strengths. In many settings there are required formats and intake information that must be gathered prior to beginning any type of treatment. In such cases, it may be possible to determine risk during an intake procedure, before moving to more strength and resource-based discussion. In cases where safety is a concern make a point to include scaling safety as a therapeutic goal, being careful to label it as the therapist's concern if it is not an identified client goal.

In some circumstances, clients may have either limited life experience or access to information and resources that might be helpful to them. Balancing a need for information with respect for the client's own knowledge and experience can be handled several ways. If clients are working in a group, they will be exposed to a wider range of possible solutions than they might generate individually. 'Modelling and role-modelling' (MRM), a nursing theory consistent with SFT, addresses the problem by providing psychoeducation only for issues about which the client indicates a desire to have additional

information.[8] Similarly, MRM looks at clients and their resources from a developmental perspective that nurses usually find helpful and that clients may find normalizing.[7]

Reflection

Accepting clients' reports of problems and possible solutions can reduce a therapist's sense of responsibility for the specifics of therapy outcomes.

What are the realistic limitations of therapist responsibility?

In what circumstances might other perspectives take precedence over client preferences?

SUMMARY

SFT is based on theoretical and practical evidence of 'what works' to help clients identify personally meaningful goals and build on clients' existing strengths and resources. Using a range of questions intended to develop an understanding of the client's perspective and encourage a positive orientation, it can be used with a wide variety of therapeutic concerns in both inpatient and outpatient populations.

REFERENCES

1. deShazer S. *Clues: investigating solutions in brief therapy.* New York, NY: W.W. Norton, 1988.

2. Barker P. Solution-focused therapies. *Nursing Times* 1998; **94** (19): 53–6.

3. Stagoll B. Gregory Bateson (1904–1980): a reappraisal. *Australian and New Zealand Journal of Psychiatry* 2005; **39**: 1036–45.

4. Barker P. The solution-focused therapies. In: *The talking cures.* London, UK: NT Books, 1999.

5. Miller S, Hubble M, Duncan B. *Handbook of solution-focused brief therapy.* San Francisco, CA: Jossey-Bass, 1996.

6. Johnson C, Webster D. *Recrafting a life.* New York, NY: Brunner/Routledge, 2002.

7. Hubble M, Duncan B, Miller S. *The heart and soul of change: what works in therapy.* Washington, DC: American Psychological Association, 1999.

8. Erickson H, Tomlin E, Swain M. *Modeling and role-modeling: a theory and paradigm for nursing.* Englewood Cliffs, NJ: Prentice-Hall, 1983.

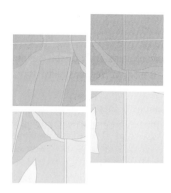

CHAPTER 45
Mindfulness

Mary E. Campbell*

INTRODUCTION

This chapter provides an introduction to mindfulness. Many different therapies are informed by or integrate mindfulness, in an effort to promote health, reduce physical and psychological distress and improve quality of life. Mindfulness is also recognized as an effective approach to stress management.

WHAT IS MINDFULNESS?

Mindfulness is *being present* with our experience as it is unfolding: knowing *what* we are doing *while* we are doing it – simply *being* or *doing*, open to the present moment. Mindfulness is characterized by attention and awareness. There is no separation between oneself and one's experience or activity. Mind and body are synchronized and one sees clearly what is happening *in the moment*. This capacity to be present in our life is natural, something that we all experience from time to time. For most of us the experience of *mindlessness* is more familiar – moving quickly from one thing to the next without paying attention, held captive by thoughts and opinions, likes and dislikes, memories of the past and plans for the future; all the while missing what is happening *now*.

The word mindfulness is also used to refer to mindfulness meditation – the practice of cultivating mindfulness.

Although mindfulness is intrinsic, and we are all mindful to varying degrees, mindfulness can be developed and strengthened through practice. The Tibetan Buddhist teacher Sakyong Mipham notes that while there is general agreement on the importance of training the body through exercise and diet, there is very little attention to developing or training the mind. Meditation practice is like working out, a way to develop the intrinsic strength and stability of mind and its ability to simply be present.[1]

The present moment has a particular potency, a kind of magic – being able to be still with whatever is going on: the magic of connecting with reality. Life unfolds in moments. Each moment has tremendous vividness and depth. As J Kabat-Zinn[2] noted, paying attention to experience from moment to moment:

> brings new ways of seeing and being in your life because the present moment, whenever it is recognized and honoured, reveals a very special, indeed magical power: it is the only time that any of us ever has.

Teachings on mindfulness originate in the Eastern meditation traditions, particularly Buddhism, where mindfulness is the path to liberation or freedom from suffering.[3] However, mindfulness does not belong to a particular religion or culture; it's universal. It's a way to look deeply into oneself and the experience of being human. Mindfulness strengthens innate human capacities for awareness, insight, compassion and skilful action.

*Mary E. Campbell RN, MSN, CS is a clinical nurse specialist in the Capital District Mental Health Program and Adjunct Professor in the School of Nursing, Dalhousie University in Halifax, Nova Scotia. Mary practises and teaches mindfulness meditation.

MINDFULNESS PRACTICE

Mindfulness practice involves placing attention on a particular activity such as *breathing* or *walking*, being present to whatever thoughts, sensations or emotions arise; noticing when the mind wanders, gently bringing it back to the object of attention. Mindfulness is 'paying attention in a particular way: on purpose in the present moment, and nonjudgmentally'.[4] We are not trying to manipulate or stop thoughts, but to be with one's experience unconditionally, without judging or trying to change it. Observing whatever enters awareness without judgement is important and common to all mindfulness practices. The attitude of *non-striving*, or dropping one's goals is also important and is one of the paradoxes of mindfulness practice.

To try mindfulness practice, the following might be useful. The instruction presented here is a *sitting* meditation practice from the Tibetan Buddhist tradition.[5] It is done in a seated position, either cross-legged on a firm cushion on the floor or in a straight back chair. When sitting in a chair, sit away from the back of the chair and place the feet firmly on the ground with the legs uncrossed.

- The posture is upright and dignified, relaxed and alert.
- Hands gently rest on the thighs, palms down.
- Eyes are open; the gaze is soft, directed slightly downward, resting on the floor, 4–6 feet in front of you.
- Mouth is slightly open and the jaw is relaxed.
- Having settled into the posture, bring your attention to the breathing, actually feel the breath.
- Breathing normally, let your attention rest on the outbreath. The breath goes out and dissolves; the in-breath happens quite naturally. There is a continual 'going out' with the out-breath and no need to follow the in-breath back in.
- Thoughts will arise, the mind will wander. When you notice that you have been lost in thought, mentally label that 'thinking' and bring your attention back to the breath.
- Continue this practice for 10 minutes.

Reflection

Try mindfulness practice using these instructions.

- What was your experience?

When people begin to practise mindfulness they are usually surprised to discover how *busy* the mind is: like a waterfall, one thought tumbling after the next. It may seem difficult to find the breath in the midst of all that mental activity. There is tremendous precision and gentleness in the practice: the precision of noticing what is happening, the waterfall of thought; the gentleness of being non-judgemental, not rejecting the busy mind. Over time, acknowledging that we *are* thinking and coming back to the breath, the waterfall gradually becomes a river and the river becomes a lake.

Relaxation and openness come with dropping the struggle of *trying* to have things be other than they are: a greater sense of ease when one is not trapped by liking and disliking. Mindfulness does not eliminate thoughts and emotions; rather, one is less likely to get caught up in them. It becomes possible to experience a state of mind that includes, but is not conditioned, by thought. Learning occurs when one is able to move into discomfort and pay close attention to it. One sees the pattern of thoughts and emotions and how they contribute to distress. In recognizing when one has been lost in thought, labelling thinking and coming back to the breath, one is letting go. Thoughts are seen *as thoughts* – rather than reality. The ability to recognize thoughts *as thoughts* frees one from the distorted reality they can create.

MINDFULNESS AND MENTAL HEALTH

Any practice that helps one recognize thoughts *as* thoughts, rather than reality, strengthens human capacities for awareness, compassion and skilful action. All these are useful in mental health. Mindfulness and Buddhist psychology have been integrated into therapeutic work in a variety of ways: mindful presence in therapy, mindfulness-informed therapy and mindfulness-based therapy.[6] In mindful *presence*, the clinician may bring a more mindful presence to his or her work, strengthening the therapeutic relationship. Mindfulness-*informed* therapy draws from mindfulness practice and Buddhist psychology while mindfulness-based therapy incorporates traditional mindfulness practices into the treatment itself.

Mindfulness practice is *not* therapy; it is an unconditional way of *being*. From the mindfulness perspective, human beings have basic sanity or intrinsic health.[7] Mindfulness is a way to connect with our inherent, basic sanity or intrinsic health. Neither is mindfulness a relaxation technique. Relaxation techniques attempt to control physical symptoms of stress or anxiety. In bringing attention to whatever is happening in the present moment, mindfulness practice *may* initially increase physical symptoms by reducing distraction. The relaxation that develops through mindfulness does so over time, as a result of dropping the attempt to control or manipulate one's experience, developing friendliness towards oneself based on genuine self-acceptance.

Mindfulness presence and nursing practice

Mindful presence in therapy refers to the way the clinician's personal mindfulness practice brings a more mindful presence to their work, strengthening the therapeutic relationship, the most potent predictor of a positive treatment outcome. Any practice that enhances the ability to be present and cultivates compassion is relevant to all therapists and care providers.

Psychiatric mental health nursing is an interpersonal process that aims to promote health and forward movement of the person in the direction of creative and productive, personal and community living.[8] Its focus is the *human response* to actual or potential health problems,[9] the *illness experience* rather than the *disease process*. Nurses meet people in times of distress and are called upon to be present. It is not easy to be present, to be open and available with the fullness of one's being. The ability to be present with oneself enables one to be present in relationship with others. Presence provides the ground for caring, empathy and compassion. Mindfulness practice strengthens the ability to be present without getting caught in one's thoughts about or emotional reactions to a situation. It enables one to see more clearly what is actually happening in the here-and-now, increasing the likelihood of a skilful response.

Reflection

- What is your experience of being present with another?
- Do you find yourself easily distracted or thinking about what you will say before the other person has finished speaking?
- What does it mean to be genuinely present?

The potential negative impact of stress, risk for burnout and the need to attend to self-care are important for nurses. In a study on the effects of a mindfulness-based stress reduction programme (MBSR) on nurse stress and burnout, nurses reported an increase in relaxation, self-awareness and self-care[10] and demonstrated a significant decrease in the emotional exhaustion subscale of the Maslach Burnout Inventory, the subscale most correlated with burnout.[11] These nurses also identified the ability to be more fully present and less reactive in relationships as one of the benefits of mindfulness practice.

Mindfulness-informed therapy

Mindfulness-informed therapy is informed by insights derived from mindfulness practice and Buddhist psychology. *Morita therapy* and the *Windhorse programme* for recovery are examples of treatment approaches informed by mindfulness and Buddhist psychology.

Morita therapy

Morita therapy[12] is a systemic psychotherapy based on Eastern psychology that was developed in 1919 by Dr Shoma Morita to treat anxiety disorders. It was original in its approach in that it did not seek causes of emotions

such as anxiety and fear. These emotions are understood as a natural phenomenon of the human psyche. Neurosis results from the secondary meanings attached to these emotional reactions rather than from the emotions themselves.

Morita viewed his therapy as a combination of rest therapy and discipline therapy. The treatment occurs over 4 weeks: week 1, bed rest; week 2, light work period; week 3, heavy work period; week 4, training for practical living. The person is supported to confront his or her problems from an objective perspective, become absorbed in the daily work of the therapeutic system and reactivate the desire to live fully. Morita therapy directs one's attention receptively to what reality brings in each moment. For example, during the period of rest, the person is encouraged to accept whatever feelings and thoughts bubble into his or her awareness. In doing so, the person learns experientially that the waves of thought and emotion come and go. The therapist does not explore the pathology. With successful treatment, the person learns to accept the internal fluctuations of thoughts and feelings and ground his or her behaviour in reality and the purpose of the moment.

Morita therapy has been used for people with depression, borderline personality disorder, alcohol dependence, childhood neurosis and schizophrenia.[13,14] It has also been applied to self-help activities and 'meaningful life therapy', an approach used for people with cancer.[13] Therapists in North America have extracted aspects of Morita's theory and method, particularly from stages 3 and 4. According to Le Vine,[15] Morita-based counselling has been well-received in North America. Le Vine herself has been administering classic Morita therapy in Australia since 1992.

The Windhorse programme for recovery

The Windhorse programme for recovery[16] provides individualized comprehensive home-based whole-person treatment for people experiencing extreme psychiatric distress. Developed by Dr Edward Podvoll and colleagues,[17] the Windhorse programme draws from Buddhist psychology, particularly Vajrayana Buddhism as taught by the Tibetan meditation master Chögyam Trungpa. Windhorse is literally the energy of basic sanity or intrinsic health, a self-existing energy that can radiate tremendous strength and healthiness in one's life.[5]

The Windhorse programme holds the view that significant recovery is possible for anyone experiencing psychosis. The mind, even when most disturbed, has what Podvoll calls 'islands of clarity',[17,p.5] when there is a sudden shift in awareness that discriminates between dream and reality. Moments of recovery are happening all the time, even in the wildest mind, and need encouragement and protection. Recovery depends on an atmosphere of simplicity, warmth and dignity. This is accomplished through creating a healing environment in the person's home.

A Windhorse team has three primary components:

- a therapeutic household with live-in housemate(s);
- several therapists providing basic attendance;
- intensive individual psychotherapy provided by a principal therapist.

There is an attempt to keep anti-psychotic medication to a minimum relying more on the healing potential of the physical and interpersonal environment. Working with a schedule brings a meaningful pattern to the day and becomes a reference point, providing a boundary between inner and outer experience or reality and delusion. The person spends several hours each day with housemate(s) sharing domestic activities. Basic attendance is provided in 3-hour shifts by a team of therapists who have trained in the practice of mindfulness awareness meditation.

Basic attendance is a way of being present that allows the other person to be present. It is paying attention to the entire situation and what the person needs to recover, doing whatever is called for – taking a walk, helping the person tidy his or her room, doing the laundry – all the while recognizing and appreciating the windows of opportunity provided by 'islands of clarity'. Basic attendance can occur in any setting – the kitchen, the laundrette, the grocery store. The activities team members do with the person become important practices in relating calmly and accurately to one's mind and developing more stability of mind. For example, playing basketball can be used to bring the mind back to the present moment. The practice of basic attendance involves 'genuine nursing of the mind'[17,p.264] and calls for a willingness to be open to learning from the person in care. It's being present in such a way that one's presence does not crowd, overpower or impose on the situation. Attending in this way supports the person and creates the necessary environment for recovery, an environment within which 'islands of clarity begin to gather and flourish'.[17,p.253]

Reflection

- How do you experience the mental health treatment settings in which you provide care?
- Consider the interpersonal and physical environment. In what ways do you notice the simplicity, warmth and dignity that is characteristic of a healing environment?

Recall a recent interaction with a person experiencing an extreme state of mind.

Were you able to notice 'islands of clarity' or moments of recovery?

- If so, describe that experience.
- If not, pay close attention the next time you have the opportunity.

Mindfulness-based clinical interventions

Mindfulness-based clinical interventions such as mindfulness-based stress reduction (MBSR) and mindfulness-based cognitive therapy (MBCT), incorporate traditional mindfulness practices. An increasing body of evidence supports mindfulness as effective in improving psychological functioning.[18]

Mindfulness-based stress reduction

Mindfulness-based stress reduction (MBSR)[19] was developed by Kabat-Zinn. MBSR is provided in a group format as an 8-week course that meets weekly for 2.5 hours and a full-day session around week 6. This programme was developed as a complement to medical treatment, to help people with chronic health problems work with the stress, pain and suffering associated with illness. Formal and informal mindfulness practices are taught as a way to strengthen the innate human capacity for awareness, insight, relaxation and behaviour change.

Formal practice involves setting aside a time to practise mindfulness following a specific set of instructions similar to the sitting meditation practice described above. Informal practice involves bringing moment-to-moment non-judgemental awareness to ordinary daily activities such as eating, washing dishes, showering and brushing teeth. The formal mindfulness practices taught in MBSR include:

1. *the body scan* – mindfulness of body sensations while moving attention through the body in a sequential fashion, done lying down with eyes closed;
2. *sitting meditation* – attention is placed on the breath while sitting quietly in an upright, dignified and relaxed posture;
3. *walking meditation* – attention is placed on the physical sensation of walking;
4. *yoga* – mindfulness of body sensations during gentle movements and stretches and while it is still, holding a posture.

Participants are given home assignments consisting of formal and informal mindfulness practice and various awareness exercises. They are expected to engage in formal mindfulness for at least 45 minutes per day, 6 days per week. An example of an awareness exercise is the pleasant events calendar in which participants are asked to bring awareness to, one pleasant event each day while it is happening and later reflect on the event using a series of questions provided; for example, 'What mood, feelings, and thoughts accompanied this event at the time?' MBSR also includes didactic content on topics such as body–mind connections, stress, relaxation, health habits and communication style.

Since its beginnings in 1979, over 15 000 people have completed MBSR training in the Stress Reduction Clinic at the University of Massachusetts.[20] There are more than 250 MBSR programmes in a variety of settings around the world – hospitals, clinics, mental health settings, correctional facilities, schools, workplaces and corporate offices.[21] MBSR has traditionally included participants with a wide range of health-related issues rather than grouping participants according to diagnosis. It has also been used with specific populations such as individuals with a diagnosis of cancer, mental illness and groups of healthcare providers.

MBSR reduces physical and psychological distress, promotes adaptive coping and improves quality of life despite chronic illness. It reduces symptoms of anxiety, panic and depression,[22–24] decreases pain and improves psychosocial adaptation in individuals with chronic pain,[25–27] decreases the number and severity of binges, anxiety and depression in individuals with binge eating disorder,[28] reduces symptoms in fibromyalgia,[29,30] increases rates of skin clearing in patients with moderate to severe psoriasis receiving phototherapy[31] and reduces mood disturbance and stress in individuals with cancer.[32]

The empirical literature on MBSR has been criticized for a number of methodological flaws: the lack of control groups, reliance on self-report measures and non-specific factors that may affect outcome such as group support. Reviewers[33,34] have identified the need for larger samples, randomized clinical trials, comparison with established treatments, isolation of active ingredients and the examination of the mechanisms through which mindfulness may create clinical change. Even so, taking the criticism into account, mindfulness-based interventions have been shown to be more effective than wait-list or treatment as usual control groups for individuals suffering from a variety of conditions including anxiety, depression and chronic pain.[33,35]

Mindfulness-based cognitive therapy

Mindfulness-based cognitive therapy (MBCT) is an adaptation of MBSR developed by Segal et al.[36,37] to prevent recurrence of major depression. MBCT combines mindfulness practice with traditional cognitive therapy strategies. Individuals who have experienced an episode of major depression are at high risk for relapse and the risk increases with each episode. In previously depressed individuals ordinary sad moods are likely to reactivate depressive thought content and ruminative thinking leading to a recurrence of depression. MBCT is a group intervention that provides training in how to disengage from depressive and ruminative thinking, reducing the risk of relapse for individuals with a prior history of major depression.

MBCT differs from MBSR in that it includes traditional cognitive strategies and the didactic content focuses on depression rather than stress, for example a discussion of automatic thoughts that are related to depression, the role of pleasure and mastery activities in lifting one's mood and

the development of an individualized relapse prevention action plan. We all have a tendency to believe our thoughts. For those who have been depressed, the tendency to believe negative thoughts can be quite strong, particularly in moments of sadness. In mindfulness practice, one begins to see thoughts and emotions as mental events that come and go rather than some kind of truth or an accurate reflection of reality.

While mindfulness practice naturally extends into daily life, this takes time. MBCT introduces a mini-meditation, 'the 3-minute breathing space'[37,p.183] that is used to provide a bridge between formal mindfulness practice and daily life. The 3-minute breathing space is a way to open to the present moment on the spot and can be used to work with challenging situations as they arise. This exercise can be done with the eyes closed and has three steps: becoming aware, gathering and expanding. One begins by taking an upright posture and bringing awareness to one's inner experience – one's thoughts, feelings and bodily sensations.

1 Ask the question 'what is my experience right now?' This is step 1, 'becoming aware', stepping out of automatic pilot and opening to the present moment.
2 'Gathering', involves bringing one's attention to the movement and sensation of the breathing, noticing each in-breath and out-breath as it occurs.
3 Next, expand awareness to include a sense of the body as a whole, including any sensations, allowing for a sense of spacious awareness.

Participants are asked to practice this mini-meditation three times per day, gradually using it as needed to work with challenging life situations.

In two randomized clinical trials,[38,39] MBCT reduced the risk of relapse for individuals with a history of three or more episodes of major depression by half. In both studies, MBCT was not found to be of benefit for individuals with two prior episodes of depression. Relapse for these individuals may be associated with major life events rather than the reactivation of depressive thought patterns by sadness. MBCT was specifically designed for individuals who are currently in remission and, as of this writing, is not recommended for treating acute depression. As with MBSR, MBCT has non-specific factors such as group support and a therapeutic alliance that may contribute to its effect.

Dialectical behaviour therapy

Dialectical behaviour therapy (DBT) is a multifaceted treatment for individuals with borderline personality disorder developed by Marcia Linehan.[40] The central dialectic in DBT is the relationship between acceptance and change. DBT combines cognitive–behavioural interventions designed to help clients change thoughts, behaviour and emotions with mindfulness skills that are taught within the context of synthesizing acceptance and change. Mindfulness 'what' skills specify what one does when being mindful – observing, describing and participating. Mindfulness 'how' skills are how one does it – non-judgementally, one mindfully and effectively. Unlike MBSR and MBCT, DBT does not prescribe specific mindfulness exercises or the frequency and duration of mindfulness practice. The individual client and the therapist develop the goals for mindfulness drawing from numerous short informal mindfulness exercises that are available.

Mindfulness has also been integrated into acceptance and commitment therapy (ACT),[41] the treatment of anxiety disorders and post-traumatic stress disorder[42] and person-based cognitive therapy for the treatment of psychosis.[43]

Mindfulness and psychosis

The traditional MBSR programme has been adapted for persons with psychosis[44] and schizophrenia[45] with positive results. Adjustments to the standard programme include a therapeutic rather than class context, fewer participants per group, shorter periods of meditation practice (10 minutes rather than 20–45 minutes), less silence and more guidance during meditation periods and encouraging but not requiring homework. Participants in one such programme[45] reported that mindfulness practice helped them to recognize and stop negative thought patterns, become less withdrawn and isolated, feel more relaxed and less frustrated, accept the good and bad aspects of oneself and gain a better understanding of self and control of impulsive behaviour. There was no increase in psychotic symptoms reported by the participants or their primary clinicians. Two participants identified the programme as helpful in managing hallucinations. One participant reported using mindfulness as 'a way of grounding' and to keep a sense of humour when things went wrong instead of becoming so upset with himself that he was unable to problem-solve effectively.

Singh and colleagues[46] introduced a simple mindfulness technique, 'meditation on the soles of the feet' to three men whose aggressive behaviour had prevented successful placement in the community. Two of the men had an Axis I diagnosis of schizoaffective disorder, the third was diagnosed with major depression with psychotic features, in remission. All had been treated with various psychotropic medications and were currently taking medication. Prior attempts at behavioural treatment for physical and verbal aggression had not been effective. They had each been discharged to the community several times and were re-admitted within weeks of discharge because of aggressive behaviour.

Meditation on the soles of the feet is a mindfulness technique that had been used successfully by a young man with mental illness and mild mental retardation to manage aggression.[47] In this technique, attention is directed from an emotionally charged thought or situation to a neutral part of the body, the soles of the feet. The participants received individual instruction in focusing on the soles of the feet while sitting, standing or walking slowly and while imagining a situation that had previously provoked an aggressive response. The participants were required to practise the mindfulness technique at least twice a day and when an incident occurred that might provoke aggressive behaviour. With this mindfulness practice, incidents of verbal and physical aggression decreased for all three men. It was noted that physical aggression decreased more quickly than verbal aggression. All three were able to return to the community where they were followed for a period of 4 years after discharge. During that time there was no evidence of physical aggression, and verbal aggression was minimal.

Mindfulness and acute care

York[48] reported on the introduction of a mindfulness group within an acute inpatient mental health unit and the results of a qualitative study. The group met weekly for 1 hour with an average of five participants. Several mindfulness techniques such as the body scan and mindfulness of breathing were introduced. Participants experienced changes in the relationship to thought, increased ability to focus, a sense of peace and relaxation, acceptance, a willingness to 'sit with' and observe discomfort and difficult feelings and increased awareness of the present. Most of the participants practiced mindfulness outside of the group and expressed an interest in continuing the practice after discharge.

MINDFULNESS AND THE BRAIN

One question currently being explored is how mindfulness changes brain structure and function. In the past it was believed that the structure and function of the brain was fixed and that the only changes that occurred after childhood were when the brain began to decline with age. Neuroplasticity,[49] the ability of the brain to change in response to activity and experience, is becoming more established in mainstream science. The connections between neurons can strengthen, new connections can be made and new neurons can be created. Learning changes the very structure of the brain and increases its capacity to learn. Neuroplastic research[49] shows that specific processing areas in the brain called brain maps can be trained so that they do more mental work. For example, the more musicians who play string instruments practise, the larger the brain maps for the left hand become. Brain scans of London taxi drivers show that the more years spent driving, the larger the volume of the hippocampus, the part of the brain that stores spatial representations. In a similar way, might mindfulness practice affect areas of the brain associated with attention and emotion?

Electroencephalography (EEG) and functional magnetic imaging (fMRI) studies have demonstrated that meditation is different from rest or sleep and that different styles of meditation lead to different patterns of brain activity.[50] Experienced meditators show increased activity in the left prefrontal cortex on EEG and fMRI.[51] The left prefrontal cortex is the area of the brain associated with positive emotional states such as joy, altruism and enthusiasm, whereas the right prefrontal cortex is associated with negative emotional states such as pessimism, depression and anxiety.

In another study,[52] experienced meditators were found to have thickening in cortical regions associated with attention and sensory processing. The differences in prefrontal cortical thickness between meditators and non-meditators were most significant in older participants, suggesting that regular meditation practice may offer protection from age-related neural degeneration. The results of this research suggest the possibility of experience-dependent cortical plasticity in adults in areas of the brain that are important for cognitive and emotional processing.

The meditators in these studies have practised meditation for many hours over 15–40 years. What about those new to meditation? Davidson and colleagues[53] looked at the effect of mindfulness practice in employees of a biotechnical corporation who participated in a mindfulness-based stress reduction programme. The employees who participated in the training and practised mindfulness showed a significant increase in left-sided anterior activation compared with the waiting-list control group of non-meditators. The meditators in this study also demonstrated a more robust immune response to the flu vaccine than the control group.

Research to date is consistent with the idea that mindfulness practice affects neurophysiology, particularly areas of the brain associated with attention and emotion.[54] Meditation is an example of a way in which purely mental training has been demonstrated to have an impact on brain function and structure. The research with meditators suggests that one can bring about changes in brain function that positively affect emotions and cognition by one's own efforts.

SUMMARY

Mindfulness is a natural, though often poorly developed, quality of mind. Mindfulness is not a technique to learn about and pass on to others; it is a way of *being in one's life*, open to and experiencing the richness and depth of the present moment. Through mindfulness practice, one develops the intrinsic strength and stability of mind and the ability to be present. One can begin with 10 minutes each day. When we are able to be present with our own state of mind, we are more likely to be present in our relationships with others. Presence can be healing. It provides the ground for caring, empathy, compassion and skilful action. The various mindfulness-based therapies presented in this chapter teach a way of paying attention to present-moment experience that has significant potential for reducing distress and enhancing health and well-being. It is essential to have experience with the practice before attempting to teach it to others. It takes experience and training to be able to guide others in the practice of mindfulness.

REFERENCES

1. Mipham S. *Turning the mind into an ally*. New York, NY: Riverhead, 2003.

2. Kabat-Zinn J. *Full catastrophe living: using the wisdom of your body and mind to face stress, pain and illness*. New York, NY: Delacorte, 1990: 29.

3. Trungpa C. *The path is the goal: a basic handbook of Buddhist meditation*. Boston, MA: Shambhala, 1995.

4. Kabat-Zinn J. *Wherever you go there you are: mindfulness meditation in everyday life*. New York, NY: Hyperion, 1995: 4.

5. Trungpa C. *Shambhala: the sacred path of the warrior*. Boston, MA: Shambhala, 1984.

6. Germer C. Mindfulness: What is it? What does it matter? In: Germer C, Siegel R, Fulton R (eds). *Mindfulness and psychotherapy*. New York, NY: Guilford Press, 2005: 3–27.

7. Trungpa C. *The sanity we are born with*. Boston, MA: Shambhala, 2005.

8. Peplau, H. *Interpersonal relations in nursing: a conceptual frame of reference for psychodynamic nursing*. New York, NY: GP Putnam's Sons, 1952.

9. American Nurses Association. *Nursing: A social policy statement*. Kansas City, MO: ANA, 1995.

10. Cohen-Katz J, Wiley SD, Capuano T. The effects of mindfulness-based stress reduction on nurse stress and burnout, part III. *Holistic Nursing Practice* 2005; **19** (2): 78–86.

11. Cohen-Katz J, Wiley SD, Capuano T. The effects of mindfulness-based stress reduction on nurse stress and burnout, part II. *Holistic Nursing Practice* 2005; **19** (1): 26–35.

12. Morita S. *Morita therapy and the true nature of anxiety-based disorders (Shinkeishitsu)*. Translated by Akihisa Kondo. Albany, NY: State University of NY Press, 1998.

13. Kitanishi K, Mori A. Morita therapy: 1919–1995. *Psychiatry and Clinical Neurosciences* 1995; **459**: 245–54.

14. He Y, Li C. Morita therapy for schizophrenia. *Cochrane Database of Systemic Reviews* 2007; **I**: CD006346, available from: www.cochrane.org/reviews/en/ab006346.html.

15. Le Vine P (ed.). Editor's introduction. In: *Morita therapy and the true nature of anxiety-based disorders (Shinkeishitsu)*. Translated by Akihisa Kondo. Albany, NY: State University of NY Press, 1998: xvii–xxvii.

16. Fortuna J. The Windhorse program of recovery. In: Warner R. (ed.). *Alternatives to the hospital for acute psychiatric treatment.* Arlington, VA: American Psychiatric Publishing, 1995: 171–89.

17. Podvoll E. *Recovering sanity: a compassionate approach to understanding and treating psychosis.* Boston, MA: Shambhala, 2003.

18. Baer RA. Mindfulness training as a clinical intervention: a conceptual and empirical review. *Clinical Psychology: Science and Practice* 2003; **10**: 125–43.

19. Kabat-Zinn J. *Full catastrophe living: using the wisdom of your body and mind to face stress, pain and illness.* New York, NY: Delacorte, 1990.

20. Davidson R, Kabat-Zinn J. Response to a letter by J. Smith. *Psychosomatic Medicine* 2004; **66**: 149–52.

21. Kabat-Zinn J. Mindfulness-based interventions in context: past, present and future. *Clinical Psychology: Science and Practice* 2003; **10** (2): 144–56.

22. Kabat-Zinn J, Massion A, Kristeller J *et al.* Effectiveness of a meditation-based stress reduction program in the treatment of anxiety disorders. *American Journal of Psychiatry* 1992; **149** (7): 936–43.

23. Kristeller J, Peterson L, Fletcher K. Effectiveness of a meditation-based stress reduction program in the treatment of anxiety disorders. *American Journal of Psychiatry* 1992; **149** (7): 936–43.

24. Miller J, Fletcher K, Kabat-Zinn J. Three-year follow-up and clinical implications of a mindfulness meditation-based stress reduction intervention in the treatment of anxiety disorders. *General Hospital Psychiatry* 1995; **17**: 192–200.

25. Kabat-Zinn J. An outpatient program in behavioural medicine for chronic pain patients based on the practice of mindfulness meditation: theoretical considerations and preliminary results. *General Hospital Psychiatry* 1982; **4**: 33–47.

26. Kabat-Zinn J, Lipworth L, Burney R. The clinical use of mindfulness meditation for the self-regulation of chronic pain. *Journal of Behavioural Medicine* 1985; **8**: 163–90.

27. Kabat-Zinn J, Lipworth L, Burney R, Sellers W. Four-year follow-up of a meditation-based program for self-regulation of chronic pain: treatment outcome and compliance. *Clinical Journal of Pain* 1986; **2**: 159–73.

28. Kristeller J, Hallett C. An exploratory study of a meditation-based intervention for binge eating disorder. *Journal of Health Psychology* 1999; **4** (3): 357–63.

29. Kaplan K, Goldenberg D, Galvin-Nadeau M. The impact of a meditation-based stress reduction program on fibromyalgia. *General Hospital Psychiatry* 1982; **4**: 33–47.

30. Goldenberg D, Kaplan K, Nadeau M. A controlled study of a stress reduction, cognitive behavioural treatment program in fibromyalgia. *Journal of Musculoskeletal Pain* 1994; **2**: 53–66.

31. Kabat-Zinn J, Wheeler E, Light T. Influence of a mindfulness-based stress reduction intervention on rates of skin clearing in patients with moderate to severe psoriasis undergoing phototherapy (UVB) and photochemotherapy (PUVA). *Psychosomatic Medicine* 1998; **60**: 625–32.

32. Speca M, Carlson LE, Goodey E, Angen M. A randomized wait-list controlled clinical trial: the effect of a mindfulness-based stress reduction program on mood and symptoms of stress in cancer outpatients. *Psychosomatic Medicine* 2000; **62**: 613–22.

33. Baer RA. Mindfulness training as a clinical intervention: a conceptual and empirical review. *Clinical Psychology: Science and Practice* 2003; **10**: 125–43.

34. Roemer L, Orsillo, SM. Mindfulness: A promising intervention strategy in need of further study. *Clinical Psychology: Science and Practice* 2003; **10** (2): 172–8.

35. Grossman P, Niemann L, Schmidt S, Walach H. Mindfulness-based stress reduction and health benefits: a meta-analysis. *Journal of Psychosomatic Research* 2004; **57**: 35–43.

36. Segal ZV, Williams JMG, Teasdale JD. *Mindfulness-based cognitive therapy for depression: A new approach to preventing relapse.* New York, NY: Guilford Press, 2002.

37. Williams M, Teasdale J, Segal Z, Kabat-Zinn J. *The mindful way through depression: freeing yourself from chronic unhappiness.* New York, NY: The Guilford Press, 2007.

38. Teasdale, JD, Segal, ZF, Williams, JMG. Prevention of relapse/recurrence in major depression by mindfulness-based cognitive therapy. *Journal of Consulting and Clinical Psychology* 2000; **68**: 615–23.

39. Ma S, Teasdale J. Mindfulness-based cognitive therapy for depression: replication and exploration of differential relapse prevention effects. *Journal of Consulting and Clinical Psychology* 2004; **72** (1): 31–40.

40. Linehan M. *Cognitive behavioural treatment of borderline personality disorder.* New York, NY: Guilford Press, 1993.

41. Hayes SC, Strosahl K, Wilson KG. *Acceptance and commitment therapy.* New York, NY: Guilford Press, 1999.

42. Roemer L, Orsillo SM. Expanding our conceptualization of and treatment of generalized anxiety disorder: integrating mindfulness/acceptance based approaches with existing cognitive–behavioural models. *Clinical Psychology: Science and Practice* 2002; **9**: 54–68.

43. Chadwick P. *Person-based cognitive therapy for distressing psychosis.* Chichester, UK: John Wiley & Sons, 2006.

44. Chadwick P, Taylor KN, Abba N. Mindfulness groups for people with psychosis. *Behavioural and Cognitive Psychotherapy* 2005; **33**: 351–9.

45. Davis L. Mindfulness as a clinical intervention for persons with schizophrenia. Paper presented at: *Integrating Mindfulness-Based Approaches & Interventions into Medicine, Health Care, and Society.* Wooster, MA, 2007.

46. Singh NN, Lancioni GE, Winton ASW, *et al.* Individuals with mental illness can control their aggressive behaviour through mindfulness training. *Behaviour Modification* 2007; **31** (3): 313–28.

47. Singh NN, Wahler RG, Adkins AD *et al.* Soles of the feet: A mindfulness-based self-control intervention for aggression by an individual with mild mental retardation and mental illness. *Research in Developmental Disabilities* 2003; **24**: 158–69.

48. York M. A qualitative study into the experience of individuals involved in a mindfulness group within an acute inpatient

mental health unit. *Journal of Psychiatric and Mental Health Nursing* 2007; **14**: 603–8.

49. Doidge N. *The brain that changes itself: stories of personal triumph from the frontiers of brain science.* New York, NY: Viking, 2007.

50. Lazar SW, Bush G, Gollub R *et al.* Functional brain mapping of the relaxation response and meditation. *Neuro Report* 2000; **11** (7): 1581–5.

51. Begley S. Scans of monks' brains show meditation alters structure, functioning. *The Wall Street Journal online* November 5, 2004. Available from: www.arcanology.com/2005/04/30/more-meditation-and-brain-scan-news/.

52. Lazar SW, Kerr CE, Wasserman RH *et al.* Meditation experience is associated with increased cortical thickness. *Neuro Report* 2005; **18** (17): 1893–7.

53. Davidson R, Kabat-Zinn J, Schumacher J *et al.* Alterations in brain and immune function produced by mindfulness meditation. *Psychosomatic Medicine* 2003; **65**: 564–70.

54. Lazar, SW. Mindfulness research. In: Germer C, Siegel R, Fulton P (eds). *Mindfulness and psychotherapy.* New York, NY: Guilford Press, 2005: 220–38.

MINDFULNESS-RELATED WEBSITES

Centre for Mindfulness in Medicine, Health Care and Society
www.umassmed.edu/cfm/mbsr/
Mindfulness-Based Cognitive Therapy
www.mbct.co.uk/
Mind and Life Institute
www.mindandlife.org/
Windhorse Community Services
www.windhorsecommunityservices.com/index.html

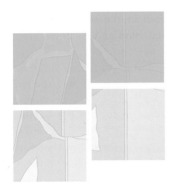

CHAPTER 46

Therapeutic communities

Gary Winship*

INTRODUCTION

It is with a second eye on the career origins of Annie Altschul and Hildegard Peplau, that this chapter positions the concept of psychosocial intervention and its therapeutic community legacy.[1] The foundations of mental health nursing, through the work of Hildegard Peplau and Annie Altschul especially, are shown to be coterminous with the emergence of the therapeutic community (TC) method. With its emphasis from the start on social inclusion and user involvement, it is argued that TC methods continue to promise radically and politically informed mental health practice, compensating the anti-therapeutic tendencies inherent in modern psychiatry.

Reflection

- What are you associations with the term psychosocial nursing?
- Are you familiar with the history of psychosocial nursing and its legacy at the Cassel Hospital?

HISTORY

A new concept of *cooperative* psychiatric therapy, the third revolution as Rapoport[2] eventually called it, emerged against the backdrop of deep social change during the Second World War. Three UK psychiatric hospitals, Northfield in Birmingham, Mill Hill in London and the 312th Military Hospital in Stafford, were involved and how they became sites for a series of innovative treatment experiments with shell-shocked soldiers is the focus of the first part of this chapter. These wartime experiments generated ideas of social participation. 'Talking therapy' and 'patient empowerment' came into sharp focus and formed the basis of social psychiatry, which remains a frame for community-based therapy today. At the time of these early experiments, however, psychiatry was mostly characterized by the use of drugs such as sodium amytol, used alongside deep insulin therapy, continuous narcosis and electroconvulsion therapy (ECT). Many soldier patients were unable to return to active service and those that returned to 'civvy street' had problems with unemployment and social disability. There was also a steady trickle of suicides.

*Gary Winship is a registered psychotherapist and Associate Professor in the School of Education, University of Nottingham, UK. He started working as a cleaner at the Bethlem Royal Hospital at 15. He was Treasurer of the Association of Therapeutic Communities (ATC) 2001–2007, and a full member of the Association of Psychoanalytic Psychotherapy in the NHS.

A general sense of dissatisfaction with conventional biological treatments in psychiatry abounded, and there was the impetus to develop some of the new talking therapies expounded by Freud and his colleagues. At Northfield Army Hospital in Birmingham, Wilfred Bion, a psychiatrist and trainee psychoanalyst took charge of a rehabilitation ward of soldiers with his colleague John Rickman. The soldier patients were known to be slovenly and undisciplined by army standards and they were affectionately referred to as the 'scallywag battalion'.[3] It appears that in the first instance Bion decided that he would not meet with any of his soldier patients on the ward until they had taken responsibility for the chaos they had created. In effect he set up a leaderless group, an idea he has previously adopted for the assessment of soldiers for officer status.[4,5] Bion hoped that the patients together would see the error of their ways, galvanize their capacities and fall into line. In fact, what happened was the contrary. The ward became even more disorganized and following a film evening the patients wrecked the dining hall, leaving broken crockery and used condoms on the floor. It is not clear at what point after these events there was a turn for the better, but over the following weeks the patients began to gather themselves into work groups. Group meetings were established on a daily basis and there were discussions held in which the analysis of conflict 'in the here and now' was examined. Bion took to strolling around the ward having discussions with patients in the corridors and kitchen. This innovative approach brought about, at the very least, modest improvements and some reports have even suggested that the ward became the cleanest and most disciplined unit in the hospital.[6]

In retrospect Bion reviewed the experiment as a sort of psychoanalytic tributary that enabled him to develop ideas about group process which culminated much later in a book about groups.[7] The analytic scope of the project at the time, however, was probably more down to Rickman, who was already established as a psychoanalyst. In many ways the free approach to the milieu resembled the psychoanalytic procedure in as much as the aim was not to relieve anxiety but rather to allow anxieties to become manifest among the soldier patients. It is clear from accounts that this approach did pay some dividends as psychological understanding of individual affliction and intra-group tensions brought about a tidy coherence to group performance.[4] However, the army hierarchy was unsettled by this radical approach and it was suspected that apart from not preparing soldiers to return to duty, a rebellious precedent had been set for free-thinking among soldiers who in army eyes were best left otherwise. The group approach also caused unease because it meant that sufferings such as bed wetting among the patients were no longer secreted by the orthodoxy of discrete or private consultation and instead became subject to open scrutiny. The provocation or permissiveness of anxiety was not reassuring to an army hierarchy that wished anxiety to be quashed in the service of blind discipline. The result was that Bion and Rickman were effectively sacked.

The Northfield experiment still continued however when Bion and Rickman were replaced by Michael Foulkes, a psychoanalyst who had already developed some original ideas about social analysis in the melting pot of the Frankfurt School of Social Research.[8] Foulkes was also a personal acquaintance of Freud and therefore commanded greater respect. He also had the mystique of being a German immigrant who had earned the accolade of being on the Nazi's hit list. Foulkes seemed better able to cajole the army establishment and was far less combative than Bion and Rickman. Influenced by the sociological ideas of Norbert Elias and Karl Mannheim, Foulkes had shifted away from Freud's psychoanalysis towards a three-body psychology of the group, and at Northfield turned his attention to seeing how far the therapeutic net would stretch to render more opportunities for therapy. Foulkes went as far to propose that the hospital itself should be treated as a whole,[9] and he believed that there were potential therapeutic gains for all parts of the organization to work cooperatively. Evolving an inclusive agenda and establishing training groups for nursing and medical staff and so forth, Foulkes, alongside other staff including Tom Main, Pat de Mare and Harold Bridger in particular, pursued an agenda of social rehabilitation that was organizationally interdisciplinary and multimodal. It was his junior colleague Tom Main who coined the term 'Therapeutic Community' as a way of describing the method in which all elements of life in the hospital community could be seen as therapeutically intentioned.

Coinciding with the experiments at Northfield, at another military hospital, this time the 312th in Staffordshire, a young newly qualified nurse called Hildegard Peplau began her work with soldier patients. Peplau had just graduated from Bennington College in the United States in 1943 with a BA in Interpersonal Psychology. At the 312th she began to put into practice what she had learned from her prior experiences at Chestnut Lodge, a hospital which at that time was well on its way to defining milieu therapy, gaining a considerable reputation as one of the most radical treatment environments yet seen in psychiatry. The psychoanalytic work of Harry Stack Sullivan, among others, had been particularly influential at Chestnut Lodge and had shaped Peplau's early expectations and capacities. At the 312th, the shell-shocked soldier patients under Peplau's care were both depressed and anxious. She took it on herself to implement formal and informal group therapy sessions with soldier casualties,[10] facilitating discussions over breakfast and in other everyday social situations taking the opportunity to engage her patients in normalizing activities as part of a community programme. Peplau might have seen some preliminary accounts of the

Northfield experiments that had been published in a special edition of the *Bulletin of the Menninger Clinic* in 1944, but it is more likely that there was a ripple effect among psychiatric practitioners, who were inclined to develop cohesive and collective approaches almost as a natural social counterpoise to the destructivity of the war. Participant group approaches and community-based ideologies were very much in the ascendant while narrow psychological and biological models of treating trauma were challenged abruptly.

This was the beginning of new orthodoxies and it is worth noting, especially in relation to the origins of mental health nursing, that while at the 312th Peplau had an affair with an officer and became pregnant. She later gave birth to her daughter while still in England. It was the outcome of her work at the 312th that Peplau saw as the base for her later professional contribution, thus England was a source for dual conception where her actual experiences of mothering informed her formulation for her *Interpersonal relations in nursing*.[11]

At the same time in London, Mill Hill was the site for evacuated patients and staff from the Maudsley. Here, a young medical psychiatrist called Maxwell Jones was experimenting with groups too. It is here that our other mental health nurse protagonist, Annie Altschul, enters the frame. In ways not dissimilar to the cooperative efforts of therapy at Northfield and the 312th, Jones found mutual learning to be beneficial in the treatment of shell-shocked soldiers at Mill Hill. Jones's approach differed from Northfield and the 312th insofar as he was not, ostensibly, working psychoanalytically,[12,13] although Jones was far from analytically illiterate having been under the guiding influence of Aubrey Lewis, his mentor and lead physician at the Maudsley, who had been keen for all his interns to be familiar with the new talking therapies derived from Freud.[14] Certainly at Mill Hill, Jones seems to have made good use of Freud's concept of conversion hysteria when, during the treatment of one soldier who was suffering from paralysis of his arm, Jones noted that the patient described the death of his friend as 'like losing your right arm'. When the conscious connection between the loss and the paralysis was articulated there was subsequent progress made in the patient's condition. And later in *Beyond the therapeutic community*[15,p.70] Jones acknowledged that 'psychoanalysis has added a great deal to knowledge of the therapeutic process'. However, Jones favoured the use of modified talking therapy in the procedure of group intervention where collective information sharing extended the orthodox model of the therapeutic dyad.

Jones noted that discussion groups were particularly effective in reducing anxiety when the physiological facts about effort syndrome were detailed and shared openly. This new open-group psycho-educative approach was modified for Jones's post-Mill Hill experiments in the rehabilitation of 300 British prisoners-of-war (POWs).

The resources for the treatment were six 'cottages' of 50 beds each, and each of the houses developed systems of group support. Attention was given to a modification of the traditional psychiatric milieu in as much as patients were involved in the business and administrative aspects of the treatment, a tangible progression from the peer involvement that had been useful at Mill Hill. The patients were encouraged to undertake tasks such as redecoration and maintenance. Annie Altschul (personal communication) worked as nurse in the Mill Hill team and she was taken with the bristling of a 'democratic ethos' in the treatment milieu both at Mill Hill and then later at Dingleton, Scotland, where she worked with Jones in the 1970s. Altschul's early contact with the idea of democratic community therapy was interwoven with her training in Vienna in the 1920s, where she had attended lectures with Alfred Adler, finding his ideas about socialism to be inspiring for her own political persuasions. Altschul must have brought some of these politics to bear at Mill Hill, exerting her own influence on the climate of social democratic therapy. Altschul later developed a renowned theory of nursing systems, theory that seemed to be well fitted to therapeutic community practice. Jones[16] later mentioned Altschul's contact with the therapeutic community at Dingleton in Scotland, when he described her as a 'well known nursing instructor'. Altschul quipped that she was one of the few dark-haired nurses who were 'allowed' to work with Jones, who had a 'preference for blond haired Scandinavian nurses' she said. Altschul was particularly impressed with Jones' use of democratic devices with the Japanese POWs. The idea was that the social and domestic engagement in ward activities helped the men return to normal functioning and prepare them for the task of finding work and employment. The diminution of symptoms of paranoia, impotency and anxiety appeared to occur not through direct attack in treatment but as a welcome offshoot of the social therapy, as Jones later recorded.[16]

The Department of Health and Labour (DoHL) was satisfied by the outcome of the rehabilitation of the Japanese POWs and asked Jones to repeat the treatment with 100 homeless men suffering with concurrent mentally infirmity. This formed the basis of the Belmont Social Rehabilitation unit in Sutton, which was established in 1947, later to become known as the Henderson Hospital.[17] Belmont and later Henderson gradually deepened the use of democratic ideas, and the emphasis on these social democratic aspects of therapy culminated in a seminal book *Social psychiatry* published in 1952 by Jones and colleagues. The book was given the sub-heading of: 'a study of therapeutic communities' at the request of the American publisher who feared that an American audience under the grip of McCarthyism would suspect anything vaguely resembling 'socialist' in the title and would therefore boycott the book.[18] The 1952 title waiver was ironic in as much as Maxwell Jones was personally far from a socialist or even a social democrat it might be said. Stewart Whitely (personal communication, 2000) described Jones as more inclined towards autocracy: a sort of 'we're-democratic-here-as-long-as-you-agree-with-me' (to use Whitely's words).

Yet there can be no doubt that democratization and the urge towards egalitarianism emanated in its earliest articulated form from the Henderson during these years. It might be argued that democracy was a *reaction* to Jones' autocracy as much as it was engendered by his own system of political beliefs. The role of other staff, such as Eileen Skellern, who went on to be an important figure in the mental health nursing profession, has often been underestimated and may have had far greater influence on the development of therapeutic democracy than is usually credited. It was not Jones, for instance, who established the formal structure of patients' involvement in the admission procedure at Henderson (voting new patients in or not) but rather one of the junior doctors.[18,p.14] Some of the tensions between Jones and his team at the Henderson at this time were highlighted in the process of the in-depth study carried out by Rapoport in the late 1950s, where the idea of therapeutic democracy became more clearly articulated.[19] There was much ill-feeling during the Rapoport study and Jones seems to have been uncertain as to the value of the study, a measure perhaps of Jones' rivalry with Rapoport.[18] Nonetheless, it was Jones who became identified with the idea of democratization and it was he who carried the message furthest. As a prolific teacher, writer and traveller, he spent much time in Europe, the USA, Africa and Australasia working as a Consultant in Mental Health for the World Health Authority (later the World Health Organization). He discovered varying degrees of fertile ground for the TC ideology and appears to have catalysed new developments in various countries.

Reflection

How do you think these formative experiences influenced the careers of Annie Altschul and Hildegard Peplau?

THERAPEUTIC COMMUNITIES AS A DOMINANT DISCOURSE

Between 1962 and 1969 Maxwell Jones returned to work in the UK as chief superintendent at Dingleton Hospital in Scotland. By then TCs following the Mill Hill lineage rather than the more analytic TCs following the hierarchical approaches of Northfield (i.e. the Cassel Hospital, the Charles Hood Unit at the Maudsley) had forged a reputation synonymous with radical social psychiatry. The intersection between therapeutic communities and the urgency towards a more liberated psychiatry was easily blended; George McDonald Bell had established Dingleton Hospital as the first 'open door' hospital in 1948 followed shortly by TP Rees at Warlingham Park Hospital in the early 1950s. David Clark likewise opened all but two of the locked psychiatric wards at Fulbourn, describing this as an 'experiment in freedom',[19] which naturally paved the way towards the concept of patient self-government. Clark later reflected on this radical time:

> Some of us began to experiment with this (self-government) – Richard Crocket at Ingrebourne, Bertie Mandelbrote at Littlemore, Denis Martin at Claybury – and began to find that you could operate a therapeutic community, certainly in a ward or a part of a psychiatric hospital. And of course we began to visit one another and talk about what we were doing, and share with one another the pains of doing something which was seen as irregular, unprofessional, shabby, lamentable, dangerous, revolutionary, by all our colleagues in the medical and nursing profession … These were the years of the student revolution. These were the years, incredible as it might seem, when a psychiatrist became a prophet for the young Ronnie Laing.
>
> Clark[20]
> *from an audio recording of*
> *conference address*

The concept of a 'therapeutic community' became synonymous with the idea of progressive psychiatry and between the late 1960s and mid–late 1970s there were 26 meetings hosted among 15 different 'therapeutic communities'[a] to discuss the development of these new ideas of empowerment and cooperation. These 'round table' meetings were heated and often turbulent.[20] It was not unusual for people to be seen 'leaping to their feet and making impassioned speeches, citing Chairman Mao and other figures like that as the way to organise things'.[20] Counter meetings were organized and where structure was instantiated in formal meetings reactionary forces would bring about drastic revisions of conference programmes. It appears the whole climate was characterized by opposition and dissonance, although Clark observed that this early period of chaos was probably functional:

> I think that the anarchic period at the beginning was quite useful for many of us, because we realised how creative an unstructured situation was, that it did allow so many things to arise.[20]

This atmosphere was in evidence at the first official psychiatric TC conference in Edinburgh in September 1969

---

[a] The hosts of these meetings (reported by Clark[20]) were as follows: Fulbourn (4), Henderson (4), Ingrebourne (3), Halliwick (2), Littlemore (2), Claybury (2), Dingleton (1), John Conolly (1), St. Bernards (1), Schrodell's (1), Charles Hood (1), Atkinson Morley (1), Marlborough Day Hospital (1), Paddington Day Centre (1), Highcroft Hall (1).

organized by the World Federation for Mental Health and the National Association for Mental Health. Clark described the events and the centrality that Maxwell Jones enjoyed at this time thus:

> It was a very important occasion for Max, because he'd just told Dingleton that he was leaving them, in fact he'd just finished at Dingleton, and in a sense it was his farewell to us in Britain before he went off once again across the Atlantic into adventures that we could only just guess of. So it was an emotionally charged conference and not uncharacteristically, like anything organised by Max, it was a shambles. The plenary sessions turned into stormy community meetings, people didn't attend the papers, there were passionate arguments and fury everywhere. There were attempts to rearrange the whole conference, and so on. Pure Max.[20]

It was at these series of chaotic meetings that the Association of Therapeutic Communities (ATC) congealed and was finally officially born in 1972[b] at a meeting at Fulbourne. Ruby Mungovan became treasurer then, and all participants were asked for a pound note by David Clark. A steady development of structure emerged with new 'officials', even though the need to have someone identified as treasurer and so forth was railed against. But Clark was philosophic about the need for formality:

> If you wanted something to go on, and be a continuing process, then you had to have some kind of structure. You had to have somebody to keep notes of what had happened, and somebody to hold the money, and some other people to plan a bit ahead. And then later one realised that if you were going to have to engage with the major world, if you were going to have to make representations to Ministries, if you were going to have to talk to charities and so on, then, alas, you had to have a formal organisation. And one of the questions I think is how in any organisation you retain the spontaneity, and yet get an effective, ongoing organisation. And I don't know whether you think the ATC has solved that now. I suspect not.[20]

In 1979 the Annual General Meeting of the Association agreed to go forward for charitable status, which meant that a chairperson had to be elected (David Clark was the first Chair). In 1980 Bob Hinshelwood started *The International Journal of Therapeutic Communities*, so the early chaos had been replaced by a formal association and an official journal. Hinshelwood[21] later noted that

the move towards standardization and conformity in TC practice during these years fell into line with an overall drift in society towards professionalization, routinization and institutional accountability. Yet he mourned the loss of the exhilaration of the political tension from which TCs had first thrived amidst the revolutionary climate of the 1960s:

> We were strengthened by being in key with society at large; but also suffered from being linked with the excesses of the permissive society. For instance revolutionary groups in Germany adopted the term 'therapeutic community' and linked with armed terrorism such as the Bader–Meinhoff group. This led to a crisp reaction against the therapeutic community in Germany, where the term is still highly unpopular.[21,p.66]

The challenge for the organized second generation of TCs was to maintain the radical edge of progress towards egalitarianism arising out of the creative chaos of a fermenting ideology while balancing the need for authoritative professional governance via standardization and statutory responsibilities. It appeared to be the challenge of applying a concept of a flattened hierarchy, as opposed to no hierarchy, where a vertical rather than horizontal system was preferred. Perhaps the closest political philosophy that resembled this new effort was the version of the drift towards the new centre left in politics that emerged under the rubric of 'Croslandism'.[22]

Although during the 1970s TCs became peripherally associated with the counter-culture movement through the anti-psychiatry work of David Cooper and Ronnie Laing, who established Kingsley Hall as a therapeutic community and later the Arbours Crisis Centre, many of the cornerstone principles of TC practice were adopted by an ever-increasing number of psychiatric hospitals who saw *Social Psychiatry* as a progressive alternative psychiatric orthodoxy. The acceptance of the TC ideology in the very hierarchical establishment of the NHS seemed something of an anathema of its radical anti-establishment roots. Anti-psychiatry itself became a dominant culture and there was fresh impetus to close the old asylums and reintegrate the mentally ill in the community under an agenda of social inclusion. TCs, which had been a sturdy haven for the interface of psychoanalysis, sociology and psychiatry, had produced a set of treatment ideologies which became embedded, to greater or lesser degrees, in all psychiatric treatments.

But this 'established' place for TCs in the network of NHS provision was found to be precariously tallied

---

[b] At an archive witness event (20 June 2003) celebrating 30 years of the ATC held at the Planned Environment and Therapy Trust (PETT) archive centre in Cheltenham, several members of the early movement gathered to reflect on the foundations of the ATC. Participants were David Anderson, David Clark, Bob Hinshelwood, David Kennard, David Millard, Melvyn Rose and Stuart Whitely (all of whom had been variably present during the early meetings between 1968 and 1971). The witness event was a rare opportunity to re-experience the collective group matrix of this group of TC innovators. One notable feature of the group discussion was the high degree of dissonance and disagreement in the flow of discussions; rarely did the narrative sequence of contributions find consonance with the previous contribution. One had a sense in observing this complex and lively combative debate that this was something of the willing quality of anarchy that might have characterized the early meetings of the ATC as David Clark describes.

to winds of political whim; when the idea of social therapy came under fire from new and mostly untested advances in pharmacology and behaviourism, the social method of TCs went out of favour. During the 1980s, the closure of the old hospital asylums, where many TCs had been rooted, saw many renowned TCs close. This drift away towards the anti-social inclinations of behaviour therapy and new biological theories saw further threats to the social type of approaches expounded by the TC method.

> ## Reflection
>
> What do you understand to be the key ingredients that linked therapeutic community practice with social psychiatry from the 1960s onwards?

THERAPEUTIC COMMUNITIES TODAY

The history of TC and milieu therapy movements usually features accounts of the key male psychiatrist figureheads like Harry Stack Sullivan, Dexter Bullard, Maxwell Jones, Michael Foulkes, Wilfred Bion, Tom Main and Ronnie Laing among others.[3,6,23–26] Suffice it to say, reports specific to nursing practice in the history of the therapeutic community tradition have been limited to a handful of accounts.[1,27–33] In reappraising the history of TCs we can glimpse the interleave of some of the most eminent founders of mental health nursing with TC evolution. Mental health nursing and TC practice emerge concurrently with the progressive traditions of user involvement and social psychiatry. So what place is there for TC practice today.

We know at present that acute psychiatric inpatient units are particularly difficult environments, which stretch the resources of even the most capable individuals.[34] The *Audit of violence*[34] drew attention to the wide array of problems encountered by staff including the unsafe atmosphere of acute wards compounded by inadequate staffing with high vacancies and inexperienced leadership. The report characterized treatments as coercive and chronic staff demoralization with 78 per cent of nurses, 41 per cent of clinical staff and 36 per cent of service users reporting that they had been personally attacked, threatened or made to feel unsafe. *Acute Care*[35] also noted high levels of boredom and inactivity reported among patients. Exposure to violence has been a key factor in low morale[36] and though it is early days yet to review changes resulting from the new management of violence guidelines in the aftermath of the Bennett Inquiry,[37] it is timely to review some of the theoretical underpinnings of ward management by mental health nurses.

There is some emerging evidence that TC group-based therapy, emerging from the traditions of TC and user involvement, is effective in producing a safe milieu.[38] And there is some persuasive evidence, albeit limited, that democratic administration and collective rule-setting in the milieu might have a positive impact on reducing levels of aggression, violence, seclusion and staff sickness and increasing staff morale.[39] It is perhaps through principles of TC practice that the transformative potential of mental health nursing practice might counter anti-therapeutic milieus. A revitalized agenda for mental health nursing might well reach to the agenda for active patient engagement espoused in the National Health Service plan,[40] aspirations that are familiar givens in TC practice.

> ## Reflection
>
> What role do you think there is for therapeutic community philosophy and practice in the future?

REFERENCES

1. Barnes E, Griffith P, Ord J, Wells D. *Face to face with distress. The professional use of self in psychosocial care.* London. Butterworth Heinemann, 1998: 5–41.

2. Rapoport RN. *The community as doctor.* London, UK: Tavistock, 1960.

3. Harrison T. *Bion, Rickman & Foulkes and the Northfield Experiment. Advancing on a different front.* London, UK: Jessica Kingsley, 2000.

4. Bion WR. Leaderless group project. *Bulletin of the Menninger Clinic* 1946; **10**; 77–81.

5. Trist E. Working with Bion in the 1940s: the group decade. In: Pines M (ed.). *Bion and group psychotherapy.* London, UK: Routledge, 1985: 1–46.

6. Main T. The concept of the therapeutic community: variations and vicissitudes. In: Pines M (ed.). *The evolution of group analysis.* London, UK: Routledge & Keegan Paul, 1983; 197–217.

7. Bion WR. *Experiences in groups.* London, UK: Tavistock, 1960.

8. Winship G. Karl Mannheim and the 'third way': the democratic origins of the term 'group analysis'. *Group Analysis* 2003; **36** (1): 37–51.

9. Foulkes S. *Introduction to group analytic psychotherapy.* London, UK: Heinemann, 1948.

10. Callaway B. *Hildegard Peplau. Psychiatric nurse of the century.* New York, NY: Springer Publishing Company, 2002.

11. Peplau HE. *Interpersonal relations in nursing.* New York, NY: G.P. Putnams Sons, 1952.

12. Jones M. Group psychotherapy. *British Medical Journal* 1942; **2**: 276–8.

13. Jones M. Group treatment. *American Journal of Psychiatry,* 1942; **101**: 292–9.

14. Lewis, A (ed.). Melancholia: a historical review. In: *The state of psychiatry.* London: Routledge and Kegan Paul 1967 [1934]: 71–110.

15. Jones M. *Social psychiatry in practice*. London, UK: Tavistock, 1968.

16. Jones M. *The process of change*. London, UK: Routledge, 1982.

17. Jones M. *The maturation of the therapeutic community*. New York, NY: Human Sciences Press, 1976.

18. Whitley SA. Community study. In: Warren F, Dolan B (eds). *Perspectives on Henderson Hospital*. Sutton, UK: Henderson Hospital, 2001 [1980].

19. Clarke DH. *Administrative therapy*. London, UK: Tavistock, 1964.

20. Clarke DH. The early days of the ATC. The Peter van der Linden Lecture, *The Association of Therapeutic Communities Windsor Conference: Crossing New Thresholds: Conservation – Adaptation – Co-operation*. 13–16 September 1999, Cumberland Lodge, Windsor, UK.

21. Hinshelwood RD. The therapeutic community in a changing cultural and political climate. *International Journal of Therapeutic Communities*, 1989; **10** (1): 63–9.

22. Crosland A. *The future of socialism*. London, UK: Cape, 1955.

23. De Mare PB, de Michael Foulkes and the Northfield Experiment. In: Pines M (ed.). *The evolution of group analysis*. London, UK: Routledge & Keegan Paul, 1983: 218–31.

24. Pines M (ed.). *The evolution of group analysis*. London, UK: Routledge & Keegan Paul, 1983.

25. Pines M (ed.). *Bion and group psychotherapy*. London, UK: Routledge, 1985.

26. Kennard D. *Introduction to therapeutic communities*. London, UK: Jessica Kingsley, 1998.

27. Main T. The ailment. *British Journal of Medical Psychology* 1957; **33**: 128–45.

28. Barnes E (ed.). *Psychosocial nursing: studies from the Cassel Hospital*. London, UK: Tavistock, 1968.

29. Dietrich G. Nurses in the therapeutic community. *Journal of Advanced Nursing* 1976; **1**: 138–54.

30. Ploye PM. On some difficulties of inpatient psychoanalytically orientated therapy. *Psychiatry* 1977; **40** (2): 133–45.

31. James O. The role of the nurse therapist in the therapeutic community. *International Review of Psychoanalysis* 1984; **11**: 151–9.

32. Clarke L. A further critical description of the therapeutic community. *Journal of Clinical Nursing*, 1994; **3**: 279–88.

33. Benbow R, Bowers L. Rehabilitation using therapeutic community principles. *Nursing Times* 1998; **94** (41): 56–7.

34. Royal College of Psychiatrists. *Audit of violence*. London, UK: Healthcare Commission.

35. Sainsbury Centre. *Sainsbury Centre For Mental Health. Acute care 2004 report*. London, UK: Sainsbury Centre, 2005.

36. Rask M, Levander S. 'Nurses' satisfaction with nursing care and work in Swedish forensic psychiatric units'. *Journal of Mental Health* 2002; **11** (5): 545–56.

37. Bennett Inquiry. *Independent inquiry into the death of David Bennett*. Cambridgeshire SHA. 2003. Available from: www.nscstha.nhs.uk.

38. Winship G, Hardy S. Perspectives on the prevalence and treatment of personality disorder. *Journal of Psychiatric and Mental Health Nursing* 2007; **14** (2): 148–54.

39. Mistral W, Hall A, McKee P. Using therapeutic community principles to improve the functioning of a high care psychiatric ward in the UK. *International Journal of Mental Health Nursing* 2002; **11** (1): 10–17.

40. DoH. *The NHS plan*. London, UK: HMSO, 2000.

SECTION
6

THE ORGANIZATION OF CARE

Preface to Section 6

After the nurse is sure that the patient can recognize and name his or her own extreme discomfort, then she can begin to help the patient to connect the anxiety and its relief behavior. She can say: 'What helps?' 'What relieves it?' 'What is relieving it right now?

Hildegard E Peplau (1964)

The practice of nursing does not take place in a vacuum, but is framed immediately by the work of other health and social care colleagues, and more broadly by policy, legislation and economics. The 'art of the possible' in nursing practice is a subtle art indeed.

All nurses need philosophies, theories and models if they are to elevate caring beyond that which could be realized by a kindly Samaritan. Once, nurses had to rely on other disciplines to provide them with 'pre-packed' theories and models. Now nurses develop their own models of practice, informed either by their own research or by their own choice of guiding philosophy. Some of these innovations in theory and practice are represented here.

In Section 6 we illustrate some of the commoner forms of organized care, beginning with acute hospital services, which remain the traditional focus for mental health services, at least in the Western world. We end with a consideration of the kind of organized support that asylum seekers and refugees might need, two groups of people who, increasingly, find themselves 'marooned' in often highly inhospitable social and cultural surroundings.

This section illustrates how many of the philosophical values and principles of practice, covered in previous sections, find expression either in the continued development of established services – like secure care, family support, or intensive care – or in more innovative services – such as crisis teams, assertive outreach and liaison psychiatry. This section also includes a consideration of the special needs of women in mental health care, illustrating the importance of assuring emotional and physical security, alongside the offer of meaningful alternatives to hospitalization.

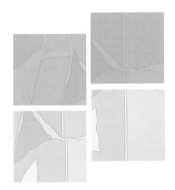

CHAPTER 47

The acute care setting

Angela Simpson*

INTRODUCTION

Mental health services have been changing rapidly, in most Western countries over the last decade. The numbers of beds available for acute psychiatric care have been reduced and the preferred treatment setting shifted into local communities. Except in the most severe cases, admission to hospital for acute psychiatric care will only be arranged once community-based treatment interventions such as crisis intervention, early intervention or assertive outreach (or local variations on such approaches) have been attempted.

Although available resources have prioritized the provision of alternative forms of supportive care based within the community, research has indicated that demand for inpatient care has remained strong. In Australia, the United Kingdom and the USA bed occupancy rates have remained high, while the duration of hospital admissions was found to be shorter.[1-3] Further, the care needs of people admitted into acute inpatient care has become increasingly complex and challenging in terms of both presentation and behaviour.[1,4] These combined factors have contributed to a climate in which it has proven difficult for psychiatric nurses and other occupational groups working within acute inpatient settings to provide therapeutic care.[2,5]

THE PURPOSE OF ACUTE INPATIENT ADMISSION WARDS

Acute inpatient admission wards provide short-term admission to hospital for the purpose of psychiatric assessment, treatment and care. Acute inpatient care is distinguished from other psychiatric support in that the person in crisis urgently requires admission to hospital, where intensive 24-hour support is provided and the person's changing condition closely observed. On admission to hospital the person is usually highly distressed and requires a more intensive form of support than that available in community settings. The primary aim of hospital admission is to assess the person's condition while also providing the human support, care environment and treatment necessary in order to re-establish emotional stability. In hospital, the person is encouraged to become involved in a collaborative helping process. Individual care needs are jointly identified and constructive helping relationships developed. On discharge, responsibility for providing care at home is transferred to a mental health worker based in the community, who continues to work with the person and his/her family or supporters.

Although this chapter focuses on the role of the psychiatric nurse working within the acute inpatient psychiatric unit, it is important to remember that nurses are

*Angela Simpson is course leader for the post-graduate diploma in Mental Health Nursing and a Research Fellow at University of York, UK. She has worked extensively in mental health nursing over a 20-year period and has a particular interest in nursing practice development in acute inpatient admission settings. Her recent research has focused the management of depression in primary care settings and recovery from self-cutting.

members of a much broader multi-professional team, including psychiatrists, occupational therapists, social workers and members of community mental health teams. Links with other support agencies (e.g. voluntary sector organizations and service user groups) are also well established. Acute care is highly team focused; this multi-professional approach allowing timely medical treatment, nursing and social care to be provided.

THE PERSON IN ACUTE DISTRESS

For the person on the brink of admission to hospital, acute crisis is characterized by significant, often overwhelming, personal distress. The distress manifests itself in different ways. The person might be highly overactive, responding to disturbing voices or profoundly withdrawn with low mood to the point of being unable to rest, eat or drink.

People who have experienced acute breakdown often talk of an experience that included a profound sense of unease and isolation. Although relationships with relatives, friends and keyworkers often become fractured in crisis, the fragmentation of relationships in acute distress extends beyond the person's external world to include the relationship that the person has with the *self*. It is not unusual for the person to withdraw, or develop an overly critical relationship with *the self* and this in turn can contribute to collapsed self-esteem. It is important to remember that the experience of acute distress whether the person is in depression, experiencing disturbing voices/ beliefs or in one of its many other forms, is often experienced as bewildering and frustrating, and these background emotions can impede the person's immediate ability to self-manage their condition.

The experience of acute crisis is life-changing. Commonly, it highlights a person's sense of identity, belonging and worth. The value of personal relationships and sense of 'future self' also tend to come to the fore. Consequently, the sense of personal instability during episodes of distress can be experienced as overwhelming. Personal crisis experienced on this scale, emphasizes the need for supportive nurse–patient relationships. Developing helping relationships with people in acute distress is an important goal for nurses working within acute inpatient settings. However, this is not easy work and can be difficult to achieve not least because of the multiple, often complex, presentations of distress.

Of all areas of mental health care, acute inpatient care illustrates the most direct collision between the raw and unrehearsed emotional distress experienced by the person in crisis, and the concerns and anxieties that this can evoke within the people charged with the responsibility of providing supportive care. People in acute distress can appear to the novice nurse to be in a condition that is difficult to understand and which (at least initially) may seem scary. Acute distress has many different presentations that are as individual as the person in distress is unique. The person's condition is changeable and spans a spectrum anywhere between profoundly chaotic to profoundly withdrawn. It is important to recognize that the often extreme nature of the presentation of acute distress can wrong-foot even the most confident and experienced nurse and it takes time to acclimatize to working with acute admission settings.

The multiple and sometimes startling presentations of acute distress can lead nurses to stand back and observe the person in distress, rather than make every possible attempt to get to know and understand them as people. Hildegard Peplau[6] reminded us that behaviour that is 'acted out' rather than discussed is unlikely to be thoroughly understood by either the person in crisis or the nurse. She also stressed the need for nurses to demonstrate a willingness to relate with the person in distress as well as a genuine curiosity regarding the nature of their experiences. This illustrates the need for psychiatric nurses working within acute inpatient settings to use every available opportunity to attempt to come to better know and understand the person. Psychiatric nurses are the mainstay providers of care in acute admission settings. They are in very close proximity to the person in crisis throughout the 24-hour period and this provides them with the opportunity to get to know something of the person's distress. An attentive and understanding nurse is able to relate with the person in distress creating a relationship in which the person might begin to feel supported enough to share their experience.

> ## Reflection
>
> Identify a nurse or professional colleague who seems to relate particularly well with people in distress.
>
> - What does this nurse/colleague do in order to develop and maintain a therapeutic relationship with people in acute distress?
> - Explore how being in close proximity to people in acute distress makes you feel.
> - How might you develop your curiosity and genuine willingness to relate with people in acute distress?

Chapter 60 describes how the nurse uses the admission interview to nurture the beginnings of a helping relationship in collaboration with the person in acute distress. Here, this theme is developed further considering what people in acute distress need from nurses in the days following on from admission, in order to best support their recovery. This process involves developing a therapeutic care environment or *milieu* in which it is possible for helping relationships to be nurtured and where individual and group support is routinely provided.

STRUCTURING CARE TO ENABLE RECOVERY

Altschul[7] recognized that the care environment is best organized when it is flexible enough to incorporate all needs. She also observed that people help each other where the supportive conditions exist for them to do so. The healing potential of the social environment has long been recognized and utilized by service users who commonly find value in meeting and talking with other people in distress.[8] The atmosphere and social surroundings of the ward is known as the milieu. Creative development of the milieu helps to provide the social conditions in which it becomes possible for people in care to undertake purposeful work, learning from each other, while living with and through individual experiences of distress. Within this supportive milieu the person in acute distress is able to:

- develop a helping relationship with a key named nurse;
- undertake individual work to develop an understanding of the experience of distress;
- share experiences with others in a similar situation both informally on the ward and through structured group work;
- contribute towards helping others through shared experience.

The milieu is best developed when there is a strong prevailing sense of purpose. To achieve this, the nursing team must provide therapeutic structure to ward-based activity supporting the nurturance of therapeutic relationships with people in acute distress and structured individual and group working. The structure that this sense of purpose brings to 'ward life' underpins a milieu in which people can share their common experiences of distress, but remains flexible and responsive enough to cater for individual needs. It is important to recognize that structuring care effectively brings a sense of purpose and organization to acute care.

Jane's story, which follows, illustrates how a key named nurse works *with* the person in acute distress. The nurse recognizes the need to work flexibly, responding to Jane's changing needs. This process involves working individually with Jane but also involving other members of the team as supports in the nurse's absence. This individualized care programme is augmented by inputs from the multi-professional team and leads, ultimately, towards the development of the discharge planning process.

The admission process is addressed in Chapter 60. Here the focus is on how a named nurse uses everyday encounters with the person in acute distress to nurture an effective helping relationship. As the person in distress begins to identify with and feel increasingly comfortable with the nursing presence and their condition begins to settle, it becomes possible for nurses to further develop this therapeutic rapport offering more intensive and structured forms of individual and group support against a backdrop of multi-professional care. These processes will now be described in more detail using Jane's story to identify the process.

Personal illustration 47.1: Jane's story

Jane was admitted to Cherry Ward 3 days ago after a concerned greengrocer contacted the police. The shopkeeper recognized Jane as previousiy being a chatty and well-presented lady, but last Thursday he found her wondering the town centre streets alone in the early morning, well before the shops were due to open. At the time she seemed perplexed and somewhat disheveled. Further, he found her unable to account for what it was that she was doing. At the police station, Jane seemed agitated and profoundly worried. She expressed concerns about her neighbours, saying that they may be trying to poison her. She also said that she left her home during the night because of this and that she feels she would be in danger if she were to return. She was seen at the police station by a doctor and reluctantly agreed to admission to Cherry Ward, a local acute psychiatric inpatient facility.

Since admission, Jane has continued to experience difficulty resting. She paces up and down and can sometimes be found peeping out of doorways. She finds it difficult to perform everyday tasks. Although she will respond to direct questions, Jane offers very little in terms of spontaneous conversation.

NURTURING THE BEGINNINGS OF RECOVERY

In the admission interview the nurse will have to begin to develop an understanding of the person in distress and the problems that they are encountering as a result of the distress (see Chapter 60). This interview provides an initial understanding of the person's immediate needs as well as aspects of the context that led up to the person being admitted to hospital. Over the coming days nurses will be concerned to build on the early rapport built during the assessment interview to develop further their knowledge and understanding of the person in distress. The nursing aim at this stage is to consolidate the emotional attachment that began to develop between the nurse and person in distress at the admission interview. Research has indicated that when the admission interview is undertaken well, that a useful and potentially productive attachment is formed between the admitting nurse and the person in distress.[7] Patients recognize the value of the admission assessment and rate highly the concern and interest extended to them at this time.[9] However, it is also the case that while the nurse's efforts to engage with the patient at the admission interview are valued by patients, nurses are less likely to develop rapport at the same level of intensity in the days following on from this.[9]

It is not unusual to find that while in acute distress the person will (at least initially) not necessarily be willing to engage in structured activity or in-depth dialogue. Jane is having difficulty resting and is experiencing problems performing basic everyday living tasks. Further she is limited in her ability to construct active dialogue in her current condition. Nurses must recognize these initial limitations and structure their own interventions around the person in a way in which the person in distress might begin to recognize the nurse as a constant and helpful presence. Nurses best demonstrate a therapeutic presence by being highly visible, spending time with and around the person in distress. Nurses achieve this when they structure time into their working day to allow themselves to be around the person in distress, participating in everyday life activities.

Following admission to hospital, Jane continues to be in a state of heightened distress. As a consequence, everyday activities have become difficult to perform. Simple procedures like washing, performing self-care and dressing are difficult to focus on and following through the task to completion can be difficult to achieve and experienced as frustrating. Recognizing this, the nurse spends time with Jane after breakfast and helps her to focus on the tasks associated with self-care and deciding what to wear. The nurse has an understanding of how difficult performing basic procedures has become for Jane. She will assist Jane where it is necessary to do so and prompt and encourage Jane to complete the task. She will achieve this without being condescending and in a way that emphasizes the need to undertake the task *with* the person rather than doing it *for*. At the same time, the nurse recognizes the need to move at the pace of the person in distress, to be patient and whenever possible use the opportunity of working alongside the person to encourage further dialogue, however minimal, about her current situation.

While undertaking tasks at this level with the person in distress, the nurse develops a detailed understanding of the person, their condition and the problems of living that they are experiencing as a consequence of their distress. Nurses will observe and document their observations of the person in distress. Structuring everyday time around the person as suggested here allows the nurse to develop a much more detailed understanding of the person and their condition. The nurse may be able to identify:

- periods of time in the day when Jane's agitation and distress appear to be heightened or decreased;
- situations in which Jane seems better able to control her condition and more able to relax;
- what Jane likes to eat and drink and periods of the day when she is better able to successfully achieve this;
- situations that appear to increase Jane's distress.

The knowledge of the person gleaned at this time forms a useful baseline. Signs of improvement are likely to be subtle at first and the observant nurse will be able to report signs of improvement to the person in crisis promoting patience and tolerance of the person's condition. By undertaking tasks alongside the person in distress in the way described, the nurse brings a positive, encouraging approach to the nurse–patient relationship and nurtures a therapeutic relationship.

Key points

1 The nurse understands that therapeutic relationships are best built by 'presencing' themselves around the person in distress.
2 By participating in routine everyday tasks *with* the person in distress the nurse is able to develop a more detailed understanding of the person, their condition and the impact their condition is having on their ability to live everyday life.
3 The nurse aims to work *with* the person in distress to ensure that basic everyday living tasks are undertaken and completed. The nurse uses this time to encourage further dialogue.
4 The nurse listens to the person in crisis and provides supportive information.
5 The nurse aims to be a constant, encouraging and caring presence, further developing rapport and a context of mutual trust.

Reflection

Identify factors that work against nurses forming close therapeutic relationships and a therapeutic milieu in acute admission settings.

- How might nurses best organize themselves to increase the therapeutic orientation of their work?
- Identify ways in which care might be better structured in order to increase the proximity of nurses at all levels to the person in care?
- Identify the philosophical nursing values that best support an emphasis of working collaboratively with people in acute distress.

Peplau[10] reminded us that during the initial stages of relationship building the person in distress is observing the nurse closely. The person might decide to 'test out' the nurse's commitment to working with them. Feelings of hopelessness or worthlessness which are very common in people with emotional distress, for example, might result in the person taking action designed to discourage the nurse from paying close attention to them or working with them. Nurses should recognize this, but importantly, continue their endeavours to presence themselves around the person. Nurses should understand that being consistent and delivering the care that has been promised to the patient are important features of further developing the helping relationship.

It is important to remember that the main nursing aim within acute inpatient care is to nurture a helping relationship within which the person in distress might feel encouraged and supported to express their emotions. As the nurse–patient relationship develops and the person's condition begins to settle, nurses' should adapt modifying their approach to helping. At this point, the person in distress might need less from the nurse in terms of direct presencing to achieve the completion of everyday living skills and more in terms of active dialogue. Nurses should be mindful that it is the supportive therapeutic relationship that helps to facilitate the development of insight and subsequent behaviour change in the patient.[10] Further, distress can be alleviated when nurses encourage the expression of emotion.[11] In Jane's case the key nurse will achieve this by structuring short periods of direct contact time into every shift. This time needs to be negotiated with the person in distress *in advance* of the meeting. The aim is to allow the person to talk in more detail about their situation and circumstances. It is essential that in acute settings, the care environment is structured to actively foster the expectation that people will have dedicated therapeutic time together, perhaps lasting half an hour, and twice a day. By so doing the nurse is creating an environment in which the person is able if they wish, to talk and be actively listened to. The nursing aim at this point is to further encourage the expression of emotions.

Key points

1 The nurse recognizes subtle changes in the patient's presentation and as the person in distress begins to settle, shifts emphasis away from presencing and managing everyday living and emphasizes instead the need for structured individual one-to-one time.
2 The nurse should arrange to meet with the person recovering from distress once or twice per day for a period of about half an hour.
3 The purpose of the meeting is to encourage further expression of the person's situation.

Using Barker's Tidal Model[12] Jane's individual sessions would focus on what was happening for Jane *here-and-now*, what she believed was *important* (in terms of her needs), and what personal knowledge or understanding she was gaining from the experience about 'what needs to happen next'. Individual sessions should emphasize collaboration. Nurses provide individual ring-fenced time for each person, but then allow the person in care to guide how 'collaborative working' might best be developed. Nurses might ask:

* What do you want from this time together now?
* How can *we* work together?

Applying the Tidal Model the record of the session is written 'live' rather than as a nursing report, after the event. This confirms the person's active role in the whole process of caring and being-in-care.

GROUPWORK

The value of sharing experience should not be underestimated as a medium for promoting shared learning and understanding. Groupwork can be very simple – organizing a venue for people to talk through issues like:

* What is going on for me today?
* How I am coping?
* What I will do if things start to go off course?

In the Tidal Model three core forms of group work are identified, which are central to the recovery process. These have a particular application in an acute setting.

The Discovery Group usually is held in the morning when people may feel at a low ebb, and may lack the motivation to engage in anything too demanding. The group is held in a relaxed atmosphere, where people have a chance to identify and discuss positive aspects of themselves, which are often overlooked in the focus on their problems. A set of questions is often used to stimulate discussion:

* What is your favorite book, film or TV show and *why*?
* What would you do if you won the lottery?
* How do you think your pets (cat or dog) would describe you?
* What is the hardest thing you have ever done … and how did you do it?

The *Solutions Group* is usually held in the afternoon and focuses on developing the participants' awareness of what positive change would mean for them. Usually, one person is encouraged to be the 'model' for difficulties that might be common to the group, which helps the 'model' identify possible solutions that already may be part of the person's repertoire, albeit perhaps at a low level.

The *Information Group* is usually held in the evening and focuses on providing people with information about their ongoing care and treatment or supporting services. Common topics include:

- medication – effects, side-effects and contraindications;
- support in the community following discharge;
- self-help groups – their form and function;
- financial matters.

A genuine 'expert' should lead this group. In the case of community-based support, often a former user of psychiatric services will lead the discussion on mutual support or self-help groups.

Reflection

Developing the therapeutic basis of acute admission care involves nurturing a productive milieu

- How might care be better organized to allow an increase of productive one-to-one time to be spent with people in recovery from episodes of acute distress?
- Identify a number of low key therapeutic groups that could potentially be organized and managed as part of the therapeutic programme in acute care. When might these be best delivered?
- Identify nursing actions that best nurture a philosophy of hope and recovery in acute inpatient admission care.

POWER AND MULTI-PROFESSIONAL TEAM MEETINGS

Team meetings are a means of reviewing progress as well as planning future care. Often, meetings are led by a consultant psychiatrist and involve a wide range of other professional groups such as social workers, occupational therapists and members of community mental health teams. Traditionally, it would not be unusual for six to eight professional staff to be involved in discussing and making important decisions about someone like Jane's ongoing care. Often, most of this group will have little direct contact with the patient. It goes without saying that Jane's involvement in these discussions is essential. Such meetings are commonly structured in a way that risks intimidating anyone, far less someone who is mentally distressed.

It is important to plan Jane's future care and treatment efficiently and this needs to involve team-wide discussion. However, traditional 'reviews' and 'ward rounds' are unlikely to allow Jane the best opportunity to express herself. Recognizing this, the key nurse must support Jane through the multi-professional team meeting ensuring that one way or another Jane's point of view is heard. To achieve this the nurse takes the following steps.

1 Identify Jane's view of her progress and the support she needs in advance of the meeting.

2 Arranges for Jane to see the doctor outside the larger meeting if she prefers to do so.
3 Encourages Jane to make a list of what needs to be said in her own words.
4 Agree with Jane that the nurse will talk through 'Jane's issues' on her behalf if she feels unable to do so.

PACING THE PERSON

For Jane, re-establishing emotional stability is a *process*, a significant element of which involves allowing sufficient time within a supportive environment for her to adjust to her changing life circumstances. Only where these features of recovery become comfortably established does it realistically become desirable for her to face the important next step of returning home. In Barker's view, the most important question that needs to be asked in acute care is 'what needs to change for the person to return home?[13] For many people the problems that were part of their admission to hospital are still awaiting them – at home or in the community. The process of discharging the person from hospital is likely to involve:

- discussing individual concerns with Jane;
- supporting her in discussions with the wider multi-professional team regarding her individual care needs on discharge;
- supported visits home;
- trial periods of leave at home prior to discharge to test out common assumptions regarding Jane's ability to cope;
- introducing Jane to the community-based key worker who takes over responsibility for coordinating care for Jane on discharge;
- working with Jane and the multi-professional team to determine a discharge plan and agree her discharge date.

Length of stay in hospital is often viewed as a measure of best practice and the desire to somehow speed up the process of caring is a seemingly constant feature of modern healthcare policy. Nurses must remain vigilant to ensure that the process of managing care does not distract nurses from the core work of providing therapeutic care. It is not unusual for people to change their 'presentation' when in hospital. The key question is, to what extent does this reflect the kind of change needed to allow the person to return home, *and* return to ordinary living? People in care need to be treated as 'people' rather than impersonal objects, processed by the healthcare system. Nurses have a responsibility to remain true to the individual care needs of the person in crisis. They might best do this by acknowledging that recovery has its own pace, a tempo that is individual to the person.

SUMMARY

The primary focus of psychiatric nursing in acute settings is to nurture close interpersonal relationships that focus on relating with the person in acute distress, attempting to understand the person's experience and the effects this has on their ability to live everyday life.[13] Psychiatric mental health nurses must also consider how to organize and structure nursing care to support this degree of human contact, inside ward environments that offer a responsive crisis service. This is best achieved when nurses work toward creating a milieu that is purposeful and structured in order that the person in care might begin to learn individually and in groups about their experience of acute distress.

REFERENCES

1. Cleary M. The realities of mental health nursing in acute inpatient environments. *International Journal of Mental Health Nursing* 2004; **13**: 53–60.

2. Sainsbury Centre for Mental Health. Acute problems: a survey of the quality of care in acute psychiatric wards. London, UK: Sainsbury Centre for Mental Health, 1998.

3. Garritson SH. Availability and performance of psychiatric acute care facilities in California Psychiatric Services from 1992–1996. *Psychiatric Services* 1999; **50**: 1453–60.

4. Richards D, Bee P, Loftus S *et al*. Specialist educational intervention for acute inpatient mental health nursing: service user views and effects on nursing quality. *Journal of Advanced Nursing* 2005; **51** (6): 634–44.

5. MIND. *Ward watch: minds campaign to improve hospital conditions for mental health patients: report summary*. London, UK: MIND, 2004.

6. Peplau H. Interpersonal relations model: theoretical constructs principles and general applications. In: Reynolds W, Cormack D (eds). *Psychiatric and mental health nursing: theory and practice*. London, UK: Chapman and Hall, 1990.

7. Altschul AT. *Patient–nurse interaction*. Edinburgh, UK: Churchill Livingston, 1972.

8. Rogers A, Pilgrim D, Lacey R. *Experiencing psychiatry*. London, UK: Macmillan, 1993.

9. Moyle W. Nurse–patient relationship: a dichotomy of expectations. *International Journal of Mental Health Nursing* 2003; **12**: 103–9.

10. Peplau H. *Interpersonal relations in nursing*. London, UK: Macmillan Education, 1988.

11. Morse JM, Miles MW, Clark DA, Doberneck BM. Sensing patients needs: exploring concepts of nursing insight and receptivity used in nursing assessment. *Scholarly Inquiry for Nursing Practice: an International Journal* 1994; **8**: 233–54.

12. Barker PJ, Buchanan-Barker P. *The tidal model: a guide for mental health professionals*. Hove, UK: Brunner Routledge, 2005.

13. Barker PJ. *Assessment in psychiatric and mental health nursing*. Cheltenham, UK: Stanley Thornes, 1997.

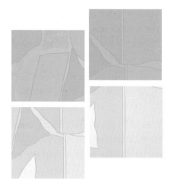

CHAPTER 48

The psychiatric intensive care unit: coercion, control or care

Cheryl Waters* and Andrew Cashin**

INTRODUCTION

Psychiatric intensive care exists to maximize safety and support while promoting independence for people who are an acute risk to themselves or others. The whole province of psychiatric intensive care is beleaguered by therapeutic conundrums and quandaries. For example:

- How is a balance struck between the caring and controlling functions of nursing?
- Is psychiatric intensive care about treatment or containment?
- How does one satisfy the competing needs for safety and privacy?
- How is the central tenet of least restriction practised in an environment where safety and risk management are crucial?

These are only some of the questions that need to be considered when nursing patients in a *psychiatric intensive care unit* (PICU). Furthermore, in no area of practice is the ability to evaluate one's own motives and desires more important for the nurse.

Here, some of these issues and challenges will be examined alongside a discussion about the nature, goals, purposes and methods of nursing care in a PICU. We will explore how one might negotiate some of these impasses and the intentions behind nursing actions and attitudes when caring for the acutely mentally ill in need of intensive treatment.

DESIGN

Given that PICUs are designed to meet local needs, there is no standard.[1] Despite general principles of design, there are large variations in how these principles are operationalized. PICUs tend to be small wards, with between eight and ten beds. They are usually locked and

*Cheryl Waters is a Senior Lecturer and immediate past Course Coordinator, Graduate Certificate Mental Health Nursing in the Faculty of Nursing Midwifery and Health, University of Technology Sydney, Australia. Her research and teaching focuses on developing innovative blended face-to-face and online methods for teaching evidence-based practice, and mental health nursing.
**Andrew Cashin occupies a clinical chair as Associate Professor in Justice Health Nursing in the Faculty of Nursing, Midwifery and Health at the University of Technology Sydney, Australia. Andrew is an authorised mental health Nurse Practitioner with a private practice on the Central Coast of NSW.

have higher staff-to-patient ratios than in other units.[2] They are also carefully furnished with attention given to covering possible ligature points, which may be used to cause self-harm. The individual's need for privacy is balanced against the need to be able to see what patients are doing to maximize safety as well as prevent absconding or elopement.[3] The unit should allow clear observation of patients at all times, while providing the semblance of privacy and an environment in which they can feel safe and supported. To make this possible the units are often structured so that patient areas surround and are visible to a central nursing area. Further, a balance is sought between a high stimulus environment that can be the result of having a number of highly acute people in the same small area, and the need for a relaxed, healing environment. Watkins[4] reported the Sainsbury centre survey of 1988, which noted that collectively the design of PICUs in the UK needs improvement to meet treatment needs and maintain a therapeutic atmosphere conducive to recovery.

FOCUS OF CARE

Even more important than the physical environment are the aims and objectives of nursing care in the PICU and how these are best achieved.

By definition the focus of care in the PICU is the intensive care of people with acute mental illness: patients who are an acute risk to themselves or others because of suicidal, homicidal or assaultive behaviour. As a rule patients in PICUs are sectioned under the local mental health act, and are there involuntarily. Voluntary patients would usually be cared for on a more open unit. The purpose of PICUs is to provide short-term or brief treatment[5,6] with a focus on risk assessment and management. Like any intensive care unit PICU patients are acutely in need of intensive care.[7] The patients have the benefit of a somewhat controlled environment until they improve and move on to a less acute unit or to the community. The spirit of all mental health acts at this time is to treat in the least restrictive environment.[8,9] Consequently, the type of person admitted is further limited to someone who cannot be treated in a less restrictive environment.

The time spent and treatment offered in PICU is only one part of an overall treatment plan and process. The PICU is not merely about containment, nor is it a punishment block that can be used to coerce patients into compliance with treatment programmes on other units.[3] The PICU is the setting for treatment during one phase of the illness experience. In Gentle's[10] study nursing staff characterized their perceptions of the patients in PICU as 'the unwanted' (by other parts of the service) and their goal as 'keeping everyone in'. Of even more concern was the description that the therapeutic environment was 'a vague goal'. This is of great concern if these views reflect a view of PICU shared by other nurses, carers, other mental health professionals and the community at large.

Such views will have an impact on care outcomes because they will influence all concerned. Staff may experience lower morale and patients a sense of hopelessness. As a result of these beliefs it could be difficult to conceive of admission to the PICU as merely a step in the recovery process or ebb in the tide of the person's illness experience.[11] If nurses are to feel valued, to value the care they give, and to achieve their therapeutic ambition of helping the person, the PICU has to be believed to be more than a 'dumping ground' for unwanted patients and nursing care more than just 'baby-sitting'. The sense of hopelessness embodied in the beliefs expressed above would infect carers and patients alike to the extent that the time in PICU would be perceived as a waste. Admission to the PICU should not remove patients from the path to achieving their therapeutic goals. Therefore, the goals for the stay in PICU need to be clear and, to the extent that it is possible, agreed upon. Clear goals make achievements obvious. Even small gains can be noticed and celebrated. The potential effect on morale and hopefulness is obvious.

Clear goals for the admission are a necessary prerequisite for effective care. The actual assessment of the patient has to be fully undertaken before admission, and needs to acknowledge a well-defined set of objectives, and a clear, recovery focused philosophy for the unit. It is necessary to be clear about why someone is being admitted, to know what must occur for him or her to have achieved the goals of the admission and not stay on any longer than required. Severimuttu[12] showed that out of 33 admissions, all of which had clear goals established prior to admission, only two admissions resulted in stays in excess of 12 days. Unfortunately, in this age of reactive clinical planning, unless clear goals and desirable outcomes are established beforehand, there is the risk that the main drive for discharge will be when the bed is required for another client with ill-defined needs.[12] This has the further effect of reinforcing negative perceptions about both PICU nursing and admission to these units.

OBSERVATION AND ENGAGEMENT

There has been much recent debate about the relationship between observation and therapeutic engagement that has arisen out of questions related to the value of close or special observation alone. A poignant critique is offered by Campbell,[13] who noted that in its most basic (and no doubt non-therapeutic) form close observation of suicidality denies 'the ability [to take one's own life] without addressing the desire'. And that this 'must be a major reason why service users find close observation unhelpful. Observation without interaction is a cold comfort'.[13]

Some of this debate took place in 2000–2001 on the Psychiatric Nursing List (a UK bulletin board for mental health nurses and others). The discussions are available on the List archives at: www.jiscmail.ac.uk/ lists/psychiatric-nursing.html. The upshot from such discussion cautions that the distinction between close observation and therapeutic engagement could be a false one, and should be an artificial one, especially in the PICU as the close contact and higher staff-to-patient ratios mean that patients are engaged with staff when they need them, and because of the higher presence and visibility there does not need to be a specially designated attentiveness.

In keeping with the characteristics of those patients who would benefit from the PICU, their condition is uncertain and unstable. Writing from a Foucauldian perspective, Stevenson and Cutcliffe noted that when people enter the PICU 'there is passing over a threshold, both physical and in terms of degree of madness, in order to become subject to special observation, ... creating a boundary across which the person is watched'.[14,p.715] The nurse in the PICU needs to develop an ongoing awareness of the potential for harm. Observation is perhaps one of the fundamentals of skilled nursing and it is a difficult intervention to carry out in a manner that is both non-intrusive and effective. As the civil rights of the person admitted to the PICU have been suspended it follows that she or he has the right to be kept safe. The premise underlying involuntary containment in a PICU is that the patient is not in the position to take responsibility for his or her actions. The legal burden for the patient's actions consequently largely falls on the hospital while they remain an involuntary patient in the PICU. People assessed as at risk in acute psychiatric wards may be placed under close observation to maintain intensified and prolonged assessment.[15] 'Close' could refer to an ongoing state of attentiveness cultivated as one of the core attributes of PICU nursing as apposed to a supposedly detached and objective monitoring presence. This attentiveness includes a continuous process of risk assessment.[3] A much debated matter in acute care and PICU nursing is this activity of close or special observation, how the patient might interpret it and what it signifies in terms of the relationship between the nurse and those in their care.

When you know what to look for, you will be struck by the craft displayed by adept and accomplished nurses when they are 'observing' patients, the fact that they always seem to be available to patients when most needed, and that when outbursts occur they have anticipated it and offer a calm and stable presence. Early in your career you might interpret the masterful ability to be present to the environment and those in it, as apparently doing nothing: hanging about, socializing with the patients and enjoying a game of pool. Years of attentive experience allow an automatic processing of the gestalt of the PICU environment and the unconscious sifting of the relevant cues from the irrelevant in an ongoing process of observation, which has become so refined it appears virtually effortless. This is an accomplishment that is at the core of mental health nursing craft, and which cannot be taught but only learned by attentive and curious involvement in the milieu (see Benner[16]). From this it can be seen how, in the hands of an expert nurse, close observation and engagement are inexorably linked.

No event or situation is by itself a stressor. What shapes our reaction to any situation is our interpretation of it, what it means for us. There is no separable reality out there as such, only events and situations that are perceived in a meaningful way peculiar to the individual. The challenge of nursing in the PICU is to develop an alliance where we can have access to this meaning through shared dialogue. It is only through the creation of this unique and privileged conversational space that we have the opportunity to assist the patient to reframe their experience and put a new perspective on it. A large part of the therapeutic work in the PICU is creating this shared space. This could be called therapeutic engagement.

Perception of admission to the PICU

1 John believes that his family and workmates are trying to put him in a government experimental programme where his organs will be replaced with mechanical devices. When the police picked him up and he was admitted under the act to the local PICU he became very distressed. Anyone who comes near him is warned not to accept any injections, food or drink, because it contains an anaesthetic.

2 Anne, who is very depressed, believes she has been locked away with these strangers because she has not appreciated or been thankful for her family. She has been sent there to languish from the incurable illness, the knowledge of which they are withholding from her.

Therapeutic in this sense broadly means any interaction that opens up a conversational space to examine the person's life story. The person who has become the patient in the PICU has a view of what is happening to them, why they are in the position of patient, why they are reluctantly in a hospital, and what is going to happen to them. The illness experience, in the initial stages of admission at least, may contribute strongly to the meanings constructed by the patient. Someone who is experiencing acute psychotic illness, by definition, will construct his or her world from this frame of reference and interpret his or her experiences in care correspondingly.

MULTI-STORIED LIVES

Once a dialogue is opened, or a conversational space has been created, then the business at hand is to work with the person's story. The space created makes room for the evolution of a new chapter in the narrative of his/her life. One function for the nurse in the PICU is to listen actively to this story. The focus is on recovery – not from the medical disease as such but from the consequences of the illness and the distress and dis-ease it creates in the person's life. One way to access this and to help rewrite this impact is through respectful attention to the stories patients tell us.

The work of Michael White and his colleagues[17–19] from the Dulwich Centre in Adelaide, South Australia, offers some insights into the role of story and narrative in the shaping of people's lives and the restructuring of people's experiences. From this work we can appreciate that the lives of people and patients are shaped by the stories they engage with to give their lives meaning: shaped in order to remain true to these internalized stories. The undertaking for the attentively listening nurse is to help deconstruct the meaning to highlight the difference between the reality of the world in which their way of being is problematic, and these internalized stories.

It is now important to consider the point of involvement in the patient's narrative in PICU and how it might be different to the goals of such an involvement in other contexts.

1 One way of thinking about *narrative* is to consider how we all use it to make sense of things. The stories we tell about our life are the expression of our experiences of a life as it is lived and how we interpret it. We can use patients' narratives to engage with them and to demonstrate respect for their experiences and interpretations. As a result we learn more about the consequences of the illness in their life and are better situated to be involved in their recovery. Without this connection we risk having inadequate comprehension for effective intervention. So patients' stories also provide us with 'frames of intelligibility' within which to make sense of their beliefs and behaviours.

2 Another reason that narrative is important relates to the idea of reality orientation. The concept of reality orientation is widely evident in mental health literature. Keltner and colleagues[2] refer to the process as acknowledging the affective component, but not the content, of delusional ideas. The concept centres on the premise of avoiding the reinforcement of delusions. In a practical sense, reality is what the person perceives it to be. The PICU nurse's goal is to orientate this reality to that which is required to allow the person to progress towards a less restrictive environment. In the long term the goal is to help the patient ultimately recreate a self-identity based on a preferred story line. In the short term there needs to be movement towards a better story line – one that is more consistent with the best explanation nurses have for culturally and historically accumulated insights about acceptable and health-promoting behaviours. In this the nurse is the mediator for sense-making. As nurses we need to listen and help people re-author their stories by inserting some well-placed questions and comments that lead the person to reflection on the utility of some of their beliefs and behaviours. Both our insights and those of the patient can be part of the search for more fitting ways of being. At the simplest level this could be called 'reality orientation' and is one of the goals for engagement through narrative approaches.

Given that the stay in the PICU is usually short term, goal-directed work on a whole life story is definitely not achievable. The issues that need immediate attention are what led up to the admission and what needs to happen here and now in terms of behavioural change and risk reduction that will allow the person to regain control of their life and move to a less restrictive environment.

3 Transitions: longer term *re-authoring* is ongoing. The narrative of a person's life is constantly evolving. The preferred story is the basis for longer term goals and the material to work on in the next setting. Taking this material into the next setting provides continuity in the person's treatment in different settings. The open ward or step-down setting may not provide enough opportunity to complete the work of re-authoring the life story and this work will need to continue into the community. The ongoing process of re-authoring and editing the narrative can form the basis of a community treatment programme and provide further continuity and connection as the person moves through the service. If she or he needs re-admission, there is some predictability that may lead to a shorter admission. If part of each admission is not about making sense of, and integrating the experience, then subsequent admissions may be as scary and unpredictable as the first admission.

Out of the telling and retelling of the story, and the reorientation to a reality that is plausible and congruent with the expectations of society, comes the possibility of the return of control and movement to a different treatment setting. The decision to legally return control is often medical. However, it is nurses, who have the most contact with patients in the PICU and have the greatest opportunity to engage the patient and do the work at hand of eliciting and editing the story.

POWER AND CONTROL

In the PICU a fundamental purpose of the nurse's involvement and engagement is to negotiate the timely and appropriate return of control to the patient. One challenge of PICU nursing is the delicate balance necessary in the separation of the controlling and therapeutic functions. Nursing negotiates this continuum continually in the PICU and the balance will change depending on the patient's ability to exercise self-control and establish achievable goals for themselves.

Medication can be a challenge to the process of engagement, particularly if administered against the person's wishes. The nurse in the PICU has a role in administering prescribed medication. This includes routine and emergency medication. The administration of medication can involve forced interaction between the person in the role of nurse and the person who has been assigned the role of patient. This can become a ritual of testing the limits and asserting the right to choice. Aggressive incidents may occur with increased frequency at this time, as the nurse must force contact. Contact is forced, as the nurse must attempt to connect even in the face of clear and overt messages from the patient that it is not their wish for contact at this time. From the standpoint of a least restrictive alternative, which endeavours to find a balance between individual rights and their need for treatment (especially in the case of impaired reality testing and impulse control[20]) forced and invasive medication and seclusion can seriously threaten the relationship between nurses and the people in their care. On first consideration it might seem that giving an atypical anti-psychotic medication (olanzapine) in a rapidly disintegrating (wafer) formulation would reduce the emergent use of intramuscular anti-psychotic drugs and seclusion. When this was tested it was not shown to improve rates of either types of interaction.[20]

The nurse can only negotiate with and for the patient within the limits defined by the law and the overall treatment plan. The challenge for the nurse is to maintain the goal of engagement and build a therapeutic alliance in the situation of having to exert coercive influence over the patient. It is the nurse who assumes these interactions: not other health professionals. These types of interactions are difficult to comprehend for reluctant patients and may have the effect of confirming their suspicions.

Reflection

- Containment, punishment and coercion – are these reasons for admission to a PICU and how could these be part of a therapeutic relationship?
- How do nurses maintain their sense of self in what are often ambiguous interactions?
- As a nurse how could you maintain your sense of safety and dissipate the sense of heightened arousal and vigilance that would be a consequence of coercive interactions with patients? What would be the consequences of such unresolved arousal on us and the people in our care?

The bottom line may be that as in any intensive care unit the patient may need to take medication to stabilize and subsequently regain control of their life. If the person is an involuntary patient the right to consent has been withdrawn. The bottom line may well involve the forced administration of medication, be it via the intramuscular or the intravenous route. (The new short-acting depot anti-psychotic medications are marketed on the basis of the need for less frequent administration. Hence, there could be less need for interactions of this sort. As is discussed above, rapidly dissolving wafers would also reduce these interactions – if the patient would take them.) Choices will need to be made about how to negotiate forced interactions around medication, and possibly food and fluid. The nurse needs to reflect on his or her investment in this power struggle, and whether decisions are based on this perceived investment. It can be difficult in the face of such interactions to maintain clear boundaries and separate out our reactions: to be sure that what is being done is a response to the patient's clinical need and not in response to fear and uncertainty. Neilson and Brennan[21,p.154] note that the 'nurses' therapeutic skills may be tested to the limit by patients' challenging behaviours, and nursing skills in observation and therapeutic engagement contribute directly to the maintenance of a safe environment and the ongoing process of risk assessment'. Patients in PICU are rarely grateful for admission and what they perceive as forced treatment. Consequently, it is important to have put some serious time, both individually and as a treatment team, into thinking about how to align oneself with and for the resistive patient: how to develop and be part of a therapeutic alliance that may be barely friendly or even civil. Social norms for behaviour and interaction cannot be used to judge the reasonableness of a patient's comportment. Before these interactions begin the goals for care need to be clear, as do the limits within which to operate. This can only occur if there is good support and communication between all members of the treatment team and if adequate opportunities exist for the development of self-knowledge and clinical practice skills. This will be touched on again before the end of the chapter.

DOCUMENTING THE JOURNEY

The nurse has a responsibility in the documentation of the patient's journey through the PICU by writing progress notes and revising the care plan or individual service plan. What is documented is the progress on the goals chosen for the patient, by the patient if possible. It is not necessarily a reflection of the progress with medical goals, or organizational goals. There are other forums for these. The notes will become a living record of the patient's personal journey during their stay in the PICU. As suggested in the Star Wards Resource Pack[22] patients might also be encouraged to maintain their own journal to map the journey and the achievement of goals and stepping-stones. Documentation will allow progress in line with the predetermined goals to be monitored in a consequential way. It allows others on the treatment team to continue the work in a meaningful and consistent way and it provides the history and description that is used to acknowledge that the time has come to leave the PICU. During a review of the patient's time in the PICU and when approaching the termination of the relationship with the primary care nurse, documentation allows an appreciation of the magnitude of the person's journey so far. This is an occasion to affirm the progress made[17] to this point. It also allows for work towards a shared understanding of what the time in the PICU has meant for the patient to help integrate this into the overall healthcare experience and their personal journey.

CHALLENGES AND OPPORTUNITIES

Working in a PICU by definition involves intensive contact with acutely ill patients. These people are often the very reluctant and hostile recipients of care. Nurses deal most frequently and most intensely with patients and they are also responsible for the overall milieu. Violence is common.[3,23] The setting poses challenges to personal resources on many levels. One of the challenges may come when we are caused to re-evaluate the source of the affirmation of our nursing worth: of the meaningfulness of our labour. As nurses, whether appropriate or not, we frequently rely on patients, or their significant others, to validate the worth of our efforts. Grateful patients and relatives often seem to make the job worthwhile. There are a number of reasons why this validation is not forthcoming in the PICU. First, when caring for reluctant patients this validation may not come at all, or if it does, it is often with hindsight on the part of the patient, and a long time after the fact.

Gratitude

It is not uncommon to meet a person some years after they have spent time with you as a patient, and to have them share with you a particular episode of care, an interaction that validated their worth as people, that meant something to them in a deep and meaningful way. At the time nothing is said as the person struggles with the acuity of their illness and the labour of finding meaning in the experience.

Second, it is not always easy to understand our own motivations in caring for patients and in wanting acknowledgement and appreciation. Without adequate preparation and support it is possible that the nurse will seek to get their own needs met through their patients. This is inevitably destructive for the relationship and for the well being of the patient. The therapeutic relationship is not a relationship of equals:[24] it exists to serve the patient.

To support nurses in plotting a course through the perils of the PICU, access to clinical supervision of nursing practice is imperative. Not only can good supervision provide the essential support necessary to restoring emotional and psychological balance, but it will also provide the essential learning context focused on challenging clinical issues.[25,26] Without support the PICU nurse is prone to burnout, followed shortly after by 'move out'. This support comes from being part of a functional team[3] and from participating in appropriate learning and restorative activities.

The PICU can cause family or friends to feel conflicted. Having a friend or family member in a PICU may not offer the same confirmation of the severity and legitimacy of illness that a medical or surgical intensive care unit may. When discussing a physically sick friend or relative the information that they are in, or were in, intensive care is used as a benchmark of the seriousness of the illness. Furthermore, in these settings it is taken for granted that the patient values the efforts made on his or her behalf to help a return to wellness. As noted earlier patients are often reluctant to receive care in the PICU.[1] Significant others are also confronted with issues of stigma and questions about cause and fault in regard to mental illness. The person in care may be detained against their will, and they are certainly conscious and verbal: they often express the belief that they should be allowed to leave or not be forced to go to hospital. Significant others are often torn between their long-term commitment to these people and their view of the benefits of hospitalization: they are often blamed for alerting mental health teams. The patient may express a very deep sense of betrayal. The responses of significant people to admission to the PICU will influence how the patient perceives of it both now and at future encounters. Accordingly, the PICU nurse has an important part to play in working with carers when they have contact with the unit.

SUMMARY

The intensity signified in psychiatric intensive care is complex. At the most basic level the acuity of illness requires a care that is intense. There is a high staff–patient ratio. This is no different to any other intensive care environments in which nurses practise. A further level of intensity is manifested in the nurse–patient relationship. In many ways this differs from other intensive care environments in which technological care is of equal importance. The only machines that go 'ding' in the PICU are the personal alarms worn by nursing personnel. The primary instrument for the nurse in the PICU is the self, and the self needs to be healthy and resilient to serve both patients and the nurse's needs well. In order to be able to participate in the nurse–patient relationship in a therapeutic manner, issues of power and control must be worked through, else the only one having their needs met may be the nurse. The privilege for nurses in the PICU is the access it enables to people in life crises who are vulnerable but who are also confronted by possibilities and opportunities. The danger is that the person may remain overwhelmed by the experience of their illness. The opportunity lies in their potential to consider their life and revise both the current and future chapters to incorporate new and more adaptive ways of being. This work of editing and rewriting is the basis of the work to continue in other settings and may underpin continuity of care.

PICU design is based around the needs of the people who will be the patients in the unit.

- The PICU is usually locked and with higher staff-to-patient ratios.
- The PICU is furnished with attention to the possibility of harm to patients or others.
- The need and right to privacy is balanced against the need to maximize safety for all.
- Balance sought between the high stimulus/high acuity environment and the need for healing.

PICUs exist for the intensive care of those who are experiencing severely impaired reality testing or impulse control, and who are seen to be a risk to themselves or others.

- Patients are usually there involuntarily.
- PICUs provide short-term care, and risk assessment and management.
- It offers a controlled and safe environment for those who apparently cannot be cared for in (benefit from) a less restrictive environment.
- It is not about mere containment and should never be used as coercion into compliance: it is one phase of planned and goal directed clinical treatment in one phase of the illness experience.
- Clear goals ensure discharge which is correlated with the patient's progress, not a reactive response to bed crises.

The key to maintaining safety and promoting therapeutic outcomes is engagement as apposed to close or special observation.

- 'Close' could refer to an ongoing state of attentiveness cultivated as one of the core attributes of PICU nursing as apposed to a supposedly detached and objective monitoring presence.
- In the hands of an expert nurse, close observation and engagement are inexorably linked.

Active engagement creates the context for dialogue and opens a conversational space for the craft of care.

- We can help rewrite the impact of dis-ease through respectful attention to the stories that patients tell us.
- Patients' narratives can be used to help us be better situated to be involved in their recovery and give us a 'frame of intelligibility'.
- The nurse in this context acts as the mediator of sense-making.
- The goal of the interaction is to help the patient to ultimately recreate a self-identity based on a preferred story line – preferred by them and consistent with a reality required for progress to a less restrictive environment.

PICU nursing is challenged to maintain the delicate balance necessary in the separation of the controlling and therapeutic functions.

- It is mainly the nurse who is challenged to pursue the goal of engagement and build a therapeutic alliance in the situation of having to exert coercive influence over the patient in relation to forced medication and seclusion.
- The nurse needs to reflect on his or her investment in this power struggle, and whether decisions are based on this perceived investment.
- In the face of forced interactions it can be difficult to maintain clear boundaries and separate out our reactions: to be sure that what is being done is a response to the patient's clinical need and not in response to fear and uncertainty.

Intense contact with reluctant and often hostile patients poses challenges to personal resources on all levels.

- The therapeutic relationship exists to serve the person in our care and can't meet our needs.
- Clinical supervision provides a buffer against burnout to restore psycho-emotional balance and provide learning opportunities.
- Carefully enacted support develops healthy and resilient staff and will ensure retention of skilled and talented practitioners.

REFERENCES

1. Clinton C, Pereira S, Mullins B. Training needs of psychiatric intensive care staff. *Nursing Standard* 2001; **15** (4): 33–6.

2. Keltner NL, Schwecke L, Bostrom C. *Psychiatric nursing*, 3rd edn. St Louis, MO: Mosby, 1995.

3. Brown K, Wellman N. Psychiatric intensive care: a developing speciality. *Nursing Standard* 1998; **12** (29): 45–7.

4. Watkins P. *Mental health nursing: The art of compassionate care*. London, UK: Read Educational and Professional, 2001.

5. Lehane M. Intensive care for acute mental illness. *Nursing Standard* 1995; **9** (36): 32–4.

6. Severimuttu A. National association of psychiatric intensive care units. *Nursing Standard* 1999; **13** (31): 31.

7. Kidd P, Wagner K. *High acuity nursing*, 2nd edn. Stanford, CA: Appleton and Lange, 1997.

8. McCoy SM, Garritson S. Seclusion: the process of intervening. *Journal of Psychiatric Nursing and Mental Health Services* 1983; **21** (8): 8–15.

9. Garritson SH, Davis AJ. Least restrictive alternative: ethical considerations. *Journal of Psychiatric Nursing and Mental Health Services* 1983; **21** (12): 17.

10. Gentle J. Mental health intensive care: the nurses' experience and perceptions of a new unit. *Journal of Advanced Nursing* 1996; **24** (6): 1194–200.

11. Barker P. The tidal model: Developing an empowering, person-centred approach to recovery within psychiatric and mental health nursing. *Journal of Psychiatric & Mental Health Nursing* 2001; **8** (3): 233–40.

12. Severimuttu A. Starting from scratch. *Nursing Standard* 1996; **10** (34): 26–7.

13. Campbell P. Commentary. In: Cutcliffe J, Ward M (eds). *Key debates in psychiatric/mental health nursing*. Oxford, UK: Elsevier, 2006: 272–7.

14. Stevenson C, Cutcliffe J. Problematizing special observation in psychiatry: Foucault, archaeology, genealogy, discourse and power/knowledge. *Journal of Psychiatric & Mental Health Nursing* 2006; **13** (6): 713–21.

15. Neilson P. A secure philosophy. *Nursing Times* 1992; **88** (8): 31–3.

16. Benner P. *From novice to expert*. Menlo Park, CA: Addison Wesley, 1984.

17. Epston D, White M. Termination as a rite of passage: questioning strategies for a therapy of inclusion. In: Neimeyer RA, Mahoney MJ (eds). *Constructivism in psychotherapy*. Washington, DC: American Psychological Association, 1995: 339–54.

18. White H. *The content of form: narrative discourse and historical representation*. Baltimore, MD: Johns Hopkins University Press, 1987.

19. White M. Narrative therapy outline. *Dulwich Centre Conference on Narrative*. Adelaide, 1999.

20. Simpson JRJ, Thompson CR, Beckson M. Impact of orally disintegrating olanzapine on use of intramuscular antipsychotics, seclusion, and restraint in an acute inpatient psychiatric setting. *Journal of Clinical Psychopharmacology* 2006; **26** (3): 333–5.

21. Neilson P, Brennan W. The use of special observation: an audit within a psychiatric unit. *Journal of Psychiatry and Mental Health Nursing* 2001; **8**: 147–55.

22. National Association of Psychiatric Intensive Care Units, Bright. *Starwards: Practical ideas for improving the daily experiences and treatment outcomes of acute mental health in-patients*. 2006. Available from: www.napicu.org.uk/starwards.htm.

23. Severimuttu A, Lowe T. Aggressive incidents on a psychiatric intensive care unit. *Nursing Standard* 2000; **14** (35): 33–6.

24. Fishwick M, Tait B, O'Brien AJ. Unearthing the conflicts between carer and custodian: implications of participation in section 16 hearings under the Mental Health (compulsory assessment and treatment) Act (1992). *Australian and New Zealand Journal of Mental Health* 2001; **10** (3): 187–96.

25. Butterworth T, Carson J, Jeacock J et al. Stress, coping, burnout and job satisfaction in British nurses: findings from the clinical supervision evaluation project. *Stress Medicine* 1999; **15** (1): 27–33.

26. Winstanley J, White E. *Clinical supervision: models, measures and best practice*. Greenacres, Australia: Australian & New Zealand College of Mental Health Nurses, 2002.

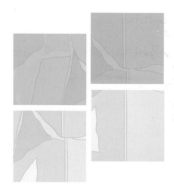

CHAPTER 49

Mental health nursing in community care

Denis Ryan*

INTRODUCTION

Psychiatric and mental health nursing are frequently used interchangeably, but the terms may well not be synonymous (see Chapter 1). Perhaps the level of professional concern relating to such issues reflects the state of flux in the profession. Psychiatric nursing began in institutional care settings[1] and has gone through various stages of development, and can be described as part of a dynamic developmental process.

The institutional origins of psychiatric nursing provide an important context for understanding the current role and function of this group of nurses, which has embraced various models of care. The term 'community psychiatric nursing' must be understood in terms of the dynamic evolution of the nursing profession. Does 'the' role of the community psychiatric–mental health nurse (here called CMHN) involve a single or a set of roles? Perhaps the situation is more complex, since nurses have moved from a single 'grade' to encompass a wider range of professional roles and activities.

From a sociological perspective, psychiatric–mental health nursing needs to be responsive to wider social health needs and policy dictates. The 'traditional' dominance of secondary and tertiary services has, until recently, been broadly accepted as the norm in Western cultures by general public, service providers and healthcare practitioners alike.

Indeed, organizational structures and professional hierarchies reflect these 'norms'. However, the international emergence of primary care poses challenges for all stakeholders, since moving to a primary care-led model involves a fundamental alteration of practice. Consequently, this is unlikely to happen rapidly, seamlessly or without influencing the roles of professional staff or existing organizational arrangements. In some countries (e.g. the UK) CMHNs are the largest single occupational group offering specialist mental health services.[2] As key stakeholders in this process, these changes are likely to affect them significantly, but they too will likely be significant contributors to the change process.

This chapter concentrates on the role of mental health nurses. It examines the milieu in which community mental health nursing services have evolved and reflects on the various policy and ideological influences on its development within the broader community, highlighting some of the key models of practice that have emerged. Finally, it discusses possible future directions for mental health nursing within the wider community.

Refection

What are the implications for CMHNs of being based within primary care ?

---

*Denis Ryan is Senior Lecturer at the University of Limerick, Ireland.

THE NEED FOR MENTAL HEALTH SERVICES

The World Health Organization has highlighted the importance of 'mental health' to the overall health agenda for the foreseeable future.[3,4] The '*burden*' of mental illness is a growing cause of concern. Within the EU, for example it is estimated that one-quarter of the population suffers from some form of mental health problem, with anxiety and depression cited as the most common disorders.[5] Approximately 15–20 per cent of the adult population, and 15–22 per cent of those below the age of 18, suffer some form of 'mental health problem'.[5]

This reflected in a high usage of health services in primary and community care by those with any mental health problem. In Finland, it has been estimated that 20 per cent of the adult population suffer from mental disorders,[6] with the same percentage of people attending their GP with common mental health problems.[7] In the UK, it has been reported that over 90 per cent of those who access the services of GPs are treated throughout the course of their illness within primary care settings, and are not referred to secondary or indeed tertiary services.[8] Similar levels of primary care service utilization are reported from Australia.[9]

Changing policy context

From the middle of the twentieth century, there has been a concerted effort internationally to shift models of care from institutional to community based. This policy shift demonstrates an ideologically driven desire to empower individuals, minimizing stigma and maximizing opportunities for social integration or reintegration.[4,10] Institutional care was also costly, inefficient, ineffective and socially undesirable. Shifting policy directions, increasing consumer demands and the requirement to demonstrate outcomes through effectiveness or efficiency measures are the basis for reconfiguring mental health services.[11] Although reasonably consistent, the solutions have been somewhat different.[12] The mid-1990s saw a reduction of 80 per cent of institution-based care in Australia when compared with the mid-1960s,[13] with similar trends internationally. It is important to consider the benefits from this shift of direction.[14,15] If the change has merely been one of location,[14] it would seem wasteful of public funding and disruptive of organizational functioning for the sake of simply changing where services are offered.

Medical model dominance and its consequences

Holistic views dominated medical practice for 1400 years,[16] whereas the emphasis on reductionism has only held sway since the rise of Cartesian Dualism, which has dominated health service thinking and practice. The dominance of the 'medical model' has hindered an appreciation of the interaction and connectedness of various facets of human functioning, as well as the relationships between man and the broader environment.

However, the influence of reductionism has had wider implications. Concentration on a 'systems approach' has led to the development of 'specialisms', which concentrate on either individual human 'systems' or 'sub-systems'. Medical practice branched into the broad areas of medicine, surgery, obstetrics, gynaecology, paediatrics and psychiatry, with further sub-divisions or sub-specialisms evolving.

Specialism and specialization

Nursing followed this trend, and has organized itself along similar lines as medical practitioners. It developed areas of specialist practice, generally being divided between adult (general) nursing, paediatric, intellectual disability, mental health nursing, as well as midwifery. Although most countries follow this generic model of practice and nurse registration, both the UK and Ireland remain examples of countries that have retained a system of segregation in nursing practice. The issue of specialization has been the subject of debate and contention both between different areas of practice in nursing as well as other disciplines. It has been part of the professional discourse in psychiatric nursing since at least the early 1950s. Hildegard Peplau argued that one of the key roles of the mental health nurse was to support the work of psychiatrists (on a voluntary basis), suggesting a complementary role between psychiatric–mental health nurses and psychiatrists.

More recently these debates have focused on the relative merits of generic health working based on integrated or collaborative working frameworks. Persuasive arguments have been made for the introduction of a generic nursing role in primary care[17] and it has also been suggested that the arguments for *post-disciplinary* work arrangements among mental health professionals are at least worthy of serious consideration.[18] The evolving dominance of primary care provides a new context for these debates and the urgency with which they must be considered are all the more pressing. Although the focus of mental health nursing practice differs from general nursing, the integration of workers into a primary care model brings with it the challenge to provide a proper evidence base for community mental health nursing.

EVOLUTION OF COMMUNITY MENTAL HEALTH NURSING

The second half of the twentieth century witnessed a sustained period of change in the organization and delivery of mental health services, marked by a decrease in the overall population of traditional psychiatric hospitals. For example, Australia recorded an 80 per cent decline in institutional care from the mid-1960s to the mid-1990s,[19] whereas in Ireland there was a 67 per cent decrease in psychiatric hospital beds from 1984 to 2004.[20]

There was a parallel development of outpatient, daycare and community-based services. In most instances, outreach services were intended to support those patients discharged from hospital to prevent re-admission. Organizationally they remained based in hospitals and clinics – partly explaining why the development of mental health nursing is in a stage of relative infancy. Most people presenting with mental health problems are treated in community settings.[21] However, there does not seem to have been a proportionate increase in, or transfer of, resources to support such services.

Although community care has been evolving since the late 1950s, there remains no consensus as to the proper role and function of mental health nurses working in community settings.[22] Much debate revolves around ideological and professional concerns, resources, and the demarcation and boundary considerations, which feature in this chapter. A recent review concluded that the types of role most commonly identified included those of *assessor, therapist, consultant, clinician, educator and manager*.[23] Considerable debate is focused on *who* CMHNs should work *with*; divided between those who believe in concentrating on people with *severe and enduring mental illnesses*, and those *common mental health problems*. However, at least one study of the community mental health nursing role reported wide variations in the interpretation of the term *serious* or *enduring* mental illnesses.[24]

It is hardly surprising, therefore, that some studies have reported that the reasons for referral to mental health nurses and the expectations for therapeutic interventions provided by community psychiatric nurses are unclear or ambiguous,[24,25] with high caseloads[23,26] that are often complex in nature.[27] The consistency of these findings across settings and time suggests that the core functions and role of CMHNs remain poorly understood or articulated. Referrals to community mental health nursing services may occur because the referring agents are unsure what else to do.

Given the burden of mental illness internationally, it is unsurprising that greater emphasis has been placed on *illness prevention* and *health promotion*, especially in primary care settings. Hildegard Peplau pre-empted later discussion by suggesting that the role of psychiatric–mental health nursing in illness prevention warranted serious consideration.[28] Her call demonstrated a shift in thinking from a curative to a preventative role. More recently, the World Health Organization emphasized mental health promotion arguing that:

> Mental health promotion increases the quality of life and wellbeing of the whole population, including people with mental health problems and their carers.[29]

Despite this, health promotion has not been a professional priority among psychiatric–mental health nurses,[30] although there are clear opportunities for professional engagement in this field.[31]

Reflection

Consider the role/s of community mental health nursing in health promotion at an individual, community or societal level.

These are some of the factors that have contributed to the difficulty of defining roles for community psychiatric–mental health nursing.[22] Indeed, considering *the role* seems inappropriate, as multifaceted roles become the norm. In addition, consideration of future roles cannot also be unrelated to the fact that there had been a variety of systems of community mental health nursing practice.[24] These seem to have evolved organically, directly related to service need and existing organizational models rather than being strategically planned in many instances.

To illustrate, the development of community mental health nursing in the UK and the Republic of Ireland is considered. Both have cultural, geographical and historical ties and mental health services evolved from shared historical origins, yet there are clear distinctions between both systems. For example, the most usual model of community mental health teams in the UK is multidisciplinary and located in the community within which they operate. While similar to the Republic of Ireland, there is a distinct difference between them. In the UK, community mental health teams normally do not have direct access to their own dedicated inpatient services,[32] whereas the Irish system has and (in most cases) remains directly a part of specialist mental health teams which provide integrated inpatient and community-based care.

While there is little doubt that community mental health teams will play a major role in developing a future framework for mental health services,[24] the current, diverse nature of definitions of *community mental health teams* prevents consensus being achieved on the contribution they might make to individual or population health. Many teams evolved to meet local needs, developing in an unstructured and fragmented manner.

Such fragmentation may, at least partly, relate to the fact that CMHNs are struggling to establish themselves as a distinct professional group.[25] The traditional work focus of CMHNs was similar to that of public health nurses or health visitors – based mainly on domiciliary care and support. CMHNs are actively trying to highlight distinctions between themselves and other specialist nurses working in community locations as well as other mental health workers such as social workers, clinical psychologists, occupational therapists, psychiatrists, etc., and hospital-based psychiatric–mental health nurses.[33]

One reason for this obsession with role and function is the atmosphere of change and uncertainty that has characterized services, internationally, since the latter half of the twentieth century.[24] The certainty associated with roles, relationships and boundaries typical of hospital care was not entirely eroded, but the variety of models, and the dynamic nature of the change which ensued, account for much of the search for meaning which has long been a feature of community mental health nursing.

Reflection

How do the key professional groups deal with mental health matters in community settings?

DEVELOPMENTS IN COMMUNITY MENTAL HEALTH CARE

The development of mental health nursing has been closely associated with the prevailing political and social ethos and philosophy of care with two core models evolving. Although separate, they are developmentally interlinked and are likely to influence future developments of this area of practice.

In the first model, community mental health nursing developed as part of a *secondary level* care initiative, segregated from other forms of nursing, and part of *specialist mental health teams*. The second model involves integrated service provision within primary care teams. This model of integrated care has been advocated in such diverse countries as Australia[19] and Ireland.[34] Although the specific operational models may differ, the emphasis on providing mental health care within a primary care framework is common.

Recently, a range of roles were suggested for mental health nurses in such settings, including various assessment functions: *mental state examination; risk assessment; functional or behavioural analysis; family and social network assessment; and 'needs assessment' including basics such as food, shelter and finances*[35] (cited in McCardle et al.[23]). Although these proposals highlight potential areas of expertise, by emphasizing assessment processes they seem more in keeping with the medical model which places a strong emphasis on diagnosis. In particular, they do not emphasize the kind of intervention, support or engagement that might articulate the unique contribution of mental health nurses in community care settings.

The specialist team approach

Since the 1950s specialist practitioners in mental health nursing began to develop community-focused care. These practitioners were drawn from a background and ethos of institutionally based care, pursuing a philosophy of supporting individuals following discharge from hospital, while seeking to prevent re-admission. Much of this work concentrated on developing supportive networks for people with a severe or enduring form of mental illness. The change from a hospital to a home-based model, or one focused on the patient's local community, involved not just a change of site, but also change in mindset and 'power' relationship between service provider and user.[36]

The predominant feature of nurse–patient relationships in hospital was one in which the locus of control and power rests firmly with the nurse. This relationship is significantly altered where the service provider is a 'guest' in the services user's home. Domiciliary and outpatient care differs from hospital-based care in the level and skills of negotiation required. In hospital the nurse's function is explicitly and implicitly understood by all concerned. However, in the community, the authority and credibility of the nurse must be established and maintained on an individual basis across different situations.

Besides power relationships, the setting in which care is provided is also important. In the community, care is made accessible as close as possible to people's own homes. With the increasing emphasis on holistic care, provision of care at a point close to the person's living environment allows for a better understanding of the person's normal world. It also has benefits from the perspective of organizing the planning, delivery and evaluation of care, and provides opportunities for long-term care initiatives and developing health promotion with families, individuals and communities. Within these types of structures, mental health nurses provide a range of services including counselling, psychosocial interventions, liaison services, depot-injection clinics, psychoeducational initiatives, with some fulfilling roles as care coordinators.

At least part of the function of the asylum system was to act as an agency of 'social control', with the right and obligation to detain individuals against their will enshrined in legislation. In some countries, such as the UK, even though the asylum system has been dismantled, recent legislation has legitimized this function in some community care environments. This implies that particular groups and individuals require 'policing' in relation to their continued care.[37] The practices within specialist care teams has, at least in part, brought with it from its original asylum base, an ethos of control, frequently evidenced through a high level of reliance on chemical methods of control and medication management and in some instances continue to be so. Evidence suggests that medication management, information giving, as well as client assessment continue to be prominent aspects of community mental health nursing.[23]

This aspect of practice is contentious from the perspectives of professional development and autonomy and is seen from two main perspectives.

1 On the one hand, the role of nurses in relation to medication management and compliance is seen as vital – with increasing calls within the profession and in the broader nursing community for an enhanced role in relation to prescribing medication.

2 On the other hand, nurse-prescribing can also be interpreted as an attempt to reassert the dominance of the medical model of care,[37] and a method of retaining nursing in a subservient relationship with medical practitioners. This move to expanding roles in medication management has been welcomed by many,[38] perhaps in part because it can be seen as a logical conclusion to the blurring of roles and the merging of skills which may occur in multidisciplinary work.

Multidisciplinary work has evolved as the norm in specialist mental health care teams.[20] Although such approaches may have been promoted on the basis of potential benefits to service users, it is equally arguable that promotion of less rigid hierarchies was attractive to the teams concerned. Despite the obvious attractions for clinically based nurses, there may be a diminution of professional autonomy and decreased efficiency through inappropriate use of specialist skills.[39] Indeed this form of working has been blamed for generating role confusion and uncertainty, with increased pressure on the staff concerned.[40]

The 'seriously mentally ill' and the 'worried well'

The concentration on issues relating to medication must also be understood within the context of the client group. Specialist and community mental health teams traditionally provided a second level service, primarily to people discharged from inpatient care or rehabilitation programmes. The traditional focus was on surveillance, supervision, intervention and support for the most severely mentally ill. More recently there has been a shift in emphasis, and a tendency in some instances to work with the 'worried well' or people with 'common mental disorders'. This can be understood as a natural progression to an illness prevention and health promotion model aimed at meeting the needs of individuals who present in primary care services with somatic manifestations, while having either underlying or co-morbid mental health conditions.

It may be argued that the dependency level of those with serious and enduring mental illness requires specialist intervention from highly competent professionals, for whom community mental health nursing resources should

be prioritized.[41,42] However, accurate operational definitions of the concept of severe and enduring mental illness have not yet been achieved. Despite conceptual confusion, it is clear that most definitions deal with the illnesses that are persistent, ongoing and are associated with a significant burden within either personal, interpersonal, family or social functioning. These types of illness, including schizophrenia, require complex psychosocial support structures. In the case of schizophrenia, social support is assumed to be associated with caring and competence.[43] However, it is not just the *level* of social support which is important, but the *type* of support available which must be considered.[44]

EVOLVING ROLES IN COMMUNITY CARE TEAMS

Within the specialist community mental health team model, several different approaches have developed. There has been increasing recognition that the original model of community mental health care, operating within normal 'business hours' was inadequate. Where the service was an extension of institutional care, operating within 'normal business hours' remained a sustainable model of practice. A pool of staff from the hospital could supplement demands for out-of-hours requirements. However, as access to inpatient care became more difficult, the requirement for out-of-hours arrangements increased. *Crisis intervention teams* and *assertive outreach programmes* emerged to support people. Although welcome initiatives, there has been criticism of the expansion of such services, on the basis that they are focused on prevention of access to inpatient services, or that they replace the models of supervision, surveillance and control which were the hallmarks of the old asylum system.[45]

Integrated care models

The debate around *where* community nurses should be based and their *legitimate role* revolves around the organization of care and the utilization of scarce resources. In most countries it is agreed that CMHNs are valued specialist practitioners. Some of the debate has focused on whether CMHNs should be a support to non-mental health specialists – such as primary care teams and other hospital-based staff – or should they be *part* of those teams.

It can also be argued that the organizational context in which community mental health teams evolved (and by association CMHNs) no longer prevails, largely born out of the deinstitutionalization movement. Later came the influence of the consumer movement, which can be credited with increasing the emphasis on accountability and transparency in health services. The logic of organizing care that places consumers at the centre demands that any expansion of services are integrated with other strands of care. Although there has been a protracted debate about the best organizational arrangements for community mental health nursing, public health policy internationally has accepted that it should be focused on primary health care.

Many mental health nursing services in such arrangements have concentrated their therapeutic engagements with the so-called 'worried well' or people with 'common mental disorders'. Partly related to resource utilization, there have been consistent calls in nursing literature to concentrate the expertise of practitioners with the most serious mentally ill. Although logical, in some instances these calls have followed negative media campaigns regarding scandals or crimes committed by former mental health service users and the perceived neglect of people with serious mental disorders. However, such responses are reactionary. If the services of CMHNs are limited in such an artificial manner, other service users are deprived of a valuable service.[27] At a more fundamental level, resources are diverted from *mental health promotion* as well as *illness prevention*, so the loss is, ultimately, to society[31,46] and the 'community'. This is ironic, given the title of these nurses. In that sense, the loss is not only a 'current' loss, but potentially a long-term loss to future generations. This dichotomy in relation to the appropriate role of CMHNs in evolving services needs resolution. Some of the arguments relate to the issue of the legitimate roles of healthcare professionals and the blurring of boundaries.

Primary care is the initial point of contact for a wide range of people requiring psychosocial interventions that can be addressed by CMHNs. However, it can be argued that the use of CMHNs with a broad range of 'common mental disorders' has more to do with overworked GPs seeking to divert unwanted areas of practice to others, rather than the best use of specialist practitioners. Another confounding factor in primary healthcare settings in countries like the UK, is the arbitrary and artificial distinction between 'health' and 'social' care. In other countries such as the Republic of Ireland, this distinction was not made, and health policies incorporated the notion of 'health and social gain' as an index of measurement – integrating these concepts in a health framework with obvious implications for practice.[34,47]

Reflection

How important is it to integrate 'social' and 'health' aspects of care for community mental health nursing practice?

THE COMMUNITY MENTAL HEALTH NURSE AND INTERDISCIPLINARY TEAMWORK

Although arguments abound about the proper areas of interest of CMHNs, there seems to be a consensus that

CMHNs fulfil a valuable role. Those who argue for the concentration of such valuable resources on meeting the greatest need believe that CMHNs are a highly qualified and skilled group of professionals who should work with those with 'serious and enduring mental illness'. This argument seems to enjoy widespread support among healthcare professionals.[48] However, there is also some support for CMHNs acting as resource agents or in a consultancy role for primary care teams[48] or as a source of specialist referral.[49] In addition there is also some support for their roles in the care and treatment of individuals who present with anxiety disorders; those who need problem-solving skills; those presenting with depression as well as psychotic disorders;[49] in other words a *range* of mental health difficulties.[27]

Traditionally, community mental health nursing services were accessed through a system of secondary referral; most commonly through either a consultant psychiatrist, another member of the specialist multidisciplinary team or GP. Although this may have protected scarce resources, it also limited integration with other non-mental healthcare professionals. The move towards integrated models of care has been progressively advanced from the 1980s. An important feature has been the development of *liaison mental health (psychiatric) teams, assertive outreach programmes* and *crisis teams* as well as *care programme approaches* in which CMHNs play a prominent role.

The fact that the role of CMHNs is evolving is evident when these types of issues are being debated. Professional boundaries were expected to become blurred through interdisciplinary work. However, there is some indication that professional boundaries remain a feature of interdisciplinary work.[40] Likewise, although the role of CMHNs is valued, it is also clear that some teams are inadequately resourced.[50] There is a danger that where roles are unclear positions may be sacrificed where team members are competing for limited resources.

The debates over the use of CMHNs highlighted the need for specialized services for a range of service users in primary care settings. It raised issues regarding who should provide these services and the skills, knowledge and background they required. Primary care teams are increasingly faced with complex mental health issues and they are not necessarily adequately skilled or experienced to deal with them.[51] This raises the issue of the CMHN acting as a skills or training resource to non-mental health practitioners, which has also been widely advocated.

CMHNs are in an excellent position to fill a range of the evolving needs within primary care settings,[27] including therapist, consultant/advisor, liaison agent and assessor.[21,35] To facilitate the removal of the arbitrary distinction between physical, psychological and social domains, the role of health educator/promoter could be added to this list.[46] However, to fulfil these roles, the educational preparation and training of future practitioners would need to be considered.[52] Specialist training and further education, while desirable are currently not an essential requirement for CMHN practice in all countries.

Although adequate educational and training preparation are essential requirements for the development and enhancement of community mental health nursing services, what is equally essential to recognize are the essential components of the psycho-educational and therapeutic roles fulfilled. The relationship between service users and healthcare professionals are the single most valued component of care as reported by patients.[53] CMHNs should be in a position to support service users through the creation or maintenance of the therapeutic milieu. To provide support, the care environment should be characterized by an ethos of acceptance; the creation and maintenance of a positive atmosphere; expectation of change; responsiveness; normalization; and an educative component.[54] Although these features require greater empirical validation, nonetheless they provide an initial framework to appreciate the requirements of community mental health nursing – including the personal and professional characteristics required of practitioners.

Reflection

What is the 'ideal' educational and practice-based preparation for CMHNs?

REFERENCES

1. Sheridan AJ. The impact of political transition on psychiatric nursing – a case study of twentieth-century Ireland. *Nursing Inquiry* 2006; **13** (4): 289–99.

2. Coffey M, Higgon J, Kinnear J. Therapy as well as the tablets: an exploratory study of service users' views of CMHNs' responses to hearing voices. *Journal of Psychiatry and Mental Health Nursing* 2004; **11** (4): 435–44.

3. World Health Organization, *WHO guide to mental health in primary care*. London, UK: Royal Society of Medicine, 2000.

4. World Health Organization. *The world health report 2001, mental health: new understanding, new hope*. Geneva, Switzerland: WHO, 2001.

5. European Commission. *Green paper improving the mental health of the population: towards a strategy on mental health for the European Union*. Brussels, Belgium: European Commission, 2005.

6. Hyvönen S, Nikkonen M. Primary health care practitioners' tools for mental health care. *Journal of Psychiatric and Mental Health Nursing* 2004; **11** (5): 514–24.

7. Goldberg D. Psychiatry and primary care. *World Psychiatry* 2003; **2** (3): 153–7.

8. Vazquez-Barquero JL, Garcia J. Deinstitutionalization and psychiatric reform in Spain. *European Archive of Psychiatry and Clinical Neuroscience* 1999; **249** (3): 128–35.

9. Australian Institute of Health and Welfare and Commonwealth Department of Health and Family Services. *First report on national health priority areas 1996*. Canberra: Department of Health and Family Services, 1997.

10. World Health Organization. *Mental health atlas 2005*. Geneva: World Health Organization, 2005.

11. Hickie I, Groom G. Primary care-led mental health service reform: an outline of the better outcomes in mental health care initiative. *Australasian Psychiatry* 2002; **10** (4): 376.

12. Secker J, Gulliver P, Peck E *et al*. Evaluation of community mental health services: comparison of a primary care mental health team and an extended day hospital service. *Health and Social Care in the Community* 2001; **9** (6): 495–503.

13. KPMG Consulting. *National mental health workforce education and training consultancy report*. Adelaide, Australia: KPMG Consulting, 1994.

14. Leff J. Can we manage without the mental hospital? *Australian and New Zealand Journal of Psychiatry* 2001; **35** (4): 421–7.

15. Cunningham G, Slevin E. Community psychiatric nursing: focus on effectiveness. *Journal of Psychiatry and Mental Health Nursing* 2005; **12** (1): 14–22.

16. Ackerknecht EH. *Ackerknecht, 1955*. New York, NY: Ronald Press Company, 1955: 47–8.

17. McKenna H, Keeney S. Community nursing: health professional and public perceptions. *Journal of Advanced Nursing* 2004; **48** (1): 17–25.

18. Holmes CA. The slow death of psychiatric nursing: what next? *Journal of Psychiatry and Mental Health Nursing* 2006; **13** (4): 401–15.

19. Australian Health Ministers' Conference. *Second national mental health plan*. Canberra, Australia: Australian Government Publishing Service, 1998.

20. Government of Ireland. *'A vision for change' report of the expert group on mental health policy*. Dublin, Ireland: Stationery Office, 2006.

21. Walker L, Barker P, Pearson P. The required role of the psychiatric-mental health nurse in primary health-care: an augmented Delphi study. *Nursing Inquiry* 2000; **7**: 91–102.

22. O'Brien LM. Nurse–client relationships: the experience of community psychiatric nurses. *Journal of the Australian and New Zealand College of Mental Health Nurses* 2000; **9**: 184–94.

23. McCardle J, Parahoo K, McKenna H. A national survey of community psychiatric nurses and their client care activities in Ireland. *Journal of Psychiatry and Mental Health Nursing* 2007; **14** (2): 179–88.

24. McKenna H, Keeney, S. Bannon D *et al*. An exploration of community psychiatric nursing: a Northern Ireland perspective. *Journal of Psychiatry and Mental Health Nursing* 2000; **7** (5): 455–61.

25. Morall PA. Murder, madness and mental health nursing: the application of realist theory. In: *RCN conference paper. Valuing mental health nursing: demonstrating its worth*. London, UK: RCN, 1997.

26. Muir-Cochrane E. The case management practices of CMHNs: 'doing the best we can'. *Australian and New Zealand Journal of Mental Health Nursing* 2001; **10** (4): 210–20.

27. Bowers L. Community psychiatric nurse caseloads and the 'worried well': misspent time vital work? *Journal of Advanced Nursing* 1997; **26** (5): 930–6.

28. Peplau H. *On beginning psychiatric nursing's second century: some unfinished business.* Presented at the Dr. Betty L. Evans Distinguished Annual Lecture in Psychiatric-Mental Health Nursing, 1983, University of Pittsburgh, PA. Cambridge, MA: The Schlesinger Library, Radcliffe Institute for Advanced Study.

29. World Health Organization. *WHO European ministerial conference on mental health; facing the challenges, building solutions.* Helsinki, Finland: World Health Organization, 2005.

30. Sheridan AJ. *Psychiatric nursing.* In: Robins J (ed.). *Nursing and midwifery in Ireland in the twentieth century.* Dublin, Ireland: An Bord Altranais, 2000: 141–61.

31. Ryan D, Deasy C. Mental health promotion. In: Morrissey J, Keogh B, Doyle L (eds). *Psychiatric Nursing.* Dublin, Ireland: Gill and Macmillan, 2008.

32. Barr W, Huxley P. The impact of community mental health reform on service users: a cohort study. *Health & Social Care in the Community* 1999; **7** (2): 129–39.

33. Morall P. *Mental health nursing and social control.* 1998; London: Whurr.

34. Department of Health and Children. *Quality and fairness: a health system for you.* Dublin, Ireland: Stationery Office, 2001.

35. Association of Psychiatric Nurse Managers. *Submission to the department of health and children on 'the psychiatric nursing component within the primary care team'.* Dublin, Ireland: APNM, 2003.

36. Muir-Cochrane E. The context of care: issues of power and control between patients and CMHNs. *International Journal of Nursing Practice,* 2000; **6** (6): 292–300.

37. Wells JS. Severe mental illness, statutory supervision and mental health nursing in the United Kingdom: meeting the challenge. *Journal of Advanced Nursing* 1998; **27** (4): 698–706.

38. Snelgrove S, Hughes D. Interprofessional relations between doctors and nurses: perspectives from South Wales. *Journal of Advanced Nursing* 2000; **31** (3): 661–7.

39. Brown B, Crawford P, Darongkamas J. Blurred roles and permeable boundaries: the experience of multidisciplinary working in community mental health. *Health and Social Care in the Community* 2000; **8** (6): 425–35.

40. Sainsbury Centre for Mental Health. *Pulling together: the future role and training of mental health staff.* London, UK: Sainsbury Centre for Mental Health, 1997.

41. Gournay K. Schizophrenia: a review of the contemporary literature and implications for mental health nursing theory, practice and education. *Journal of Psychiatric and Mental Nursing* 1996; **3**: 7–12.

42. Audit Commission. *Finding a place: a review of mental health services for adults.* London, UK: HMSO, 1994.

43. Buchanan J. Social support and schizophrenia: a review of the literature. *Archives of Psychiatric Nursing* 1995; **9** (2): 68–76.

44. Clinton M, Lunney P, Edwards H *et al.* Perceived social support and community adaptation in schizophrenia. *Journal of Advanced Nursing* 1998; **27** (5): 955–65.

45. Godin P. A dirty business: caring for people who are a nuisance or a danger. *Journal of Advanced Nursing* 2000; **32**: 1396–402.

46. Ryan D, McNamara Mannix P, Deasy C. *Health promotion in Ireland: principles, practice and research.* Dublin, Ireland: Gill and Macmillan, 2006.

47. Department of Health. *Health strategy: shaping a healthier future.* Dublin, Ireland: Stationery Office, 1994.

48. Bruce J, Watson D, van Teijlingen ER *et al.* Dedicated psychiatric care within general practice: health outcome and service providers' views. *Journal of Advanced Nursing* 1999; **29** (5): 1060–7.

49. Badger F, Nolan P. General practitioners' perceptions of community psychiatric nurses in primary care. *Journal of Psychiatry and Mental Health Nursing* 1999; **6** (6): 453–9.

50. Shanley E, Watson G, Cole A. Survey of stakeholders' opinions of community psychiatric nursing services. *Australian and New Zealand Journal of Mental Health Nursing* 2001; **10**: 77–86.

51. Russell G. Potter L. Mental health issues in primary healthcare. *Journal of Clinical Nursing* 2002; **11**: 118–25.

52. Bugge C, Smith LN, Shanley E. A descriptive study of multidisciplinary mental health staff moving to the community: the demographic and educational issues. *Journal of Psychiatric and Mental Health Nursing* 1997; **4**: 45–54.

53. Solomon P, Draine J. Satisfaction with mental health treatment in a randomised trial of consumer case management. *Journal of Nervous and Mental Disease* 1994; **182**: 179–184.

54. Evans IM, Moltzen NL. Defining effective community support for long-term psychiatric patients according to behavioural principles. *Australian and New Zealand Journal of Psychiatry* 2000; **34**: 637–44.

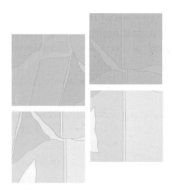

CHAPTER 50

Crisis assessment and resolution

Clare Hopkins* and Julie Mackenzie**

INTRODUCTION

We all know what it is to be in crisis. We are faced with a problem for which we do not have a solution and that is not responsive to any of our usual coping strategies. For example, you miss the last bus home and are stranded in an area where you feel at risk. You have no money for a taxi and no means of contacting friends or relatives (your usual coping strategies). The reader will be able to think of many similar examples of being in crisis.

When people experience a mental health crisis:

- they may be having feelings and experiences that are completely new to them and which may be extremely frightening;
- they and those around them may perceive the person as being 'different' leading to isolation for the person in crisis and anxiety, fear, guilt and hostility in others;
- this in turn may mean that others keep their distance and withdraw their support. They too may be in crisis;
- if this is their first experience of such a crisis, they may have limited ways of coping. If they have experienced this kind of crisis before and were unable to find a way to cope, they may feel helpless.

Mental health crises take many forms and can be seen by professionals as having differing degrees of severity.

However, if the person and their family are in crisis because of a mental health problem, these differing degrees will be irrelevant, they will simply be in crisis and in need of help. Much will depend upon their previous experience of mental health problems and their own coping styles.

CRISIS THEORY AND THE PERSON IN MENTAL HEALTH CRISIS

In 1942 Erich Lindemann[1] and his colleagues in Boston, USA, were the first to develop specific ways of working with people who were in crisis because of trauma (a fire in a night club). Lindemann and Caplan[2] set up a community programme based on crisis theory and using brief crisis intervention techniques to prevent later distress and psychopathology.

According to Caplan[2] the experience of crisis is universal. People face crisis when they encounter an 'obstacle to important life goals': one that is not amenable to the person's usual coping strategies. 'A period of disorganization ensues, a period of upset during which many abortive attempts at solution are made.' Caplan identified three phases of crisis.

1 Onset: The immediate increase in tension as the individual realizes that the problem cannot be resolved quickly.

*Clare Hopkins is a Primary Care Mental Health Worker with Newcastle Primary Care Trust. She works with adults of working age suffering from common mental health problems. Her interests are in family therapy, crisis work and suicide/self-harm.
**Julie Mackenzie has been a psychiatric nurse for over 20 years and works predominantly in acute psychiatry. She is Nurse Consultant in the Crisis Assessment and Treatment service in Newcastle and North Tyneside, UK. She has a Masters in Systemic Practice and also practices Brief/Solution-Focused Therapy.

2 Breakdown/disorganization: Tension and anxiety quickly rise to intolerable levels and all of the person's coping strategies become exhausted. This is often the point at which the person's behaviour changes – they may stop meeting their responsibilities or cease caring for themselves.

3 Resolution: Because crises are often passing events, a resolution of some kind may occur. However, this resolution may be positive or negative. If the outcome is positive then the person may have learned new, positive ways to help themselves in the future; alternatively, they may develop ways of coping that are harmful.

The aim of crisis resolution is to help the person during the phases of 'breakdown' or 'disorganization' when they may be amenable to finding or learning new, positive ways of coping with difficulties.

Although crisis theory was built around the experiences of people who are normally psychologically healthy but exposed to extraordinary events, it has been successfully applied to people in mental health crisis. It is important to stress that mental health crisis is not a description of a specific event but an individual and subjective response to an event or circumstance that may lead to longer term mental health difficulties such as depression or adjustment disorder if not resolved.

Mental health crisis and psychiatric emergency are essentially different. A psychiatric emergency is when the person has gone beyond the breakdown phase and has adopted a maladaptive solution. A psychiatric emergency may require a more formal response if the maladaptive strategy involves risk to the person or to those around them and these formal responses may include invoking mental health legislation or involving the police.

Reflection

Think about times when you have been in crisis.

- What did you do to try to deal with it?
- What helped to resolve the crisis and what did you do that turned out not to be helpful?

EVOLUTION OF CRISIS SERVICES IN THE UK

The introduction of crisis resolution and home treatment teams has been one of the key factors in the modernization of mental health care in the UK. In 1998, the Department of Health set out its agenda for change[3] which emphasized the need to offer care in the least restrictive environment and provision of alternatives to hospital. The NHS Plan[4] made a commitment to establish 335 crisis teams and that all people in contact with specialist mental health services should be able to access crisis resolution services at any time.

The model for crisis resolution and home treatment (CRHT)

- Service availability 24 hours a day, 365 days a year;
- provide an alternative to hospital admission for those experiencing acute mental health difficulties;
- multidisciplinary team working;
- provision of care to the person in their own homes by a mobile workforce;
- provision of intensive support. Visits may occur two or three times each day in the acute phase of the crisis and the team will stay involved until the crisis is resolved;
- aim of intervention to help the person to learn and develop helpful coping strategies from the crisis;
- offer support to family/carers intensively from the point of assessment;
- care planning and coordination with other mental health services;
- act as gatekeepers for inpatient beds;
- work collaboratively with inpatient services to reduce the length of admission when this has been necessary.

However, the evolution of crisis resolution and home treatment teams in the UK has been slow and erratic, there has been little consistency of approach in providing services and there is often lack of fidelity to the recommended CRHT model. A survey of CRHT provision carried out in 2006[5] identified 243 crisis resolution teams of whom just over half offered a 24-hour, 7-day per week home visiting service.

The mental health policy implementation guide[6] recommends that a standard team will cover a population of approximately 150 000 and have a caseload of 20–30 service users at any one time while being responsive to the needs of the local population. A standard team of 14 is recommended for a caseload of 25 people requiring home treatment at any one time.

The impact of CRHT services

Crisis services have radically changed the experience of mental health crisis and a number of people are admitted to psychiatric units unnecessarily.[7] Crisis teams have had a significant impact on the number of people who are admitted to hospital.[8–10] Most importantly, they reflect the increasing power of the voices of those who use the services for a wider range of options for treatment and care which are available and responsive around the clock.[11,12] It can also offer individualized and culturally sensitive care and treatment to people from diverse cultures.[13] Acute units have been criticized as being stigmatizing and promoting institutionalization; ward environments may be run-down, cramped and dirty; and that there is often little opportunity for the person to spend individual time with a member of staff.[14-16]

For the person in crisis, being able to stay in their own environment can lead to new and helpful ways of coping. Any mental health crisis is at least in part a social event and may be perceived in a variety of ways. Admission to hospital could lead to friends and family reframing the need for admission in terms of the individual rather than their circumstances.[17] Once in hospital, the person's diagnosis and perceived level of risk become the overriding concern. Removing a person in crisis from their family and social environment risks 'closure', a process of emotional withdrawal by friends/family as an act of self-protection, resulting in dehumanization of the person in crisis.[18]

There will always remain occasions when treatment at home becomes impossible. Having support from family or friends may be what the person in crisis needs most, but, by the time CRHT team becomes involved, a great deal of stress may have occurred and the strain in relationships may be evident.[19] If the relationship with the person in crisis is already fragile and full of conflict, or if the family are at the end of their tether and do not know how to cope, then being a carer may seem like an unbearable burden.[20]

It is important to remain vigilant for those occasions when support at home cannot be fostered because friends and family are exhausted by the emotional labour of caring. The family's personal circumstances may make care at home impossible or the person's behaviour while in crisis may have caused a serious schism in either close personal relationships or within the wider community.[21] When people from black and minority ethnic groups are in mental health crisis, the option of treatment at home may offer a culturally acceptable response to the needs of the whole family.[22] This may be especially true for refugees or asylum seekers who may have been exposed to severe physical and psychological trauma.

Personal illustration 50.1

Stacey is a 36-year-old married woman living with her husband and 5-month-old daughter, Amy. She is referred to the CRHT by her GP, who was concerned about her talk of suicide, depressive symptoms and inability to relate to others.

After assessment by the team, Stacey is offered urgent medical review by a psychiatrist who prescribes medications to help her mood, relieve her anxiety and to help her sleep. It is arranged that a member of the team will visit Stacey at her home every day, to monitor her mood, level of suicidality and to discuss any problems with medication. It is also planned that the nurses visiting will help Stacey and her husband understand more about depression and find their own ways of solving the problems they are facing. Stacey and her husband are offered access to a 24-hour telephone line, which enables the couple to request more urgent visits, seek advice about medication as

well as knowing that there was always someone available to offer either of them support.

Another level of work occurred 'behind the scenes', which includes liaison with the other health professionals involved with the family – the health visitor, the peri-natal community mental health team and the family GP. In particular, the health visitor expresses concern that she does not know enough about depression and the risk of suicide and the team offers her informal training about these.

ASSESSMENT AND TREATMENT

Working with people in crisis offers very special opportunities, but also represents very special responsibilities. Crisis theory holds that at the point of crisis, the person is more than usually open/vulnerable to change – either positive or negative – and this opportunity should be used to its maximum positive effect. The process of crisis assessment may be divided into five phases. However, this is not to suggest that they necessarily occur neatly or sequentially:

- speedy assessment;
- helping the person and their family/carers to describe and examine what is happening;
- assessment of risk;
- developing problem-solving skills, identifying strengths and supports, generating solutions and maintaining hope;
- negotiating a plan.

Speedy assessment

Crises merit a speedy and timely response. Once the CRHT has accepted the referral, assessment will occur rapidly.[23] If there are no indicators of risk to staff this assessment will probably take place in the person's home. Members of their family, friends or professional carers may be present when members of the team arrive. Nurses in crisis situations need to be calm, responsive and thoughtful, enabling them to gather information from multiple sources and to make knowledgeable judgements about the situation and the level of risk it presents.

Offering a full and clear explanation of their role, the reason for the visit and an explanation of the alternatives that the team can offer should help to diffuse tensions caused by assumptions about contact with mental health services. Those people who have previous experience of admission to hospital compulsorily may make assumptions or have fears that jeopardize the therapeutic relationship.[24]

A respectful, warm, empathic but professional manner is essential as is a keen awareness and observation of social and cultural etiquette, which is congruent with being in another person's home. This positively changes the balance of authority from that which is usual in inpatient settings.[25]

This becomes especially important when the person in crisis is from a different religious group or culture.[13]

Observation of the person: Does the person appear malnourished, dehydrated, dirty, dishevelled? Do they smell of alcohol? Are they behaving in an unusual way – are they guarded, suspicious, fearful, anxious, agitated, restless, elated, grandiose, angry, depressed or perhaps confused, disorientated, sedated? Do they behave in a manner suggestive of unusual thought processes?

Observation of the environment: Does the environment give any clues to the person's state of mind – is it untidy and chaotic? Is it obsessionally neat, suggesting compulsive traits? Does the person's home suggest that they have financial difficulties (little furniture, no evidence of any food or drinks)? Is there physical evidence of alcohol or drugs? Does the environment give clues about the person's interests, beliefs or spirituality? Is there anything about the environment that might betray unusual thought patterns (notices pinned up, windows/doors sealed up and curtains permanently drawn, unusual decoration, unwillingness to use electricity or gas)?

What evidence is there of the person's mood state? What does their body language betray – agitation, euphoria, irritability, hopelessness or helplessness? What do they say? Can they concentrate on the interview? Is their speech accelerated, disjointed or slowed, affectless, preoccupied, obsessional? Is there evidence of rhyming, punning, loosening of association or any other evidence of a psychotic process? Do they describe disturbance in sleep, appetite, thought, libido and energy levels? Are they experiencing thoughts of harming themselves or others?

Does the person have any physical difficulties? Do these need attention and do they impact negatively on their mental health or level of risk?

Relationships: If any other people are present, how does the person relate to them and to the crisis workers and how do others relate to the person in crisis? What cultural issues are influencing the person in crisis and their relationship with others? Are there tensions, anger, threats of violence between them or against others? Is there an absence of any effective communication? If there are children present or resident in the house, issues of safeguarding their well-being will also be an important consideration.

Stephen and Margaret who are nurses with the CRHT call to meet with Stacey, her husband James and Amy. Although Stacey is initially very hesitant about expressing her feelings and seems extremely preoccupied, their ability to be patient and remain calm, eventually provides her with the reassurance she needs that they can be trusted.

Because they have managed to gain good rapport with Stacey and James, the team ensure that they are the crisis workers who call twice a day; that Margaret is present when Dr Jones calls to see Stacey and that she and Stephen are the ones who bring Stacey's medication each day.

During these visits they use their observational skills to note not only Stacey's behaviour and the way she expresses her thoughts but also the relationship between Stacey and James, being watchful for any tensions being created by the crisis as well as Stacey's ability to relate to Amy.

Helping the person to describe and examine the crisis

Helping people tell their story is one of the basic skills for nurses working in crisis services. The following skills are particularly important:

- the ability to listen;
- the ability to ask questions which open up the conversation;
- helping the person to identify the difficulty;
- helping the person and their carers to develop problem-solving skills, identifying strengths, skills, supports and to generate solutions and maintain hope.

Listening: Listening is not a passive activity. If you, as a stranger, are to be trusted with the intimate details of another person's life, it is vital to quickly establish a trusting relationship. Active listening demonstrates not only attention but also respect for the story that is unfolding and can help the person to 'discharge' uncomfortable feelings and is a vital part of crisis resolution.[26]

Asking questions: It is not only essential to know what information to gather (see Box 50.1) but also to know how to ask questions, working flexibly around this structure, constantly seeking opportunities to promote expression and ventilation of feelings. Questions that require the person in crisis to reflect upon their current predicament, on ways in which they have coped with similar difficulties in the past as well as enquiring about the perspectives of those around them, will promote hope and open up possibilities.

Important people in the person's life may be present by agreement. If the person is part of a different religious or cultural group then great sensitivity will be required to ensure that the proprieties are observed. The crisis worker, through questioning and listening, may act as a catalyst to the forging of new joint understandings and empathy.[27] Seeking to gain an understanding of how the crisis is being defined by all concerned – the person themselves, their family and friends and wider society – will also provide information on the meaning of the crisis. The words which are being used to describe what is happening are important too – is the person in crisis being talked about in blame-laden language? For example, is Stacey's failure to take the medication prescribed for her being seen as making her responsible for the distress and disruption to the whole family? By being prepared to listen patiently, rather than seeking to 'fix' the problem, the crisis worker can open up, rather than restrict the options for the person in crisis and their carers.[28]

Reflection

Think of people you have known in mental health crisis.

- What role might those around them have played in the crisis?

Assessment of risk

In the context of crisis care, the following factors are important.

- Do the person in crisis and her/his family accept the feasibility of treatment at home?
- Has it been possible to establish a high level of rapport and trust with the person in crisis? This will give an indication of whether the client would feel able to contact the team for support at times of (increased) risk?
- Are there any aspects of the client's behaviour (including drug and alcohol use), which indicate that they could act impulsively to harm themselves or others?
- Will the client and her/his family feel confident in their ability to offer support? Has the client's family become exhausted or lost empathy with the client, because of high levels of stress?

Direct, though sensitive questioning, must be used to check on the changing level of risk. Constant reappraisal of risk is especially important when the person is being treated at home. Subtle changes in the level of commitment to safety may occur unobserved and the means to harm may be more readily acquired. Direct telephone access to the CRHT should be offered whilst under their care for both the person in crisis and their family/carers.

Shneidman's[29] early model of suicide risk assessment is a helpful and rapid aid to crisis workers. He identified that vigilance should be maintained for three key signs which might predict a growing risk of any individual's harm to themselves. These key signs are:

- perturbation – a high level of uncontained, expressed or unexpressed but visible emotion;
- cognitive constriction – being able to think in only one way (usually negatively) and an inability to think about alternative strategies or perspectives;
- lethality – does the person have access to the means with which to harm themselves and how lethal is that means?

When Stephen or Margaret call to see Stacey they always ask about her level of hopelessness and thoughts about suicide. She has become quite used to these questions, which are asked calmly and gently, and, at times, seems relieved to be able to talk about the thoughts. After 5 days of regular visits, Stacey starts to talk about having plans to kill herself. She is agitated and seems unable to sit down, has started to talk very negatively about her life and seems to have lost contact with any of her previous pleasure and joy. Eventually she confides to Stephen that she has plans to drive the family car into a wall with the intent of killing herself.

Reflection

How might being in mental health crisis affect a person's thoughts about suicide or harm to themselves?

Developing problem-solving skills, identifying strengths and supports, generating solutions and maintaining hope

People in mental health crisis may have lost contact with their skills in solving problems. The symptoms they are experiencing may be new to them or they may be facing a situation that they have faced previously when the 'solution' to their dilemma was that other people intervened and took control of their lives. This may have been seen to be the only course of action that was possible at that time. Crisis resolution – especially when linked to the possibility of home treatment – offers the opportunity to help people in crisis and their family to find positive ways of coping with the crisis, that include remaining in the 'least restrictive environment' of their home[4] and of harnessing cultural and community resources.

Seeking opportunities and solutions: how do we assist?

Working with people in crisis requires flexibility, ingenuity and the ability to think laterally about possible solutions, for example:

- asking questions about ways in which they have coped with difficulties in the past and applying this knowledge to their current crisis;

- where the crisis represents a totally new experience then an exploration of coping strategies used successfully in other circumstances is helpful;
- asking questions about exceptions to the difficulty and how these are experienced;
- remaining solution-focused rather than problem-saturated during discussions about the crisis and ways of dealing with it. There is a fine balance to be kept in doing this, avoiding becoming a 'Pollyanna', or being captured by the person's sense of despair. The use of appreciative comments when positive strategies are identified amplifies the resources/competencies of the system;
- giving information that is sufficient, reliable, timely and hope-mediating;
- fostering collaboration between the team, the person in crisis and their support network. Facilitating support from others for the person in crisis and development of a sense of ownership of the crisis phase rather than a sense of being overwhelmed by it;
- negotiating small, achievable, measurable goals within a limited time frame, involving all relevant parties, together with an agreed review date is very important in adopting a solution-focused approach;
- remaining aware of the issues of power, dominance and potential oppression that has traditionally existed between nurses and people classified as mentally ill, crisis workers can actively work to prevent the risk of 'bringing the institution into the community'.[27] Crisis workers must have a highly attuned awareness of issues of cultural and social difference.

Since Stacey has been in crisis because of depression, her parents-in-law have been overtly blaming of her. Her mother-in-law commented to Margaret, 'What has she got to be depressed about, Amy is a lovely baby'. This gave Margaret an opportunity to give some information about the effects of depression upon the person and how best to provide support.

On one visit which Margaret and Stephen make to see Stacey and her family, they become aware of her rapidly deteriorating mood state and decreasing level of activity, wishing to return to bed whenever possible.

Stephen: How are you feeling this morning Stacey?

Stacey: Awful, totally awful.

Stephen: I wonder if there have been any moments when you felt less bad? For example, I know you have told me that you get great comfort from having that first cup of tea.

Stacey: But that is just a moment.

Stephen: I wonder if, between us, we might think about ways of making those moments happen at other times too.

James: When your sister comes you seem just a bit brighter Stacey.

Stephen: Is she due to come today?

Stacey: She usually does – but I don't see what difference it will make.

Stephen: What about if James were to telephone and ask her if she would take perhaps a short walk with you, maybe as far as the shop. How would that be?

Stacey: [resigned sigh] Well, I'll try but it won't make any difference.

Stephen: Well, when I come tomorrow perhaps we can talk about what happened.

Negotiating a plan

Negotiating with the client and carers is essential if home treatment is to be offered. The key areas of negotiation are:

- the willingness of both client and carers to engage in home treatment;
- a plan to manage risk, which is negotiated jointly between the person, their family or friends and the team;
- the accessibility of the team by telephone;
- arrangements for visits to the client at home, identifying who will be visiting (being sensitive to issues of gender) and who may (or may not) be present;
- the length of the involvement of the team (short term);
- the fact that the nurse will be liaising with other professionals/helping agencies involved in that person's care and negotiation around the information to be discussed with others.

Following discussion among the multidisciplinary CRHT team involved in Stacey's care and with full consultation with the other agencies who are also involved, it is decided that issues of risk have become too great to manage whilst she is at home and concerns are raised that James is becoming exhausted with the task of caring for her and for Amy.

Stephen and Margaret visit the family at home to negotiate her admission to the Mother and Baby Unit of a local hospital.

Margaret: Stacey, we have all become very worried about what your thoughts of killing yourself, and we think that being in hospital for a short while might help you and also help James. How would you feel about that?

Stacey: But what about Amy?

Margaret: She would go to hospital too and they have special nurses there who would help you to look after her. James would be able to come to see you every day if that is what you would both like.

Stacey: What about Jane (health visitor)?

Margaret: Jane knows about us suggesting this to you, and agrees that it would be the best thing. She will come to the hospital to see you and Amy if you would like.

Stacey: I won't have to stay there long will I?

Margaret: Once you are feeling better and don't need to be in hospital any more, Stephen and I will come to see you here again. Would that be OK with you both?

James: Yes, that would be fine. Love, I think this is the best thing too and I will come up every day, you know that …

SUMMARY

Crisis resolution and home treatment services provide a responsive, timely alternative to traditional hospital care, where it is safe to do so. They represent a response to political and economic factors and the demands of users and carers. However there is little consistency between CRHT teams, many of which do not have fidelity to the recommended model for CRHT. Crisis theory suggests that the person who has reached the stage of 'breakdown/disorganization' will seek help and will be at the point where interventions (good or bad) will have the optimum effect. The role of CRHT is to mitigate the impact of the crisis on the person and their family/carers as well as fostering positive culturally sensitive ways of coping that not only enhance the recovery process but mitigate the possibility of future crisis responses.

The main points covered in this chapter are listed below.

- CRHT offer not just 'psychiatric' care and treatment but also offer brief psychological approaches and social interventions. CRHT are uniquely privileged in working with people and their families during difficult times, upholding respectful attitudes and maintaining awareness of social and cultural difference.
- CRHT teams endeavour to view individuals as retaining competency, in order to preserve the integrity of not just the individual but also their family system, using a strengths-based model of intervention.
- The burden of stress of significant others caring for the person in crisis is continually considered and monitored.
- Assessment of risk in all forms – self-neglect, self-harm or risk of suicide of the person in crisis as well as consideration of the well-being of others, especially safeguarding the well-being of children and vulnerable adults are an essential part of the work of CRHT and may lead to a decision to promote admission to hospital for the person in crisis.
- Workers in CRHT require specialized training in the CRHT model, assessment, brief interventions and a comprehensive knowledge of risk assessment.

- CRHT teams can only work effectively if they are part of a comprehensive and closely linked system of other mental health services with whom they have a well-established system of communication.[14]
- Although CRHT can be of help to many people in mental health crisis, for some there will always remain the need for true 'asylum' of admission to hospital if caring relationships within the home or the community have broken down.

REFERENCES

1. Lindemann E. Symptomatology and management of acute grief. *American Journal of Psychiatry* 1944; **101**: 141–8.

2. Caplan G. *An approach to community mental health*. London, UK: Tavistock, 1964.

3. Department of Health. *Modernising mental health services: safe, sound and supportive*, London, UK: HMSO, 1998.

4. Department of Health. *NHS Plan*. London, UK: HMSO, 2000.

5. Care Services Improvement Partnership. *A national survey of crisis resolution teams in England*. 2006. Available from: www.mentalhealthobersvatory.org.uk.

6. Department of Health. *The mental health policy implementation guide*. London, UK: HMSO, 2001.

7. Protheroe D, Carroll A. Twenty-four hour crisis assessment and treatment teams: too radical for the UK? *Psychiatric Bulletin* 2001; **25**: 416–17.

8. Glover G, Arts G, Babu K. Crisis resolution/home treatment teams and psychiatric admission rates in England. *British Journal of Psychiatry* 2006; **189**: 441–5.

9. Johnson S, Nolan F, Hoult J *et al.* Outcomes of crises before and after introduction of a crisis resolution team. *British Journal of Psychiatry*, 2005; **187**, 68–75.

10. Keown P, Tacchi M-J, Niemiec S, Hughes J. Changes to mental healthcare for working age adults: impact of a crisis team and an assertive outreach team. *Psychiatric Bulletin* 2007; **31**: 288–92.

11. Cohen M. Users' movement and the challenge to psychiatrists. *Psychiatric Bulletin* 1998; **22**: 155–7.

12. Mental Health Foundation and the Sainsbury Centre for Mental Health. *Being there in a crisis: a report of the learning from eight mental health services*. London, UK: Mental Health Foundation, 2002.

13. Department of Health. *Delivering race equality in mental health care. An action plan for reform inside and outside services*. London, UK: HMSO, 2005.

14. Smyth M. Crisis resolution/home treatment and in-patient care. *Psychiatric Bulletin* 2003; **27**: 44–7.

15. Rethink. *Behind closed doors*. London, UK: Rethink, 2004.

16. Quirk A, Lelliott P. What do we know about life on acute psychiatric wards in the UK? A review of the research evidence. *Social Science & Medicine* 2001; **53**: 1565–74.

17. Bridgett C, Polak P. Social systems intervention and crisis resolution. Part 1: assessment. *Advances in Psychiatric Treatment* 2003; **9**: 424–31.

18. Reed A. Manufacturing a human drama from a psychiatric crisis: crisis intervention, family therapy and the work of R. D. Scott. In: Barker P, Stevenson C (eds). *The construction of power and authority in psychiatry*. Oxford, UK: Butterworth Heinemann, 2000: 151–61.

19. Sutherby K, Szmukler G. Community assessment of crisis. In: Phelan M, Strathdee G, Thornicroft G. (eds). *Emergency mental health services in the community*. Cambridge, UK: Cambridge University Press, 1995: 149–73.

20. Fulford M, Farhall J. Hospital versus home care for the acutely mentally ill? Preferences of caregivers who have experienced both forms of service. *Australian and New Zealand Journal of Psychiatry* 2001; **35**: 619–25.

21. Östman M, Kjellin L. Stigma by association: psychological factors in relatives of people with mental illness. *British Journal of Psychiatry* 2002; **181**: 494–8.

22. Dean C, Phillips J, Gadd E *et al.* Comparison of community based service with hospital based service for people with acute, severe psychiatric illness. *British Medical Journal* 1993; **307**: 473–6.

23. Brimblecombe N. Assessment in crisis/home treatment services. In: Brimblecombe N (ed.). *Acute mental health care in the community. Intensive home treatment.* London, UK: Whurr, 2001: 78–102.

24. Brimblecombe N, O'Sullivan G, Parkinson B. Home treatment as an alternative to inpatient admission: characteristics of those treated and factors predicting hospitalisation. *Journal of Psychiatric and Mental Health Nursing* 2003; **10**: 683–7.

25. Brimblecome N. Community care and the development of intensive home treatment services. In: Brimblecombe N. (ed.). *Acute mental health care in the community. Intensive home treatment.* London, UK: Whurr, 2001: 5–28.

26. Szmukler G. The place of crisis intervention in psychiatry. *Australian and New Zealand Journal of Psychiatry* 1987; **21**: 24–34.

27. Rosen A. Crisis management in the community. *The Medical Journal of Australia* 1998; **167**: 633–8.

28. Kolberg, C. Creating conversations in times of crisis. *Gecko* 1999; **2**: 10–17.

29. Shneidman E. Suicide thoughts and reflections 1960–1980. In: *Suicide and life threatening behaviours.* New York: Human Sciences Press, 1981: 195–364.

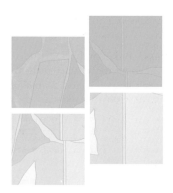

CHAPTER 51

Assertive outreach

Mervyn Morris* and Mike Smith**

INTRODUCTION

Although many people are satisfied with the care they receive, for various reasons we fail to reach a significant number of people. Assertive outreach services are not so much a new form of therapy, but a more intensive arrangement of services for people who, whether because of choice or circumstances, have not developed a helpful relationship with services, resulting in greater distress and frequent re-hospitalization. Where there is a lack of relationship, medication often becomes the only (and often very problematic) option and, critically, the person's needs are no longer at the centre of care as professionals attempt to take control of the situation.

Assertive outreach provides an opportunity to break this pattern and move beyond focusing on monitoring and medication compliance; assertive outreach teams have the resources and time to create opportunities for recovery for even the most difficult to engage people with complex needs. Working as part of an assertive outreach team is an ideal situation for nurses who want to make a difference. Where it works well, there is a very low staff turnover because of high levels of job satisfaction.

THE POLICY CONTEXT

Assertive outreach services can be seen as a culmination of policy development in mental health, wherever greater emphasis has been placed on effective multi-professional and inter-agency working. In England, the most notable report is Building Bridges[1] from 1995, which brought in to sharp focus problems of services for people with 'severe mental illness' in the community, and it is the needs of a small number of people within this broader group that has driven the implementation of this model.

This smaller group of people can be understood in two ways. First, the service recipients are those who service

*Mervyn Morris trained in the 1970s, working in a range of residential settings, including therapeutic communities and academic units. With additional training in psychodynamic, family and community interventions, Mervyn worked in a community-based team with older adults and people with severe mental illness, as well as liaison work in GP practices. Mervyn is Professor and Director of the Centre for Community Mental Health at Birmingham City University, and a Visiting Professor at University College Buskerud, Norway.
**Mike Smith is an independent trainer and author of a number of books and articles on self-harm, voice hearing, suicide, psychiatric first aid and the process of recovery from mental distress. He was awarded the overall nurse of the year award in 1997 for his work and also won the Bethlem & Maudsley 750th anniversary award for the advancement of mental health. Mike is formerly a Director of Nursing in the NHS and director of the International Mental Health Network, an active member of Intervoice and a research fellow at the Centre for Community Mental Health at Birmingham City University.

providers would describe as including at least some of the following characteristics:

- experiencing a particularly disruptive and enduring illness, resulting in significant problems in daily living;
- a history of psychiatric services having difficulty sustaining engagement, reflected by a pattern of regular and compulsory admission to hospital;
- reluctance to comply with treatment plans, primarily medication;
- 'co-morbid' presentation of a drug or substance misuse problem, homelessness and involvement with criminal justice systems;
- multi-professional and multi-agency interventions in their lives.

Second, assertive outreach (AO) can be seen as a means to better responding to the needs of society and care providers. There have been a number of events involving tragic deaths of professionals,[2] members of the public (perhaps most notably the death of Jonathan Zito in 1992),[3] as well as service users (though perhaps most notable is Ben Silcock, who was mauled by lions in London Zoo in 1992). These and many similar incidents created significant press interest and political lobbying related to the community treatment of people with 'severe mental illness'. Resulting inquiries, reports and pressure groups have highlighted failures in the coordination of assessment for and provision of services, and also raised the question of compulsory treatment extended beyond the hospital setting.

AO offers a comprehensive, more intensive, consistent, personalized and sustaining relationship with services, so that the events that lead to compulsory treatment are minimized. From a service recipient's perspective these services are valued if provided in such a way where the relationship offers choice and empowerment, enhances personal well-being and goal attainment, and as a result minimizes circumstances that lead to avoidable tragic events.

HISTORY

AO as it is commonly known in the UK arose out of the work in the early 1970s in the USA, where it is more generally known as assertive community treatment (ACT) or programme of assertive community treatment (PACT). The pioneers in this work were Arnold Marx, Leonard Stein and Mary Ann Test.[4] The service evolved out of the closure and retraction of state facilities in the de-institutionalization era of the 1970s in America and was probably the first systematic move to re-provide more appropriate new services in a community rather than just withdrawing services or replicating the old in a different setting.

Discharge from long-stay hospitals was based on the idea that many people's illness had become 'stable' or 'manageable' in hospital, and thus they could be returned to the community if 'rehabilitated'. However it became clear that successful rehabilitation in hospital was a poor predictor of success after discharge, and specifically the lack of community support for many led to the repetitive cycle of hospital admission and discharge: the so-called 'revolving door'. ACT was developed as both a more cost-effective way of intervening as well as a humane attempt to respond to people whose lives were obviously unsatisfactory for themselves and everyone around them. Stein and Test's work is seen as seminal in the field and essential reading for the background of assertive outreach.[5–7] As new programmes developed across the USA, a tool was developed to specify characteristics that demonstrated the degree a service had fidelity to a model ACT team.[8]

It is the most extensively evaluated model of community care for the 'severely mentally ill' and has become policy for many states in the USA, and has become a global model, from Moss in Norway to Townsville in Australia. In England it is now a standard component of services as part of the National Service Framework for Mental Health,[9] following which over 200 teams have been developed.

There was a flurry of activity around developing a UK evidence base that initially created some concerns about the efficacy of the teams.[10] This raised awareness of an important fidelity component of the 'team approach', having the opportunity to engage with many different team members, rather than using 'intensive case management' where the person works intensively with only one professional.

Perhaps the most influential evidence about AO is the Cochrane meta-analysis review, which supported the importance of fidelity, concluding that:

> ACT is a clinically effective approach to managing the care of severely mentally ill people in the community. ACT, if correctly targeted on high users of in-patient care, can substantially reduce the costs of hospital care whilst improving outcome and patient satisfaction. Policy makers, clinicians, and consumers should support the setting up of ACT teams.[11]

This arrangement of services contrasts with previous psychiatric community services in many ways, most notably in that they have much smaller staff–service recipient ratios, and actively involve the whole team rather than a single professional key worker, so that intensive engagement and complex care packages become more easily achievable.

AO teams also provide a role in supporting such community mental health teams, by accepting people who have gained little or nothing from services, and negatively experienced by professionals as 'difficult', 'disruptive', 'exhausting' and 'time-consuming'.

In some services including Northern Birmingham Mental Health Trust, the development of assertive outreach has been part of a wider reconfiguration of community services, including home treatment teams. The effective working relationship between community teams is an important influence on the effectiveness of AO.

Reflection

What is the demand for an AO service for the people you work with?
How does it, or how would it, integrate with existing service provision?

WHAT ASSERTIVE OUTREACH DOES

AO services are provided by a multi-professional and multi-agency team. This can include employment/vocational workers, sports/recreation specialists, befrienders, advisors/counsellors, community activists and also experts by experience; people who have recovered from a psychiatric illness themselves and who can help by using their experiences of recovery with others.

The aim is not only to enable access to helpful professional resources provided in a coordinated and consistent way, but also acting as a gateway for reaching into the wider network of community services and supports; in the longer term it is this that provides the more permanent relationships and usual life opportunities for personal development and achievement. Connecting people to non-professional relationships and away from mental health services is crucial to success; developing personal connections in the community, friendship and love bring expectations and commitment that can be far more meaningful and influential in helping people get back on top of their lives.

AO teams provide a single point for case management (hence the range of skills in a team); holistic assessment and psychiatric intervention; employment and housing assistance; family support and awareness; substance abuse services; and other supports critical to an individual's ability to live successfully in the community. Teams ideally offer a round the clock service for every day of the year in the community, particularly as evenings and weekends are often times of crisis and emergency hospitalization, with the consequent distress for the person and disruption to relationships and plans.

These teams are more effective the better they are able to communicate a belief in recovery, and then facilitate and support this by working creatively with a person over time both when they are well and when they are in difficulty. In our experience, AO works best where

it offers and supports the belief that a person can accommodate their experiences and play a valuable role in their community. This takes time and commitment from both parties, the latter developed through the person building confidence in themselves and services.

CHARACTERISTICS OF AN ASSERTIVE OUTREACH TEAM

There are several fidelity[8] characteristics that are evident in assertive outreach teams that together differentiate them from other community mental health teams. The following are thought to be the essential components:

- There is a *core team* with a breadth of skills to address all of a person's needs in a timely way, thus minimizing the risks inherent in having a large number of separate teams involved in supporting someone. As the *main provider of* services, a full mental health professional team is required (psychiatrist, nurses, social workers, occupational therapists) with a small service recipient to staff ratio to minimize the need for referral to other mental health service providers.
- The AO team share a single base, with an emphasis that *staff are interchangeable* in a range of roles to ensure that services are not disrupted because of shift systems, leave or illness.
- Unlike most other areas of service provision, *team rather than individual engagement* is a paramount aim, though of course team members will have differing relationships and thus have potentially different opportunities for helping.
- The team is also continually aware of *safety*, and the level of risk that the person may present to themselves and others. Visiting people in pairs minimizes risk to both the professional and the vulnerable individual, particularly where a person has either threatened or attacked others in the past.
- *Engagement* is an essential part of the work of AO teams, and may take many years to fully establish. The early focus of the team is primarily to develop rapport, build trust, and demonstrate both a consistent and persistent desire to work with the individual. The more willing the service is to meet the person to address their agenda, work flexibly, to demonstrate integrity and most importantly to remain supportive when problems or conflict arises, the more likely a positive relationship will emerge.
- AO is described as an *in vivo service* in that it takes place where the person is and where the most useful resources are available, i.e. in their community. Services are not provided in offices, i.e. as outpatients or in day centres and other mental health centres, but in the home or community. This approach maximizes the service's ability to match intervention to the actual situation of

the person, and use the person's potential to maintain and develop their identity in the community. Should someone be admitted to hospital, the team remains fully engaged and involved during this time, as a means to facilitating discharge at the earliest opportunity.

- Care is *highly individualized*, recognizing that people and relationships change over time, emphasizing a flexible and dynamic approach, engaging with the person in such a way that allows them to take and retain personal responsibility, maximizing choice and self-advocacy, and working through disagreement without coercion or rejection. Hope is a fundamental component of any therapeutic relationship, and all interventions should encompass the possibility of recovery, to aim to help the person to reclaim their lives, rather than maintain them as ill people in perpetuity.

- Treatment and support are *ongoing* rather than time limited; it is not a curative process but rather a form of support which enables the person to maintain their community links when they are unwell and to be in the best position to grow and recover when they are well.

- There is an *assertive approach*, where teams are committed to meeting that person's needs, and so do not look to hand over care, avoid intervention or regard 'doing nothing' as an option. People are engaged with wherever they are, be it at home, at a friend's, the local pub or wherever the individual feels safe and comfortable.

- A focus upon *meaningful occupation and employment* where the team encourages and facilitates all service users to pursue interests and gain employment, providing most 'vocational rehabilitation' services directly without referring on to other teams. This has perhaps the most substantial benefits in terms of independence and destigmatizing people, but also requires significant support to deal with issues of confidence as well as shifting often long-established negative self-perceptions.

- Many of the people using the service have complicating *substance use and misuse problems*. The more effective approach is where the mental health team leads on these interventions, and coordinates if not provides the substance abuse component of care.[12] To achieve this, services should include at least one team member with expertise in dual diagnosis working.

- A '*psycho-educational*' approach is taken that allows people to become collaborative partners in their treatment. People are encouraged to reflect upon, be aware and learn about themselves as well as their illness experiences, and also develop life skills both in managing symptoms as well coping with daily living. This of course is a two-way process and requires the staff to have a broad view of how individuals make sense of and bring meaning to their lives. Employing 'experts by experience' (i.e. recovered service recipients) is particularly valuable in this area, helping staff to challenge their professional views of the nature and impact of mental distress.

- *Family support and awareness with the active involvement of the service user*: AO staff include the person's support systems (family, 'significant others') as part of the recipients of an AO service. Families are no less important to service recipients than anyone else, and often more important where there is a need to improve negative and emotionally charged relationships, particularly to reduce conflict, increase autonomy and restore a more positive role. This work includes discussions about relationships as well as working with family goals and strategies, facilitating better understanding of illness experience and developing the ability to help each other.

- *Community participation*: The team supports and where appropriate facilitates people to be less socially isolated and more integrated into their local community through engaging with neighbours, local facilities, groups and organizations of their choice.

- The team pays attention to meeting all *healthcare needs*, offering support and guidance on essential health matters that improve well-being, as well as encourages and facilitates access to health education and other related services in the local community. Mental health service recipients also have some of the highest rates of untreated physical disease morbidity, which not only increase psychiatric symptom experience, but also undermine any sense of hope and aims for personal achievement.[13]

- To ensure their continued fidelity and success AO teams above all must have clearly stated *values that are evident in practice*. These values include relationship building, being person centred rather than treatment focused as the basis for personal recovery, with individualization of services as central building blocks for their work, as well as a commitment to evaluating and responding to the person's experiences of the service.

CAPACITY OF AN ASSERTIVE OUTREACH SERVICE

There is a balance to be struck between minimum caseloads to make this service cost-effective, as well as a maximum to ensure that the necessary time that people need is offered, and studies suggest a target ideal ratio of 1:10, that is one member of staff to every 10 service users. Assertive outreach teams should slowly build up their caseloads, as the early stages of engagement with services are more intensive and thus more time-consuming. The overall capacity is limited by team dynamics and the amount of people a whole team can effectively engage with, certainly no more than 100 service recipients served no less than 10 WTE case managing staff. Densely populated areas are able to focus teams still further, such as working with younger people in early intervention or working primarily with specific communities such as the

African-Caribbean population. However services are configured, it is essential that the team composition reflects the community within which it works, to ensure a full grasp of social and cultural issues for service users, as well as enabling effective community networking.

It is important to recognize that doctors and administrative staff are extra to these figures as they do not in most events case manage. There should be a dedicated psychiatrist on a full-time or part-time basis for a minimum of 16 hours per week for every 50 service users.

TARGET GROUP FOR ASSERTIVE OUTREACH

The criteria suggested for selection are listed below.

1 People between the age of 16 and 65 with 'severe and persistent mental illnesses', invariably experiencing symptoms within the range of psychotic illness diagnoses (individuals with a *primary* diagnosis of a substance use disorder, personality disorder or learning disability are not regarded as appropriate).

2 People with significant problems in community living, as demonstrated by at least one of the following criteria:

   a inability to consistently perform the range of practical daily living tasks required for basic functioning in the community (e.g. maintaining personal hygiene; meeting nutritional needs; caring for personal business affairs; obtaining medical, legal and housing services; recognizing and avoiding common dangers or hazards to self and possessions) or persistent or recurrent failure to perform daily living tasks except with significant support or assistance from others such as friends, family or relatives;

   b inability to be consistently working at a self-sustaining level or inability to consistently carry out a role at home (e.g. household meal preparation, washing clothes, budgeting, or childcare tasks and responsibilities);

   c inability to maintain a safe living situation (e.g. repeated evictions or loss of housing).

3 People with histories of high use and demand for psychiatric services characterized by:

   a high use of acute psychiatric hospitals (e.g. two or more admissions per year, or a hospital stay of more than 6 months, or detention under the mental health act at least once in previous 2 years) or psychiatric crisis resolution services such as home-based treatment;

   b intractable (i.e. persistent or very recurrent), severe major symptoms (e.g. affective disorders, psychotic, suicidal);

   c co-existing substance use disorder of significant duration (e.g. greater than 6 months);

   d high risk or recent history of criminal justice involvement (e.g. frequent arrests and imprisonment);

   e inability to meet basic survival needs due to living situation; residing in substandard housing, homeless, or at imminent risk of becoming homeless;

   f residing in an inpatient bed or in a supported community residence, but clinically assessed to be able to live in a more independent living situation if intensive services are provided, or requiring a residential or institutional placement if more intensive services are not available;

   g inability or unwillingness to participate in residential or traditional office-based services.

TEAM ORGANIZATION

The development of a team ethos is fundamental to assertive outreach, where close working overcomes the many professional and agency boundaries that exist within services. The team structure is very much a flattened hierarchy, where each member has a valuable role. Although there are legal aspects to the responsibility of the medical consultant, the most effective decision-making is based on a shared responsibility for care. However the role of team manager or leader (often a nurse) is crucial in facilitating a strong team ethos and promoting the philosophy of care that must be consistent as service users will meet and engage to some degree with the whole team. Expert (fidelity) opinion highlights that services work best where the manager is an integral member of the care-providing team, ideally contributing 50 per cent of their time as an active practitioner.

Another core fidelity criterion is that all members of the team meet every day, to share information, agree visiting and intervention arrangements, and maintain morale through mutual support and team supervision. As an extension to this, it is also important for the team to reflect more expansively on the care provided to each service user, and the overall service expectations. It is important to ensure not only regular reviews of individual clients, but also the development of the team's range of engagement strategies and interventions, as well as team dynamics, inter-team and inter-agency working, community relationships and networks.

As with all services, identifying areas for development of individuals and the team, regular review of policies and procedures, perhaps most notably how 'risk' is worked with, and identifying service and user outcomes, each contribute to ensuring consistency and confidence among all staff. Each team should be able to identify a strategic plan against which it can measure its effectiveness, and through formal reporting identify measurable areas of success but also limitations, both of which are essential to identifying future resource issues and priorities.

A service's focus shifts as it develops, so for example a team that is in the early stages of setting up and taking on its first service users will have a very different agenda to those running for years with its service user number at capacity, and perhaps some individuals looking to move on from psychiatric care.

Optimally there is a service available from the team 24 hours of the day 365 days of the year, although active and routine hours of operation are two 'shifts' each day to provide contact, treatment, rehabilitation, and support activities 7 days per week (some services are more limited at weekends). It is recommended as a minimum that services should be active 12 hours per day on weekdays, and 8 hours each weekend day and every holiday. There are various arrangement for an after-hours service where teams do not work 7 days or over 24 hours, including support from home treatment teams.

The AO team has the ability and capacity to provide multiple contacts per week, maybe as frequent as two or three contacts per day, 7 days per week, depending on individual need. Many if not all staff shall share the responsibility for addressing the transient needs of service users requiring frequent contacts. The AO team has the capacity to rapidly increase service intensity when required, but as a guide the mean number of visits over a year should be around three per week.

CARE AND TREATMENT IN ASSERTIVE OUTREACH

Within the aforementioned organization of the service, AO teams offer specific approaches to treatment that should be discrete, and particularly in the engagement process should not be prioritized over the need to establish a relationship. Medication is cited as a significant reason for disengagement.[14] The early aim of treatment can be oriented to harm minimization rather than focusing on treating illness. In Northern Birmingham, the development of the service used available literature and access to existing service providers in the USA to develop comprehensive policy and procedure documentation.[15]

First, the team revolves around a case management approach. Each service user is allocated a case manager (may be referred to as keyworker or lead worker for example, but they must operate to case management principles). The allocation of the case manager is dependent on a number of factors within the team, but most significantly determined by the relationship with the person. The professional is responsible for the coordination of the assessments and care plans of the individual, and is also able to take the lead in the engagement with the person and coordinating the care offered by the team. The case manager is also responsible for ensuring review of care plans and the timeliness and accuracy of information gathered. They must also ensure that the

person's rights and desires are advocated for within the team and that the individual has access to independent advocacy and representation where possible.

If a crisis develops then the case manager is responsible for the implementation of any crisis plan and to ensure that appropriate care and support is offered, and should be the lead person in working with the person's social support and family.

ASSESSMENT

Initial assessment

An initial assessment and care plan is done at the time of the service user's admission to the AO by the team leader or the psychiatrist, with the participation of designated team members.

Comprehensive assessment

A comprehensive assessment is initiated and completed within one month of the person commencing receipt of service according to the following requirements.

1 Each assessment area shall be completed by AO team staff with skill and knowledge in the area being assessed and shall be based upon all available information, including self-reports, reports of family members and other significant parties, and written summaries from other agencies, including police, courts, and outpatient and inpatient facilities, where applicable.
2 The comprehensive assessment shall include an evaluation of the following areas:
   a psychiatric symptomatology and mental state;
   b risk and vulnerability, particularly experience of abuse, exploitation, and also aggression and violence toward others, including service providers;
   c psychiatric history, including adherence to and response to prescribed medical and psychiatric treatment;
   d family and social networks and relationship skills;
   e medical, dental and other health needs;
   f extent and effect of any drug or alcohol use;
   g housing situation and activities of daily living (ADL);
   h vocational and educational skills, experience;
   i extent and effect of criminal justice involvement;
   j life events, current and past that may account for current experiences;
   k personal goals, ambitions, expectations and priorities.

While the assessment process shall involve the input of most, if not all, team members, a team member will be allocated to take responsibility for preparing the written assessment, and ensuring that a comprehensive treatment plan is completed within 1 month of the person commencing receipt of service. The case manager and individuals who have a specific contribution to make will be assigned by the manager of the service at the end of the assessment period.

RECOVERY PLANNING

The team aims to encourage hope through an ongoing commitment to support the person toward their own recovery, commencing from first contact, with the formulation of a care plan that aims to meet or clarify the person's own aspirations and desires to recover. Motivational interviewing techniques can help the individual (and the relationship) become future rather than problem orientated.

CRISIS ASSESSMENT AND INTERVENTION

Crisis assessment and intervention is available from the team. This can include telephone as well as face-to-face contact, though it may be provided in conjunction with the local 24-hour crisis/home treatment team if available and needed. This includes developing crisis plans, which include agreement about intervention preferences and what action is not helpful. For example, this can include who needs to be informed and who is willing to become involved as a support, what places provide safety and comfort, and medication preferences.

SYMPTOM ASSESSMENT, MANAGEMENT AND THERAPY

Symptom assessment, management and individual supportive therapy helps service users cope with and gain ownership and accommodation of their symptom experiences. This therapy should include but not necessarily be limited to the following:

1 ongoing assessment of the person's 'symptom' experiences and response to interventions;
2 awareness of the person regarding his or her illness and the effects and side-effects of prescribed medications, where appropriate;
3 symptom management efforts directed to help the person identify the symptoms and occurrence patterns, including early warning signs of his or her illness experience and develop a range of strategies to help lessen their effects. This information also forms the basis for drawing up a crisis plan as outlined above;
4 a full range of psychological interventions, both on a planned and as-needed basis, to help resolve life events

that have triggered symptoms, adjust to secondary problems of involvement with mental health services, as well as developing and accomplishing personal goals and coping strategies for successful day-to-day living.

Reflection

We have not discussed in this chapter any specific psychological interventions the team might use.
What strategies do you consider most appropriate for the people who use this service?

Medication

1 The team psychiatrist and medical team role includes:
   a assessing each person's psychiatric status, symptoms and related behaviour, and prescribing appropriate medication where useful;
   b monitoring general health, particularly where individuals are not engaged with primary care services, as this can influence the impact on symptom experience as well as response to medication. This is a critically important part of a person's needs from the team;
   c regularly reviewing the individual's physical and psychiatric status, as well the response to prescribed medication treatment;
   d aiming to raise awareness regarding the person's health status, both physical and psychiatric, from a medical perspective, and the effects and side-effects of medication and substance use.
2 All team members are involved in the continuous assessment of the person's symptom experiences and responses to any medication, including monitoring for side-effects.

PROVISION OF SUBSTANCE ABUSE SERVICES

Substance use and misuse is particularly complex with people who have severe mental illness, particularly where used to help manage symptoms. The complex relationship between these two sets of problems requires time, resources and experience beyond that available to substance misuse services, and are thus primarily provided by a dual diagnosis specialist 'in-house'. Provision of a substance abuse service includes a range of interventions:

1 identify substance use, effects and patterns;
2 recognize and individually evaluate the relationship between substances used, symptoms and psychotropic medication;

3 develop motivation for stopping or decreasing substance use as appropriate;
4 develop coping skills and alternatives to minimize substance use;
5 achieve sustainable periods of abstinence or stability in use.

In some areas there are specialist services for the treatment of people with a serious mental illness and who also use and misuse substances, providing a valuable source of advice and supervision. However, the management and intervention work remains the responsibility of the team.

WORK-RELATED SERVICES

Work-related services to help service users find and maintain employment in the community. Areas will include but not necessarily be limited to:

1 assessment of job-related interests and abilities, through a complete education and work history assessment as well as on-the-job assessments in community-based jobs;
2 assessment of the effect of the person's health on employment, with identification of emotional, lifestyle as well as behaviour that interferes with work performance, developing strategies to build confidence and deal with problems;
3 development of an ongoing job plan to help each person establish the skills necessary to find and maintain work;
4 individual supportive therapy to assist people to identify and cope with symptom experiences that may interfere with their work performance;
5 on-the-job or work-related support and crisis planning;
6 other support such as personal presentation, time-management and transport.

ACTIVITIES OF DAILY LIVING

Services to support activities of daily living in community-based settings. Developing problem-solving and other practical skills, alongside offering emotional and practical support so that the person can take responsibility for:

1 achieving a level of self-care sufficient to create acceptance, dignity as well as self-respect;
2 creating a good home environment, including cleaning, cooking shopping, and laundry, and also décor, furnishing and layout to reflect personal preferences for home;
3 finding and maintaining housing that is safe and affordable (may include finding someone to lodge with or a flat, dealing with landlords, cleaners, purchasing household goods and necessities (telephone, linens) getting services connected, e.g. gas, electricity;

4 developing or improving money management skills, including banking and financial advice;
5 using public transport;
6 registering with and using primary care services, e.g. GP and dentist, as well as any specialist health care.

SOCIAL SUPPORTS, RELATIONSHIPS AND LEISURE TIME EXPERIENCE

Many people are not just disengaged from services, they also have been excluded or alienated for parts of their lives from social networks that provide the many life opportunities and experiences for personal development and achievement. A critical part of care is reintroducing people to everyday activities and relationships in order that they can make friends, meet people and enjoy themselves. Practical skills may be developed in a variety of ways to help people in this aspect of their lives, particularly building confidence and personal responsibility.

The aims of these experiences should be to:

1 improve communication skills, develop assertiveness and increase self-esteem as necessary;
2 develop social skills, increase social experiences, and where appropriate, develop meaningful and reciprocal personal relationships;
3 plan appropriate and productive use of leisure time;
4 relate to landlords, neighbours, professionals and other service providers positively;
5 familiarize themselves with available social and recreational opportunities and increase their use of such opportunities;
6 make use of local community facilities such as advice and welfare support agencies.

AWARENESS, SUPPORT AND CONSULTATION TO SERVICE USERS' FAMILIES AND OTHER MAJOR SUPPORTS

Family interventions should aim to create a normal family role rather than turn family members into professionals and treating their loved one as a patient. Services should actively seek to engage with families and other major supports, with the person's agreement and involvement, and include:

1 awareness about the service user's symptom and illness experience, and the role of the family in providing support, particularly allowing personal responsibility and offering hope through recognizing potential for recovery;
2 interventions to resolve areas of day-to-day problems, family conflict and crises;
3 ongoing communication and collaboration, face-to-face and by telephone, between the team and the

family, particularly to deal with personal difficulties of family members where these are problematic for the service user, or where the service user can be helpful.

DISCHARGE FROM ASSERTIVE OUTREACH TEAMS

Discharge from AO ideally occurs where the person, the team and the person's support network believe the level of service is no longer required. More often it is due to a permanent or an extended move outside the geographic area of AO responsibility. In such cases, the team shall arrange for transfer of mental health service responsibility to a provider wherever the service user is moving. The team will aim to maintain contact with the service user until this service transfer is completed and engagement established. It also may be that the person requests discharge, despite the team's best efforts to develop a relationship and care plan acceptable to them. It is important that where discharge is requested that this process is undertaken to maximize the opportunity for success, and allows the option for people to return.

CRITICISMS

The development of ACT has also raised concerns about creating circumstances where teams become risk averse and over-vigilant, emphasizing medication compliance.[15] Service recipients may feel staff become aggressive rather than assertive. The primary aim of these services is to develop a care package that enables the potential for recovery, and this usually includes medication but as only one component. It is the person-centred focus that provides the grounds upon which the professional can engage and negotiate the best decision where compliance becomes an issue.

As already highlighted, there have been questions over the validity of the evidence and concern to ensure transfer of the original model appropriately to other cultures and settings. Although the model is said to be preferred by families and service users, there have been a number of criticisms from service users in the UK of the aggressive use of the model and its singularity of approach in assertively providing medical treatment.[16,17] We believe most of these concerns are about implementation and not the model and could be addressed by adhering to basic principles, and is the reason national organizations (National Forum for Assertive Outreach, www.nfao. co.uk/Homepage/Home.htm) attempt to ensure a degree of fidelity to team composition, organization and interventions outlined in this chapter.

There are real concerns where services and team membership do not reflect the population they serve, particularly in terms of cultural competence, and this is compounded where there is ineffective building of bridges with community leaders and resources. However, this is not a problem unique to assertive outreach.

REFLECTION

What are the key personal qualities required to work in an Assertive Outreach team?

SUMMARY

Dealing with people who are vulnerable and who may also present as a risk to themselves or others is a regular dilemma for practitioners in these services, and the philosophy of the team is perhaps most evident around its decision-making in this area. We take it as axiomatic that people can only recover by getting a life together in the community and being allowed to make decisions wherever and whenever possible, and of course this includes consideration of others. For professionals there is thus a balance to be struck between giving the person the opportunity to move on, test themselves and learn through taking risks and making mistakes, and avoiding situations that can very rapidly and seriously change to crisis. For some people this is only possible through the intensive sustained and meaningful contact that an assertive outreach can offer. Assertive outreach is ultimately about a climate of hope, respecting individuality, finding potential and facilitating opportunity for people where these essentials for recovery are least likely to exist.

REFERENCES

1. Department of Health. *Building bridges: a guide to arrangements for inter-agency working for the care and protection of severely mentally ill people*. London, UK: Department of Health. 1995.

2. Blom-Cooper L. *The falling shadow: one patient's care in the mental health system*. London, UK: Duckworth, 1995.

3. Ritchie J, Dick D, Lingham R. *The report of the inquiry into the care and treatment of Christopher Clunis*. London, UK: HMSO. 1994.

4. Marx AJ, Test MA, Stein L. Extrahospital management of severe mental illness. *Archives of General Psychiatry* 1973; **29**: 505–11.

5. Stein LI, Test MA. Retraining hospital staff for work in a community programme in Wisconsin. *Hospital and Community Psychiatry* 1976; **27**: 266–8.

6. Test MA, Stein L. *The clinical rationale for community treatment: a review of the literature. Alternatives to mental hospital treatment*. New York, NY: Plenum, 1978.

7. Stein LI, Test MA. Alternatives to mental hospital treatment: 1. Conceptual model, treatment programme and clinical evaluation. *Archives of General Psychiatry* 1980; **37** (4): 392–7.

8. Bond GR, Drake RE, Mueser KT, Latimer E. Assertive community treatment for people with severe mental illness: critical ingredients and impact on patients. *Disease Management and Health Outcomes* 2001; **9** (3): 141–59.

9. Department of Health. *National service framework for mental health*. London, UK: The Stationary Office, 1999.

10. UK 700 Group. Comparison of intensive and standard case management for patients with psychosis: rationale of the trial. *British Journal of Psychiatry* 1999; **174**: 74–8.

11. Marshall A, Lockwood A. *Assertive community treatment for people with severe mental disorders*. The Cochrane Library, 3, Chichester, UK: Wiley 2004.

12. Department of Health. *Mental health policy implementation guide: dual diagnosis good practice guide*. London, UK: The Stationary Office, 2002.

13. Cooley C, Morris M. Mental health and cancer: is there a missing link? *British Journal of Nursing* 1999; **8**: 1478.

14. Priebe S, Watts J, Chase W, Matanov A. Processes of disengagement and engagement in assertive outreach patients: a qualitative study. *The British Journal of Psychiatry* 2005; **187**: 438–43.

15. Northern Birmingham Mental Health Trust. *A model operational policy for assertive outreach services*. Birmingham, UK: Northern Birmingham Mental Health Trust, 2001.

16. Spindel P, Nugent JA. Polar opposites: empowerment philosophy and assertive community treatment (ACT). *Ethical Human Sciences and Services* 2000; **2**: 93–100.

17. Smith M, Coleman R, Allott P, Koberstein J. Assertive outreach: a step backwards. *Nursing Times* 2000; **95** (30):46–7.

ADDITIONAL READING

Stein LI, Santos AB. *Assertive Community treatment of persons with severe mental illness*. New York: Norton, 1998.
Burns T, Firm M. *Assertive outreach in mental health: a manual for practitioners*. New York: Oxford University Press, 2002.

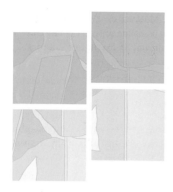

CHAPTER 52

Family support: growing the family support network

Chris Stevenson* and Evelyn Gordon**

This chapter explores how to widen the person's support network by involving their family and professional network in care and treatment. We propose a systemic approach[1] to care as more holistic, providing a potentially richer resource network to the patient and treatment system, and facilitating more coherence in the planning and delivery of care.

FROM INDIVIDUAL TO SYSTEM

There has long been a tradition in Western society to locate problems within the person because of an emphasis on individual independence and responsibility rather than on collective and community social processes. This approach is reflected in mental health care whereby mental illness is viewed as primarily located within the person's psyche and/or biology and to a lesser extent social system. Consequently, there is a lack of attention to the perspective of other people who have been involved in the process of moving towards being a psychiatric patient. People are often stripped of their existing connections when diagnosed with a psychiatric illness and on entering treatment systems.[2]

Scott and Ashworth[2] describe a kind of 'closure' that arises when treatment focuses on the individual perceived to be ill disregarding the wider family or social system. This kind of closure occurs at a number of levels resulting in the person losing their connectedness with their social world. When a crisis develops those connected to the person in distress may experience conflicting emotions such as distress and relief. The family may be faced with an unbearable sense of hurt and pain and feel isolated from the patient and treatment system. In the face of this, family members may cut off from the person who is ill.[3] This does not usually lead to family members abandoning one another in a physical sense, but rather a kind of dehumanizing process may follow whereby the person is viewed more and more through a diagnostic lens, while their individual personhood fades into the background. There may also be a sense of relief from relatives and sometimes from psychiatric and non-psychiatric professionals who have been struggling to find an appropriate way to help the person in distress. Hence, a form of community closure takes place whereby the hospitalization is viewed as the end-point or solution rather than an event on a continuum, and a defeat or limitation rather than a therapeutic opportunity.

*Chris Stevenson is Chair of Mental Health Nursing at Dublin City University, Dublin, Ireland. Previously she was Reader in Nursing at the University of Teeside, UK. Her doctoral research focused on the processes inherent in family work.
**Evelyn Gordon is a lecturer in Mental Health Nursing and Psychotherapy at Dublin City University, Dublin, Ireland. Her doctoral research is in suicidology.

Closure can be a point of no return. A symptom represents a partial death of that person as a social being, and being in the psychiatric space makes this death official. In effect this amounts to a 'treatment barrier'[4] as people's social context both contributes to and is affected by the process of being diagnosed.

We propose that this treatment barrier can be prevented or broken down by engaging with a person's social network, and moving from professional monologue to open dialogue[5] and trialogue[6] between those connected to the person in mental health distress. This is based on the premise that the person is part of a social network which influences their way of being and interacting in the world and to which they contribute, a recursively influencing engagement that gives meaning to living, life and self.

Actively involving families, and significant others including professionals, requires an approach to organizing assessment and intervention meetings that aims to create dialogic exchange between all concerned. Some practical ideas for making this a workable process are addressed in the sections on convening family meetings, and engaging and joining. Similarly, ongoing use of this systemic approach requires sustaining open dialogue as described in the section on collaborative approaches to change.

CONVENING FAMILY MEETINGS

Thinking about involving families in work with individual clients/patients can be daunting. For example, deciding how to invite and engage with them, and ensuring that this work is beneficial to the patient and family and that it enhances the treatment programme offered. Questions that might arise include:

- To whom should a letter of invitation be addressed?
- Is it better to write or phone?
- What needs to be said?
- Where is it best to meet with families?
- Who should attend to carry out family work?
- What information might be helpful to know?

There are no conclusive answers as each family is different. However, the family therapy literature in particular, offers much guidance in relation to making such 'opening moves'. Although some early family therapists refused to undertake therapy unless all family members were present, this is a less rigidly held position today as it is acknowledged that influence on any part of the system will produce a ripple effect across the entire system.[1] Currently, there is more attachment to thinking systemically when working with individuals and there is a growing interest in seeing families in their 'natural' milieu, rather than in the unreal context of the professional's domain. Carpenter and Treacher[7] provide more detail on these issues, but some 'rules of thumb' are noted below. It is important that in adopting this systemic approach that you negotiate this with the client/patient, explaining that it is your preferred way of working, and that you obtain their consent to involve other family members in this way.

To whom should the letter be addressed?

Sometimes it is sensible to send a letter to the entire family, especially where there is already commitment from the family members to attend. For instance, on admission, some family members will indicate to staff that they want to be involved as much as possible. A more personalized address is needed when you are requesting attendance of someone less well 'known'. This allows you to include specific information relevant to each person. For example, 'I understand from Joe that you have particular concerns about how he will manage at school/work since he has been having problems'. You will need to contact people in the wider network separately.

Is it better to write or phone?

Sometimes it is easier to make a phone call which involves a two-way exchange, providing space for questions about the meeting to be asked and answered, which can be helpful. However, you are then only communicating with one family member and this exchange can set the scene for future patterns of communication. This may become problematic if certain people are 'elected' to speak on behalf of others.

What needs to be said?

Box 52.1 (p. 446) shows a 'standard' letter, although it is important to consider what needs to be included for each family/family member. For example, are particular family members aware that their relative is receiving care for a mental health problem? A phone call would have a similar content, although the discussion could take place immediately. It is useful to include an information leaflet which sets out the reasons for a family meeting, how it is conducted, etc.

Where is it best to meet with families?

Overall, choose somewhere with which family members are comfortable. There are times when a health service facility is useful, for example, if video recording and viewing technology are required for team involvement and review purposes. It can be important to choose somewhere that is non-stigmatizing – not everyone wants to attend a psychiatric clinic. It is sometimes good to see family members in their own living circumstances, gaining a flavour of family life. However, more creativity may be needed in facilitating a home meeting as family life is a rich ecology, but that very richness can get in the way of talking.

Box 52.1: Standard convening letter

Dear …

Since I have been involved with Joe, I have become very aware of how important you, his family (and/or named friends and professionals), are/is to him, and I imagine that there is much concern for you around how his situation arose, what is happening now and what the future holds.

I have found that it is often useful to bring together the important people when someone's life is interrupted in order to discuss how we might move forward. With this in mind, I want to invite you to a 'family' meeting on … at … I enclose some information about the venue, and how to get there.

The meeting would involve the family team. This is made up of a group of people who work for … and who have a special interest in the wider context of people's problems. Having a team makes it easier to hear all the information people have to offer and allows more ideas to be generated about what might be helpful.

I would like to offer you the opportunity to discuss my invitation in more detail. I am contactable on … The best time to reach me is usually … , or you can leave a message … and I will get back to you. I look forward to speaking and to meeting with you.

Yours sincerely,

Who should attend in order to carry out family work?

There are ongoing debates about what constitutes a family system or social network. As a general rule, speak to the person in distress about whom they think it would be helpful to involve. There may be very good reasons why someone is not welcomed, and/or why someone does not think it is useful to attend. As mentioned earlier, while early family work operated on the principle that therapeutic work could only occur in the session or outside the meeting by people who are regular attendees, there has been recognition that families can communicate with people who do not attend, taking the story of the meeting back home. Practically, it may be better to meet with part of a network than not to meet at all.

What information might be helpful to know?

Before meeting with the family it is useful to consider what information would help the treating team understand the patient and their situation better so that care and treatment can be organized and delivered in a relevant and effective manner. This preparation helps to focus the meeting around practitioner initial hypotheses, leaving space for other questions and ideas to emerge.

Reflection

Think about the challenges you might encounter in setting up a family meeting in your own work context.

What resources are available to you to manage these challenges?

ENGAGING AND JOINING

Once you have successfully invited family members to attend a meeting, it is important to make them feel sufficiently attached to the event. Remember that most families will not have any understanding of what they might contribute to the meeting. They may feel vulnerable, for example fearing that they will be blamed for the problem, or that they will be given responsibilities that they are unable to enact. In a study a family member said:[8]

> … because I think we both (parents) came here, both of us before we came, came with a preconceived idea that, as I say, we were in some way being made to feel guilty, the guilty party. It was quite a relief … to be told that we weren't to blame ourselves … I think it's nice to voice our opinions and not feel under any pressure …

Engaging with families is like being a good host: offer to shake hands with everyone; invite people to come in and find a comfortable seat; enquire about how they found the journey to the meeting; offer drinks; use 'small talk' (which is big in its effect of relaxing people).

At this point, you will need to explain to the family members how the session will unfold so that they know what to expect. You may have already sent out an information leaflet, but it is still worth reiterating important aspects of the process so that you can be sure that everyone is consenting to participate and does not feel coerced into this. You may want to ask the family's permission to audio or video record the meeting, in which case you will need to explain that the purpose of this is to enhance your work together, and follow the consent procedure that the organization has in place. It is best to try to accommodate their particular needs. For instance, some families are happy to have the meeting taped if they have the opportunity to review the tape and if they can ask for tapes to be wiped at any time. When working with an observing team family members may prefer to meet the team who are positioned behind a one-way mirror before the meeting begins.

It has been argued by family therapists that if you want to effect change in families, then the therapist and family need to be 'joined'. Minuchin and Fishman state:[9]

> Joining is more an attitude than a technique, and it is the umbrella under which all therapeutic transactions occur. Joining is letting the family know

that the therapist understands them and is working with them and for them ... under her protection ... the family [can] have the security to explore alternatives, try the unusual, and change. Joining is the glue that holds the therapeutic system together.

These authors identify three joining positions that can be taken by the practitioner.

- In the *proximal* position, the interviewer relates closely to the family, at times making alliances with some family members. They use positive ways of looking at the family's functioning. Carpenter and Treacher[7] see this as particularly advantageous when working with families where blame and negativism are plentiful. The male therapist might say, 'It is particularly good to see you here today Mr Brown. It is not always easy for us men to talk about family issues'.
- In the *median* position, the interviewer listens actively but tries to stay neutral. They do not enter into alliances, but prompt the family to tell their story. The interviewer might say, 'Who would like to begin to tell me how come we are meeting here today?'
- In the *disengaged* position, the interviewer takes the stance of an expert fixer, while trying to create a sense of competence or hope of change with the family. They are a gatherer of information, finding out about how families explain their experiences and about patterns of communication. There is a strong leadership role for the interviewer in this position. They might ask, 'When the problem is around, who is the most able to ignore it?'

How the nurse positions themselves depends greatly on the therapeutic stance and framework that they prefer and deciding when it feels right to shift position with the family to maintain therapeutic engagement or gain therapeutic leverage. Thus, they may position themselves as the expert by being distant from the family and taking the role of leading the family to new understandings and insights about the problem that has beset them – therapist-led approaches. Alternatively, the interviewer and team may take a more collaborative approach and be close to the family and involved in a two-way exchange, or dialogue.

Although we advocate the latter approach, it is important that the practitioner(s) decide what approach is more fitting in each particular context and when this might need to be shifted. Some specific practices for maintaining this collaborative dialogic stance are elaborated below in addition to some more therapist-led and covert techniques described first.

Reflection

Take a moment to reflect upon your own preferred position and the ways that this both helps and hinders therapeutic engagement with clients/families.

THERAPIST-LED APPROACHES TO CHANGE

A number of techniques can be used by the practitioner to promote therapeutic change by perturbing the systems way of thinking and behaving, some of which are outlined below.

Reframing

The purpose of reframing is:

To change the conceptual and/or emotional setting or viewpoint in relation to which a situation is experienced and to place it in another frame which fits the 'facts' of the same concrete situation equally well or even better, and thereby changes its entire meaning.[10]

For example, when a person characterized as depressed says she is struggling to spend time with her children the interviewer might respond, 'So the children have some space to develop their own independent playing'. This can have the effect of releasing the mother figure from feeling guilty, because the meaning of 'mothering' has been altered. There are many powerful examples of reframing, for example the review by Richard Bandler and his colleagues.[11]

Messages and task-setting

Sometimes it is useful to give the family a message that is prepared by the team that shares the team's perceptions of their situation. For example, the team may choose to convey its respect for the way in which the family has been trying to deal with the problem. Messages can be given informally or the interviewing practitioner may read from a script. Messages may contain a task-setting component, that is the interviewer may ask the family to complete some task within or between the sessions. For example, a family 'at verbal war' with one another may be asked to experiment with finding some time each day when they can 'debate' (reframe) the family issues. They might be requested not to discuss those issues at any other time and are invited to report back during the next family meeting. Thus, the problem of out of control conflict is reorganized/ordered within a manageable pattern of necessary debate.

Paradoxical intervention

Some strategic family therapists have developed 'paradoxical intervention'.[12] In relation to systems theory, some family therapy approaches take the view that symptoms in one or more family members are a means to keep the family in a steady state wherein change is difficult. This 'homeostatic' state is safe, if unfulfilling. For example, the young person who begins to eat differently does not have to face the

---

Personal illustration 52.1

Jean has been an inpatient on an acute, psychiatric admission ward for 6 months. Recently, there have been discussions about alternative accommodation for her. The options have ranged from going back to her own flat to supported hostel accommodation or group living. From a systemic perspective, Jean has become part of the ward system. She has a function there, e.g. organizing shopping for staff and other patients, and feels that the nursing staff are, in her words, 'like family'.

Contemporaneously to the discussions about accommodation, Jean has begun to scream for periods of time, ranging from a few minutes to half an hour. This occurs both in the main ward area and at the ward entrance. The screaming is loud and is clearly distressing for the other patients as well as for Jean herself. The nursing staff have engaged her in conversations about the screaming, but these have not allowed Jean to act differently. She says that she cannot control the screaming at all, but is concerned that it upsets others. From a systemic perspective, the symptom can be seen as a way of keeping the system in balance as the screaming means that Jean is less likely to be discharged to alternative living and the ward staff are obliged to focus on Jean's needs, making her feel more attached.

Following a case discussion with the ward nursing team, a paradoxical intervention was chosen. Although the team was sceptical about whether such an approach would work, they were aware that the behaviour they were trying to treat was very entrenched. A message was prepared. Jean was to be advised that the ward team had been very concerned about her and decided that the screaming was obviously very important and a way in which she could release her feelings. Therefore, she should try to scream even more, even if she does not feel like it. For the next 4 days she would have access to a room where she could go to scream in private without disturbing others. She should do this four times a day at 09.00, 12.00, 15.00 and 18.00 hours. She was advised that she must scream as loudly as possible for at least 20 minutes. Of course, the screaming might occur outside these times, but that was to be expected.

For the first day, Jean followed the prescription. There was no screaming outside. Then she approached staff to say that she would be unable to scream any more because her throat was too sore. At this point, it is important to reinforce the paradoxical message. The staff advised Jean that it was even more important that she should scream, as her feelings would be bottling up by the minute. Therefore, she should continue to go into the room and practice screaming silently. She should adopt the position for screaming and open her mouth and scream without making any noise. This led to a cessation of the screaming. This illustrates an important facet of paradoxical prescription. There must be no room for the patient/family to escape from the paradox.

---

prospect of leaving home, and their parents do not have to face an 'empty nest' and the prospect of relating to each other as partners rather than parents. As the fear of change can be greater than the desire for change strategic therapists recognize that encouraging families to change may lead to resistance. This allows an argument for paradoxical intervention – the person wants to change and gives messages to this effect, for example, 'I am sick of being unable to go out'. This is taken as permission for the therapist to work covertly without contravening ethical codes. In order to push the family in a 'therapeutic' direction, the therapist uses the family resistance that is directed at the therapist as the agent or energy for change. The therapist gives a message that is seen as paradoxical by the family: directing the family to continue with the very behaviour that is problematic; acknowledging the dilemma in which they find themselves while hoping they will resist the prescription and establish a different pattern of relating and behaving. A case example is provided in Personal illustration 52.1. It is important that such interventions are thoroughly considered and delivered in a compassionate manner; otherwise they may be viewed as flippant or arrogant. As Watzlawick and colleagues[13] put it:

> The choice of an appropriate paradoxical injunction is extremely difficult and … if the slightest loophole is left, the patient will usually have little difficulty in spotting it and thereby escaping the supposedly untenable situation planned by the therapist.

For this reason, and because the intervention is covert, it is usually better to take a team approach in using paradoxical intervention and be guided by a therapist experienced in this technique.

COLLABORATIVE APPROACHES TO CHANGE

Sustaining dialogue requires more than the use of techniques. The practitioner needs to adopt a 'reflexive' position with the family, which is enhanced through the use of reflecting processes and a narrative approach.

Reflecting processes

Reflecting processes are characterized by transparency in relation to ideas and concerns held by all. Andersen[14] developed a reflecting team process, whereas Rober[15] describes methods that can be used by the lone practitioner. Clients hear what professionals say about the client's situation, rather than the professional network being secretive. The openness is achieved by various methods. The interviewer, family and team, real or imagined, can move between speaking and listening positions. As there is no desire to uncover the 'real truth' about a problem, it is possible to construct layers of meaning through reflection upon reflection upon reflection. Deciding when to change position, from talking to listening and vice versa, is negotiable. There may be a pause in the flow of conversation that invites a change, or a family member, interviewer or team may request it, although it is never demanded. One way is for clients to meet with a team of professionals. One professional talks with the family for a while with the team listening to that talk. At an appropriate moment, the listening members of the team talk about what they saw, heard and thought when they listened to the family talk. Thereafter, the family members have a turn in responding by talking about what they were thinking when they listened to the team's talk.[16] The lone practitioner may choose to reflect aloud in the presence of the client/family and/or incorporate other perspectives by pondering about what others might think about the issues being discussed. In relation to interviewing, there are some guiding principles that assist the practitioner with this reflecting process.

Adopting 'a not-knowing' stance

A 'not-knowing approach' advocates that the interviewer not presume that they have superior expertise in relation to the situation; rather they have a potentially useful contribution to make to the therapeutic conversation. For example, Anderson and Goolishian[17] describe the case of a 40-year-old man who chronically felt that he had a contagious disease and was perpetually infecting others, even killing them with it. Multiple medical consultations and psychotherapies had failed to relieve the man of his conviction and fear about his infectious disease, hence a consultation was arranged. Early in his story, wringing his hands, he told about being diseased and infectious. The consultant (Goolishian) asked him, 'How long have you had this disease?' Looking astonished and after a long pause, the man began to tell his story. He had sought help for his problem and had always been told that he was in excellent physical health but that he did have a mental condition, and he was referred on several occasions for psychiatric consultation. He felt misunderstood. As the consultant continued to show an interest in his dilemma by viewing this as an authentic concern, if not an objective reality, the man became more relaxed and he elaborated his story. The consultant did not simply take a history or recollect events of the static past. His curiosity remained with the man's subjective reality (the disease and contamination problem). The intent was not to challenge this or his personal story, but rather to learn about it, and to let it be retold in a way that allowed new meaning and new narrative to emerge. In other words, the consultant's intent was not to talk or manipulate the man away from his ideas, but rather through not-knowing (non-negation and non-judgement) to provide a starting point for dialogue and the opening of therapeutic conversational space. Colleagues viewing the interview were quite critical of this collaborative position. They feared that such questions might have the effect of reinforcing the patient's 'hypochondriacal delusions'. Many suggested

that a safer question would have been, 'How long *have you thought* you had this disease?' However, to have asked this question would only have served to impose the consultant's predetermined or 'knowing' and 'paradigmatic' view that the disease was a figment of the man's imagination or a delusion or distortion in need of correction. The most likely outcome is that the man would have again felt misunderstood and alienated.

It is useful to distinguish between a not-knowing approach and other ways of utilizing practitioner expertise. In the not-knowing position, the practitioner is informed by their professional and personal expertise and tentatively shares this with the client/family, whereas taking a position of 'ignorance' suggests that this is withheld or denied. Alternatively, engaging in 'professional monologue' may lead the practitioner to impose their expert view on the client/family.

Radical listening

The interviewer and team listen attentively. They try to hear what the person says while temporarily suspending their preferred ways of understanding. This radical listening can open up possibilities for creative reflection. For example, as a reflecting team member said, 'When I heard Sylvia say that she is the Duchess of Kent, I imagined how she might walk and talk and dress differently, and I wondered how other people might respond to her then'.[8]

Use of systemic/relational questions

Questions of a different order are used in systemic work. These are described as circular questions. Circular questioning is a system of questioning that helps to reveal new information and people's different perceptions of the problem and its resolution. They allow the interviewer to explore hypotheses about what is happening in, for and around the family. Examples of systemic questions are given in Chapter 13 of this book. Attentive listening can be enhanced by using the language of the client/family rather than professional jargon, and using client/family feedback to guide your next move in the interview. For example,

Client: I have been low for a long time now.

Interviewer: Can you recall when you first began to feel low … and what was happening in your life at that time?

Attention to our own personal and professional beliefs/prejudices

What is offered as a reflection is often accompanied by the reflector's own consideration of why they have offered the particular reflection rather than another. For example, a team member encountered a couple when working as an 'observer' on a family team. The couple had been on the brink of divorce and this was attributed to the husband's long-standing depression. However, he had strong negative beliefs about marital breakdown, thinking that the couple would have to grin and bear the situation for the sake of his two sons. He seemed uncomfortable at being in the meeting and was vocal in his dislike of feminists and social scientists who made claims that divorce was often a humane alternative to inharmonious family life. Behind the screen, CS felt that she was being personally attacked by a 'chauvinist' with a vested interest in keeping the status quo within the family. However, since working in a reflecting team she had become accustomed to listening attentively to what people say and examining her own prejudices alongside that. As the meeting unfolded, she discovered that the man's father had died when he was a boy and he had struggled to gain an identity in the context of a female household. She wondered if this man interpreted 'evidence' from social science and feminism through the lens of his own experience and found it wanting. Thus, his antagonism to such theory was *understandable* once the broader context of his life was included. By the end

of the meeting she found herself in admiration of someone who would sacrifice himself for the sake of providing a role model for his sons. Recognizing her own prejudices assisted CS in constructively challenging these and shifting her position with the client/family.

Reflection

You may wish to consider what prejudices might emerge for you in working with a similar scenario.

How would you respond if a client/patient challenged your professional knowledge?

Generating ideas to reflect back to family and interviewer can be difficult especially when you first begin to work in this way. Although there are some general guidelines for producing feedback, it is important to remember that sometimes intuition gives us ideas about what to offer. The 'helpful ideas', shown in Box 52.2, encourage us to think about what was *actually* said and different possible versions. Having thought about what was said, by whom, to whom; the range of ideas; the nature of silence; and how things could be interpreted differently, feedback needs to be given to the family in a sensitive manner. Some guidance is provided in Box 52.3.

Box 52.2: Helpful ideas when reflecting: guidelines

Content

How were things described? For example, I noticed that when Mary refers to herself she always says 'just' – like 'It's just my opinion'.

How could things be described? For example, I wondered whether when John says he is tired of living it could be that he is tired of fighting the problem?

How were things explained? For example, it caught my attention that there was a lot of talk about how tablets work or don't work.

How could things be explained? For example, I know that a lot of people make sense of what's happening for them in relation to changes in their physical body. I have a different idea that how we talk about problems can make them grow smaller or larger.

What relationships *seemed* to exist between issues? For example, I noticed at several points in the session that when Joan becomes tearful Jean looks away.

What relationships may exist between issues? For example, I found myself making connections between Gail's angry outbursts and Neil's needs to have a bit of space.

What may have happened if something else was attempted? For example, I heard the family say that when Harry has a drink they all start to nag at him. I was wondering what would happen if someone in the family asked him whether there was anything upsetting him?

Process

Who talked?

Who talked with whom?

How many different ideas were expressed?

Silences: When? Who broke these?

Box 52.3: Guidelines for reflecting back

Use of language (non-prejudicial, not jargon laden). For example, 'I noticed that being a person described as having alternative ways of thinking has meant that Don has had to put his life on hold'.

Use of metaphor/imagery. For example, 'I wondered whether this family know the story of Alice in Wonderland – Alice is asked by the Caterpillar "Who are you?" and Alice can hardly answer for she has undergone so many changes since being in Wonderland'.

Conversational style. The reflecting space is not about scoring points off one another as practitioners, i.e. seeing who can come up with the best reflection which mirrors some reality of the family's distress. Rather it is about opening up different versions of how life is or can be played out.

Remain positive. For example, 'I was impressed that Hilary was able to share her tears with the rest of her family and the team'.

Remain within the context set by the conversation listened to. For example, 'I heard Frank say that he was "horrified" by what has been happening at his work'.

Tentative advice in third person. For example, 'I just wondered whether it would be worthwhile to try …'

5–10 minutes uninterrupted: a longer period of reflection risks losing the listeners' attention.

Narrative approaches: theory, principles and practice

A narrative approach promotes a different mode of understanding, one more concerned with subjective understanding and less concerned with objective explanations. From this perspective, we need to hear and understand a person's personal stories or narrative in order to understand them. Narrative carries the weight of context and so, for Bruner,[18] it is a more suitable medium for relating human experience. It is through the fictions and stories that we tell ourselves and others that we live our lives, in other words they help to create and represent us. Stories allow us self-protection, to find a way to be with others, but also can create tangles and interrupt the flow of life.

There is a growing interest in narrative in health disciplines. In a series in the *British Medical Journal*, Greenhalgh and Hurwitz[19] offer the following summary points in relation to narrative-based medicine.

- The process of getting ill, being ill, getting better (or getting worse), and coping (or failing to cope) with illness, can all be thought of as enacted narratives within the wider narratives (stories) of people's lives.
- Narratives of illness provide a framework for approaching a patient's problems holistically, and may uncover diagnostic and therapeutic options.
- Taking a history is an interpretive act; interpretation (the discernment of meaning) is central to the analysis of narratives (for example, in literary criticism).
- Narratives offer a method for addressing existential qualities such as inner hurt, despair, grief, and moral pain which frequently accompany, and may even constitute, people's illnesses.

Launer[20] offers some case material of a narrative approach in action. When a narrative approach is favoured within family work the members of the team remember that there are many versions of the family's story, authored by each member, while also accepting that the practitioner creates their own narrative about the patient and family narrative which informs their actions.

In the field of family therapy, Epston and colleagues[21] have used narrative approaches extensively. These authors state that stories are created to make our life experiences meaningful and, in turn, such stories shape our lives. Sometimes a particular story becomes so well rehearsed that it is difficult to step outside of the text and act in a more productive, creative or less pathologizing way. In therapy, there is a space for revising (re-visioning) stories and the life practice that follows from them. For Epston and White, the therapist and family member(s) can work to re-author life events and co-create an alternative story. They describe a client, Rose, who had been struggling with a demanding job in advertising and was insecure in her sense of self. She met with Epston, who invited her to tell her story. He followed this up with a letter that re-storied her life experience as an odyssey involving overcoming the legacy of neglect and oppression through her special wisdom, determination and ability to self-protect. She was described as having 'grit' and a 'survival instinct' (re-frame). A month after receiving the letter, Rose had found a job in her ideal career, felt her life was on the right track, had renewed her relationship with her mother, and had established the validity of her abusive experience through checking with her siblings. 'Rose was radiant and witty as she contemplated the future she was now anticipating'.[20]

Box 52.4 indicates the principles that guide interviewing when taking a narrative approach. These are similar to the guidelines for sustaining reflective dialogic processes discussed above.

> ### Reflection
>
> You may wish to consider how these fit with your own practice and identify those that you would like to develop further.

> ### Box 52.4: Principles that guide interviewing within a narrative approach
>
> Adoption of a 'not-knowing' approach. The practitioner does not believe and/or act as if they have all the answers. Rather the family members are seen as the experts in relation to their predicament.
>
> Radical listening. The practitioner attends to channels of communication that are not routinely followed, e.g. the use of a particular grammatical style, the use of metaphor, etc.
>
> The use of systemic/relational questions.
>
> Reflective practices and formats for the sessions.
>
> Attention to personal and professional beliefs and prejudices.

SOCIAL NETWORK MEETINGS

When people come into hospital the social network will have generated a variety of accounts, sometimes conflicting, about the problem and how it should be addressed, and, as mentioned, there are frequently strong and conflicting emotional responses to the event. There may be a feeling that there can be a cooling off period during which the person admitted can 'settle down' on the ward. However, coming into hospital can also be an awkward and unsettling experience. When individuals and relatives are asked about the process of coming into hospital they tend to identify several challenges. Patients have to find a way to relate to the ward staff and understand how they operate individually and in terms of the ward routine. They state the need to feel some sense of control about what is happening and what is going to happen. They are concerned that they will never 'get out of hospital'. The relatives state that they feel excluded from decisions and that the valuable information they have is not gathered and/or used. Other professionals who have played a significant role in the patient's life are frequently excluded. Given this sense of confusion and lost opportunity, what is the evidence for engaging with the social network around crisis and admission?

Finnish colleagues have been working with people in crisis and at risk of hospital admission and with people newly admitted to hospital.[5] The team found that it was worthwhile to make the boundary between hospital and community more open through a dialogic process between all concerned. They convened a meeting of the key people to create a space in which treatment can be discussed openly. In other words, all decisions are made with respect for the opinions of the patient and their family and the professional network. The aim is to come to an agreement, if not a complete consensus, about the way forward, to which all parties sign up. This has the benefit of circumventing the possibility of different agendas being played out. The evaluation of the Finnish team's approach is summarized as follows: in a sample of 30 people with a psychotic diagnosis, only 9/30 had more than 31 hospital days in 2 years' follow-up; 9/30 used neuroleptic drugs, but six out of these nine discontinued without detriment; 20/30 patients had no psychotic symptoms at follow-up, 7/30 had mild symptoms and three had severe symptoms.

These ideas have been expanded, for example, into the reception or social network meeting, instigated by Reed and colleagues[22] to promote more collaborative and open working relationships between professionals, and between professionals and families. Such meetings are organized around the idea that families are agents of change, not objects of change. The family members, including the member in distress, are seen as the experts about their own family and social lives. Meetings are organized to be as warm and welcoming as possible. For example, participants are offered a drink. The professionals concerned actively try to avoid using professional jargon that is exclusive and to adopt a more conversational style. The people who convene and facilitate are careful that the family members are not made to feel that they are being called to account for something. Nor is the agenda to make the family aware of what is medically best for their relative, or to arrive at and convey a diagnosis. The meetings are organized in such a way that people are encouraged both to speak and listen or engage in open dialogue and trialogue rather than monologue.

SUMMARY

This chapter has provided a theoretical framework and some practical guidelines to how meetings with families and others can be organized and conducted. Research, theory and personal practice experience support the idea that a systemic orientation promotes opportunities for creative change. This approach is sensitive to the wider context of the individual and facilitates families and significant others in their social and professional network to open up possibilities for collaborative working relationships. A word of warning, however; it is important to acknowledge that different families are made up of different individuals, in varied personal and emotional circumstances. Although the guidance offered here is a starting point for family and network work, the particular context will inform how these meetings proceed. Therapeutic recipes can be fruitfully adapted.

REFERENCES

1. Dalos D, Draper D. *An introduction to family therapy: systemic theory and practice*. Maidenhead, UK: Open University Press, 2000.

2. Scott RD, Ashworth PL. 'Closure' at the first schizophrenic breakdown: a family study. *British Journal of Medical Psychology* 1967: **40**: 109–45.

3. Reed A. Manufacturing a human drama from a psychiatric crisis: crisis intervention, family therapy and the work of RD Scott. In: Barker P, Stevenson C (eds). *The construction of power and authority in psychiatry*. Oxford, UK: Butterworth Heinemann, 2000: 154.

4. Scott RD. The treatment barrier: Part I. *British Journal of Medical Psychology* 1973; **46**: 45–55.

5. Seikkula J, Sutela M. Co-evolution of the family and the hospital: the system of boundary. *Journal of Strategic and Systemic Therapies* 1990; **9**: 34–42.

6. Amering M, Rath I. The first Vienna trialogue: experiences with a new form of communication between users, relatives and mental health professionals. In: Lefley H, Johnson D (eds). *Family interventions in mental illness: international perspectives*. Westport, CT: Praeger, 105–24.

7. Carpenter J, Treacher A. *Marital and family therapy*. Oxford, UK: Blackwell, 1989.

8. Stevenson C. Negotiating a therapeutic context in family therapy. Unpublished PhD thesis, University of Northumbria, 1995.

9. Minuchin S, Fishman C. *Family therapy techniques*. Cambridge, MA: Harvard University Press, 1981: 31–2.

10. Watzlawick P, Weakland J, Fisch R. *Change*. New York, NY: Norton, 1974: 95.

11. Bandler R, Grinder J, Andreas S. *Frogs into princes: neurolinguistic programming*. Moab, UT: Real People Press, 1979.

12. Cade B. The use of paradox in therapy. In: Walrond-Skinner S (ed). *Family and marital psychotherapy: a critical approach*. Boston, MA: Routledge and Kegan Paul, 1979.

13. Watzlawick P, Beavin AB, Jackson DD. *Pragmatics of human communication*. New York, NY: Norton, 1967: 242.

14. Andersen T. Reflections on reflecting with families. In: McNamee S, Gergen K (eds). *Therapy as social construction*. London, UK: Sage, 1992: 54–68.

15. Rober P. The therapist's inner conversation in family therapy practice: some ideas about the self of the therapist, therapeutic impasse, and the process of reflection. *Family Process* 1999; **38** (2): 209–28.

16. Andersen T. The reflecting team. *Family Process* 1987; **26**: 415–28.

17. Anderson H, Goolishian H. The client is the expert: a not-knowing approach to therapy. In: McNamee S, Gergen K (eds). *Therapy as social construction.* London, UK: Sage, 1992: 25–39.

18. Bruner J. *Acts of meaning.* Cambridge, MA: Harvard University Press, 1990.

19. Greenhalgh T, Hurwitz B. Why study narrative? *British Medical Journal* 1999; **318**: 48–51.

20. Launer JA. Narrative approach to mental health in general practice. *British Medical Journal* 1999; **318**: 117–19.

21. Epston D, White M, Murray K. A proposal for re-authoring therapy. In: McNamee S, Gergen K (eds). *Therapy as social construction.* London, UK: Sage, 1992: 96–115.

22. Reed A, Wilson M, Stevenson C. Social network meetings ease trauma of psychiatric admission. *Nursing Times* 1998; **94** (42): 52–3.

CHAPTER 53

The liaison psychiatric service

Chris Hart*

INTRODUCTION

Over a half century ago, *The work of nurses in hospital wards*[1] noted a difficulty in meeting specific patient needs. It attributed this to the allocation of nursing care in the form of separate tasks carried out by different nurses, which meant little time was given to emotional care.[2] This thesis eventually led to the introduction of the nursing process from the United States in the late 1970s and early 1980s, and more explicit attempts to address the patient's care on a holistic basis. The preeminence of the nurse–patient relationship peaked with primary nursing in the late 1980s, but both that approach to nursing and the holistic care of the individual has declined over the past decade for a variety of educational, organizational and political reasons.[3]

In mental health, the growing scandal at the recognition of premature death for people with serious mental health problems has led to renewed attempts to address this group's physical health needs.[4] However, both physical and mental health is still viewed as distinct rather than interdependent.

Liaison psychiatry conceptualizes the relationship between the mind and body as wholly entwined and relates itself to the health of the individual. Its practitioners concern themselves with meeting the mental health needs of the patients in the general hospital and integrating an understanding of those with the individual's physical health care. This could be said to come into conflict with aspects of medical and psychiatric practice, as well as healthcare organizations that still reflect the dualistic concepts of philosophers such as Descartes, who conceived of a separation of mind and body.[5]

This approach echoed the work of Peplau,[6] who viewed the holistic needs of the patient as being central to the nurse–patient relationship, arguing it was demonstrated by the nurse 'bringing all her capacities, talents and competencies to bear upon the life of another person', requiring a closeness, 'Not so much … to the person who is ill, but rather one of being "closer to the truth" of that person's current dilemma.'

Reflection

What factors increase or lessen the extent to which you work with patients on a more holistic basis, addressing their psychological, social, physical and spiritual needs?

How does this affect your relationship with the person?

*Chris Hart is a nurse consultant in liaison psychiatry, based at South West London & St George's Mental Health NHS Trust and a Principal Lecturer at the Faculty of Health & Social Care Science, Kingston University & St George's University of London. He is currently working on the second edition of his book, Nurses and Politics and co-editing a book on relational management in health care.

- It has been estimated that 20–40 per cent of all people attending a general hospital, either as an inpatient or outpatient, will have psychological disorders or mental health problems in addition to the physical disorders that prompted their original referral or admission.[7]
- It has been estimated that 20–30 per cent of people attending A&E departments will have psychiatric problems co-existing with physical disorders and 5 per cent will have presented due to mental health problems alone.[8,9]
- Approximately 150 000 people are identified as self-harming each year in the UK, most presenting to an A&E department.[10]
- Self-harm is the commonest reason for the admission of young people to hospital and one of the top five causes of acute admission of all adults.

TABLE 53.1 Levels of service

Level	Components of the service
Level 1	24-hour service provision to whole hospital, including A&E department, inpatient wards and outpatient departments
Level 2	Limited hours service provision to whole hospital, including A&E Department, inpatient wards and outpatient departments
Level 3	24-hour service provision to A&E department and inpatient wards
Level 4	Limited hours service provision to A&E department and inpatient wards
Level 5	24-hour service provision to A&E department
Level 6	Limited hours service provision to A&E department

Box 53.2: A comprehensive range of services provided by a liaison psychiatry service to an acute hospital

1 Mental health assessments, including assessments under the Mental Health Act (1983).
2 Risk assessment and assistance with risk management.
3 Assistance with diagnosis of particular disorders.
4 Assistance with assessments of a patient's capacity to consent.
5 A range of psychological, psychosocial and pharmacological treatments.
6 Support to carers.
7 Referral to appropriate agencies following assessment, including specialist services within mental health trusts.
8 Advice and assistance in the management of common mental health problems and serious behavioural disorders in a mental health context.
9 Mental health promotion and training and education in the recognition, understanding, treatment and management of common mental health problems and related issues.
10 The study of psychiatric morbidity in the physically ill.

problem-solving and improving staff understanding and skills for dealing with similar patient presentations for the future.[15,16]

Although the demand is well documented, the range and organization of service provided by liaison psychiatry teams to meet it is inconsistent. Ideally, a team would be resourced to be able to provide a comprehensive service (Box 53.2 and Table 53.1) but this is rarely the case.

BRIEF HISTORY

The practice of liaison psychiatry is relatively young. Its genesis, first in the United States and then in the UK, has been quite different and is worth comparing. The first seminal paper was published in the late 1920s in the United States, but progress only really took root in the post-war years through collaborations between physicians and psychiatrists as a result of psychiatric units being placed in general hospitals, bringing the two groups together.[17]

A range of factors made it possible for nurses to follow psychiatrists into areas of physical health care, especially once clinical specialist roles were developed and accepted. As the value of the service crystallized, psychiatrists could not keep pace with demand. American nurse education had moved into the universities in the 1960s, giving it a solid academic foundation, and base from which senior academics ventured out to provide clinical input. With a generic training, nurses were used to working in the general hospital setting, with a body of nursing literature developing about the psychosocial needs of patients as well as a more recent emphasis on the 'interplay of mind and body in wellness and illness in the context of an explosion in neurobiological knowledge by the American psychiatric nursing community'. Despite initial misgivings on the part of some physicians and surgeons, through a combination of clinical competency, political skills and determination, a handful of pioneering psychiatric consultation–liaison nurses (PCLNs) established

The need for liaison psychiatry services is underlined by the fact that the general hospital patient group will have higher rates of psychological difficulties than people in the wider community (Box 53.1).

Left untreated, depressive disorders delay rehabilitation from disabling physical illness, diminish pain tolerance, affect the individual's ability to seek help and treatment and are predictors of poor outcomes 1 year after myocardial infarction.[11–13] Interventions from liaison teams are argued to be cost-effective for hospitals needing to maintain a steady 'throughput' of patients, as well as prevent relapse or re-presentation to services.[14] Equally, the value of working proactively and alongside clinical teams in the general hospital has been recognized in immediate themselves. Some worked alongside psychiatrists but many practised autonomously. Graduate programmes in psychiatric consultation–liaison nursing were established in the early 1970s, with published nursing research and articles following, addressing the nursing role and practice. Contemporary psychiatric consultation–liaison nursing is provided by advanced practice registered nurses educated to at least master's level.[15,18]

Lipowski[19] described a division of labour between nursing and medical members of liaison psychiatric teams, with nurses taking referrals from nurses while psychiatrists could take referrals from either nurses or medical colleagues. However, the realities of service demand meant such a neat separation was rarely maintained, most particularly as not all hospitals had psychiatrists on the staff. More usefully, Robinson[15] explored the differences in roles in practice. Although these were complex and not always consistent, she noted the PCLN's emphasis on the health of the patient, assisting nurses in the patient's overall care and management and working with psychosocial issues, in contrast to the psychiatrist's focus on symptom management and diagnosis.

The evolution of the service was very different in the UK. There were similar alliances of like-minded physicians and psychiatrists but Morriss and Mayou[20] attribute the early demand for liaison psychiatry services to the decriminalization of suicide in 1961, after which the Ministry of Health advised that all people who had attempted to kill themselves be seen by a psychiatrist before leaving hospital. A clearer division of labour emerged in the UK largely because, as nurses were gradually recruited into expanding teams, they enjoyed neither the established relationship with the general hospital of their US counterparts, nor the status that came from having academic qualifications as advanced practitioners or clinical specialists. The closure of large swathes of mental health beds in the late 1980s and 1990s and a shortage of community mental health services only served to increase the importance of having nurses able to assess patients presenting at the general hospital who had self-harmed or were attending with a mental health emergency.

The discipline only found recognition in the Department of Health's *Mental health nursing review*, which recommended that nursing posts be established in liaison services.[21] Relatively little has been published by UK nurses and no educational framework identified as essential for the role. Only two universities have established a module in liaison psychiatry.[22]

MODELS OF SERVICE

Liaison psychiatry exists in a policy vacuum at a national level. Few policy initiatives directly reference it, although many have clear implications, demanding mental health and risk assessment,[23] easy access to mental health clinicians,[24] mental health promotion,[25] reduction in suicide rates[26] and support for carers.[24] Despite liaison psychiatry services being a main gateway for patients and their carers into mental health services, it has been denied the funding for development and implementation programmes provided by government for initiatives such as assertive outreach, early intervention and crisis services. Nor, to date, has a single, coherent model of liaison psychiatry service or nursing role emerged.[23] Some hospitals have separate adult, older age, child and adolescent, and drug and alcohol services. Others provide a more integrated service but, despite more recent published material and texts on the organization and structure of liaison psychiatry services, e.g. Harrison and Hart,[27] there is no apparent rationale to the way in which many ser-vices have developed. Determinants are likely to be available funding, individual lobbying and/or alliances or inquiry recommendations. A model for understanding the range of service levels is provided in Table 53.1.

Twenty-four-hour services have become more common, prompted by – often spurious – arguments about clinical effectiveness and choice. Yet, in reality, without additional resources, it often means depth being sacrificed for breadth, i.e. no more clinical time is available for patients and clinical activity is simply spread throughout the 24-hour cycle. This means fewer clinicians are rostered on at any one time, and those on duty are more likely to be limited to emergency assessments, with little time available for follow-up sessions and more proactive work.

Whichever model of service is in operation, however, the way in which the team works together will be essential to the quality of care provided to patients, particularly given that much of the clinical work is undertaken individually and there will be few opportunities for working together. Key components to team working in liaison psychiatry are:

- triaging referrals and then discussing them as a team before allocating to an individual clinician;
- having mechanisms for group and individual clinical supervision;
- conducting clinical reviews together;
- team training;
- adopting a problem-solving approach, based on openness, transparency in decision-making with a clear, agreed focus about the work of the team.

THE CLINICAL ROLE

Lipowski[17,19] described the essential role of the liaison psychiatry practitioner as working with:

1 the distressed and/or disturbed patient;
2 the crisis in the relationship with the doctors, nurses and others in the clinical team created by this disturbed behaviour;

3 the effects of those relationships on the patient. The clinician from the liaison service will try to assist both the patient and the team to resolve the crisis and any issues that arise out of it.

To these three elements can be added a fourth category, which is far more typical to British services. This is the specialist assessment, initial care and treatment of people with mental health emergencies and/or presenting with episodes of self-harm beyond the scope of practice of the A&E team.

Much of the core role and work of liaison mental health nurses (LMHNs) is similar to that of mental health nurses as a generic group. However, some key areas of practice are far more particular to the general hospital and its varied patient group. The expansion of the role of the LMHN into psychiatric assessment, risk management, capacity assessments and more complex areas of cognitive–behavioural treatments moves it a long way from a more traditional view of the work of a nurse.

In some respects, it is easier for medical staff to maintain clearer boundaries to their role. Royal College of Psychiatry guidelines describe the clinical work junior doctors should undertake when on a liaison psychiatry placement, while their work is also subject to strict guidelines about accommodation, interview rooms and clinical activity.[8,28] Nothing similar exists for nurses. There is also some logic to psychiatrists accepting referrals for medically complex cases or seeing patients for whom medication is likely to be the key treatment factor. A discrete, 'pure' nursing role is harder to define and develop. The issues arising from the direct, face-to-face consultation aspect of the role are contingent upon the context of the hospital and how relationships are developed.

Although ward or unit nursing staff are usually the most affected by Lipowski's so-called 'crisis in the relationship',[19] British LMHNs – unlike their American counterparts – rarely develop the liaison component which involves the clinician working with the relevant clinical team rather than seeing the patient.[29] This might involve providing supervision around the care and management of a patient presenting with challenging behaviours, breaking bad news or issues related to the care of a patient with a pre-existing mental illness. This is particularly relevant given the generalized anxiety and dysfunction experienced by nurses in the general hospital as a consequence of the tensions in working with the sick and dying.[30,31]

Reflection

What behaviours do you think of as challenging?

What response do you see from healthcare professionals towards people exhibiting challenging behaviours in your clinical area?

Personal illustration 53.1

Referral

Hazel is a 30-year-old woman on a haematology unit having difficulty in accepting her prescribed treatment. She is described as angry, tearful and lacking in motivation, often refusing to cooperate with nursing staff. She has threatened to discharge herself without completing her treatment.

Assessment

Hazel has a history of poor family relationships, particularly with her mother. Marrying young, she has a 5-year-old daughter but became depressed after the birth, separating from her husband a year later. She lived with her daughter in a small flat until she began to experience symptoms of acute myeloid leukaemia (AML). Her daughter is now staying with her mother, some distance from the hospital.

It emerges she was sexually abused as a child by a male friend of her mother and has been ruminating on past events while being nursed in isolation in order to minimize the risk of infection to Hazel. These feelings were brought into the 'here and now' by what she perceived as increasingly intrusive and unpleasant physical treatments and a sense that she had no control over her own body, treatment and care. Highly anxious, low in mood, not sleeping, Hazel has no appetite, finds it difficult to concentrate, and is unable to look forward to things, even her weekly visits from her daughter.

Treatment interventions

Hazel says she wants to get a sense of 'control'. An open-ended number of sessions are offered while she is an inpatient, with the aims of teaching her some relaxation techniques and helping her develop cognitive and behavioural strategies to adapt to her time on the ward, particularly being nursed and treated in isolation.

Within this framework, Hazel explains a range of experiences relating to her fear of a loss of control and issues related to her illness, treatment and prognosis. She also articulates her increasing fears of dying and losing her relationship with her child, which underpins her generalized anxiety. Able to challenge negative thoughts and adapt more to her illness and its effects, she feels calmer. Explaining to the nurses and medical staff something of Hazel's background, with her permission, allows them to understand her behaviour rather than see it as 'difficult' or 'irrational'. Adjusting their interventions, explaining when and why they have to do certain things and negotiating what can be changed alters the relationship between the clinical team and Hazel.

Discussion

Some form of differential diagnosis is perhaps more important in liaison psychiatry than in other spheres of nursing. For example, a person's apparent 'bizarre' behaviour may be due to psychosis, related to personality and/or situational issues or organic causes such as infection or brain injury, whereas low mood can have a variety of causes.

The nurse assessing someone with AML presenting with apparent biological changes has to take into account the progress of the disease as well as the effects of chemotherapy, possible steroid and any other pharmacological treatments before considering a depressive disorder.

Nonetheless, the detailed biographical history, knowing something of the individual, how he/she sees him or herself, coping mechanisms, psychological strengths, as well as all the other components of assessment, will be vxital in determining, with the person, what is happening and why, with psychosocial input likely to be at least as much value as any pharmacological intervention. Equally, having the knowledge and skills to develop a dynamic understanding of the patient's predicament and how that affects the interaction with the ward team, can further aid the LMHN's work with the patient by promoting a constructive, consistent and containing response from the team.

Reflection

What type of behaviours do you think patients might use to demonstrate their perception of having little or no control over their environment?

How do you think healthcare professionals respond to these behaviours?

ASSESSMENT

This forms the main bulk of the work in liaison psychiatry, as most hospital patients will only require short-term interventions and patients attending the A&E department who require longer term treatment and care will be referred onto CMHTs.

Barker has identified that assessment should have four overall objectives:

1 measurement – gaining information on the scale or size of a problem;
2 clarification – understanding the context or conditions of the problem;
3 explanation – exploring the possible cause, purpose or function of the problem;
4 variation – explores how the problem varies over time, its seriousness and how it affects the individual.[32]

However, if a nurse is the only clinician to see the patient, there is usually an implicit expectation that the more formal elements of a 'psychiatric assessment' will be included, most particularly the mental state examination (MSE). This involves a series of linear questions aimed at eliciting changes in the individual's cognitions, perceptions and affect, for example, intrusive negative thoughts, auditory hallucinations, diurnal variation of mood, etc. that would indicate or exclude symptoms of a

mental disorder as defined by either the DSM-IV[33] or ICD-10.[34] As nurses are not educated in conducting MSEs during their preregistration training they are often reliant on learning this from psychiatrists either in the form of supervision and observation or more formalized teaching.

It requires considerable skill, confidence and experience to use a philosophical and clinical approach that attributes distress and disturbance to a more complex process than biological changes and alterations to an individual's mental state, yet still assess the latter in the process.

WORKING WITH PEOPLE WHO SELF-HARM

Assessing and working with people who have presented following an episode of self-harm remains one of the principle aspects of the LMHN's work. Jeffrey identified that A&E department patients were classified as 'good' and 'bad', or 'interesting' and 'rubbish', with patients who had presented following a self-harm or suicide attempt being classified as 'the normal rubbish'.[35] 'Interesting' or 'good' patients would have a more unusual medical presentation that, in addition, would be beneficial to medical staff in developing knowledge and practice skills helpful in passing exams. The negative response of staff to 'bad' and 'rubbish' patients noted by Jeffrey was explored further by Roberts[36] and Hemmings,[37] who attributed these attitudes to the high levels of anxiety such patients arouse in A&E nurses. However, this can be addressed through educational programmes aimed at helping A&E department nurses be more self-aware, have a better understanding about mental health issues and the reasons for particular patient presentations, knowing where their own role begins and ends and improving communication skills.[37]

Reflection

What attitudes do you hear reflected by healthcare staff about people who self harm?

How do you think this affects their treatment and care?

Although there is insufficient evidence to recommend a specific clinical intervention after self-harm, limited ongoing engagement, with the intention of providing brief psychological interventions and problem-solving, can be effective in reducing both suicidal ideation and further episodes of self-harm.[38,39] It is also key for services trying to meet the national targets set for the reduction of suicide rates[26] as well as meet the objectives set out in the *Essence of care*.[40]

Personal illustration 53.2

Referral

Steve is 42 years old. He was brought to the local A&E department having ingested approximately 18 paracetamol tablets while intoxicated, but vomited the tablets. His sister called an ambulance after calling unexpectedly at his flat and finding him unwell. She informed the A&E Department staff that he had been drinking heavily for several months and feeling 'very low'. Steve has had a triage assessment and been referred directly by the triage nurse, who has identified him as being at high risk of further self-harm.

Assessment

Steve had lost his job 6 months previously and not worked since. Financially dependent on his girlfriend, this had placed more strain on an already problematic relationship. As he was drinking more heavily, his girlfriend ended the relationship. Denying any suicidal ideation, he says he took the tablets impulsively, 'wishing to go to sleep for a while' to 'get away' from his 'miserable feelings', but acknowledges he feels hopeless about his future. He also says he sometimes has vague ideas that people are watching him, think he's a loser and know he is 'inadequate'.

A full biographical history is taken. Academically bright, he dropped out of university, feeling he 'didn't fit in'. He hints at difficulties at key maturational developmental points, saying he has always found relationships 'hard work' as an adult. His girlfriend leaving him, coupled with his financial difficulties, was the 'last straw.' He says he was depressed several years previously but recovered without any treatment.

Distinguishing whether or not this was a suicidal attempt or episode of self-harm is crucial. There are concerns that, despite his view that he took the tablets impulsively, there was an element of planning, in that he had purchased the tablets that day and took them not expecting anyone to come to the house. Moreover, his gender, age, financial status, being unemployed, recently separated, drinking heavily, social isolation and hopelessness are high clinical risk indicators. He is assessed as being a high suicide risk, particularly if he continues to drink.

Treatment

Offered a follow-up appointment for the next day, Steve doesn't want to visit a CMHT but agrees to meet for six sessions. He opts for a solution-focused approach, setting his initial goals as reducing his drinking, rebuilding his confidence and keeping himself safe.

Discussion

With clear benefits to providing interventions for patients who present with self-harm and/or suicide attempts,[38,39] this is a key element of the work of the LHMN. Working with A&E staff who have been provided with mental health training by the liaison team builds both mutual confidence and a shared understanding of each other's work. Using an agreed mental health screening tool[41] to conduct a brief mental health assessment, enables the triage nurse to categorize risk as low, medium, high or very high and refer direct from triage, thus substantially cutting the waiting time for the patient and reducing the problems about patients having to repeat their story several times over.

THE ADVANCED NURSING ROLE IN THE GENERAL HOSPITAL

Although the parameters of nursing might be expanding, the actual role of many nurses working in services such as liaison psychiatry could be argued to be narrowing. Taking on new, specific tasks means abandoning at least some elements of the emphasis on the 'holism of patient health promotion, maintenance and restoration',[42] as well as nurturing any continuing relationship with the patient that would underpin it. Once integral elements that supported nursing practice, such as the writing of care plans, objective setting and defined nursing interventions, have had to be adapted. Nor are the nurse's interventions necessarily documented in the nursing notes. Referrals might be made by doctors or nurses, but, despite this, a LMHN will almost always record their assessment and/or interventions in the medical notes, and often using a medical framework.

However, although the medical model as an ideological construct may have been created by the medical profession and predicated on the supremacy of the psychiatrist, it became a system of treatment and care adhered to by whole multidisciplinary teams, who were also accepting a view of mental illness as being a result of certain biological changes creating a variety of symptoms that can be classified and codified into a medical diagnosis,[43] albeit one that is actually based on little more than observation and subjective judgements.

This is exacerbated by the complexity the work in the general hospital setting poses. Clinical presentations can have a variety of causes and consulting with doctors and/or discussion with the referring clinician is an essential part of assessment and overall clinical practice. Although psychiatrists will be able to draw upon their own medical training and education and feel comfortable doing this, nurses can be perceived – and may perceive themselves – as 'seeking advice' in such situations, thus perpetuating a subordinated role. Equally, because of the short-term nature of the clinical work with many patients in the general hospital, the pressure to produce rapid change can create an even greater reliance on pharmacology rather than problem-solving or psychosocial interventions, which again emphasizes a particular philosophical view and skills' set, different to that of mental health nursing and its core values, leaving LMHNs potentially further adrift from the stated aims and ambitions of their wider peer group, even if they are able to prescribe in their own right.

Nonetheless, the 'medical model' cannot be said to be a static, functional approach. Although a psychiatrist's traditional assessment would try to seek symptoms and phenomena, in many cases there has been a gradual shift within their paradigm and practice towards the nurses' focus on a biopsychosocial model, both in assessment and treatment, paying particular attention to interpersonal issues as much as psychiatric symptoms.

The most common reason for referrals to liaison psychiatry services from wards is when doctors cannot be definitive about diagnosis.[44] Uncertainty about the reason for the referral and what it is the referrer is seeking from the liaison psychiatry services is inevitably problematic and can be the cause of the referral being rejected. However, while describing how to make an effective referral and the need to consider referrals carefully, Harrison[22] has argued that liaison psychiatry practitioners should be willing to maintain a low threshold for referral in terms of detail and a clear expression of what is required precisely because of the difficulties the referring team may have in clarifying these issues without initial recourse to specialist help.

Indeed, there is an argument that a liaison clinician provides 'added value' for referrers by taking a 'step back' from the inadequacies of a referral and helping the referrer think about why they had not gathered the necessary information or been clear in their mind about the problem to which a solution is being sought. This might be designed to assist in helping them work out how the patient's mental health problems are impacting on attempts to treat and care for their primary physical illness, about how this is affecting the clinicians themselves, or how it might have led to a less than full referral.

Reflection

Managing one's own anxiety is a key skill for psychiatric nurses. What leads to you feeling anxious in relation to your own clinical work and how do you manage it?

SKILLS NEEDED

As stated above, core components of liaison mental health nursing include:

- a range of assessments;
- risk management;
- consultation, education and advice;
- a range of short-term treatments;
- administration, documentation and management;
- audit and research.[45]

The broad range of skills required to deliver these is summarized in Box 53.3.

Box 53.3: Skills needed by nurses working in a liaison psychiatry service

- Excellent communication skills, both oral and written.
- The ability to gather data and information from available sources and put it to therapeutic use.
- Being able to create as safe and confidential an environment as possible, even in the difficult circumstances of a busy, noisy, hospital ward.
- Establishing a rapport and collaborative relationship with the patient within a short space of time, specific to the task and to facilitate the function of assessment and treatment.
- Carrying out a variety of assessments, where a singular approach is both unhelpful and inappropriate.
- Developing a formulation about the presenting problem in a biographical context, identifying risk and unmet needs either in collaboration with, or incorporating the patient's own perspective.
- Adopting either a solution-focused or problem-solving approach to managing risk.
- Being able to take an eclectic but evidence-based approach, wherever possible, to treatment, identifying a clear rationale for actions taken.

Given the short-term nature of the work, terminating contact in a healthy and helpful way is both difficult but important. This involves liaising with other healthcare staff, as well as carers, and making referrals to specialist agencies where necessary, while involving the patient in all decisions about their care.

Gradual role blurring, as well as a greater reliance on advanced nursing knowledge and skills – sometimes in areas unfamiliar to nurses – means there has been a need to identify core competencies or capabilities. Although this has not been done at a national level and there is no advanced qualification as a LMHN, more recently, groups such as the London Liaison Mental Health Nurses' Group, and nurses at the Avon & Wiltshire NHS Trust, have designed and developed competency frameworks,[46] assessment tools,[41] educational packages and integrated care pathways, all aimed at helping define and develop the nursing role. In part, this has led to LMHNs being recognized as 'highly specialist nurses', in some NHS Trusts under the new pay system, *Agenda for change*.

SUMMARY

Nurses working within liaison psychiatric services have developed an advanced role in the last 15 years. Yet, while UK nurses have followed much of the clinical practice of their American counterparts, they lack the academic framework to their work and, consequently, much of their status and independence. This has crucially affected their direction and, to a degree, the clinical content of their work. The nursing role still stands within the shadow of the psychiatrist but has also influenced it in more recent years so that both roles could be said to have been blurred by their close relationship.

Contradictions and tensions remain as nurses try to preserve the key principles of holistic practice with the more specific and technical demands of the service but its importance is underlined by the identified needs of the general hospital population. As work is done to identify and develop the core competencies, skills and knowledge required for the role, liaison mental health nursing stands at the forefront of clinical practice, facilitating both innovation and, to a degree, the more 'traditional' nursing values of holism, as well as a patient-, and health-centred, focus.

Reflection

* How are nurses prepared for the clinical role expected in a liaison psychiatry service?
* What is the tension between advanced practice and adopting a holistic approach to patient care?
* What is the clinical and organizational impact of role blurring between nursing and psychiatry?

REFERENCES

1. Goddard HA. *The work of nurses in hospital wards* (*The Horder Report*). London, UK: Nuffield Provincial Hospitals Trust, 1953.

2. White R. *The effects of the NHS on the nursing profession 1948–1961*. London, UK: King's Fund, 1985.

3. Hart C, Williams L. The provision of holistic care. In: Harrison A, Hart C (eds). *Mental health care for nurses: applying mental health skills in the general hospital*. Oxford, UK: Blackwell, 2006.

4. Department of Health. *From values to action: the chief nursing officer's review of mental health nursing*. London, UK: DoH, 2006.

5. Turp M. *Psychosomatic health*. Basingstoke, UK: Palgrave Macmillan, 2001.

6. Peplau HE. Professional closeness. *Nursing Forum* 1969; **8** (4): 342–60.

7. Benjamin S, House A, Jenkins P (eds). *Liaison psychiatry: defining needs and planning services*. London, UK: Gaskell, 1994.

8. Royal College of Physicians and Psychiatrists. *The psychological care of medical patients: recognition of need and service provision*. London, UK: The Royal College of Physicians Publication Unit, 1995.

9. Storer A. The accident and emergency department. In: Peveler R, Feldman E, Friedman T (eds). *Liaison psychiatry: planning services for specialist settings*. London, UK: Gaskell, 2000.

10. Richardson C. Self-harm: understanding the causes and treatment options. *Nursing Times* 2004; **100** (15): 24–5.

11. Robinson R, Bolla-Wilson K, Kaplan E *et al*. Depression influences intellectual impairment in stroke patients. *British Journal of Psychiatry* 1986; **148**: 541–7.

12. Morriss RK. Physical illness and depressive disorders. *Opinion in general and elderly medicine*, 1999: 8–12.

13. Mayou RA, Gill D, Thompson DR *et al*. Depression and anxiety as predictors of outcome after myocardial infarction. *Psychosomatic Medicine* 2000; **62**: 212–19.

14. Maguire P, Haddad P. Psychological reactions in to physical illness. In: Guthrie E, Creed F (eds). *Seminars in liaison psychiatry*. London, UK: Royal College of Psychiatrists and Gaskell, 1996.

15. Robinson L. Psychiatric consultation liaison nursing and psychiatric nursing doctoring: similarities and differences. *Archives of Psychiatric Nursing* 1987; **1** (2): 73–80.

16. Egan-Morriss E, Morriss R, House A *et al*. The role of the nurse in consultation-liaison psychiatry. *In:* Benjamin S, House A, Jenkins P (eds). *Liaison psychiatry: defining needs and planning services*. London, UK: Gaskell, 1994.

17. Lipowski Z. Review of consultation psychiatry and psychosomatic medicine. *Psychosomatic Medicine* 1967; **29**: 1–3.

18. Minarek PA, Neese JB. Essential educational content for advanced practice in psychiatric consultation-liaison nursing. *Archives of Psychiatric Nursing* 2002; **16** (1): 3–15.

19. Lipowski Z. Liaison psychiatry, liaison nursing and behavioural medicine. *Comprehensive Psychiatry* 1981; **22**: 554–61.

20. Morriss R, Mayou R. International overview of consultation-liaison psychiatry. In: Guthrie E, Creed F (eds). *Seminars in liaison psychiatry*. London, UK: Gaskell, 1996.

21. Department of Health. *Working in partnership. The report of the mental health nursing review team*. London, UK: HMSO, 1994.

22. Harrison A. Mental health liaison team. In: Harrison A, Hart C (eds). *Mental health care for nurses: applying mental health skills in the general hospital*. Oxford, UK: Blackwell, 2006.

23. Department of Health. *Saving lives: our healthier nation*. London, UK: HMSO, 1999.

24. Department of Health. *The national service framework for mental health*. London, UK: HMSO, 1999.

25. Department of Health. *Making it happen: a guide to delivering mental health promotion*. London, UK: HMSO, 2001.

26. Department of Health. *National suicide prevention strategy for England: annual report on progress*. London, UK: DoH, 2002.

27. Harrison A, Hart C (eds). *Mental health care for nurses: applying mental health skills in the general hospital*. Oxford, UK: Blackwell, 2006.

28. Royal College of Psychiatrists. *Psychiatric services to accident and emergency departments* (*Council Report 43*). London, UK: The Royal College of Physicians Publication Unit, 1996.

29. Brendon S, Reet M. Establishing a mental health liaison nurse service: lessons for the future. *Nursing Standard* 2000; **14** (17): 43–7.

30. Menzies IEP. *The functioning of social systems as a defence against anxiety*. London, UK: Tavistock, 1970.

31. Hart C. *Nurses and politics*. Basingstoke, UK: Palgrave Macmillan, 2004.

32. Barker P. *Assessment in psychiatric and mental health nursing: in search of the whole person*. Cheltenham, UK: Stanley Thornes, 1997.

33. American Psychiatric Association. *Diagnostic and statistical manual of mental disorders*, 3rd edn, revised. Washington, DC: APA, 1987.

34. World Health Organization. *Mental disorders: glossary and guide to their classification in accordance with the Ninth Revision of the International Classification of Diseases*. Geneva, Switzerland: WHO, 1978.

35. Jeffrey R. Normal rubbish: deviant patients in casualty departments. *Sociology of Health and Illness* 1979; **1** (1): 90–108.

36. Roberts D. Suicide prevention by general nurses. *Nursing Standard* 1996; **10** (7): 30–3.

37. Hemmings A. Attitudes to deliberate self-harm among staff in an accident and emergency team. *Mental Health Care* 1999; **2** (9): 300–2.

38. Hart C. *Nurses assessing risk in the emergency department*. 20th Annual Conference of the American Psychiatric Nurses Association, Orlando, FL, 2007.

39. Guthrie E, Kapur N, Mackway-Jones K *et al.* Randomised controlled trial of brief psychological intervention after deliberate self poisoning., *British Medical Journal* 2001; **323**: 135–7.

40. Department of Health. *The essence of care: patient-focused benchmarking for healthcare practitioners*. London, UK: HMSO, 2001.

41. National Institute for Clinical Excellence. *Self-harm, the short term physical and psychological management of and secondary prevention of self harm in primary and secondary care*: London, UK: NICE, 2004.

42. Hart C, Harrison A, Colley R. *Risk assessment matrix*. London, UK: St George's Hospital, 2004.

43. Royle JA, Walsh M. *Watson's medical surgical nursing and related physiology*, 4th edn. London, UK: Baillière Tindall, 1992.

44. Rogers A, Pilgrim D. *Mental health in Britain: a critical introduction*. Basingstoke, UK: Macmillan, 1996.

45. Gomez J. *Liaison psychiatry, mental health problems in the general hospital*. London, UK: Croon-Helm, 1987.

46. Hart C, Eales S (eds). *A competence framework for liaison mental health nursing*. London, UK: London Liaison Mental Health Nurses Special Interest Forum, 2004.

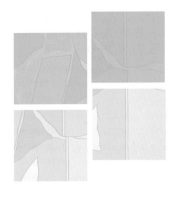

CHAPTER 54

Services for people requiring secure forms of care: a global problem

Colin Holmes*

INTRODUCTION

This chapter provides an overview of services available for people receiving psychiatric care in secure settings, principally those representing a significant danger to themselves or others, or who are detained in connection with an offence in law. The focus is on the services rather than on the roles of nurses and other health professionals, although I note some of the key challenges facing those who work in such settings. The organization and management of services differ greatly between jurisdictions, and the chapter focuses mainly on the UK, since it is well represented in published literature and provides well-documented illustrations. To understand secure psychiatric services, and the problems they face, it is important to understand how they evolved.

HISTORICAL CONTEXT

The beginnings of secure provision

In the early nineteenth century, when institutional care for 'lunatics' started to become widespread across Europe,

North America and the British colonies, almost all facilities were 'secure'. Wards or blocks were locked, patients were monitored and escorted at all times, the whole complex was surrounded by high walls, and entry and exit were through a single imposing 'main gate' controlled by the gatekeeper. The asylum therefore typically constituted an appropriate destination for people who had committed minor offences and were found to be insane. From the very beginning, most asylums had a number of 'criminal lunatics', and acquired special facilities to accommodate patients detained under criminal or lunacy legislation.

Special verdicts and/or sentencing arrangements had long existed in Europe, and evidence that courts recognized the diminished responsibility of some people with mental disorders appears in the earliest Greek literature and the works of Aristotle and Plato. Legislation in respect of lunatics appeared in Britain in 1800, when the Criminal Lunatics Act enabled courts to detain 'at His Majesty's Pleasure' persons found to be 'insane on arraignment', that is at the time they appear in court. The courtroom was an important, highly public site for testing and legitimating the emerging psychiatric expertise and, not surprisingly, the medical superintendents of European and North American asylums led the ground-breaking

*Colin Holmes is Professor at James Cook University, Townsville, Australia. Previously he was Professor of Mental Health Nursing at the University of Western Sydney, Sydney, Australia.

debates about the legal implications of insanity. The case which set the standard for determinations of insanity in homicide cases was that of Daniel McNaughtan (there is much dispute over the correct spelling of this name), who attempted to shoot the British prime minister in 1843, but missed and killed his secretary. McNaughtan was found to be insane, and out of his trial came a principle, 'the McNaghtan Rules', based on the ability to distinguish right from wrong. The case been explored in great depth by Moran.[1] This led to the development of the 'Not Guilty by Reason of Insanity' verdict, temporarily replaced in 1883 by the Trial of Lunatics Act, which enabled courts to return a verdict of 'Guilty But Insane'.

In Scotland, 'diminished responsibility' because of mental disorder, although rarely used, has been a defence to murder since at least the eighteenth century, reaffirmed in the case of *R.* v *Dingwall* in 1867, and upheld again in *Galbraith* v *HMA* (Her Majesty's Advocate) in 2004. It was not until the Homicide Act of 1957 that it was introduced into English law, which nevertheless continued to resist the notion of a defence based on 'irresistible impulse', long accepted in most other European countries. In the United States, a strict application of the M'Naghten Rules has tended to prevail in most states, despite the formulation of modern alternatives, notably the 'Durham Rules' of 1954. There are several detailed histories of the insanity defence and its evolution.[2–4]

Alongside the development of the legal basis for special consideration of mentally disordered offenders have developed options for disposal, and of associated services. The first asylums catering primarily for criminal lunatics were those built in Australia, settled as a penal colony for the UKs most undesirable and dangerous offenders. There is some evidence that transportation to Australia was more likely if the offender exhibited signs of 'degeneracy', such as madness, drunkenness or sexual perversion but the deprivations of the journey to Australia undermined the mental and physical health of even the fittest transportees. There was, therefore, a high level of lunacy among the convicts arriving in the colony, and most of the patients of the colony's early asylums were convicts. They were subject to especially harsh and neglectful treatment since they were considered to be especially dangerous. Australia's first psychiatric facility, Castle Hill Asylum in Sydney, New South Wales, opened in 1811 for 30 patients, with medical services provided by Dr William Bland, who was himself serving a sentence for causing death by duelling. Much of the direct care was provided by the most troublesome convicts as a form of punishment, a practice not officially abandoned until late in the century. In Tasmania, the site of Australia's second penal colony, facilities likewise initially catered for the convict population, with New Norfolk Asylum taking its first lunatic convict patient in 1829. Interestingly, the medical officer at New Norfolk at this time was Dr John Meyer, who later became Medical Superintendent at Broadmoor Criminal Lunatic Asylum in England. By the 1850s, New Norfolk was notorious for its use of electric shocks, blistering, cold showers and emetics, both to treat and punish its patients: it was Tasmania's last institutional psychiatric facility, closing in February 2001.

Thus, although not the first to provide separate facilities, Australian asylums were among the first to cater primarily for mentally ill offenders, and as the proportion of colonists increased in relation to convicts, it became important to distinguish between the criminal insane, insane convicts and the general insane, and to resolve questions as to where they should be cared for and under whose authority. This prompted the establishment of some designated facilities for criminal and convict lunatics, but these distinctions and the need for separate facilities have remained contentious.[5,6]

The first separate facility for criminal lunatics anywhere in the world appears to have been Dundrum Criminal Lunatic Asylum, near Dublin, Ireland, which opened in 1850 at the urging of Lord Chancellor Sugden. Today, Dundrum offers a national forensic service to the Republic of Ireland. Its more famous English equivalent, Broadmoor Criminal Lunatic Asylum, was not opened until 1863, but was much larger and by 1882 had some 500 patients. Until 1949 it was under the jurisdiction of the Home Office, which administered Britain's prisons, and then became part of the National Health Service. In Scotland, both male and female criminal lunatics were housed in a special wing of Perth Prison from 1865, and no other special facilities appear to have been developed until the opening of Carstairs State Hospital in 1957, when patients were transferred from Perth Gaol.[7]

In Canada, Rookwood Asylum in Kingston, Ontario, was built by convicts and opened specifically for criminal lunatics in 1856. It was part of the penitentiary system until 1877, when its name was changed to Kingston Asylum for the Insane. The first American facility specifically for the criminal insane appears to have been the New York State Asylum for Insane Convicts at Auburn, New York, which opened in 1859, initially for 80 patients. In 1891 it moved to new, larger premises, known as the Matteawan State Hospital, but this also became overcrowded and in 1900 another facility was opened, the Dannemora State Hospital. Although the history of psychiatry is a massive scholarly industry, little attention has been paid to the history of forensic psychiatry, and there are almost no published resources devoted specifically to the history of day-to-day care.

The lessons and legacy of history

The origins of secure services for mentally ill people in the English-speaking world are emblematic of a time when secure services were the norm. Although 'secure' or 'forensic services' are today reserved for a very special and challenging group of patients, they continue to reflect these origins, and many of the issues and dilemmas faced in the nineteenth century still face us today. The early Australian lunacy services, for example, immediately faced the question of whether separate provision should be made for the criminal insane and the convict insane, i.e. those found to be insane *prior* to sentencing, and those who *become insane* while serving a sentence, and whether this provision should be separate from that for the civil insane. This entailed the question of who should have responsibility for these various services, and where they should be located. Many colonial authorities felt that the convict insane should remain the responsibility of the prison department and cared for in prison, while the criminal insane should be the responsibility of the health department and cared for in asylums. The less popular view was that all insane persons, of whatever origin or status, should be cared for in the health system. This view was championed by many who worked in the prison system and saw psychologically disturbed prisoners as disruptive, dangerous or vulnerable, and a negative influence on other prisoners and the smooth running of the prison. An outspoken supporter of this approach was William Neitenstein, the head of the New South Wales prison department at the turn of the century, who argued as early as the 1880s that sex offenders should be located in asylums rather than in prisons, so that they could receive appropriate treatment. In practice, services in Australia, and most countries, developed in an 'ad hoc' fashion, subject to the preferences and interests of successive political, medical and other authorities, and were a victim of their generally negative and neglectful approach to both offenders and the mentally ill. As a result, some services have remained prison based, some are exclusively based in the health system and yet others are located within prison facilities but serviced by health system personnel. In Britain, the question of who provides health services to prisoners was carefully reconsidered in 2000–2001, in the light of scandalous conditions and unacceptable standards; in 2000 it was decided they would be handed over in their entirety to the Department of Health, and this took place in April 2006.

Associated with these questions about the location of, and responsibility for, services for mentally ill offenders, have been difficulties with legislation, which has generally failed to keep track of advances in the understanding and treatment of people with mental illnesses, with increased understanding of offender behaviour, and with developments in penological thinking and practice. This continues to create difficulties for today's forensic psychiatric services, and now involve the added problem of how legislation can facilitate rather than inhibit continuity of care in the community, and enable professionals to operate effectively in and across a variety of services and settings.

Another group of questions that arose in the early days of the asylum system concerned the appropriate level of security for different types of patient, and how the special precautions necessary for dangerous criminal and convict patients could be reconciled to the therapeutic aspirations of the asylum and to the comparatively less intrusive security needs of other patients. In recent times, the relationship between therapy and security, or care and custody, persists as a practical and psychological problem facing those who plan, manage and provide care, and has been debated almost ad nauseam. As discussed below, the issue of varying levels of security is also raised today in response to the expectation that each patient will receive individualized care appropriate to their particular needs.

The historical record is also relevant because early lay and professional discussions concerning this group of patients used evaluative language expressive of attitudes which would today be widely considered discriminatory, demeaning and politically incorrect, but which was entirely acceptable in its day. This highlights several continuing but neglected problems.

1 It testifies to the fact that the patients concerned are, indeed, sometimes extremely obnoxious or morally repulsive, and that relating to them therapeutically, might be problematic.
2 It raises the problem as to the relationship between 'madness' and 'badness', how these are conceived, and how society should respond when they are met in the same individual.[8]
3 It illustrates the problem of public and political negativity toward mentally ill offenders, who are still liable to be seen principally as criminals, for whom punitive, prison-like conditions are appropriate; most obviously, this means that care has long been expected to be delivered in facilities built a century or more ago, when such attitudes were the norm, and this has significantly undermined efforts to create therapeutic environments with graduated levels of security, and to reintegrate patients back into the community.
4 Finally, the early history is important because it rehearsed the difficult question as to the extent to which criminal behaviours are, of themselves, legitimate targets of professional psychiatric intervention, and Neitenstein's call for the removal of sex offenders to asylums is a case in point. Furthermore, during the early part of the nineteenth century, protracted disputes occurred concerning the extent to which evidence presented by psychiatrists, or 'alienists', regarding a person's actions should be taken into account in determining questions of guilt and sentencing. In fact, the courts tended to prefer 'commonsense' explanations of defendants' behaviour, and of their level of culpability, and it took many years for medicine to establish authority in presenting such evidence. These disputes also revealed

the ways in which the two powerful discourses of law and medicine interact in the highly charged context of the courtroom, exposing the limitations of psychiatric explanation and evoking fears that it seeks to undermine the pursuit of justice. Precisely these phenomena still operate today whenever psychiatry is transported into the courtroom, and its authority continues to be challenged from a range of public and professional sources.[9–12]

Reflection

How are mentally disordered offenders represented in the popular media, such as films, television programmes and newspapers?

In what ways do the attitudes and assumptions they display reflect the history of forensic psychiatry and the problems of determining the effect of mental disorder on guilt?

TERMINOLOGY

The terminology which characterizes the discourses of forensic and secure psychiatric care can be confusing. It is inconsistent between jurisdictions and disciplines, and has its origins in the development of psychiatry as a medical specialty. A simple strategy to help medicine establish its authority in relation to lunacy during the early nineteenth century, particularly in the courtroom, was to develop a technical discourse, with a plethora of obscure terms, the aim being to give the appearance of precision and certainty as to the nature of the problem, and to exclude and confuse those outside the profession. This discourse was initially chaotic and haphazard, with each 'alienist' preferring his own particular descriptive terms, but the level of standardization gradually increased, even though competing theories and diagnostic systems persisted, and today forensic psychiatry mostly employs the terminology of the *Diagnostic and statistical manual of the American Psychiatric Association* (DSM-IV-R). It also uses many terms and phrases that are rarely encountered elsewhere, or which have unclear or special meanings. For their part, nurses need to understand terminology that has developed in three contexts – organizational, clinical and legal – and it is important to be clear about the basic terms.

Forensic – has its origins in the Latin word meaning 'forum', that is a court or debating chamber. Except in classical studies, where it is still used to refer to such forums, it now means 'relating to courts of law'.

Forensic patient is widely used to distinguish patients coming under the jurisdiction of forensic services from other service users, and usually refers to patients who have come into conflict with the law and require psychiatric care while serving their sentence, or are subject to the jurisdiction of a court and require care in a secure setting in virtue of the danger they pose to themselves or others. The term should be used with caution because not all facilities providing forensic services restrict their clientele to such individuals, and neither are such individuals or the services that care for them always designated as 'forensic'. When they are in transitional accommodation prior to, or are living in the community following, discharge from a health facility, or are serving a non-custodial sentence, or no longer serving a custodial sentence, they may be absorbed into the caseloads of non-forensic services. The State of New South Wales, Australia, is perhaps unique in defining the term in law.

Forensic psychiatry – that form of psychiatry relating to courts of law. Since law has civil and criminal aspects, the term can be used to refer to involvement in civil cases, such as the provision of expert opinion in divorce and child custody proceedings, insurance and damages cases, employment law, challenges to wills, and the regulation of professions: this usage is common in the United States. In other countries it is generally reserved for psychiatry applied to criminal cases. Nevertheless, it is rare in practice for forensic psychiatric services to be reserved exclusively for people who have appeared in a court of law. Most services assume a much wider range of responsibilities, notably in assessing, advising on, and sometimes managing, patients who present with especially challenging or dangerous behaviours, either transiently or chronically; and, the policies of many forensic units allow for such individuals to be admitted as local needs dictate.

Forensic psychiatrist usually refers to a psychiatrist who works with forensic patients, although it guarantees no specialist qualifications and its use is a matter of custom and practice. Specialist training is available to psychiatrists in some countries, but is not mandatory.

Forensic psychologist may refer to a psychologist who provides a service to clients who have come into conflict with the law, specializes in the psychology of the courtroom and the justice process, or provides expert testimony in the courtroom. Specialist training is widely available at postgraduate level and the term is increasingly protected by professional organizations that, in Australia and the United States, have significant forensic sections.

Forensic nursing should be used to refer to all forms of nursing provided as part of forensic health or correctional services, although job descriptions do not generally include the word 'forensic'. Appropriate post-registration courses for nurses have become available during the last decade, but its use still tends to characterize the setting in which forensic nurses work, rather than their qualifications. In North America, the term is used almost exclusively to refer to the care of victims of crime, especially victims of sexual assault. However, it is gradually being extended to include nursing care of victims of a wide range of traumas, including natural and man-made disasters, terrorist violence and domestic abuse. Elsewhere, however, the offender is the focus of forensic nursing, and engagement with victims, or even offenders' significant others, is unusual. Specialty areas within American forensic nursing include forensic clinical nurse specialist, forensic nurse investigator, nurse coroner or death investigator, sexual assault nurse examiner, legal nurse consultant, forensic gerontology specialist, correctional nursing specialist and forensic psychiatric nurse. Outside North America, forensic nursing is widely distinguished from forensic psychiatric–mental health nursing, which is regarded as a specialty in its own right and not a specialty within forensic nursing. These kinds of distinctions reflect the ways in which education and registration of nurses takes place in each jurisdiction. Major texts on 'forensic nursing' have appeared in recent years.[13–15]

Forensic mental health nursing, or *forensic psychiatric nursing*, should be reserved for the forensic branch of mental health or psychiatric nursing. It is widely thought to be important to make a distinction between forensic and non-forensic roles, and to identify the distinctive skills and expectations of those working in forensic settings.[16–21] An extensive study of nursing in secure environments conducted by the Faculty of Health, University of Central Lancashire, on behalf of the United Kingdom Central Council for Nursing, Midwifery and Health Care[22] suggested the roles and competencies of the forensic mental health nurse. The former Scottish National Board produced extensive documents on the enhancement of the role,[23] but the Scottish Prison Service has since adopted a detailed generic statement of competencies for all nurses working in prisons.[24] The case for a separate identity for forensic psychiatric nurses appears at least as strong as that for other specialties within nursing, and a recent literature review confirms a number of enduring distinctive features.[25] Most obviously, the client group comprises primarily forensic patients and, whether in an institutional or community setting, the problems being managed are significantly linked to criminal offending, unlike those normally faced by non-forensic mental health nurses. A flood of high-quality texts, addressing forensic psychiatric nursing issues, appeared around 1999–2001,[26–32] but this has reduced to a trickle.[33,34] Whereas texts on 'forensic nursing' are North American, all these books originate in the UK.

Corrections nursing is a term used in the United States and Australasia to refer to all forms of nursing provided within the prison system. Such services may be the responsibility of the health system, the penal system, or a mixture of both. *Prison nursing* is the equivalent term in the United Kingdom, Ireland and Canada. However, since correctional services are increasingly extending care to settings other than prison facilities, including a variety of periodic detention centres, and the community, the term 'prison nursing' could be viewed as a specialty within corrections nursing.

Reflection

What titles are used to refer to nurses who work in secure psychiatric facilities where you live?

How do they differ in different work settings, and how does this usage relate to the organization of services?

Mentally ill offender, although most obviously referring to a mentally ill person convicted of an offence, is sometimes defined in criminal legislation, each statute wording the definition in slightly different ways. In some contexts, it refers to those people once called 'criminal lunatics', that is people found to be mentally ill prior to sentencing, but in others it includes the 'convict insane', that is those found to be mentally ill whilst serving a custodial sentence. 'Mental illness' for these purposes is usually taken to be as defined in civil legislation, notably Mental Health Acts, though not all such Acts refer to 'mental illness', preferring other terminology. The phrase is problematized by the *Diagnostic and statistical manual of the American Psychiatric Association*, since this abandons the term 'mental illness' completely, in favour of 'mental disorder'. In any case, it should not be used to describe all people who use forensic services, because many of these people are not convicted offenders, but may have been remanded for pre-trial assessment. Furthermore, forensic services frequently include services to people who have just been taken into custody and are being assessed at a police station, prior to any court appearance; and, in some places, the clientele includes non-forensic patients for whom appropriate secure provision is otherwise unavailable.

Mentally disordered offenders is a term used in some jurisdictions where the distinction between 'mental illness' and 'mental disorder' is incorporated into civil or criminal legislation. It often includes people who have a psychological problem not amounting to a mental illness, such as may arise as a result of post-traumatic brain damage, intellectual disability, or transient drug-induced organic states. In some countries, such as Britain, forensic psychiatric services for those suffering from personality disorder, or a sexual abnormality, are made available through the health system, whilst in others, such as Australia, they are provided, if at all, exclusively within the penal system.

Court liaison nurse/officer (mental health court support worker) refers to a nurse who conducts psychiatric assessments of defendants, presents their findings in court, and makes recommendations as to the appropriate disposal of defendants.[35,36] Despite the demonstrated effectiveness of these roles as part of the diversion of mentally disordered offenders from prison, they are reported to be in decline.[37]

Forensic terminology is developing as services expand, new roles emerge and the language of professionals become more precise, and the short descriptions given above should be regarded only as a starting point. Although tending to concentrate on forensic environments, this chapter is intended to be relevant to all situations in which care is provided in secure conditions.

Types of secure provision

There are a number of ways of organizing or distinguishing secure psychiatric services. They may be multifunctional and organized around geographic areas, areas of population or legal jurisdictions; they may be distinguished according to clinical speciality, or the characteristics of the clientele (e.g. age, gender, source of admission), or according to their size or the organizational system that runs them (e.g. health, correctional, independent). In Australia, mental health and relevant criminal legislation is state and territory based, and services are thus organized at state level. There is no formal system distinguishing types of facility or levels of security, and services have developed in a largely ad hoc fashion around population centres. In the UK, services are distinguished according to the level of security they are supposed to provide, namely high, medium and low, and these are briefly described.

High secure

High secure services in England and Wales are provided by the National Health Service and comprise three hospitals, Ashworth, Broadmoor and Rampton, previously called 'Special Hospitals' with a total capacity of approximately 800. In Scotland, high secure services are provided by the State Hospital at Carstairs, which also serves Northern Ireland. People admitted to these hospitals are deemed to pose a grave and immediate danger to the public, although they may continue to reside in the hospital after that danger has subsided.

Medium secure

Together, the NHS and the independent sector provide some 3500 places in medium secure facilities across England and Wales, catering for people who pose a serious danger to the public. Medium Secure Units (MSUs), which typically have 30–60 beds, may serve a local area or a region, with regional facilities including those designated Regional Secure Units (RSUs), which were formerly distinguished from MSUs as offering a higher level of security. Northern Ireland's RSU, the Shannon Clinic in Belfast, opened in 2005, and others are planned; Scotland has two MSUs. Within this category, three Women's Enhanced Medium Secure Services (WEMSS) are being piloted, which aim to offer gender-sensitive

intensive care. The first of these is the 45-bed facility, The Orchard, which opened in West London in September 2007. MSUs may subsume a range of specialized services, such as a pre-discharge low security area, and a psychiatric intensive care unit.[38]

Low secure

Although often difficult to distinguish from general psychiatric services, low secure facilities in England and Wales are provided by the NHS and the independent sector for patients who pose a significant danger to themselves or others. Patients include those who are gradually moving down from higher levels of security, some may be voluntary patients, and many are admitted directly from the community. The recommended maximum length of stay in UK low secure settings is 8 weeks.[39] The term 'Therapeutically Enhanced Secure Services' is now being used to refer to low secure services for men and women with learning disability.

Prisons

Once largely ignored, mental health problems in prisons have become a major concern in recent years. In all countries around the world, regardless of legal and sentencing characteristics, the prison population exhibits high rates of psychiatric disorder. In some countries, including Australia, at one extreme there may be no on-site psychiatric services, and at the other there may be a dedicated specialist service, including a psychiatric hospital, operating within the prison complex. In the UK, health care in prisons was the responsibility of HM Prison Service but concern over the quality of care led to a number of initiatives, including the development of prison 'in-reach' teams to provide mental health services. These multidisciplinary teams are employed by the NHS and have had a major impact.[40–43] They are supposed to serve a variety of functions:

- reaching out to the wings of the prison where the prisoners reside;
- focusing on prisoners with severe and enduring mental health problems;
- working with healthcare and primary care practitioners in prisons;
- raising mental health awareness, particularly among prison staff;
- offering evidence-based interventions (such as cognitive–behavioural therapy);
- offering a similar multidisciplinary service and model of care to that which a community mental health team provides outside prison.[44]

However, the reality may be rather different. It has been found that nurses are often the only members of the team, and the range of interventions offered is very limited.[42,44] Since the responsibility for management of prisons in England and Wales was transferred from the Home Office to the new Ministry of Justice in 2007, and responsibility for health care was transferred to the Department of Health in 2006, prison mental health services are in a transitional state, spurred on by a number of key policy statements and initiatives.[45–48]

THE CORE PRINCIPLES OF A QUALITY FORENSIC SERVICE

The equivalence principle

Nurses working in forensic settings *must* accept that mentally ill offenders are entitled to receive care of the same standard as they could reasonably expect were they not offenders. This simple principle, sometimes called 'the equivalence principle', has its origins in statements of the United Nations Organization in relation to the care of prisoners, and has gradually been formally or indirectly adopted in many countries and organizations.[49] It has been endorsed by the World Health Organization in its 'Health Care in Prisons' project, and in related reports[50] entered into documents produced under the auspices of the Council of Europe, and reflected in the criteria for health service accreditation in the United States and elsewhere. It has been enshrined in UK Home Office statements since 1990[51] and is reasserted in the UK's Prison Service healthcare performance standard.[52] It remains a key theme in statements on prison health care around the world, including the standards for Australian and New Zealand corrections services. The Australian standards, for example, state that 'Every prisoner is to have access to evidence-based health services provided by a competent, registered health professional who will provide a standard of health services comparable to that of the general community.'[53] It is the first principle in the Australian *National statement of principles for forensic mental health*,[54] and is embodied in State policies. The *Queensland forensic mental health policy*, for example, states that 'People who have a mental disorder or severe mental health problem and have been charged with an offence shall have equitable and timely access to a range of high quality, mental health services and shall be free from any form of discrimination or stigma related to their criminal behaviour.'[55]

The equivalence principle provides a legal and ethical basis for the provision of services for mentally ill offenders,

and the delivery of care by clinicians of all disciplines. It means that all the standards and conditions of care, all the ethical and professional codes, practice guidelines, accreditation criteria, quality assurance expectations, legal safeguards, and so forth, which apply in non-forensic settings must apply in forensic ones; and that care must be provided in accordance with local, national and international covenants, conventions and laws. The overwhelming majority of the literature champions the equivalence principle, but it might be useful here to acknowledge some of the problems that it might present.

First, it has been widely recognized that the equivalence principle may not be realizable in the context of the limited resources which tend to characterize secure settings, especially health services within prisons.[56] This includes financial resources, the physical facilities and appropriately qualified staff. Second, equivalence may not be possible for reasons of security. Applying the equivalence principle in relation to the confidentiality of patient information, for example, can be especially problematic. A key issue in this connection is the tension between patient or inmate confidentiality and the need for collaboration with the large number of stakeholders often involved in managing mentally disordered offenders and those people needing secure psychiatric care or presenting a risk to themselves or others. If psychiatric professionals and other stakeholders wish to enjoy public confidence and respect, it is essential that information is shared in ways that are professionally, ethically and legally responsible, and that this is part of a collaborative approach to managing significant risks.

Security demands and the effective management of risk must also be set against the principle that treatment and care will be provided in the 'least restrictive environment' compatible with the legitimate right of the community to be protected from unacceptable levels of danger, and the protection of the individual patient from unacceptable risks of serious damage to self or serious deterioration. This is embodied in a wide range of standards and policies. The Queensland policy states that 'Assessment and treatment for mentally ill offenders is provided by a mental health service which balances the rights of the individuals to optimal care, provided in the least restrictive setting, with the rights of the public to protection against risk of harm.'[55] Deciding what constitutes the most appropriate level of security in individual cases is thus an essential task, and an important contribution can be made by a well-founded and continuous risk assessment process. There is some difficulty in defining particular levels of security, and although it is common in many countries to distinguish distinctions between low, medium and high security services, there has been little effort to specify what these comprise. Only in recent years have the practical issues of establishing, maintaining and reviewing security in forensic settings been the subject of publication.[57] The Scottish Forensic Network has developed a brief 'matrix of security' which attempts to formalize some of the distinctions between levels.[58]

The conflict between the custodial functions of secure settings and the therapeutic nature of nursing[59] continues to be an issue for nurses,[60,61] and more work needs to be done to help nurses view care and security as part of a single coherent management strategy,[62] rather than as a characteristic of a facility. The World Health Organization (WHO) concept of the 'health-promoting prison' offers one example of how custody and care can work together.[50,63,64]

Another problem with the equivalence principle is that nurses in particular may find it difficult to provide equivalent care when they know that the patient's offending behaviour has been particularly unpleasant or horrendous. Nurses may find it psychologically difficult, or even morally repugnant, and may consciously challenge the equivalence principle. This issue has received little acknowledgement in the literature, and yet some resolution is necessary if nurses are to avoid consequences harmful to all parties concerned.

Finally, there are a number of philosophical objections to equivalence; the commonest of these concern the following claims:

1 Differential rationing of scarce health care resources is unavoidable, some groups are more deserving than others, and it is difficult to justify funding services for mentally ill offenders when considered alongside the needs of others, such as sick children.

2 It is impossible to establish what constitutes 'equivalent' mental health services when care is being provided to different client groups, in significantly different environments, and there are distinctly different therapeutic challenges and objectives; in particular, there does not appear to be a standard quality of general psychiatric care to which the care in a particular secure setting can be compared.

3 Since offenders have broken the 'social contract' they can no longer claim rights equal to those of law-abiding citizens.

4 Some offenders have no commitment to normal moral conventions, do not belong to the community of moral beings, and are therefore not owed the moral respect that membership of that community entails.

Individuals who provide health care in secure and forensic settings must ponder these and similar puzzles and come to a reconciliation or understanding which allows them to comfortably maintain their professional and therapeutic roles.

Standards for a quality forensic service

Assuming, then, that mentally ill offenders are entitled to a quality service, we might ask exactly what such a service should be like. Clearly, it should reflect international and national covenants establishing standards of services for mentally ill people, and these may apply to services located in the community, in health facilities or in correctional settings.[65] In Britain, the international statements are reflected in the seven evidence-based standards listed in the *National service framework for mental health* (September 1999),[66] which is still in force and fleshes out the policies announced in the paper *Modernising mental health services* (1998).[67] Some specific targets have been achieved. For example, the framework noted the commitment of the British Government to work toward the elimination of mixed sex accommodation in all National Health Service facilities,[67,p.106] and this was reported by the Chief Nursing Officer to have been largely achieved by the end of 2004, although no separate figures for mental health facilities are provided.[68]

In Australia, standards were laid down as part of the National Mental Health Strategy, comprising the *Mental health statement of rights and responsibilities*, the *National mental health policy*, and the Australian Health Ministers' *Second national mental health plan*.[69–71] The last document explicitly stated that it 'is relevant for the whole system of mental health service delivery',[71,p.6] and thus includes forensic services. The plan identified 'forensic populations' as one of several 'target groups for whom improved service access and better service responses are essential'.[71,p.10] The third plan, covering the period 2003–08,[72] reaffirmed these positions. The 1996 *National standards for mental health services* went into further detail and is currently being updated.[73] In addition, the health departments of some Australian states have developed their own standards and sets of expectations for mental health services. The New South Wales Health Department's *Charter for mental health care*,[74] for example, is a concise statement as to the level of service that the public can expect. In Canada, there are a number of statements establishing standards of service for mentally ill offenders, notably the *Standards for health care* published in 1994.[75] In New Zealand, a detailed framework for forensic mental health services appeared in March 2001[76] with a strong emphasis on the integration of community and institutional care, but says little about the standard of service that clients can expect in the future. Indeed, even its two-page statement of the underlying philosophy of care is presented as a list of questions.

There are many examples of excellence in forensic care, both in health service settings and in correctional facilities. Specific examples of good practice in prison mental health care in the UK can be found in the Department of Health's 2007 report *Good practice in prison health*.[46] In relation to high security services, aspirations to good practice are well illustrated by the State Hospital at Carstairs in Scotland. In 1998 it published its *Health improvement programme*, which described specific clinically oriented targets, and although no longer in force they illustrate the issues that need to be considered. The hospital was:

- developing a systematic and comprehensive approach to the assessment of dangerousness and offending behaviour;
- developing a treatment approach to the management of anger;
- developing a range of specialist treatment interventions covering sexual and other behaviour problems such as fire raising;
- developing structured treatment and education programmes in drug and alcohol abuse;
- developing a more coordinated approach to women's services;
- reviewing the clinical, environmental and social configuration of every ward;
- developing more scientific risk assessment and risk management;
- promoting best practice to ensure clinical effectiveness through the development of research and audit, and clinical guidelines;
- developing and implementing a health promotion strategy;
- introducing an independent arm to advocacy;
- improving external collaboration to encourage the development of a nationally integrated framework of forensic psychiatric and social services;
- reviewing the needs of patient's relatives and friends, with a view to providing them with better support and information;
- implementing quality human resources, information and estate strategies to support all of the above;
- ensuring the above developments represent sound value for money for the public purse.

Although the hospital's new *Local delivery plan 2007–08*[77] is strategic, and therefore policy and performance oriented, it refers to many of the activities listed above and explains what strategies are in place or planned. In relation to health promotion, for example, the plan states that the hospital is 'implementing a Weight Management Strategy and a Nutritional Policy' and goes on to describe the relevant initiatives, such as 'designing an appropriate nutrition screening tool'; similarly, there are specific initiatives aimed at increasing physical activity, smoking cessation and managing chronic disease.

Such plans and initiatives reflect several key UK policies described elsewhere in this text, including:

- integrated care pathways (ICPs);
- the care programme approach (CPA): A number of documents laid down that prisoners, as well as those receiving care in secure psychiatric facilities, should be managed according to the CPA, which is currently the subject of review.[78,79] Telfer (2000) describes her experiences of developing CPA for prisoners in a top security prison;[80]
- concern for 'clinical effectiveness', a new regard for physical health and well-being, and continuing concern for groups with special needs.

In 2007, clear and detailed guidance for the conduct of adult medium-secure services was issued in the UK by 'Offender Health', a partnership between the Ministry of Justice and the Department of Health,[81] and the Royal College of Psychiatrists published a set of quality standards.[82] Although careful to reflect existing governmental recommendations and standards, neither document refers to the evidence supporting its specifications. A set of clinical practice standards for forensic psychiatric nursing has now been published for discussion.[83] In relation to ethical and professional practice, clinicians in forensic settings are subject to those which regulate their profession at local and national level but there may be additional requirements. In New South Wales, for example, Justice Health has adopted a new multidisciplinary code that comprises the Health Department's Code of Conduct and additional provisions specific to Justice Health staff.[84]

In accordance with the equivalence principle, a quality service for mentally ill disordered offenders and others in secure settings must be 'appropriate to their needs', and this raises important challenges.[85,86] Much of the early research concerned the mental health needs of the prison population as a whole rather than the needs of offenders with a mental disorder, and needs assessments are now conducted at a local level to inform the development of local services. There is a gathering body of evidence regarding the needs of specific groups, notably women[87] and young people.[88,89] A small literature addressing the needs of members of ethnic and cultural minorities has developed,[90–93] some of which are seriously over-represented in forensic settings, not least in Australia. Resolution of some of the problems will hopefully take place within the context of the many policies and strategies aimed at establishing non-discriminatory practices, as they apply to the wider correctional and healthcare services.

Recognizing vulnerability and responding to abuses

A quality forensic service should acknowledge that its clientele will include many vulnerable individuals, and it should have a strategy for recognizing, and dealing quickly and effectively with, suspected cases of abuse, as well as strategies for minimizing, monitoring and learning from actual cases of abuse. A quality service will have clear and accessible procedures for staff and patients, indicating how to respond to abuse or suspected abuse, including appropriate lines of communication and options relating to disciplinary or criminal proceedings. Most importantly, it should be recognized that mentally ill offenders enjoy the same legal protections and resources as any other person, and this must be scrupulously observed: they should have unhindered access to legal advice, for example, and be able to institute appropriate inquiries and proceedings. The history of prisons and secure psychiatric institutions, along with recent studies, suggest that because of significant power differentials and perceived role functions, nurses in such settings are prone to engage in abusive relationships with patients.[94] There must be policies and procedures which minimize the risk that patients will be abused, but which also protect staff and others from wrongful accusations. Nurses should be fully aware of these procedures and adopt an advocacy role in relation to their use by patients and colleagues. Adopting such a role is sometimes not easy and there must also be a system in place for the protection of any person, staff or patient, who could be considered a 'whistleblower' and therefore at risk. It is significant that because of the seriousness of this risk, formal procedures for the protection of whistleblowers are a legal requirement for health services in many countries.

Clear and carefully observed policies relating to patient confidentiality are highly relevant to the issue of protecting potentially vulnerable patients, as the disclosure of sensitive personal information may heighten their vulnerability and place them, and staff, at increased risk. Lastly, the vulnerability of any particular patient must feature in assessments of risk, and be taken into account in treatment programmes, in day-to-day management and in discharge planning. Needless to say, the nurse is a key player in the conduct of these processes, and in the protection of vulnerable individuals.

Risk assessment and management

Protecting vulnerable patients and ensuring patient safety relates to the role of nurses in risk management. 'Risk' here covers risk to one's own safety, health and quality of life – material, cultural and spiritual – as well as risk to others. It may apply to the patient's further offending, accidental or deliberate self-harm, suicide, homicide and violence to others, vulnerability to sexual abuse, stalking and harassment, material exploitation, property damage, public nuisance, neglect or abuse of or by dependants, intimidation and threats to others, and reckless behaviour such as dangerous driving, and multiple drug abuse with consequent exacerbation of mental disorder and offending risk. There are a wide variety of ways of evaluating these various risks and a correspondingly vast and diverse literature. Forensic psychiatric services worldwide are attempting to place clinical and management decision-making on a sound evidence-based footing, and this includes assessments of the risks posed by mentally ill offenders to themselves and the community. In a quality

forensic service, risk assessment procedures are formally developed and conducted, and based on a subtle blend of multidisciplinary clinical judgement, research evidence and standardized tests, for which staff are appropriately trained. Authorities are now acknowledging that risk can never be eliminated, but rather must be managed in light of the potential harms and benefits. Such an approach is called 'positive risk management'. Detailed advice on best practice in risk management in mental health, as it relates to many of the issues listed above, has recently been provided by the UK Department of Health.[95]

Reflection

What are the arguments for and against distinguishing the category of 'forensic psychiatric nurse'?

Would you prefer to see the forensic psychiatric nurse as a specialist within 'forensic nursing', as a specialist within 'psychiatric nursing', or simply as some other category of forensic mental health worker?

How should nurses working in non-forensic secure facilities be designated?

PROBLEMS, CURRENT DEVELOPMENTS AND FUTURE PROSPECTS

Secure psychiatric services are finally beginning to shake off the legacy of the past. Since the first edition of this text, in several countries there have been dramatic increases in funding, a plethora of multidisciplinary policies and strategies, new state-of-the-art facilities, and a culture change characterized by optimism and increased mutual respect, perhaps nowhere more so than in the UK. Disputes over authority and legitimacy have diminished as a result of the relaxation of medical domination, and a shared concern as to the quality of care being provided. Clinical governance and the care programme approach or a similar system have been widely embraced in Australia, New Zealand and the UK,[96,97] with nurses playing a significant role. Clinical supervision and evidence-based practice, have become a norm for many forensic settings. There are now well-established national and international forums and networks, of varying formal status, aided in great part by Internet communications and desktop publishing, which bring together clinicians and interest groups to share information and experiences and contribute to policymaking. Another development has been the gradual increase in the involvement of patients in their own care planning, and of service users and ex-users in policy and practice development.

Although a multidisciplinary approach to care is now widely accepted,[34] and post-disciplinary approaches are increasingly common,[98] there remains a need to create a professional identity for clinicians who work in forensic settings. There are continuing problems in the recruitment and retention of high quality staff, and educational opportunities remain limited. Partnerships between the various stakeholders in secure care have been formalized in many jurisdictions, fuelled by a realization that continuity of care between agencies is essential. There is cooperation between public and private providers, but continuing concern over the proliferation of private prisons and the emergence of private secure psychiatric services. Arguments over the role of psychiatry in assessing and managing dangerousness remain, and proposed new mental health legislation in England and Wales, particularly as it concerned people with a personality disorder, drew a strident response apparently based on the view that clinicians should not be party to 'anti-therapeutic' activities such as incarcerating dangerous individuals, and forcing medication upon people in the community. Like many others hinted at in this review of services, these are controversial and complex issues but ones to which nurses, in whichever countries they work, should give careful thought, form an opinion and give expression.

REFERENCES

1. Moran R. *Knowing right from wrong: the insanity defence of Daniel MacNaughtan*. New York, NY: Free Press, 1981.

2. Fingarette H. *The meaning of criminal insanity*. Berkeley, CA: University of California Press, 1972.

3. Robinson D. *Wild beasts and idle humours: the insanity defence from antiquity to the present*. Cambridge, MA: Harvard University Press, 1996.

4. Boland F. *Anglo-American insanity defence reform: the war between law and psychiatry*. Aldershot, UK: Dartmouth Publishing, 1999.

5. Barclay W. *Discussion paper: a study of corrections mental health services in New South Wales*. Sydney, Australia: Corrections Health Service, 1997.

6. Bluglass R. *Review of forensic mental health services, New South Wales*. Matraville, NSW: Corrections Health Service, 1997.

7. McComish AG. The development of forensic services in Scotland 1800–1960. *Psychiatric Care* 1996; **3** (4): 153–8.

8. Feinberg J. Sickness and wickedness: new conceptions and new paradoxes. *Journal of the American Academy of Psychiatry and Law* 1998; **26** (3): 475–85.

9. Barton WE, Sanborn CJ (eds). *Law and the mental health professions: friction at the interface*. New York, NY: International Universities Press, 1978.

10. Dershowitz AM. *The abuse excuse: and other cop-outs, sob stories, and evasions of responsibility*. Boston, MA: Little Brown & Company, 1994.

11. Arrigo BA. *The contours of psychiatry: a postmodern critique of mental illness, criminal insanity, and the law*. New York, NY: Garland, 1996.

12. Buchanan A. *Psychiatric aspects of justification, excuse and mitigation: the jurisprudence of mental abnormality in Anglo-American criminal law*. London, UK: Jessica Kingsley, 2000.

13. Hammer R, Moynihan B, Pagliaro EM (eds). *Forensic nursing: a handbook for practice*. Sudbury, MA: Jones & Bartlett, 2005.

14. Lynch V (ed.). *Forensic nursing*. St Louis, MO: Mosby, 2005.

15. Pyrek KM (ed.). *Forensic nursing*. Boca Raton, FL: CRC, 2006.

16. Burrow S. An outline of the forensic nursing role. *British Journal of Nursing* 1993; **2**: 899–904.

17. Burrow S. The role conflict of the forensic nurse. *Senior Nurse* 1993; **13** (5): 20–5.

18. Royal College of Nursing. *Buying forensic mental health nursing: an RCN guide for purchasers*. London, UK: Royal College of Nursing, 1997.

19. McCourt M. Five concepts for the expanded role of the forensic mental health nurse. In: Tarbuck P, Burnard P, Topping-Morris B (eds). *Forensic mental health nursing: policy, strategy and implementation*. London, UK: Whurr, 1999: 149–61.

20. Robinson D, Kettles A (eds). *Forensic nursing and multidisciplinary care of the mentally disordered offender (forensic focus 14)*. London, UK: Jessica Kingsley, 1999.

21. Kettles AM, Woods P, Collins M. Introduction. In: Kettles AM, Woods P, Collins M, Rae M (eds). *Therapeutic interventions for forensic mental health nurses*. London, UK: Jessica Kingsley, 2001: 13–20.

22. Faculty of Health, University of Central Lancashire. *Nursing in secure environments: a scoping study conducted on behalf of the United Kingdom Central Council for Nursing, Midwifery and Health Visiting*. London, UK: UKCC, 1999. Available from: www.fnrh.freeserve.co.uk/docs/Nursing%20in%20Secure%20Environme.pdf. Accessed 8 January 2008.

23. National Board for Nursing, Midwifery and Health Visiting for Scotland. *Continuing professional development portfolio – a route to enhanced competence in forensic mental health nursing*. Edinburgh, UK: National Board for Nursing, Midwifery and Health Visiting for Scotland, 2000.

24. Scottish Prison Service. *Competency framework for nursing staff working within the Scottish Prison Service*. 2005. Available from: www.sps.gov.uk/multimediagallery/B256945F-A411–49C2-A44A-065D60FBA90C.pdf. Accessed 11 January 2008.

25. Bowring-Lossock E. The forensic mental health nurse – a literature review. *Journal of Psychiatric and Mental Health Nursing* 2006; **13**: 780–5.

26. Chaloner C, Coffey M (eds). *Forensic mental health nursing: current approaches*. Oxford, UK: Blackwell, 1999.

27. Robinson D, Kettles A, Rae M (eds). *Forensic nursing and multidisciplinary care of the mentally disordered offender (Forensic focus 14)*. London, UK: Jessica Kingsley, 1999.

28. Dale C, Thompson T, Woods P (eds). *Forensic mental health: issues in practice*. Edinburgh, UK: Baillière Tindall & The Royal College of Nursing, 2001.

29. McClelland N, Humphreys M, Conlon C, Hillis H (eds). *Forensic nursing and mental disorder: clinical practice*. Oxford, UK: Butterworth-Heinemann, 2001.

30. Tarbuck P, Burnard P, Topping-Morris B (eds). *Forensic mental health nursing: policy, strategy and implementation.* London, UK: Whurr, 1999.

31. Kettles A, Woods P, Collins M, Rae M (eds). *Therapeutic interventions for forensic mental heath nurses.* London, UK: Jessica Kingsley, 2001.

32. Mercer D, Mason T, McKeown M, McCann G (eds). *Forensic mental health care: a case study approach.* Edinburgh, UK: Churchill Livingstone, 1999.

33. Forensic Nurses' Research and Development Group. *Forensic mental health nursing: forensic aspects of acute care.* London, UK: Quay Books, 2007.

34. Wix S, Humphreys S (eds). *Multidisciplinary working in forensic mental health care.* Edinburgh, UK: Elsevier, 2005.

35. Hillis G. Diverting people with mental health problems from the criminal justice system. In: Tarbuck P, Burnard P, Topping-Morris B (eds). *Forensic mental health nursing: policy, strategy and implementation.* London, UK: Whurr, 1999: 36–50.

36. New South Wales Law Society. Justice and mental health systems cheer new court liaison program. *Law Society Journal* 1999; **37** (8): 12.

37. NACRO. *Findings of the 2004 survey of court diversion/criminal justice mental health liaison schemes for mentally disordered offenders in England and Wales.* London, UK: National Association for the Care and Resettlement of Offenders, 2005.

38. Dolan M, Lawson A. A psychiatric intensive care unit in a medium-security unit. *The Journal of Forensic Psychiatry* 2001; **12** (3): 684–93.

39. Rutherford M, Duggan S. *Forensic mental health services: facts and figures on current provision.* London, UK: Sainsbury Centre for Mental Health, 2007. Available from: www.scmh.org.uk. Accessed 10 January 2008.

40. Meiklejohn C, Hodges K, Capon D. 'Work in Progress' – community mental health in-reach into prison: lessons from HMP Gloucester. *Mental Health Nursing* 2004: **24** (6): 8–10.

41. Brooker C, Ricketts T, Lemme F *et al.* An evaluation of the Prison In-Reach Collaborative. Sheffield: School of Health and Related Research, University of Sheffield, 2005. Available from: www.nfmhp.org.uk/MRD%2012%2046%20Final%20Report. pdf. Accessed 10 January 2008.

42. Sainsbury Centre for Mental Health. *Mental health care in prisons.* Briefing paper No. 32. July, 2007. London, UK: Sainsbury Centre for Mental Health. 2007. Available from: www.scmh.org.uk. Accessed 10 January 2007.

43. Steel J, Thornicroft G, Birmingham L *et al.* Prison mental health in-reach services [Editorial]. *British Journal of Psychiatry* 2007; **190** (5): 373–4.

44. Durcan G, Knowles K. *Policy paper 5: London's prison mental health services: a review.* London, UK: The Sainsbury Centre for Mental Health, 2006. Available from: www.scmh. org.uk/80256FBD004F3555/vWeb/flKHAL6N3GV4/$file/po licy5_prison_mental_health_services.pdf. Accessed 10 January 2008.

45. Department of Health. *Changing the outlook: a strategy for developing and modernising mental health services in prisons.* London, UK: Department of Health, 2006. Available from: www.dh.gov.uk/publications. Accessed 2 January 2008.

46. Department of Health. *Good practice in prison health.* London, UK: Department of Health, 2007. Available from: www.dh.gov.uk/publications. Accessed 2 January 2008.

47. Offender Health. *Improving health, supporting justice: a consultation document.* London, UK: Department of Health, 2007. Available from: www.dh.gov.uk/publications. Accessed 10 January 2008.

48. Royal College of Psychiatrists. *Prison psychiatry: adult prisons in England and Wales.* Available from: www.rcpsych. ac.uk/publications/collegereports/cr/cr141.aspx. Accessed 10 January 2008.

49. Niveau G. Relevance and limits of the principle of 'equivalence of care' in prison medicine. *Journal of Medical Ethics* 2007; **33**: 610–3.

50. Moeller L, Stöver H, Jürgens R *et al.* (eds). *Health in prisons: a WHO guide to the essentials of prison health.* Copenhagen: WHO, 2007.

51. Wilson S. The principle of equivalence and the future of mental health care in prisons. *British Journal of Psychiatry* 2004; **184**: 5–7.

52. HM Prison Service. *Performance standard 22. Health services for prisoners:* Issued May 2004. London, UK: HM Prison Service, 2004. Available from: www.hmprisonservice.gov.uk/assets/documents/10000305_22HealthServicesforPrisoners.pdf. Accessed 3rd January 2008.

53. Australian Corrective Services joint publication. *Standard guidelines for corrections in Australia.* Revised 2004. Place of publication not stated: Corrective Services Departments of the States and Territories of Australia, 2004: 20. Available from: www.aic.gov.au/research/corrections/standards/aust-stand.html. Accessed 3 January 2008.

54. Commonwealth of Australia. *National statement of principles for forensic mental health.* Canberra: Commonwealth of Australia, 2002. Available from: www.health.wa.gov.au/mhareview/resources/documents/FINAL_VERSION_OF_NATIONAL_PRINCIPLES_FOR_FMH-Aug_2002.pdf. Accessed 11 January 2008.

55. Queensland Health. *Queensland forensic mental health policy.* Brisbane: Queensland Health, 2002. Available from: www.health.qld.gov.au. Accessed 6 January 2008.

56. Birmingham L, Wilson S, Adshead G. Prison medicine: ethics and equivalence. *British Journal of Psychiatry* 2005; **188**: 4–6.

57. Dale C, Gardner J. Security in forensic environments: strategic and operational issues. In: Dale C, Thompson T, Woods P (eds). *Forensic mental health: issues in practice.* Edinburgh, UK: Baillière Tindall & The Royal College of Nursing, 2001: 251–73.

58. Scottish Forensic Network. *Matrix of security. 2006.* Available from: www.forensicnetwork.scot.nhs.uk/documents/reports/Matrix%20of%20Security.pdf. Accessed 10 January 2008.

59. Dale C, Woods P. *Caring for prisoners: RCN prison nurses' forum roles and boundaries project.* London, UK: Royal College of Nursing, 2001. Available from: www.fnrh.freeserve.co.uk/docs/prison%20final%20report.PDF. Accessed 9 January 2008.

60. Weiskopf CS. Nurses' experience of caring for inmate patients. *Journal of Advanced Nursing* 2005; **49** (4): 336–43.

61. Isherwood T, Burns M, Rigby G. A qualitative analysis of the 'management of schizophrenia' within a medium secure service for men with learning disabilities. *Journal of Psychiatric and Mental Health Nursing* 2006; **13**: 148–56.

62. Tarbuck P. The therapeutic use of security: a model for forensic nursing. In: Thompson T, Mathias P (eds). *Lyttle's mental health and disorder*, 2nd edn. London, UK: Baillière Tindall, 1994: 552–70.

63. Gatherer A, Moller L, Hayton P. The World Health Organization European Health in Prisons Project after 10 years: persistent barriers and achievements. *American Journal of Public Health* 2005; **95** (10): 1696–700.

64. Whitehead D. The health promoting prison (HPP) and its imperative for nursing. *International Journal of Nursing Studies* 2006; **43**: 123–31.

65. Blaauw E, van Marle HJ. Mental health in prisons. In: Moeller L, Stöver H, Jürgens R et al. (eds). *Health in prisons: a WHO guide to the essentials of prison health*. Copenhagen: WHO, 2007: 133–46.

66. Department of Health. *National service framework for mental health*. London, UK: Department of Health, 1999. Available from: www.dh.gov.uk/en/Publicationsandstatistics/Publications/PublicationsPolicyAndGuidance/DH_4009598. Accessed 3 January 2008.

67. Department of Health. *Modernising mental health services*. London, UK: Department of Health, 1998. Available from: www.dh.gov.uk/en/Publicationsandstatistics/Publications/PublicationsPolicyAndGuidance/DH_4003105. Accessed 3 January 2008.

68. Chief Nursing Officer. *Privacy and dignity – a report by the CNO into mixed sex accommodation in hospitals*. London, UK: Department of Health, 2007. Available from: www.dh.gov.uk/publications. Accessed 3 January 2008.

69. Australian Health Ministers. *Mental health statement of rights and responsibilities*. Canberra: Mental Health Branch, Commonwealth Department of Health and Family Services, 1991. Available from: www.health.gov.au/internet/wcms/publishing.nsf/Content/mental-pubs. Accessed 7 January 2008.

70. Australian Health Ministers. *National mental health plan*. Canberra: Mental Health Branch, Commonwealth Department of Health and Family Services, 1992. Available from: http://www.health.gov.au/internet/wcms/publishing.nsf/Content/mental-pubs. Accessed 7 January 2008.

71. Australian Health Ministers. *Second national mental health plan*. Canberra: Mental Health Branch, Commonwealth Department of Health and Family Services, 1998. Available from: www.health.gov.au/internet/wcms/publishing.nsf/Content/mental-pubs. Accessed 10 January 2008.

72. Australian Health Ministers. *National mental health plan 2003–2008*. Canberra: Australian Government, 2003. Available from: www.mentalhealth.gov.au. Accessed 10 January 2008.

73. Australian Council on Healthcare Standards. *Review of National standards for mental health services* (Webpage). Available from: www.achs.org.au/StndsMentalHealth. Accessed 7 January 2008.

74. New South Wales Health Department. *Charter for mental health care*. Sydney: New South Wales Health Department, 1998. Available from: www.health.nsw.gov.au/policy/cmh/legal/mhcharter.pdf. Accessed 7 January 2008.

75. Correctional Service of Canada. *Principles and standards for health care*. Revised 1994. Ottawa: Correctional Service of Canada, 1994. Available from: www.csc-scc.gc.ca/text/prgrm/fsw/hlthstds/toc_e.shtml#TopOfPage. Accessed 10 January 2008.

76. Ministry of Health (New Zealand). *Services for people with mental illness in the justice system: framework for forensic mental health services*. Wellington: Ministry of Health, 2001. Available from: www.moh.govt.nz/moh.nsf/pagesmh/771?Open. Accessed 7 January 2008.

77. The State Hospitals Board for Scotland. *The State Hospitals Board for Scotland local delivery plan 2006–2007–2008–2009, updated for 2007–2008*. Carstairs, Lanark: The State Hospitals Board for Scotland, 2007. Available from: www.tsh.scot.nhs.uk/FreedomOfInformation/policyframework.htm. Accessed 8 January 2008.

78. Department of Health. *Reviewing the care programme approach*. London, UK: Department of Health, 2006. Available from: www.dh.gov.uk/publications. Accessed 2 January 2008.

79. The State Hospitals Board for Scotland. *Review of care programme approach guidance for restricted patients in Scotland: draft for consultation*. Carstairs, Lanark: The State Hospitals Board for Scotland, 2006. Available from: www.tsh.scot.nhs.uk/FreedomOfInformation/policyframework.htm. Accessed 10 January 2008.

80. Telfer J. Balancing care and control: Introducing the care programme approach in a prison setting. *Mental Health Care* 2000; **4** (3): 93–6.

81. Jobbins C, Abbott B, Brammer L et al. *Best practice guidance: specification for adult medium-secure services*. London, UK: Department of Health, 2007. Available from: www.dh.gov.uk/publications. Accessed 3 January 2008.

82. Tucker S, Hughes T. Standards for medium secure units. *Quality network for medium secure units*. London, UK: Royal College of Psychiatrists' Centre for Quality Improvement, 2007. Available from: http://www.rcpsych.ac.uk/msu. Accessed 10 January 2008.

83. International Association of Forensic Mental Health Services. Special Interest Group for Forensic Mental Health Nurses, Newsletter. March 2007: 6–13. International Association of Forensic Mental Health Services. Available from: www.iafmhs.org/files/NewsletterMarch2007IAFMHSNsingNews1.pdf. Accessed 10 January 2008.

84. Justice Health (NSW). *Code of conduct, 2006*. Matraville, NSW: Justice Health, 2006. Available from: www.justice-health.nsw.gov.au/pubs/code_of_conduct_new.pdf. Accessed 11 January 2008.

85. Marshall T, Simpson S, Stevens A. *Health care in prisons: a health care needs assessment*. Birmingham: Department of Public Health and Epidemiology, University of Birmingham, 2000.

86. Cohen A, Eastman N. *Assessing forensic mental health needs: policy, theory and research*. London, UK: Gaskell, 2000.

87. Lart R, Payne S, Beaumont B et al. *Women and secure psychiatric services: a literature review*. Bristol: School for Policy Studies, Bristol University, 1998. Executive Summary. Available

from: www.york.ac.uk/inst/crd/report14.htm. Accessed 11 January 2008.

88. Bailey S, Dolan M (eds). *Adolescent forensic psychiatry.* London, UK: Butterworth-Heinemann, 2002.

89. Schekty DH, Benedek EP. *Principles and practice of child and adolescent forensic psychiatry.* Washington, DC: American Psychiatric Press, 2002.

90. Fernando S, Ndegwa D, Wilson M. *Forensic psychiatry, race and culture.* London, UK: Routledge, 1998.

91. Kaye C, Lingiah T (eds). *Race, culture and ethnicity in psyc-hiatric practice: working with difference.* London, UK: Jessica Kingsley, 1999.

92. McKeown M, Stowell-Smith M. Language, race and forensic psychiatry: some dilemmas for anti-discriminatory practice. In: Mason T, Mercer D (eds). *Critical perspectives in forensic care: inside out.* London, UK: Macmillan, 1998: 188–208.

93. Byrt R, Aiyegbusi A, Hardie T, Addo M. Cultural and diversity issues. In: *Forensic Nurses' Research and Development Group. Forensic mental health nursing: forensic aspects of acute care.* London, UK: Quay Books, 2007: 219–33.

94. Holmes D. Governing the captives: forensic psychiatric nursing in corrections. *Perspectives in Psychiatric Care* 2005; **41** (1): 3–13.

95. Department of Health. *Best practice in managing risk.* London, UK: Department of Health, 2007. Available from: www.dh.gov.uk/publications. Accessed 2 January 2008.

96. Department of Health. *Clinical governance in prison health care: a discussion document.* London, UK: HM Prison and the Department of Health, 2001. Available from: www.dh.gov.uk/en/Publicationsandstatistics/Publications/PublicationsPolicyAndGuidance/DH_4084148. Accessed 6 January 2008.

97. Duffy D. Clinical governance: a framework for quality in forensic mental health care. In: Dale C, Thompson T, Woods P (eds). *Forensic mental health: issues in practice.* Edinburgh, UK: Baillière Tindall & The Royal College of Nursing, 2001: 53–60.

98. Holmes CA. Postdisciplinarity in mental health-care: an Australian viewpoint. *Nursing Inquiry* 2001; 8: 230–39.

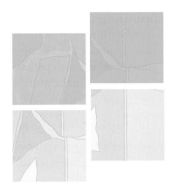

CHAPTER 55

Services for children and young people

Sue Croom*

RIGHTS OF CHILDREN AND ADOLESCENTS

There is still considerable stigma attached to child mental health.[1] Children, as developing individuals, can be disempowered by mental health services and by society. All professionals who work directly with children and young people or who work with parents/carers, have a duty to be aware of and respond to the United Nations Children's Rights Convention[2] and to ensure that these principles are meaningfully integrated into their strategies and care packages. In doing so, they are required to maintain an ethical and therapeutic balance between providing developmentally appropriate care and recognizing the growing autonomy and potential of children and young people. Article 23.1 of the CRC stipulates that a mentally or physically disabled child should enjoy a full and decent life, in conditions, which ensure dignity, promote self-reliance and facilitate the child's active participation in the community. The rights of children, young people and parents as users of services should be carefully considered, particularly in relation to issues of consent and confidentiality. The right to participate in the evaluation and development of services is also crucial and child and youth advocacy can play a useful role in developing and implementing policies that are respectful, empowering and confidential.[3]

Article 3 pf the CRC stipulates the principle of the best interest of the child. Child and adolescent mental health (CAMH) nurses and all involved professionals working with children and their families have a duty to make an informed judgement of what is 'in the best interest' of the child. Any child protection issues must be assessed and responded to, as the child's safety will always be paramount. In collaboration with the child, the family, other professionals and relevant agencies, an assessment must be made of the social, emotional and cognitive development of the child and their capacity to make decisions. Where there are child protection issues, nurses and other professionals must abide by their local and national protocols to ascertain the physical and emotional safety of the child and the capacity of their carers to keep the child in their family setting.

DEVELOPMENTAL PSYCHOLOGY AND PSYCHOPATHOLOGY

The definitions of child and adolescent mental health, developmental norms and developmental psychopathology are social constructs, which are culture bound[4] and will change over time and in different circumstances.

*Sue Croom is Lead Nurse for Northumberland and North Tyneside Mental Health Trust. Over her 25 years' experience in CAMH she has combined clinical work with university teaching and research in order to develop clinically relevant degree/masters programmes and participative action research focused on improving partnership with young people and carers. She had received two international fellowships and has lectured widely including in Canada and Russia.

However, CAMH services tend to employ current globally agreed key properties that can be summarized in definitions of CAMH and CAMH disorders.

Mental health in children and young people can be defined as:

- a capacity to enter into and sustain mutually satisfying personal relationships;
- continuing progress of psychological development;
- an ability to play/engage in recreation and learn so that attainments are appropriate for age and intellectual level;
- a developing sense of right and wrong;
- the degree of psychological distress and maladaptive behaviour is within normal limits for the child's age and context.[5–7]

A significant CAMH problem/disorder is characterized by:

- a change in the child's usual behaviours, emotions or thoughts;
- persistence of the problems (as a minimum 2 weeks);
- being severe enough to interfere with the child's everyday life;
- disability to the child and carers.

The above criteria must however take into account the child's stage of development and their social and cultural context.

Prevalence of CAMH problems and implications for services

Although there is variation in the global prevalence rates, there appears to be a worldwide consensus that there is significant CAMH need.[8,9] Diagnosable psychopathology annually accounts for five of the top 10 leading causes of disability in the world for those aged 5 years and over.[5] Recent analyses of the burden of disease associated with CAMH problems provide evidence of the lifelong societal costs associated with disorders beginning in childhood and adolescence.[8,10]

A national study of children in the UK found that 9.5 per cent of children aged 5–16 had a 'mental disorder', i.e. a problem of sufficient severity that it had a daily impact on the child's function and relationships.[11]

Although similar profiles are found globally,[12] CAMH services in the UK can extrapolate from these statistics to predict that in any secondary school of 1000 pupils there are likely to be 100 pupils with problems serious enough to be given a CAMH diagnosis.

However, it is estimated that only one in five children, who have a diagnosable disorder and need CAMH services actually receive them.[7,9] Nurses and other CAMH professionals working in the community must be aware of the national and local incidence when planning their workload and identify opportunities for promotion, prevention, screening and identification of significant CAMH problems. Nurses in key position, for example adult community psychiatric nurses working with parents with mental health problems, can play a significant role in the prevention of problems and early intervention through the recognition of a child's level of distress.

It is not within the scope of this chapter to discuss the range of CAMH problems and disorders in detail, but an overview of internationally agreed CAMH disorders will now be provided.

CAMH disorders

As infants are totally dependent on their caregivers, disorders in infancy are related to the infant's rapid development and also to the carer–child relationship. Disorders, which can arise at this stage, include attachment disorders and autistic spectrum disorders (ASDs). Although autism can usually be picked up and identified in infancy, ASDs comprise a range of lifelong developmental disorders characterized by difficulties in social interaction, communication and imagination. ASD disorders represent a spectrum of problems ranging from children with learning disabilities, who may have profound language disabilities to those with average or above average intelligence such as Asperger's syndrome, who have difficulties in recognizing others' feelings and may appear insensitive and present with profound difficulties in being sensitive to and cooperating with others.

A range of disorders can arise in childhood including conduct and oppositional defiant disorders, anxiety disorders, ASD (which may or may not have been identified in infancy), speech and language disorders, attention deficit and hyperactivity disorders. Conduct disorders are characterized by a repetitive pattern of antisocial, aggressive and/or defiant conduct.[13]

Hyperkinetic disorders (such as attention deficit hyperactivity disorder or ADHD) are characterized by restlessness, over-activity, inattentiveness, concentration difficulties, impulsivity and disruptive or destructive behaviour across more than one context.[11] These children can have significant problems in peer interactions that can affect their social and emotional development. Without support, children with hyperkinetic disorders suffer a high risk of moving onto the more difficult and intractable conduct disorders.

Children with depression can present with acting out type symptoms as well as the classical symptoms of sadness. Irritability, loss of interest in activities, appetite changes, sleeps disturbances, difficulties in concentration and feelings of loss of self-worth.

Disorders in adolescents can be considered under three headings (although this can be an artificial categorization) and include unresolved childhood disorders, e.g. conduct disorders and autism and pervasive development disorders; disorders arising in adolescence such as depression, anxiety disorders; disorders specifically related to adolescence such as drug and alcohol misuse; and adult mental health problems and disorders such as suicidal behaviour and major affective disorders such as depression and psychosis.[14]

Suicide rates are low in children but start to increase from the age of 11.[14] Boys and young men are most at risk, although there this has started to fall in the last few years.[7] Attempted suicide is primarily a problem of adolescence and is higher for girls and is related to depression, serious mental health problems and drug misuse and the risk increases with any previous attempt.[14]

Eating disorders (discussed earlier in this volume) are primarily a problem of adolescence although there is a growing incidence in pre-pubescence. The average age of onset of anorexia is 15 years and of bulimia, 18.[15]

Psychotic disorders increase in adolescence and include schizophrenia and bipolar disorder, which are discussed in previous chapters of this volume.

Reflection

- What are the opportunities and challenges for using diagnostic categories in CAMH?
- Given that diagnostic categories drive the commissioning of services, how might nurses use them in the provision of person-centred care?
- What are the implications for nursing of gender difference in the incidence of types of CAMH disorders?

LOCATING CAMH PROBLEMS AND SERVICES IN A DEVELOPMENTAL CONTEXT

As development is a core construct of CAMH, professionals and providers of CAMH services strive to ensure that services are socially, emotionally and cognitively relevant for a range of developmental stages including infancy and early childhood, middle childhood, early adolescence and late adolescence. The different stages can be distinguished by different developmental tasks. However, this can be over-simplistic, as development is a complex, continuous process and the transition between stages takes place over a period of time. Furthermore, all children and young people will follow their individual developmental pathway and children with learning disability, for example may physically be undergoing adolescent changes while still operating cognitively at a much earlier stage.

CAMH services during infancy and early years

In infancy the major developmental task is the development of a secure attachment with the caregiver.[16] Lack of appropriate stimulation in the early years may result in social, physical, cognitive and language delay. In these early years, the child cannot be separated from the family system. Any factor, which reduces the parent's capacity to be cognitively, emotionally and physically available to their infant/young child, such as mental illness, trauma or socioeconomic difficulties can impact on the development of the attachment relationship unless the parents/carers are able to find or can be provided with additional support. The child's sense of a secure attachment forms a platform for developing mental health through a positive sense of worth and a growing ability to regulate their emotions[17] and thus to grow and learn from their experiences.

The young child builds upon the sense of trust, which they learn through a secure attachment, to begin to value developing a sense of control as a way of pleasing their carers and so begin to adopt their carer's rules regarding what is right and wrong. Particular support may be required for parents who are ill (including those with mental illness) or who have a disability and this necessitates that CAMH services work closely with primary care services, adult mental health services and early years support services. CAMH services expertise in family work and parenting groups and in supervision can support the work of a range of community professionals and parents/carers through behavioural programmes and therapeutic work on the attachment relationship.

CAMH services between early childhood and adolescence

In middle childhood, a key task is to develop a sense of self-competence and of social rules including the rules of right and wrong in order to begin to develop their social and individual conscience and the related social rules outside of the home.[18] These rules enable the child to engage positively with school, peers and extracurricular activities.[19] Positive engagement with school and prosocial activities such as sport thus becomes a particular protective factor at this stage. If a child has developed a sense of trust in infancy and early childhood, they are more likely to trust that adults will keep them safe and they can thus build on the confidence in their growing set of competencies in order to engage in activities, which will promote peer relationships.

CAMH services can liaise with and support professionals involved in the growing number of systems with which the children at this age begin to interact with such as schools, extracurricular sports/activities and community centres. Support to the child and the family can be offered through groups such as social skills and to parents through parenting groups. Parent groups that are held simultaneously with child/young person groups have been found to be more effective than when provided alone.[20,21]

A child who is supported to achieve their developmental tasks in middle childhood is more likely to build on their developing sense of competence and trust in peers and adults in order to achieve their adolescent tasks.

CAMH services for adolescents

In adolescence, the general developmental tasks are to develop a positive sense of identity, to develop their set of values so that they can contribute as citizens and form the intimate relationships of adulthood.[18] Adolescents can suffer from mental health problems, e.g. ADHD or autistic spectrum disorders that were identified in childhood; they may develop a CAMH problem such as conduct disorder in adolescence; they may develop adolescent-related mental disorders such as anorexia or they may develop adult mental illnesses such as psychosis.

Adolescents with mental health problems need to be cared for, as far as possible in their community context. On the minority of occasions when this is not feasible because of safety or therapeutic reasons, then they can be admitted into an inpatient milieu, which is orientated to the unique stage of adolescence and to the shifting balance of autonomy and nurture that characterizes adolescence.

CAMH services need to take into account the resources required to meet the increasing incidence of severe mental illness in adolescence, e.g. by responding to vocational and social issues, which can support the young person's transition to adulthood and reduce the likelihood of social exclusion, that can be a secondary consequence of mental illness. CAMH services also need formal arrangements with other services, who offer specific approaches to dealing with a range of co-morbidities, e.g. problems with drug and alcohol misuse, learning difficulty, youth offending, and related problems such as school exclusion and teenage pregnancy.

Reflection

- How could you ensure that a CAMH service is responsive to the developmental needs of the children and young people it serves?
- How do you think developmental theories can help you as a practitioner, when working with parents and/or children?

Consider a parent you are working with:

- How do you think their previous development has impacted on how they function as a parent?

Consider a child/adolescent you are working with:

- What current developmental tasks are they negotiating?
- How can their previous developmental history provide an insight into how they are currently functioning?

RISK AND RESILIENCE

Developmental psychopathology can arise from a combination of congenital, constitutional, environmental, family or illness factors. There is a significant body of research in CAMH, which identifies the relative impact of risk and protective factors at an individual, family and community level that differentially impact across the developmental stages.[19,22]

Risk factors are individual or environmental variables, which increase the probability of a negative developmental outcome or disorder. Protective factors are individual or environmental factors that help to prevent or attenuate the development of negative developmental outcomes or disorders. The relative risk of any single risk is relatively small and it is the accumulation of risks, which have an impact on developmental progress and CAMH or developmental psychopathology and ill health, e.g. a child with three risk factors is at substantially higher risk than a child with one. However, CAMH services can use risk and resilience research to guide work with children and families by identifying their individual profile of risk and protective factors and offering a menu of evidence-based strategies to reduce the risk and protective factors in ways, which are both feasible according to the resources available and individually and culturally acceptable to the child and family in their context.[23]

The risk factors at an individual, family and community level will now be summarized.

Risk factors

Individual factors

- Genetic influences such as depression in the family or autistic spectrum disorders in the family can increase the risk of a related child developing the conditions.
- Children with learning difficulties are at increased risk. This is particularly so with reading and literacy.[19] Collaboration with education services is therefore essential.
- Any kind of developmental delay including language or neurological delay can increase the risk of developing CAMH problems.
- Mismatch between the child and carer's temperament. This term refers to the pattern or 'style' of the child's behaviour. Such style is fairly stable during infancy and early childhood. Children with an 'easy' temperament tend to be happy, regular in feeding and sleeping patterns, and adapt well to new situations. Children with a 'challenging' temperament tend to be irritable, unhappy, intense, irregular and have difficulty adjusting to change and are at a higher risk for emotional and behavioural problems if their temperament does not 'match' the temperament of their significant caregivers, e.g. in infancy their mother, and in middle

childhood their teacher. A temperamental match occurs when the caregiver can respond positively to the child and meet their needs, e.g. a very quiet father can meet the needs of his impulsive, highly active child by responding positively to their level of energy.

- Children with physical illnesses, especially chronic illnesses such as diabetes are at higher risk of developing mental health problems and disorders. Liaison and collaboration with paediatric services is crucial.
- Academic failure.
- Low self-esteem.
- Maltreatment (physical or sexual abuse, harsh discipline, neglect) has a marked influence on development, and often results in significant psychopathology.

Family risk factors

- Children of families suffering from socioeconomic disadvantage, family discord and particularly overt family/parental conflict and violence have a higher risk and this is more likely to occur if parents are unemployed or homeless.
- Family environment: development is influenced by the quality of the family environment in which the child is reared. Family environments which foster adaptive psychological development are characterized by the family's ability to provide physical and emotional care, secure attachment relationships, consistency, and appropriate, non-punitive limit setting. Secure attachment relationships are those that reduce anxiety and provide emotional protection in stressful situations. Family environments that have a negative effect on psychological development tend to be characterized by lack of affection, parental conflict, overprotection, and inconsistent rules and discipline and difficulties adapting to a child's changing developmental needs.
- Abuse: physical, sexual and or emotional.
- Parental ill health: mental illness (including maternal depression) and drug and alcohol abuse in parents are risk factors for the emotional well-being of the child.
- Parental criminality, alcoholism and personality disorder.
- Death and loss including friendships.

Environmental risk factors

- Socioeconomic disadvantage.
- Homelessness.
- Disaster.
- Discrimination also significantly increases risk and this is affected by local and national attitudes and values.[19]

Resilience

Mental health is not just the absence of a problem, but also the resilience to cope despite adversity, e.g. higher intelligence is usually associated with a decreased risk and a better prognosis.[19]

Research has shown three groups of factors which appear to protect children and adolescents in situations of adversity:

- at an individual level: self-esteem, sociability and autonomy;
- at a family level: family compassion, warmth and absence of discord;
- at a community level: social support systems that encourage personal effort.[19,22]

Reflection

Consider a parent, child or young person you are working with.

- Identify the risk and protective factors at an individual, family and community level.
- How could you work with the child/family to gain a joint understanding of their risk and protective factor profile?
- How could you work in partnership with the child/family to decide on the risks to be reduced and the protective factors to be promoted?
- What strategies could you offer the child/family to reduce the risks and promote the protective factors in ways that might be effective, feasible and acceptable to the family?

PRINCIPLES OF A COMPREHENSIVE CAMH SERVICE

All children must be seen as part of their family and wider community and social systems,[22,24] and therefore the goal of a comprehensive child and adolescent mental health service is to deliver seamless, culturally sensitive multi-sectoral mental health services for children, adolescents and young people and their families in a way that maximizes the total set of resources and partnerships in the community.

Partnership working

Effective partnership working can improve children and young people's experience of services and lead to improved outcomes.[22] Once a child or young person has been referred to specialist CAMH services, nurses and other professionals must ensure that effective partnerships are continued or that they are established across all of the systems with which the child and family need to interact.

A CAMH SERVICE MODEL

A tiered model of care for CAMH services is in operation in the UK.[6,7] The tiered model is based on the principle that CAMH services should be structured to provide the

---

Personal illustration 55.1: Partnership working

Sheila, a community psychiatric nurse is currently working with Emma, who suffers from bipolar disorder. Emma has two children aged 9 and 11. Emma is a single parent, living in rented accommodation on state benefit. Sheila is aware that children of parents with mental illness have an increased risk for developing CAMH disorders, particularly when in it combined with poverty. She has worked with Emma and with social services to provide family support. Although Sheila's assessment indicates that the children appear to be functioning well on a day-to-day basis, she is aware that they are both becoming increasingly anxious and confused about their mother's illness.

With Emma's permission, she contacts the CAMH primary mental health worker to discuss ways of promoting the children's mental health and their understanding of their mother's experiences. Through this, they identify that there is a gap in services for children of parents suffering from a mental illness. The CAMH service set up a group in collaboration with the school health advisor for children, whose parents have mental health problems. The group aim is to provide health education about mental illness, share anxieties, and provide support and to help the children to recognize when they feel stressed and how to seek support.

Evaluation of the group indicated that the children felt that they developed a better understanding of mental illness, their anxiety was reduced and they felt less isolated. The group thus succeeded in promoting the children's skills and understanding of mental health and promoted their future resilience for coping with any further parental episodes of mental illness and also how to recognize their own stress/mental health problems and how to seek support for this. Emma described how she felt that participation in the group had helped her to communicate with her children and to feel supported as a parent. Through sharing experiences with others, Emma began to feel less guilty about how her illness may have impacted on her children and had become more aware of her own strengths as a parent.

Sheila, the school nurse and the social worker worked in partnership with the participating parents and children to put together a proposal for joint funding to mainstream the children and parents group across adult mental health, CAMH, social services and primary care services. They used their evaluation as well as literature on risk and resilience and the importance of supporting parents with mental illness and their children[25] to underpin their proposal.

---

health visitors/public health nurses and general practitioners. These non-CAMH specialist staff can (with support from specialist CAMH staff in the other tiers) identify mental health problems early in their development, offer general advice and in certain cases provide treatment for less severe mental health problems and pursue opportunities for promoting mental health and preventing mental health problems.

Tier 2 refers to individual professionals including clinical psychologists, child psychiatrists, occupational therapists, psychotherapists and community CAMH nurses. In England, CAMH primary mental health workers (PMHWs) lead on tier 2 work by offering training and consultation to other professionals in tier 1, providing consultation for professionals and families, offering outreach to identify severe or complex needs when children of families are unwilling to use specialist services and providing assessment which may trigger treatment at another tier.

Tier 3 refers to specialist multidisciplinary community and outpatient services and includes social work, clinical psychologists, community psychiatric nurses, child psychiatrists, psychotherapists, occupational therapists, play therapists, family therapists, art, music and drama therapists. They provide multidisciplinary assessment and treatment of CAMH disorders, assessment for referral to tier 4 services and consultation to other tiers as well as participation in research and development projects.

Tier 4 CAMH services refer to highly specialist tertiary services such as day units, highly specialist outpatient clinics and inpatient units for older children and adolescents who are severely mentally ill or at suicide risk. Admission to tier 4 inpatients represents a last resort service as taking a child or adolescent away from their family and social milieu should be avoided whenever possible.

Admission for treatment may be indicated when the child/young person's behaviour is so disturbed that management elsewhere cannot be practically sustained. The main reasons for someone going into inpatient care are to make sure the young person is safe, and to provide intensive treatment to reduce their level of distress.

Day patient services are offered to children, whose problems are too complex or do not respond at tier 3 and require that the children/young people spend large parts of their waking day in a therapeutic milieu, where they can receive an in-depth assessment across settings and receive therapy, education and joint work whilst work with their families is undertaken.

least invasive care in the least intensive setting, commensurate with effectiveness. Children should only be referred to the next tier if it is evident (through rigorous assessment) that a less invasive tier cannot meet their needs.

Tier 1 refers to primary care CAMH, which provides universal services, i.e. available to all children and families by professionals such as school nurses, teachers,

---

Reflection

- Why is it important to have an optimum combination of universal, targeted and specialist CAMH services?
- What do you mean by a comprehensive CAMH service?

Personal illustration 55.2:   Tiered CAMH

Jim, aged 16, was seen as an emergency by the 24-hour crisis assessment team. The police had prevented him from jumping off the roof of the local library. Jim was convinced he had been given a special gift from God that he could fly and was invincible. If not closely supervised, he attempted to run away and find a higher roof in an attempt to demonstrate his powers and he became increasingly agitated by and suspicious of those who attempted to stop him. He was referred to the Early Intervention in Psychosis (EIP) team, who felt that his persistent and deeply routed delusions meant that he was a significant danger to himself. Because of his age, they decided that he needed to be cared for by professionals with an in-depth understanding of adolescent development and mental health disorders.

They assessed that he was intellectually able to engage in discussions, despite his delusional beliefs. With the help of his mother and his grandparents, Jim was persuaded to be admitted to the specialist adolescent inpatient unit, without the need for a section, to begin an in-depth assessment and provision of care to ensure his safety. In the unit, Jim responded to his medication and in the safe, predictable milieu of the unit, he was helped to understand his experiences and to develop coping mechanisms to deal with his distress. He was soon discharged from inpatient care to the community EIP service.

Through liaison with Jim, his mother, his GP and teacher, it was possible to gain an in-depth assessment and greater understanding of his behaviours and distress. Jim had suffered a range of life crises and had been subject to a cumulative set of risks. His parents had divorced a year ago and he had moved with his mother to a new city 6 months ago. He had always had difficulties making friends, although in his previous location, he had enjoyed the company of two special friends, whom he had known from primary school. He struggled academically and appeared to be underachieving at school. A psychological assessment was organized and this indicated that he had profound literacy problems, which had not been previously picked up.

In his new school, Jim was quiet, had not caused any problems and was considered to be of lower academic ability. The academic difficulties and his sense of failure gradually increased Jim's sense of isolation. He tried cannabis 4 months ago and finding that this helped him to relax, he progressively increased his use of it as a way of self-medicating. His mother was unaware of this.

To formulate a long-term strategy with Jim, a joint assessment of his risk and protective factors were completed at an individual family and community level.

At an individual level, Jim had an increased risk of developing psychosis. His uncle had suffered a number of psychotic episodes. He had low self-esteem because of his academic difficulties and temperamentally he had never adapted well to change. However, prior to his illness, Jim had been an excellent golfer and when he was younger had been a good gymnast.

At a family level, His mother was well educated and worked as a personal secretary before they moved. She felt more supported as she was nearer to her parents, who doted on Jim and this was reciprocated. Jim's father visited when he could but because of the acrimonious divorce, contact tended to be stressful for all concerned.

At a community level, Jim was isolated and beginning to identify with peers involved in drug misuse, which posed a major community problem.

As a result of the assessment, a plan was agreed with Jim and his parents to reduce the risks and capitalize on his strengths. Through family work, Jim's parents and grandparents were helped to understand and work together to meet Jim's needs for predictability and routine, particularly around access to his father.

A community nurse from the EIP team became his case manager and met him on a weekly basis. The EIP service provided specialist education and support to help Jim and his parents to understand psychosis, medication and Jim's need to be in a predictable routine. A drug worker from the adolescent team agreed to meet with Jim to discuss his use of cannabis and to help to stop using skunk. Jim agreed to attend a group with other adolescents recovering from a psychotic episode and found that sharing his experiences made them feel less frightening. From this group, the young people were supported to meet a youth worker and to gradually take part in community activities in which they felt safe and interested. Jim's mother responded well to education about psychosis and represented a major source of strength for Jim and also increased the understanding of the grandparents. Jim's father agreed to take more responsibility for Jim by planning a predictable visiting schedule.

With the permission of Jim and his mother, a meeting was organized in school and plans were made to support him with his literacy and to encourage him with sports and English. His mentor in school arranged a meeting to discuss employment opportunities with Jim, who had mentioned that he would like to work in a golf club. The school health adviser agreed to meet Jim every 2 weeks, initially in school, in order to support him and to intervene quickly with any signs of stress or relapse indicators.

The coordination of services across tier 4 CAMH inpatient, community EIP service, tier 1 and the universal services provided in school, employment services, youth services, tier 2 services to provide education to Jim and his family, CAMH drug and alcohol services all helped Jim to balance his risks with protective factors and to develop sufficient resilience to begin to return to school. Continued work to build his self-esteem through literacy classes and sports, in which he excelled, helped him to address his developmental tasks of adolescence. The sports activities were particularly useful in helping Jim to engage with a small group of peers, to develop a more positive image of himself and begin to return to his developmental trajectory. The combination of his increased resilience and his increased understanding about psychosis and early signs helped to attenuate the risk of a further damaging psychotic episode.

Transition to adult mental health services

Mental health problems in young people have been found to be a clear predictor of problems in adulthood[26] and therefore networks between CAMH services and adult mental health services (AMHS) are essential.

Protocols should be in place to ensure that if required, young people experience a smooth transition of care between child and AMHS. Training for adult mental health staff on the developmental needs of young people is crucial. If a young person goes to an adult ward, services must ensure that child protection and safeguarding of young people is adhered to and the dignity and safety of young people cared for in adult psychiatric beds is met.

Reflection

How would you ensure a smooth transition for a young person from a CAMH service to an adult mental health service?

What skills and knowledge do adult mental health services need to take care of young people aged 18–25?

SUMMARY

Children and young people are members of a number of interrelated systems and networks including families, schools, youth work and employment. This chapter has explored how *collaboration across agencies* as well as *partnership* with children, young people and their families, is necessary for holistic care.

An awareness and appreciation of the rights of children and younger people is fundamental to CAMH services.

CAMH services need to develop a philosophy and working practices, which develops, values and respects young people, and acknowledge the important role they play in their own health and well-being. Services should be offered to children, young people and their parents in ways that are respectful of their own culture and appropriate to the developmental stage of the young person.

REFERENCES

1. Timimi S. *Pathological child psychiatry and the medicalisation of childhood*. Hove, UK: Brunner Routledge, 2002

2. UN. *The United Nations Convention on the rights of the child*. Geneva: United Nations, 1989.

3. Mental Health Foundation. *Turned upside down*. London, UK: MHF, 2001.

4. Prillitensky I. Value-based praxis in community psychology: moving towards social justice and social action. *American Journal of Community Psychology* 2001; **29**: 747–78.

5. World Health Organization. *Child and adolescent mental health resources. Global concerns: implications for their future*. Geneva: World Health Organization, 2005.

6. Health Advisory Service (HAS). *Together we stand: thematic review*. CAMH. London, UK: HMSO, 1995.

7. Department of Health. *National services framework for children, young people and maternity services. The mental health and psychological well being of children and young people*. *Core*. London, UK: HMSO, 2004.

8. World Health Organization. *Caring for children with mental disorders: setting WHO directives*. Geneva: World Health Organization, 2003.

9. Offord DR, Chmura Kraemer H, Kazdin AE *et al.* Lowering the burden of suffering from child psychiatric disorders: trade offs among clinical, targeted and universal interventions. *Journal of American Academy of Child and Adolescent Psychiatry* 1998; **37**: 686–95.

10. Scott S, Knapp M, Henderson J *et al.* Financial cost of social exclusion: follow up study of anti-social children into adulthood. *British Medical Journal* 2001; **322**: 191–5.

11. Office National Statistics. *Mental health of children and young people in Great Britain, 2004*. London, UK: HMSO, 2005.

12. Waddell C, Offord D, Shepherd C, Hua J. Child psychiatric epidemiology and Canadian public policy making: the state of science and the art of the possible. *Canadian Journal of Psychiatry* 2002; **47**: 825–32.

13. World Health Organization. *The ICD-10 classification of mental and behavioural disorders: diagnostic criteria for research*. Geneva: WHO, 1993.

14. British Medical Association. *Adolescent mental health*. London, UK: BMA, 2003.

15. Young Minds. *Mental health services for adolescents and young adults*. London, UK: Young Minds, 2002.

16. Sroufe LA. *Emotional development: the organisation of emotional life in the early years*. New York, NY: Cambridge University Press, 1996.

17. Sroufe LA. Psychopathology as an outcome of development. *Development and Psychopathology* 1997; **9**: 251–68.

18. Bee H, Boyd D. *The developing child: Pearson international edition*. New York, NY: Pearson Education, 2006.

19. Haggerty RJ, Sherrod LR, Garmezy N, Rutter M. *Stress, risk and resilience in children and adolescents*. Cambridge, UK: Cambridge University Press, 1996.

20. Henggeler S, Rowland MD, Schoenwald SK. *Serious emotional disturbance in children and adolescents: multisystemic therapy*. New York: Guilford press, 2002: 24–60.

21. Cunningham C, Bremner R, Boyle M. Large group community based parenting program for families of pre-schoolers at risk of disruptive behaviour disorders: utilisation of cost effectiveness and outcome. *Journal of Child Psychology and Psychiatry* 1995; **36**: 1141–59.

22. Swenson CC, Henggeler S, Taylor IS, Addison OW. *Multisystemic therapy and neighbourhood partnerships: reducing adolescent violence and substance abuse*. New York, NY: Guildford Press, 2005.

23. Croom S, Procter S. The Newcan Practice Framework: using risk and resilience to work at the interface between professional expertise and parental knowledge and experience in child and adolescent mental health. *Practice* 2005; **2**: 114–26.

24. Brofenbrenner U. Ecological systems theory. In: Vasta R (ed.). *Six theories of child development: revised formulation and current issues.* London, UK: Jessica Kingsley, 2005: 197–249.

25. Place M, Reynolds J, Cousins A, O'Neill S. Developing a resilience package for vulnerable children. *Child and Adolescent Mental Health* 2002; **7**: 162–7.

26. Koot HM. Longitudinal studies of general populations and community samples. In: Verhulstand FC, Koot HM (eds). *The epidemiology of child and adolescent psychopathology.* Oxford, UK: Oxford University Press, 1995: 337–65.

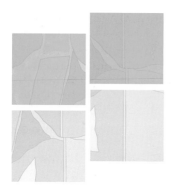

CHAPTER 56

Services for older people with mental health conditions

Trevor Adams* and Elizabeth Collier**

INTRODUCTION

Demographic studies show that because of increased life expectancy and declining fertility rates there is likely to be a global increase of older people in the future, particularly those over the age of 75 years. The World Health Organization estimates that there will be 1.2 billion older people worldwide by 2025.[1] Epidemiological studies show that the incidence of various forms of dementia increases with age, although depression is the most common mental health problem in later life with a prevalence of around 15%.[2] This has two important implications. First, the majority of older people do not have mental health problems; and, second, despite this, there is likely to be an increased number of older people in society who *do* have mental health conditions. Quite clearly, there is an urgent need to develop effective and appropriate services to older people who have a range of mental health conditions.

Mental health nurses work within different policy contexts in different parts of the world. However, a number of key principles appear to be similar, namely mental health promotion, healthy living, independence, integrated services and challenging age discrimination. The differences appear to be largely dictated by where older people mental services are located, i.e. whether older people with mental health conditions benefit from a general mental health policy that includes access, for example, to early intervention services, crisis services and psychological therapies, or are addressed within an older person's generic policy that focus on the *older person context* rather then the mental health context. In some places, such problems have created an inadvertent discriminatory policy towards older people with mental health problems.

AGEISM AND SERVICE PROVISION

The provision of services to older people, including people with mental health conditions has been affected by *ageism* and is a significant issue for health care in which direct age discrimination – such as the rationing of treatment – is

*Trevor Adams lectures in mental health nursing at the University of Surrey, Guildford, UK. He has specialized in dementia care nursing for 25 years within practice, education and research. He has authored over 50 chapters and papers and edited three books.
**Elizabeth Collier is a lecturer in mental health at the University of Salford, UK. She is currently a PhD student researching the effect that long-term mental ill health has on the achievements and goals of older adults.

recognized and addressed through policy documents and research. In the UK the Healthcare Commission[3] identified age discrimination as one issue where there has been a lack of progress in service provision, and indirect age discrimination is particularly problematic.[4] Indirect age discrimination is more subtle and often goes unchallenged as individuals perpetuate society's acceptance of this through their use of language, fuelled by advertising and the media. These phenomena have entered nursing, reinforcing stereotypical attitudes in nursing practice. Butterworth[5,p.39] for example, states:

> working with elderly confused and dementing patients was, in my own training lifetime, used as a punishment for nurses who had overstepped the mark or committed an organisational misdemeanour.

Also there is a medical legacy that may influence attitudes to older people with mental health problems. Mental illnesses, other than dementia, were not recognized in older people until the 1950s, and diagnoses such as schizophrenia relevant for older people, were not written into diagnostic manuals until the 1980s. Beekman et al.[2,p.213] stated:

> older people with serious depression do not have symptoms that fit current classification of mood disorders which have been generated to reflect symptoms in younger people. Older people may have insufficient symptoms to meet the threshold for the disorder and presentation differs because of ageing, physical illness or both.

Reflection

What examples of ageism have you seen in mental health nursing?

Adams[6] argues that mental health nursing in the UK primarily focused on 'severe and enduring mental illness' (i.e. psychoses) in the 1990s, and was only really interested in younger people with functional psychoses such as mania and schizophrenia, not older people or people with organic psychoses, such as dementia. Increased funding was made available and psychosocial interventions (PSI) were developed and formed part of the work of many mental health nurses. These services and interventions however, largely followed an ageist agenda and typically did not deal with older people, particularly those with dementia.

More recently, Collier[7] illustrated how indirect age discrimination could affect the appropriate provision of care for an older woman through a vignette presented to student mental health nurses. Groups identified the issues and the help that they thought a woman who has been married for 40 years and who is confused about her sexuality

and failing marriage would need. Despite the nature of her concerns, it has been common belief among students that she misinterprets her feelings for lack of friendship and needs referring to psychiatric or neurological services for assessment for dementia. This reflects 'the Alzheimerization of ageing' in which all older people are thought likely to develop dementia, and there is a reverse discrimination for younger people with dementia who may not receive a timely or appropriate diagnosis of early onset dementia. One suggestion has been for services to address the question: 'Are you working with health promotion to reduce stigma and discrimination around older people with mental health problems and the early recognition of dementia?'[8]

This chapter, written in the spirit of the inclusive approach, applies ideologies and language used in services for people of 'working age' to services for older people, in the belief that this will reduce the dichotomy between services for older people and those for people of working age, and help stop the differential provision of services to older people with mental health conditions.

WORKING WITH DIFFERENCE

Recent developments within the social sciences have highlighted how dominant groups establish whatever is considered 'normal'. Often expert knowledge, such as that of medicine, identifies what is normal by defining 'the other' as abnormal. There is a need to respect other people's differences and understand the value their contribution can make within society. Within mental health nursing there is a strong tradition of accepting people as they are, and adopting a non-judgemental approach. All mental health services need to adopt this approach.

There is a tendency to treat older people as a homogeneous group despite the fact that, with longer life, there may be two generations of a family over the age of 65. Can we assume that our ways of working with a 65 year old are going to be based on the same model of care as for a 90 year old? Clearly, the principles will be similar, and individual differences will dictate how we proceed, but this question is rarely examined. On what evidence do we base our practices? Attention to equality and working with difference remains of utmost importance. However, unmet needs can be found in services for older people. One group who has perhaps not received the same attention as others are people who are deaf. Older deaf people (sign language users) who are in need of care may be placed with people with dementia, without access to sign language-speaking staff, whether or not they have dementia themselves. This has serious implications for the care of a group of people whose needs are not being met.

People with learning disability have particular needs in relation to their care. People with Down's syndrome, for example, commonly develop Alzheimer's disease, and as they are living longer these issues become more prevalent for services. They often fall between services as they may not be accepted in a mental heath service or a learning disability service, both believing they belong in the other.

Sexuality issues are gaining increased recognition for older people. The Alzheimer's Society recognizes particular needs of gay and lesbian partners. Many older people will have lived through times when homosexuality was illegal and as such may not have disclosed their sexuality until late in life. Also, stereotyped ideas about old people and sex has prevented acceptance of this as an issue for older people.

In addition, different cultural perspectives may affect access to mental health services. Marwaha and Livingstone[9] found that older black African Caribbean people were more likely to identify 'depression' and 'psychosis' as a spiritual issue and turn to a faith leader for help. In their study, mental health services were considered only relevant for violent people and irrelevant to them.

The examples are particular 'minority' issues. However, we would support this understanding of *difference* in society and would recognize and value difference in older people with respect to gender, sexuality, ethnicity and disability.

In addition to recognizing and acknowledging difference, we also argue that mental health services for older people should not only focus on the individual but should also affirm their identity and enhance their well-being. We support Kitwood's[10] approach, in his development of person-centred care, but believe that this approach should not be restricted to people with dementia, but extended to all older people with a mental health condition. Within the UK this approach has been developed in social policy that supports the maintenance of dignity and the promotion of respect to older people. It is perhaps the nearest framework for understanding how we can work with people with dementing illnesses, however, the more recent emergence of a 'recovery' framework (see Box 56.1) for understanding mental health has emerged. There has been little debate to date as to how the ideas associated with recovery apply to people with dementing illnesses, as Woods[11] notes, although he points out that definitions incorporating 'living with (limitations)', hope, and developing meaning and purpose within any experience of ill health, has resonance with how people with dementia might describe their situations. One illustration of a dementia service that has used this approach to underpin care is described later. It is perhaps easier to see how it could be applied with older adults who have mental health conditions that do not have an organic origin such as those diagnosed with clinical depression, anxiety or schizophrenia. In practice however, it is possible that thinking in terms of older people needing only 'care', rather than

applying 'recovery' thinking and exploring personal development and citizenship in the same way as for younger people appears to remain challenging.

Reflection

Are the needs of older people with mental health conditions, who do not fit into mainstream groups, addressed by mental health nurses?

PROMOTING RECOVERY

Recent interest within mental health nursing has concerned the idea of 'recovery'. Deegan[12] sees 'recovery' as the lived or real life experience of people as they accept and overcome the challenge of a disability, and this corresponds with a disability perspective towards mental health in which therapeutic engagement with clients is concerned with facilitating acceptance and growth about their condition and/or situation. At first sight, the idea of recovery might not appear to fit well with some older people with mental health conditions, such as people with dementia. But this view is dependent on a medical rather that a disability perspective, and assumes that recovery means cure. However, within the approach, recovery is not the same as cure and although people may never be cured, they are able to attain an acceptance and growth about their condition and/or situation.

Box 56.1

Recovery in mental health nursing with older people is:

- the lived or real life experience of people as they accept and overcome the challenge the disabling effect of having dementia and physical, emotional and social hardship of providing care;
- not the same as cure;
- about growth: does not refer to an end-product or a result;
- not limited to a particular theory about the nature and causes of dementia;
- not specific to people with dementia and includes family carers;
- about taking back control over one's life;
- not a linear process;
- different for every person and is deeply personal.

Adapted from Repper and Perkins.[13]

Reflection

How do you think 'recovery' ideas apply to mental health nursing with older people?

PROMOTING PARTICIPATION

We also would see older people as making an active contribution within local communities. This approach draws on an activity approach towards older people and also that older people should have the responsibility, wherever possible, for their own health and social care decisions. We would argue that nurses should take the view that older people, even those with cognitive impairments, have views and opinions and that it is the responsibility of nurses to do whatever they can to hear what older people are saying. We would thus see nurses and other health and social care professionals as helping older people with mental health conditions making choices about the services that they receive. In addition, we would argue that older people should be involved in each service development that includes commissioning, design, development and evaluation of services.

VOICE OF SERVICE USERS

People with dementia have views and opinions and there is a moral obligation upon family members and nurses to hear what people with dementia want to say and make their views and choices known. The idea of 'voice' used here has a more political connotation than how it is generally used in everyday speech. It is the voice of the weaker person, in this case someone weakened by cognitive impairment, and is closely associated with having or not having power. Often people with dementia find that their views, interests and agendas are passed over and that those of other family members, medical practitioners, nurses and informal carers are given priority. Sometimes the stories that are shared within dementia care situations offer people with dementia a subject position in which they are represented as having little ability to say anything worthwhile and gives rise to their disempowerment. Stories therefore provide more than just insights into the experience of the person with dementia and family carers, they also offer people a subject position in which they are seen as having particular expectations, responsibilities and obligations.

Brooker and Dinshaw[14] suggest that staff in old age psychiatry can feel as disempowered as the patients they serve. A 5-year research study to hear the voice of both service users *and* staff on psychogeriatric inpatient assessment wards, gave a powerful message that they hold the key to quality improvement themselves. They conducted interviews with 75 patients (on discharge) and 85 staff. The patients and staff identified different issues such as, from staff, timing of meal times, afternoon tea as a social occasion; and from patients, condiments on tables at meal times and staff to wear names badges. Interestingly, however, there was an increased dissatisfaction amongst the nurses during this process due it seems to their empowerment and changed expectations.

Reflection

How is the voice of older people with mental health conditions heard within mental heath nursing ?

MENTAL HEALTH SERVICES FOR OLDER PEOPLE

There is a range of services that work with older people who have mental health conditions, located in primary, secondary and tertiary settings. These are offered by health and social care agencies and calls for good collaboration between the two agencies. This collaboration is necessary because many older people have multiple health and social difficulties and it is necessary to offer packages of care that draw on health and social care resources. Primary care may be offered by a range of agencies such as GPs and practice nurses. Secondary services may include agencies that are part of the mainstream such as acute general units and respite care and those that are specialist services for older people with mental health conditions, such as community mental health nurses, home care, day care, respite care and specialist housing offering extra care provision. Tertiary care may be offered by residential and nursing care homes and inpatient services.

It is important to note that because older people with mental health conditions are frequently in mainstream, non-mental health services, they can find themselves in services that are unable to meet their needs. This is a growing difficulty as the number of older people increases. There is thus an urgent need to enhance the ability of non-specialist health and social care workers to assess and appropriately implement care to people with mental health conditions. In addition, there is an increasing need for mental health nurses in specialist agencies to liaise with agencies offering non-specialist care to older people with mental health conditions.

It is also worthwhile to note that much of the support and care given to older people with mental health conditions arises in informal settings such as families, friends and neighbours. However, it is usually the family that is able to provide a sustainable means of support, though this often breaks down when the physical and emotional demands of providing care becomes too great. Often the provision of informal care within families falls along gender lines with female family members finding that there is an expectation amongst the rest of the family that they should be the primary provider of care to its dependent members. However, it is often the case that men find giving care difficult and are ill prepared to deal with such a role. Mental health nurses can offer carers a range of interventions that are aimed to promote the carer's well-being that includes information and support through individual meetings and relative support groups and help gaining access to different agencies.

Mental health nurses working in crisis teams, assertive outreach or early interventions services often find themselves working with people of 'working age'. This is because these services are largely influenced by age-related service models of care provision as described earlier. These services are therefore not available to older people, even though the first onset of mental ill health in later life is just as common for older people as for any other age group. Cooper et al.[15] found that only 25 (31.6%) of the 79 English NHS Trusts providing acute mental health services with at least one crisis resolution team offered this service to older people. People with dementia had access to crisis services in only 1 in 10 cases. One example of a service that has attempted to redress this issue through creative interpretation of national policy is the specialist mental health intermediate care team within Cambridgeshire and Peterborough Mental Health Partnership NHS Trust. This team provides a rapid/crisis response and intensive home treatment for people with acute mental health problems, and enables avoidance of unnecessary admissions to hospital or attendance at A&E departments. This service is independent of the younger adult crisis resolution home treatment service in the locality (N Joy, personal communication).

> ## Reflection
>
> Should older people share the same mental health services as younger people?

CARE HOME EDUCATION AND SUPPORT SERVICE, NORTH CUMBRIA, UK

One community mental health team for older people that incorporates many of the ideas that we have outlined is the Care Home Education and Support Service (CHESS) based in North Cumbria, UK. The service offers a rolling programme of education for residential home care workers and supports the transition of people to care homes from hospital services and from care homes to other community settings. The broad aim of CHESS is to improve the quality of life of older people with mental health problems by integrating and developing inpatient and community services so that a seamless service is provided that meets people's individual needs. Underpinning CHESS is the idea that the integration of care may be achieved by improving the knowledge and skills of staff in care homes and is based on the belief that it will limit the need to transfer clients to other settings and will therefore reduce the distress on older people and their relatives. CHESS illustrates its philosophy by adopting a logo comprising chess pieces and develops the analogy that the initial position of clients is like that of a pawn in the game with little influence on the outcome of the game. The vision of CHESS is that the patient becomes the king and that the

other pieces in the game work together to protect the king throughout his mental health journey. The recovery approach is central to service provision within CHESS. This approach aimed to realize people's potential, not to focus on their ill-being or medical diagnosis, and provided a clear link between their past, present and future. Instead, the focus of client care was on their maximizing well-being, strengths and promoting how they or others could cope with the differing consequences of each part of the client's mental health experience.

The project adopted a two-pronged approach towards achieving its overriding aim. The first was through the development of a rolling education programme for staff in care homes and the second was the development of an outreach service that offered practical support with individual patients and offers support through skilled interventions and therapeutic activities. In addition, CHESS offers staff in care homes knowledge and the skills that will enable them to understand and manage mental health issues through the use of person-centred care and a range of therapeutic approaches that included use of life story work, cognitive stimulation, specific interventions such as psychological therapies. Moreover, an important part of the work of CHESS is by working with the care homes and the inpatient services to provide a structured staged discharge for patients from the ward to the care home.

CHESS has been very successful and its benefits have affected not just external services but its own. It was found that following the introduction of CHESS there was a substantial reduction in admissions to hospital from care homes because of care homes being able to manage residents with mental health issues. Moreover, there was an increased recognition of staff in care homes to recognize when residents were experiencing mental health difficulties and also improved use of psychological skills to address issues that arose. The project has improved and developed knowledge about mental health and has developed the skill of care staff in the homes and has helped create a transition from task orientated to person-centred care. 'Pledges' have been used to monitor what changes staff will make in their practice following attendance at the education programme. These are then signed off by members of the CHESS team and the care home manager to try to influence change. CHESS has consistently seen improvement in recognition and management of mental health issues among care home staff.

'GRADUATES'

There are two distinct groups of people in terms of mental heath and older people – those who experience mental ill health for the first time in later life, and those that have experienced mental ill health through a long period of their lives, often from their early twenties. These people are often referred to as 'graduates' within the medical literature.[16] This is a particularly important group of clients as it has been suggested that many people thought to be 'lost' to services when they 'graduate' has been due to death by natural causes or suicide, or homelessness.[17] However the lack of records means that we do not know for sure how many people are affected. It is also interesting as people who lose contact with services after 65 were potentially people who previously had or were perceived as needing (and were receiving) highly supportive packages of care (particularly those diagnosed with schizophrenia). The needs of 'graduates' have been rarely investigated in the literature, although Dadswell[18] found four themes relating to the move from 'adult' services to 'old age' services. These relate to 'connectivity', where the relationship was more important than where the care was received; 'dichotomy of self', where being moved to 'old age' services without consultation made them face an issue that they had not previously found significant, that is being considered 'old'; 'meaningful life', where occupational type activity was lost when leaving 'adult' services; and 'done unto', where there was a resigned acceptance. Although there is very little published evidence about this issue, in the UK many services have now implemented 'transition' policies as a response to anti-discriminatory and needs-based health policy, where people who reach their 65th birthday no longer are automatically moved from 'adult' services to 'old age' services but remain with the team they may have been with for some time, only moving to an old age team if they develop significant changes related to dementia or physical ill health.

One service model that has been implemented in Shropshire is shown in Box 56.2.

Box 56.2: Shropshire model (Marpole[19])

- Specialist nurse practitioner role (specific study at degree level)
- Oversee the transition of patients from adult services to services for older people
- Patient referred by adult team at age 64
- Comprehensive review with adult services care coordinator for one year
- Review includes diagnosis, physical and mental health, social care needs
- Patient included in planning care
- Patient carers and statutory or voluntary agencies included
- Nurse-led outpatient clinical for patients run by specialist practitioners
- Clinics act as a way of remaining in contact with patients who are at risk of relapse
- Clinics ensure continuity of care
- Those unable to attend clinics are visited at home

SUMMARY

Not all types of services available for older people have been reflected here; however, a range of issues have been discussed and examples provided. As can be seen in the examples, local innovations and the commitment of the teams involved are often at the centre of meaningful developments. This should encourage nurses to challenge any current provision that restricts access to older people. Although policy for older people addresses mental health, it does not assist in addressing the context for older people with mental illness, and as such they tend to remain relatively excluded from benefiting from general developments in mental health services. Age-defined services utilize an arbitrary age of 65 (in some places 75) to organize services and this potentially contributes to a misunderstanding of over 65s as a homogeneous group.

The mental health of older people is one of the most complex and interesting areas of nursing as an understanding of ageing processes as well as rigorous examination of personal attitudes and beliefs is required. The willingness of mental health nurses to meet this challenge will ensure effective services will continue to be developed for the future.

Reflection

- How is the individual diversity of older adults reflected in services offered?
- Why are older people largely thought of in 'care' terms?
- What are the barriers to working with older people as people and citizens rather than 'service users'?

REFERENCES

1. WHO. *The world is fast ageing – have we noticed?* www.who.int/ageing/en/. Accessed 10 January 2008.

2. Beekman AT, Copeland JR, Prince MJ. Review of community prevalence of depression in later life. *British Journal of Psychiatry*. 1999; **174**: 307–11.

3. Healthcare Commission, Audit commission, CSCI. *Living well in later life*. London, UK: Commission for Healthcare Audit and Inspection, 2006.

4. Department of Health. *National service framework for older people: interim report on age discrimination*. 2002. Available from: www.dh.gov.uk/en/Policyandguidance/Healthandsocialcaretopics/Olderpeoplesservices/DH_4001924.

5. Butterworth T. Breaking the boundaries. *Nursing Times* 1988; **34**: 36–9.

6. Adams T. *Dementia care nursing*. Basingstoke, UK: Palgrave Macmillan, 2008.

7. Collier E. Approaches to help support and care. In: Neno R, Aveyard B, Heath H (eds). *Mental health nursing and older people. A handbook of care*. Oxford, UK: Blackwell Publishing, 2007.

8. CSIP (Care Services Improvement Partnership). *Supplementary guidance for older peoples mental health services.* Colchester, UK: CSIP, 2007.

9. Marwaha S, Livingstone G. Stigma racism or choice. Why do depressed ethnic elders avoid psychiatrists. *Journal of Affective Disorders* 2002; **72** (3): 257–65.

10. Kitwood T. *Dementia reconsidered.* Buckingham, UK: Open University Press, 1997.

11. Woods B. Recovery – is it relevant to older people? *Signposts* 2007; **12** (1): 2–3.

12. Deegan P. Recovery as a journey of the heart. *Psychiatric Rehabilitation Journal* 1996; **19** (3): 91–7.

13. Repper J, Perkins R. *Social inclusion and recovery a model for mental health practice.* Edinburgh, UK: Ballière Tindall, 2003.

14. Brooker DJ, Dinshaw CJ. Staff and patient feedback in mental health services for older people. *Quality in Health Care* 1998; **7**: 70–6.

15. Cooper C, Regan C, Tandy AR *et al.* Acute mental health care for older people by crisis resolution teams in England. *International Journal of Geriatric Psychiatry* 2007; **22**: 263–5.

16. Kalim S, Overshott R, Burns A. 'Older people with chronic schizophrenia'. *Aging and Mental Health* 2005; **9** (4): 315–24.

17. Campbell P, Ananth H. Graduates. In: Jacoby R, Oppenheimer C (eds). *Psychiatry and the elderly*, 3rd edn. Oxford, UK: Oxford University Press, 2002.

18. Dadswell RA. 'What does it feel like to be transferred from adult mental health services, to services for older people on reaching the age of 65 years? The lived experience is explored using a phenomenological approach'. Unpublished thesis in part fulfilment of MSc Advanced Practice (Mental Health). University of Surrey, 2005.

19. Marpole A. Specialist nurse practitioners in mental health: the Shropshire experience. *Nursing Older People* 2005; **17** (2): 20–2.

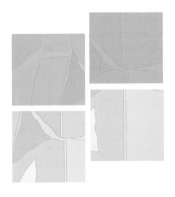

CHAPTER 57

Early interventions in psychosis

Paul French*

INTRODUCTION

Each year in the UK about 7500 people will develop a first episode of psychosis (FEP), the onset usually occurring in young people (aged 16–30). Often, they can experience lifelong problems, leaving them on the margins of society, struggling to maintain relationships, or employment, an income or a home. As many as 1:10 die by suicide often within the first 5 years. Families, friends and communities often carry huge burdens of care.

A growing body of research shows that the early phase of psychosis is well understood and underpins secondary prevention strategies translated into specific programmes for early intervention within the UK and internationally. Prior to these developments, on average, people could wait up to 2 years before getting meaningful and effective help. Access to early intervention in psychosis (EIP) services is still variable by country and by region. Where no service exists, about half these young people can expect their first contact with mental health services via the police, or by compulsory hospitalization, their situation having deteriorated greatly before there is any useful action.

It does not have to be like this. The first 3 years appear critical,[1] when treatment response is very good, and all the important things that give life meaning and stability, home, work, relationships, are still intact. Working with this group can lead to significant impacts.

It is also recognized that a group can be identified even before the onset of psychosis,[2] using the so-called at risk mental state or ARMS, identifying those with a significant disability from a complex array of psychological, emotional and social problems. Despite evidence that this group may be particularly responsive to phase-specific interventions, they may not fit neatly into conventional service configurations and typically are passed from one service to another, or fall between services.

WHAT IS EARLY INTERVENTION?

Early intervention is a set of phase-specific interventions for people in the early stages of a developing psychosis. Central themes run through these phases around the provision of recovery, diagnostic uncertainty and symptom rather than diagnostic management. However the approach falls into two main categories of interventions: (1) people considered to have an ultra-high-risk mental state for developing a psychosis; and (2) people in the first 3 years of a psychosis.

Reflection

How would you identify someone at risk of psychosis? Do you think this would have any implications?

*Paul French is Associate Director of the Early Intervention Services based at Bolton, Salford and Trafford Mental Health Trust, UK. He has worked in mental health since 1986 with a particular interest in services for people with psychosis.

Early intervention in ultra-high-risk groups

This approach is potentially one of the most exciting developments in psychosis research and intervention of recent years and has seen an explosion of research and clinical interest during that time. The idea is not a new one. Harry Stack Sullivan discussed the possibility of this in 1927, and Ian Falloon undertook a study to see whether the prevalence of schizophrenia could be reduced in Buckingham, UK, before the recent excitement about early intervention.

It is important, first, to clarify the terminology used to describe this population. The term *prodromal* is used, retrospectively, if someone has developed a psychosis. However, until we can predict with certainty who will develop psychosis the term prodromal should not be used for people *before* they develop psychosis, but reserved for those with experience of a psychotic episode to describe the build-up to psychosis. For those considered to be 'at risk' of developing a first episode of psychosis, other terms such as ultra-high-risk (UHR) and ARMS should be used.

The possibility of prevention relies on the ability to identify factors that contribute towards the development of psychosis. The aetiology of schizophrenia and related psychotic disorders is unknown, but there is a consensus among researchers and clinicians that a *stress vulnerability* model best accounts for the available evidence.[3-5] This suggests that there is a biological vulnerability to the disorder but that transition to psychotic illness is mediated by environmental stressors.

The biological vulnerabilities associated with psychosis have attracted a great deal of attention over the years. Till now the most effective method of identifying groups vulnerable to schizophrenia has been to identify children whose parents had a diagnosis of schizophrenia and follow up their children, thus identifying an 'at-risk' population. However, the majority of people who develop a psychosis have no family history. Therefore, large numbers of individuals will be missed if this alone is used as an identification strategy.

There has been increased interest in the initial prodrome since a study in Australia, where 40 per cent of an initial prodrome population made the transition to psychosis.[6] This indicates that the identification of high-risk individuals is a possibility and further work is being undertaken to improve the ability to predict who will develop psychosis through the use of specific measures. There are now several measures specifically designed for this population.

The *structured interview for prodromal symptoms* (SIPS) and the *scale of prodromal symptoms* (SOPS)[7] were developed to identify people in the ARMS category. These have been widely utilized in clinical trials and services internationally. The *comprehensive assessment of at risk mental states* (CAARMS) was developed by Alison Yung and her team at the PACE clinic in Melbourne.[8] This very useful measure uses an interview to highlight factors which have been shown to accurately identify this 'at risk'

group. The tool's scoring system helps the clinician to judge if someone is at risk of an impending psychosis or has already become psychotic.

Accurate identification of clients in the initial prodromal phase of psychosis may indicate that an intervention aimed at this population could result in primary prevention of psychosis, as Falloon[9] attempted. There are a range of treatment options available for schizophrenia and by far the most common and generally accessible treatment for psychosis is medication. However, the drugs used to treat psychosis have a range of side-effects and even the atypical anti-psychotic drugs are still associated with a number of unpleasant side-effects. Using medication as a treatment option for this high-risk group, would mean exposing the majority to side-effects of neuroleptic medication when they may never go on to develop psychosis. This clearly has ethical considerations and little or no justification.

One solution would be to employ a treatment strategy with minimal side-effects that targets the problems causing concern. In this case a psychological intervention would, therefore, be indicated. Cognitive–behavioural therapy (CBT) for psychosis has been around for almost 50 years, starting with a single case study[10] and now with a number of clinical trials supporting its use.[11-13] CBT is also widely used in treating mood disorders and would appear the most appropriate treatment strategy to be offered during the initial prodrome in an effort to minimize symptoms and possibly prevent the transition to psychosis.

There is good evidence to suggest that identification of high-risk groups is possible;[6,14,15] however, there have been only a small number of clinical trials which have attempted to intervene with this ARMS group. One trial in Melbourne utilized medication, CBT and case management, comparing this with 'treatment as usual', over 6 months of intervention and 6 months of follow-up. At the end of treatment transition to psychosis was reduced in the treatment group (10 per cent transition to psychosis) compared with the treatment as usual group (36 per cent transition to psychosis).[16] However, these results were not maintained at 6-month follow-up. They concluded that this demonstrated the ability to *delay* rather than *prevent* psychosis. The researchers wondered if they had maintained the intervention over a longer period would this have more effect. They also concluded that medication might have been the important factor although they had very little data to support this. A second trial in the United States used medication only as their intervention in a double blind trial of olanzapine.[17] This trial experienced major difficulties in recruitment and retention primarily due to their intervention and they found a small trend at the end of their study towards medication having an effect on reducing transition to psychosis.

Another study has utilized the possibility of CBT alone to minimize transition to psychosis in this high-risk population. This form of intervention would generally require a radical change in the clinician's view of the concept of psychosis. However, a range of evidence suggests that psychological processes have a large part to play in the development and maintenance of symptoms. Hallucinations are not specific to psychosis, and are found in a wide range of presentations and in certain circumstances are considered absolutely normal.

For example, let us consider the death of an elderly man who has been married for 50 years to his childhood sweetheart. When his wife tells us that she frequently hears him calling her name and has seen him sitting in his favourite chair, we do not immediately consider the prescription of neuroleptic medication. Rather we spend time normalizing this experience.

However, to fully embrace the concept of *normalization* we should believe that psychotic symptoms are understandable. Formulation-driven approaches, which promote the understanding of symptoms, should apply.

Utilizing this approach a treatment manual has been devised[18] and tested[19] specifically for use with ARMS clients. This study adopted a similar strategy to McGorry, where one group received CBT the other monitoring and 'treatment as usual'. The treatment was applied over 6 months and followed up for a further 6 months. Interestingly a significant difference was found at the end of follow up phase, as well as treatment.[20] These benefits were maintained at 3 years.[21] The 3-year data have very small numbers, but suggest the possibility of prevention. Further work is being undertaken and the manual is being used in a number of clinical trials internationally, including a large multi-site randomized controlled trial in the UK with over 300 ARMS clients (see also Bechdolf's[22] study).

Reflection

If you felt that someone was an ultra-high-risk for developing psychosis, how would you explain this to the person?

Practical application

What can be offered to this at risk group?

- The identification of at risk cases.
- Identification and monitoring.
- Identification and treatment.
- What criteria will be used to classify a case as high risk?
- What will treatment consist of?
- If psychological interventions are to be used, are there sufficiently qualified staff who will be able to deliver these interventions?
- Will this be carried out by a dedicated ARMS team through an existing early intervention team?

These questions should all be considered when developing a strategy for 'at risk' populations.

Teams should take stock of their existing resources, links and networks, building upon links with primary care in the initial stages. However, it is important to remember that identification of existing cases is hard enough, identifying at risk groups even harder. The primary care teams can be helped to make referrals. It is then up to the specialist team to come to a decision whether or not the referred person fits into a high-risk criteria or not. If the person is unsuitable, the client should be offered other options. If suitable, the person should be monitored, to observe whether they make the transition to psychosis. If they do, treatment should begin as discussed above. If treatment is going to be offered to people in the high-risk group prior to transition to psychosis, this should *not include* anti-psychotic medication, as this would be unethical. If pharmacological treatments are to be considered they should target the symptoms for which the person is seeking help, such as anxiety, depression, sleep disturbance.

The treatment of choice at this stage should be cognitive therapy designed specifically for this group. This is structured, time limited, problem and goal orientated and has proven efficacy in treating psychotic and non-psychotic symptoms. Psychological interventions with this client group are especially challenging not only in terms of necessary skills, but also in terms of changing our perceptions of psychosis as being an understandable process amenable to psychological intervention. Key aspects associated with provision of 'at-risk' services are shown in Table 57.1.

FIRST EPISODE CARE

One of the most important issues associated with early intervention is the move away from diagnostic labelling, e.g. schizophrenia, to the umbrella term of 'psychosis'. This is due to the difficulties of making a diagnosis in the early stages of an illness. Many clients will have multiple diagnoses throughout their history and, typically, several other 'differential diagnoses'. Diagnostic ambiguity is an important aspect of early intervention and a real challenge to some clinicians. However, many find that it fits with a needs-based approach which has been utilized in mental health services for a number of years. Also important is the adoption of a recovery-based model. Again, many would claim that this has been part of general services for some years. EIP has however taken the idea of recovery and embraced it to the full.

Reflection

If you or a member of your family developed psychosis, what help would you want?

TABLE 57.1 Key aspects associated with provision of 'at-risk' services

Key components	Key elements
Raising awareness of psychosis and early warning signs indicative of an 'at-risk mental state'	Active participation in community-based programmes to reduce stigma associated with mental health issues
	Educational programmes for primary care, education institutions, social services and other relevant agencies
Focus on client-identified problems and signs common to an 'at-risk mental state'	Professionals need to understand the various risk factors which may lead to the development of 'at risk mental states' as well as an awareness of 'normal' changes which may occur during adolescence/early adulthood
	Referrers should be aware of those signs which may indicate an 'at risk mental state' and refer in accordance with their concerns for the young person rather than them having knowledge that the young person is definitely at risk of developing psychosis
	Those problems identified by the young person as being the most distressing should be targeted first in therapy while also focusing on other key engagement factors
Age-, culture- and gender-sensitive services	Services should effectively engage services for young people in the local area and need to be recovery focused
	Access to translation services should be made available and thought given to how the service can be made available to those whose first language is not English
	Gender-sensitive services should be provided
Early detection	Education and training should be provided to GPs, primary care clinicians and other key agencies including connexions staff, youth offending teams and education staff about potential signs of an 'at risk mental state' and how to refer those people who fit these criteria
	Routine audit of effectiveness of referral pathways and training packages offered
Assessment	Service user-centred assessment with an identified key individual taking a lead
	Allowing enough time to develop trust while ensuring that an early assessment is completed as soon as possible
Care plan	Initial care plan produced within a week of assessment
	Initial care plan reviewed at 3 months
	Use of care plans at an appropriate level
Early and sustained engagement	Case management should be provided through the team
	Assessment should take place in an appropriate low-stigmatizing setting, i.e. client's own home, primary care setting, youth service
	Sustained engagement using an assertive outreach model so that service users do not become lost to follow-up
	Service users should not be discharged if fail to engage with interventions
Psychological therapies	Use of cognitive therapy to prevent transition to psychosis and target other co-morbid difficulties
	Normalization and psycho-education
	Service user involved in decision-making and monitoring effects of therapy
	Therapists should work collaboratively with clients and tackle the problems that the clients themselves identify and wish to work on in order to achieve their goals
Family/carers/significant others involvement and support	Family/carers/significant others should be involved in assessment and interventions as early as possible
	Provision of psycho-education and family therapy and support
	Involvement with other key agencies such as connexions
Case management	Assessment and interventions should reflect all aspects of daily living
	Care plan should address how these needs will be met
	It is important to locate the case management within the team promoting independence at every opportunity, be wary not to foster dependence
Providing pathway to involvement in valued education and occupation	An education, training or vocational plan/pathway should be produced within 3 months
Treating co-morbid difficulties	Regular assessment of common difficulties including:
	Substance misuse
	Depression

(Continued)

TABLE 57.1 Continued

Key components	Key elements
	Anxiety disorders
	Interventions
Staying well plan	Assessment and interventions should yield an individual staying well plan for the service user and their file
	Plans should incorporate service user and significant others
Monitoring of mental state	Assessments should be regularly repeated to ensure the effectiveness of interventions and to monitor mental state over time
	Monitoring should be offered for up to 3 years even where the service user has not engaged with other aspects of the service
Crisis plan	Service user/family/significant others know how to access help if necessary
	Intensive support in the community provided by the team during crisis
	If acute care is required then joint assessment should take place between the at-risk team, crisis team and/or acute care team so that the least restrictive/stigmatizing setting for care is arranged
Discharge	The following discharge possibilities could be considered:
	If well – discharge to GP with regular monitoring and final discharge post-3-year monitoring
	If no longer meeting 'at risk' criteria but may require further care in relation to other difficulties consider referral onto appropriate team, e.g. primary care psychology, while still offering monitoring
	If the service user moves out of area during the period of intervention care should be transferred over to an appropriate team. Where there is no appropriate early detection team transfer of care should be thoughtful with detailed information about plans of care and the rationale for this along with consultation if necessary

Why early intervention in psychosis

Several studies have indicated that a longer duration of untreated psychosis (DUP) is associated with poorer prognosis,[23–25] one finding it to be the most important predictor of treatment response in first admission patients.[26] One study examined the occupational activity of 163 first episode psychosis clients and found that a shorter DUP was significantly associated with increased occupational activity at 3-year follow-up.[27] Concerns have been raised that the association between DUP and poor treatment response may merely represent a difference in the illness itself with longer DUP being associated with a more insidious onset and shorter DUP associated with an acute presentation. It is also uncertain whether early detection programmes recruit more people with higher DUP.[28] One review of DUP[29] found some tentative evidence to suggest a relationship between initial response to treatment and DUP, although they found no evidence to suggest a relationship to longer term outcomes while a more recent review of the data did indicate evidence of an association between DUP and outcome.

However, the main clinical implication is that minimizing DUP would be advantageous to the client, family and treatment team even if this were by a few weeks rather than months. Whatever definition is used, it is obvious that there are clear difficulties in being able to identify people who are in the early stages of psychosis, although a shorter DUP is associated with more frequent GP attendance in the 6 years before the onset of psychosis.[30] One study[31] interviewed people who had experienced their first psychotic episode and found that there may be factors associated with the symptoms themselves that contribute to the DUP. In this study, two themes were associated with a reluctance to disclose symptoms: fear about *disclosing symptoms* because of what may happen; and people becoming *preoccupied with the symptoms*. Fear and preoccupation can accentuate the DUP, preventing people from seeking help. However, it is not only the symptoms themselves that serve to prolong DUP. The Northwick Park Study[32] suggested that if things are not managed in the early stages then deterioration continues until finally a crisis occurs, which frequently involves the police. This study found that people do try to access help for their symptoms, with an average of eight 'help-seeking' contacts prior to appropriate treatment. Unfortunately, the police are often the final help-seeking contact. This will frequently involve taking the person for assessment, often involving admission to hospital. These hospital admissions may be involuntary, requiring the use of the Mental Health Act in the UK. This can be extremely traumatic for the individual, family and friends, and there is evidence that such admissions can lead to the development of post-traumatic stress disorder.[33,34]

DUP is considered to end when someone starts taking medication. This reliance on a medical intervention could be seen as counterproductive in that it may encourage clinicians to prescribe earlier, to minimize DUP. However, it is important to remember that alternative treatments are important in the treatment of psychosis. One study found that delay in the provision of psychosocial treatments may be more important for the long-term prognosis of negative symptoms than medication alone.[35]

Practical application

Once new cases are identified at an early stage then it becomes a priority to engage with the individual and also their family or carers. Engagement has been recognized as a vital component of many aspects of psychiatric care including case management and there is a wealth of literature on engagement strategies. These will not be discussed in detail here. People working within community mental health teams (CMHTs) generally have excellent engagement skills and have experience of working with clients with existing mental illness, although they need to be aware of the specifics of working with people with early-onset psychosis. The person may not wish to discuss matters associated with their illness, adopting a sealing over recovery strategy.[36] This may well affect the way in which the person engages with all aspects of their treatment from psychological interventions to medication. An ability to recognize different recovery styles and work within these styles can be useful. Typically, the most effective way of engaging people is to work on problems they themselves identify and not on a service-based agenda of needs.

Reflection

If you had problems, what would make you want to stay involved with a service?

Treatment should have its emphasis within community settings, attempting to minimize hospital admissions, as this can lead to trauma. Managing episodes through the least restrictive environment, possibly through joint work with home treatment teams, may minimize this trauma. Early intervention teams should be well educated, motivated and positive about outcomes and potential ways to impact upon prognosis. Ideally these teams should be distinct from other services, with members focusing their efforts towards first episode care. In the early stages

diagnosis is frequently uncertain and a symptom orientated approach to management may prove more fruitful. In terms of medical treatment, the newer atypical drugs, which have minimal side-effects (compared with typical anti-psychotic drugs), should be utilized. However, side-effects, such as weight gain and sexual dysfunction, are still present. Pharmacists can offer expert advice, although they are not always used. Alongside pharmacological management of symptoms, comprehensive psychological management should take place. CBT has been the most widely researched psychological intervention for psychosis with significant evidence indicating the efficacy of this form of intervention. There is a range of potential CBT interventions that could be employed at this point. Also, family interventions should be offered and not just to high expressed emotion (EE) families but also to low EE families as well.

Personal illustration 57.1

John, a 17-year-old man, is referred to psychiatric services from his GP because of concerns from his family that his behaviour is becoming increasingly 'odd'. He finally agreed to be seen by his GP and appeared sullen, withdrawn and preoccupied although he denied any present concerns. His family said he spent more time isolated in his room and they occasionally heard him talking to himself. He was eating very little and tended to sleep during the day rather than at night. John admits to smoking cannabis frequently in the past but denies any current use. No other drug or alcohol use. Until recently he had a girlfriend and used to go out with her and his friends, although since the break-up with his girlfriend he hardly goes out and does not see his friends. They ring him less and less as time passes.

John is sent an appointment to attend an outpatient appointment at his local mental health unit. On receiving this he becomes angry and increasingly withdrawn from his family. John does not attend the appointment, causing further tension in the family. Another appointment is arranged and his family takes him to the appointment. He is finally assessed and it is felt that he may depressed with some paranoid ideas, related to his drug use. He is given a prescription for antidepressants, a follow-up appointment and the number of a local voluntary organization that works with young people.

John does not contact the voluntary organization or take medication and he does not attend his follow-up appointment. Things become steadily worse within the family home as John's behaviour deteriorates to the point where he assaults one of his elderly neighbours and the police are involved. They take him to a local casualty department where he is thought to be experiencing a psychotic episode and is formally admitted. Unfortunately, the local unit has no beds and he is sent to another unit some distance away, making it difficult for his family to visit. All this impacts upon how John and his family view the services, and they feel as though they have been let down.

Discussion

John's story illustrates some of the difficulties associated with the onset and development of psychosis. It can be hard to define the difference between adolescent behaviour, drug-induced symptoms and the onset of psychosis. Frequently clinicians do not consider the development of psychosis for many reasons such as their unwillingness to stigmatize individuals. However, offering non-stigmatizing services, which target people's problems and engages them and their family with services, can overcome this. John displays some potential risks and engaging with John and his family at this stage could be extremely beneficial. If services can be geared towards a 'wait and see' approach, with more emphasis on engagement of the person, offering flexible appointments, this might affect how services are perceived and used. Unfortunately, many services are geared towards *crisis provision* rather than prevention. This may not only affect how people engage with services but also the effectiveness of any help on offer, whether pharmacological or psychological.

SUMMARY

Exciting opportunities exist to minimize the chances of developing psychosis. However, these require a range of interventions. In the prevention of heart disease, there exists a wide range of interventions, addressing diet, exercise and smoking. Further layers of intervention are provided through primary care, and specialist services exist to treat more severe presentations. Finally, despite this range of services some people die because of the severity of their condition. Psychosis is similar. However, we have had no access to any of the public education or primary care interventions, relying on the specialist end of the spectrum. We need to consider psychosis as everyone's business. A clinical staging model of understanding may enable this.[37]

REFERENCES

1. Birchwood M, Todd P, Jackson C. Early intervention in psychosis. The critical period hypothesis. *British Journal of Psychiatry* 1998; **172** (Suppl. 33): 53–9.

2. Cannon TD, Cornblatt B, McGorry P. Editor's introduction: the empirical status of the ultra high-risk (prodromal) research paradigm. *Schizophrenia Bulletin* 2007; **33** (3): 661–4.

3. Zubin J, Spring B. Vulnerability – a new view of schizophrenia. *Journal of Abnormal Psychology* 1977; **86** (2): 103–26.

4. Gottesman II, Shields J. *Schizophrenia: the epigenetic puzzle.* Cambridge, UK: Cambridge University Press, 1982.

5. Gottesman II, Wolfgram DL. *Schizophrenia genesis : the origins of madness.* New York, NY: W.H. Freeman, 1991.

6. Yung AR, Phillips LJ, McGorry PD *et al.* Prediction of psychosis. A step towards indicated prevention of schizophrenia. *British Journal of Psychiatry* 1998; **172** (Suppl. 33): 14–20.

7. Miller TJ, McGlashan TH, Woods SW *et al.* Symptom assessment in schizophrenic prodromal states. *Psychiatric Quarterly* 1999; **70** (4): 273–87.

8. Yung AR, Phillips L, Simmons J *et al.* Comprehensive assessment of at risk mental states. Unpublished manuscript 2006.

9. Falloon IR. Early intervention for first episodes of schizophrenia: a preliminary exploration. *Psychiatry* 1992; **55** (1): 4–15.

10. Beck AT. Successful outpatient psychotherapy of a chronic schizophrenic with a delusion based on borrowed guilt. *Psychiatry* 1952; **15** (3): 305–12.

11. Tarrier N, Yusupoff L, Kinney C *et al.* Randomised controlled trial of intensive cognitive behaviour therapy for patients with chronic schizophrenia. *British Medical Journal* 1998; **317** (7154): 303–7.

12. Drury V, Birchwood M, Cochrane R, Macmillan F. Cognitive therapy and recovery from acute psychosis: a controlled trial. I. Impact on psychotic symptoms. *British Journal of Psychiatry* 1996; **169** (5): 593–601.

13. Sensky T, Turkington D, Kingdon D *et al.* A randomized controlled trial of cognitive-behavioral therapy for persistent symptoms in schizophrenia resistant to medication. *Archives of General Psychiatry* 2000; **57** (2): 165–72.

14. Morrison AP, French P, Lewis SW *et al.* Psychological factors in people at ultra-high risk of psychosis: comparisons with non-patients and associations with symptoms. *Psychological Medicine* 2006; **36** (10): 1395–404.

15. Yung AR, Phillips LJ, Yuen HP, McGorry PD. Risk factors for psychosis in an ultra high-risk group: psychopathology and clinical features. *Schizophrenia Research* 2004; **67** (2–3): 131–42.

16. McGorry PD, Yung AR, Phillips LJ *et al.* Randomized controlled trial of interventions designed to reduce the risk of progression to first-episode psychosis in a clinical sample with subthreshold symptoms. *Archives of General Psychiatry* 2002; **59** (10): 921–8.

17. McGlashan TH, Zipursky RB, Perkins D, *et al.* The PRIME North America randomized double-blind clinical trial of olanzapine versus placebo in patients at risk of being prodromally symptomatic for psychosis. I. Study rationale and design. *Schizophrenia Research* 2003; **61** (1): 7–18.

18. French P, Morrison AP. *Early detection and cognitive therapy for people at high risk of developing psychosis: a treatment approach.* Chichester, UK: Wiley, 2004.

19. Morrison AP, Bentall RP, French P *et al.* Randomised controlled trial of early detection and cognitive therapy for preventing transition to psychosis in high-risk individuals. Study design and interim analysis of transition rate and psychological risk factors. *British Journal of Psychiatry* 2002; (Suppl 43): s78–84.

20. Morrison AP, French P, Walford L *et al.* Cognitive therapy for the prevention of psychosis in people at ultra-high risk: randomised controlled trial. *British Journal of Psychiatry* 2004; **185**: 291–7.

21. Morrison AP, French P, Parker S *et al.* Three-year follow-up of a randomized controlled trial of cognitive therapy for the

prevention of psychosis in people at ultrahigh risk. *Schizophrenia Bulletin* 2007; **33** (3): 682–7.

22. Bechdolf A, Veith V, Schwarzer D et al. Cognitive-behavioral therapy in the pre-psychotic phase: an exploratory study. *Psychiatry Research* 2005; **136** (2–3): 251–5.

23. Marshall M, Lewis S, Lockwood A et al. Association between duration of untreated psychosis and outcome in cohorts of first-episode patients: a systematic review. *Archives of General Psychiatry* 2005; **62** (9): 975–83.

24. Crow TJ. The continuum of psychosis and its implication for the structure of the gene. *British Journal of Psychiatry* 1986; **149**: 419–29.

25. Loebel AD, Lieberman JA, Alvir JM et al. Duration of psychosis and outcome in first-episode schizophrenia. *American Journal of Psychiatry* 1992; **149** (9): 1183–8.

26. Drake RJ, Haley CJ, Akhtar S, Lewis SW. Causes and consequences of duration of untreated psychosis in schizophrenia. *British Journal of Psychiatry* 2000; **177**: 511–5.

27. Norman RM, Mallal AK, Manchanda R et al. Does treatment delay predict occupational functioning in first-episode psychosis? *Schizophrenia Research* 2007; **91** (1–3): 259–62.

28. Friis S, Vaglum P, Haahr U et al. Effect of an early detection programme on duration of untreated psychosis: part of the Scandinavian TIPS study. *British Journal of Psychiatry* 2005; **48** (Suppl): s29–32.

29. Norman RM, Malla AK. Duration of untreated psychosis: a critical examination of the concept and its importance. *Psychological Medicine* 2001; **31** (3): 381–400.

30. Skeate A, Jackson C, Birchwood M, Jones C. Duration of untreated psychosis and pathways to care in first-episode psychosis. Investigation of help-seeking behaviour in primary care. *British Journal of Psychiatry* 2002; **43** (Suppl): s73–7.

31. Moller P, Husby R. The initial prodrome in schizophrenia: searching for naturalistic core dimensions of experience and behavior. *Schizophrenia Bulletin* 2000; **26** (1): 217–32.

32. Johnstone EC, Crow TJ, Johnson AL, MacMillan JF. The Northwick Park Study of first episodes of schizophrenia. I. Presentation of the illness and problems relating to admission. *British Journal of Psychiatry* 1986; **148**: 115–20.

33. Frame L, Morrison AP. Causes of posttraumatic stress disorder in psychotic patients. *Archives of General Psychiatry* 2001; **58** (3): 305–6.

34. McGorry PD, Chanen A, McCarthy E et al. Posttraumatic stress disorder following recent-onset psychosis. An unrecognized postpsychotic syndrome. *Journal of Nervous and Mental Disease* 1991; **179** (5): 253–8.

35. de Haan L, Linszen DH, Lenior ME et al. Duration of untreated psychosis and outcome of schizophrenia: delay in intensive psychosocial treatment versus delay in treatment with antipsychotic medication. *Schizophrenia Bulletin* 2003; **29** (2): 341–8.

36. McGlashan TH. Recovery style from mental illness and long-term outcome. *Journal of Nervous and Mental Disease* 1987; **175** (11): 681–5.

37. McGorry PD, Hickie IB, Yung AR et al. Clinical staging of psychiatric disorders: a heuristic framework for choosing earlier, safer and more effective interventions. *Australian and New Zealand Journal of Psychiatry* 2006; **40** (8): 616–22.

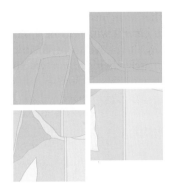

CHAPTER 58

Services for women

Penny Cutting*

Women's health is inextricably linked to their status in society. It benefits from equality, and suffers from discrimination. Today, the status and well being of countless millions of women worldwide remain tragically low. As a result, human well-being suffers, and the prospects for future generations are dimmer.[1]

INTRODUCTION

Although almost 10 years old, this World Health Organization (WHO) quote remains relevant. Across cultures women currently face major inequalities in all aspects of life. As I write, the daily papers provide examples of the extremes of prejudice against women: the appalling rate of detection and conviction of perpetrators of rape;[2] the extent of domestic violence;[3] that women still earn less than men for doing the same job; the subsequent greater impoverishment of women;[4] the lack of women in positions of power across all professions;[4] the trafficking of women from various countries to the UK and elsewhere for forced prostitution.[5] Today's newspaper reports that 10 million baby girls are aborted or killed soon after birth in India because they are valued less than boys, who are seen as an asset to the family.[6]

Why should psychiatric–mental health nurses be concerned with these social issues? There are many reasons but the recent reviews of psychiatric–mental health nursing in the UK explicitly called for nurses to do what they can so that all groups in society receive an equitable service[7,8] and to ensure that 'rights' are respected.

Society's treatment of women is reflected within the psychiatric and mental health system, which continues to be dominated by patriarchy, with the service user generally at the bottom of the power hierarchy. However, with the rise in the service user group movement and survivor groups, women's voices have begun to be heard. Many excellent service user survivors/campaigners, researchers, mental health workers and groups such as MIND (a UK mental health non-statutory campaigning and service user-led group) have drawn attention to the fact that in the UK mental health services for women are unacceptable because they are unsafe,[9] traumatize and perpetuate the gender discrimination suffered by women in society.[10,11]

WOMEN'S EXPERIENCES OF PSYCHIATRIC/MENTAL HEALTH SERVICES

Previous UK research has highlighted women's negative experiences of particularly psychiatric hospital admission.

*Penny Cutting is Manager of the Croydon Women's Service, which is part of South London and Maudsley Trust.

Qualitative data from focus groups and interviews with female service users[12] suggest that for many women the psychiatric–mental health environment is detrimental to their well-being and in particular women in the study had a specific difficulty sharing the environment with men (staff and service users), and felt that the psychiatric and mental health services that they had encountered had:

- left them feeling dehumanized;
- made them fearful for their safety across inpatient and community outpatient settings;
- exposed them to unacceptable levels of violence from men (as witness and victim) mostly in inpatient settings;
- forced them to share living and therapeutic space with men making them feel uncomfortable and unhappy about the lack of privacy;
- exposed them to sexual harassment, sexual assault, intimidation and on reporting this they were not believed;
- required them to participate in mixed-sex groups where they could not talk about intimate problems, were judged, made to feel ashamed or guilty as they felt unable to talk with men present;
- rendered them powerless. They felt silenced by the system, and 'unheard'.

These findings are replicated across much of the UK mental health system with a few notable exceptions.[10] For these reasons there is a move in the UK to provide women-only inpatient and community mental health services, seeking to work with women in partnership, to actively tackle discrimination and issues of inequality within the system and to really listen to what women say they want and need.

WOMEN-CENTRED MENTAL HEALTH CARE: CHALLENGING THE SYSTEM

So what does working in a women-centred way look like? In the National Health Service in the UK this has taken, first, the form of providing women-only inpatient facilities and some women-only community services. The development of women-only inpatient units has, so far, involved turning mixed-sex environments into 'women-only' by changing admission policies. There is a risk that services taking this approach will see no benefits for women and that the women themselves will be as unhappy with this as they were with the mixed-sex environment. What must be done is to craft the culture of the care environment to make it safe, effective and empowering for women, helping them focus on recovery rather than just surviving the experience of hospitalization. Later, I will describe a service that has developed as an alternative to psychiatric hospital for women. Unfortunately, these are rare within the NHS. However, research into their effectiveness is beginning to demonstrate service user preference and good clinical outcomes.[13] Hopefully, more services will base their approach on this philosophy.

Among the critical issues is the balance of power on the unit. The multidisciplinary team needs to model democratic working relationships where every voice is heard and all team members are valued and respected by one another. The old model of having a 'consultant' in charge will not work as it maintains the imbalance of power that women experience in their lives disempowering staff and service users. Where institutional traditions are maintained change can be very difficult to implement. There has been much resistance to the idea of women-only services. Many staff argue that housing male and female 'patients' together reflects 'normal' society. However, there is nothing 'normal' about having to go into a ward, possibly against your will, after living on your own or with a partner, where unknown men can wander in and out of your bedroom.

Another challenging debate involves the place of male staff on a women-only unit. I have argued against this,[14] believing that negative gender stereotypes about work in an all-female environment partly fuel resistance to this new model. Although women should be exposed to good men, to discover that not all men risk doing them harm, as previously noted,[14] the point of crisis requiring an acute hospital admission is not the time to do this. This view is not in any way intended to undermine male colleagues but is raised only for the reader to consider. Some women-only services have chosen to have mixed-sex staff and others have not. No conclusive research has been published that identifies the 'right' gender mix, if indeed there is such a thing. What is important is that women-sensitive and knowledgeable staff are recruited and that women are given a choice about the gender of staff working with them.[15]

Reflection

Who holds the most power where you work?

How would you feel as a man or woman to be forced to share your living space with strangers from whom you could not escape and who frightened you?

What might be the benefits and drawbacks of having an all-female staff? Are any of the things you have thought about as a result of your own gender stereotypes?

What are some of the differing needs of men and women?

WOMEN'S MENTAL HEALTH

Women are diagnosed with mental health problems more often than men.[16] However, it is important to identify what *types* of mental illnesses are more common among women, which might explain why women are over-represented in the statistics.

The rates of conditions like bipolar disorder and schizophrenia are similar for men and women. However, women are twice as likely as men to develop depression and for this to be a more long-term or recurring problem. There also exists a positive relationship between the childhood sexual abuse, domestic violence, rape, experiences of violent conflicts and other gender-based inequalities and the frequency and severity of conditions such as depression in women.[17] To address women's mental health we need to focus not only on the latest treatment but the reasons why the woman became ill in the first place.

It is accepted that the onset, duration, and course of mental illness in women differs from men. For example women tend to develop schizophrenia later on in life than men.[18] This means that the woman may well have a partner, children, a job, have formed close social relationships, achieved her educational goals and be in a caring role either for children or other family members. Having a multiplicity of roles has also been identified as a stressor or added burden, negatively impacting upon women's mental health.[10]

The development of schizophrenia in men is quite different: they tend to be much younger and as such have not developed socially, emotionally or interpersonally, and so have different needs from women. This illustrates that the impact of developing schizophrenia, although devastating both sexes, has very different consequences for each sex. However, when women enter the mental health system the 'treatment' offered is the same as that offered to men.

It is here that psychiatric mental health nurses can really make a difference in addressing the issues that make recovery difficult for women.

WOMEN-CENTRED APPROACHES TO PSYCHIATRIC–MENTAL HEALTH NURSING

It can be seen, therefore, that attention needs to be paid to the specific stresses that women experience. It is useful to consider what can be done to diminish the factors known to increase the risk of mental health problems as outlined previously, and to build upon a woman's strengths, bolstering the aspects of her life that are known to be help protect against mental ill health. Three

main protective elements for women's mental health have been identified.[19]

1 Having sufficient *autonomy* to exercise some control in response to severe events.
2 Access to some *material resources* that allow the possibility of making choices.
3 *Psychological support* from family, friends or health providers.

We will first consider assessing the factors known to *harm* women's mental health and will then explore building upon the protective factors.

ASSESSMENT OF FACTORS THAT CAN HARM WOMEN'S MENTAL HEALTH

Modern psychiatric–mental health nurses must do all they can to ensure that they provide an equitable service. To do so they need to consider those aspects of women's lives that have either led to the development of mental health problems or are exacerbating them. The following outlines some of the key factors that are problematic for women, followed by suggested questions that the psychiatric–mental health nurse should consider.

Multiple roles: What roles does the woman fulfil? Which of these roles does she find rewarding and which does she find draining and stressful?

Caring roles: Who is the woman responsible for other than herself? Does she have family expectations placed upon her that require her to put others before herself? Is she expected to 'drop everything' and attend to extended family matters at any time? How does she rate her parenting skills? Does she need more support in her role as parent? Can she get time to herself and a break from her children? Does she need help with child care? Has anyone assessed her children's needs thoroughly; are they at risk in any way?

Financial independence: Where does her money/income come from? Does she have enough money to live on? Does she control her money or does someone else do this? Does she have her own bank account? Does she have access to advice/help regarding all her entitlements to welfare/extra financial support? Is she in debt? Has she contacted anyone to help her work through the management of her finances/debts? Is there anyone demanding money from her?

Work within and outside the home: What work does she do within the home? Is she expected to do all the housework and clean up after others? Does anyone help her with this? Does she work outside of the home, and if so do her employers support her? Has she disclosed that she has mental health problems? Is she being unfairly treated or discriminated against at work? Does she have good working relationships with her colleagues? Is she being exploited by anyone or bullied at work? Does she need help to plan for returning to work or finding employment?

Educational aspirations: What is her educational level? Does she speak enough English to make her needs and wishes understood, and can she understand all that is being said to her? Would she like help to further her education? Does she know what is available to her locally in terms of educational facilities?

Physical well-being: Has she seen her GP recently and has she attended a well-woman clinic? Does she regularly check her breasts for changes? When was her last cervical smear? Has she any injuries internal or external (make sure these are documented very thoroughly in her notes in case they are needed to support her when/if she reports assault)? Does she feel physically well? Does she eat enough/comfort eat? If taking any medicines does she have any side-effects? What effects does she notice from the medicines she takes? Have the medicines had any specific effect on her menstrual cycle/or caused changes in libido?

Interpersonal relationships: Who are the significant people in her life? How would she describe her relationships with them? Is she in a relationship where she is powerless or feeling helpless/overwhelmed/bullied or victimized in any way? Does she feel supported by her relationships or not? Is she always putting other people and their needs before her own?

The following assessment requires a great deal of tact and sensitivity. It is important to let the woman know that you will be asking very personal questions and that she only need tell you what she feels able to. It is helpful to let her know that experiences of childhood and adult abuse and violence are major contributors to mental ill health in women and are commonly experienced by women/girls. Also, that you will not just be asking questions but that you will ensure that she gets the help and support she needs to begin to recover from these experiences.

Experiences of domestic violence including emotional, psychological abuse: Between 50 and 60 per cent of women mental health service users have experienced domestic violence. In addition, up to 20 per cent will be experiencing current abuse.[20] It is vital to ask difficult questions around these areas. The psychological and physical consequences of domestic violence are great and are known to be implicated in the development of many mental health difficulties.

When asking these questions it is important to remember that the woman is seen on her own (unless she requests otherwise). Asking a woman in front of friends/partners or other family members will not help her to feel able to disclose. Also, for women who require

an interpreter it is important to consider not using a family member. This person may be abusing her or if discussing abuse is taboo or shameful for her, she may be unable to disclose such matters to others.

If a woman discloses domestic violence, the assessment is not the time to discuss how to help her leave. However, there are fundamental issues that you need to help her with, including ways to stay safe and providing information about local domestic violence services that can help her in the short and long term. A woman who discloses that she is being abused in any way should not be expected to return to the abusing person/environment without adequate safety planning/protection and support. Does she know about services such as women's aid and refuge that could help her? When domestic violence is disclosed you will need to talk with the woman about your duty under the safeguarding children laws to ensure that her children are safe.

If you are working with a woman on a long-term basis, then working with other agencies may enable you to help her plan her way out of this situation if this is what she wants. However, this needs to be done very carefully and with the help of several other agencies. What are the risks involved? What would need to happen to help her and her children leave safely?

Rape: As with domestic violence this needs very careful questioning. Again, it is vital to this area as such an experience has an ongoing impact upon all aspects of a woman's life. Her physical, psychological and spiritual well-being can be severely damaged by rape. Posing the question needs careful thought and tact, for example:

> has anyone ever hurt you in a sexual way or has anyone ever forced you to have sexual contact with them when you have not wanted this?

It is very important that the woman who discloses that she has been raped feels listened to, believed, and understands that you are aware that this has had a major impact upon her mental health and her ongoing distress.

Forty-five per cent of women reporting rape have been raped by their husband or partner; 9 per cent by their ex-husband or partner; 29 per cent by a man known to the woman; 4 per cent are date rape; and 9 per cent by a stranger.[2,3]

As a result, you will need to ask whether she is with the person who raped her and how safe she feels currently.

Childhood sexual abuse: As before a gentle approach is needed. However, we know that up to 50 per cent of women service users are struggling to survive the experience of sexual abuse and that staff are reluctant to ask the question. However, to avoid this is to deny the woman's lived reality. Any help you offer without knowledge of abuse risks being ineffective and potentially damaging. It is important to be matter of fact about the question. We are not asking about something rare or unheard of. Up to half of service users have been abused. Helping them to recover from this should be the core of our working practice. Making women aware that their distress, and the way they have coped with abuse, has been their way of surviving, and is not a sign of weakness, failure or madness, is key to helping them learn new and safe ways of coping.

You need also to ask about the identity of the abuser. If the woman was abused by her parents and if those same parents are now grandparents to her children, they may be looking after them while she is in the mental health services. Steps will need to be taken to ensure that the children are safe and alternative arrangements made.

Other traumatic incidents: Many women have experienced other traumatic incidents such as witnessing murder, war, terrorism or other violent conflict. They may be asylum seekers who have fled the most terrifying of experiences. It is important that we understand these circumstances so that we can ensure that they get the help that they need.

PROTECTIVE FACTORS FOR WOMEN'S MENTAL HEALTH

To illustrate how nursing practice may provide protective factors, I will discuss a women-only service that I have been working in for the last 10 years. I will use a personal illustration (see p. 506) to give an example, which hopefully will help readers see what is possible. Providing a good service to women is really not difficult, and I have found that during the years I have been able to apply the skills I learned in my basic training to full effect in this service more than anywhere else that I have worked.

The 'Women's Service' is an NHS unit offering an alternative to admission for women with enduring mental health problems in crisis. The service was developed in partnership with the local mental health service user group and local women's organizations as well as from research carried out with the current women service users.[12] It has eight bedrooms and a large garden, designed by women users of the service, to ensure that the space reflected what women would find therapeutic and useful.

The unit is a nurse-led unit staffed by women psychiatric–mental health nurses and health care assistants, with support from a visiting woman consultant psychiatrist once or twice a week. Recognizing its high value by service users and their carers, local services wanted to replicate this unit on their hospital inpatient wards. In the last year, following reorganization, a women-only inpatient ward

was created, which works in partnership with the 'Women's Service'. Both services have team leaders but are managed overall by the 'Women's Lead' – a senior mental health nurse with an in-depth knowledge and experience of gender-specific care for women.

The two units have a women-centred philosophy and ward staff are being trained in gender-specific theory and practice. Opportunities exist for staff to cross-over between the two units, extending the range of their experience. This ongoing project demonstrates the potential of creative thinking. Women needing admission can still receive women-centred care within a safe and therapeutic environment.

The personal illustration illustrates how the unit works to promote the protective factors for women's mental health: autonomy and control, resources and choices, and psychological support. To ensure confidentiality this case study is a 'typical' picture of various different women's journeys through this service.

A brief note about vicarious traumatization

Rates of violence and abuse against women are extreme to say the least. When staff really listen to women recount their life stories, it is easy to be overwhelmed by the horror and the pain of their lives. As women working with women, you may well have had the same, or a similar, traumatic experience as the service user. Nurses may even avoid service users or avoid talking about violence and abuse, because it is too traumatic for them to hear. Nurses may find it difficult to switch off from work. Some women staff, working with women who have been raped, may find themselves having difficulties in being intimate with their partners. This vicarious traumatization is an avoidable consequence of this type of work. Staff need to take care of themselves and find healthy ways of leaving work at work. Each person needs to find a way that is right for them. If you find that your own traumas are resurfacing then you need to find your own psychological support. Frequent, regular, clinical supervision, which explores in detail the interpersonal relationship development and dynamics, between nurse and service user, is essential if the nurse is to remain effective in working with traumatized women.

Reflection

If you could ask 'Laura' one question, what would that be?

When, during your contact with her, would you have asked this question?

Why would you have asked it, at that point?

Personal illustration 58.1

Laura is a 40-year-old woman with two teenage children. She lives on her own with them and has no family or support close by. She has been diagnosed with bipolar affective disorder for 5 years and for the last 2 weeks has been spending money beyond her means, and has been contacting local businesses trying to establish a 'fantastic money-making opportunity'. She has been unable to care for her children, who have been asking neighbours for food. Laura has been staying up all night, singing loudly and generally has been behaving out of character. She refuses to take any of her prescribed medication. Her psychiatrist and community psychiatric nurse (CPN) want her to go into hospital. She refuses. No one asks why. She had been assaulted previously on a ward. Many times in the past she has been 'sectioned' under the Mental Health Act. The approved social worker, who is aware of the 'Women's Service' in the community, asks Laura if she would consider this as an alternative to hospital. She helps Laura phone the Service, to describe what she is experiencing at present. Staff ask what she wants to do and what has helped in the past. She is offered an immediate face-to-face assessment and is given a choice when she could come. Staff ensure that she understands what is on offer, so that she feels in control of the care she receives. She agrees to an admission to the 'Women's Service' and once she has established trust with staff she sees that she needs extra help.

Working with a primary nurse, Laura drew her 'life line', plotting significant life events both positive and negative alongside her extremes of mood. This helped Laura see that there was a pattern to her mood swings.

Together Laura and the nurse identified what was causing most difficulty at present. Laura disclosed that she was being forced to have sex by a man who loaned her money. Over time, she revealed that this was not the first person to abuse her. She was helped to look at ways of keeping herself and her children safe from this man. Although Laura wanted to talk in detail about her earlier abuse, the nurse helped her contain this, focusing on her basic safety needs. The team recognizes the importance of avoiding exploring issues of sexual abuse too soon. The woman needs a firm safety foundation first. This includes basic issues such as having enough money, food, sleep and rest, a safe place to live, trustworthy supportive people in her life, and a period of relative mood stability.

The nurse explained to Laura the relationship between this traumatic experience and her present mental health, helping her look at how she was being affected right now. Laura was having flashbacks to scenes of earlier abuse that other staff had disregarded as part of her 'illness'. With her nurse she learned how to ground herself, learning how to control her response to these flashbacks, lessening her anxiety.[21] The nurse also explained that this time of crisis was not the safest time to work in depth on her earlier abuse, but that she would make sure that psychological support would be available to her when she left, on a longer term basis. Laura felt safer in the knowledge that she could tackle things one at a time and that she would get on-going support.

Together the nurse and Laura drew up a care plan, discussing this with her CPN and psychiatrist. Laura was helped to lead this discussion, making clear what she needed, and what was acceptable and unacceptable to her. Her nurse also helped her to explain to her children about her mental health problems. To make sure they received the help they needed, the children were put in touch with the local Young Carers group.

During her time at the 'Women's Service' Laura attended the daily support group[22] where she discovered that sharing her experiences with other women in a safe, supportive group was therapeutic. She felt less isolated, and was able to give and receive support. She was also able to participate in the daily creative groups which provided opportunities to explore (e.g. music, art, sand tray work, creative writing, role play) the main theme from the morning support group. This gave her the chance to explore and express herself and her feelings in new ways.

As part of her basic safety work she was helped to look at her dietary intake and learned about foods that can help her mood. She helped to plan the weekly menu for the service and was able to join in the cooking. (It is not just expected that as a woman she would want or enjoy to cook!) She then became interested in planning a weekly menu for her and her children.

In preparation for discharge, the 'Women's Service' helps women to draw up a health maintenance and well-being plan. This is based upon what has been described as a WRAP (wellness recovery action plan) plan.[23] Laura was helped to identify what helps, what hinders, what resources she needs, what do to if she starts feeling unwell, where she can get support from, how she can help herself and what help she can expect of the services. She also wrote a care plan for her own use at home to help her plan and structure her days. She was helped to contact the police who spoke to the man who was forcing her to have sex. (She decided against the trauma of prosecuting him.) The police were happy to help and the abuse stopped.

This brief sketch illustrates how working in partnership with Laura made a significant difference to her well-being. This helped her avoid being detained under the Mental Health Act and, over the years, she has been able to contact the service herself when she feels she needs it. She sometimes phones for support or visits the service, e.g. when they are celebrating International Women's Day, and says that just knowing it is there helps her. She has stayed in touch with some of the other women who were staying at the time and now has a network of supportive friends. She has been able to help when we are interviewing for new staff – her opinion and insights are extremely helpful. She has not required an admission under the Mental Health Act for 8 years.

SUMMARY

Women face highly specific difficulties, both in mental health services and in society at large. Here I have outlined the rationale for women-only inpatient and community services in the UK illustrating one such service.

The reader has been invited to consider the wider aspects of the life of a woman 'service-user', and examples have been provided of the kind of questions that might help to determine the present factors that may be harming her mental health.

I hope that readers can see that to work with women in a holistic way, they need to work across agencies and traditional working boundaries, tackling discrimination, challenging stereotyped views and opening themselves up to hearing what service users are saying. This is not easy, requiring commitment, stamina, considerable self-awareness and self-care. However, this is not so hard when compared to the courage and strength required by the women service users we are privileged to work with.

REFERENCES

1. World Health Organization. *Executive summary the World Health Report 1998 – life in the 21st century – a vision for all.* Geneva, Switzerland: World Health Organization, 1998.

2. Myhill A, Allen J. *Rape and sexual assault of women the extent and nature of the problem: findings from the British Crime Survey.* Home Office Research Study 237. London, UK: Home Office, 2002.

3. Walby S, Allen J. *Domestic violence, sexual assault and stalking; findings from the British Crime Survey.* Home Office Research Study 276. London, UK: Home Office, 2004.

4. Equal Opportunities Commission. *Completing the revolution: the leading indicators.* London, UK: Equal Opportunities Commission, 2007.

5. Kelly L, Regan L. *Stopping traffic: exploring the extent of, and responses to, trafficking in women for sexual exploitation in the UK.* Home Office Police Research Series Paper 125. London: HMSO, 2000.

6. Ramesh R. Foetuses aborted and dumped secretly as India shuns baby girls. *Guardian* 28 July 2007: 25.

7. Department of Health. *From values to action: the Chief Nursing Officer's review of mental health nursing.* London, UK: Department of Health, 2006.

8. Scottish Executive. *Rights, relationships and recovery – the report of the National Review of Mental Health Nursing in Scotland.* Edinburgh, UK: Scottish Executive, 2006.

9. National Patient Safety Agency. *With safety in mind: mental health services and patient safety.* London, UK: National Patient Safety Agency, 2006.

10. Department of Health. *Women's mental health: into the mainstream – strategic development of mental health care for women.* London, UK: Department of Health, 2002.

11. Department of Health. *Mainstreaming gender and women's mental health: implementation guidance.* London, UK: Department of Health, 2003.

12. Cutting P, Henderson C. Women's experiences of hospital admission. *Journal of Psychiatric and Mental Health Nursing* 2002; **9**: 705–9.

13. Meiser-Stedman C, Howard L, Cutting P. Evaluating the effectiveness of a women's crisis house: a prospective observational study. *Psychiatric Bulletin* 2006; **30**: 324–6.

14. Cutting P. The problem with psychiatry: a woman's perspective. In: Henderson C, Smith C, Smith S, Stevens A (eds). *Women and psychiatric treatment: a comprehensive text and practical guide.* London, UK: Routledge, 2006: 9–21.

15. Kohen D, McNicholas, S, Beaumont K. Inpatient psychiatric services for women. In: Henderson C, Smith C, Smith S, Stevens A (eds). *Women and psychiatric treatment: a comprehensive text and practical guide.* London, UK: Routledge, 2006: 47–7.

16. Kohen D (ed.) *Women and mental health.* London, UK: Routledge, 2000.

17. World Health Organization. *Women's mental health: an evidence based review.* Geneva, Switzerland: World Health Organization, 2000.

18. Zolese G. Women and schizophrenia. In Kohen D (ed.). *Women and mental health.* London, UK: Routledge, 2000: 133–53.

19. World Health Organization. *Gender and women's mental health.* Geneva, Switzerland: World Health Organization, 2007.

20. Women's Aid. *Principles of good practice for working with women experiencing domestic violence: guidance for mental health professionals.* London, UK: Women's Aid, 2005.

21. Ainscough C, Toon K. *Breaking free workbook*, 2nd edn. London, UK: Sheldon Press, 2000.

22. Williams J. Women's mental health; taking inequality into account. In: Tew J (ed.). *Social perspectives in mental health: developing social models to understand and work with mental distress.* London, UK: Jessica Kingsley, 2005: 151–67.

23. Copeland ME. *Wellness recovery action plan.* Dummerston, VT: Peach Press, 2000.

CHAPTER 59

Services for asylum seekers and refugees

Nicholas Procter*

INTRODUCTION

This chapter aims to describe practical steps in meeting the mental health needs of refugees and asylum seekers. In providing such services, nurses may work with people at the very point of their distress – often during the processes attendant upon gaining asylum or, depending upon the outcome of the claim, a pernament protection visa. Although services may be provided outside of or external to immigration detention facilities, there is scope for mental health nurses to act as consultants to the multidisciplinary team working directly with asylum seekers. Practical strategies are presented in this chapter for the generation of trust and supportive counselling with implications drawn for nurses working across a range of practice settings, such as in accident and emergency departments, psychiatric clinics, community health centres and as general practice nurses. Continuity and integration of mental health nursing care is achieved by bridging discrete elements in the asylum seeker journey through legal reviews, news from home and ongoing psychosocial stressors, in the context of different episodes, interventions by different providers or changes in illness status. Also important will be therapeutic actions that build resilience intrinsically over time, such as the asylum seeker's values, sustained supportive interpersonal relationships and therapeutic care plans. The central argument of this chapter will be that no single organization or individual working alone can achieve the improvement of mental health care and the prevention of mental illness for asylum seekers and/or refugees.

ASYLUM SEEKERS AND GLOBALIZATION

In January 2003, 20.6 million people were registered globally with the United Nations High Commission for Refugees[1] as 'Persons of Concern', approximately one in every 300 people on the planet. More recently, it is estimated that about 1 per cent of the world's population has been displaced either from home or from their home country.[2]

A majority of people seeking asylum come from countries with history of war, conflict and persecution. An

*Nicholas Procter PhD RN is Associate Professor and domain leader for mental health research in the School of Nursing and Midwifery at the University of South Australia. He has a long-standing interest in mental health care and multicultural mental health in particular, and has published widely in these areas.

asylum seeker is described by the United Nations as someone who has made a claim that he or she is a refugee and is awaiting the determination of his or her status. At the time of publication several regions, such as Sudan, Iraq and Afghanistan, are receiving extensive news coverage with fierce and explosive fighting, non-existent to unstable law and order, and hostage-taking being commonplace. A subtle but significant feature of horrors being beamed into our living rooms from these countries is that they represent globalization whereby the compression of the world as Robertson[3,p.25] observes, 'increasingly invokes the creation and incorporation of locality processes which largely shape the world'. Far from people's lives being distanced from what is happening in their homeland, mental health and well-being and a fear of being forced to return are blended in the wake of expanding telecommunications, regulated and non-regulated people movements and the increasing global influences over personal and social life.[4]

With countries such as New Zealand, the UK and Australia being home to asylum seekers, there is an increasing diversity of connections among phenomena once thought disparate and worlds apart. These connections involve ideas and ideologies, people and futures, images and messages, information technologies and techniques that are inevitably interrelated but not homogeneous.[5]

This chapter has been developed within this global context, simultaneously incorporating the fundamental beliefs that prevention of mental health problems, mental illness and suicide should take account of:

1 understanding the factors that heighten the risk of these occurring and the factors that are protective against them;
2 inclusive decision-making and collaborative partnerships between relevant organizations;
3 identifying the groups and individuals likely to benefit from interventions;
4 developing, disseminating and implementing effective interventions that are culturally and linguistically appropriate.[6]

REFUGEE AND ASYLUM SEEKER MENTAL HEALTH

On the basis of 7 years developing clinical response plans on depression and suicidal thinking for people released on 3-year *temporary protection visas* (TPVs) from Immigration Detention Centres across Australia, I have come to appreciate the therapeutic merits of social connectedness as an integrated mental health promotion and suicide prevention activity that is inclusive of interdisciplinary collaboration.[7] Social connectedness is, in this sense, an external 'protective factor' promoting resilience, sense of belonging and purposeful being with others.

There have been some high-profile suicides of asylum seekers in Europe and Australia when the sense of belonging has broken down. On Friday 18 May 2004, Zekria Ghulam Salem Mohammed committed suicide in Glasgow just days after he had been told by the British Home Office that his claims for asylum had been rejected and he must return to Afghanistan. Electronic and print media reports surrounding the death indicate that, after exhausting all legal attempts to stay in Britain, he was told that he would have to leave his flat, and his £38 per week allowance for food and other essentials was stopped. Informal, non-government supports failed to arrive and he was 'too proud to beg and scavenge for food in bins'.[8] Forbidden to work or study, starving, ashamed and broken, he felt there was no hope left. He smashed a glass panel above a door, looped a rope around it and hanged himself. As one of his close friends, who found his body, told Scottish television, 'They first killed his heart and drove him to such a condition that he took his own life'.[9]

The uncertainty of their existence and strongly held beliefs that it is unsafe to return to their country of origin has taken an enormous physical and psychological toll on some. This was highlighted in a very profound way in South Australia in February 2003 when Habib Vahedi, a TPV holder, hanged himself from powerlines after receiving a letter from immigration officials requesting him to return to Afghanistan. His suicide note blamed 'mental pressure'.[10] Habib Vahedi's death exposed the depression and hopelessness many asylum seekers on TPV feel. An educated man, believed to have had a good command of the English language, his death was the subject of much public discussion and debate. In the months following Habib Vahedi's death, men detained in the same conditions as he had been remained silent, fearful that anything they said could adversely affect their visa status. Concern about speaking out was for some overtaken by desperation and a sense of having nothing to lose.

Such anecdotal reports are not uncommon and supported by studies from the United States that have placed prevalence rates for mental ill health among refugees at 40–50 per cent.[11] In the United Kingdom it is estimated that prevalence rates are around 40 per cent.[12] Closer scrutiny of this literature reveals post-traumatic stress disorder (PTSD), depression and anxiety are diagnosed most frequently among refugee children and young people,[13] although a range of other mental illnesses and social and behavioural problems are also widely reported.[14]

It is estimated that several thousands of refugees living in Western countries are believed to be suffering from PTSD.[15] Among those affected, PTSD has been found to be most closely associated with past trauma and elevated stress (re-traumatization) during resettlement, whereas depression has been found to be related to more recent life stresses.[16] Past trauma may take the form of events experienced or witnessed and where lives have been threatened or people have been killed. Also significant for children and young people (as well as adults) is the loss of family, friends, relatives, personal belongings and possessions, livelihood, country and social status. PTSD with co-morbid depression and anxiety is relatively common, but PTSD alone is more likely to sustain over time.

Refugees also suffer from significant conflict-related exposures. The risk factors most commonly found to increase the likelihood of suicide among refugee children and young people include exposure to violence and trauma, lack of family support, living with a mentally ill parent, family stress, being unaccompanied, prolonged (more than 6 months) incarceration in immigration detention centres,[17] poor coping skills and resettlement stress. Within these broad categories, unaccompanied minors, asylum seekers and former child soldiers are at increased risk of mental health problems and mental illness.[18]

Reflection

Imagine that you were required to leave your homeland, fleeing persecution or other intolerable living conditions. What kind of experiences would you be carrying and how might these affect your everyday life?

CULTURAL CONSIDERATIONS OF MENTAL HEALTH

With awareness of how we live in a globalizing culture, we can look more deeply at how different cultures have different views of what constitutes mental health and mental illness. This is largely dependent upon on what each particular culture and individuals within regards as 'normal' or 'abnormal' thought, feeling and/or behaviour, and the influence of other factors such as the immediate social environment, gender, socioeconomic status, education, religion or spiritual beliefs. In many cultures, the Western view of mental illness is a foreign concept. If it is understood at all, it may be seen through explanatory models of spiritual ancestry. At the same time, it may be heavily stigmatized and the Western idea of recovery is almost unknown.

If mental illness is a factor – a person's beliefs about this is important – they can affect all aspects of care, collaboration and partnership. For some, the Western notion of mental illness may be rejected and if so this will have implications for understanding the cause of mental ill health (broadly and culturally defined) to adherence to treatment. Our understanding of these issues in practice helps develop cultural competence. Cultural competence is, in this sense, a set of behaviours, attributes and policy infrastructure that come together in a system or organization or among professionals and enable that system, organization or those professions to work effectively in cross-cultural situations.[19]

Cultural competency for assessment and treatment of mental health problems across cultures requires services to understand the concept of culture, its impact on human behaviour, and the interpretation and evaluation of thought, actions and behaviour. Cultural competency also implies recognition of other issues sometimes associated with working with people from different cultures. These include stigma, isolation, communication and language difficulties, and sensitivity to specific problems experienced by people from diverse cultural backgrounds, clinicians and service providers when working with interpreters in the health setting. Cultural competency in health service delivery also includes the practitioner's ability to understand the emphasis many cultures place on the involvement of family in the client's care and an understanding of the role of family and its implications, particularly in relation to confidentiality and gaining trust.

Based upon the work of Kleinman and Seeman[20] this means examination of the way in which symptoms of mental distress are understood and presented, the way help is sought, and the way care is interpreted and evaluated by those who receive it. This process links the mental health experiences of relocation and settlement as they are held by refugees and asylum seekers, their leaders, healers and other concerned people with health professionals' interpretation of them. The clinical work of mental health nurses – no matter how willing or keen to help – will be compromised if it does not take account of the persons' understanding of health difficulties and what practitioners themselves see as different perceived causes of ill health, optimal care and culturally appropriate support and treatment.[21]

Achieving cultural competence will depend upon the practitioners' openness and flexibility around cultural awareness. The cultural awareness questions listed below are adapted from Multicultural Mental Health Australia's Cultural Awareness Tool[22] and designed to help mental health nurses respond to clients in the context of their mental health problems and/or mental ill health.

- Can you tell me about what brought you here? What do you call this problem? (*Use the client's words for their problem.)
- When do you think it started, and why did it start then?
- What are the main problems it is causing you?
- What have you done to try and stop/manage this * to make it go away or make it better?
- How would you usually manage this * in your own culture to make it go away or make it better?
- How have you been coping so far with this *?
- In your culture, is your * considered 'severe'? What is the worst problem this * could cause you?

- What type of help would you be expecting from me/our service?
- Are there people in your community who are aware that you have this condition?
- What do they think caused this *? Are they doing anything to help you?

When providing services to people from culturally and linguistically diverse backgrounds it is important to communicate clearly. Wherever possible, clients should be able to use their preferred language, especially in stressful situations. If the client requests an interpreter or has inadequate language skills, a professional interpreter should be used. The following tips will help discover how well and to what extent a client speaks and understands English.[23]

- Ask questions the person has to answer in a sentence. Avoid questions that can be answered by 'yes' or 'no'. What? Why? How? When? questions are best.
:• Ask the person to repeat in their own words some information you have just given them.

If the person cannot answer the questions easily, or can't repeat back information accurately, use a professional interpreter. When working across cultures it is important to remember:

- asking people their name, address, date of birth and other predicable information is not an adequate test of English language skills;
- having social conversation skills in English does not always mean a person understands complex information in spoken or written English;
- verbal skills do not always equate with reading and writing skills. Remember the need to tell people their rights and get informed consent;
- people often lose their second language skills in stressful situations, for example, when talking about mental health problems or seeking help.

> ### Reflection
>
> *Imagine that you are interviewing a refugee or an asylum seeker, who appears to have some significant 'mental health problems'.*
>
> - Apart from the questions suggested above – what would you want to ask this person?

MIGRATION AGENT AND/OR LAWYER CONSULTATION

An important part of providing mental health services to refugees and asylum seekers is associated with processes surrounding claims for asylum. Beginning with a selective review of the nature of suicide for migrants and refugees,

I will argue that the structure of individual mental health support should be built around the processes of seeking asylum and coping with rejections and set backs during lengthy and at times complex legal processes. Similarly, the function of supportive mental health counselling during migration agent/lawyer consultation has the potential to help refugees and asylum seekers prepare for the 'next stage' of their (application) journey, helping to build resilience and understand personal reactions to (for example) rejection, fear, frustration and disappointment.

BACKGROUND ISSUES FOR MIGRATION LAW SUPPORT

Although asylum seekers frequently face periods of suffering and periods of calm, individual suffering has become increasingly intolerable at times of re-interviewing and rejection of refugee claims by immigration officials. When people seek asylum their application is considered in light of the information they can supply and any facts known about the country they are fleeing. Some people in immigration detention and at times of re-applying for permanent protection suffer a denial of credibility because of inconsistencies in their story, and this may lead to claims being dismissed on grounds of minor discrepancies. This situation appears at times to have a flow-on effect whereby it is difficult for therapeutic trust to be developed between mental health provider and person in or released from immigration detention.

People value and connect with organizations they trust and this is critical in a system known to push people back into the community without adequate support. From this perspective, the need for valuing human connectedness between organizations and asylum seekers who seek support is consistent with a recent and extensive review of literature about treating possible suicide and life-threatening behaviour. The reviewers concluded that it is the trust inherent in the therapeutic relationship that allows the person to take the necessary risks, do things differently, reach out during periods of acute and excruciating vulnerability, and experiment with new skills, all essential for progress and recovery.[24]

Also important is the knowledge that mental distress and emotional problems can and will impact upon the quality of information people can remember. Where the experience is highly traumatic (for example, a situation involving serious injury to the person) the situation is considered even more complex. There may be important differences between traumatic and non-traumatic memories. For example, initial recall of traumatic events by people with PSTD typically does not involve normal narrative memory. In other words, the story of what happened may be fragmented and therefore appearing inconsistent. Recent research in the UK has found that people seeking asylum who have post-traumatic stress at the time of their interviews are systematically more likely to have their claims rejected the longer their application takes.[25]

To make clinical mental health matters worse, not all countries and jurisdictions provide advanced notice of review procedures. In some settings there is no way of knowing well in advance the precise date and time when interviews to assess claims, invitations to interview or rejection letters will arrive, what questions will be asked or what will be the primary data source used to determine whether a homeland country is safe to return to. The level of distress reported among asylum seekers is significant.

Also significant as a background issue is the knowledge that suicide by people born overseas represents 25 per cent of all suicides.[26] Of these, 60 per cent are by people from non-English-speaking backgrounds.[27] Although suicide is not a mental illness (rather, it is a behaviour), it is strongly associated with mental illness, and the risk factors pertinent to both mental illness and suicide for refugees and asylum seekers are overlapping and inter-related. Thus, the issue of mental health support and suicide prevention necessarily requires an integrated prevention response that acknowledges both the separateness of mental illness and suicide, and the association between the two.

Visa reviews for refugees and asylum seekers are handled by immigration authorities. Procedural delays and at times the fragmented way reviews are being undertaken leaves many asylum seekers disillusioned and suspicious of the processes and sceptical of the outcome. Knowledge of these and other stressors impacting upon refugees and asylum seekers is important for both mental health professionals and migration agents/lawyers because prevention of mental health problems, mental illness and suicide for asylum seekers should incorporate:

- understanding the factors that heighten the risk of these occurring and the factors that are protective against them;
- identifying the groups and individuals likely to benefit from interventions;
- developing, disseminating and implementing effective interventions that are culturally and linguistically appropriate.[28]

Fundamental to the delivery of clinically relevant integrated services will be appreciation of the way in which cultural beliefs guide and inform communication of health problems, the way symptoms are presented, the way stressors are received and when, how and why help is sought and evaluated.

MENTAL HEALTH SUPPORTS WITH MIGRATION AGENT/LAWYER CONSULTATION

With the nexus between mental health need and migration support so apparent, advocacy is an increasing feature of a coordinated response to assist asylum seekers in particular cope with their situation. Up-to-date information about individual claims speaks to the urgent need for coherence and that support is available. For this reason, it is recommended that asylum seekers who are given mental health services have them provided in conjunction with their migration agent/lawyer consultation. Indirect questioning and more attention being given to asylum seekers' expression and explanation of personal narrative, metaphor and symbolism will help articulation of feeling and promote a caring, supportive framework. This framework can provide an important backdrop for feelings to be received, lives revealed and cultural injunctions towards building resilience in order to continue moving forward through legal processes.

The structure of supportive counselling during and after migration agent/lawyer consultations should be built around the processes of seeking asylum and coping with rejections, frustrations and setbacks during what is frequently a lengthy legal process. Similarly, the function of supportive counselling will help asylum seekers prepare for the 'next stage' of their (application) journey, helping to build resilience and understand personal reactions to (for example) rejection, fear, frustration and disappointment. Mental health support with migration agent/lawyer consultation will help in a variety of ways.

- Providing asylum seekers with a confidential relationship within which they are able to disclose personal circumstances in privacy without fear that others may use such information to their detriment. Asylum seekers report that they are particularly anxious concerning how others, for example in group settings, would react to their disclosures. Such anxiety may preclude their productive participation in that setting and exacerbate mental health symptoms.
- Providing opportunities for a closer relationship to develop between the counsellor, migration agent/lawyer and asylum seeker. This factor is particularly important for those who have developed close relationships with significant people in their lives since arriving in Australia and these relationships, by their nature and scope, are fragmented and need clarification and understanding.
- Providing an important forum for discussing how relationships with others (such as volunteer support workers during application and review processes) can be strengthened, strategically focused and, as appropriate, sustained with the intensity they sometimes require over a lengthy, indefinite period of time.[29]

In addition to these matters, individual mental health support and migration agent/lawyer consultation can be conducted to match the asylum seeker's pace of learning what practical help is needed to advance legal processes. This is particularly suited to asylum seekers who, due to their length of time since being released from immigration detention, cope poorly with re-interviewing by immigration authorities and struggle to attain new ways of coping; such issues can be difficult for both counsellors and migration agent/lawyer. This is particularly important for asylum seekers who are contemplating suicide, suffering from poor concentration and who may be distracted by the complexity of interactions that can take place in group settings.

Finally, individual mental health support and migration agent/lawyer consultation may be useful for individuals who feel they need to differentiate themselves from others in group situations in order to feel they can be understood and helped – for example, those who have different political views or English language skills better than those of other asylum seekers.

Reflection

What effect has the information contained so far in this chapter had on your feelings about asylum seekers or refugees?

COMMUNITY MENTAL HEALTH SUPPORT: OVERVIEW OF GENERAL PRINCIPLES

This section uses the term 'social intervention' for interventions that primarily aim to have positive social effects, and the term 'mental health intervention' is used for interventions that primarily aim to have positive mental health effects.

The World Health Organization in its constitution defines health as a state of complete physical, mental and social well-being, and not merely the absence of disease or infirmity.[30] This chapter uses this definition as an anchor point and, at the same time, acknowledges that social interventions have secondary mental health effects and that mental health interventions have social effects as the term 'psychosocial' suggests.

1 Preparation beforehand should involve (i) development of a system of coordination with specific focal persons responsible within each relevant organization; (ii) design of detailed plans to prepare for adequate social and mental health response; and (iii) education and training of relevant personnel in indicated social and psychological interventions.

2 Assessment and planning for the local context (i.e. cultural beliefs, setting, history and nature of mental health problems, family perceptions of distress and illness, ways of coping, resources within community network, etc.). Planning should include quantitative assessment of disability and/or daily functioning as well as qualitative dimensions of context. When assessment uncovers a board range of needs that are unlikely to be met, assessment reports should specify urgency of needs,

local community resources and potential external resources.

3 Collaborative interventions involving consultations and engagement between migration lawyers and/or agents, mental health workers and immigration officials and its contractors, non-government organizations and supporters working in the area is essential to ensure sustainability. A multitude of agencies operating in a synchronized fashion will prevent wastage of valuable resources and help bring benefit to the asylum seeker.

MANAGING INTER-AGENCY CONFLICT

An important consideration regarding mental health services for refugees and asylum seekers is the potential conflict over assessment and care planning. This makes breakdown of communication and deadlock between people and organizations a very real possibility. The implications of this can be catastrophic – especially when the issue (e.g. admission to hospital) is time sensitive. But resolving the problem early on is ultimately more desirable in a health service where many issues have significant implications for inter-related parts of service provision. When people collaborate more freely and openly, they are more likely to trust each other. When people trust their organizations they are more likely to give of themselves now in anticipation of future change and reward.[31]

Knowledge of these and other interventions for people released from immigration detention are important for human service and health professionals because they are fundamental to the delivery of clinically relevant integrated services. To this end it is crucial that there is an appreciation of the way in which cultural beliefs guide and inform communication of health problems, the way symptoms are presented, the way adverse stressors are received and when, how and why help is sought and evaluated.

EMERGENCY MENTAL HEALTH STRATEGIES WHEN APPLICATION FOR ASYLUM IS REJECTED

In the event of the asylum being rejected, evidence of previous behaviour may indicate that the impact on individuals or the family will be negative and place them at risk. The choice of intervention will vary with the phase and personal impact/severity of the rejection. The acute emergency phase is here defined as the period where the crude morbidity rate is elevated and the risk of self-injurious behaviour or harm to others is extreme. This period is followed by a reconsolidation phase when fundamental needs are again at a level comparable to that prior to the emergency.[32] There are a number of valuable early mental health interventions in the acute phase.

1 Establish and maintain contact with interpreter, emergency mental health worker to manage urgent psychiatric crises (i.e. dangerousness, to self or others, psychoses, severe depression, mania). If an individual has any pre-existing mental illness sudden discontinuation of medication should be avoided.

2 Acute interventions due to exposure to extreme stressors may be best managed without medication by following the principles of 'mental health first aid' in order to preserve life where a person may be a danger to themselves and/or others; prevent major or permanent damage to a person's emotional health and well-being, and prevent deterioration and promote recovery.[33] These principles include listening, convey compassion, assess needs, ensure basic physical needs are met, do not force talking, provide or mobilize company from significant trusted others, encourage but do not force social support, protect from further harm.

3 Being cautious in the approach to an individual or family, particularly if the person is not known to the worker or interpreter, or the situation or environment is unfamiliar. Speak in a calm voice saying that you are not here to hurt anyone and your actions are to help this person. Ask yourself the following questions:[33] 'Am I in immediate danger?' 'Is the person in any immediate danger?' (e.g. standing near a road or a dangerous object – actual or potential). 'Is anyone else in immediate danger – especially children or other vulnerable people?' 'Can you safely remove a third person from danger?' 'Can you safely communicate with this person in his/her preferred language?'

Valuable early social interventions may include establishing and disseminating an ongoing reliable flow of credible accurate written and verbal information on (i) the application process; (ii) efforts to establish physical safety of self and family (if a family situation); and (iii) information on efforts being made by each organization/individual to help and support the asylum seeker. Information should be disseminated according to the principles of being uncomplicated and in a language most familiar to the individual and their family (i.e. understandable to a local 12 year old) and empathic (showing understanding of the situation of the family member).

Assuming availability of trusted others it may be useful to organize non-intrusive emotional support and personal safety built around the above principles of mental health first aid. Because of the possible negative effects, it is not advisable to organize forms of single session psychological debriefing that push people to share personal experiences beyond what they would naturally share.[34]

RESEARCH WITH REFUGEES AND ASYLUM SEEKERS

An important consideration when providing services to refugees and asylum seekers is research and evaluation of clinical effectiveness. Research that adopts an iterative consent process[35] is recommended as it is participatory in nature. This means that at each point of the research and evaluation process refugees and asylum seekers as community participants are active in reviewing the aims and objectives of the project and consent to participation is confirmed or rejected. Revising the aims, purposes and permissions of a research project with refugee and asylum seeker clients provides additional opportunity to discuss and clarify information in an incremental and participative way as required. This open and participatory approach keeps the 'door open' for community participants to make informed choices about whether or not to continue with the project, decline to participate further or withdraw all together at any time.

When engaging refugees and asylum seekers in research projects, it is also important to take into account the way in which past experiences can have a profound impact on the way they perceive services now and in the future. For this reason, a non-probing, gentle and supportive inquiry[36] is the preferred method used for clients. For clients who have first-hand experience of system interaction with family or significant others there may also be particular needs and considerations such as feeling marginalized or let down.[37] Special care should be taken by the researcher to prevent distressing symptoms or experiences (previous trauma) from resurfacing. Support and advocacy should be given as required. This may take the form of making a referral to a collaborating transcultural and/or community mental health centre.

> ## Reflection
>
> What specific skills or qualities do you think people need who work with refugees or asylum seekers?
> To what extent do you have these skills and qualities?
> How might you develop them further?

SUMMARY

Globalization and the mass movement of people worldwide is an unavoidable side-effect of war, trauma and regional dislocation. The provision of adequate resources in the form of the delivery of clinically relevant integrated mental health support services is fundamental to prevent risk to refugees and asylum seekers. Continuity and integration of mental health care involving key stakeholders is best achieved by bridging discrete elements in the asylum seeker journey through preparing for visa appeals, visa reviews, news from home and ongoing psychosocial stressors – in the context of different episodes, interventions by different providers, and changes in mental health and well-being. Input from supportive networks that build resilience intrinsically over time is crucial, as it sustains, for example supportive interpersonal relationships and therapeutic care plans. To help strengthen continuity and integration of mental health supports for refugees and asylum seekers, well-resourced care must be experienced as culturally competent and appropriate. This will help provide refugees and asylum seekers with a sense of mental health care as connected and coherent. Fundamental to this will be the ability to synthesize different viewpoints to create workable solutions.

REFERENCES

1. United Nations High Commissioner for Refugees. *Refugees by numbers 2003 edition*. Geneva: UNHCR, 2003.

2. Ringold S, Burke A. Glass RM. Refugee mental health. *The Journal of the American Medical Association* 2005; **294**: 646.

3. Robertson R. Glocalisation: time-space and homogeneity-heterogeneity. In: Featherstone M, Lash S, Robertson R (eds). *Global modernities*. London, UK: Sage, 1995: 25–44.

4. Giddens A. *Runaway world: how globalisation is reshaping our lives*. London, UK: Profile Books, 1999.

5. Appardurai A. Globalisation and the research imagination. *International Social Science Journal* 1999; **51**: 229–38.

6. Australian Health Ministers. *Australian Health Ministers National Mental Health Plan 2003–2008*. Canberra: Australian Government, 2003.

7. Procter NG. Paper plates and throwaway cutlery: aspects of generating trust during mental health initiatives with asylum seekers released from immigration detention centres. *Synergy* 2004; **4**: 8–9.

8. Kelbie P. The life and death of an asylum seeker. *Independent* 2004; **29 May**: 1–2.

9. Procter NG. They first killed his heart (then) he took his own life. Part 1: a review of the context and literature on mental health issues for refugees and asylum seekers. *International Journal of Nursing Practice* 2005; **11**: 286–91.

10. Ashford K. Seeking trust in asylum. *Adelaide Review*. 2003; Nov (2–3). Available from: www.adelaidereview.com.au/archives/2003_11/issuesandopinion_story1.shtml. Accessed 21 October 2007.

11. Sack WH, Him A, Dickason D. Twelve-year follow-up study of Khmer youths who suffered massive war trauma as children. *Journal of the American Academy of Child and Adolescent Psychiatry* 1999; **38**: 1173–9.

12. Hodes M. Psychologically distressed refugee children in the United Kingdom. *Child Psychology and Psychiatry Review* 2000; **5**: 57–68.

13. Hodes M, Tolmac J. Severely impaired young refugees. *Clinical Child Psychology and Psychiatry* 2005; **10**: 251–61.

14. Hodes M. Children of war [Editorial]. *Clinical Child Psychology and Psychiatry* 2005; **10**: 131–76.

15. Frazel M, Wheeler J, Danesh J. Prevalence of serious mental disorder in 7000 refugees resettled in western countries: a systematic review. *Lancet* 2005; **365**: 1309–14.

16. Sack WH, GN Clarke, Seeley J. Multiple forms of stress in Cambodian adolescents refugees. *Child Development* 1996; **27**: 107–16.

17. Steel, Silove D, Brooks R *et al*. Impact of immigration detention and temporary protection on the mental health of refugees. *British Journal of Psychiatry* 2006; **188**: 58–64.

18. Lustig SL, Kia-Keating M, Knight WG *et al*. Review of child and adolescent refugee mental health. *Journal of the American Academy of Child and Adolescent Psychiatry* 2004; **43**: 24–36.

19. Eisenbruch M. *The lens of cultural, the lens of health: toward a framework and toolkit for cultural competence*. Sydney, Australia: Centre for Ethnicity and Health, University of New South Wales, 2004.

20. Kleinman A, Seeman D. Personal experience and illness. In: Albrecht GL, Fitzpatrick R, Scrimshaw SC (eds). *Handbook of social studies in health and medicine*. London, UK: Sage, 2000.

21. Procter NG. *Mental health and human connectedness for all Australians*. 55th Annual Oration, The Great Hall, University of Sydney: Sydney, Australia: The College of Nursing Australia, 2007.

22. *Cultural Awareness Questions*. Multicultural Mental Health Australia, 2004. Available from: www.mmha.org.au. Accessed 21 October 2007.

23. *Language Competency Tips*. Multicultural Mental Health Australia, 2004. Available from: www.mmha.org.au. Accessed 21 October 2007.

24. Rudd MD, Joiner T, Rajab MH. *Treating suicidal behaviour: an effective, time limited approach*. London, UK: Guilford Press, 2001.

25. Herlihy J, Scragg P, Turner S. Discrepancies in autobiographical memory – implications for the assessment of asylum seekers: repeated interviews study. *British Medical Journal* 2002; **324**: 324–7.

26. Cantor C, Neulinger K, Roth J, Spinks D. The epidemiology of suicide and attempted suicide among young Australians. In: *Setting the evidence-based research agenda for Australia: a literature review. National youth suicide prevention strategy*. Canberra: Commonwealth Department of Health and Aged Care, Commonwealth of Australia, 2000: 1–12.

27. Hassan R. *Suicide explained: the Australian experience*. Melbourne: Melbourne University Press, 1995.

28. Australian Health Ministers. *Australian Health Ministers National Mental Health Plan 2003–2008*. Canberra: Australian Government, 2003.

29. Procter NG. Support for temporary protection visa holders: partnering individual mental health support with migration law consultation. *Psychiatry, Psychology and Law* 2004; **11**: 110–12.

30. World Health Organization. The World Health Report 2001. *Mental health: new understanding, new hope*. Geneva: WHO, 2001.

31. Weiss J, Hughes J. Want collaboration? Accept and actively manage conflict. *Harvard Business Review*, 2005; **March**: 92–101.

32. World Health Organization. *Mental health in emergencies, mental and social aspects of health of populations exposed to extreme stressors*. Geneva: Department of Mental Health and Substance Dependence, World Health Organization, 2003.

33. Myhill K, Tobin M. *Mental health first aid for South Australians*. Adelaide, Australia: Mental Health Unit, Department of Human Services, 2001.

34. McFarlane AC. Debriefing: care and sympathy are not enough (Editorial). *Medical Journal of Australia* 2003; **178**: 533–4.

35. Procter NG. *Speaking of sadness and the heart of acceptance: reciprocity in education*. Sydney, Australia: Multicultural Mental Health Australia, 2004.

36. Mitchell TL, Radford JL. Rethinking research relationships in qualitative research. *Canadian Journal of Community Mental Health* 1996; **15**: 49–60.

37. Marshall SL, While AE. Interviewing respondents who have English as a second language: challenges encountered and suggestions for other researchers. *Journal of Advanced Nursing*. 1994; **19**: 566–71.

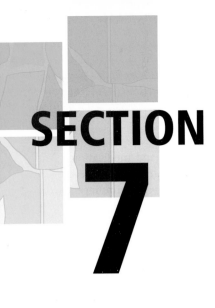

SECTION 7

SOME STANDARDIZED PROCESSES OF NURSING PRACTICE

Preface to Section 7

Students need to learn what makes people tick in a human sense. Even if people end up working in a highly medicalized area, it is vital that students recognize the importance of social, psychological and spiritual perspectives. This is, after all, what brought the patient into contact with the services in the first place.

Ed Manos

As members of the multidisciplinary team, nurses have discrete responsibilities. In earlier sections, some of the broad principles and the value base of nursing practice were illustrated. In this section, we consider how nurses might fulfil more specific roles in the development or delivery of specific *aspects* of mental health service provision.

The section begins with the process of admission to hospital and ends with the emerging role of nurses in the prescription and overall management of medication. These two chapters illustrate both the tradition of care and treatment – hospitalization and medication – and how practice is changing, as a result of political, economic and philosophical factors, all of which impinge on our appreciation of the quality of care.

This section also includes considerations of how nurses might approach the assessment and engagement with people who represent a risk to themselves, through suicide or self-harm. We also consider how care is documented, through record-keeping and as preparation for discharge. And we consider the highly specific role of the nurse in the electroconvulsive therapy delivery programme in which caring and clinical expertise must achieve a perfect balance.

This section also includes a thorough examination of the emergent role of the nurse in mental health promotion and prevention. This chapter clearly signals the future of genuine mental health care, with its many challenges and potential rewards.

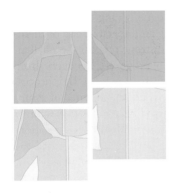

CHAPTER 60

Admission to a psychiatric unit

Angela Simpson* and Jerome Wright**

THE CRISIS AND OPPORTUNITY OF HOSPITAL ADMISSION

The person on the brink of admission to an acute inpatient unit is invariably frightened. This fear is commonly compounded by the growing realization of the need for admission to inpatient psychiatric care. For the person in crisis, the scale of personal change can seem overwhelming. It is not uncommon for the person to feel as if a breaking point has been reached, destabilizing the 'self' and the person's perception of themselves in the future. Following such a breakdown, people commonly find themselves in a situation in which they need to redefine themselves and their relationships, and begin to question the direction of their lives.

Nurses working in acute inpatient settings are in close contact with people in distress. As a result, they can find the experience of working *with* people in crisis unnerving. People in crisis respond in different ways to distress, so the ward environment is often characterized by uncertainty and unpredictability. In these conditions, nurses may begin to question their ability to respond effectively and may even doubt their skill in supporting people in crisis. A gap between what the person in crisis needs and what nurses

feel able to provide can lead nurses to question their purpose, role and potential usefulness. A reaction to this occupational stress may lead nurses to seek to *control* the environment, leading to criticism that acute admission wards provide custodial rather than therapeutic care.[1-3]

Failing to recognize acute admission wards as highly complex and innately 'fear-full' places is a fundamental error when seeking to create and sustain a caring and therapeutic environment. Fear has positive as well as negative effects. It frees us from complacency, stimulates action and, above all, brings us face to face with our shared humanity or common human experience. From this starting point, acute admission wards might be freed from the presence of overwhelming fear and control, and the development of fundamentally humanizing, and caring, environments may be realized.

THE FUNCTION OF ACUTE ADMISSION WARDS

Although available resources have prioritized delivering mental health care in the community over the last decade, research has indicated that demand for inpatient

*Angela Simpson is course leader for the Post Graduate Diploma (Mental Health Nursing) and a Research Fellow at the University of York. She has worked extensively in mental health nursing over a 20-year period and has a particular interest in nursing practice development in acute inpatient admission settings. Her recent research focused on the management of depression in primary care settings and recovery from self-cutting.

**Jerome Wright is a Lecturer in Nursing at the University of York, UK. He has a clinical nursing background in a variety of care specialties including acute mental health care and community psychiatric nursing and as a Clinical Nurse Specialist in liaison psychiatry. He has a particular interest in the care of people in acute distress and for those with concurrent physical health problems, and currently teaches and researches on HIV/AIDS and mental health.

psychiatric care remains strong.[4] Further, demographic, economic and societal changes, and the widening gap between the rich and poor, have a major impact on people's mental health. The nature and organization of existing mental health services also significantly affect the role and functioning of the acute admission unit. Expansion of community-based treatment interventions, such as crisis intervention, early intervention and assertive outreach, not only influence the severity and complexity of patients' problems and length of stay on the unit but also highlight the perspective of the role that the acute inpatient unit serves within the context of mental health care. This perspective renders incompatible the 'hospital-centric' view of service provision in favour of one that reinforces inpatient care as a brief supportive intervention within a range of mental health services that are flexible enough to meet the individual and changing needs of patients. Such a move encapsulates the shift from 'what services offer' to 'what people need'. From such a perspective, support is offered through respect and active engagement, helping people to interpret and make sense of their own experiences, offering choice, information and a continuity of care.[5–8] Incorporating these human conditions into the milieu of acute inpatient care shifts the focus away from the ward as a repository for the most troubled and vulnerable to a place of healing and recovery where caring relationships can be established.

NURSING ALONGSIDE THE PERSON IN ACUTE DISTRESS

Mental health nurses should be 'natural allies' of people in emotional crisis.[9] The close proximity of the nurse to the person in crisis affords an opportunity to develop close alliances with people in care, establishing relationships that foster hope and growth, while also providing practical and emotional support. Two core nursing values – empowerment and curiosity – allow nurses to develop such close rapport.

The nurse who seeks to actively empower the person in crisis acknowledges the person as 'an expert of the self', and as such identifies strongly with the need to place the person at the centre of decision-making. To empower the person, nurses demonstrate an awareness of the person's needs, the need to promote personal choice, to provide information, to allow time to complete tasks and to discuss future care options.[10]

Maintaining a fundamental sense of curiosity about the person and his or her experiences is also necessary. Peplau[11] spoke of a 'gentle curiosity', which is a willingness to relate to people and a concern to provide people with the support they need to free themselves from their distress. This is more than a fleeting attention, offered only when the person's speech or actions demand it, but is an active engagement and dialogue, seeing the task of the person in crisis as developing an understanding of themselves. For people in acute distress, this can be challenging and traumatic 'work in progress'. Recovery from psychological or emotional distress is not a tidy process and it does not necessarily involve the absence of symptoms,[12] since the person might resolve to live with or work through distress. Thus, individual caring relationships that are established in crisis might best instil the prospect of limitless possibilities within the person.

The first 72 hours of any person's admission to an acute inpatient ward are pivotal to the establishment of the helping relationship and are likely to have a significant impact on the person's experience of crisis and his or her view of the prospect for recovery. Here, a case illustration follows Jon and his family through the first 3 days after admission to an acute psychiatric unit.

Personal illustration 60.1

Jon is 17 years old. He has recently returned to live in the family home after spending a year living in a shared house with fellow students. He has dropped out of his studies and spends his time isolated in his bedroom. Contacts with his friends have deteriorated. There is growing tension between Jon and his brother. Unlike Jon, Andy has graduated from college, has found himself a job which he enjoys and has a wide circle of friends. This growing tension resulted in an incident in which Jon threatened and physically assaulted his brother. Jon's family is becoming increasingly concerned about him, especially his irritability and growing emotional distance. They seek advice from their general practitioner (GP). Jon admits to the family doctor that he has been hearing voices since he left home and that these are scary because they are critical and derogatory. The situation between Jon and his brother continues to deteriorate and the family is at breaking point. The GP arranges for a psychiatrist to visit, and it is recommended that Jon be admitted to hospital for further assessment.

MEETING THE PERSON IN CRISIS

The decision to admit Jon to an inpatient admission unit is medically led, but is made in collaboration with Jon, his family and the nursing team. In preparing to meet Jon, the nurse takes the opportunity to discuss what is already known about him, seeking the views of the medical team regarding the purpose of the hospital admission. In Jon's case the family situation is vital so, where possible, the nurse takes the opportunity to discuss the wider social situation, with the team, which has been involved recently. This background information gives the nurse some idea of what to expect from Jon and his family on admission. More especially, the nurse develops early insight into Jon's own view of his admission to hospital, helping the nurse to gauge whether Jon is likely to be a willing, or reluctant, participant.

Medical colleagues are likely to have already begun to form a 'working hypothesis' regarding an early diagnosis of Jon's condition, which will be reflected in conversations with the nursing team and records relating to the admission. While taking into account the views of medical colleagues, it is important that nurses remain open-minded. The nursing focus will place considerable emphasis on attempting to understand Jon's experience of distress, identifying strongly with Jon's interpretation of his own experience.[13]

Although acute inpatient units offer a responsive crisis service, there is usually always a time interval between the ward receiving notification of the need for admission to hospital and the person arriving on the ward. This time is put to good use by nurses who, in preparing to meet Jon:

- collate all available information about Jon and his family, liaising with other members of the multiprofessional team who have already established contact – such as medical and primary care colleagues;
- make appropriate preparations on the ward, creating a comfortable bed space for him.

Prior to admission, the nursing team should identify the nurse who is best placed to be Jon's key nurse. This will involve:

- providing a consistent source of contact for Jon and his family
- working closely with Jon, providing the conditions in which a constructive, helping relationship might be developed
- accepting responsibility for coordinating Jon's care
- liaising with the nursing team and wider multiprofessional team to coordinate Jon's care while he is in hospital.

Prior to admission nurses concern themselves with creating the conditions in which Jon might experience a strong sense of 'togetherness' or 'attachment'. The nursing team should be aware that Jon is likely to identify closely with the nurse undertaking the admission interview,[14] so in most cases this nurse becomes best placed to further develop the key nurse relationship.

Reflection

- Explore how being in close proximity to people in acute distress makes you feel.
- Identify philosophical values that might best underpin the beginnings of a helping relationship.
- How might the nurse best demonstrate the philosophical values to the person who has become the patient?

Arrival at the unit

People react in different ways to the experience of hospital admission. Typical responses can include a sense of hopelessness questioning 'What good is this going to do?' Others sometimes feel rejected by family or those close to them. Some people, especially those compulsorily admitted, feel angry or irritated by the prospect. Whatever the view of the person about their admission, the nurse must accept the person as they are within the crisis, and allow this to be the starting point of constructive helping.

Taking an interest in how the person presents on arrival to the ward will inform the key nurse about the level of the person's discomfort and distress. This distress should be acknowledged by the key nurse who:

- introduces themselves to Jon, explaining that they are a nurse on the ward who has special responsibility to work closely with him
- empathizes with Jon's situation
- seeks guidance from Jon about what can be done now to make him more comfortable
- recognizes the social discomfort experienced by Jon, who is clearly outside of his usual environment.

The key nurse is well aware that the experience of being admitted to hospital, or having a family member/close associate admitted to hospital, is stressful. As such, the key nurse communicates interest in Jon, his family and friends and his situation and is careful to demonstrate respect. Although the situation is far from 'normal', commonly nurses are able to break this difficult 'social ice' by gently normalizing the situation. Nurses do this by remaining relaxed (although quietly confident) and paying immediate attention to the comfort needs of Jon and his family who need:

- private space on the ward to talk with each other, and the nurse
- refreshments
- to know where Jon's bedroom is located
- to be shown where the bathroom/toilets are located
- to identify with the key nurse as a consistent and helpful presence.

Orientating the person to his new surroundings helps Jon to feel at ease on the ward. These early attempts to ease the distress of the admission process can be likened to friendship building. The person in distress expects nurses to function as both friend and professional.[15] Admitting Jon to hospital allows the nurse the opportunity to extend simple kindness, in a genuine attempt to develop a personable relationship characterized by mutual understanding and warmth. Jon and his family might find some comfort in the fact that, although the situation is an unusual one for them, it is not unusual for the key nurse.

The ward as a safe haven

Jon needs to be reassured that the ward is safe. The nurse communicates this in two ways. Firstly, interpersonal safety and trust are nurtured through the beginnings of the helping relationship. Here, the nurse develops a personable relationship with Jon and his family and provides information in an easy and relaxed manner, but is also competent and responds to situations requiring professional knowledge and expertise. Secondly, the nurse communicates issues of wider personal safety directly to the person on admission. Jon's attention is drawn to some basic ground rules that maintain the safety of everyone, whether residing, visiting or working within the unit. These usually include:

- the need to store all medications in a clinical room
- the need for every person to hand in sharp objects
- no alcohol to be drunk or stored on the ward
- no illicit substances to be used or stored on the ward
- the need for everyone to treat each other with courtesy and respect.

While these ground rules help to instil confidence that the ward is safe, the nurse should also discuss with Jon the team's expectations that everyone will treat one another, and the environment, with respect. Although people will experience episodes of distress from time to time, the nursing team should clearly articulate the importance and expectation that everyone concerned will attempt to support each other through extending concern and respect. When distressed, the person is expected to extend the same degree of concern for others that they would expect for themselves, while also being respectful of the environment. These are the conditions that will help the person to best support himself and support others, while allowing nurses to provide support to Jon and other people admitted to the ward.

Reflection

- How does the nurse best orientate the person in care to the acute ward environment?
- Identify ways in which the nurse creates the conditions in which a helping relationship might start to be developed.

Preparing for the admission interview

The nurse begins, tentatively, to develop an understanding of Jon and his wider family situation. However, it is important to note that these impressions remain 'impressions' until they are carefully explored with Jon. The nurse uses the admission interview to explore Jon's perceptions of his experience. The timing of the admission interview itself is important. Although most people admitted to hospital like Jon are willing and able to talk through their situation in more detail, on admission some are initially unwilling or unable to engage in this process. It is important to recognize that the quality of the interview and the opportunity within it for constructive engagement is pivotal to therapeutic helping. The admission interview is best undertaken as a collaborative process, so the nurse seeks to create the conditions in which Jon might become a willing and active participant in the process.

The nurse takes the time to discuss with Jon what he might expect from the admission interview, gauging his willingness and potential ability to collaborate. At this early stage, the nurse needs to demonstrate a willingness to work with Jon as a person, responding to his individual needs. This means allowing time and space to make decisions, but, more especially, allowing personal choice whenever it is possible to do so. These conditions help to reduce fear. As Jon retains control and independence, autonomy is promoted and respected. This also means, however, that in some respects the nurse is following the lead of the person in care.

While the process of conducting the admission interview necessarily involves the nurse asking questions and recording supporting information, it is important that the interview does not descend into a remote, impersonal 'tick box' exercise. The nurse is challenged to overcome the organizational need to collate specific information and the nursing aim of striving to meet with the person, developing an increased understanding of Jon the 'person' and his experience of crisis. Creating the conditions in which such human contact can occur requires a degree of preparation. Jon needs to understand why the admission interview is necessary, and also must be informed that information collected and written down will be shared with other members of the multi-professional team. To prepare Jon for the admission interview and win collaborative support for the process, the nurse:

- explains the interview process
- gives Jon copies of the paperwork to be completed
- encourages him to ask questions
- counters concerns that it is a lengthy process by reassuring him that it can be completed at his pace, allowing time for a break if necessary
- understands that Jon might not be able to complete the interview in one attempt; if this occurs it is the nurse's responsibility to continue to attempt to create the conditions in which Jon might settle to this collaborative task.

THE ADMISSION INTERVIEW: THE PATIENT AS A PERSON

The admission interview provides the nurse with a valuable opportunity to make human contact with Jon. This is the forum in which the skillful nurse begins to sow the seeds of a constructive helping relationship. At the admission interview, the nurse listens carefully to Jon's account of his experience of distress and investigates with him how this affects his ability to live everyday life.[13] Adopting this approach allows the nurse to demonstrate early concern and understanding for Jon as a person. It also helps to instil early confidence in Jon that his perceptions and concerns might best be addressed within a constructive and supportive relationship as opposed to facing this alone.

The admission interview is not a routine chore and is best approached by nurses who possess a keen interest and an open mind. According to Barker[13,p.43] the admission interview serves the nurse with opportunity to:

- develop a relationship with the person
- establish trust
- promote professional closeness and collaboration
- start to identify problematic patterns in the person's actions
- identify how the person's personal resources might help the person to overcome distress.

The admission interview achieves its optimum potential when both parties experience it as a 'human-to-human' activity. For nurses, this might mean accepting the need to leave their 'professional' status to one side, choosing instead to give something of themselves, placing emphasis on attempting to understand Jon's 'human crisis' in a 'human way'. In developing this line of enquiry, the nurse will explore:

- Jon's perception of the circumstances that have resulted in the hospital admission
- how Jon views himself now within the crisis
- how it feels to be Jon
- how things have changed for Jon and how he feels about this
- Jon's view on the family crisis.

In finding out more about Jon and his situation, the nurse is likely to begin to gauge the extent of his personal distress. Assessing the extent to which people might be a risk to themselves or other people is an important feature of the admission interview. The nurse will have developed an awareness of how Jon's experience and situation are affecting his ability to live and will also have developed some understanding of the extent to which Jon feels his situation to be inside or outside of his own control. During the admission interview, the nurse will develop a sense of how Jon sees himself in the future. The extent to which he feels optimism or hopelessness are important elements of this process. Felt hopelessness is strongly associated with personal risk.[16] The admitting nurse therefore needs to question Jon sensitively with regard to the issue of personal safety, discussing how Jon

and the ward team can work together to maintain and maximize meaningful interpersonal engagement while seeking also to maximize personal safety.

At some point, the nurse will need to look beyond the immediate *felt* need of Jon's experiences and seek to explore wider health needs or concerns. Although it is unlikely that Jon's mental health difficulties will have resulted in severe physical ill health, this cannot be assumed. Personal neglect and preoccupation with particular thoughts and worries may have reduced Jon's ability to ensure he receives adequate diet, nutrition, rest, etc. His deteriorating mental state may also have led to him engage in behaviours that may affect his physical health such as drug-taking, sexual behaviour or being the victim of violence.[17,18] It is also not uncommon for patients to have pre-existing, concurrent or indeed previously unidentified physical health problems that are affected by the acute mental health crisis. The nurse therefore needs to create the opportunity for Jon to explore such issues, to identify any health risks or vulnerabilities and, with Jon's consent, to initiate any appropriate investigations or treatments. Attention to such physical health needs and their relation to mental health reflects a holistic approach to care and encourages Jon to view himself as a 'whole' person with unique and interrelated needs.[19]

The nurse needs to:

- seek permission from Jon to explore other areas of his lifestyle that may affect his health;
- listen to Jon's perspective of health concerns and behaviour;
- if necessary, at an appropriate time, initiate discussion on the risk behaviours commonly related to mental health problems;
- provide a rationale for and perform routine health observations such as blood pressure, pulse, respirations, temperature, weight and urinalysis;
- assess with Jon and other members of the multidisciplinary team the priority of attending to any concerns;
- organize any necessary investigations, examinations or specialist referral.

> ## Reflection
>
> - Describe the role of the psychiatric nurse when carrying out an admission interview.
> - How does the nurse best convey a sense of individual understanding to the person in care?
> - How does demonstrating individual understanding help to embed the helping relationship?
> - Consider ways in which personal/physical neglect may contribute to the overall health of the person in distress.

Recording the interview collaboratively

During the interview the nurse begins to formulate an understanding of Jon, his condition and his situation. Having listened carefully and made observations, the nurse checks their perceptions and understandings with Jon to clarify their accuracy and to avoid making assumptions. Striving to achieve this degree of accuracy helps to convey genuine concern and respect. At some point, the observations made by the nurse and Jon will need to be recorded. Progressive nursing teams will recognize the value of offering Jon the opportunity to write down his own experience in his own words.[15] If Jon does not feel able to do this, the nurse agrees the language to be used within the documentation and writes this down on his behalf. The nurse might choose to use direct quotes made by Jon, as his language is likely to closely reflect his experience. Undertaken in this way, the admission interview has the potential to be fundamentally empowering, as the person in care is involved in a transparent documentary process, which is inherently collaborative. More especially, by completing the admission assessment with Jon, he retains a degree of control within the process.

Negotiating care

Jon needs to maintain a sense of purpose regarding the hospital admission. This is achieved when a plan of care for the next 72 hours is developed collaboratively. The nurse discusses with Jon what he might expect to happen over the next few hours and days. Jon needs to be informed of the degree of individual contact that he can expect from his key nurse and also any structured group activity he might be expected to attend. Jon needs to understand that these opportunities exist so that he might learn through his own experience, but also through the wider experience of others. It is not uncommon for people in distress to feel as though they are not worthy of help themselves, but they can invariably be persuaded to offer support to others. This is a highly constructive starting point for people who are reluctant to share their experiences with others.

Beyond this, Jon also needs to know how to access nursing support quickly should he begin to feel a growing sense of unease and distress. The nurse must also ensure that Jon receives support without needing to ask for it. Jon needs to develop an awareness at this early stage that the primary purpose of the admission to hospital is for him to find the words to articulate his distress. Jon needs to get to know and understand his distress while being supported in a safe and purposeful care environment.

As the admission interview draws to its natural conclusion, the nurse takes the opportunity to thank Jon for working through the process and acknowledges that the task may well have been a difficult one for Jon to undertake. The nurse remains optimistic, indicating a willingness to continue to work constructively with Jon.

Summary

The nurse conducting the admission interview:

- views the admission process as a unique opportunity to make 'human contact' with Jon; this is not a routine, menial or paper-based task, rather it provides the nurse with the opportunity to develop awareness of Jon's experience of distress and how this affects the way he lives;
- provides simple, practical support to enable Jon to become comfortable within the ward surroundings;
- is quietly, but authoritatively, supportive, mixing informal friendly support with practical expertise;
- looks beyond diagnostic labels, developing a keen interest in Jon's view of what is happening for him;
- is keenly attentive, listening to Jon, allowing him time to identify with his experience and feelings, while remaining watchful;
- recognizes that helping relationships are developed over time in small steps; the developing sense of 'togetherness' helps to create the conditions in which Jon might begin to feel safe and emotionally supported;
- avoids making assumptions about Jon's experience; rather, the nurse demonstrates interest and respect by carefully checking Jon's interpretation of his experience;
- ensures a collaborative assessment of need over time that enables related health concerns or risk behaviours to become identified and addressed.

The nurse conducting the interview will have obtained a large amount of information about Jon, his experience of distress and his view of his current situation. This will be communicated to other nurses and the wider multi-professional team. Shared awareness of Jon and his situation helps the team to plan purposeful and constructive care for the next few days.

Reflection

- Consider ways in which the nurse might actively collaborate with people in acute distress.
- How might nurses best create the conditions in which people are supported to articulate their distress?

CHANGING PRESENTATION OF THE PERSON IN CRISIS

Although the nurses will have worked carefully with Jon collecting further information regarding his situation and condition, they need to recognize that this assessment represents a snapshot of Jon's experience and is subject to continual change. Jon's changing needs are illustrated as his story of distress continues to unfold.

During the night Jon again experiences some scary voices, which he said were telling him that his life was worthless. He briefly talks to the nursing staff on duty about this but is not willing to talk at length. The following day, Jon is observed packing his belongings and says that he is leaving. He seems distracted and single-minded.

Working with the person in acute distress involves responding constructively and purposefully to meet the person's needs. Such help is best constructed when nurses accept the person when they are emotionally seeking to expand their knowledge of the person's unique experience of distress.

The primary focus of nursing involves attempting to understand the experience of the person in crisis as opposed to attempting to explain it.[13] This is an important distinction. Here, the nurse who seeks to explain Jon's experience is likely to focus on Jon's recent voice hearing and view this in a restricted way, regarding this as a feature of his illness that might best be managed through increased observation and perhaps medication. This limits Jon's involvement in the potential solution and restricts his ability to learn through his experience of distress. It also reinforces the view that Jon is ill and therefore in need of medical attention.

The nurse who seeks to understand Jon and his experience, and views this as the primary (although not exclusive) focus of nursing, will avoid applying diagnostic criteria to Jon's experience of distress, but instead will focus attention on:

- recognizing Jon's increasing distress as a human response to crisis
- providing Jon with a safe space to articulate his experience
- accepting his experience of distress, without judging him
- seeking further clarification about what is happening now
- allowing Jon to talk through his distress, exploring what is happening for him
- exploring all of the options available, discussing the likely consequences of proposed actions
- identifying Jon's strengths that might help him manage this crisis.

In seeking to understand the person's experience, the crisis and the situation, nursing employs a shift in emphasis away from the medicalization of the life problems. This involves caring with the person, within which the experience of distress is openly shared and available strengths and opportunities are explored and utilized. There may be a need for medical treatment within this situation, but equally there may not. To gauge this need with compassion and understanding of Jon's human needs, nurses must retain their caring focus, viewing nursing as unique and valued in its own right. By seeking to understand Jon's human experience, the nurse creates the opportunity for Jon to discuss his distress. This involves the person in identifying with a range of opportunities that exist within the crisis and seeks to support the person through the process. The range of opportunities available to the person in crisis is expanded rather than restricted and, wherever possible, the nurse maximizes opportunities for the person to make his or her own choices. More especially the person in crisis begins to acknowledge that the solution to the crisis and the problems of living rests within themselves. Thus, caring retains an empowering and optimistic focus and the person in crisis is supported throughout the experience of distress. The nurse shares the journey towards recovery with the person in crisis.

Summary

The nurse works with the person in crisis, empathically and pragmatically. Nurses avoid over-reacting to the crisis situation, seeking instead to develop their understanding of the person and his or her situation through constructive dialogue.

- The nurse approaches crisis situations with openness and curiosity.
- The nurse does not jump to early conclusions and keeps calm, allowing the person to articulate his or her distress.
- Where possible, the nurse promotes choice.
- The nurse gently points out possible limitations within the person's own thinking.
- The nurse seeks to de-escalate the situation while minimizing whenever possible the need for the use of control.

REFERENCES

1. Sainsbury Centre for Mental Health. *Acute problems: a survey of the quality of care in acute psychiatric wards*. London, UK: Sainsbury Centre for Mental Health, 1998.

2. Muijen M. Acute hospital care: ineffective, inefficient and poorly organised. *Psychiatric Bulletin* 1999; **23**: 257–9.

3. Barker S. *Environmentally unfriendly: patients' views of conditions on psychiatric wards*. London, UK: Mind, 2000.

4. Cleary M. The realities of mental health nursing in acute inpatient environments. *International Journal of Mental Health Nursing* 2004; **13**: 53–60.

5. Lewis SE. A search for meaning: making sense of depression. *Journal of Mental Health* 1995; **4**: 369–82.

6. Deegan P. Recovery as a journey of the heart. *Psychiatric Rehabilitation Journal* 1996; **19**: 91–7.

7. Read J. What do we want from mental health services? In: Read J, Reynolds J (eds). *Speaking our minds*. Milton Keynes, UK: Open University Press, 1996.

8. Faulkner A. Evidence of what? *Mental Health Nursing* 2000; **20** (6): 3.

9. Repper J. Adjusting the focus of mental health nursing; incorporating service users' experiences of recovery. *Journal of Mental Health* 2000; **9** (6): 575–87.

10. Faulkner M. Empowerment and disempowerment; models of staff/patient interaction. *Nursing Times Research* 2001; **6** (6): 936–48.

11. Peplau H. *Interpersonal relationships in nursing*. New York, NY: Putnam, 1952.

12. Anthony WA. Recovery from mental illness: the guiding vision of the mental health service system in the 1990s. *Psychosocial Rehabilitation Journal* 1993; **12**: 55–81.

13. Barker PJ. *Assessment in psychiatric and mental health nursing*, 2nd edn. Cheltenham, UK: Nelson Thornes, 2004.

14. Altschul AT. *Patient–nurse interaction*. Edinburgh, UK: Churchill Livingstone, 1972.

15. Jackson S, Stevenson C. What do people need psychiatric and mental health nurses for? *Journal of Advanced Nursing* 2000; **31** (2): 378–88.

16. Barker P, Buchanan-Barker P. *The tidal model: a guide for mental health professionals*. New York, NY: Brunner Routledge, 2005.

17. Smith MD. HIV risk in adolescents with severe mental illness: literature review. *Journal of Adolescent Health* 2001; **29**: 320–9.

18. Hercus M, Lubman DI, Hellard M. Blood-borne viral and sexually transmissible infections amongst psychiatric populations: what are we doing about them? *Australian & New Zealand Journal of Psychiatry* 2005 **39**: 849–55.

19. Department of Health. *From values to action: the Chief Nursing Officer's review of mental health nursing*. London, UK: Department of Health, 2006.

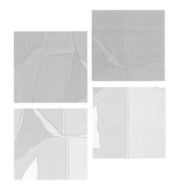

CHAPTER 61

Assessing risk of suicide and self-harm

John Cutcliffe*

INTRODUCTION

Suicide and self-harm, although by no means exclusive to the population, are often associated with people with mental health problems. Indeed, the commonality of self-injurious behaviour is such that psychiatric–mental health nurses (PMHNs) are highly likely to encounter people who present with an increased risk of suicide and/or self-harm. This chapter will thus not belabour the obvious need for PMHNs to be competent in risk assessment of *both* suicide risk and risk of self-harm. Although risk assessment is only the beginning and, to be effective, must lead to evidence-based interventions,[1,2] the possibility of prevention arguably lies in the veracity of risk assessment and the judicious application of these findings to each individual situation.

However useful, risk assessment is a complex and imperfect science; one bedevilled with conceptual difficulties, methodological limitations and operational problems. This chapter outlines some ways of enhancing nurses' risk assessment through the use of empirically based risk assessment instruments. The limitations of such instruments are acknowledged and situated within the broader context of risk assessment per se.

DEFINITIONS

Distinctions between *self-harm* (sometimes called parasuicide) and *suicide* are problematic, not least because of the practical difficulties in determining the person's intent,[3] the historical conflation of the phenomenon in the associated literature and the related problems of producing a shared nomenclature (and resultant definition) for suicide.[4] As a result, construction of a precise definition that clearly differentiates between self-harm and suicide is difficult, though this may be helped by the recently published proposed nomenclature for the study of suicide.[5] Nevertheless, previous attempts at definitions have been made. Shneidman's[6,7] undeniable contributions to suicidology include early work towards a definition. His 1973 definition[6] stated that suicide is the human act of self-inflicted, self-intentioned cessation of life. In 1985 he declared that[7,p.3]

suicide is a conscious act of self-annihilation, best understood as a multi-dimensional malaise in a needful individual who defines an issue which suicide is the best solution.

*John Cutcliffe holds the 'David G. Braithwaite' Professor of Nursing Endowed Chair at the University of Texas (Tyler), USA. He is also the Associate Dean: Psychiatric Nursing, Stenberg College, Vancouver, Canada, and Adjunct Professor of Nursing, University of Ulster, UK. John is an Associate Editor for the International Journal of Mental Health Nursing and Assistant Editor for the International Journal of Nursing Studies. His principal research interest is suicide and the care of the suicidal person.

Whereas *self-harm* has been defined as[8]

> any non-fatal act in which an individual deliberately causes self-injury or ingests a substance in excess of any prescribed or generally recognised therapeutic dose.

And more recently[9] as the deliberate alteration of body tissue without conscious suicidal content or intent:[10]

> Self-harm is commonly defined as an individual's intentional damage to a part of his or her body, without a conscious intent to die, although the result might be fatal.

Some authors continue to conflate the terms, proposing that they are 'one and the same'; merely different points on a continuum of lethality.[11,12] Most contemporary theoretical and empirical work clearly distinguishes self-harm from suicide and suicidal ideation. These differences were captured succinctly by Maris *et al.*:[13]

> as a starting point, we must distinguish indirect self-destructive behaviors from behaviors more directly suicidal … In marked contrast, there are, however, a vast number of behaviors that are self-harmful, frequently injurious, self-negating, and self-defeating in which the individual engages but in which there may be no intention to die.

There are significant differences between suicide and self-harm, and not only in the outcome. Self-harm is not necessarily a failed suicide attempt. Reduced to their most fundamental differences, self-harm is a *life-orientated*, coping-related act, whereas suicide is death-orientated. Furthermore, while self-harm questions have been included in some suicide risk instruments,[14] this can be misleading, not only for the subject/client but also for the interpretation of the results. Therefore, this chapter acknowledges the differences between self-harm and suicide and deals with them separately.

However, by differentiating between suicide and self-harm, I am not suggesting that the issues are not linked or that any person who self-harms is, by the nature of the differences, not at risk of suicide. Indeed, numerous studies continue to highlight the significantly increased risk of eventual suicide for people who engage in self-harm.[10,15] However, a wealth of empirical evidence shows that more than 95 per cent of people who engage in self-harm do *not* go on to take their own lives.[10,16,17]

Reflection

In the practice settings you have experience of, what evidence have you seen of the conflation of suicide and self-harm?

ASSESSING RISK OF SELF-HARM

Several variables appear to be linked to increased risk of self-harm.[17] These include:

- being single or divorced
- being unemployed
- having a recent change in living situation
- having a so-called mental disorder
- having a previous self-harm incident.

While acknowledging the methodological limitations of this study the most significant risk factors identified were younger age and being female. In a related study,[18] the risk factors identified were:

- high incidence of psychiatric illness (affective disorders in particular)
- psychiatric co-morbidity
- family distress
- sexual abuse
- physical abuse.

The findings from studies such as these offer a useful starting point for risk assessment, although the following caveats should be considered. Firstly, rates of self-harm in populations are not static; patterns of self-harming behaviour change over time.[3,15,19,20] The often cited stereotypical image of a self-harmer as a white, middle class, teenage girl is far from the reality of the situation. Accordingly, it would be imprudent for PMHNs to 'lock themselves in' to these stereotypical views of the key at-risk populations. Secondly, while these studies provide valuable information regarding 'conventional risk factors', there is a growing recognition that assessing for conventional risk factors alone is likely to be insufficient, potentially misleading and is unlikely to improve the current predictive criteria, given the heterogeneous nature of the population who engage in self-harm.[21]

A study of the specificity of risk assessment for self-harm found that the most potent short-term predictor of self-harm repetition was the Beck Hopelessness Scale, whereas in the longer term the number of previous self-harm incidents was the major predictor.[21] Indeed, numerous other studies report that previous incidence of self-harm is perhaps the clearest indicator of current/future risk of self-harm.[22,23] However, compelling and widely confirmed evidence indicates that a history of childhood sexual abuse appears to be the clearest indicator of increased risk of self-harm, particularly if the duration of the abuse is long, if the perpetrator is known to the victim and if force/penetration are used.[10,24–28] Accordingly, there appears to be a firm consensus that these two variables represent the most significant predictors of further incidences of self-harm.

Importantly, additional work[22] has concluded that patients' characteristics alone are an insufficient explanation of the risk of self-harm and that alternative considerations are available. This is an argument supported by Anderson,[29] who offers a cogent case for consideration of the internal and external factors and their interactions in the person's life, in that they allow shape and depth to be added to the assessment. Thus, checking for the presence of certain risk factors should form one part of a more composite and thorough clinical assessment.

Further, self-injurious acts have a symbolic meaning; the form of self-harm should not be regarded as a random act. As a general rule, self-injurious behaviour, particularly when people have been given the diagnostic label of 'multiple personality disorder' or 'borderline personality disorder', is a coping-orientated (and communication-orientated) act rather than a death-orientated act.[30] Although it would be unwise for the practitioner to adopt a 'cavalier' attitude towards suicide attempts in such clients, these clients have offered a range of reasons for self-harming behaviour and each of these dynamics has been repeatedly shown to have a strong association with a history of self-harming. Thus, assessment of the future risk of self-harm should determine the presence and influence of the following intrapersonal dynamics of whether self-harming is used:

- as a means to release intrapersonal tension
- as an expression of 'letting the badness flow out'
- to assuage a sense of guilt
- to harm the rejecting object (e.g. the abuser) by harming what is dear to them, i.e. the self-harmer
- as a way to interrupt the person's feelings of 'internal deadness' or 'invisibility'; a way of still 'feeling alive'[31]
- as a metaphor for 'blood letting'[32]
- as a means of exercising control in a life that otherwise feels out of control.[31]

ASSESSING RISK OF SUICIDE

Since suicide is a multifaceted, complex phenomenon, it clearly needs a pluralistic, multidimensional and multiprofessional response, especially within mental health care.[2,33] This complexity and multifactorial nature is mirrored in the assessment of suicide risk wherein precise assessment of the extent of risk is extremely difficult to achieve.[34,35] This is particularly the case when practitioners adopt simplistic and 'isolated' assessment tools in the hope that these provide enough accurate information to gauge suicidal risk. According to Morgan,[35] traditionally, at least in clinical psychiatry, this simplistic and 'isolated' approach was concerned with matching the client with a set of risk factors, each of which has been shown to have a statistically positive correlation with increased suicide

risk. Considering the complexity and interplay of the biopsychosocial processes and dynamics of suicide,[36] and the individual nature of each suicidal person, it is unsurprising that, in isolation, this simplistic approach has many limitations. While such tools can be accurate over the long term, they can be very unspecific and insensitive over the short term,[35] creating a large number of false positives (people regarded to be at high risk of suicide when they are not) and false negatives (people regarded to be at low risk of suicide when they are actually at high risk).

As a 'golden rule', the fundamental basis of risk assessment must be a full and thorough clinical evaluation of each individual.[34,36] While I support this position, I would add a two-stage caveat.

1 Full and thorough clinical evaluations require a degree of 'clinical judgement'. If they are to develop this clinical acumen, inexperienced clinicians need time and 'first-hand' experience of clients deemed to be at high risk of suicide.
2 The current emphasis on 'evidence-based practice' would suggest that full and thorough clinical evaluations of individuals are perhaps best served when they are underpinned with evidence.

Although the limitations of any/all suicide risk assessment instruments are well documented,[33,35,37] and thus their utility can be questioned, as Shea[33] purports, 'assessing for the presence of risk factors can alert the clinician to suspect that the client *may* [original emphasis] be at higher risk'. This is a view supported by Morgan,[35] who asserts that instruments can provide useful check lists and can help guard against complacency and overconfidence. Consequently, in keeping with these arguments, and considering the two-stage caveat described above, the remainder of this chapter focuses on the Nurses' Global Assessment of Suicide Risk instrument.

BACKGROUND TO THE DEVELOPMENT OF THE NURSES' GLOBAL ASSESSMENT OF SUICIDE RISK[a]

Studies with a noted vintage[38,39] and more contemporary work[40] have shown that the detection of suicide risk in populations of psychiatric clients poses many problems. Perhaps mindful of these problems, PMHNs based at a mental health provider unit wished to enhance their assessment of suicide risk with the introduction of an evidence-based tool and, yet, were simultaneously mindful of the need to develop clinical judgement, particularly in the less experienced PMHNs. Importantly, given their

---

[a] For a more comprehensive explanation of the background and development of the risk assessment tool, see Cutcliffe JR, Bassett C. Introducing change in nursing: the case of research. *The Journal of Nursing Management* 1997; **5**: 241–7.

clinical judgement based on years of experience,[41] the tool would not replace the experienced clinician's own judgement but serve to augment it. As Motto *et al.*[42] point out,

> a scale can only be a supplement to clinical judgement and should not, on its own, override contradicting information.

On its own, risk assessment does not necessarily constitute evidence-based practice. However, as noted, specific variables are associated with increased risk of suicide,[37,42–44] with some having a stronger statistical correlation than others.[37] A risk assessment tool that enabled the PMHNs to assess for the presence and influence of these predictor variables then means that part of their assessment becomes evidence based. Importantly, regarding Shea's view,[33] this had the influence of raising the nurses' awareness of the problem of suicide and factors associated with increased risk, and a corresponding increase in their vigilance. A crucial problem in constructing any suicide risk assessment tool lies in the fact that high-risk issues for an individual cannot be generalized into a larger population. Similarly, high-risk factors for large populations do not necessarily translate and apply to the individual.[42,45] However, even an imperfect instrument can serve a useful purpose, especially for those who are less confident or experienced with their suicide risk assessment skills, and especially if the instrument could then be rated (and validated) in practice by means of a variety of methods.

The Nurses' Global Assessment of Suicide Risk (NGASR) takes the form of a simple scoring scale with 15 items (Table 61.1). The tool was designed so that all the information necessary to score each of the predictor variables could be extracted during the admission interview. By highlighting the predictor variables that the clinician feels are pertinent to the client, and totalling the scores, a single final score or rating is arrived at. This score then correlates with an (estimated) indication of the level of potential suicide risk and also corresponds to a suggested level of engagement (Box 61.1). Additionally, subsequent risk assessment ratings, aided by the use of the tool, mean that all the formal and informal collection of data (e.g. observations of the client's mood and behaviour, records of interactions with nurses, other clients and additional healthcare staff) could be 'summarized' and repeated on a regular basis, providing an indication in changes in apparent risk of suicide.

The NGASR was based on a review of the relevant empirical literature, which indicated that the presence (and influence) of some variables appeared to suggest a higher degree of risk than others.[37] Thus, unlike many other suicide risk assessment instruments, not all indicators of suicidal risk were given the same 'weighting' or score. The most potent predictors in the NGASR – those with a

TABLE 61.1 Nurse's Global Assessment of Suicide Risk

Predictor variable	Value
Presence/influence of hopelessness	3
Recent stressful life event, e.g. job loss, financial worries, pending court action	1
Evidence of persecutory voices/beliefs	1
Evidence of depression/loss of interest or loss of pleasure	3
Evidence of withdrawal	1
Warning of suicidal intent	1
Evidence of a specific plan for suicide	3
Family history of serious psychiatric problems or suicide	1
Recent bereavement or relationship breakdown	3
History of psychosis	1
Widow/widower	1
Prior suicide attempt	3
History of socioeconomic deprivation	1
History of alcohol and/or substance misuse	1
Presence of terminal illness	1
	Total = (a maximum score of) 25

Box 61.1: NGASR and corresponding levels of risk and suggested engagement

Score of 5 or less = low level of risk estimated. Suggested level of engagement = *level 4*.

Score between 6 and 8 = intermediate level of risk. Suggested level of engagement = *level 3*.

Score between 9 and 11 = high level of risk. Suggested level of engagement = *level 2*.

Score 12 or more = very high/extreme level of risk. Suggested level of engagement = *level 1*.

---

reported higher statistical correlation with suicide – are weighted with a score of 3, the remainder being allocated a score of 1.[33,35,37,38,42,43–48]

An additional difficulty in designing risk assessment tools involves determining the demarcations between degrees of risk. As previously noted, suicide is a complex phenomenon and models which suggest that one can either be at risk or not at risk of suicide are simplistic and inappropriate. As a result of a study involving attending over 75 formal suicide coroner's inquests, reviewing each set of case notes and in-depth interviews with the families, the author[49] felt that there should be four discrete levels of risk for suicide. Two polarized opposite levels of risk were clear: very high or extreme risk and very little risk. Extreme risk refers to that state of being that might be likened to a state of 'psychiatric emergency'.

The person is extremely vulnerable, requires the highest degree of engagement and input from the PMHN, and presents with a number of high-risk factors (variables) and perhaps some other risk factors too. Since it would not be prudent for PMHNs to claim that a client presents with no risk of suicide, the category that represents the least risk is termed low risk of suicide. These individuals would thus score low and present with few (if any) of the risk factors. A further two categories were added: intermediate and high risk. Again, given the complexity of suicide and the multiple factors that can be involved in predicting risk, a single third category was felt to be rather simplistic and did not allow for the interplay of risk factors and the cumulative degree of risk that multiple factors combined indicated.

EMPIRICAL EVIDENCE AND RATIONALE TO SUPPORT THE 15 KEY INDICATOR VARIABLES IN THE NGASR[b]

1 There is a well-established body of empirical evidence that indicates how feelings of hopelessness are highly correlated with increased suicide risk.[43–45] These studies indicate that feelings of hopelessness, often associated with a depressive state, are a more accurate indicator of increased risk than the depressive state itself. Moreover, hopelessness is not isolated or unique to depressive states; people with recurrent forms of mental and/or physical distress or personal or social problems can develop a sense of pervasive hopelessness. If PMHNs wish to assess this area in more detail, in order to verify the initial assessment, they might draw upon one of the well-established and validated instruments for estimating hope/hopelessness.

2 Holms and Rahe[50] produced a list of life events which appeared to 'carry' a certain degree of associated stress. In certain circumstances, and particularly if there are cumulative stressful life events, these can usher the individual into thinking about suicide as a 'way out'. Details of these events can be determined during the admission interview and/or from any existing professional reports, e.g. social work reports.

3 Although not associated exclusively with diagnosed mental health problems,[51] some formal diagnoses are associated with auditory hallucinations ('hearing voices') and/or delusional beliefs. When such 'voices' take on a persecutory tone or content, this can contribute to the person's sense of hopelessness. Furthermore, some voices/beliefs may contain more explicit messages of self-harm or destruction. When this is the case, there can be an increased risk.[33]

4 There is a relationship between depression and suicide.[52] Additionally, when this depression manifests in the form of loss of interest or pleasure, this can be regarded as further indication of potential suicidal risk.[43] These phenomena are not only manifest in people with a formal diagnosis of depression, but may also be evident in people with other severe forms of mental or physical distress.

5 Some studies into predictive risk factors in suicide have indicated that a withdrawal from interpersonal and social interactions can be associated with increased risk.[53] Such withdrawal can be one of the first warning signs that the person is experiencing difficulty in maintaining the pattern of everyday living. That is not to suggest that anyone who spends time alone should automatically be considered to be at risk of suicide. It is more a matter of changes in patterns of interpersonal and social interaction, i.e. a change in the balance of time spent alone against time spent with others.

6 Although the verbalization of suicidal intent is not always conclusive evidence of genuine intent,[35] such warnings should not be ignored, and can indeed be genuine and clear indications of increased thoughts about suicide. Some studies have indicated that a number of 'cries for help' have passed by unnoticed.[39,40] Yet, such warnings can also be evidence of clients 'reaching out' for help.

7 Any evidence of a specific plan to commit suicide represents a major risk factor, especially if the person attempts to keep the plan secret.[33,37,42] Such plans may be uncovered by accidental discovery of physical evidence, or perhaps by way of something(s) that the person says which either alludes to such a plan or reveals part of it.

8 A further predictor that needs to be considered is that of a family history of serious psychiatric problems or suicide.[48] Such a history can compound the person's sense of hopelessness and inevitability. When significant family members (or even close friends) have died by suicide, this can, inadvertently, serve as a role model and lead to the so-called 'contagion effect'.

9 A recent bereavement or relationship breakdown should be considered as another significant risk factor.[42,43,48] Loss and bereavement affect the person in many different ways, yet one frequently reported commonality of unresolved bereavements appears to be loss of hope.[54] Consequently, the person may be left feeling like ending his or her life in response to the loss, and these feelings can be compounded by the concomitant loss of hope. This may particularly be the case when the person has lost his or her primary source of human, interpersonal support.

[b] Owing to space and word limitations, references for each of these risk factors have been restricted. For a more comprehensive explanation of the supporting literature, see Cutcliffe JR, Barker P. The Nurses' Global Assessment of Suicide Risk (NGASR): developing a tool for clinical practice. *Journal of Psychiatric/Mental Health Nursing* 2004; 11: 393–400.

10 When the person has a history of psychosis, then the risk of suicide appears to be slightly increased.[33,48,52] Although it is accepted as an axiom that not all people who endure and live with psychosis also experience suicidal thoughts, the person's process of reasoning can be impaired/altered.

11 Previous empirical studies have shown that when the person is a widow/widower, then the risk is slightly increased.[42] This is particularly the case if people have not reached any 'resolution' to their bereavement or have not 'adapted' to their loss. It is important to remember that, in contemporary society, this predictive variable also includes the loss of 'common law' spouse and the loss of a homosexual life partner.

12 Any indication or evidence of a prior suicide attempt, and thus the 'acquired ability to make a serious attempt on one's life', should be taken to be a significant indicator of current/future risk of suicide.[33,37,55]

13 Suicide is a multifactorial event that does not happen in isolation from the world in which the person lives.[36] Thus, it can be precipitated by both internal phenomena and external events, in addition to external circumstances. For example, a history of socioeconomic deprivation (e.g. poor housing, unemployment, low quality of life) appears to be associated with increased risk of suicide.[55]

14 Further studies have supported the findings of Barraclough et al.,[52] and continue to suggest that a history of alcohol and/or substance misuse is associated with a higher risk of suicide.[33,37] This may particularly be the case when the concept of 'spontaneous act' suicides and people using alcohol/drugs in order to gain the courage to go through with the suicidal act is taken into account.

15 Finally, some people who are suffering from a terminal illness consider suicide.[56] This can be a means of dealing with physical pain, a means of taking an element of control/dignity or a way of dealing with the prospect of further holistic deterioration and loss (euthanasia).

Reflection

What formal education and/or training have you received (before and after registration) in assessing the risk of suicide or self-harm? Was this sufficient?

DEVELOPING AN EVIDENCE BASE FOR SUICIDE RISK ASSESSMENT

Formal assessment tools for estimating the risk of suicide constitute only a part of the assessment process. Nevertheless, they are a useful component of the 'bigger picture'

and perhaps have particular value for less experienced staff. In addition to formal risk assessment tools, a full clinical assessment may include some (or all) of the following.

- The clinical judgement of all practitioners involved. Particular value may be attached to the judgement of a clinician who has established a strong/close relationship with the client, or someone who has spent long periods of time in the company of the client.
- Ongoing assessment evaluations (whether based on a risk assessment tool or not) that piece together to form a cumulative 'picture' of the person's potential risk.
- Data/information gained during the initial admission interview and subsequent interviews with the client, family and/or significant others.

Having identified that formal interviews (admission interviews and subsequent assessment interviews) can also play a key part in more accurate assessments of a person's risk of suicide, it is necessary to consider some of the questions that might be asked in such interviews (Box 61.2). Each interview will have to be conducted with extreme sensitivity and empathy, and should conclude with an emphatic declaration of support, care and concern for the individual. Also, each interview is likely to be unique, since it will involve a unique situation and unique personality and unique presenting needs of the particular client. Therefore, the questions included in Box 61.2 should be regarded as guidelines and not as a 'checklist' of questions that the PMHN should follow unthinkingly.

Box 61.2: Suggested questions for suicidal risk assessment interviews (adapted from references 34, 35, 57)

- When you think about your current situation and difficulty, do you think that it can improve, that things can turn out well?
- Where does it hurt? Are you in psychological pain (psychache)?
- How much pleasure do you gain from your life, from those activities and relationships that used to give you pleasure?
- How hopeful do you feel? Do you feel that you still have hope on a day-to-day basis?
- At the start of the day, how do you feel about the day to come and how you will be able to cope?
- Does your current situation make you question the point or purpose of it all? Of your situation or even your life/existence?
- Would you describe yourself as feeling desperate or experiencing a sense of despair?
- How does the thought of having to face another day make you feel?
- Have you ever thought or felt that you are a burden, and, if so, could you say in what way? A burden to whom?
- Have you ever thought about or wished that it would all end?

- Have you ever thought that death would be a relief? That it would provide an end to your psychological pain or that death would present a way out? Have you ever wished that you were dead?
- Have you ever thought about ending your life? How often do you have these thoughts and are you having them at the moment? How compelling or pressing are they?
- Have these thoughts ever led you to make an attempt to take your own life? When did this happen? Have you made more than one attempt?
- Have you ever made a plan about how you would take your own life? Do you have such a plan at the moment?
- If you experience pressing thoughts about taking your own life, how are you able to resist them? How might we be able to help you when you experience such thoughts?
- How serious are your thoughts, your intent to harm yourself?
- Do you feel the need for extra interpersonal support and security right now? What would this look like? Please tell me what you need.
- How easy is it for you to ask for help, particularly when you are feeling vulnerable to harming yourself?
- How do you feel right now?
- How can I help you right now?
- What degree of interpersonal support and security do you feel you need right now?

Reflection

What evidence do you see of the increasing focus on risk assessment and why do you think that is?

SUMMARY

It is important to be realistic and to recognize the limitations of self-harm and suicide prevention.[56] A number of authors have pointed out that, because of the ubiquitous nature of suicide and its omnipresence throughout history,[2,58] the complete eradication of suicide is highly unlikely. Nevertheless, methodological limitations notwithstanding, historical and contemporary epidemiological data with regard to suicide and self-harm clearly indicate that there is a great deal more that formal mental healthcare services (including PMHNs) can do to reduce the rate of suicide, and better manage a person's self-harming behaviour; both of which are prefaced by accurate risk assessment. While acknowledging that risk assessment tools are only one aspect of a more thorough assessment of risk, the NGASR provides PMHNs with an instrument which can greatly assist them with this assessment process, and it may be of particular worth to less experienced (and student) nurses. The NGASR is now utilized in the UK, Canada, Australia, the USA, New Zealand and Switzerland. It has been translated into German for use in Europe, is increasingly used in accident and emergency rooms[59] and is woven into the Tidal Model.[60]

REFERENCES

1. Maris RW. Foreword. In: Cutcliffe JR, Stevenson C (eds). *Care of the suicidal person*. Edinburgh, UK: Elsevier, 2007: xii–x.

2. Cutcliffe JR, Stevenson C. *Care of the suicidal person*. Edinburgh, UK: Elsevier, 2007.

3. Kinmond KS, Bent M. Attendance for self-harm in a West Midlands A&E department. *British Journal of Nursing* 2000; **9** (4): 215–20.

4. Silverman MM. Current controversies in suicidology In: Maris RW, Silverman MM, Canetto SS (eds). *Review of suicidology 1997*. New York, NY: Guildford Press, 1997: 1–21.

5. Silverman MM, Berman AL, Sandadal N *et al.* Rebuilding the tower of Babel: a revised nomenclature for the study of suicide and suicidal behaviors. Part 2. Suicide-related ideations, communications, and behaviors. *Suicide and Life-Threatening Behaviors* 2007; **37** (3): 264–77.

6. Shneidman ES. Suicide. In: *Encyclopaedia Britannica*. Chicago, IL: Williams Benton, 1973; **21**: 383–5.

7. Shneidman ES. *Definition of suicide*. New York, NY: John Wiley, 1985.

8. Krietman N. *Parasuicide*. Chichester, UK: Wiley, 1977.

9. Favazza AR. *Bodies under siege*. Baltimore, MD: John Hopkins University Press, 1996.

10. Santa Mina EE, Gallop R. Childhood sexual and physical abuse and adult self-harm and suicidal behaviour: a literature review. *Canadian Journal of Psychiatry* 1998; **43** (8): 793–800.

11. Anderson M, Jenkins R. The national suicide prevention strategy for England: the reality of a national strategy for the nursing profession. *Journal of Psychiatric and Mental Health Nursing* 2006; **13**: 641–50.

12. Claassen CA, Trivedi MH, Shimizu I *et al.* Epidemiology of nonfatal deliberate self-harm in the United States as described in three medical databases. *Suicide and Life-Threatening Behavior* 2006; **36** (2): 192–212.

13. Maris RW, Berman AL, Silverman MM, Farberow N. Indirect self-destructive behavior. In: Maris RW, Berman AL, Silverman MM (eds). *Comprehensive textbook of suicidology*. New York, NY: Guildford Press, 2000: 427–55.

14. Stuart G. Self-protective responses and suicidal behaviour. In: Stuart G, Laraia MT (eds). *Principles and practices of psychiatric nursing*, 7th edn. New York, NY: Mosby, 2001: 381–400.

15. Cooper J, Kapur N, Webb R *et al.* Suicide after deliberate self-harm: a four year cohort study. *American Journal of Psychiatry* 2005; **162** (2): 297–303.

16. Anderson R. Assessing the risk of self-harm in adolescents: a psychoanalytic perspective. *Psychoanalytic Psychotherapy* 2000; **14**: 9–21.

17. Welch SS. A review of the literature on the epidemiology of parasuicide in the general population. *Psychiatric Services* 2001; **52** (3): 368–75.

18. Read GFH. Trends in adolescent and young adult parasuicide population presenting at a psychiatric emergency unit: a descriptive study. *International Journal of Adolescent Medicine and Health* 1997; **9** (4): 249–69.

19. Hawton K. Attempted suicide. In: Clarke DM, Fairburn CG (eds). *Science and practice of cognitive behavioural therapy.* Oxford, UK: Oxford University Press, 1997: 285–312.

20. McLoone P, Crombie IK. Hospitalisation for deliberate self-poisoning in Scotland from 1981–1993: trends in rates and types of drugs used. *British Journal of Psychiatry* 1996; **169**: 816.

21. Sidley GL, Calam R, Wells A *et al.* The prediction of para-suicide repetition in a high-risk group. *British Journal of Clinical Psychology* 1999; **38** (4): 375–86.

22. Burrow S. The deliberate self-harming behaviour of patients within a British special hospital. *Journal of Advanced Nursing* 1992; **17** (2): 138–48.

23. Kreitman N, Casey P. Repetition of parasuicide: an epidemiological and clinical study. *British Journal of Psychiatry* 1988; **153**: 792–800.

24. Berliner L, Elliott DM. Sexual abuse of children. In: Briere J, Berliner L, Bulkey J *et al.* (eds). *The APSAC handbook on child maltreatment.* Newbury Park, CA: Sage, 1996.

25. Gratz KL, Conrad SD, Roemer L. Risk factors for deliberate self-harm among college students. *American Journal of Orthopsychiatry* 2002; **72**: 128–40.

26. Van der Kolk BA, Perry JC, Herman JL. Childhood origins of self-destructive behavior. *American Journal of Psychiatry* 1991; **148**: 1665–71.

27. Zlotnick C, Mattia JI, Zimmerman M. Clinical correlates of self-mutilation in a sample of general psychiatric patients. *The Journal of Nervous and Mental Disease* 1999; **187**: 296–301.

28. Zlotnick C, Shea MT, Pearlstein T *et al.* The relationship between dissociative symptoms, alexithymia, impulsivity, sexual abuse, and self-mutilation. *Comprehensive Psychiatry* 1996; **37**: 12–16.

29. Anderson M. Waiting for harm: deliberate self-harm and suicide in young people. A review of the literature. *Journal of Psychiatric and Mental Health Nursing* 1999; **6** (2): 91–100.

30. Marmer SS, Fink D. Rethinking the comparison of borderline personality disorder and multiple personality disorder. *Psychiatric Clinics of North America* 1994; **17**: 743–71.

31. Fitzpatrick C, Dunne M, Power R, Moore C. *The other side of childhood: self-harm.* Available from: www.rte.ie/radio1/theothersideofchildhood/programme1.pdf. Accessed 2 February 2007.

32. *Self-Injury and Related Issues.* Available from: www.siari.co.uk/Self-injury_The_significance_of_seeing_ the_blood.htm. Accessed 2 February 2007.

33. Shea SC. *The practical art of suicide assessment: a guide for mental health professionals and substance abuse counsellors.* New York, NY: John Wiley, 1999.

34. Shneidman ES. *Autopsy of a suicidal mind.* Oxford, UK: Oxford University Press, 2004.

35. Morgan G. Assessment of risk. In: Jenkins R, Griffiths S, Wylie I *et al.* (eds). *The prevention of suicide.* London, UK: Department of Health, 1994: 46–52.

36. Maris R. Social forces in suicide: a life review. In: Maris RW, Silverman MM, Canetto SS (eds). *Review of suicidology 1997.* New York, NY: Guildford Press, 1997: 42–60.

37. Joiner T. *Why people die by suicide.* Cambridge, MA: Harvard University Press, 2005.

38. Goldstein RB, Black DW, Nasrallah A, Winokur G. The prediction of suicide: sensitivity, specificity and predictive value of a multivariative model applied to suicide among 1906 patients with an affective disorder. *Archives of General Psychiatry* 1991; **48**: 418–22.

39. Morgan HG, Priest P. Suicide and other unexpected deaths among psychiatric in-patients. The Bristol confidential inquiry. *British Journal of Psychiatry* 1991; **158**: 368–74.

40. Thomas S, Ferrier N, Watkinson H *et al. Avoidable deaths: five year report of the National Confidential Inquiry into Suicide and Homicide by People with Mental Illness.* Manchester, UK: University of Manchester, 2006.

41. Menghella E, Benson A. Developing reflective practice in mental health nursing through critical incident analysis. *Journal of Advanced Nursing* 1995; **21**: 205–13.

42. Motto JA, Heilbron DC, Juster RP. Development of a clinical instrument to estimate suicide risk. *American Journal of Psychiatry* 1985; **142**: 680–6.

43. Fawcett J, Scheftner W, Clark D *et al.* Clinical predictors of suicide in patients with major affective disorders: a controlled prospective study. *American Journal of Psychiatry* 1987; **144**: 35–40.

44. Weisharr ME, Beck AT. Hopelessness and suicide. *International Review of Psychiatry* 1992; **4**: 177–84.

45. Young MA, Fogg LF, Schefter WA, Fawcett JA. Interactions of risk factors in predicting suicide. *American Journal of Psychiatry* 1994; **151**: 434–5.

46. Beck AT, Weissman M, Lester D, Trexler L. The measurement of pessimism: the hopelessness scale. *Journal of Consulting and Clinical Psychology* 1974; **42**: 861–5.

47. Pokorny AD. Prediction of suicide in psychiatric patients: report of a prospective study. *Archives of General Psychiatry* 1983; **40**: 249–57.

48. Powell J, Gedde, J, Hawton K. Suicide in psychiatric hospital in-patients. *The British Journal of Psychiatry* 2000; **176**: 266–72.

49. Cutcliffe JR, Ramcharan P. Levelling the playing field: considering the 'ethics as process' approach for judging qualitative research proposals. *Qualitative Health Research* 2002; **12**: 1000–10.

50. Holms TH, Rahe RH. The social readjustment rating scale. *Journal of Psychosomatic Research* 1968; **11**: 213–18.

51. Romme M, Hoing A, Noorthoorn E, Escher A. Coping with hearing voices: an emancipatory approach. *British Journal of Psychiatry* 1992; **161**: 99–103.

52. Barraclough B, Bunch J, Nelson P, Sainsbury P. A hundred cases of suicide: clinical aspects. *British Journal of Psychiatry* 1974; **125**: 355–73.

53. Charlton J, Kelly S, Dunnell K *et al.* Trends in suicide deaths in England and Wales. *Population Trends* 1992; **69**: 6–10.

54. Cutcliffe JR. *The inspiration of hope in bereavement counselling.* London, UK: Jessica Kingsley, 2004.

55. Gunnell D, Frankel S. Prevention of suicide: aspirations and evidence. *British Medical Journal* 1994; **308**: 1227–33.

56. Hawton, K. Causes and opportunities for prevention. In: Jenkins R, Griffiths S, Wylie I *et al.* (eds). *The prevention of suicide*. London, UK: Department of Health, 1994: 34–45.

57. Barker P. *Developing the security plan: guidance notes*. Newcastle: Newcastle City Health Trust, 1999.

58. Alvarez A. *The savage God: a study of suicide*. New York, NY: WW Norton, 1974.

59. Mitchell AM, Garand L, Dean D *et al*. Suicide assessment in hospital emergency departments. *Topics in Emergency Medicine* 2005; **27**: 302–12.

60. Barker P, Buchanan-Barker P. *The tidal model: a guide for mental health professionals*. Hove, UK: Brunner-Routledge, 2005.

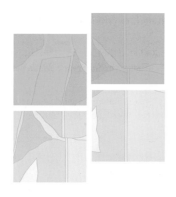

CHAPTER 62

Engagement and observation of people at risk

John Cutcliffe*

Suicide is a form of behaviour as old as man himself but the phenomenon has been described in differing ways according to the attitudes prevalent within society at various times in history.

Rosen[1]

THE GROWING PROBLEM OF SUICIDE: THE POLICY CONTEXT

Although suicide as a public health problem is by no means exclusive to contemporary society,[2,3] epidemiological evidence indicates alarming rises in rates during the last 50 years.[4] As a result, public and mental health policy documents reflect the growing public concern. In the UK, the documents *Health of the nation*,[5] *Modernising mental health services: safe, sound and supportive*[6] and the *National service framework for mental health*[7] each drew attention to the increased risk of suicide in people with mental health problems, and the need for services to

address this. Following these, the production of a *National suicide prevention strategy for England*[8] indicated six goals, the first of which was to reduce risk in key high-risk groups. Furthermore, it is noteworthy that the first of the high-risk groups to be identified included people who are currently, or have recently been, in contact with mental health services.

Although caution needs to be exercised when interpreting epidemiological studies of suicide given the well-documented methodological limitations,[9] recent evidence suggests a downward trend in suicide rates in the UK.[10] However, when one examines the international data,[4] this is not the case for the majority of countries. Numerous sources of evidence indicate that people with mental health problems continue to be at a significantly higher risk than members of the general population.[10,11] Though suicide is not a mental health problem per se and there is no formal diagnosis for *being suicidal*,[12] mental health services in the UK (and elsewhere) have a long history of providing services for suicidal people. Within these, one

*John Cutcliffe holds the 'David G. Braithwaite' Professor of Nursing Endowed Chair at the University of Texas (Tyler), USA. He is also the Associate Dean: Psychiatric Nursing, Stenberg College, Vancouver, Canada, and Adjunct Professor of Nursing, University of Ulster, UK. John is an Associate Editor for the International Journal of Mental Health Nursing and Assistant Editor for the International Journal of Nursing Studies. His principal research interest is suicide and the care of the suicidal person.

can locate the extensive history of psychiatric–mental health nurses (PMHNs) working with suicidal people. Consequently, these nurses continue to have an important role in providing care for suicidal people, particularly, though not exclusively, in inpatient settings and thus have the potential to have a major therapeutic influence.

Given the associations between PMHNs and suicidal people, it is perhaps counterintuitive that there is a paucity of suicidology-focused literature produced by PMHNs; exactly how PMHNs should go about providing care to suicidal clients is not well understood. Most of the previously published work has focused on attempting to keep the person physically safe; more specifically, on close or 'special' observation (or other vernacular expressions of this practice). A more recent literature has emerged that has a distinctly different focus, and it behoves any PMHNs who works with the suicidal client to be conversant with these bodies of work.

THE BIOLOGIZING OF THE HUMAN DRAMA OF SUICIDE

Within the international suicidology academe it is regarded as axiomatic that suicide is a complex, multidimensional phenomenon; one that often requires sophisticated and integrated approaches to care. Indeed, one of the leading suicidologists of his generation, Maris[12,13] captures this multidimensionality with his biopsychosocial model of suicide. Despite this well-documented consensus, some texts continue to inappropriately conflate suicide with depression and, as a result, emphasize the need to 'treat' the underlying affective mood disorder.[14] For example, Rawlins[15,p.281] suggests that a suicidal client needs to be

given anti-depressant medication to elevate his mood and make him more amenable to treatment. Electroconvulsive treatment (ECT) is an additional treatment that has proved effective.

And, more recently, Anderson and Jenkins[16] purport that

the medical practitioner is able to select from a range of common anti-depressants, mood stabilizers or anti-psychotic medication that are currently used to treat people who are suicidal.

There is further evidence of this conflation in the recently published *National suicide prevention strategy for England: annual report on progress 2006*[10] in which future reductions in the suicide rate are predicated by increasing and enforcing compliance with pharmacological regimes. Schneidman,[17] the creator of suicidology as a discrete area of study (and clinical practice), is critical of the automatic alleged isomorphic relationship between depression and suicide. He asserts,[17,p.73]

Converting suicide into depression is a kind of methodological sleight of hand. The central fact about depression is that one can lead a long happy life with depression ... suicide and depression are not synonymous.

A more comprehensive examination of the evidence pertaining to the efficacy of pharmacological agents as an effective treatment for 'suicide' indicates that the evidence is equivocal. However, there are data that indicate there is some utility in certain antidepressant medications for some suicidal people.[18] Other evidence indicates the suicide risk-reducing value of atypical anti-psychotics for some people given a diagnosis of 'schizophrenia'.[19] On the other hand, there is evidence that selective serotonin reuptake inhibitors continue to be associated with increased rates of suicidal thinking and behaviour; most specifically in children and adolescents.[20,21] Likewise, Gunnell and Frankel[22] point out that several retrospective reviews of the treatments received by psychiatric patients provided no consistent evidence that these pharmacological treatments reduced the likelihood of suicide. Accordingly, positing such pharmacological interventions as the effective mainstay of treatment for suicidal people appears to be misrepresenting our current knowledge base and may constitute evidence of the 'biologizing' of suicide. This prompts Shneidman to assert[17,p.73]

the biologizing of suicide is an integral part of the medicalization of what is essentially – so I believe – a phenomenological decision of the mind.

Despite the attempts of some to make the multidimensional experience of suicidality into little more than 'a depressed brain in need of a chemical' and the associated emphasis on pharmacology, a more balanced representation of the evidence suggests that we are far from having an effective pharmacological treatment for all suicidal people. Indeed, Maris *et al.* declare,[12,p.525]

Psychopharmacotherapy does not target suicide per se. There simply is no anti-suicide pill.

Furthermore, ignoring the questionable efficacy of these therapies with respect to 'treating' the suicidal client, it is fair to say that they do not appear to offer much to PMHNs by way of how they might interact, support, help and work with suicidal people on a day-by-day, hour-by-hour or minute-by minute basis.

PRINCIPAL APPROACHES TO THE PSYCHIATRIC NURSING CARE OF SUICIDAL PEOPLE: OBSERVATION

Some authors appear to advocate a 'masculine' approach to caring for suicidal clients, when they suggest 'interventions' including removing harmful items (such as belts, socks!) and placing the client on 24-hour-a-day observation on a one-to-one basis.[15,23] Others purport that the observation can be carried out in the form of a disconnected and dehumanized 'gaze'. Bowers and Park, for example, argue,[24,p.777]

> Although some authors decry the nurse who sits in the doorway of a patient's room reading a newspaper, even this might be appropriate at times and temporarily offers the patient a form of privacy of solitude.

Even a cursory examination of the literature will show that it has become de rigueur to place suicidal clients 'under' or on 'close or special observation'. These increased levels of observation are determined and ordered or 'set' by psychiatrists, often a junior doctor[25] and enshrined in hospital policies. Numerous authors have drawn attention to the significant variation that exists in not only how close observation is captured in policy documents[24,26] but additionally how it is undertaken in clinical practice.[24,27–30] As a result it is difficult to provide precise direction to PMHNs on how they should participate in close or special observation. Nevertheless, close observation is purported to focus on the short-term management of people in crisis who require a higher than normal degree of supervision, usually because they present a risk to themselves or others. Perhaps as an attempt to minimize the variation between individual observation policies, the Standing Nursing and Midwifery Advisory Committee[31] provided a robust example of such a policy.

OBSERVATION: SAFE AND EFFECTIVE?

Despite the current widespread use of observation, there is very little empirical evidence that supports its use for suicidal people. It should be noted that no study has hitherto tried to examine whether 'being under' certain levels of observation actually reduces the number of suicide attempts (although audit data exist showing the number of people who still manage to complete suicide while under observation). Similarly, no randomized controlled trial has been undertaken to compare psychiatric care units that use close observation with units without constant observation in terms of rates of suicide. As a result, the only 'comparative' data that we have in this area conceivably come from audits and evaluatory 'studies' following on from changes in service delivery.[32–34]

Also, while some continue to champion and emphasize 'observation' as the modus operandi for the care of the suicidal person, it is increasingly being called into question, and as a result alternative models of care are being considered. Key figures in the international suicidology academe have added their voices to this debate; for example, Links[35,p.xi] refers to the

bareness of thought that has been applied to our understanding of the nursing care of the suicidal client. As a clinician and a psychiatrist, I have ordered one-to-one nursing care for many acutely suicidal patients; much as one would request valet parking: Please return my patient in one piece.

The practice of observation was developed as a means to inform medical staff of the status of the patient; it served the function of assuring the absent doctor of the physical safety of the patient. Close observation is undeniably concerned with preventing a person from causing physical harm to himself or herself. Yet even in this most central function, the empirical evidence is both telling and disturbing. The *Safety first*[34] report highlighted that 18 per cent of all completed mental health inpatient suicides occurred while people were under observation. The latest and most comprehensive data on the UK contained in the *Five year report of the National Confidential Inquiry into Suicide and Homicide by People with Mental Illness*[10] is highly concerning and speaks directly of the failure of close observation to maintain even the physical safety of suicidal people. It reports that,[10,p.66]

> Twenty two percent of the patients (185 cases) were under special (non-routine) observation, similar to the 23% in the previous inquiry report. Of those who died on the ward, 48% (117 cases) were under special observation.

It continues,

> In this sample, 18 cases (3%) were under one-to-one observations. The number of deaths under observation has not fallen since 1997, which means that they have increased as a proportion of inpatient suicides.

The case for maintaining close observation as the principal form of care for suicidal people in inpatient units is further diminished when one considers what happens after the observation is removed. Numerous sources of UK and international evidence have reported that the time period representing the highest risk of suicide for people with mental health problems is immediately following discharge.[10,36,37] These data indicate that suicide attempters who present to hospital services are at a much greater risk of dying from suicide in the first year following the attempt, which is 66 times the annual risk in the general population.

OBSERVATION: THE EXPERIENCES OF SERVICE USERS AND PSYCHIATRIC NURSES

A small number of studies have attempted to investigate both the clients' and PMHNs' experiences of observation, and have similarly tried to extrapolate that the experience is either therapeutic or not therapeutic. Caution should be exercised when interpreting these findings because, tragically, the experiences of those people who were under observation and still managed to complete their suicide will never be available to us. Even the most junior researcher would thus recognize that this will skew any sample of clients who have been under observation. However, critical examination and synthesis of this literature clearly indicates that the findings are equivocal.

Several studies have identified and repeatedly reported how 'being under' close observation is experienced as non-therapeutic.[26,29,30,32,33,38–43] This body of work purports that non-therapeutic aspects of close observation include lack of empathy, lack of acknowledgement, disinterested practitioners, lack of information provided, lack of privacy, invasion of personal space, observers reading newspapers/books/magazines while observing the client, and confinement.

Interestingly, some of these studies also report that some clients have identified certain therapeutic aspects to close observation.[39,41–43] The therapeutic aspects have been described as observer intentions, optimism, acknowledgement, distraction, emotional support and protection. Worryingly, there is also evidence in this body of literature of how some people who are placed under observation *lied about their degree of suicidality in order to hasten the termination of constant observation*. Thus, an intervention allegedly used to help people not complete suicide actually leads 'at-risk' people to offer purposefully misleading information, false assessments of suicidal risk and adds another layer of psychache to the already psychologically burdened suicidal person.

Interestingly, when one examines this literature in more detail, it becomes clear that it is certain attitudes and practices of the PMHN within (or during) the observation that appeared to be experienced as therapeutic and not the being observed per se. For example, in an often cited study, one participant stated,[41,p.1068]

> I think having somebody speak to you makes a more positive experience. I mean a million times more positive. It's beyond qualification how important it is. Just come in and talk to you.

Similar evocative statements occur with conspicuous regularity throughout this body of work; for example,

> Some do closes [observation] nicely. They talk to the patient like a friend and still carry on with their other duties. But others are like robots. When the patient moves they follow like zombies.[44]

> They didn't actually ask me if I was feeling suicidal. Just went everywhere with me.[42]

> Most of the staff I got lumbered with did not, could not or would not make even small talk with me, let alone discuss my illness … it always amazed me that the least experienced staff were given the most distressed patients to work with … There have got to be ways of helping a person feel safe and supported without reducing them to victims of voyeurism and seriously eroding away their basic human rights.[33,p.256]

THE 'WHO' QUESTION

Inextricably linked to the alleged value (or otherwise) of observation is the matter of who undertakes it. The literature is unswerving in showing that there is significant variation in who undertakes close observation. According to the literature, close observations have been undertaken by the following groups: experienced, qualified psychiatric nurses;[45] inexperienced, qualified psychiatric nurses;[25,32,33] licensed practical nurses;[27] nursing students/medical students;[25,26] care aids;[42] volunteers;[46] family members;[47] sitters;[39,41] security guards;[48] and close circuit TV cameras.[48,49]

There is also evidence of a strong degree of consensus within this literature that close observations are regarded as a 'low-skill', unpleasant and unpopular activity.[24,25,43,50,51] As a result, close observations are often delegated to junior and/or untrained staff. This situation is exacerbated by the extensive and 'global' shortage of qualified psychiatric nurses and the resultant reliance on 'bank' or agency staff.[52] Such a position is counterproductive[32] because it contributes little in the way of risk assessment and effective intervention for suicidal people within acute wards. Indeed, this situation leaves such nurses in reactionary, custodial roles and, despite the rhetoric of 'supportive observation', nurse are often construed as custodians, if not doormen.[29]

PRINCIPAL APPROACHES TO THE PSYCHIATRIC NURSING CARE OF SUICIDAL PEOPLE: 'ENGAGEMENT'

If one were to invoke a simplistic form of logic, it would appear to be counterintuitive (and an ill-advised choice) to 'treat' or 'care' for people with sophisticated, complex, multidimensional problems by preventing the physical means of attempting suicide and hoping that the suicidal person simultaneously, spontaneously resolves whatever problems (and psychache) ushered them towards suicide in the first instance. Furthermore, in these days of 'evidence-based practice', psychiatric nurses are increasingly analysing the evidence (or more accurately – lack of it) that supports the use of close observation for suicidal people. As a result, for many PMHNs, there is a growing recognition that the nursing care of people who are at risk of suicide needs to re-focus on a more manifest form of care and support, rather than upon tightening up the 'policing' strategy of observation.

Robust support for this position is found in the seminal works of key figures within the international suicidology academe. As he does so often, Shneidman[53] eloquently captures the essence of this message when he states,

> When dealing with a highly suicidal person, it is simply not effective to address the lethality directly. We can address thoughts about suicide by working with this person and asking why mental turmoil is leading to feelings of lethality.[53,p.25]

> There is a basic rule to keep in mind: We can reduce the lethality if we lessen the anguish, the perturbation. Suicidal individuals who are asked 'Where do you hurt?' intuitively know that this is a question about their emotions and their lives, and they answer appropriately, not in biological terms but with some literary or humanistic sophistication, in psychological terms. What I mean by this is to ask about the person's feelings, worries and pain.[53,p.29]

> To understand suicide we must understand suffering and psychological pain and various thresholds for enduring it; to treat suicidal people (and prevent suicide) we must address and then soften and reduce the psychache that drives it.[53,p.29]

Views highly congruent with Shneidman's are expressed by Maris *et al.* when they assert[12,p.13]

> As important as the biological treatment of hopelessness is, any treatment of a suicidal patient that relies solely on impersonal therapies (e.g. psychoactive medication, seclusion, restraint, and 15 minute checks [observations]) may be second rate … Many psychiatrists argue that the heart of the treatment of suicidal individuals is the relationship of the therapists and the patient.

Recent findings from studies undertaken by PMHNs about the psychiatric nursing care of suicidal people add further empirical depth to these views. These studies (re)affirm the central or core process(es) of such nursing care and these interpersonal processes are perhaps best captured under the term 'engagement' (or paraphrases/synonyms for this process).

In the largest study of its kind yet undertaken,[4,54] an account is given of the psychosocial processes (and interventions) that PMHNs use to help move suicidal people from a 'death-orientated' position to a 'life-orientated' position. This study posits the core aspect of the psychiatric–mental health nursing care of the suicidal person as re-connecting the person with humanity. This work describes a three-stage process of healing: reflecting

an image of humanity, guiding the individual back to humanity, and learning to live. PMHNs achieved this re-connection through re-establishing the person's trust in humanity. These authors show that, through gaining trust in the nurse, the person is then re-connecting with a person; taking the first tentative steps towards re-connecting with the wider community of 'humanity'. The suicidal person is further guided back to humanity through the nurses' nurturing of additional insight and understanding in him or her, through supporting and strengthening the person's pre-suicidal beliefs and as a result of experiencing the additional sense of security offered within the novel relationship. The re-connection with humanity is also brought about by the person gaining understanding of, and beginning to make sense of, his or her suicidality.

Highly congruent findings to these are evident in closely related international studies. In papers that attempt to explore the psychiatric–mental health nursing of suicidal people in Taiwan, Sun *et al.*[55,56] describe a four-stage model consisting of holistic assessment, provision of protection, provision of basic care and provision of advanced care. Unfortunately, they do not appear to explain how restraining or secluding suicidal people helps address suicidal ideation or suicidality per se. Interestingly, Sun *et al.* conclude,[55,p.281]

> The emergent findings … indicated that psychiatric nurses should have the skills and qualities required to provide advanced care for suicidal patients, the compassionate art of nursing was generated as the overarching principle.

Talseth *et al.*[57,58] report insightful work on the processes and experiences of the care of suicidal people in Scandinavia. In these studies, PMHNs confirmed rather than criticized the suicidal clients' emotions and feelings, and PMHNs conveyed and communicated an acceptance of the suicidal person and created time for them. In so doing, PMHNs ensured that they listened, without prejudice, to the clients. There are obvious and clear parallels between Cutcliffe *et al.*,[54] Cutcliffe and Stevenson,[4] Sun *et al.*[55,56] and Talseth *et al.*;[57,58] most especially, the necessity and subsequent therapeutic value of co-presencing (and all the microskills and qualities that such a phrase captures) in care of the suicidal person.

Earlier, though mostly theoretical and case study focused, work has when engaging with suicidal clients similarly espoused the importance of:

- forming a relationship: a human–human connection, conveying acceptance, tolerance and hearing and understanding;[30]
- the value of compassion and emotional identification when caring for the suicidal client, in addition to the

trust that is built through regular contact between client and nurse;[59,60]

- the need to consider one's own attitudes towards suicide in order that nurses can ensure they do not distance themselves from the client (a finding further supported in Carlen and Bengtsson's study;[61])
- the importance of relating to suicidal clients;[62]
- the value of engaging in twice weekly counselling sessions with some suicidal clients;[57,58,62]
- the value of nurses initiating contact with suicidal clients, and attending to clients' basic needs (including the value of physical contact with suicidal clients);[57,58]
- the unconditional acceptance, tolerance, empathy and positive regard of the suicidal client, as opposed to all too commonly encountered disapproving attitudes from some formal care staff;[63,64]
- the therapeutic value of listening, hearing and understanding.[63,64]

ENGAGEMENT AS A MEANS TO INSPIRE HOPE

There is an abundance of evidence that indicates hopelessness is a key element in determining whether or not a person will take their own life rather than merely considering it,[65] and that suicidal people need hope. PMHNs who operationalize the 'engagement' approach are ideally placed to be one such source of hope. It should be noted that, at present, there is no specific theory of how PMHNs can inspire hope in suicidal clients. There exists, however, a parallel literature(s) of hope inspiration in related client groups.[66,67]

Cohen and Cutcliffe conclude their review by stating that[66,67]

Epistemological prudence notwithstanding, tentative conclusions can be drawn and the evidence, such as it is, points to the possibility of a formal level theory of the inspiration of hope in P/MH [psychiatric–mental health] nursing that transcends individual substantive areas. Furthermore, this formal level theory appears to ground the inspiration of hope in P/MH nursing in the relationship established between nurse and person in need of hope; an emerging empirical finding that has obvious congruence and synchronicity with the philosophy and theory of a Peplauvian based approach to P/MH nursing.

Accordingly, PMHNs who wish to consider hope inspiration in suicidal people might benefit from mining this parallel literature for additional possible therapeutic interventions but should also be mindful of grounding these in a meaningful, interpersonal relationship. Where people at risk of suicide are concerned, the caring relationship must

be developed as a 'hope-inspiring' form of engagement. Only through engaging with the person will the nurse come to understand the nature of the person's psychache and what might need to be offered to address this. The nurse's engagement with the suicidal person must therefore be dedicated to understanding the person's suicidal lived experiences and the nature of his or her psychache and to developing the means to re-instil hope. The value of this hope-inspiring form of engagement for the suicidal client is further reinforced by the following personal illustrations.

Personal illustration 62.1: Walter

History and context
Walter was a 24-year-old man with a history of cutting and self-mutilation. He had experienced over 10 previous admissions. Walter had been diagnosed with 'multiple personality disorder', schizophrenia, a sociopathic personality disorder and demon possession! He expressed having some difficulty with close interpersonal relationships and described himself as homosexual. He had had several previous 'suicide attempts', although, on each occasion, he was always 'found in time'.

Overview of care provided
At the beginning of Walter's care episode, the nursing staff carried out an assessment of his suicide risk using the NGASR (see Chapter 61) and determined that he presented with a low risk of suicide. However, this potential risk was identified as a need and, together with Walter, a care package was negotiated. A range of interventions/practices, all of which were based on the 'engagement' approach for care of the suicidal client, were implemented and these are summarized as follows.

- 'One-to-one' sessions with Walter and his nurse were arranged. These occurred three times a week, in a quiet room. This formal, structured, undisturbed time provided Walter with the chance to experience the undivided attention of someone who was willing to work with him. Walter would use this time however he wanted; he would set the 'agenda', but most commonly he would turn to talking about his particular outlook on the world.
- On every day, one of the nurses involved in Walter's care would discuss with him how Walter intended to use the day and what (if any) activities Walter would like to participate in. Additionally, the nurses would explore how the nursing team could assist him with those activities (e.g. share a meal together, attend and participate in any ward-based groups).
- When Walter was feeling vulnerable, it was negotiated that a nurse would make a purposeful contact with Walter every hour. Frequently, this purposeful contact was subsumed within some larger interpersonal contact, e.g. going for long walks or enjoying a cup of coffee together.

Personal illustration 62.2: Johnny

History and context

Johnny was a 62-year-old man who had been married to the same woman for nearly 40 years. He had two grown-up children and three grandchildren. Over the previous 2 years he had been experiencing what he described as 'funny turns'. His appetite appeared to be good but he often woke up very early in the morning and could not get back to sleep. He ran a local gymnasium, which he said he enjoyed but it also caused him a lot of pressure and stress. He had recently started taking antidepressant medication, prescribed by his GP. When things were bad, he would say, 'Sometimes I feel like ending it all', but he was looking forward to his retirement. On admission, he said he felt 'hopeless' at the time and that his thoughts about 'ending it all' were more frequent and pervasive.

Overview of the care provided

As with Walter's care episode, Johnny's care began with an assessment of his suicide risk using the NGASR (see Chapter 61) and it was determined that he presented with a high risk of suicide. Therefore, for the first few days of his care, a 'package' of care was negotiated with Johnny and it was agreed that this would be reviewed after 3 days. As with Walter, a range of interventions/practices, all of which were based on the 'engagement: hope inspiration' approach for care of the suicidal client, were implemented, as follows.

- The nurses agreed that, because of concern about Johnny's well-being, he would not be left alone during this 3-day period. They felt that he needed a high level of engagement; thus, there would always be a nurse very close to him (physically close). The nurses explained to Johnny that this physical closeness was a gesture of concern for him, not a custodial intervention. Furthermore, this physical closeness would provide a range of opportunities for Johnny and his nurse to engage in dialogue or activities.
- This high level of engagement was used purposefully to encourage Johnny to talk about his thoughts and feelings, to enable him to vent his painful emotions, for the nurse to listen to these verbalizations, and to provide unconditional acceptance and support.
- Each day his level of suicidal risk was assessed using the same assessment tool, and, owing to the high level of engagement and the relationship that was being established, the assessment was felt to be highly accurate.
- The nurses would occasionally sit quietly together with Johnny.
- The nurses would read together with Johnny and play board games.
- More latterly, the nurses began to look at his choices and options and started to challenge, subtly, some of his more 'hopeless' or 'negative' constructs.

After several days of this high level of engagement, Johnny's risk assessment showed that his level of suicide risk was declining, and therefore his care was renegotiated accordingly.

SUMMARY

The two current approaches to care for suicidal people can be categorized as 'close or special observation' and 'engagement'. Despite the widespread use of observations, the UK and international data are compelling: 'observation' is a woefully weak intervention and fails between 23 and 48 per cent of the people it is supposed to protect. It lacks an empirical evidence base and the 'supportive' evidence, such as it is, suggests that it is certain attitudes and practices of the PMHN within the (or during) observation period that appear to be experienced as therapeutic, and not the being observed per se.

Engagement is concerned with inspiring hope through the interpersonal relationship. It is concerned with exploring and attempting to understand the nature of the person's psychache. While it also contains elements of attending to the person's safety, it does so by facilitating the person's reconnection with humanity. Accepting the axiomatic complexity and multidimensionality of suicide and, at the same time, the undeniable fact that suicide is a *human drama* played out in the everyday lives, minds, brains and interactions of people, it may not be entirely surprising that, for PMHNs at any rate, caring for suicidal people must be an interpersonal endeavour, and one personified by talking and listening.

Reflection

- Which of the two broad approaches covered in this chapter has the most congruence with your own philosophy and approach to psychiatric–mental health nursing?
- What kind of help do you think you would need/want if you were feeling suicidal?
- Why do you think some PMHNs are reluctant to let go of defensive practices and engage in a more interpersonal, engagement-focused form of care for the suicidal person?

REFERENCES

1. Rosen G. History in the study of suicide. *Psychological Medicine* 1971; **1**: 267–85.

2. Aldridge D. *Suicide: the tragedy of hopelessness.* London, UK: Jessica Kingsley Publishers, 1998.

3. World Health Organization. *Depression/suicide.* 2002. Available from: www.int/health_topics/suicide/en/. Accessed 2 February 2007.

4. Cutcliffe JR, Stevenson C. *Care of the suicidal person.* Edinburgh, UK: Elsevier, 2007.

5. Department of Health. *Health of the nation.* London, UK: HMSO, 1990.

6. Department of Health. *Modernising mental health services: safe, sound and supportive.* London, UK: HMSO, 1998.

7. Department of Health. *National service framework for mental health.* London, UK: HMSO, 1999.

8. Department of Health. *National suicide prevention strategy for England.* London, UK: HMSO, 2002.

9. Tanney B. Psychiatric diagnosis and suicidal acts. In: Maris RW, Berman AL, Silverman MM (eds). *Comprehensive textbook of suicidology.* New York, NY: Guilford Press, 2000.

10. Department of Health. *National suicide prevention strategy for England: annual report on progress 2006.* London, UK: HMSO, 2007.

11. Canadian Association for Suicide Prevention. *Blueprint for a Canadian National Suicide Prevention Strategy.* 2004. Available from: www.suicideprevention.ca. Accessed 2 February 2007.

12. Maris RW, Berman AL, Silverman MM. *Comprehensive textbook of suicidology.* New York, NY: Guildford Press, 2000.

13. Maris R. Social forces in suicide: a life review. In: Maris RW, Silverman MM, Canetto SS (eds). *Review of suicidology.* New York, NY: Guildford Press, 1997: 42–60.

14. Pritchard C. Psychosocioeconomic factors in suicide. In: Thompson T, Mathias P (eds). *Lyttle's mental health and disorder,* 2nd edn. London, UK: Baillière Tindall, 1998: 276–95.

15. Rawlins RP. Hope-hopelessness. In: Rawlins RP, Williams S, Beck AT (eds). *Mental health nursing: a holistic life cycle approach,* 3rd edn. St Louis, MO: Mosby, 1993: 257–84.

16. Anderson M, Jenkins R. The national suicide prevention strategy for England: the reality of a national strategy for the nursing profession. *Journal of Psychiatric and Mental Health Nursing* 2006; **13**: 641–50.

17. Shneidman ES. *Comprehending suicide: landmarks in 20th-century suicidology.* Washington, DC: American Psychological Association, 2001.

18. Jick H, Kaye JA, Jick SS. Antidepressants and the risk of suicidal behaviors. *Journal of the American Medical Association* 2004; **292**: 338–43.

19. Wagstaff A, Perry J, Caroline M. Clozapine: in prevention of suicide in patients with schizophrenia or schizoaffective disorder. *CNS Drugs* 2003; **17** (4): 273–80.

20. Healy D, Whitaker C. Antidepressants and suicide: risk–benefit conundrums. *Journal of Psychiatry and Neuroscience* 2003; **28**: 331–7.

21. Healy D. *Psychiatric drugs explained,* 4th edn. Edinburgh, UK: Elsevier, 2005.

22. Gunnell DJ, Frankel S. Prevention of suicide: aspirations and evidence. *British Medical Journal* 1994; **308**: 1227–33.

23. Stuart GW. Self-protective responses and suicidal behaviors. In: Stuart GW, Laraia MT (eds). *Principles and practices of psychiatric nursing,* 8th edn. St Louis, MO: Mosby, 2005.

24. Bowers L, Park A. Special observations in the care of psychiatric inpatients: a literature review. *Issues in Mental Health Nursing* 2001; **22**: 769–86.

25. Duffy D. Out of the shadows: a study of the special observation of suicidal psychiatric in-patients. *Journal of Advanced Nursing* 1995; **21**: 944–50.

26. O'Brien L, Cole R. Close-observation areas in acute psychiatric units: a literature review. *International Journal of Mental Health Nursing* 2003; **12**: 165–76.

27. Moore P, Berman K, Knight M, Devine J. Constant observation: implications for nursing practice. *Journal of Psychosocial Nursing* 1995; **33** (3): 46–50.

28. Horsfall J, Cleary M. Discourse analysis of an observation 'levels' nursing policy. *Journal of Advanced Nursing* 2000; **32**: 1291–7.

29. Barker P, Cutcliffe JR. Clinical risk: a need for engagement not observation. *Mental Health Care* 1999; **2** (8): 8–12.

30. Cutcliffe JR, Barker P. Considering the care of the suicidal client and the case for 'engagement and inspiring hope' or observations. *Journal of Psychiatric and Mental Health Nursing* 2002; **9** (5): 611–21.

31. Standing Nursing and Midwifery Advisory Committee. *Practice guidance. Safe and supportive observation of patients at risk: mental health nursing – addressing acute concerns.* London, UK: Department of Health, 1999.

32. Dodds P, Bowles N. Dismantling formal observation and refocusing nursing activity in acute inpatient psychiatry: a case study. *Journal of Psychiatric and Mental Health Nursing* 2001; **8**: 173–88.

33. Bowles N, Dodds P, Hackney D *et al.* Formal observations and engagement: a discussion paper. *Journal of Psychiatric and Mental Health Nursing* 2002; **9** (3): 255–60.

34. Department of Health. *Safety first – five year report of the National Confidential Inquiry into Suicides and Homicides by People with Mental Health Problems.* London, UK: HMSO, 2001.

35. Links P. Foreword. In: Cutcliffe JR, Stevenson C (eds). *Care of the suicidal person.* Edinburgh, UK: Elsevier, 2007: x–xi.

36. Geddes JR, Juszczak E, O'Brien F, Kendrick S. Suicide in the 12 months after discharge from psychiatric inpatient care, Scotland 1968–92. *Journal of Epidemiology and Community Health* 1997; **51**: 430–4.

37. Desai RA, Dausey D, Bosenheck R. Mental health service delivery and suicide risk: the role of individual patient and facility factors. *American Journal of Psychiatry* 2005; **162**: 311–18.

38. Younge O, Sterwin LL. What psychiatric nurses say about constant care. *Clinical Nurse Research* 1992; **1**: 80–90.

39. Pitula CR, Cardell R. Suicidal inpatients' experiences of constant observation. *Psychiatric Services* 1996; **47**: 6491–51.

40. Moorhead S, Langenbach M, Kennedy J *et al.* Observations of the observed: a study of inpatients' perceptions of being observed. *Irish Journal of Psychological Medicine* 1996; **13**: 59–61.

41. Cardell R, Pitula CR. Suicidal inpatients' perceptions of therapeutic and non-therapeutic aspects of constant observation. *Psychiatric Services* 1999; **20**: 1066–70.

42. Fletcher RF. The process of constant observation: perspectives of staff and suicidal patients. *Journal of Psychiatric and Mental Health Nursing* 1999; **6**: 9–14.

43. Jones J, Ward M, Wellman N *et al.* Psychiatric inpatients' experiences of nursing observation: a United Kingdom perspective. *Journal of Psychosocial Nursing* 2000; **38** (12): 10–19.

44. Barker P, Walker L. *A survey of care practices in acute admission wards*. Report submitted to the Northern and Yorkshire Regional Research and Development Committee. Newcastle, UK: University of Newcastle, 1999.

45. MacKay I, Paterson B, Cassells C. Constant or special observations of inpatients presenting a risk of aggression or violence: nurses' perceptions of the rules of engagement. *Journal of Psychiatric and Mental Health Nursing* 2005; **12**: 464–71.

46. Bowers L, Gournay K, Duffy D. Suicide and self-harm in inpatient psychiatric units: a national survey of observation policies. *Journal of Advanced Nursing* 2000; **32**: 437–44.

47. Heyman EN, Lombardo BA. Managing costs: the confused, agitated or suicidal inpatient. *Nursing Economics* 1995; **13**: 107–11.

48. Cutcliffe JR. The differences and commonalities between United Kingdom and Canadian Psychiatric/Mental health nursing: a personal reflection. *Journal of Psychiatric and Mental Health Nursing* 2003; **10**: 255–7.

49. Holmes D, Kennedy SL, Perron A. The mentally ill and social exclusion: a critical examination of the use of seclusion from the patient's perspectives. *Issues in Mental Health Nursing* 2004; **25**: 559–78.

50. Buchanan-Barker P, Barker P. Observation: the original sin of mental health nursing? *Journal of Psychiatric and Mental Health Nursing* 2005; **12**: 541–9.

51. Stevenson C, Cutcliffe JR. Problematizing special observation in psychiatry: Foucault, archaeology, genealogy, discourse and power/knowledge. *Journal of Psychiatric and Mental Health Nursing* 2006; **13**: 713–21.

52. Gournay K, Ward M, Thornicroft G, Wright S. Crisis in the capital: inpatient care in inner London. *Mental Health Practice* 1998; **1**: 10–18.

53. Shneidman ES. The suicidal mind. In: Maris RW, Silverman MM, Canetto SS (eds). *Review of suicidology, 1997*. New York, NY: Guildford Press, 1997: 22–41.

54. Cutcliffe JR, Stevenson C, Jackson S, Smith P. A modified grounded theory study of how psychiatric nurses work with suicidal people. *International Journal of Nursing Studies* 2006; **43**: 791–802.

55. Sun FK, Long A, Boore J, Tsao LI. Nursing people who are suicidal on psychiatric wards in Taiwan: action and interaction strategies. *Journal of Psychiatric and Mental Health Nursing* 2005; **12** (3): 275–82.

56. Sun FK, Long A, Boore J, Tsao L. A theory for the nursing care of patients at risk of suicide. *Journal of Advanced Nursing* 2006; **53**: 680–90.

57. Talseth AG, Lindseth A, Jacobson L, Norberg A. Nurses' narrations about suicidal psychiatric inpatients. *Nordic Journal of Psychiatry* 1997; **51**: 359–64.

58. Talseth AG, Lindseth A, Jacobson L, Norberg A. The meaning of suicidal in-patients' experiences of being cared for by mental health nurses. *Journal of Advanced Nursing* 1999; **29**: 1034–41.

59. Sainsbury Centre for Mental Health. *Acute problems: a survey of the quality of care in acute psychiatric admission wards*. London, UK: Sainsbury Centre for Mental Health, 1998.

60. Davidhizar R, Vance A. The management of the suicidal patient in a critical care unit. *Journal of Nursing Management* 1993; **1**: 95–102.

61. Carlen P, Bengtsson A. Suicidal patients as experienced by psychiatric nurses in inpatient care. *International Journal of Mental Health Nursing* 2007; **16** (4):257–65.

62. Rogers P. Assessment and treatment of a suicidal patient. *Nursing Times* 1993; **90** (34): 37–9.

63. Long A, Reid W. An exploration of nurses' attitudes to the nursing care of the suicidal patient in an acute psychiatric ward. *Journal of Psychiatric and Mental Health Nursing* 1996; **3**: 29–37.

64. Long A, Smyth A. Suicide: a statement of suffering. *Nursing Ethics* 1998; **5**: 3–15.

65. Weisharr ME, Beck A. Hopelessness and suicide. *International Review of Psychiatry* 1992; **4**: 177–84.

66. Cohen C, Cutcliffe JR. Hope and interpersonal psychiatric/mental health nursing: a systematic review of the literature – part one. *Journal of Psychiatric and Mental Health Nursing* 2007; **14** (2): 134–40.

67. Cutcliffe JR, Cohen C. Hope and interpersonal psychiatric/mental health nursing: a systematic review of the literature – part two. *Journal of Psychiatric and Mental Health Nursing* 2007; **14** (2): 141–7.

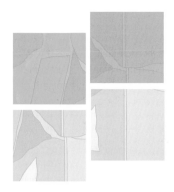

CHAPTER 63

Record-keeping

Martin F. Ward*

INTRODUCTION

It is probably fair to say that, of all the clinical, administrative and professional activities that nurses are involved in, the process of writing and maintaining effective clinical records is the one most fraught with problems but the one which few nurses ever really give any serious thought to once they have achieved their registration. Something carried out so repetitively ceases to attract much attention because it lacks stimulation. It is a little like the first time we buy a new personal fragrance, it smells wonderful and we wear it all the time. After a while we put more and more on because we cannot smell it ourselves, whereas others who come into contact with us are overpowered by it. Nurses who read clinical records for the first time often see things that the experienced writer has missed during their production, and writers would probably be annoyed at having their mistakes pointed out to them.

The fact is that most nurses are exposed to good record-keeping principles as students and receive no more instruction, coaching or guidance for the rest of their careers, unless a crisis occurs, precipitating a management-led insistence that they review local policies or seek the guidance of national standards.[1] Considerable evidence suggests that most practising nurses find it difficult to reconcile their professional ideals with the way that they regularly record information concerning patients' progress. When questioned closely, research participants regularly express doubts about the efficacy of their written communications, frustration with the systems they have to use and the limitations of the infrastructures they see as inhibiting this vital aspect of their work.[2,3] Audits, both local and national, and public inquiries continue to highlight record-keeping as a major factor in the escalation of serious and untoward incidents into tragedies.

THE FUNDAMENTALS OF GOOD RECORD-KEEPING

Among other things, records should be clear, concise and legible. However, such principles are not enough because the written record of one professional – as a source of information for another – involves more than having a clean and legal document. Such simplicity confuses the differing needs for a *complex* 'professional record' with the more straightforward requirements of a 'legal document'.

Records have to serve a purpose. In health care, that purpose may involve more than just a communication about the state of a person's well-being. By first identifying the *purpose* of record-keeping we can describe what needs to be done to make it effective, while at the same time disentangling the *legal* from the *professional* requirements. This will also help us to identify the different forms of records required to meet our different purposes. In doing so, this raises the status of record-keeping from a mundane activity to one of sophistication, requiring high levels of professional skill.

*Martin Ward has been a psychiatric nurse, tutor and researcher for over 30 years. He was the Director of the Royal College of Nursing's Mental Health Nursing Programme at Oxford and presently is an Independent Consultant in Mental Health.

Record purpose and integration of care

If a nurse records information quickly, merely as an end product to some other activity, then record-keeping risks becoming a secondary process, with no great significance. As a first principle, record-keeping should be:

> Integral to the overall process of care; carrying equal status to any other component; needing to be considered with the same attention to detail as the intervention itself.

The reason for this is quite clear. Records are part of the intervention. Nurse–patient contact time needs to be planned if it is to be effective. It has to fit an operational process that builds up into a picture of care. Each contact has to be evaluated and its impact measured. Finally, it has to be recorded, not just because protocol dictates that it should, but as part of this overall picture. Change or progress cannot be measured without baselines, from which comparisons can be made. If we do not record details of what has taken place, historically, in our various contacts with the patient, how else can we know when we need to revise our interventions? How can continuity between practitioners be maintained unless everyone has access to details of what happened in their absence? How can the memory of one observation endure, clearly, over weeks or even months? How can patients make a real contribution to their own care if there is no record that will help them to see themselves as others do? Finally, how can care be truly evaluated if there are important gaps in the chain of recorded events, or if lack of precision blurs all events into a single story of everyday routine?

Seeing the recording process as secondary to – or divorced from the care process – devalues nursing and dilutes the impact of concerted teamwork. None of the above outcomes from the recording process can be achieved successfully without the attention to detail demanded by good record-keeping. Recognizing that recording and care are on the same continuum enables the practitioner to appreciate the importance of identifying the purpose of the recording.

In Personal illustration 63.1, previous care records highlighted key and significant information that could be used as a way of ensuring that others could work for the patient's benefit. Primary concerns about the patient's response to perceived threats were the main purpose of the written record and, as a result, were integral to the care itself.

It could be argued that an experienced nurse would have the skills to work all this out for himself or herself while on the phone with Archie. However, why should the nurse have to experiment and risk prolonging or exacerbating Archie's difficulties? The recorded information helped Janine to resolve the situation quickly and then Archie was calm enough to return to the unit safe in

---

Personal illustration 63.1

Janine, a nurse on a busy inpatient acute unit, receives a telephone call from a patient who has gone home to collect some personal belongings. Archie tells the nurse that his home has been burgled. He is distraught and abusive on the phone. He resists her first attempts to calm him down and threatens to hurt himself unless something is done to help him, immediately. As his primary nurse, Mike, is off duty, Janine has no direct responsibility for Archie. As no one else is available, Janine must handle the situation herself. Archie is becoming increasingly agitated and starts shouting down the phone. Janine asks him to describe what has happened in his home and, while he is talking, she opens his care record. Carefully documented records of his care plan outcomes highlight that Archie responds well to active listening. Further reading gives two examples of previous incidents. However, the primary nurse has underlined a section which tells that analysis of previous conversations indicates that Archie does not like to be given the option of making difficult decisions. Janine manages to defuse the situation by prompting more controlled discussion and by offering to phone the police once Archie has returned to the unit, where he can give an interview.

---

the knowledge that someone understood and cared enough to help. More importantly, Archie received care that lessened his distress, reducing the possibility of the situation escalating into a real emergency. The continuity between responses of his primary nursing team and this 'outsider' would only reinforce his confidence in his care programme.

Good record-keeping has to be seen as having a specific purpose and integrated with the process of care delivery. The production of appropriate records is, therefore, a state of mind and is as philosophically bound as any model of care. This mindset has been referred to as a 'symbol of professionalism'.[2] However, as such, it can cause conflict and tension when set against organizational requirements. In his ethnographic research, Allen[2] described nurses on a surgical ward having difficulty reconciling their professional ideals about the quality of their records with the way that they were viewed by their employing organization, the time available to complete them, and the credibility with which they were viewed by other members of the clinical team. In the USA, tension between nurse-driven documentation and the perceptions of that work by other disciplines was seen – in one case – as a cause for a breakdown in support between different working groups, to the detriment of patients.[4] In that study, the nurses were advanced psychiatric practitioners and the problems were resolved by increasing the amount of significance that their records had to the process of care. Further examples of this way of thinking can be found in Japan,[5] Sweden[6] and Norway[7] as well as the UK.[8,9]

Reflection

- Is record-keeping integral to your work or something ancillary to it?
- Do your colleagues agree with you on this matter?

Professional development

In the same way that individual practitioners need to update themselves in relation to changes in healthcare attitudes and techniques, so too it is important that they regularly review how they record information generated by those changes. If we accept the link between recording and care delivery we also accept that developments in each area are interdependent. Research has shown that not only does an ongoing programme of reviewing personal record-keeping improve the efficiency of this activity but it also raises awareness of the necessity to view such work as central to clinical effectiveness.[10] This pilot scheme included 6-monthly updates and evaluations of nurses' adherence to a documentation system, linked to their care delivery process, and demonstrated the benefits of attributing continued importance to the recording process. Another project exploring the effects of a 30-week multidisciplinary mental health education programme carried out in the UK identified communication as part of the core skills of mental health workers. However, it was concluded that participants in the programme tended to overestimate their skills in the two key areas of care planning and record-keeping.[11]

In work carried out in Granada, Jimenez *et al.*[12] developed a specific recording tool whereby treatment methods were recorded by means of previously designated numerical codes corresponding to the interventions carried out. Nurses had to be trained to use this tool and research had to be used to underpin its design, but it was so successful that the records were subsequently computerized and made available for analysis and audit. Similar work undertaken in Germany[13] clearly shows the links between well-developed documentation, the training to use it and powerful quality management systems within psychiatric settings.

Practice-based research from the UK identifies the links between the application of research within a clinical environment and the absolute necessity of modifying the supporting recording activities.[14] However, the two processes in this study, *care delivery* and *record-keeping*, were not separate entities, but part of the same process, with one equally informing the other. In all the above studies the need for educational development within record-keeping was identified as a prerequisite for change.

Formal education programmes can account for only a small proportion of the professional development of any practitioner during the course of his or her career. Conversely, record-keeping is a daily event. Likewise, the growth in understanding of a way of doing something, or the increase in personal technology, is a cumulative process with each day building on the last. Formal education can usually address only primary issues relevant to a group or section of the working community, identified by stage of training, exposure to specific working methods or seniority, etc. In effect, these educational programmes aggregate knowledge to create standardized development. While the ability to generate summative improvements in care quality is important, it is not designed to meet the needs of individual practitioners. Record-keeping itself is not a static thing, and improvements in computer technology, for example, have created a whole new generation of documentation possibilities, with software packages enabling multilayered record-keeping to follow patients throughout the whole of their care.[15]

Ongoing professional development can benefit from an exploration of individual records in a far more dynamic way. Cutcliffe[16] outlined the need to record information from clinical supervision sessions. If one takes his discussion to its logical conclusion, it also shows the importance of using written records as a method of supervision itself. Reviewing evidence of actual clinical work through the written record of the supervisee, then jointly developing strategies for understanding both the clinical work and its subsequent recording would seem to have benefits for both activities. Discussions about what nurses did in given circumstances or how they did or did not resolve conflict can easily be shrouded by poor memory or preconceived ideas about their own effectiveness. The written record can be used as an aide-memoire for reflective discussion. Exploring the ways in which information is recorded would be the first step in improving the performance of the nurse.

Take, for example, the situation involving Archie. If Janine was concerned about her responses to him on that day, or perhaps the outcome of the event had not been so positive, then some form of reflective activity might highlight areas she could develop or practise later. To be able to use the written record of the event to support this mentoring process, it would need to show a clear picture of both what took place and how each of the players was involved. By doing so, it would also show the importance of matching recording purpose to that of clinical intention. Hence, in this case, the record would be both a clinical and an educative purpose. Significantly, it would also highlight the loop within which these two elements exist; the quality of one being interdependent upon the quality of the other. This is not to suggest that clinical recording be undertaken merely for staff reflection, but surely the two things are linked if the record itself is to have meaning after the event. Matching a recording process to fit the requirements of clinical actions calls for different forms of recording. The more skilled nurses become at recognizing this, the more sophisticated and effective they become at responding appropriately to the changing needs of individual patients.[17]

This need to identify different forms of record-keeping for different purposes has far-reaching implications. One failing of the current hierarchy within psychiatric–mental health nursing (at least in the UK) is the accepted convention that junior nurses act as key workers or primary nurses, while more senior clinical staff act as managers or consultants. Consequently, documents supporting the work of a clinical team are often the products of the junior staff. Additionally, senior staff may provide clinical supervision, but this is not standard practice. Unless junior staff seek advice and/or regular supervision, their own record-keeping becomes the benchmark or 'standard' and they have limited opportunities to develop this important professional skill. Record-keeping is only as good as the person who makes the record. If there are no quality goals, or the quality remains static, the value of those records will gradually diminish. Dimond[18] points out that there are enough lessons on record-keeping standards which can be drawn from reports of the Health Service Commissioner (ombudsman) to enable any quality conscious organization to improve the way that material concerning patients is recorded. Clearly, senior practitioners need to contribute regularly to the recording process, even if this requires a change in the infrastructure within which the nurses work.

To this situation one must also add the problems associated with the implementation of certain models or ways of delivering nursing. If the philosophical basis of care centres on a high degree of patient autonomy, the recording process for contact with that patient needs to reflect this. Fowler[19] offered a good example in relation to the application of Peplau's theory of interpersonal relations, about interpersonal working with patients and the difficulty of recording these interactions. In Fowler's view, the holistic nature of Peplau's work did not easily fit with a record-keeping system. While acknowledging this fact, the author recommended that nurses develop a recording style, in the form of a commentary that best suited the approach, i.e. the clinical contact being reflected in the recording purpose.

Reflection

- Who should be responsible for the day-to-day record-keeping associated with nursing care?
- Should those individuals be properly prepared for this and, if not, how do you think this might be improved?

LEGAL REQUIREMENTS AND GOOD PRACTICE

Practitioners need to recognize the difference between professional and legal accountability. In countries where there is specific mental health legislation (such as the UK, Canada, Australia and New Zealand), the process of care delivery is provided within a framework that sets parameters for the circumstances under which that care can be delivered.[17,20] For example, determining when they can be treated against their wishes, the period of their hospitalization, and their access to appeal protects patients' rights. Other medicolegislation combines with this to ensure confidentiality and access to patients' records. Increasingly, legislation demands that care should:

- be appropriate to the needs of the individual
- be of the highest quality
- comply with new ideas and technology.

In effect, such legislation sets the scene for care delivery but does not prescribe the nature of the care to be delivered. It leaves clinical decision-making to the clinician. Professional accountability, therefore, is very much a personal choice, albeit guided by standards of professional conduct.[21]

Conversely, the nature of medically related record-keeping is determined by strict rules that have to be complied with to ensure not only confidentiality but also the maintenance of standards.[22,23] Although decisions concerning these issues should not be left to individual choice, evidence from service reviews suggests that this is not always the case.[24] While nurses have choice over the care that may be offered, and therefore determine the purpose of the associated record-keeping, they do not have choice about the framework of the records themselves, nor the standards that have to be met to make them an accepted legal document. Separating the legal from the professional requirements of good record-keeping enables nurses to identify clearly the framework upon which they base the choice element of the work. Only once nurses are aware of what has to be done to comply with legal standards can the construction and design of the records, which fit the purpose of care, proceed.

The following is a summary of the key points governing legally acceptable records and standards of good practice. All recorded entries *must* be:

- *legible*, i.e. written in the national language and readable
- *written in blue or black ink* – both for necessary copying purposes and to make the text bold
- *signed and dated by the recorder* – initials are only acceptable when a code is provided to enable auditors to clearly identify the recorder
- *signed and dated where there are deletions* – mistakes or crossings out within the text have to be sanctioned by the recorder
- *originals* – photocopies of documents fade or discolour over time and can seriously hamper the reader's ability to decipher what is written; entries must be made on original documents; when it is necessary for a copy

of notes to be made this fact must be clearly stated on the file itself

- *given in full without abbreviations* – abbreviations can mean different things to different readers, and nothing at all to others; they may cause confusion and are generally the result of sloppy unidisciplinary professionalism
- *stored in a locked cabinet or safe place* – access must be only for those who have direct responsibility for patients or for those who need to have information about the patient for legal or professional reasons, i.e. multidisciplinary team members in clinical decision-making roles
- *available to those who have legal access to them* – where appropriate this will include the patient's legal representatives with permission given by the patients' representatives of the Mental Health Act Commission or similar bodies and authorized auditors.

Entries should:

- *involve patients* – when possible patients should be involved in documenting the impact of the care they receive, as well as designing and evaluating it
- *be relevant to the patient in whose file they are being made* – complicated observations about the interactions between different patients should be divided into sections and placed in each patient's records, thus ensuring that all the patients involved have a record of the event and not just one patient
- *be concise* – accurate and to the point; more words do not necessarily mean more information and health professionals need to know the facts as quickly as possible; if the facts are hidden in rhetoric they are likely to be missed or the record itself ignored
- *record progress* – repeat entries of 'slept well' and 'no change' are pointless; it should be assumed that if no entry is made in a progress record there is no change from the previous entry; only things that are different need to be reported
- *be information sensitive* – key or significant information that influences care decisions should be highlighted or placed on a separate data sheet for ready access
- *be systematic* – all entries for a particular patient should follow a pattern as determined by the purpose of the recording
- *be sequential* – if entries have to be made in retrospect they should be clearly marked accordingly
- *be recorded on the appropriate document* – most case files contain any number of different documents and entries need to be in the right place
- *be coded* – in a way that enables a reader to see which pieces of the total record fits with other entries
- *not be repeated* – if it is necessary to place the same entry on a different document, either use an accepted coding system to refer the reader to the original entry, as with care plans and evaluation records, or review the use of the documents themselves to avoid over-reporting

- *be multidisciplinary* – although this may not always be possible, systems that encourage different disciplines to use their own records have been shown to be poor communicators of relevant healthcare information and this can be a key factor in the event of complex care failing to support individual patients.

PROBLEMS ASSOCIATED WITH GOOD RECORD-KEEPING

Patient involvement

While most practitioners accept the principle of involving patients in the design, delivery and evaluation of their care as a fundamental part of contemporary psychiatric care, for many it remains unclear as to how such ideals can be operationalized. When considering the possibility of patients helping to construct their own care record alarm bells often go off because such records are seen to be the domain of practitioners. However, this can only be the case if sensitive information is to be withheld from patients or if they are too disturbed to be able to make either a genuine contribution or appreciate what is being asked of them. Of course, there are more sinister reasons, such as that the entries themselves are derogatory to the patient as a person, badly written or patently incorrect.

With the growth in discreet computer software that enables different aspects of patients' files to be displayed at any given time[25] it is possible to restrict the amount of access that a patient has. Even with traditional paper records, access should not be a problem. Patients should already have access to their own care plan; indeed, they should have been encouraged to help construct it. Why then should they not have access to the reporting data charting the impact and progress of that care plan? If individual practitioners are having difficulty in finding ways of reducing the tokenism of patient involvement, sharing the responsibility for completing some of the patients' records with the patients themselves may be a good place to start. There is some evidence within the literature that shows it is possible not only for patients to participate in this activity but also to be the ones who initiate the recording process itself. Rosenbloom *et al.*[26] developed a computerized note-capture tool which was used solely by service users. Their research showed that it was possible for users to fully undertake their own recording process provided that they had a choice in how they recorded information. Something of this order, implemented within an outreach or a rehabilitation setting, would require considerable training and support from nursing staff for it to be successful, but it would certainly link the purpose of care with its integration. The problems of such an approach are probably not those of the patients but those of the staff, who might well see such a 'progressive' development as undermining one of their key professional roles, i.e. maintaining a clinical record. However, there appears to be no ethical, moral or even legal reason why patients should not at least share in this responsibility.

Reflection

- Are you comfortable with a patient for whom you have responsibility being able to read what you have written about him or her and being party to writing this?
- If not, why not?

Multidisciplinary record-keeping

Multidisciplinary or joint record-keeping has been the focus of much debate over the past two decades. Despite evidence to suggest that it *reduces* duplication, *increases* practitioner reporting effectiveness, *enhances* transfer of data across teams, *raises awareness* of the contributions of individual team members and provides a clearer picture of care overall,[27,28] the approach is still resisted by many. Several factors may be involved, not least the possible poor quality of individual disciplines' record-keeping. However, as Rigby *et al.*[29] reported, modern technology and new ways of recording dictate that all members of a care team use similar recording mechanisms. Yet, other members of the team may need to be convinced of the effectiveness of such a radical move. One way of achieving this is for nurses to tailor their recording so that it fits with both the purpose of the care offered and is written in such a way as it becomes accessible to other disciplines. Adherence to the recording principles described within this chapter would also improve the overall quality of nursing records and thus make their inclusion in joint records a valuable asset. One way of achieving this would be through the clinical governance agenda, using audit processes to monitor the impact of multidisciplinary records but using the nurse lead as the person responsible for them. This makes sense, if only because nurses need to monitor their own clinical actions and should be held responsible within clinical governance for activities over which they have clinical responsibility.[30]

'Organizational straightjackets': the documents themselves

In this era of quality improvement, clinical governance, audit and cost-effectiveness many organizations have demonstrated their desire to improve efficiency by developing standardized recording documentation. While there are obvious benefits for an organization to implement such schedules within a psychiatric setting, say for audit and quality assurance purposes, they tend to ignore the nature and purpose of some of the more interpersonal and reflective aspects of mental health care. It could be argued that the recording purpose has to dictate the

record, not the other way around. Liberto and colleagues[31] posed the question as to what happens to the anecdotal information gathered during a conversation, an observation or an incident. They suggested that individual practitioners adapted their recording style to fit with that of the organization, but that they included more subjective and anecdotal data within a commentary. This would then be accessed readily by others, but not confused with factual reporting. What takes place between patients and nurses is not always clear. Standardized recording demands answers and requires the recorder to make quick decisions about what is experienced or observed. This challenges much conventional wisdom in contemporary psychiatric–mental health nursing and, as a result, more open reporting styles need to be developed. Such a style of reporting may get 'messy' from an audit perspective, but reducing complex patient information into checklists is clinically counterproductive.

Consider a clinical environment in which all disciplines use the same recording device, patients are encouraged to write in their own records, record-keeping is regarded as a part of the care process and is, therefore, commensurate with care actions, and nurses are encouraged to explore more personalized approaches to documentation. The record for the event described at the beginning of this chapter might read that shown in Figure 63.1.

This example offers only a snapshot of what is possible. There is no 'rocket science' here, just good sense and clear recording. What is important is that the record itself is part of what actually happened, not an afterthought.

SUMMARY

Record-keeping is a complex and dynamic process and cannot be relegated to the status of an 'also-ran'. If care is to be regularly tested against outcomes, measured for its effectiveness, modified or even totally changed to reflect new ideas and technology, ideology or philosophy, it has to be supported by a recording process which is both fit for the purpose and as robust as the clinical intervention itself.

The written records of any professional group testify to the working activities of that group. There will always be problems associated with maintaining high-quality, informative and practical records, within a work environment that may be stressful, complex and time-consuming. Nonetheless, if the nurses' contribution to this process is disjointed, lacks depth and is poorly prepared it will diminish the contribution that nurses make to the delivery of care. In effect, this will devalue the contribution of nursing generally within the mental health care team. While nursing will no doubt attempt to find other ways of preserving its reputation, the real losers in this situation are the patients. Failure to see the importance of good record-keeping by nurses that is targeted to its

Entry 45, 18th April 2002 15:30 hrs	Archie phoned the unit in an agitated state shouting that his flat had been burgled. I found it difficult to calm him down and he threatened to harm himself if I did not do something to help him. He was genuinely upset, and for obvious reasons. Referred to <u>Entry nos. 27 and 31</u> for some idea of how to deal with this. Mike's notes enabled me to ask Archie to come back to the unit and I would phone the police for him. He agreed and is on his way. Janine Wilson, Staff Nurse (Janine Wilson)
Entry 46, 18th April 2002 16:20 hrs	Archie has returned (refer <u>Entry 45</u>). Still upset but calmer and no longer shouting. Contacted police on 01865 123456 and spoken with PC Wilson. They will send someone to interview Archie this evening. Will talk to Archie to see if anything else can be done. Janine Wilson, Staff Nurse (Janine Wilson)
Entry 47, 18th April 2002 17:00 hrs	*Thank you Janine, I feel a lot better now. Can someone sit with me when the police come?* *Archie Raymond*
Entry 48, 18th April 2002 11:00 hrs	*Can Janine, Archie and Mike meet with me tomorrow, 19th April, at about 17:30 hrs to see if* *we can alter Archie's support programme please (refer <u>Entry 45</u>)?* *Alan Bennett, Senior Reg.* (Alan Bennett)
Entry 49, 18th April 2002 18:20 hrs	Meeting arranged (refer <u>Entry 48</u>). Janine Wilson, Staff Nurse (Janine Wilson)
Entry 50, 18th April 2002 20:15 hrs	*Archie Raymond interviewed Re: break-in.* *Malcolm Wilson* (M. Wilson PC 234)
Entry 51, 18th April 2002 21:00 hrs	*I want to talk tomorrow about how I can deal better with these situations (refer <u>Entry 45</u>).* *I was very frightened when I got home and if it had not been for Janine I would have done something stupid.* *Janine says there are several ways we can approach this so I will be better prepared in the future.* The meeting should be good. Janine Wilson, Staff Nurse (Janine Wilson) **and** *Archie Raymond*

Figure 63.1 Example of record-keeping

purpose and intrinsically linked to care delivery is a failure to see the importance of nursing in the relief of suffering for those with mental health problems.

REFERENCES

1. Rodden C, Bell M. Record keeping: developing good practice. *Nursing Standard* 2002; **17**: 40–2.

2. Allen D. Record-keeping and routine nursing practice: the view from the wards. *Journal of Advanced Nursing* 1998; **27**: 1223–30.

3. Taylor H. An exploration of the factors that affect nurses' record keeping. *British Journal of Nursing* 2003; **12**: 751–8.

4. Glair-Gajewski C, Trigoboff E. Formulation of a systematic method of documentation for nurse-led mental health groups. *Journal of New York State Nurses Association* 1993; **24**: 16–18.

5. Kataoka K. Evaluation of mental health, psychiatric care, and welfare planning at a public hospital. *Seishin Shinkeigaku Zasshi* 1996; **98**: 865–9.

6. Andersen T, Johansson BM, Lindberg M, Stenwall R. New documentation routines in psychiatry in Vasterbotten: unified structure for better quality of care. *Lakartidningen* 1999; **96**: 2102–6.

7. Am T, Riaunet A. Integrated psychiatric care planning. *Tidsskrift for Den Norske Laegeforening* 1997; **117**: 1759–62.

8. Briggs M, Dean KL. A qualitative analysis of the nursing documentation of post-operative pain management. *Journal of Clinical Nursing* 1998; **7**: 155–63.

9. Moloney R, Maggs C. A systematic review of the relationships between written manual nursing care planning, record keeping and patient outcomes. *Journal of Advanced Nursing* 1999; **30**: 51–7.

10. Bernick L, Richards P. Nursing documentation: a program to promote and sustain improvement. *Journal of Continuing Education in Nursing* 1995; **25**: 203–8.

11. Parsons S, Barker P. The Phil Hearne course: an evaluation of a multidisciplinary mental health education programme for clinical practitioners. *Journal of Psychiatric Mental Health Nursing* 2000; **7**: 101–8.

12. Jimenez GF, Pareja IM, Jimenez LP, Sanchez CM. How to evaluate nursing procedures for bedsores, or decubitus ulcers by means of a codified and computerized record-keeping system. *Revista de Enfermeria* 2005; **28**: 23–6.

13. Mann K, Muller MJ, Hiemke C, Benkert O. Standardized documentation procedure as a basis for improvement of process quality of treatment in psychiatric hospitals. *Der Nervenarzt* 2003; **75**: 235–44.

14. Dowding D. Examining the effects that manipulating information given in the change of shift report has on nurses' care planning ability. *Journal of Advanced Nursing* 2001; **33**: 836–4.

15. Teale L. Automated record keeping gives time back to busy clinicians. *Australian Nursing Journal* 2006; **14**: 25.

16. Cutcliffe JR. To record or not to record: documentation in clinical supervision. *British Journal of Nursing* 2000; **9**: 350–5.

17. McGeehan R. Best practice in record-keeping. *Nursing Standard* 2007; **21**: 51–5; quiz 58.

18. Dimond B. Exploring common deficiencies that occur in record keeping. *British Journal of Nursing* 2005; **14**: 568–70.

19. Fowler J. Taking theory into practice: using Peplau's model in the care of a patient. *Professional Nurse* 1995; **10**: 226–3.

20. Dimond B. Exploring the principles of good record keeping in nursing. *British Journal of Nursing* 2005; **14**: 460–2.

21. Nursing and Midwifery Council. *Code of professional conduct*. London, UK: NMC, 2002.

22. Squelch J. Good record-keeping. *Nursing Standard* 2007; **21**: 59.

23. Dents K. Record keeping: just for the fun of it? *Paediatric Nurse* 2005: **17**: 18–20.

24. Sainsbury Centre for Mental Health. *National Visit 2. A visit by the Mental Health Act Commission to 104 mental health and learning disability units in England and Wales: improving care for detained patients from black and minority ethnic communities.* London, UK: Sainsbury Centre for Mental Health, 2000.

25. Ammenwerth E, Eichstadter R, Haux R *et al.* A randomized evaluation of a computer-based nursing documentation system. *Journal of the American Medical Informatics Association.* 2001; **40**: 61–8.

26. Rosenbloom S, Grande J, Geissbuhler J, Miller R. Experience in implementing Inpatient Clinical Note Capture via a Provider Order Entry System. *Journal of the American Medical Informatics Association* 2004; **11**: 310–15.

27. Keenan G, Yakel E. Promoting safe nursing care by bringing visibility to the disciplinary aspects of interdisciplinary care. In: *Proceedings of the 2005 American Medical Informatics Association Annual Symposium.* Washington, DC: AMIA, 2005: 385–9.

28. Ettner S, Kotlerman J. An alternative approach to reducing the costs of patient care? A controlled trial of the multidisciplinary doctor–nurse practitioner (MDNP) model. *Medical Decision Making* 2006; **26**: 9–17.

29. Rigby MJ, Roberts R, Williams JG. Objectives and prerequisites to success for integrated patient records. *Computer Methods and Programs in Biomedicine* 1995; **48**: 121–5.

30. Ward MF. Clinical governance and nurse leadership. In: James A, Worrall A, Kendall T (eds). *Clinical governance in mental health and learning disability services: a practical guide.* London, UK: Gaskill, 2005: Chapter 20.

31. Liberto T, Roncher M, Shellenbarger T. Anecdotal notes. Effective clinical evaluation and record keeping. *Nurse Education* 1991; **24**: 15–18.

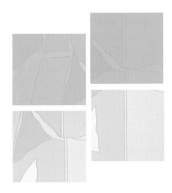

CHAPTER 64

Discharge planning

Martin F. Ward*

INTRODUCTION

Imagine that you board a plane, sit in your seat for hours, being offered an endless supply of refreshments and indigestible meals, yet have no idea where you are going nor how long it would take. Then, when you land, you are not told where you are but are herded from the aircraft and left in the terminal building.

Imagine that you had been admitted to a psychiatric unit and that the same level of information had been offered to you. The analogy may seem like a strange one, but whereas few of us have ever been admitted to a psychiatric unit, most of us have flown. Even on short flights we crave information about where we are, how long before we land and what the weather is like at the destination. We have some sort of travel arrangements and our destination is usually something we can visualize and, as a consequence, feel comfortable with. It has a purpose and we feel safe. Conversely, the patient in the psychiatric unit, given none of the relevant information, finds it difficult to make sense of the journey (the admission) and probably feels very insecure about the destination (the discharge)!

If we would not accept the consequences of a meaningless and blind journey, why do we so often accept for our patients the clinical limitations imposed by unplanned discharge[1] and/or poor communication about the transition between care and discharge?[2] The point of a journey is to arrive. Equally, the purpose of a hospital or community admission is to be discharged in a state of health that enables the person to sustain himself/herself as independently as possible. One is part of the other. Both constitute the reason and both are part of the outcome. To divorce one from the other risks leaving nurses incapable of delivering appropriate interventions during the admission period that will lead, eventually, to discharge.

However, the emphasis in contemporary psychiatric practice throughout most of the world is placed upon risk, and its assessment has created something of a paradox for nursing. On the one hand, nurses accept that, theoretically, the purpose of admission is successful discharge. Yet, on the other, they are confronted with the constraining influences of insufficient inpatient facilities that are prone to generating unplanned discharge for certain patients, supervised discharges that require significant and, often incomplete, community resources, the requirement of a seemingly endless supply of suitably trained key workers and, for many patients, the absence of any meaningful lifestyle once discharged.[3] Is it any wonder, therefore, that many nurses find it difficult to rationalize harsh reality with high professional expectations?[4] To fully understand the complexity of the discharge process as the rubric for clinical efficacy it is necessary to explore both the nature of different care continuums and the roles and values of those involved.

*Martin Ward has been a psychiatric nurse, tutor and researcher for over 30 years. He was the Director of the Royal College of Nursing's Mental Health Nursing Programme at Oxford and presently is an Independent Consultant in Mental Health.

DISCHARGE GOALS

There are five basic forms of discharge from an inpatient mental health unit.

1 *Short stay or acute*. Anything from a few days to a few weeks, possibly repeated several times within a care sequence but always with the purpose of reducing dependence upon care staff before it takes place.
2 *Rehabilitation or long stay*. Often referred to as continuing care, but this does not fully do it justice for the discharge itself is based around reversing a long-term trend of dependence upon staff and producing independence of them. The goal here is not so much the maintenance of a level of self-sufficiency but more the reacquisition of lost skills and the confidence to use them.
3 *The so-called 'revolving door'*, often a combination of the above two. Goals will vary according to patients' needs but will nearly always involve programmes to enable patients to achieve a level of concordance with community treatment and the implementation of skills for self-determination.
4 *Against medical advice*. Always clinically unplanned and often caused because of patient dissatisfaction with treatment or conditions of care, whether warranted or not. The patient's goal is usually based upon frustration with progress, a sense of infringement upon personal space or conflict with treatment targets. For those requiring care, there is usually a very poor outcome from such a discharge.
5 *Completion of treatment*. Although the concept of cure has little or no meaning within mental health care, patients do achieve levels of self-determination, decision-making and absence of symptoms that demand absolute discharge. They are recognition of personal success and their goal is simply to allow people to lead their own lives.

With the exception of the last form, the goals of these discharges are predicated upon the assumption that professional support will be needed over time after inpatient care. In other words, the inpatient process is only part of the overall package of care. However, there is another form of discharge, with a different goal, that usually occurs only from a community source.

Some authors describe generic goals for discharging patients who fall into the categories listed above. Gibson[5] identifies the goals of a rehabilitation service as being linked specifically to those of patients, and particularly those suffering the effects of severe and enduring mental health problems such as schizophrenia. Producing measurable gain in functioning, promoting independence and self-direction and implementing care designed to help patients live a meaningful life in the least restrictive environment are the central goals upon which discharge is based. Gibson, along with most other authors and researchers, also suggests that treatment concordance within the community reduces recidivism and therefore includes work that promotes this as part of the discharge goal.

These goals would seem to be consistent with the outcomes of planned discharge,[6] as can be seen when considered against outcome research carried out to explore the lives of patients currently living in the community. A longitudinal comparative study carried out in Berlin[7] demonstrated that the main gain for patients who had worked through a planned discharge programme designed to meet their individual needs was in the area of social functioning. Significantly, the presence of psychiatric symptoms was the same for both the inpatient control group and those in the community. Similar findings were established in studies carried out in both Japan[8] and Denmark.[9] The main goals for discharge for these long-term patients had been to mobilize community resources in the areas of accommodation, employment and social interaction, described in other German research as 'vocational rehabilitation'.[10] The results of the study by Hoffmann *et al.*[7] were also supported by work carried out to explore the impact of mental health case managers on social functioning[11] as well as that undertaken enabling patients to evaluate the effectiveness of their own care in the community.[12]

What is important about these studies is that they show how linking inpatient therapeutic processes to rehabilitation activities designed to meet discharge goals, then resourcing the ongoing support of these goals once patients are discharged, has a better chance of bringing about a successful conclusion to the care package. They also demonstrate that planned discharge does not occur by accident but by design, and the Canadian study[1] pointed out that unplanned discharges more often result in readmission. In Australia, Owen *et al.*[13] showed that the readmission rate to an inpatient acute unit within 6 months of discharge was as high as 38 per cent even when the community resource was well financed and integrated between health and social care agencies. The major determining factor for readmission was not so much the quantity of the community resource, but the quality of the planning prior to discharge in mobilizing resources that would most successfully meet the needs of the individual patient. A failure on the part of inpatient care staff to use discharge goals as determinants for treatment packages will inevitably result in disjointed movement between the two parts of the service.

Reflection

What are the key things to consider when a patient is being discharged?

ADMISSION TO DISCHARGE: THE CARE CONTINUUM

Readmission rates for psychiatry are important indicators because they provide us with some clues as to the effectiveness of the original discharge. However, reliance upon them alone may actually weaken the case for improving the planning that goes into a discharge. For those requiring intensive support and hospitalization, being discharged does not mean that they are well, it simply means that a new stage in the care process has been reached. Patients are discharged from care for a variety of reasons to meet discharge criteria. This can range from anything such as being recovered to simply being 'more well' than another person needing an admission. Although this last may seem reprehensible given the limited supply of beds in most psychiatric establishments worldwide, and the even more limiting lack of available mental health nurses, there is often little else that hard-pressed practitioners can do in such circumstances. This does not mean that individuals have to be discharged in such a way as to contravene their care packages because even this criterion for discharge can be handled both sympathetically and in support of the patient. However, people have to return to hospital in all walks of medicine and for all sorts of reasons. For the same reasons that people move from inpatient care to community care, they may well need to move back again. The problem is not so much the readmission but the inference that the care, or indeed the patient, has in some way failed within the community. Statistics detailing readmission rates tell us only that X per cent of patients had to return to hospital, they do not provide information about why, nor do they tell us anything about the discharge planning during the preceding admission. Predicting readmission seems a rather futile exercise unless the work is designed to establish what needs to be done to improve the rates, or, better still, explain them.

Consider the example in Personal illustration 64.1.

Personal illustration 64.1

A young male patient, diagnosed as suffering the effects of schizophrenia, is admitted to his local acute inpatient unit for the third time in 12 months. Staff on the ward refer back to his case records for information about previous admissions and discharge activities. Having read the research that shows historical knowledge about prior readmissions is a main indicator for predicting future readmission, they conclude that the patient will more than likely return to hospital following this admission. They construct a care package in line with that which he received during previous admissions because while in hospital he responded well to it. After 3 weeks he is deemed well enough to return to the care of the community team and is discharged. Two months later, he is readmitted and the staff show no surprise at his reappearance.

Question: Who failed in this situation?
Answer: It's not that simple!

Why? Well for a start the patient may well have received the correct care while in hospital and the discharge package may well have been appropriate for his needs. Second, as a young man he may have encountered new threats to his personal integrity that could not have been predicted within any care package, and, third, spending small amounts of time being hospitalized may have been the right way to help him through this phase of his illness. On the other side of the coin, no one checked to see what the contextual problems associated with the requirement for readmission were; second, no subsequent alterations were made to either the treatment or discharge patterns in the absence of key community data; and, finally, the staff simply assumed he would return and his readmission affirmed their clinical judgement. No one failed, but no one succeeded either. Unfortunately, staff decision-making (and to a certain degree, prejudice) was reinforced, and consequently beliefs about the patient's ability to sustain himself within the community diminished. If the balance of failure shifts further towards the patient from the care staff, so their desire to individualize his care will begin to fade.

Consider again the work of Owen *et al.*[13] in 1997. They concluded that readmission was necessitated as a result of a poor fit between patients' needs and aftercare facilities. However, their project was undertaken against the backdrop of a large hospital closure programme with established health and social aftercare facilities. What is not explicit within this work is how the patients were prepared prior to discharge nor how the aftercare quality was evaluated in relation to the requirements of individual patients. Discharge begins with admission and ends if, and when, the patient has to be readmitted when the cycle begins once again. What the predictive qualities of psychiatric readmission tell us are several things:

1 many patients may need readmission, and for a variety of reasons;
2 the preparation for discharge has to fit the patient's individual requirements;
3 community resources have to fit the goals of discharge;
4 much can be learnt from exploring the effectiveness of previous inpatient episodes and associated discharges but this should not be seen as always predicting similar outcomes in the future;
5 care and discharge for each subsequent admission has to be tailored to fit individual requirements at that time, not those of previous admissions;
6 patients who are poorly prepared for discharge are more likely to require readmission and staff must evaluate their previous performance accordingly.

Admission, for a community team, will mean something different from that for an inpatient team, yet the same principles apply to both groups. The real difference is that the point of care contact is altered, thus admission means being supported by a community nurse, discharge, albeit temporary, means transferring to the inpatient facility. In both cases, links between the care teams and the patient should remain intact especially if readmission is anticipated, perhaps even planned for in the case of the community team.

Viewed from this perspective it is easier to understand the concept of discharge being the starting point for admission. When a patient begins the supportive period attributed to community care, the community nurse should already have been party to developing the inpatient discharge programme. The community nurse may be identified as a key worker or case manager and his or her responsibilities for that patient will have begun during the inpatient stay. The unplanned or hurried inpatient discharge produces severe problems for community staff, but so too does the planned discharge that did not have involvement from the staff having to implement it. Similarly, patients who are readmitted to inpatient facilities should return with careful records of progress from the community team, enabling a thorough analysis of the circumstances that brought about the event.

However, this does not fully explain the situation experienced by staff receiving a new admission, which is, to all intents and purposes, an unknown entity. In this case, the whole purpose of admission will be to resolve immediate problems and return the individual back to his or her own life, with as little negative impact on that life as possible. The nurse has to develop a picture of what that life looks like, and discharge has to be considered in the light of that information. Thus, care delivered to that patient has to be delivered with one eye on what, for them, is considered to be normal. As we will see later, probably the main source of this information is the patient himself/herself, but, for now, suffice to say that the goal of discharge has to fit what patients think they need to be able to return to their own home. Although objectives of care set within the nursing process may well be small and immediate, there has to be a wider view of the reasons for those objectives. Remembering that much of the rehabilitation process is geared towards sociological as well as psychological functioning, the provision of clinical therapies or therapeutic activities has to be made in order to operationalize those areas. Certainly, symptoms have to be addressed, especially those that produce fear, risk and misery, insecurity and the will to live, but they need not necessarily be the sole determinants for discharge. Indeed, many ex-users of mental health services lead relatively successful lives, yet still experience psychiatric symptoms that would confound the majority of society.[14] It is the patients' ability to deal with these symptoms that is important, and very often this requires very sophisticated personal strategies on their part. Ironically, Often the successful support required by these individuals is far

less sophisticated, being simply an understanding person who appreciates what the individual is doing and is there for them on a regular basis or when needed. One Danish study shows that although discharged patients' general level of life satisfaction tends to be lower than that of the general population, one factor that increases this level is the close relationship that develops between themselves and a healthcare professional who genuinely appears to care about them.[15] This is confirmed by a similar study in The Netherlands.[16]

Reflection

How can the relationship between the patient being prepared for discharge and the responsible care worker influence the quality, effectiveness and sustainability of the discharge package?

PATIENTS' INVOLVEMENT

As already mentioned, the key source of information about expectation of care is the patients themselves. Yet, it would minimize the involvement of patients if we only view their role within care as providing information alone. The construction, delivery and evaluation of that care all fall within their remit. In the context of this chapter, their commitment to the construction of a dedicated plan of their own discharge would seem to be an ideal way of achieving this. There are, of course, always going to be potential problems that may hold up or delay a patient's discharge, such as a lack of community resources, but involvement of patients in planning their own discharge may in fact enable some of these problems to be overcome.[17] Such collaboration may allow for higher levels of risk and subsequently creative and/or novel approaches to care delivery and support for patients.[18] There are other issues to consider.

For many years, data concerning patients who absconded from inpatient care were regarded as proof simply that some patients would leave against medical advice. However, Bowers et al.[19] undertook a series of 52 interviews in the East End of London with patients who returned following absconding. The reasons given for leaving were both rational and in the main contextual to the care process. Within the clinical area, they described being bored, frightened by other patients and feeling trapped and confined, while extraneous factors included feeling cut off from relatives and friends, having household responsibilities or being worried about the security of their home or property. Psychiatric symptoms, though mentioned, were not usually the primary cause for leaving. Of course, some patients left impulsively often following bad news about anticipated leave or discharge. Collectively, these described causes provide us with a clue to the admission activities of these patients. It is unlikely that they were actively involved in the development and delivery of their own care because, had they been, so much of this absconding may have been averted. An example of this is given in Personal illustration 64.2.

Personal illustration 64.2

Tony is becoming agitated because he needs to get home to sort out bills that he tells his primary nurse are accumulating on his doorstep. Having been an inpatient on the unit for nearly 2 weeks he has had no opportunity to check this fact, but logic tells him that life is going on outside and he has responsibilities that have to be met. The primary nurse tells him that she will get Tony's social worker to go to his house and sort things out. Tony is happy with this. Two days later, having had no feedback and becoming increasingly concerned, he asks again for news of the social worker's visit, only to be told that the nurse has not been able to contact him yet but will try again later. Twenty minutes later, Tony goes missing.

Question: Who failed in this situation?
Answer: The system.

The 'system' here is the organizational structure that excluded Tony from his own care activities and the bureaucratic processes that gave personal responsibility to others that should have been his. Had the nurse and Tony been working together the nurse would have appreciated the importance of the home situation for Tony's ability to concentrate on his mental health problems, and indeed may even have concluded that they were one and the same thing. One of the key recommendations of the work carried out by Bowers et al.[19] was that serious consideration be given to the patient's meaning of an admission. If it could be argued that effective return to the community was the main objective, it is clear that the work of the care team is to deliver care that is designed to promote this. If Tony has no say in this aspect of the care package, when exactly does he have involvement? If he is in a position to be accompanied to his home, either by his primary nurse or by a community nurse working in an inreach capacity, the immediacy of such action would reduce the anxiety he feels and working with the nurse would enable him to resolve the problems created by the bills.

However, the 'system' has to be designed so that it places the patient at the heart of the care team, and not the care staff. To paraphrase Bowers et al.,[19] serious consideration has to be given to the patient's meaning of being *discharged* from hospital, and the only person who can tell you that is the patient. If the discharge begins with admission then surely the patient has to be actively participating in clinical decision-making from the very

beginning, not at the point of discharge when all the decisions about him have already been made.

Similarly, when the patient has returned to the community as part of a planned package of care and is now working with community staff, the issue of involvement remains paramount. For a discharge package to work, it has to be agreed by all parties. Compromise may be required but this is all part of individualizing care. However, concordance (or at the very least collaboration) as opposed to mere compliance has to be the aim of any potentially successful discharge plan and the nurse has to consider many factors that may inhibit the patient's ability to achieve this. High levels of risk, including the possibility of suicide, unrealistic views about their life outside the hospital and non-viable demands placed upon the care providers may all play a part. Additionally, the lack of involvement by patients in their care package during their inpatient stay, or support within the community, could easily affect the so-called collaborative approach adopted at the terminal stage of the admission. We know that recidivism has been shown to be reduced when patients are able to see the necessity of continuing with treatment regimes following discharge, but unless they are involved in the process of developing this understanding for themselves their discharge may seem like nothing more than being told what to do. Patients have to see the importance of the treatment long before they return home, so the process of discharge begins with the admission or at the start of their rehabilitation programme.

Reflection

Given what has been said above, if patients do not want to engage in their own discharge does this mean that they are not really ready for discharge?

MULTIDISCIPLINARY WORKING

Joint patient–care staff planning using carefully described rehabilitative goals can only truly be said to function properly when the care staff themselves are working as an integrated team. It is not the purpose of this chapter to address the issues of multidisciplinary or multiagency working in its widest sense but careful examination of the literature reveals that one aspect of the discharge process can be heavily influenced by effective team working – that of risk consideration. Undoubtedly, the decision for patients to leave the protective confines of an inpatient facility to re-establish themselves in the community can be a period of high risk within their overall care package. Research exploring the nature of delayed discharges,[20] previous vulnerability, including attempted suicide,[21] those who had been compulsorily admitted,[22] violence after discharge,[23] the complex problems associated with dual diagnosis,[24] drug and alcohol problems[25] and levels of social disability[26] are testament to this. Risk screening on admission not only speeds up discharge but targets potential difficulties long before discharge decisions are reached, thus reducing the necessity for possible readmission. However, such screening requires input not just from the inpatient team but also from multiagency staff working in the community. The 'system' in this situation needs to have cooperation and coordination consistent with one organization, not the polemicism associated with traditional arguments about inpatient versus community. It also requires staff to work together with patients irrespective of professional boundaries.

When all of these factors are put together an example of a planned discharge might look like that described in Personal illustration 64.3.

Question: Who failed in this situation?
Answer: No one! And certainly not Christine.

SUMMARY

Effective discharge has to be considered the optimum for all admissions, whether they be inpatient or community. The process of discharge has to be targeted to a goal or series of goals with individual patients determining the specific nature of these goals. The patient's involvement with the rest of the multidisciplinary team is a major determinant for the success of both the admission and its discharge, and readmission need not necessarily be seen as a failure of care if the work that went into the original discharge was appropriate and patient centred. How these criteria are operationalized within any given service will ultimately depend upon the skill of the practitioners and the motivation of the patients. However, some things are clear.

Nurses have a key role to play in the provision of appropriate discharge and aftercare. Their unique position as the main point of professional contact for patients places the burden of care firmly on their shoulders and, in the twenty-first century, one of their key roles will be the coordination of aftercare. They have the skills, and with the right resources should also have the opportunity, to affect the implementation of evidence to support their work. Similarly, medical staff need to realize that the presence or absence of clinical symptoms is only one factor within a patient's discharge profile, and not necessarily a primary one. Patients themselves place far more emphasis on the quality of their life and its social orientation than do healthcare professionals.

All sorts of factors will come into play in determining whether a patient is equipped for discharge, many of them beyond the control of care staff and not least of them whether the patient should have been in hospital

---

Personal illustration 64.3

Christine was readmitted to an acute inpatient unit accompanied by both her daughter and Mike, the community psychiatric nurse, having had a relapse in her ability to cope with daily living activities at home. There was a substantial increase in expressed clinical symptoms that had, in part, been brought about by a deterioration in the relationship between Christine and her husband. Mike had been working with Christine over a 4-month period and had been in regular contact with both social care staff helping with accommodation and finance issues and Christine's psychiatrist at the outpatient clinic. Mike was able to feed back to the inpatient primary nurse relevant information concerning Christine's changing need pattern, and a review of the multidisciplinary records provided a picture of the progress of care to date. Christine had previously been discharged with a minimum supervision package under the terms of the care programme approach, meaning that Mike had acted as her key worker both prior to discharge as well as afterwards. Mike's original inreach work had enabled him to work with Christine on developing discharge goals, but the relationship between the patient and her spouse had not been targeted at that time.

Within the first few days, a discharge plan was developed based on Christine's own perception of what she felt she needed to achieve and she was screened for risk factors that might impede her once back in the community. These included self-harm after arguments with her husband and wandering off on her own when she could not contact her daughter. Christine set cognitive targets for herself that included personal strategies and seeking help. When met, these would indicate that she had both overcome the risk factors and reached a point at which she felt she was ready for discharge. Over a hospitalization period of 5 weeks the immediate problem of expressed symptoms was dealt with, enabling Christine to concentrate on her relationship difficulties. She worked with her primary nurse and the psychologist to construct and practise strategies for dealing with her identified relationship problems, and both her daughter and her husband were invited to take part in this work when appropriate. In the meantime, Mike met with the social worker and these family members and discussed ways of working together with professional support once Christine was discharged.

Finally, a discharge letter was faxed through to Christine's GP as the primary care team would later play a crucial role in monitoring the impact of her care package. Following a series of team meetings, which Christine attended, the decision was made for her to have a trial period at home on leave to see how her new strategies and the overall support package functioned. Additionally, the social worker had secured more suitable rented accommodation for the family. At the end of a controlled discharge period Christine was discharged, with Mike providing regular weekly feedback both to the community mental health team and to the inpatient primary nurse. Christine was readmitted 18 months later following the complete breakdown of her marriage.

in the first place. Finally, just because community after-care is provided it does not necessarily mean that it is appropriate, or that patients should take advantage of it. Irrespective of the organization, the resources and the 'system' in place, if nurses and care staff generally do not have a mindset that sees discharge planning as integral to the total package of care they provide patients will continue to suffer the effects of poor professional insight.

REFERENCES

1. Gillis K, Russell VR, Busby K. Factors associated with unplanned discharge from psychiatric day treatment programs. A multicenter study. *General Hospital Psychiatry* 1997; **19**: 355–61.

2. Rotondi AJ, Sinkule J, Balzer K *et al.* A qualitative needs assessment of persons who have experienced traumatic brain injury and their primary family caregivers. *Journal of Head Trauma Rehabilitation* 2007; **22**: 14–25.

3. Moore C. Discharge from an acute psychiatric ward. *Nursing Times* 1998; **94**: 56–9.

4. Ward MF, Cutcliffe J, Gournay K. *The nursing, midwifery and health visiting contribution to the continuing care of people with mental health problems: a review and UKCC action plan.* London: UK Central Council for Nursing, Midwifery and Health Visiting, 2000.

5. Gibson DM. Reduced rehospitalizations and reintegration of persons with mental illness into community living: a holistic approach. *Journal of Psycho-social Nursing and Mental Health Services* 1999; **37**: 20–5.

6. Marsen-Luther Y. Reforming the appeals process. *Mental Health Today* 2007; **Feb**: 18–22.

7. Hoffmann K, Kaiser W, Isermann M, Priebe S. How does the quality of life of long-term hospitalized psychiatric patients change after their discharge into the community? *Gesundheitswesen* 1998; **60**: 232–8.

8. Naoki K, Nobuo A, Emi I. Randomized controlled trial on effectiveness of the community re-entry program to inpatients with schizophrenia spectrum disorder, centering around acquisition of illness self-management knowledge. *Seishin Shinkeigaku Zasshi* 2003; **105**: 1514–31.

9. Nielsen LF, Werdelin G, Petersen L, Lindhardt A. The staff's knowledge of patients' social function and needs: in connection with discharge planning. *Ugeskrift for Laeger* 2000; **162**: 786–90.

10. Kallert TW, Leisse M. Rehabilitation concepts of schizophrenic patients treated in community psychiatry. *Rehabilitation (Stuttgart)* 2000; **39**: 268–75.

11. Ward MF, Armstrong C, Lelliott P, Davies M. Training, skills and caseloads of community mental health support workers involved in case management: evaluation from the initial UK

demonstration sites. *Journal of Psychiatric and Mental Health Nursing* 1999; **6**: 187–97.

12. Lelliott P, Beevor A, Hogman G *et al.* 'Carers' and users' expectation of services: user version CUES-U, a new instrument to measure the experience of users of mental health services. *BMJ* 2001; **179**: 67–72.

13. Owen C, Rutherford V, Jones M *et al.* Psychiatric rehospitalization following hospital discharge. *Community Mental Health Journal* 1997; **33**: 13–24.

14. Campbell P. Caring for the suicidal patient – the modus operandi: engagement or observation? In: Cutcliffe JR, Ward MF (eds). *Key debates in psychiatric/mental health nursing.* Edinburgh, UK: Churchill Livingstone, 2006: Commentary in Debate 7.

15. Folker H, Jensen BM. Study of selected methods of self-assessment of health, quality of life and satisfaction with treatment. Use among patients four weeks after discharge from a psychiatric ward. *Ugeskrift for Laeger* 2001; **163**: 3347–52.

16. Monden MA, Duindam JM. Conditional discharge of three committed psychiatric patients, the ambulatory practice. *Nederlands Tijdschrift voor Geneeskunde* 2000; **144**: 1548–51.

17. Langan J, Lindow V. *Living with risk: mental health service user involvement in risk assessment and management.* London, UK: The Policy Press, 2004.

18. Barker P, Buchannan-Barker P. Bridging: talking meaningfully about the care of people at risk. *Mental Health Practice* 2004; **8**: 12–15.

19. Bowers L, Jarrett M, Clark N *et al.* Absconding: why patients leave. *Journal of Psychiatric and Mental Health Nursing* 1999; **6**: 199–205.

20. Paton JM, Fahy MA, Livingston GA. Delayed discharge: a solvable problem? The place of intermediate care in mental health care of older people. *Ageing and Mental Health* 2004; **8**: 39–9.

21. Qurashi I, Kapur N, Appleby L. A prospective study of non-compliance with medication, suicidal ideation, and suicidal behavior in recently discharged psychiatric inpatients. *Archives of Suicide Research* 2006; **10**: 61–7.

22. Kan CK, Ho TP, Dong JY, Dunn EL. Risk factors for suicide in the immediate post-discharge period. *Social Psychiatry and Psychiatric Epidemiology* 2007; **42**: 208–14.

23. Duncan JM, Short A, Lewis JS, Barrett PT. Re-admissions to the State Hospital at Carstairs, 1992–1997. *Health Bulletin (Edinburgh)* 2002; **60**: 70–82.

24. Farren CK, Mc Elroy S. Treatment response of bipolar and unipolar alcoholics to an inpatient dual diagnosis program. *Journal of Affective Disorders* 2008; **106**: 365–72.

25. Timko C, Sempel JM. Intensity of acute services, self-help attendance and one-year outcomes among dual diagnosis patients. *Journal of Studies on Alcohol* 2004; **65**: 274–82.

26. Rymaszewska J, Jarosz-Nowak J, Kiejna A *et al.* Social disability in different mental disorders. *European Psychiatry* 2007; **22**: 160–6.

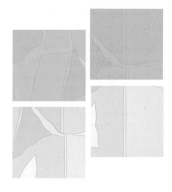

CHAPTER 65

The nurse's role in the administration of electroconvulsive therapy

Joy Bray*

INTRODUCTION

Electroconvulsive therapy (ECT) remains one of the most controversial treatments in psychiatry. However, in the last 5 years several influential publications have emphasized the importance of taking into account service users' viewpoints, thus ensuring their understanding of the process, including a detailed appreciation of unwanted effects such as memory loss.[1–3] To fully appreciate their role, nurses need to be aware of the contemporary evidence base supporting ECT, relating this to the service users' wishes.

> I know ECT works well for me when I am seriously depressed and unable to do anything for myself. I have a right to choose to have it. It is the only way I have of regaining myself and my life quickly when I am seriously depressed. If I don't have it I am unable to do anything for around 6 months – with ECT it is over in a few weeks. Without ECT I would have lost my job and most of the things I value in life.
>
> **Woman – ECT in last 2 years**

> The ECT affected my memory long term, has slowed down my thinking process and has damaged my ability to associate words and ideas. Because of this my speech is sometimes not as fluent as it was before I had ECT. I cannot recognize some of the faces of people I have known for some time. My confidence and self-esteem are very low and the ECT treatment has contributed to this.
>
> **Woman – ECT in last 2 years**

These directly opposing statements are taken from a Mind survey of experiences of having ECT.[4] Some find it a life-saving procedure and are grateful to be offered it; others find it degrading and distressing, leaving them with permanent side-effects – usually memory loss. Mental health professionals should be able to discuss the benefits and difficulties of any treatment with those involved and

*Joy Bray is a Mental Health Specialist Nurse working for Cambridge University Hospitals NHS Foundation Trust. She has had training in psychotherapy, groupwork and cognitive–behavioural therapy. She was employed as a senior lecturer for many years and has recently returned to practice working across the general hospital giving mental health nursing care to inpatients.

their relatives or carers. However, ECT can be prescribed as an emergency in most countries, and administered *without* patient consent framed by the Mental Health Act 1983. This can make the administration ethically and emotionally difficult.

This chapter focuses on the service user's experience and associated distress. The evidence base underpinning the administration of ECT will also be considered, alongside contraindications and alternative treatments. The key issues around consent, and the procedure itself, will be discussed using electronically available UK guidelines.

ECT AS TREATMENT

The Department of Health[5] has defined ECT as:

> … a treatment involving the passage of an electric current across the brain. The treatment is only administered to an anaesthetized patient who has also been administered a muscle relaxant. The electric current induces seizure activity in the brain which is necessary for the therapeutic effect of treatment.

In the UK, an independent agency, the National Institute for Health and Clinical Excellence (NICE), assesses treatments available in the National Health Service (NHS). Published guidelines for the administration of ECT state:[2]

> ECT is used only to achieve rapid and short-term improvement of severe symptoms after an adequate trial of other treatment options has proved ineffective and/or where the condition is considered to be potentially life-threatening, in individuals with
>
> - Severe depressive illness
> - Catatonia
> - A prolonged or severe manic episode.

NICE took specific note of evidence from service users concerning the adverse, unwanted effects of ECT, in which cognitive impairments discounted the benefits of ECT. This led to their decision to restrict the use of ECT to situations where all alternatives had been exhausted, or where the illness was considered life-threatening. As the longer term benefits and risks of ECT are not clearly established, it is not recommended as maintenance therapy in depressive illness.

A systematic review of ECT for schizophrenia, considering quantitative research only, has been carried out.[6] Although ECT should remain a potential treatment option for people with psychosis, drugs remain the preferential treatment for schizophrenia, and there is no suggestion that ECT should be used alone *or* that it should be the treatment of first choice in schizophrenia.[a]

The decision to administer ECT should be based on documented assessment of the risks and potential benefits to the individual, including the risks associated with the anaesthetic, co-existing conditions, anticipated adverse effects (particularly cognitive impairment) and the risks of not having treatment.[1]

Although one of the commonest reasons given for administering ECT is that it prevents suicide, this assumption can be challenged. On reviewing the literature, Challiner and Griffiths[7] were unable to definitively endorse this assumption and presented evidence to the contrary, i.e. that ECT does not necessarily prevent suicide in those with severe depression.

The Department of Health survey (January to March 1999)[5] illustrates the use of ECT. Of 2800 patients who received ECT, 900 were men and 1900 women; 44 per cent of the men and 36 per cent of the women were 65 years or over. Notably, there is a preponderance of use of ECT in women and people over 65 years of age.

Fink[8] suggested that ECT is favourably accepted by professional bodies in countries outside the UK. In addition to reviews in the USA, professional organizations in Denmark, The Netherlands, Germany, Austria, India, Canada and Australia found on balance that ECT was effective and safe and have produced professional guidelines for its use. Fink[8] noted in 2006 the increased interest in ECT from Belgium, Hungary, India, Japan, Australia, Russia, Pakistan and Greece shown by publications in the *Journal of ECT*.

Some patients will always choose ECT as a first-line treatment, citing that it has decreased a fear of having depression again and that it worked.[9] However, contrasting evidence suggests that up to one-third of individuals experiencing ECT find it deeply and lastingly traumatic. It may exacerbate feelings of shame, failure and badness, which are already features of depression. Many wish to avoid ECT if offered again. An apparently successful outcome may simply indicate compliance and powerlessness, allied to a fear of confiding one's true feelings to staff.[10]

ECT: THE EVIDENCE

Although ECT continues to have controversial status, there is a shift in the professional perspective which now maintains that service users must be fully informed of the potential risks and benefits of ECT before giving consent.[1] While a nurse can expect the prescriber to give the service user this information, it will be important to be aware of contemporary evidence so that the individual

---

[a] A copy of the review Electroconvulsive therapy for schizophrenia can be obtained from *The Cochrane Library* 2007, issue 2. Available from: www.thecochranelibrary.com.

and carers can discuss the implications of consenting to ECT with an informed nurse.

When the Royal College of Psychiatrists was developing *The ECT handbook*[1] systematic reviews from both professional and consumer perspectives were considered[3,11] alongside evidence apart from randomized controlled trials. Consequently, the handbook had a much wider evidence base, including service users' viewpoints. A study found that nurses with a more positive response to ECT had a greater knowledge base, but that nurses' knowledge of ECT in general is inadequate and needs some improvement.[12] This is important since, arguably, all nurses require a sufficient understanding of ECT to be able to discuss fully its nature and purpose and possible adverse effects, and to negotiate consent to treatment.

Three areas of evidence need to be considered:

1 the experience of individuals having ECT
2 the evidence suggesting the efficacy of ECT
3 known adverse effects.

Surveys by Mind in 2001[4] and the United Kingdom Advocacy Network (UKAN)[13] in 1995 presented the individual's experience of receiving ECT. The respondents' comments made difficult reading as many had found ECT emotionally and psychologically damaging: 60.5 per cent of recipients stated that they had not received information about adverse effects; 84 per cent described the experience of adverse effects; and 34 per cent were not told that they could refuse to give consent. In the short term, 36 per cent found the treatment helpful or very helpful and 27 per cent unhelpful or damaging. These were disturbing findings. A systematic review[11] carried out predominantly by service users in 2003 noted that service users' evaluations of the 'success' of the treatment involved more criteria than simply the relief of symptoms. Also of importance was the loss of autobiographical memory, which has been widely described but insufficiently investigated.[11] These important considerations have been included in subsequent guidelines and there is increasing recognition that ECT should be a treatment of choice for an individual. Donahue's[14] description of her experience of ECT shows how difficult it is to weigh up 'benefits' against 'adverse effects'.

> Occasionally, I feel bitter. More often, it is a sadness, a sense of deep loss that may not even have had to happen. It is a grief that keeps deepening over time, because there is hardly a week that goes by that I do not discover yet another part of my life that is lost somewhere in my memory cells.
>
> Despite that, I remain unflagging in my belief that the electroconvulsive therapy I received in the fall of 1995 and then the spring of 1996 – 33 treatments, initially unilateral and then bilateral – may have saved not just my mental health but my life. If I had the same decision to make over again, I would

> choose ECT over a life condemned to psychic agony and possible suicide. Like a heart patient who has to choose the risks of surgery over the risk of heart attack or stroke; like the cancer victim who must choose the horrible side effects of chemotherapy over certain death to the disease – I live with and accept the price I paid to break the stranglehold of a seemingly intractable and severe depression.

Philpot *et al.*[15] reported on research by a service users' group, in which a self-report questionnaire asked about experiences of bilateral ECT. Of 108 questionnaires, 44 were completed (41 per cent response rate). Four themes emerged.

1 If the respondent had previously received ECT, 14 (74 per cent) said they would have it again. Only four of the total of 19 people who had it for the first time would definitely have it again.
2 A feeling of compulsion was evident in which recipients did not feel fully informed before giving consent or were not fully aware of their right to refuse the treatment.
3 Persistent adverse effects were noted: 45 per cent of respondents reported persistent memory loss and 55 per cent reported general persistent adverse effects including memory loss, flashbacks, headaches, tremor and dizziness.
4 'Putting one's trust in doctors'. A significant minority felt that there was no alternative to ECT, as it was the only treatment that had worked in the past, or they felt too ill or confused to make a decision. Consequently, they trusted the psychiatrist to do what was best.

A qualitative analysis of service users' views[16] concluded that views about health interventions – such as ECT – are complex. People who report benefit from ECT are in the minority. However, those who feel the treatment works are not silenced by those who oppose it. Such respect for diversity of opinion in service users' discourse is noteworthy.

The implication for nursing is that we need to be open with service users when discussing ECT and provide adequate information that is accessible to each individual, considering education level, culture and disability, to ensure genuine informed consent.

Reflection

Think about a time when you worked with a service user who had ECT.

What was the experience like for that person?

Did you ask about side-effects and wonder how you could help with these?

How well prepared and confident did you feel?

If it was a poor experience – for either yourself or the service user – what would have empowered you both and altered the experience?

The effectiveness of ECT

ECT remains controversial. The service user research cited above suggests that the effectiveness of ECT is not predictable. Although its mode of action remains unknown, a great deal is known about its effects on the central nervous system, and this knowledge is rapidly developing. Reid[17] suggested that ECT modulates monoamine systems in the brain, such as the serotonergic and norepinephric pathways, in the same way as chemical antidepressants. This enhances the activity of the dopaminergic systems, explaining some of its effectiveness in Parkinson's disease as well as depressive disorders. ECT has anticonvulsant properties that it shares with the anticonvulsant drugs now used to treat bipolar disorder. ECT affects many systems in the brain, and the effects on individual transmitter systems may be more specific and focused than those induced by chemical antidepressants. It is increasingly acknowledged that chronic depression is associated with atrophy of brain structures in the frontal and temporal lobes and ECT may work to arrest or even reverse these degenerative effects.[17]

The therapeutic action of ECT may derive from the induction of a generalized seizure of adequate quality and duration. Short generalized, missed, focal or unilateral seizures have little or no therapeutic effect. If an ECT-induced seizure is to have a therapeutic effect, the stimulus given must induce seizure activity throughout the whole brain, which is a generalized seizure.[1]

Four weeks is the usual duration of the artificial euphoria that commonly follows a closed head injury. This may explain the therapeutic effects of ECT, although this also means recognizing that some brain damage is a consequence of ECT.[18] While it is generally accepted that ECT causes a certain amount of brain damage, the amount and severity is continuously debated. However, the *definitive* therapeutic action of ECT remains unknown.

The UK ECT Review Group[3] suggested that a substantial body of evidence supports the efficacy of ECT in short-term treatment of depression. When compared with drug therapy, ECT is more effective, possibly for the reasons cited above.[3] Other factors influencing effectiveness are bilateral versus unilateral administration, frequency, dose and the number of sessions.

Historically, *bilateral* placement was preferred when speed of recovery was the priority, and *unilateral* when minimizing cognitive adverse effects. Now, no generic statement can be made about the placement of choice. The final selection should follow an estimation of the risks and benefits and be informed by the wishes of the service user. Where treatment is not urgent, unilateral placement is indicated to minimize adverse cognitive effects, and should be given over the cerebral hemisphere that is *not* dominant for writing and using a tool.[1]

In both bilateral and unilateral ECT, the optimal frequency is twice weekly. Rather than prescribe a set number of treatments, the person should be assessed after each to see whether further treatments are necessary. If no clinical improvement is evident after six properly administered bilateral treatments, the course should be abandoned. Where there is slight improvement the course can be extended to 12 before being abandoned.[1] This is significant for nursing staff, who should participate in the assessment of clinical improvement as they spend the most time with the service users, and will be able to judge changes in cognition, demeanour and affect.

Although ECT is thought to be effective in severe depressive psychosis or psychomotor retardation, more recent evidence suggests that it generates early improvement in all subtypes of depression. ECT could be considered as a first-line treatment in all emergencies, but not for general depression. However, clearly informed consent remains a critical consideration alongside the following factors:

- the speed and efficacy of ECT
- a history of treatment-resistant depression
- medication intolerance
- a previous positive response to ECT
- medical status.[1]

Continuation of antidepressant drug treatment is essential after successful ECT. Van Beusekom *et al.*[19] carried out a small, long-term follow-up of patients with depression who had responded to ECT following failure to respond to drug treatment. They concluded that continuation of medication started immediately after the last ECT session is an important factor in preventing recurrence of the depression, even in individuals previously unresponsive to antidepressant drugs.[19] However, there is no place for continuing ECT as an aspect of relapse prevention. In a large study, more than half of the patients either relapsed or left the study, leading to the conclusion that more effective relapse prevention was needed.[20]

OTHER VOICES

So far, discussion has focused on evidence relevant to the person who chooses to have ECT. However, many individuals will not make that choice and should be supported in their decision.

From a sociological perspective, mental illness is a social phenomenon rather than biologically determined, and ECT is seen as a method of effectively *silencing* people, thereby legitimizing the lack of attention paid to our malfunctioning society.[21]

Burstow[22] reframed ECT as a form of violence against women. Drawing on personal testimonies and scientific research, she argued that ECT is more frequently prescribed for women, resulting in cognitive and physical impairment. It functions, and is therefore experienced, as a form of assault and social control that silences women.[22] Certainly, the prescription of ECT obviates the necessity to engage with individuals and to sit with them in their distress, effectively silencing them. However, this applies to men also.

Read[23] noted that the prescription of ECT has steadily declined worldwide, and suggested that psychiatrists who do prescribe it believe that it is a medical procedure treating an illness. Nevertheless, he suggests that the research evidence indicates that ECT is a contemporary example of simplistic theories being used to suggest that punitive and damaging treatments are beneficial to 'mad' people; a futile attempt to bully distressed people back to sanity.[23]

Social learning theory characterizes ECT acts as a *negative reinforcer* resembling early theories of punishment. Although this view is now largely discarded, some people obviously feel *as if* they are being punished or threatened.

Although how ECT works remains unclear, the seizure is fundamental to the process. The apparent efficacy of chemically induced seizures suggests that electricity itself, with its barbaric undertones, is not essential.[24]

ECT: adverse effects

Ann Watkinson,[25] a former nursing student, consented to ECT when depressed, and wondered why she agreed so willingly. She concluded that it was because she felt uninvolved in her treatment and also because everything happened so quickly: only a couple of days between her psychiatrist suggesting it and treatment commencing. She suffered severe adverse effects, and memory loss and regrets the treatment. She lost her 'autobiographical' memory for almost 2 years before her ECT. She cannot remember her two daughters' weddings nor the birth of her grandchild – a personal cost she deeply regrets.[25] Memory loss is difficult to quantify as patients do not know what they do not remember.

The recognition of adverse effects has altered radically since the publication of the UK reviews of ECT. These include the Service User Research Enterprise (SURE), the first ever systematic review of service users' views on ECT.[16] Some of the conclusions from these reviews suggest that at least one-third of service users experience permanent amnesia and newer methods of ECT have not resulted in reduced adverse effects.[3] This new evidence provides opportunities to fully delineate the nature of the permanent adverse effects of ECT and to develop relevant assessment tools in order to provide consent which is fully informed.[26] Memory loss should not be dismissed as merely a transient symptom of depression, which is now an outdated notion.

The following extracts illustrate how memory can be damaged.

> I can remember very little of this year, after having ECT in September. I found once I came home I would meet people while out, knew them but could not place them or remember their names.
>
> **Woman – Wales**

> I found myself unable to play the guitar and sing songs and tunes I had been playing for 25 years.
>
> **Man – Yorkshire**

> Creativity, reading and things that I enjoyed and was patient in doing went down sharply.
>
> **Woman – London**

> I have long- and short-term memory impairment, I have serious cognitive damage. I cannot do any work with figures, numbers mean nothing to me. I have great difficulty reading. I was a taxi driver for 20 years. Now I can only find my way if I have my carer present to give directions. I do not know my left from my right.
>
> **Woman – Yorkshire**[4]

Terminology used for adverse effects of ECT

Memory

- *Autobiographical memory*, one's store of knowledge of past experiences and learning; amnesia, the loss of autobiographical memory, cannot be accessed by effort or reminders.
- *Retrograde amnesia*, amnesia for the time before ECT.
- *Anterograde amnesia*, amnesia for the time after ECT.
- *Working memory*, the ability to store and access information in daily life; memory disability is the loss of working memory.[26]

Nurses need to understand the many kinds of memory loss when assessing a person's functioning between ECT doses. The following deficits need to be noted:

- patients cannot hold on to information
- their memory is not as good as before or for someone of the same age
- they forget where they have put items (e.g. keys)
- they have to make lists all the time
- they cannot remember faces or names
- they forget what they were about to say or do.

Monitoring the adverse effects relating to memory is of critical importance and will be discussed in the nursing care section. However, adverse cognitive effects can be detected 6 months following an acute treatment course.[27] In hospital, service users are not using living skills such as shopping and driving and so may be unaware of deficits until some time after treatment ends.

If patients are already taking various psychotropic medications, this will have an effect on seizure duration and may raise the seizure threshold.[28]

Mortality associated with ECT is similar to that of general anaesthesia in minor surgical procedures (approximately two deaths per 100 000 treatments). Despite the use of ECT for people with physical illnesses (which render them unsuitable for antidepressant treatment) and the prevalence of use with elderly patients, many believe that ECT carries a lower mortality rate than the use of antidepressant drugs. Johnstone[29] argues against this and suggests that mortality is consistently under-reported.

ALTERNATIVE TREATMENTS

The importance of psychological therapies, medication and bereavement counselling is acknowledged by the UK ECT Forum. Indeed, it advocates the use of adjunct therapies, stating that the positive effects of ECT are short-lived (H Baldwin, personal communication, July 2001; Chair of the ECT Nurses' Forum, UK).

NICE guidelines[30] clearly state that psychological therapies followed by medication are the treatments of choice for depression, including treatment-resistant forms. NICE advises that older people should be offered the same range of psychological therapies, including cognitive–behaviour therapy (CBT), as younger people, outlawing ageist discrimination.

Repetitive transcranial magnetic stimulation (rTMS) is a relatively new treatment involving the focal application of magnetic energy to the cerebral cortex, thus inducing small electrical currents. *Subconvulsive rTMS* does not involve loss of consciousness, loss of memory or seizure, and so avoids the difficulties around administering ECT. On comparing treatments, both were associated with a degree of improvement in refractory depression; this treatment may become more available in the future.[31]

There is much current interest in *deep brain stimulation* for individuals with chronic treatment-resistant depression. Here, an implanted pacemaker sends currents to two electrodes that reach deep into the brain, stimulating area 25. Anecdotal reports have been very positive with negligible side-effects, but further work is being carried out and this remains an area of development.[32,33]

Finally, there is considerable evidence showing that exposure to family and social disadvantage (particularly multiple) during childhood can predispose individuals to major depression in adulthood.[34,35] This is not to suggest that ECT is always inappropriate. However, there is a need to consider preventative methods which might help this vulnerable population to live a more healthy life.

INFORMED CONSENT: THE ETHICAL DIMENSION

The legal framework of the relevant state or country frames the concept of informed consent. Professional guidelines exist for use in conjunction with the relevant mental health legislation, to enable best practice from clinicians.[36,37]

To practise ethically, informed consent is of paramount importance. The first stage involves an assessment of the person's capacity to give (or refuse) consent. In the UK, the current legal test of capacity requires a person to:

- understand and retain the information relevant to the decision in question
- believe that information
- weigh that information in the balance to arrive at a choice.[38]

The Royal College of Psychiatrists and NICE advise that the potential for cognitive impairment is highlighted during the consent process – the service user should be told that ECT may have serious and permanent effects on both memory and non-memory cognition. Robertson and Pryor[26] rightly suggest that service users are encouraged to speak with or read accounts written by people who have experienced amnesia (some are found in the reports of SURE,[16] NICE[2] and Mind[4]). Also, service users should be encouraged to interact with online forums, for example at www.ect.org, where they may be able to ask questions of former recipients.

The capacity to consent and the person's expression of consent are dynamic, with the potential to change throughout the course of ECT. The assessment of capacity is complex. Vaughn McCall[39] differentiates refusal and reluctance, suggesting that reluctance is often seen on the morning of treatment and can be a combination of issues, such as fear of anaesthesia and fear of the procedure. Working with this is an aspect of nursing care in which the aim is to help individuals to make an *informed choice* that is right for them at that particular time. When refusal is stated, the competent person should not proceed to ECT.

As obtaining consent involves assessment of capacity, a senior clinician, usually the person's consultant, should undertake this. As part of the process, alternatives to ECT must be discussed and it should be made clear that refusal will not compromise further care. Also, individuals consent to a course of treatments rather than to each treatment separately, and so they must understand that *they can withdraw from treatment at any time*. The Capacity Act 2005 is clear that except in an emergency (when a person will be sectioned under the Mental Health Act) ECT may not be given to anyone who has the capacity to refuse consent, and may be given to an incapacitated person only when it does not conflict with any advance directive or decision of a deputy or of the Court of Protection.[40]

If individuals refuse ECT but are sufficiently mentally ill not to understand why they are offered the treatment, ECT may be given under the auspices of the appropriate mental health legislation.

In England during the period January to March 1999, 2800 patients received ECT treatment. Of these, 700 patients were formally detained while receiving the treatment, 59 per cent of whom did not consent to treatment.[5] If a patient cannot consent to ECT, the proper course of action is to use the Mental Health Act 1983, Sections 2 and 3. Administration of ECT is covered by Part IV of the Mental Health Act, Sections 58 ('treatments requiring the patient's consent or a second opinion') and 62 ('urgent treatment'). Consent to ECT should always be sought by the *responsible medical officer* (usually the patient's medical consultant) and the patient may withdraw consent at any time. If the patient refuses or withdraws consent, a second medical opinion is sought, appointed by the Mental Health Act Commission, who will interview and assess the patient. In emergencies, compulsory ECT may be given (under Section 62) without the second opinion safeguard if it is necessary either to save the patient's life, because their physical condition is so fragile, or prevent deterioration of such. In this case, the Commission should be informed so that a second opinion may be provided as soon as possible.[41]

However, these safeguards appear, at times, to be disregarded. Some of the survey respondents noted above said that they had consented 'under duress' or had felt 'coerced'. A number said they had been threatened with the use of the Mental Health Act if they did not comply. Consequently, they felt pressured and lost the second opinion safeguard.[4]

The role of advocates and advanced directives are central to the future resolution of this issue.

NURSES' DILEMMAS OVER ECT

ECT remains controversial. In some US states, the treatment is banned and the public's perception of the treatment is negative.[42] An important ethical aspect of ECT is whether the therapeutic benefits outweigh the risks and adverse effects. Given that there is no conclusive evidence to identify ECT as the treatment of choice in major depression, each case needs individual assessment. This means that nurses have a responsibility to care for and support the patient during the whole process of deliberation and treatment. It can be argued that there are suitable alternatives to the prescribing of ECT; these include intensive nursing care, CBT and psychotherapy, which seem to be rarely considered. This may be because of the extra cost involved. However, the patient group most frequently prescribed ECT are older women who do not have a strong political voice.

Current guidelines state that unless it is a life-threatening situation ECT should not be given *without* fully informed consent, including full details of adverse effects. When the patient has had full information *and* freely consents to the treatment there is no dilemma, as we acquiesce to the patient's wishes.

THE NURSING ROLE AND FUNCTIONS

The nurse's role in ECT involves three distinct but related areas:

1 preparation of the patient
2 care during the procedure
3 care following recovery.

Although general principles may be outlined for each area, there is a need to individualize care through carrying out a comprehensive assessment[43] using standardized assessment tools where relevant, e.g. within the Tidal Model, which is a collaborative nursing framework.[44]

Each mental health service should possess relevant practice and procedure guidelines, framed within state/national directives from relevant professional bodies. ECT should take place in a purpose-built clinic within a hospital, with a waiting area, treatment clinic, and *separate* lying recovery and sitting recovery areas.

ECT in the UK takes place in designated areas or, increasingly, in day surgery facilities. There should always be a nurse employed who is a specialist in ECT in charge of the whole process for outpatients and responsible for inpatients while undergoing treatment. The employed time should be adequate to carry out the following responsibilities:

- spending time with service users and their carers in order to provide support and information
- liaising with the prescribing teams and ECT team
- assisting in treatment sessions
- updating protocols and policies
- performing audit and risk assessment
- training of staff and updating own skills and knowledge.[37]

The ECT nurse responsible for care during treatment is supported by the escorting nurse and the nurse in charge of recovery. Although the escorting nurse is not a specialist she or he should *always be a trained nurse* and should know the service user. Each service user should be individually escorted. The nurse should have:

- up-to-date training in life support and be competent in the practice
- a good knowledge of the ECT process, especially the side-effects and the nursing actions required
- familiarity with the clinic and the emergency equipment.

One patient's experience of ECT (Personal illustration 65.1) sets the scene for an overview of the procedure.

Preparation of the patient

Psychological preparation

- Education of, and discussion with, service users and their family/carer. This should be repeated as often as requested. Video and written information should be

Richard is in his thirties with a diagnosis of schizophrenia from 5 years ago. He is a striking, vibrant man with an appealing, arresting voice and an obvious sense of humour.

When first prescribed clozapine, this coincided with the beginning of a severe autoimmune illness. Richard had a depressive element to his schizophrenia. However, he was prescribed ECT partly because the medical opinion was that continued administration of atypical anti-psychotic medication constituted an unwarranted physical danger. ECT was administered on an outpatient basis and he had two treatments out of the 10 prescribed. When asked 'What helped?', Richard said: 'The ECT nurse had been there for years, she was called Electric Annie. She was a real nurse, very caring but appropriately so. She was calming and reassuring, you felt you were the most important thing. This was important because the process itself is very scary. She had a generally friendly and reassuring manner, she said things like "Don't worry you won't know anything about it". But she was honest, and that was the most important thing. She said I'd have a stinking headache after and would feel quite unpleasant. And I did! Afterwards I got the king of all migraines. She made sure I got a cup of tea after (a hot one would have been nice) and later I got two paracetamol, which didn't touch the headache.

The worst thing was being wheeled on a trolley through the hospital. This hadn't been explained to me, and the anaesthetist was late and couldn't find the veins. But I don't remember a great deal. The nurse was very good with my mum as well. She came with me and the nurse calmed her down, as she was very apprehensive. My mum came because Caroline [long-term partner] wouldn't come. She was against me having it [ECT]. It's not good to do it without the consent of the nearest and dearest, it was so damaging for us. Caroline hasn't participated in any of my treatment since, which has been awful for me. It had a real impact.'

The treatment was stopped after two sessions because of the partner's fears and a different atypical anti-psychotic was commenced.

- Memory diaries can be used as a way of helping individuals reorientate themselves following treatment; these contain information which the patient finds meaningful and can contain current or old material. This work can be done collaboratively with service users and their carers. The aim is for individuals to have a fund of material which will help prompt the memory because the adverse effect of memory loss is very serious. When discussing this with patients, they may have an idea of what they would like in their diary, e.g. photos, favourite pieces of writing, lists of favourite music and memories associated with these, a narrative/plan of their daily or weekly routines. If a service user is too incapacitated to do this work the carers may find it helpful to carry this out.

As an aspect of helping with memory the service user might use the WRAP[b] (wellness and recovery action plan) to help recognize and develop their own coping strategies.

Following treatment the person can use the diaries to recall life before, or between, episodes of illness to help orientation. If events or diary descriptions cannot be recalled, this indicates memory deficit and should be reported to the multidisciplinary team, and should become part of the multidisciplinary care plan.

Physical preparation

- Tests need to be done to ensure physical fitness prior to a general anaesthetic: chest radiograph, electrocardiogram (ECG), baseline electroencephalogram (EEG), blood count and erythrocyte sedimentation rate (ESR). For an extensive list, refer to Bowley and Walker.[45] (Cardiovascular complications are the major cause of death associated with ECT. Blood tests assess current health and consider any other relevant pathology.)
- Ensure that patients understand they need to fast for 6 hours before the general anaesthetic (to prevent regurgitation and inhalation of undigested food during anaesthesia). A low-fat meal is advised the evening before.
- Patients prescribed cardiac and antihypertensive drugs may take these with sips of water only.

offered that might be viewed or read afterwards. Time must be spent discussing the possibility of adverse effects with service users, and encouraging them to read accounts of having ECT and access online discussion forums. Fact sheets are available online (e.g. from the Royal College of Psychiatrists or Royal Australian and New Zealand College of Psychiatrists). The patient's anxiety can be overwhelming and will need to be understood within the context of a potentially threatening procedure. Best practice suggests that preparation be carried out by the patient's primary nurse.

- Many clinics offer educational and orientation visits to relatives/carers prior to treatment.

---

[b] A copy of this is available from www.mentalhealthrecovery.com (or by typing WRAP Copeland into an Internet search engine), and is a useful self-help tool which asks individuals to write down triggers for illness but also what keeps them well.

Care during the procedure

- Ensure that the patient has fasted.
- Property should be deposited for safe keeping (e.g. rings, necklaces).
- Loose, comfortable clothes should be worn, which can be readily opened at the front for monitoring equipment to be positioned (e.g. ECG leads).
- Spectacles may be worn, but not contact lenses.
- Hair must be clean and dry for optimal electrode contact, and hair ornaments removed to prevent contact with the electrodes.
- Nail varnish and make-up should be removed to allow monitoring of changes in colour, which may indicate cardiovascular functioning.
- Measure the patient's temperature, pulse, respiration rate and blood pressure to provide a baseline measure.
- Immediately prior to treatment ask the patient to visit the toilet to empty their bladder.

The escorting nurse should always be a trained nurse and may use a checklist to ensure that preparation is complete. The key role is to act as the service user's advocate by offering support and reassurance, ensuring that privacy and dignity are maintained, and relaying any anxieties, if expressed, to the core team. Some service users benefit from being accompanied by a relative/friend throughout treatment. If clinic staff consider that the service user will benefit, the relative/friend may remain present throughout all treatment stages. The service user may request information at any time, and this is provided to reduce anxiety. *The service user may withdraw consent at any time before anaesthesia commences.*[c]

Care following recovery

- People take differing times to recover and should not be rushed. The escorting nurse should provide frequent reassurance and reorientation, repeating the information until the person can remember. The relative or friend may wish to take this role. Confusion may be an unwanted effect. The nurse may be able to use material from the memory diary to help orientation. It is important to document the presence of confusion.
- Service users who are fully conscious and responsive to verbal commands and willing to move should be accompanied to a quiet area in the ECT suite and given refreshment, an important consideration for comfort and rehydration.
- The person should be asked if there are any unwanted effects such as headache, muscle aches or nausea (they may not always say so, spontaneously). Prescribed medication should be administered and checked for efficacy.
- Accompany the person back to the ward where they may well want to rest. The primary nurse will be responsible for monitoring the patient's condition, including vital signs, for a reasonable interval (usually 4 hours) following their return.
- Night staff will continue to observe the person during the night following treatment.
- Service users may well want to discuss their experience of treatment, issues which were disturbing and also what was helpful; this information can usefully be integrated into the care plan.
- Continued monitoring and discussion of side-effects and adverse effects is important and may indicate a need to alter prescribed treatment, e.g. increased dosage of analgesia.
- An assessment of mental state between treatments is essential to monitor improvement or deterioration. Standardized assessment tools are used, such as the Beck Depression Inventory. Memory will also need to be assessed, but is the responsibility of the multidisciplinary team.[26]

SUMMARY

ECT continues to be a controversial and emotionally difficult area of nursing care. Since ECT is not beneficial for all patients, the prescribing of ECT and its administration warrants careful consideration and monitoring, focused on the service user's wishes. Poor practice in ECT administration has been evident in systematic audits carried out in the UK. It is important, therefore, that nurses involved in its administration have specific training and are professionally accountable for their actions.

One aspect of care which has a poor record is providing information to the person and family/carer about both the procedure and possible adverse effects. The evidence base is now quite clear and guidelines recommend that all service users should be informed of adverse effects. It is vital that any nurse involved with the administration of ECT is well-educated in all aspects of the treatment. By involving independent advocates throughout the process, any perceived lack of information can be rectified and the individual will be able to give a true informed consent. Working collaboratively means that individuals who choose, or request, ECT should be enabled throughout the process. Supporting the person in making an informed choice for treatment with ECT, in full awareness of all appropriate alternative effective treatments available, is the most reasonable basis for care.

---

[c]In *The ECT handbook* there is an excellent section (Appendix VII: Nursing guideline for ECT) which describes the responsibilities of the ECT nurse, the recovery nurse and the escorting nurse. It is recommended that this detailed account is accessed (available from www.rcpsych.ac.uk or by typing Royal College of Psychiatrists ECT Handbook into an Internet search engine).[37]

REFERENCES

1. Scott AIF (ed.). *The ECT handbook*, 2nd edn. Council Report CR1 28 of the Royal College of Psychiatrists. London, UK: RCP, 2005.

2. National Institute for Health and Clinical Excellence. *Guidance on the use of electroconvulsive therapy*. Technology Appraisal 59. London, UK: NICE, 2003. Available from: www.nice.org.uk.

3. UK ECT Review Group. Efficacy and safety of electroconvulsive therapy in depressive disorders: a systematic review and meta-analysis. *Lancet* 2003; **361**: 799–808.

4. Pedler M. *Shock treatment, a survey of people's experiences of electro-convulsive therapy*. London, UK: Mind, 2001.

5. Department of Health. *Electroconvulsive therapy: survey covering the period from January 1999 to March 1999, England*. Statistical bulletin. London, UK: Department of Health, 1999.

6. Tharyan P, Adams CE. Electroconvulsive therapy for schizophrenia. *Cochrane Database of Systematic Reviews* 2005; Issue 2, Art No: CD000076.

7. Challiner V, Griffiths L. Electroconvulsive therapy; a review of the literature. *Journal of Psychiatric and Mental Health Nursing* 2000; **7**: 191–8.

8. Fink M. Challenges to British practice of electroconvulsive therapy. *Journal of ECT* 2006; **22**: 30–2.

9. Perkins R. My three psychiatric careers. In: Barker P, Campbell P, Davidson B (eds). *From the ashes of experience*. London, UK: Whurr Publishers, 1999.

10. Johnstone L. Adverse psychological effects of ECT. *Journal of Mental Health* 1999; **8**: 69–85.

11. Rose D, Wykes T, Leese M *et al*. Patients' perspectives on electroconvulsive therapy: systematic review. *BMJ* 2003; **326**: 1363–7.

12. Gass JP. The knowledge and attitudes of mental health nurses to electro-convulsive therapy. *Journal of Advanced Nursing* 1998; **27**: 83–90.

13. United Kingdom Advocacy Network. Ukan's national user survey. *Openmind* Dec 1995/Jan 1996; **78**.

14. Donahue A. Electroconvulsive therapy and memory loss: a personal journey. *Journal of ECT* 2000; **16** (2): 133–43.

15. Philpot M, Collins C, Trivedi P *et al*. Eliciting users' views of ECT in two mental health trusts with a user-designed questionnaire. *Journal of Mental Health* 2004; **13** (4):403–13.

16. Rose D, Fleischmann P, Wykes T. Consumers' views of electroconvulsive therapy: a qualitative analysis. *Journal of Mental Health* 2004; **13** (3): 285–93.

17. Reid I. How does ECT work? In: Scott A (ed.). *The ECT handbook*, 2nd edn. London, UK: RCP, 2005: Appendix 1.

18. Breggin P. *Brain disabling treatments in psychiatry*. New York, NY: Springer, 1997.

19. Van Beusekom B, van den Broek W, Birkenhager T. Long-term follow-up after successful electroconvulsive therapy for depression: a 4 to 8 year naturalistic follow-up study. *Journal of ECT* 2007; **23**: 17–20.

20. Kellner C, Knapp R, Petrides G *et al*. Continuation electroconvulsive therapy vs pharmacotherapy for relapse prevention in major depression. *Archives of General Psychiatry* 2006; **63**: 1337–44.

21. Wallcraft J. ECT: effective, but for whom? *Openmind* 1993; **62**: 14.

22. Burstow B. Electroshock as a form of violence against women. *Violence Against Women* 2006; **12**: 372–92.

23. Read J. Electroconvulsive therapy. In: Read J, Mosher L, Bentall R (eds). *Models of madness*. Hove, UK: Brunner Routledge, 2004.

24. Fitzsimmons LM, Mayer R. Soaring beyond the cuckoo's nest: health care reform and ECT. *Journal of Psycho-Social Nursing* 1995; **33**: 10–13.

25. Watkinson A. ECT: a personal experience. *Mental Health Practice* 2007; **10** (7): 32–5.

26. Robertson H, Pryor R. Memory and cognitive effects of ECT: informing and assessing patients. *Advances in Psychiatric Treatment* 2006; **12**: 228–38.

27. Sackeim H, Prudic J, Fuller R *et al*. The cognitive effects of electroconvulsive therapy in community settings. *Neuropsychopharmacology* 2007; **32**: 244–54.

28. Taylor D, Paton C, Kerwin R. *The South London and Maudsley NHS Trust Oxleas NHS Trust 2005–2006 Prescribing Guidelines*. London, UK: Taylor & Francis, 2005.

29. Johnstone L. *Users and abusers of psychiatry*, 2nd edn. London, UK: Routledge, 2000.

30. National Institute for Health and Clinical Excellence. *Depression: management of depression in primary and secondary care*. Clinical Guideline 23. London, UK: NICE, 2004.

31. Rosa M, Gattaz W, Pascual-Leone A *et al*. Comparison of repetitive transcranial magnetic stimulation and electroconvulsive therapy in unipolar non-psychotic refractory depression: a randomized, single-blind study. *International Journal of Neuropsychopharmacology* 2006, **9**: 667–76.

32. Dobbs D. Turning off depression. *Scientific American Mind* 2006; **August/September**.

33. Mayberg H, Loano A, Voon V *et al*. Deep brain stimulation for treatment-resistant depression. *Neuron* 2005; **45**: 651–60.

34. Sadowski H, Ugarte B, Kolvin I *et al*. Early life family disadvantages and major depression in adulthood. *British Journal of Psychiatry* 1999; **174**: 112–20.

35. Read J, Mosher L, Bentall R (eds). *Models of madness*. Hove, UK: Brunner-Routledge, 2004.

36. The Royal Australian and New Zealand College of Psychiatrists. *College statement – electroconvulsive therapy explained*. August 2001. Available from: www.ranzcp.org/ statements/ps/ps40.htm.

37. Cullen L. Nursing guidelines for ECT. In: Scott A (ed.). *The ECT handbook*. London, UK: RCP, 2005: Appendix VII.

38. Barnes R, Dyer J, McCelland R, Scott A. The law and consent to treatment. In: Scott A (ed.). *The ECT handbook*. London, UK: RCP, 2005.

39. Vaughn McCall W. Refusal versus reluctance. *Journal of ECT* 2006; **22** (2): 89–90.

40. Kinton M. *Mental Health Act Commission Policy Briefing for Commissioners*, issue 17. 2007. Available from: mat.kinton@mhac.org.uk.

41. Department of Health and the Welsh Office. *Code of Practice Mental Health Act 1983*. London, UK: HMSO, 1993.

42. Whitaker R. *Mad in America*. New York, NY: Basic Books, 2002.

43. Barker PJ. *Assessment in psychiatric and mental health nursing*, 2nd edn. Cheltenham, UK: Stanley Thornes, 2004.

44. Barker P, Buchanan-Barker P. *The tidal model*. Hove, UK: Brunner-Routledge, 2004.

45. Bowley J, Walker H. Anaesthesia for ECT. In: Scott A (ed.). *The ECT handbook*. London, UK: RCP, 2005.

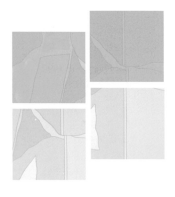

CHAPTER 66

Mental health promotion and prevention

Jon Chesterson*

Somewhere within, the child is watching,
A picture of symbols, a journey of choice,
Remember the one in your past life who told you,
The gift in yourself, their innocent voice.
They're waiting …

Canberra 1996[a]

INTRODUCTION

The World Health Organization (WHO) at the Ottawa Charter in 1986[1] identified five objectives that form the basis for improving mental and physical health:

1 build healthy public policy
2 create supportive environments
3 strengthen community action
4 develop personal skills
5 reorient health services.

To achieve these objectives and effectively improve the health of the population, many organizations need to work together. While health and social services have an important role to play, their work is most effective when complemented by other sectors such as education, recreation, environment, central and local government, commerce, industry and the non-government and voluntary sectors. Social inclusion and support, involvement of community organizations and individual members of local communities is vital. Health is best understood in a holistic sense, as defined by the WHO in 1948:[2]

Health is a state of complete physical, social and mental wellbeing, and not merely the absence of disease or infirmity. Within the context of health promotion, health can be expressed as a resource, which permits people to lead an individually, socially and economically productive life.

Reflection

How fundamental is mental health to our existence, our lives and our livelihood, our health?

*Jon Chesterson works in promotion and prevention for Hunter New England Mental Health (NSW Health) Newcastle, Australia, and Chairs the NSW Branch and Board of Credentialing, Australian College of Mental Health Nurses. He is a past Board Director for Lifeline (Newcastle-Hunter) and PRA (Psychiatric Rehabilitation Association); past president of the Australian & New Zealand College of Mental Health Nurses; and a founding member of the Mental Health Council of Australia.

[a] Wherever the asterisk appears in the text, this is intended to refer the reader to the verse at the beginning of this chapter.

The historical development of mental health promotion has over the years been piecemeal and limited in any clear national strategies of what constitutes mental health and how to maintain it in a society that places innumerable pressures on individuals in all aspects of our lives. Mental health promotion has clear links with public health concerns, such as the environment we live in, with poverty, inequality and all those pressures that are both seen and felt by all of us throughout the life cycle. We know that the experience of oppression dampens the spirit and psyche and can lead to major mental health problems at any stage of life.[3]

Today, within the developed world there is a growing focus on mental health promotion, prevention and recovery paradigms, part driven by human rights, socio-economic realism (cost-effectiveness) and scientific enquiry (empirical evidence) on the one hand and constrained by fiscal management (economic rationalism) and social control measures (government legislation, defensive bureaucracy, safety/risk management) on the other. In many developing and particularly Third World countries, which represent two-thirds of the planet's population, mental health promotion and prevention in terms of government policy and service intervention is practically non-existent, as are mental health services, despite mental disorders not being culturally bound. To understand this we need to recognize that promotion and prevention and mental health may be defined in a completely different way, by different cultures, values, beliefs, religious–social norms, societal infrastructures, sociopolitical agendas and economic realities. Whether we view mental illness as a consequence or trigger for social problems may be derived from our understanding – social drift theory asserts that people with a mental illness decline in social status and capacity; social determinants of mental illness indicate otherwise. Box 66.1 includes research findings on prevalence and impact of mental disorders highlighting the need for prevention on multiple levels.

> ### Reflection
>
> What factors determine a society's response to mental illness or promotion of mental health and well-being?

Mental health services and nurses have a vital role and are well placed to incorporate promotion and prevention into their practice and service delivery. Mental health nurses need to adopt a population-based approach to do this effectively, and such an approach requires that many other sectors in society be involved. What is effective and how can this be done successfully? The real challenge is how can this be done in societies where mental health services and mental health nurses do not exist? This suggests that we may need to adopt alternative strategies and resources and/or use them in a different way, while recognizing

> ### Box 66.1: Prevalence of mental disorders: rationale for prevention[4–12]
>
> *Mental disorders: 11 per cent of total disease burden in 1990; 15 per cent by 2020*
>
> - Depression is the second leading cause of disability after ischaemic heart disease
> - Mental disorders affect 1 in 5 people (20 per cent); > 25 per cent aged 18–24 years
> - 25 per cent co-morbidity among mental disorders; high use of alcohol and drugs
> - Risk/vulnerability in childhood increases risk in adulthood
> - Association between poverty and mental disorders appears to be universal
> - Socioeconomic costs of mental ill-health estimated at 3–4 per cent of gross national product
>
> *Most psychoses begin in late adolescence/early adulthood*
>
> - 43 per cent experience chronic illness and incomplete recovery
> - 72 per cent unemployed; 85 per cent reliant on welfare benefits
> - 45 per cent in temporary/supported accommodation or homeless
> - 84 per cent single, separated, widowed, divorced; high rates of loneliness
> - More than 50 per cent report physical abuse by others or self
> - 67 per cent smoke nicotine, more than three times general population
> - Physical health problems significantly higher than general population

others in any given society may already be championing this cause by another purpose, identity or means.

DEFINITIONS

> ### Reflection
>
> What norms, assumptions and values underpin your definition and understanding of mental health and mental illness? How does this differ between cultures?

Prevention is an approach adopted by the WHO and the national mental health policies and strategies of numerous countries and has its roots in preventive psychiatry. The classic and commonly accepted definition divides prevention into three categories or levels: *primary, secondary* and *tertiary*.[13]

- *Primary prevention* is concerned with decreasing the incidence and prevalence of mental disorders, one aspect of which is considered to include the promotion of mental health. This is more clearly differentiated later.

- *Secondary prevention* is concerned with early diagnosis, prompt and effective treatment or intervention to reduce duration and impact of mental disorders, and preventing development of lifetime disorder and/or disability.
- *Tertiary prevention* is concerned with reducing long-term disability and social disadvantage associated with mental disorders. This is reflected in approaches to care such as psychiatric rehabilitation and recovery.

Definitions of mental health promotion are a starting point for understanding but are also 'value loaded'.[14] They reflect the philosophy and practice of mental health promotion, personal or professional style, and influence the choice of intervention. The approach may reflect a particular focus or have a combination of discrete features: medical or preventive; behavioural change; educational; empowerment; and social change.[2]

Mental health promotion

- Mental health promotion aims to enable people to manage life events, both predictable and unpredictable, by increasing self-esteem and a sense of well-being. This is achieved by working with individuals, groups and communities to improve life skills and quality of life as well as trying to influence the social, economic and environmental factors that can have an impact on mental health.[15]
- Also, it involves any action to enhance the mental well-being of individuals, families, organizations or communities.[16,17]
- Mental health promotion is about developing positive mental health both for and with the community in general and individuals who may have mental health problems. It includes self-help, service provision and organizational skills. The concept of mental health promotion recognizes that people's mental health is inextricably linked to their relationships with others, life-style, environmental factors and the degree of power they can exert over their lives.[3]

Definitions of mental health promotion also depend on our definition of mental health:

> **Mental health** is a state of emotional and social wellbeing in which the individual realizes his or her own abilities, can cope with the normal stresses of life, can work productively and fruitfully, and is able to make a contribution to his or her community
>
> **WHO[18]**

This definition is consistent with the broader 1948 definition of health at the beginning of this chapter,

which underpins the slogan *there is no health without mental health*.

Reflection

Whose responsibility is it to carry out promotion and prevention at each of the three levels mentioned?

MODELS AND FRAMEWORKS

Boxer[19] summarizes three models of health promotion, drawing from the following theoretical constructs and approaches:

- radical humanist and structuralist, humanist and traditional
- health persuasion, legislative action, personal counselling and community development
- disease management and prevention, health education, and politics of health involving social action, policy and economic management.

Together with the five strategic approaches for health promotion identified – medical, behaviour change, educational, empowerment and social change – these constructs and approaches illustrate how individuals and countries have tried to develop an understanding of the context of mental health in different parts of the world, and be proactive. The balance between a medical and social paradigm is a desired outcome as to how different countries tackle mental health problems as part of a wider framework of health and social care delivery.[4,5]

Mental health promotion today is understood within a context of a public health paradigm – from a whole of population approach. While the 1980s marked the emergence globally of the 'new public health' philosophy, population health has emerged as a more useful term, which in part alleviates the confusion with publicly funded health service structures, e.g. public hospital systems:

> **Population health** attends to the health status and health needs of whole populations. It encompasses population needs assessment, developing and implementing interventions to promote health and reduce illness across the whole population and/or in particular population groups, along with monitoring trends and evaluating outcomes. Population health recognises that health and illness result from the complex interplay of biological, psychological, social, environmental and economic factors at personal, local and global levels.
>
> **Commonwealth Department of Health and Aged Care[17]**

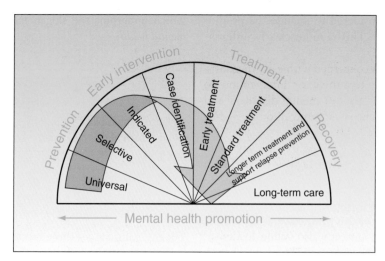

Figure 66.1 Spectrum of interventions 1: mental health promotion and prevention. Adapted from Commonwealth Department of Health and Aged Care;[17] Mrazek and Haggerty[21]

There are four key domains of a population-based service model, each interconnected and overlapping.[20]

1 *Focus*: population–community/organizational–family/individual.
2 *Spectrum of interventions*: prevention–treatment–recovery.
3 *Life span*: infancy–adulthood–old age.
4 *Level of prevention*: primary–secondary–tertiary.

Mrazek and Haggerty[21] describe a spectrum of interventions for mental health including prevention, treatment and maintenance or continuing care (including rehabilitation and long-term care). Mental health promotion (and prevention too) is applicable across the spectrum, not just at one end of the continuum. The prevention of mental disorders is just one level; secondary and tertiary prevention includes early intervention, relapse prevention, prevention of disability, suicide and self-harm, physical illness, family or social breakdown. This adapted model provides a broad operational framework for mental health promotion and prevention, with a clear focus and target for intervention within existing service delivery structures (Figure 66.1).

It is useful to distinguish between mental health promotion and prevention. Mental health promotion is concerned with the promotion of emotional and social well-being. Consequently, it is concerned with people who are well, people with minimal risk of mental illness, those at risk and vulnerable, and those experiencing mental illness. The primary purpose of mental health promotion is to:

- protect, support and sustain emotional and social well-being
- promote mentally healthy life-styles and living – support productive and meaningful lives
- increase sense of belonging, social awareness and connectedness

- promote healthy communities, schools, workplaces and social supports
- strengthen personal, family, educational, occupational, economic growth and functioning
- build community acceptance, tolerance and understanding of personal, social, cultural and spiritual differences/preferences
- improve coping skills, capacity and adaptation of individuals and communities, particularly in response to adversity
- build resilience – increase/strengthen protective factors, reduce risk factors/behaviours that threaten emotional and social well-being, and health
- improve mental health literacy.

Mental health prevention is defined as an intervention that occurs prior to onset in order to prevent development of a mental disorder (or illness).[17,21] Interventions may be targeted at specific times across the life span to prevent specific disorders and reduce prevalence associated with life cycle transitions and age-related onset, such as children, young adults, perinatal, mid-life, retirement and ageing. It may be focused on the population or on an individual, and divided into three levels – primary, secondary and tertiary prevention. Promotion of mental health and well-being may improve resilience to mental illness, but unlike prevention not defined by it. The primary purpose of prevention is to:

- reduce incidence (new people presenting) and prevalence (number of people presenting) of specific mental disorders – *primary and secondary prevention*
- reduce and/or delay recurrence of mental disorder (frequency and/or interval) – *relapse prevention*
- reduce time spent with, or severity or impact of, symptoms including immediate harm, distress, pain and suffering – *treatment, recovery, secondary and tertiary prevention*

- reduce risk factors, high-risk behaviours and/or social/environmental conditions associated with mental disorders – *all levels*
- reduce impact of mental disorder on the person, their family and society (minimize psychiatric disability, social burden and disadvantage) – *treatment, maintenance, clinical rehabilitation, recovery, secondary and tertiary prevention.*

Prevention also aims to:

- reduce morbidity, including loss of productive employment, economic and social capacity, independence, quality of life – *disability support*
- reduce mortality (death/premature death) associated with suicide, self-harm, disease and physical illness, accident, neglect
- reduce incidence and prevalence of drug and alcohol problems (co-morbidity)
- reduce incidence and prevalence of physical health problems and illnesses – *all levels*
- reduce violence, aggression, emotional and sexual abuse, domestic violence
- reduce restrictive practices and violation of human rights, freedom and choice
- reduce vulnerability, poverty, loneliness, socioeconomic, cultural and educational alienation – *social determinants and consequences, stigma, social inclusion, tertiary prevention.*

Table 66.1 summarizes key strategies and actions for promotion and prevention at a population and individual level across the spectrum of interventions using our model adapted from Mrazek and Haggerty.[21] It provides definitions for universal, selective and indicated prevention, which helps distinguish between primary and secondary prevention in mental health.

Relapse prevention is an important function of helping people to stay well following a first or subsequent episode of mental illness. In a medical or psychiatric context it is concerned with preventing or reducing recurrence of mental illness and exacerbation of symptoms. It is best understood in terms of promoting awareness, recovery and resilience – not only medication adherence and education. What happens during remission – life experiences, growth and development, risk and protective factors, and social circumstances – has a significant impact on prevention. Box 66.2 highlights components of a relapse prevention plan.

RESILIENCE

Box 66.2: Components of a relapse prevention plan

- Engagement and rapport
- Awareness – recognition, acceptance, motivational change
- Relapse signature – identify triggers and early warning signs
- Individual and family education
- Division of responsibilities – mutual collaboration, who does what
- Advanced directives – identify personal preferences, future options
- Self-help support and social inclusion (connectedness)
- Maintenance – what to continue, what to avoid
- Early intervention – self-action, access, re-engage, stabilize
- Empowerment in remission – build resilience

The capacity to cope with adversity and to avoid breakdown when confronted by stressors differs tremendously among individuals. Not all responses to stress are pathological and they may serve as coping mechanisms. Numerous researchers have studied healthy mechanisms of defence and coping. Rutter[22] conceived resilience as a product of environment and constitution that is an interactive process. Protective factors can modify a person's responses to an environmental hazard so that the outcome is not always detrimental, and these may become detectable only in the face of a stressor.

Risk factors are commonly identified as part of psychosocial and mental health assessments in early case identification and treatment. They are useful in determining risk management, level and scope of intervention and care planning, while identification of clinical symptoms of mental disorder provides the basis for correct diagnosis and treatment. The risk factors identified in Box 66.3 relate to primary prevention and might be useful to incorporate into selective and indicated prevention programmes, screening for vulnerable at-risk groups, targeted mental health literacy and education programmes, social interventions and strengthening resilience at a community or individual level.

Box 66.3: Reducing risk factors

- Poor or interrupted development or maturity
- Unstable or dysfunctional relationships
- Overwhelming adversity, grief and loss
- Absent or poor parenting and role modelling
- Family discord, domestic violence and abuse
- Parent(s) with serious mental disorder and disability
- Loneliness, lack of friends, peer and social support
- Persistent physical illness, disability or distress
- Drugs or excess alcohol use, poor nutrition and sleep
- Social exclusion, disadvantage, injustice, poverty, stigma

TABLE 66.1 Spectrum of interventions 2: strategies for mental health promotion and prevention at population and individual level

Spectrum	Approach	Definition	Population strategy	Individual* strategy	Lead agency
Prevention *(Primary)*	Universal	Targeted at general public or whole population group not identified on basis of risk[14,p.24]	Mental health awareness campaign; Use of multi-media – people's stories; Community education and stigma; Bullying prevention programme; Mental health literacy; Government policy and social action	Mental health promotion; Healthy life-style education; Teach resilience; Emotional intelligence; Self-awareness; Meet people with mental illness	Government and public service; Schools/higher education; Employment/workplace; Non-governmental organization (NGO) sector; Mental health NGOs; News media and TV
	Selective	Targeted at subgroup of population whose risk of developing mental disorders is significantly higher than average[14,p.25]	Mental health literacy in schools; Parenting and early years; Children of parents with mental illness; Indigenous and ethnic groups; Refugees and asylum seekers; Mentally healthy ageing; Carer support and respite programmes	Anger management; Grief and loss counselling; Bereavement support; Mental health promotion; Healthy life-style education; Teach resilience; Risk and protective factors	Government and public service; Schools/higher education; Mental health NGOs; Community services; Social services; Indigenous/ethnic groups; Aged care services
	Indicated	Targeted for people with high risk – minimal detectable signs and symptoms or markers indicating predisposition to mental disorders – do not meet DSM diagnostic criteria[14,p.25]	School counselling support programme; Employer counselling service; Mentally healthy workplace/practices; Prenatal and postnatal support; Parenting programme for parents of troubled preschool children; Phone counselling service – children's phone line; Web resource and information services; self-help support groups	Mental health screening and advice; Family support/counselling; Mental health promotion; Risk and protective factors; Healthy life-style education; Stress management	Counselling services; Schools/higher education; Employment/workplace; Maternal/child/family health; Mental health NGO; Other indicated agencies
Early Intervention *(Secondary)*	Case identification	Early identification of mental health problems or diagnosis in clinical settings or outreach – early and reliable recognition of mental disorders[9,p.33]	General practitioner (GP) support, consultancy and liaison; GP education and partnerships; GP enhancements and incentives; Access mental health professionals; Outreach programmes and clinics; Early psychosis programmes; Community mental health provision	Engagement; Physical health screening; Mental health/risk assessment; Identify risk/protective factors; Case coordination; Short targeted therapies; Supportive counselling; Mental health education; Medication education	General practices; Health centres; Outreach clinics; Emergency departments; Crisis and community mental health teams; Specialist mental health services; Counselling services; Other indicated agencies

	Description	Services/Programmes	Activities	Agencies
Early treatment	Early access and engagement – targeted, evidence-based, short-term treatments, therapies and support to achieve quick effective recovery	Crisis intervention and after hours; Referral pathways; Mental health nurses in primary health care and general practice; Mental health nurse practitioners; Practitioner-led support groups	Drug and alcohol education and motivational change; Suicide prevention; Prevention of self-harm; Mental health promotion; Healthy life-style education, referral and follow-up	Mental health services; General practice; Legal services; Consumer/carer organizations; Other indicated agencies
Standard treatment	Access and engagement with specialist clinical and support services – routine, effective, least restrictive, evidence-based treatments, therapies, care and support to achieve fullest possible recovery	Inpatient and community mental health; Outpatient clinics; Comprehensive mental health service; Clinical practice guidelines; Model legislation; Legal representation; Mental health advocacy; Navigator: user/carer guide to mental health service; Consumer and carer support groups	Medication monitoring; Shorter term therapies; Supportive counselling; D&A education and motivational change; Case management; Mental health promotion; Healthy life-style education; Discharge plans/follow-up; Relapse prevention	
Treatment — Longer term treatment and support	Targeted for people at risk of relapse, whose mental disorders continue or recur – optimal clinical treatment, therapies, care and support with key focus on recovery and relapse prevention	Inpatient and community psychiatric rehabilitation; Disability support programmes; Personal support programmes; Housing/accommodation; Supported and open employment; Recreational and community access; Voluntary support programmes; Stigma, social inclusion and citizenship; Inter-agency partnerships; Social capital investment	Relapse prevention; Mental health promotion; Healthy life-style education; Living skills training; Social skills training; Vocational training; Regular health checks; GP access; Quit smoking; D&A education and motivational change	
Recovery — Long-term care	Targeted for people with mental disorders whose health and social well-being is at significant risk of decline, neglect, alienation or exploitation – continuing care, treatment and support with key focus on social and occupational functioning, quality of life and social inclusion	Building NGO sector capacity; Public mental health policy; Model legislation; Legal representation; Mental health advocacy; Consumer-led support groups; Media monitoring	Medication management; Case management; Therapies; Supportive counselling; Social support networks; Hope and empowerment; Support and advocacy	Mental health services; General practices; Mental health NGOs; Consumer/carer organizations; Disability support agencies; Housing; Employment agencies; Educational institutions; Government: national and local; Other indicated agencies

---

Box 66.4: Building resilience: protective factors

- Nurturing, affectionate, secure family relationships
- Positive/rewarding school and work environments
- Personal and shared opportunity and achievements
- Social 'connectedness' and belonging
- Reliable friendships and social support networks
- Positive 'temperament', humour, patience, tolerance, hope
- Presence of mind, emotional intelligence, expression
- Self-awareness, esteem, acceptance, courage
- Mentors or personal encouragement (past or present)*
- Healthy life-style

Protective factors are less frequently identified in routine clinical practice. The protective factors identified in Box 66.4 relate to mental health promotion and primary prevention. Anti-bullying programmes in schools, promoting healthy working environments, parent education and training, promoting healthy life-styles, self-help and social support groups, personal growth and development courses, teaching of emotional intelligence and resilience, mental health literacy, and connecting people in the community including ethnic minorities and those who are socially disadvantaged contribute to building resilience to mental illness and the promotion of emotional health and well-being in society. At the clinical level, incorporating protective factors into routine practice helps promote optimum recovery, coping skills, higher level of functioning, prevention of recurrence (relapse prevention), psychiatric disability and social isolation, consistent with recovery and strengths models.

The primary goal is to reduce risk and strengthen protective factors, maintaining balance with something in reserve to cope with adversity and the unexpected. We can predict times of increased stress and vulnerability, but our ability to cope is often compromised when confronted with and overwhelmed by unexpected or multiple events. This is not dissimilar to the 'ABC' of coping with stress: awareness/recognition; balance/stability; and control/manage. Athletes in the sporting world prepare and train to build their stamina and *endurance*, helping them to go the extra mile when they need to. This concept might be useful in understanding resilience, having something extra in reserve when needed, increasing our capacity to adapt to life situations and circumstance. Teaching resilience is about:

- accepting and understanding yourself*
- getting to know, understand and live with others
- taking responsibility for ourselves and our health
- recognizing and learning to cope with stress and adversity, adaptability
- understanding our illness when it is present, learning to accept it and live with it

- protecting ourselves from unnecessary risk and harm
- talking to others when we have a problem and being around to help others.

Resilient people:

- are able to set attainable goals and remain focused, open and decisive
- express their emotions and control them
- are proactive, reflective and creative, not just reactive
- are not easily distracted or defeated, have endurance
- can support and comfort others in compassionate and helpful ways
- handle risk, conflict and stress in a variety of ways
- have the capacity to get the best out of life for themselves and others.

Reflection

A mentor may be a parent, teacher, friend, mature, older, wise person. Their encouragement of us becomes part of our self-talk, our image, our values and who we strive to be.* How might 'mentoring' be used in the design of a mental health promotion project or programme?

MENTAL HEALTH LITERACY

Jorm *et al.*[23] define mental health literacy as the ability to recognize specific disorders; knowing how to seek mental health information; knowledge of risk factors and causes, self-treatments and professional help available; and attitudes that promote recognition and appropriate help-seeking. This has given rise to the development of mental health first aid training programmes in countries such as Australia, which can be usefully conducted to raise awareness and competence around mental illness among the general population and targeted at specific population groups, communities, agencies and services that come into contact with either people at risk or people with a mental illness, such as the non-governmental organization (NGO) sector, welfare and social services, education sector, police, employment agencies, housing departments, refuges, aboriginal and ethnic minorities and migrant services. The concept of mental health first aid is one which embraces the notion that a wider range of people in the community can offer and benefit from initial support and assistance, provide information and links to specific services, and improve positive health-seeking behaviour. It challenges myths and social stigma around mental illness that inhibit community recognition, acceptance, use of mental health services and access to other community-based services by a person with a mental illness and their family, owing to ignorance or feeling unwelcome.

SOCIAL INCLUSION

Historically, and even today, people with a mental illness frequently remain isolated at home, through massive unemployment rates and low incomes, by loss of socio-economic livelihood, with limited access to education, compromised by lower levels of confidence and social skills, and higher levels of social stigma in the community. People with a mental illness have often encountered a diminishing circle of friends and find it difficult to develop and maintain adequate social support networks, with higher rates of single living, separation and divorce, grief and loss, and homelessness. Access to community infra-structures and resources are barely affordable for people on low incomes, disability support or unemployment benefits and they are less mobile and less likely to own a private vehicle or able to use public transport. Living at home is either a solitary affair or there is little choice who you share with, if living in supported accommoda-tion, hostels or group homes. Not surprisingly, people with a mental illness express and encounter prolonged and lifelong loneliness, poor quality of life and greater vulnerability to major depression, poorer general health and physical illnesses. Public myths and fear of people with a mental illness, violence and dangerousness, often exaggerated and sensationalized in the press and mass media, poor media representation and understanding of people with a mental illness, lack of public compassion, imagination, negative portrayal and stereotypes do little to ease the burden of social isolation.

In a rapidly changing world of globalization, corporati-zation, greater dependence on technology for human interaction, competitive employment and living, large urban and remote rural populations, diminishing natural resources, and vanishing or disempowered local commu-nities, loneliness and social isolation is increasingly an issue for other socioeconomically disadvantaged groups, notwithstanding that of the general population, along-side increasing global prevalence of depression. More people are at risk than ever before, and this includes carers and families who usually share and shoulder this burden, becoming increasingly vulnerable themselves.

Mental health promotion and prevention involves addressing social isolation and related social determin-ants at both primary and tertiary prevention level. The former has already been discussed, the latter requires strategies and programmes specifically designed to increase access, social inclusion and participation of people with a mental illness in the community and for communities to be more inclusive. Fuller participation in the local community and society is a matter of citizen-ship: the right to be considered and included; the right to be productive, make a contribution, earn one's own keep; the right to share responsibility and benefits; the right to fair treatment and equal opportunity; the right

to self-determination, freedom and choice. The focus can be on the individual, community, population or public policy level:

- assertive community and social outreach
- improved access and provision of public transport
- supported and open employment, rapid job searching and matching
- job support/maintenance programmes targeting employers and employees
- range of supported, public and private housing includ-ing joint service agreements
- improved access to vocational, secondary and tertiary education
- access and incentives to recreation and leisure facilities
- social connection and community supports
- intersectoral collaboration, partnerships, memoranda of understanding
- responsible media coverage and reporting in relation to mental illness and suicide
- strengthening civil rights and responsibilities, model mental health legislation
- social skills training
- training in mental health literacy for general public and targeted sectors/agencies.

Mental health promotion and prevention is not the unique province of mental health services and mental healthcare professionals, neither is it the unique respon-sibility of people with mental illness or their families. The degree to which each sector or level of society and individuals within it accept this charge with positive atti-tudes towards people with mental illness strengthens its own culture, the communities within it and the mental health and well-being of all citizens.

Reflection

What is the relationship between citizenship, mental health and mental illness?

EVIDENCE FOR MENTAL HEALTH PROMOTION AND PREVENTION

Most of the available evidence for mental health promo-tion and prevention has been generated from wealthy developed nations. There is substantial evidence at the individual level but less at the levels of population and public health and policy evaluation. Traditionally, best available evidence comes from randomized controlled trials, usually restricted to high-income countries. There are many questions around mental health promotion, programme design and implementation and evaluation, especially at a population level, that cannot be answered by singular experimental approaches. There is a need for combined research designs that incorporate qualitative and ethnographic approaches that are conducted in areas of the world which would be more relevant to a larger proportion of the world's population, i.e. where public service infrastructures and diversity of culture differ and socioeconomic conditions, poverty, war and famine have greater impact and where less is known about mental health, how people maintain their mental health, and the most effective means of promoting mental health and preventing mental illness. There is no doubt that the promotion of mental health is closely linked with human rights and relies heavily on identifying social determinants and easing the burden of socioeconomic disadvantage and poverty at both individual and national economic levels, and there is a growing body evidence of effectiveness of interventions at local community level. Box 66.5 provides examples of effective universal interventions from around the world.[24,25]

WHO identifies three strategies for effective mental health promotion in low-income countries:[25]

1 *Advocacy* aims to generate public demand for mental health and to persuade all stakeholders to place a high value on mental health.
2 *Empowerment* is the process by which groups in a community who have been traditionally disadvantaged in ways that compromise their health can overcome these barriers and exercise all rights that are due to them, with a view to leading a full, equal life in the best of health.
3 *Social support strategies* aim to strengthen community organizations to encourage healthy life-styles and promote mental health, and intersectoral alliances are effective.

SUSTAINABILITY

Goodman and Steckler[26] followed up and reviewed a range of programmes to identify factors which predicted whether programmes 'lived' or 'died', 10 years after initial funding and support had ceased. A key factor that was identified was the presence of a champion higher up in the host organization who acted as an advocate for the programme in key decision-making forums, and a later study concluded how a programme is set up in the first place affects the likelihood of its continuation.[27]

Main features associated with programme sustainability are:[25]

- evidence of the programme's effectiveness
- consumers, funders and decision-makers involved in the development
- host organization is mature, stable and resourceful with a history of innovation

---

Box 66.5: Universal prevention: evidence of effective interventions. Reproduced from Hosman et al.[24] and WHO[25,pp.35-41]

Macro-interventions with mental health impact: supportive environments and public policy

- Improving nutrition (WHO, UNICEF) – combining nutrition and psychosocial care, iodine supplements
- Improving housing – systematic review
- Improving access to education (India, Pakistan, World Bank) – literacy, numeracy, gender
- Strengthening community networks (USA, UK, The Netherlands, Australia)
- Reducing misuse of addictive substances – impact on early childhood development
- Intervening after disasters (WHO)
- Preventing violence (WHO)

Meso-/micro-interventions for mental health promotion: across the life cycle

- Early stages of life (UNICEF)
  - Home visiting in early childhood (USA, Europe)
  - Preschool educational and psychosocial interventions (USA)
  - Reducing violence, improving emotional well-being in school setting (WHO, CASEL www.casel.org/index)
  - Effective school-based interventions for mental health (Australia, New Zealand)
  - Changing school ecology (WHO) – child-friendly schools, positive school environment
  - Multicomponent programmes (USA)
- The adult population
  - Reducing the strain of unemployment (USA, China, Finland, Ireland)
  - Stress prevention programmes in the workplace – coping skills, workplace environments, stress management, social skills training, fitness, roles, conflict, relationships
- Improving mental health of the elderly
  - Socializing care and promoting health of older people (Vietnam)
  - Social support, community empowerment, healthy life-style, befriending, hearing aids

---

- host organization provides real or in-kind support from the outset
- potential to generate additional funds is high
- programme and host organization have compatible missions
- programme not separate – policies, procedures and responsibilities integrated into the organization
- someone other than the programme director acts as a champion at a high level in the organization
- programme has few 'rival providers' who would benefit from discontinuation
- value and mission of the programme fit well with the broader community

- community champions who advocate or lobby to ensure continuation
- other organizations copy and/or develop.

Box 66.6 outlines specifications for a project proposal in designing a mental health promotion intervention or programme.

Box 66.6: Mental health promotion intervention: project based on the Great Idea Planning Tool, Mental Health Promotion Network, Northern Region, Hunter New England AHS, NSW

Project proposal

- Project title and outline
- Identify need, gap and evidence for effectiveness of approach
- What you hope to achieve, who will benefit (target group)
- Local/national strategic priorities met by project
- Proposed timeline, milestones, strategies
- How will you know the project works, evaluative measures
- Use of existing resources, availability, host organization/employer support
- Funding, resources, support required and potential sources
- Identify partners, collaborators, stakeholders, champions
- Consultation and feedback from consumers, carers, relevant parties
- Indicators of sustainability built into project
- Disseminate results, capacity to replicate project elsewhere

---

PUBLIC HEALTH POLICY AND POPULATION APPROACHES

WHO places great importance on the community as a resource and setting for tackling the causes and effects of mental health problems. This ranges from self-help and mutual aid, through lobbying for changes in mental health care and resources, carrying out educational activities and participating in the monitoring and evaluation of care, to advocacy to change attitudes and reduce stigma. Consumer groups have emerged as a powerful, vocal and active force, often dissatisfied with the established provision of care and treatment. These groups have been instrumental in reforming mental health.[2]

The WHO views mental health in a social and medical context, recognizing that successful health and mental health promotion requires change at a number of levels: individuals, family, organizations, communities and society. This is translated at macro-governmental level to policy and action designed to actively support the right of all citizens to good health. Health promoters have come to perceive health in socioecological terms, recognizing the fundamental link between health and conditions in economic, physical, social and cultural environments. Policy-makers are looking beyond traditional healthcare illness-oriented systems to improve population health, in recognition that, in addition to biological factors, health is determined by external factors such as poverty, housing, environment and social support. Investment in mental health service reform, designing model mental health services and delivery of effective treatment services is a dreadful waste of money (not in itself), if it is not accompanied by social change and addressing the social determinants of mental health in society.

Reflection

What terms, phrases and portrayals in the media stereotype or stigmatize people with mental illness? What can you do about it?

In 2005 the National Institute for Mental Health in England released a best practice guideline to improve mental health and well-being and outlining nine priorities for action: marketing mental health and well-being, equality and inclusion, violence and abuse, early years, schools, employment, workplace, communities, and later life.[28] It provides a framework for raising the public's awareness of how to look after our own mental health and other people's, involving all communities, organizations and sectors in taking positive steps to promote and protect mental well-being, and meeting the requirement of standard 1 of the *National service framework for mental health*.[29] It states that there is sufficient evidence to demonstrate the benefits and effectiveness of promoting mental health with an emphasis on local needs and action. Good practice at a local level includes:

- local needs assessment
- clear statement of what success would look like and how to measure it
- cross-sector ownership, governance and resourcing
- links to wider initiatives to improve health and social outcomes
- evidence-based interventions
- building public mental health capacity
- developing public mental health intelligence [literacy].

Similar public health policy and action has been developed in other countries, including a policy for Europe[6] and global policies established by WHO.[25] In Australia, current mental health promotion and prevention policies and initiatives can be traced back to the priorities laid down in three consecutive 5-year national mental health plans, since 1992, preceded by a chain of historical events, commissions and inquiries. Much of the consciousness raising and lobbying for social action and change over the years was from the consumer, carer and

NGO sectors as a result of outrage by how people with a mental illness were treated, resulting in human rights abuses, poor treatment, maltreatment, Aboriginal deaths in custody, high rates of suicide (especially in young adults), drug and alcohol use, homelessness, unemployment, disability and neglect.[30] The catalyst for change was not medical science, research or psychiatry, deinstitutionalization, government policy or action, mental health services or mental health professionals. It was largely personal action from those most affected by mental illness, triggering public mental health inquiries, public consciousness and government action, which has since supported the research and the knowledge we have today. Having translated the research into economic terms and disease burden, it has become a matter of national concern and priority, but much more is needed to recover lost ground during the mid- to late twentieth century, in which there was (and still is) a fundamental lack of public financial and social investment in mental health. Since 1992, a considerable body of work has been accomplished through funded research: evidence on the prevalence and impact of mental disorders,[7–9] identification of needs and vulnerable groups,[31,32] effectiveness of mental health promotion and prevention, and a generation of targeted programmes at local, state and national level to improve mental health and well-being.[33,34] These initiatives have occurred in tandem with major mental health service policy reforms such as mainstreaming. In 2000, the Commonwealth government released a monograph and national action plan for promotion, prevention and early intervention, outlining the need for action, the burden of mental disorders, the policy context, definitions and concepts, and adopting a population health approach across the life cycle, targeting priority and special needs groups.[17,35]

CASE EXEMPLAR

Suicide and mental illness in the media is a Mindframe resource developed in Australia for the mental health sector to strengthen knowledge, skills and confidence of healthcare professionals and others working in the mental health sector in reporting and working with the media.[36] An updated companion resource kit was developed for media professionals and journalists.[34,37] This was a Commonwealth government-funded initiative arising out of the National Mental Health Strategy and Action Plan to reduce the social stigma of mental illness, operating on a variety of project and sector levels, which included development of: practice guidelines for media health professionals and mental health professionals; curriculum resources for journalist students and teachers (*ResponseAbility*); evidence of how mental illness and suicide were portrayed in the media and its impact; research and statistics on mental health, illness

and suicide in Australia; and development of a community action site to promote accurate and respectful portrayal. It has also led to media watch and monitoring projects conducted by two independent non-government organizations – SANE Australia and the Mental Health Council of Australia (MHCA).

This initiative is a good example of effective mental health promotion and prevention at a universal level, supported by a public health policy and action plan. It is a clearly targeted multilevel intervention with a wide impact on the general public in terms of promoting mental health literacy and health, and in improving social stigma and conditions that affect people and their families with a mental illness. It demonstrates key elements of sustainability: scope of project and set up; relevance to the needs of the community; gathering of evidence including programme effectiveness, resourcefulness and mission compatibility of host organizations; organizational and community champions; other organizations taking up the cause; and built-in evaluative outcomes and reporting. It also addresses the ongoing education and training needs of mental health professionals, journalists, NGOs, consumer consultants, people with a mental illness, carers and members of the general public.

Reflection

What are the mental health needs of the future and are there ecological determinants and consequences to consider? What will this mean for mental health promotion and prevention in the future?

SUMMARY

One in five are affected by a mental health problem or disorder. The prevalence of mental disorders and their impact on people's lives and the socioeconomic costs to society are indicative of the need for a major shift in mental health towards promotion and prevention, a trend that has been gathering momentum over the past 10–15 years. Mental health promotion is primarily concerned with strengthening the mental health and well-being of all people in society. Prevention is concerned with reducing the incidence and prevalence of mental illness and its sequelae. Both require culturally appropriate strategies and actions targeted at the individual, family, organizational, local community and population level, across the life span and intervention spectrum of service delivery. Social determinants, inequalities of poverty, housing, education, health, unemployment, living, access to services, citizenship and human rights are critical threats to mental health and well-being in all societies. Strengthening resilience and the promotion of public mental health literacy play a vital role in prevention and, together with interventions to reduce social isolation and stigma, help to mitigate the lives of people with a mental illness and their families. Early intervention and relapse prevention are important functions of mental health practice and have a significant impact on treatment outcome and recovery.

Mental health promotion and prevention is everyone's business and not the sole function of specialist mental health services. It involves a treatment approach that incorporates promotion and prevention into the routine practices of all healthcare professionals. It requires education, advocacy, empowerment, social action, community development, intersectoral collaboration, networking, partnerships and coherent public health policy. Mental health promotion and prevention is a specialist function and the core business of effective mental health nursing practice. To be sustainable, programmes and practices need to be incorporated into individual, organizational and professional values and missions, they need to be effective and relevant to people's needs and they need champions. Mental health promotion and prevention is strategically supported by the WHO and public health policy. There is a substantial body of knowledge and evidence which can be sourced from research literature, government policies, national mental health strategies, funded projects and reports, and the Internet hosts an impressive range of organizational resources, research and public information. No treatment approach or craft of caring can do without it. The relationships among mental health and well-being at an individual/family level, healthy functioning communities and human society in the context of a future socio-ecological sustainable world is yet to be imagined.*

The key messages of this chapter are as follows:[25,pp.10–11]

- There is no health without mental health.
- Mental health is more than the absence of mental illness: it is vital to individuals, families and societies.
- Mental health is determined by socioeconomic and environmental factors.
- Mental health is linked to behaviour.
- Mental health can be enhanced by effective public health interventions.
- Collective action depends on shared values as much as the quality of scientific evidence.
- A climate that respects and protects basic civil, political, economic, social and cultural rights is fundamental to the promotion of mental health.
- Intersectoral linkage [and networking] is the key for mental health promotion.
- Mental health is everybody's business.

ACKNOWLEDGEMENT

This chapter incorporates some text from Chapter 57: Mental health promotion by Judy Boxer, Senior Lecturer in the School of Health and Social Care, Sheffield Hallam University, UK, in the previous edition.[19]

REFERENCES

1. World Health Organization. *Ottawa Charter: the first international conference on health promotion*. Geneva, Switzerland: WHO, 1986.

2. Naidoo J, Wills J. *Health promotion: foundations for practice*. London, UK: Baillière Tindall, 1994.

3. McCulloch G, Boxer J. *Mental health promotion: policy, practice and partnerships*. London, UK: Baillière Tindall, 1997.

4. World Health Organization. *Investing in mental health*. Geneva, Switzerland: WHO, 2003.

5. World Health Organization. *The state of mental health in the European Union*. Geneva, Switzerland: WHO, 2001.

6. Jane-Llopis E, Anderson P (IMHPA). *Mental health promotion and mental disorder prevention: a policy for Europe*. Nijmegen, The Netherlands: Radboud University Nijmegen, 2005. Available from: www.imhpa.net.

7. McLennan A. *Mental health and wellbeing: profile of adults, Australia 1997*. Canberra, Australia: ABS, 1998.

8. Jablensky A, McGrat J, Herrman H *et al*. People living with psychotic illness: an Australian study 1997–98. Canberra, Australia: Commonwealth of Australia, 1999.

9. Teeson M, Burns L. *National comorbidity project (National Drug & Alcohol Research Centre)*. Canberra, Australia: Commonwealth Department of Health and Aged Care, 2001.

10. Patel V, Kleinman A. Poverty and common mental disorders in developing countries. *Bulletin of the World Health Organization* 2003; **81**: 609–15.

11. Lawrence D, Holman D, Jablensky A. *Duty to care: preventable physical illness in people with mental illness*. Perth, Australia: University of Western Australia, 2001.

12. World Health Organization. *Mental health: new understanding, new hope*. World Health Report. Geneva, Switzerland: WHO, 2001. Available from: www.who.int/whr/2001/en/.

13. Caplan G. *Principles of preventive psychiatry*. New York, NY: Basic Books, 1964.

14. Tudor K. *Mental health promotion*. London, UK: Routledge, 1996.

15. Macdonald G. *Promoting mental health: a report for the health education department*. London, UK: HEA, 1994.

16. Department of Health. *Making it happen: a guide to delivering mental health promotion*. London, UK: HMSO, 2001: 27.

17. Commonwealth Department of Health and Aged Care. *Promotion, prevention and early intervention – monograph*. Canberra, Australia: Mental Health and Special Programs Branch, Commonwealth Department of Health and Aged Care, 2000: Chapter 3.

18. World Health Organization. *Strengthening mental health promotion*. WHO Fact Sheet No. 220. Geneva, Switzerland: WHO, 1999.

19. Boxer J. Mental health promotion. In: Barker P (ed.). *Psychiatric and mental health nursing: the craft of caring*, 1st edn. London, UK: Arnold, 2003: 476–87.

20. Raphael B. *A population health model for the provision of mental health care*. Canberra, Australia: Commonwealth of Australia, 2000.

21. Mrazek PJ, Haggerty RJ. *Reducing the risks for mental disorders: frontiers for preventive intervention research*. Washington, DC: National Academy Press, 1994.

22. Rutter M. Resilience in the face of adversity. *British Journal of Psychiatry* 1985; **147**: 598–611.

23. Jorm AF, Korten AE, Jacomb PA *et al.* Mental health literacy: a survey of the public's ability to recognize mental disorders and their beliefs about effectiveness of treatment. *Medical Journal of Australia* 1997; **166**: 182–6.

24. Hosman C, Jané-Llopis E, Saxena S (eds). *Prevention of mental disorders: an overview on evidence-based strategies and programs*. Oxford: Oxford University Press, 2004.

25. World Health Organization. *Promoting mental health – concepts, emerging evidence, practice: summary report*. A report from the World Health Organization, Department of Mental Health and Substance Abuse, in collaboration with the Victorian Health Promotion Foundation (VicHealth) and the University of Melbourne. Geneva, Switzerland: WHO, 2004. Available from: www.who.int/mental_health/evidence/en/promoting_mhh.pdf.

26. Goodman RM, Steckler AB. A model of institutionalization of health promotion programs. *Family and Community Health* 1987; **11**: 63–78.

27. Shediac-Rizzkallah MC, Bone LR. Planning for the sustainability of community-based health programs: conceptual frameworks and future directions for research, practice and policy. *Health Education Research* 1998; **13**: 87–108.

28. National Institute for Mental Health. *Making it possible: improving mental health and wellbeing in England: best practice guidelines – priorities for action*. Leeds, UK: NIMHE, 2005.

29. Department of Health. *National service framework for mental health: modern standards and service models*. London, UK: DoH, 1999.

30. Human Rights and Equal Opportunity Commission. *Human rights and mental illness (Burdekin): report of the National Inquiry into Human Rights of People with Mental Illness*. Canberra, Australia: Australian Government Publishing Service, 1993.

31. Raphael B. *Promoting the mental health and wellbeing of children and young people. Discussion paper – key principles and directions*. Canberra, Australia: National Mental Health Working Group, 2000.

32. Australian Infant Child Adolescent and Family Mental Health Association. *Children of parents affected by a mental illness: scoping project report*. Canberra, Australia: Department of Health and Aged Care, 2001.

33. Commonwealth Department of Health and Aged Care. *Learnings about suicide (LIFE): a framework for prevention of suicide and self-harm in Australia*. Canberra, Australia: Commonwealth of Australia, 2000.

34. Commonwealth Department of Health and Aged Care. *Achieving the balance: a resource kit for media professionals for the reporting and portrayal of suicide and mental illness*. Canberra: Commonwealth of Australia, 1999.

35. Commonwealth Department of Health and Aged Care. *National action plan for promotion, prevention and early intervention for mental health*. Canberra, Australia: Mental Health and Special Programs Branch, Commonwealth Department of Health and Aged Care, 2000.

36. Hunter Institute of Mental Health, AUSEINET and SANE Australia. *Suicide and mental illness in the media: a Mindframe resource for the mental health sector*. Canberra, Australia: Commonwealth of Australia, 2006.

37. Australian Government Department of Health and Ageing. *Reporting suicide and mental illness: a Mindframe resource for media professionals*. Canberra, Australia: Commonwealth of Australia, 2006.

FURTHER READING

Alliston C (ed.) *Challenges and triumphs: a mosaic of meanings*. Adelaide, Australia: AUSEINET, 2002. Available from: www.auseinet.com.

Cootes A, Wilson G. *My brush with depression: the Greg Wilson story*. Essendon, Australia: Pennon Publishing, 2005. Available from: www.gregwilsongallery.com.

Edwards J, McGory PD. *Implementing early intervention in psychosis: a guide to establishing psychosis services*. London, UK: Martin Dunitz, 2002.

Ewles L, Simnett I. *Promoting health: a practical guide*, 4th edn. London, UK: Baillière Tindall, 1999.

Hamilton C. *Broken open*. Sydney, Australia: Bantam, 2004.

McCulloch G, Boxer J. *Mental health promotion: policy, practice and partnerships*. London, UK: Baillière Tindall, 1997.

McMurray A. *Community health and wellness: a sociological approach*. Sydney, Australia: Harcourt, 1999.

Morrow L, Verins I, Willis E. *Mental health work: issues and perspectives*. Adelaide, Australia: AUSEINET, 2002. Available from: www.auseinet.com.

Rowling L, Martin G, Walker L (eds). *Mental health promotion and young people: concepts and practice*. Sydney, Australia: McGraw Hill, 2002.

Rutter M. *Helping troubled children*. London, UK: Penguin Books, 1975.

Wass A. *Promoting health: the primary health care approach*, 2nd edn. Sydney, Australia: Harcourt, 2000.

Wright RH, Cummings NA. *Destructive trends in mental health: the well-intentioned path to harm*. New York, NY: Routledge, 2005.

WEBSITES

AUSEINET: www.auseinet.com

BeyondBlue – Depression: www.beyondblue.org.au

Clifford Beers Foundation UK: www.cliffordbeersfoundation.co.uk/

Commonwealth Mental Health and Wellbeing Australia: www.mentalhealth.gov.au

COPMI – Children of Parents with Mental Illness: www.copmi.net.au

DOH UK – Mental Health: www.dh.gov.uk/en/Policyandguidance/Healthandsocialcaretopics/Mentalhealth/index.htm

IMHPA Europe: www.imhpa.net

Mental Health Commission NZ: www.mhc.govt.nz

Mental Health Council of Australia: www.mhca.org.au

Mental Health Media Europe: www.mhmedia.com

Mindframe – Media Resource for Mental Health Sector and Journalists: www.mindframe-media.info

MindMatters – Program for Secondary Schools: http://online.curriculum.edu.au/mindmatters

National Social Inclusion Programme – NSIP UK: www.social inclusion.org.uk

ResponseAbility – Mental Health/Suicide for Teachers and Journalists: www.responseability.org

Sainsbury Centre for Mental Health UK: www.scmh.org.uk

SANE Australia: www.sane.org SANE UK: www.sane.org.uk

World Federation for Mental Health: www.wfmh.org

World Health Organization – Mental Health: www.who.int/mental_health/en/

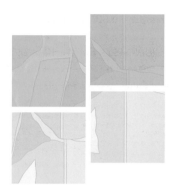

CHAPTER 67

Mental health nurse prescribing

Steve Hemingway* and David Scarrott**

INTRODUCTION

This chapter uses the UK context as an exemplar of nurse prescribing to develop the US perspective offered in the first edition.[1] Mental health nurse (MHN) prescribing now has been in situ in the UK for a number of years, and there exists a growing body of evidence of the effect on the outcomes of MHNs prescribing interventions for the service user.[2] Firstly, a brief historical overview of nurse prescribing in the UK is offered. Secondly, we explore why MHN prescribing has developed. Thirdly, we establish the requirements for MHNs to prescribe safely, competently and lawfully. The fourth section provides evidence of *how* and *where* mental health prescribing is utilized in practice using four personal illustrations. Finally, a summary of the future of MHN prescribing is offered.

MHNs AND THEIR ROLE IN PRESCRIBING PSYCHOTROPIC MEDICATION

MHNs have always played a major role in the delivery of physical treatments, but this was usually subject to the direction of the medical superintendent.[3] Nolan[3] found that Victorian asylum attendants had some significant autonomy in deciding which treatments to utilize when faced with severely disturbed patients. However, historically, the care of the mentally ill has been dominated by scandals and abuse of patients, with an emphasis on control rather than care.[3,4]

The emergence of treatments for symptoms of the major mental illnesses of depression, schizophrenia, bipolar affective disorder and anxiety in the 1950s changed the face of mental health care and validated the role of the psychiatrist,[4] with MHNs administering these new treatments. Rather than becoming a long-term hospital patient, many people could be diagnosed and prescribed medication, enabling them to manage their mental illness at home. Alongside these new treatments, community care was championed as the way forward for mental health care, bringing it into the mainstream of society rather than hidden away.[4]

Although it took four decades to develop the more comprehensive inpatient and community-based specialist services found today, the MHNs who emerged from the 'asylum' system had to adapt to a new context of care. The emergence of community psychiatric nurses saw MHNs working autonomously, helping patients manage their

*Steve Hemingway is a Lecturer in Mental Health Nursing at the University of Huddersfield, UK. He has a background in acute mental health care, both inpatient and home treatment. He has written extensively on both medication management and nurse prescribing. He is studying to doctorate level in the subject.
**David Scarrott is Team Manager of the Crisis Resolution and Home Treatment Team in Rotherham, UK. He has a background in acute psychiatry and liaison psychiatry. He has been supplementary prescribing within his role for the past 2 years.

predicament in the home setting, liaising as appropriate with other services providing care in the community.[3]

Alongside these roles, MHNs played a major role in prescribing decisions regarding psychotropic medication, especially in primary care liaison with GPs and in discussion with junior doctors.[5,6] Until recently, this unauthorized role had no legal back-up and was known as 'de facto' prescribing. As the largest workforce in the field, it was a natural development to formalize such unregulated prescribing for MHNs. Where there is a shortage of psychiatrists, this would prove economic but would also increase choice and flexibility of prescribing for people with mental illness.[7]

Reflection

Think of your experiences of the MHN's role regarding prescribed medication? Why do you think MHNs should adopt the role of prescribing drugs?

Do MHNs have the requisite knowledge and skills to prescribe? Would service users welcome nurses prescribing for them?

THE DEVELOPMENT OF NURSES AS NON-MEDICAL PRESCRIBERS

In England, the potential of nurses' prescribing was first mooted in a report by the Department of Health and Social Security on the future of community nursing.[8] This accepted that nurses should be able to prescribe from a limited range of medicines, appliances and dressings relative to district nursing practice. Following further consultation, nurse prescribing was seen to offer the potential of reducing time spent waiting for a doctor's signature, and a real alternative for the patient while validating existing nursing expertise. In 1994, eight pilot sites involved district nurses and health visitors in using a limited formulary to evaluate nurse prescribing.[8] These pilot studies succeeded in improving the service with more effective use of resources.[8] Although there were worries over the possible cost of implementation, the argument was made in a report commissioned by the government that this would be a better use of resources, and the case was made for prescribing to be broadened to be within nurses' scope of practice.[9] Although mentioned in the first Crown report,[9] prescribing was extended to mental health nurses only in 2001.[10]

Prescribing from a limited formulary was soon replaced by *extended formulary prescribing* (prescribing from an original list of 200 medicines) and *supplementary prescribing* (based on a clinical management plan once the doctor had assessed, diagnosed and prescribed medication for a patient). More recently, nurses can qualify and independently prescribe all drugs from the *British national formulary*,[11] with the exception of controlled drugs, and in the near future following a Home Office consultation independent prescribing of controlled drugs is expected.[12] Prescribing by MHNs has developed with over 600 out of

approximately 40 000 nurses trained on the independent/supplementary prescribing programme (N. Brimblecombe, personal communication, 2007). Guidance regarding the implementation has already been published,[7] and MHNs as prescribers have been mentioned as one of the new developing roles in the recent Chief Nursing Officer's (England) review for MHNs to make a difference.[13,14] There is growing evidence of prescribing by MHNs,[2,15–17] although there have been differing opinions as to why prescribing by nurses in mental health care has developed. These are explored below.

Progress chart

- 1990s: limited formulary prescribing
- 2001: extended formulary prescribing
- 2002: supplementary prescribing for nurses and pharmacists permitted, subsequently extended to physiotherapists, podiatrists, radiographers and optometrists
- 2005: supplementary prescribing of controlled drugs allowed
- 2005: independent prescribing for nurses and pharmacists announced
- 2008: full independent prescribing of controlled drugs for nurses and pharmacists expected

WHY HAS NURSE PRESCRIBING DEVELOPED?

Given that the health service is overstretched, there are political attractions in nurse prescribing, not least in relation to potential savings.[6,8,9,18] Today, some people with schizophrenia, depression, bipolar affective disorder and dementia are not receiving appropriate medical treatment. The reasons for this include the shortage of psychiatrists[6,16] and the failure of general practitioners (GPs) to diagnose and prescribe appropriately.[19] There exists also a pandemic of depression[20] and some service users feel disempowered because their non-medical needs are not being taken into consideration.[21] In this situation, appropriately trained MHNs could make a significant difference.

In seeking to improve the mental health prescribing service, non-medical prescribing would:[7]

- allow service users quicker access to medication, i.e. utilizing the greater number and expertise of appropriately trained MHNs so that medicine can be provided at the time of need;
- provide services more efficiently and effectively, i.e. utilizing a specialist MHN in primary care could provide expert and appropriate prescribing;
- increase service user choice, i.e. rather than one source of prescribing the service user has more flexibility to access appropriate interventions;
- make better use of nurses' skills and knowledge, i.e. validating the MHN intervention with medication, something which has been a major part of their role.

In principle, there are sound reasons for nurse prescribing. However, it has been argued[22] that nurse prescribing has been used by government to challenge the power of the medical profession. By diluting the doctors' prescribing power, there is a danger of 'dumbing down' prescribing. James and colleagues[23] saw the development of nurse prescribing as a quest for professionalization of their role rather than relying on the medical profession for professional legitimacy. Jones[18] highlights the ways in which nurse prescribing was kept on the government's agenda, suggesting that it may be a way of 'female nursing' asserting itself alongside 'male medicine'. McCann and Baker[24] allude to the 'care or cure' debate and the fact that prescribing by MHNs could mean that caring qualities could be lost to emphasis on the curing, diagnostic activity. Daniels and Williams[1] suggest prescribing by MHNs challenges nurses to work within a more holistic framework, with psychobiologic perspectives being as important as psychotherapeutic approaches. For some, biological interventions by MHNs is an area that mental health nurses have needed to address for some time in terms of skill and knowledge.[6,19,20] Keen[25] suggested that the increased emphasis on psychopharmacological approaches ensued from the decade of the brain (1990s) and was a result of pharmaceutical companies increasing their influence.

Despite these debates and, in England, the fallout from the Shipman inquiry, nurses and pharmacists will hopefully be able to prescribe controlled drugs from spring 2008. This will include MHNs in substance misuse services independently prescribing potent drugs. This represents a major shift from the limited formulary in the first wave of prescribing.[7,26]

Reflection

After reading the above section do you think that nurse prescribing has developed for 'therapeutic reasons', or will nurses be fulfilling doctors' roles on the cheap, effectively diluting care?

THE LAW PERTAINING TO THE PRESCRIBING OF MEDICINES (Box 67.1)

The Medicines Act of 1968, i.e. 40 years ago, remains the legislation guiding the prescribing of medicines. The Act restricts the prescribing of 'prescription only' medicines to 'appropriate practitioners' – originally doctors, dentists and veterinarians. The Medicines Act was amended by the Medicinal Products: Prescription by Nurses etc. Act 1992 to allow nurses to prescribe from a limited formulary. This was required to be followed by amendments to the Pharmaceutical Services Regulations 1994 to enable pharmacists to dispense prescriptions written by nurses. Supplementary prescribing rights were enabled by statute by The Health and Social Care Act (2001), therefore non-medical prescribers including MHNs can,

Box 67.1: Legislation relating to prescribing of medicines in the UK

- The Medicines Act (1968)
- The Medicinal Products: Prescription by Nurses etc. Act (1992)
- The Pharmaceutical Services Regulations (1994)
- The Health and Social Care Act (2001)
- The Misuse of Drugs Act (1971) modification order (2001)
- The Misuse of Drugs alterations (2005)

after undertaking the appropriate independent/supplementary prescribing programme, prescribe within their scope of practice. With the enactment of the Mental Capacity Act (2005), the changes to the Mental Health Act 1983 and with the added responsibility prescribing brings for the MHN who is adopting the role, a sophisticated understanding of the complex issues of consent also will be paramount.[27] Further exploration of this important topic is beyond this chapter, but this issue has been explored previously in depth.[27]

THE AUTHORITY TO PRESCRIBE

The two modes of prescribing open to the MHN are:[12]

1 Independent prescribing, in which any licensed medicine including some controlled drugs can be prescribed within the competence and scope of practice of the non-medical prescriber.
2 Supplementary prescribing, in which the non-medical prescriber in partnership with the doctor (independent prescriber) and service user are able to prescribe any medicine including controlled drugs and unlicensed medicines that are listed in a clinical management plan.

The mode of prescribing that the MHN will adopt in practice is dependent on the context and service users' presentation. At the time of writing, it appears that most mental health nurses will be more likely to be supplementary rather than independent prescribers. Some MHNs have stated that they would feel more comfortable working within a clinical management plan, which would allow novice prescribers to establish their new practice under the supervision of a psychiatrist.[20] In contrast to this, MHNs have identified where acting as an independent prescriber is more appropriate for contexts and service users' needs.[28] MHN prescribers also need to work within their own scope of practice and within their respective trust/organizational policy and seek appropriate union cover.[7,27,29]

Prescribing competence

Do MHNs have the appropriate assessment, diagnosis and consultation skills as well as the deep understanding of psychopharmacology needed to prescribe psychotropic drugs?[9,16,20] This has been discussed at length with doctors questioning nurses' capacity to prescribe safely.[30,31] It has also been debated whether or not the independent/supplementary prescribing course, with its 27 days of theory and 12 days of supervised practice, adequately prepares the MHN to practise as a prescriber, by contrast with the Master's prepared programmes in the USA.[20] Questions have also been raised over the need for a mental health specialist prescribing module,[32,33] and whether a mandatory module on management of medicines and psychopharmacology should pre-empt the existing course. We believe that MHNs will develop competence in prescribing according to their individual experience and knowledge attainment. Key components, however, are:

- pre-course confidence regarding knowledge of medication
- appropriate, supportive supervision by a psychiatrist
- accessing management of medicines and psychopharmacological education opportunities
- developing practice within a supportive and well-organized environment (one of the authors has developed his prescribing practice within such a context as part of a team development).

The context of mental health nurse prescribing

There is growing evidence that MHNs can prescribe safely, competently and to the satisfaction of the service user.[2,15,16] MHN prescribing appears to reflect MHN

TABLE 67.1 MHNs' areas of work following prescribing training

Area of work	Percentage (n)
Old peoples services	30 (14)
Early intervention and psychoses	20 (9)
Acute mental health	17 (8)
Substance Misuse	11 (5)
Crisis & Liaison Psychiatry	9 (4)
Forensic and prison services	4.33 (2)
Child and adolescent	4.33 (2)
Primary Care Liaison	4.33 (2)
Total	**100 (46)**

services across the lifespan,[17] although mostly in services provided in secondary care community and clinics[17] but with significant developments in inpatient care[15,17] and forensic, prisons and primary care settings.[7,17]

Hemingway and Harris[17] found that, following prescribing training, MHNs worked in a variety of areas (Table 67.1).

PERSONAL ILLUSTRATIONS

Although not fully representative of the services represented in Table 67.1, the personal illustrations below offer a picture of how nurses are applying prescribing in their day-to-day interventions.[a]

Personal illustration 67.1

Provided by Simon Greasley, Specialist Nurse in Substance Abuse, Sheffield Road Surgery, Barnsley; simon.greasley@gp-c85009.nhs.uk

Mark, a 32-year-old separated father of two, attended clinic for a new patient appointment after being referred by a needle exchange. Mark disclosed a 10-year heroin addiction, and was spending £150 per day; he was unkempt and malnourished, seldom having enough money for food. Mark reported being low in mood and was poorly motivated and could not see a way out of his situation.

Mark funded his habit by stealing electrical equipment from shops and was banned from the town centre. Mark reported living in a Ford Escort as his family had disowned him; he has children but rarely saw them as he was often dirty and he did not like his children to see him in the 'State I'm in'.

Mark was seen jointly by a GP and a nurse prescriber who specializes in substance misuse. It was decided that Mark would go on a methadone maintenance programme as he had tried this in the past by buying some on the streets and had found it helpful. A clinical management plan was agreed between the GP, nurse prescriber and the patient. Mark was started that day on methadone mixture at a dose of 40 ml.

Mark's methadone was increased by the nurse prescriber at following appointments; he was initially seen three times a week and settled on a dose of 110 ml of methadone. The patient felt comfortable on the dose and did not have to use heroin. He was supervised Monday to Friday in a community pharmacy for the first 3 months of treatment. In that time he quickly stabilized and started building bridges with his family and secured a property. After being in treatment for 6 months Mark had progressed to once a week pick-up of his methadone and started working full-time as a fork lift truck driver at a local distribution centre.

Mark now sees his children regularly and they stay at his house every weekend when it is his day off. Mark also plays football for a team of service users, and they now play in a local league. He feels the exercise has helped lift his mood and self-esteem, and training twice a week gives him a great feeling of achievement. Mark has made excellent progress and reports not having used heroin since being in treatment and has no desire or cravings to do so.

The availability of the nurse prescriber in the primary care setting meant that Mark's progress could be monitored regularly, which is something that was beyond the resources of the GP, plus it enabled the nurse to titrate his dose according to his needs and wishes.

---

[a] Permission was granted by all service users whose cases are presented. Pseudonyms have been used to protect confidentiality.

Personal illustration 67.2

Provided by Richard Clibbens, Nurse Consultant for Older People's Mental Health, Wakefield Memory Service, South West Yorkshire Mental Health Trust; Richard.Clibbens@swyt.nhs.uk

Phillipa is a 76-year-old woman referred to the memory service by her GP owing to increasing forgetfulness. The nurse consultant from the memory service arranged a home appointment to confirm a diagnosis following completion of a comprehensive health and social care needs assessment, CT brain scan, cognitive blood screening tests, ECG and identification of Phillipa's wishes relating to diagnosis disclosure. Phillipa received a diagnosis of mixed picture dementia, with features of probable Alzheimer's disease and vascular dementia. Information on available acetylcholinesterase anti-dementia medication was provided and discussed, including potential side-effects and benefits. Supplementary nurse prescribing was discussed and agreed with Phillipa and an information leaflet was provided on supplementary prescribing.

A clinical management plan was completed to enable supplementary nurse prescribing of acetylcholinesterase anti-dementia medication, agreed with Phillipa, the medical consultant (independent prescriber) and nurse consultant (supplementary prescriber). The nurse supplementary prescribing role enables the nurse monitoring the person's response to an anti-dementia drug to titrate the dose or discontinue it or to swap to an alternative acetylcholinesterase drug within the bounds of the clinical management plan. This enables quicker access to prescriptions and clearer lines of clinical accountability, without the need to wait for a doctor to write a further prescription when he or she has not personally assessed or monitored the person prescribed for. The nurse consultant diagnostic role has enabled the memory service to significantly increase the number of specialist diagnostic appointments available each week, in addition to providing greater choice and flexibility of where the appointment takes place with the provision of home diagnostic appointments in addition to hospital-based clinic appointments.

The nurse consultant issued a supplementary nurse prescription for donepezil 5 mg for a 6-week supply, together with service user information on the drug, possible side-effects and monitoring. Phillipa's progress was monitored 4 weeks later and the dose titrated up to 10 mg. Four weeks later, this was again reviewed by the nurse consultant and, as Phillipa was satisfied that this dose was well tolerated with no reported further deterioration in cognitive function, the GP was requested to take over shared care prescribing of this medication in accordance with the locally agreed shared care guidelines. Phillipa was invited by the nurse to attend an 8-week 'memory support group' together with a friend, partner or relative. This is facilitated by the Alzheimer's society and memory service nursing staff to promote effective coping with memory problems and dementia diagnosis, with additional ongoing access to a drop-in dementia cafe and service user/carer-organized social and support network of past group attendees.

Further 6-monthly monitoring appointments were arranged to review Phillipa's progress and enable discussion of issues such as advance decision-making. The dementia assessment and diagnosis pathway experienced by Phillipa was designed to provide information, choice and control during the difficult period of diagnosis and potential anti-dementia treatment. Good quality written information is crucial to support all stages of this experience, together with the opportunity for structured post-diagnostic support, access to service user support groups and networks and the availability of cognitive rehabilitation whether anti-dementia drugs are prescribed or not. Memory service users have identified that they value continuity of contact with a known member of staff and choice and flexibility in where and when assessments take place. Prescribing by the nurse consultant ensured continuity of contact from diagnosis through to the monitoring of medication, minimizing time delays and promoting choice and timely information for Phillipa.

Personal illustration 67.3

Provided by Michael Shaw, Senior Practitioner, Community Treatment Team (Calderdale), South West Yorkshire Mental Health NHS Trust; michael.shaw@swyt.nhs.uk

Tony is a 22-year-old single man. He was referred to a psychiatric outpatient unit by his GP when he threatened his mother with violence. Tony lives with his parents, and recently dropped out of his full-time college course. For several months the family has noticed that he is becoming more and more isolated and seems to be talking to himself in his bedroom. He no longer participated in the activities he used to enjoy, such as playing football and going out with his friends. He would spend the majority of his day in his bedroom watching TV or dosing.

Tony was seen by the consultant psychiatrist and was diagnosed as suffering from a psychotic illness of a schizophrenic type. There was no evidence of illicit drug use and he drank alcohol only on an occasional, social basis. He admitted to experiencing auditory hallucinations, and further assessment confirmed he was experiencing

fixed delusions of a persecutory nature and feelings of paranoia. On the whole, he did not present as aggressive and other than one episode of threatening to hit his mother there was no significant history of aggression, either physical or verbal. However, his relationship with his parents had deteriorated further since the GP referral and he was now living with his grandparents.

Tony did have some insight into his mental health problems in that he agreed that his behaviour was inappropriate and that he had lost touch with his friends and family and was becoming isolated and unapproachable. He agreed that he would accept the help from a mental health worker from the community mental health team and would consent to psychotropic medication. He had refused the offer of medication from his GP.

The consultant psychiatrist prescribed olanzapine 15 mg/day. For some weeks he was concordant with this treatment but eventually stopped taking the tablets. Following further outpatient assessment he was prescribed a depot anti-psychotic drug, flupentixol decanoate 40 mg every 2 weeks, and to continue the olanzapine at 10 mg. At this stage, he was referred to the medication and monitoring clinic for routine administration of the depot and for physical and side-effect monitoring.

After 6 months he eventually became asymptomatic in terms of psychosis; however, following observation and side-effect monitoring it became evident that he was experiencing akathisia (motor restlessness, an extrapyramidal side-effect) and weight gain. He had gained nearly 2 stones in weight and had an obese body mass index. As a supplementary precriber for Tony, using a clinical management plan devised by myself and the consultant (independent prescriber) and agreed by Tony, I discontinued the flupentixol decanoate and decreased the olanzapine to 7.5 mg/day and introduced depot risperidone at 25 mg (every 2 weeks). The rationale for this was that the olanzapine and flupentixol combination (which is polypharmacy) was probably the cause of the weight gain, and the flupentixol was the likely reason for the akathisia. Tony agreed to this prescribing decision, which was reached after considering and discussing all the alternatives with him.

He also attended a healthy living group, which he found helpful both in terms of peer support and advice and in terms of helping the gradual resocialization process.

He experienced a remission of the symptoms of akathisia and also gained no further weight. He was starting to see his friends again and was now living in his parents' home.

However, he was not losing weight despite dietary modification and exercise. Therefore, using the clinical management plan he agreed to discontinue the olanzapine. After several weeks he reported fluctuating feelings of paranoia and so the depot risperidone was increased to 37.5 mg (every 2 weeks).

Some months later, using the clinical management plan, this dose was reduced back to 25 mg. He has remained well in terms of mental health and experiences only very minimal side-effects, mainly occasional tiredness. His prolactin levels have remained within the normal range, as confirmed by routine blood monitoring every 6 months (research shows that anti-psychotic-induced hyperprolactinaemia is associated with risperidone use).

Using the clinical management plan, and following assessment of his concordance with medication (using the Drug Attitude Inventory), I have recently switched the route of the drug from the intramuscular preparation to oral. I continue to see Tony to monitor his progress and offer any support he needs.

In Tony's case, using supplementary nurse prescribing has enabled him to have quicker access to treatment and treatment changes.

Personal illustration 67.4

Provided by David Scarrott, Clinical Nurse Specialist, Crisis Resolution and Home Treatment Team, Rotherham; david.scarrott@rdsh.nhs.uk

Ruth is a 32-year-old married mother of two young children referred by her GP for admission into the acute assessment ward with a possible postnatal psychosis.

At the first assessment, she was very upset, scared and concerned for the safety of her youngest child.

She had a very fixed belief that this child's death was imminent, owing to her own inability to parent. She held a belief that it was God's way of punishing her for being a poor parent.

She described her own childhood as difficult – her own parents were very authoritative and demanded the highest of standards. Ruth was using these same high standards to judge her own parenting skills.

Her sleep pattern was poor, appetite had gone and she had no insight into her current situation. She had an episode of depression following the birth of her son 2 years ago. She saw the immediate situation as hopeless, but could concede that the situation could improve.

The consultant psychiatrist from the intensive home treatment team had given Ruth a diagnosis of postnatal psychosis and was in full agreement with the commencement of a clinical management plan.

This was completed using the Department of Health template for when the supplementary prescriber and the independent prescriber have access to the medical notes.

Ruth agreed to the home treatment nurses prescribing the medication regime and a management plan was formulated for the nurse to use drugs from the antidepressant and atypical anti-psychotic groups from the *British national formulary*.[11] The aim of the treatment was the alleviation of the symptoms, and it was agreed that the plan would be reviewed on a weekly basis at the home treatment team review.

Ruth and her family were relieved that an admission to hospital could be avoided and were committed to a community approach to the care.

Initially, this was very intensive with three visits a day needed, including a night call. Ruth was commenced on olanzapine 10 mg and mirtazapine 30 mg daily. She discussed her concerns at the possible side-effects of weight gain from the olanzapine, so using a direct payment we referred Ruth to join a local mainstream gymnasium. This helped to engage her medication regime and encouraged concordance.

Ruth initially took the medication, although she was convinced that there was nothing wrong with her and that it was her daughter's health that was being neglected. She was very fixed that her daughter's death was imminent.

Being in home treatment and implementing a clinical management plan allowed the medication regime to be very responsive to the patient's needs, with the people who knew her best making the small changes to her medication without involving doctors who might not know the patient or the background of the long-term objectives of a treatment plan.

Ruth responded very quickly to the introduction of olanzapine and shortly began to regain insight that the concerns about her baby's health could be a false belief. The clinical management plan finished when she was discharged to the community mental health team and the responsibility for prescribing passed back to primary care.

The home treatment team now has three qualified nurse prescribers, and two are undertaking the training. The team is working towards all registered nurses prescribing within a clinical management plan. It has proved a popular initiative with patients, their families, the nurses and medical staff, allowing patients real choice and flexibility with their medication and care.

These illustrations show that nurse prescribing in mental health is supportive of recovery principles, helping service users to gain control over their life.[34] Each case shows how the MHN prescriber enabled recovery based on individual and family needs, and that prescribing was only one part of service provision.

What stands out is that the MHN prescriber shows how the original brief of the introduction of non-medical prescribing can be met, therefore increasing choice, flexibility and accessibility of prescribing services and making better use of nurses' skills and knowledge.[7,29]

Reflection

After reading these illustrations, do you think that the nurses' roles met the criteria set out as the *benefits* of nurses developing a prescribing role?[7]

These are all examples of *supplementary* prescribing; however, three of the practitioners in these personal illustrations are actively planning to begin independent prescribing.

MENTAL HEALTH NURSE PRESCRIBING IN THE FUTURE

Prescribing by nurses in mental health is here to stay and has been proposed by two reviews of mental health nursing in England and Scotland[13,34] as central to MHNs improving their contribution to service user recovery.

Recommendation 13 of *From values to action*[13] stated:

Service providers to put in place arrangements to support the implementation of nurse prescribing, based on local need, taking into account the potential for service redesign and skill mix review, using both supplementary and independent prescribing arrangements.

MHN prescribing has also been recognized as a way of making existing posts available to focus on other aspects of care.[14] In essence, MHNs will be taking some of the medical roles of psychiatrists, allowing them to concentrate on complex and demanding cases. This could be seen as the dumbing down of some aspects of care provision, as forecast by McCartney *et al.*[22] However, as shown in the personal illustrations, MHNs can make a difference when involved in the prescribing of medication for service users in their care in an inclusive way.

The challenge is for MHNs to embrace this new role and to play a part in empowering service users to manage their prescribed medication effectively and individualized to their wishes and life-style as appropriate.

The introduction of the potential of independent prescribing by MHNs presents challenges for future educational provision. Independent prescribing can be seen as an advanced practice, and part of autonomous practice, including assessment/diagnosis/ordering tests and retests.[34] How universities facilitate MHNs' skills and knowledge attainment for advanced practice will be an important step for nurses to truly be prepared appropriately for the role of prescribing and allied interventions.[20,34] The future of educational provision may well need to be Masters-level advanced practice courses similar to the preparation of MHNs in the USA.[20,34]

SUMMARY

Mental health nurse prescribing is developing across the lifespan, from adolescents to older people, from inpatient to community and primary care.[17] Questions about this new service provision continue to be critically debated,[20,25,29,35] challenging MHNs to provide robust evidence of the efficacy of their prescribing interventions, safety of prescribing and improvement in the satisfaction of the service user. Only time will tell whether this will be the case, but studies have shown promise in the way that mental health nurses can make a difference in this context.[2,14,15] Indeed, the national evaluation of mental health supplementary prescribing in the UK by Norman and colleagues[2] showed no significant difference in the health and social care outcomes, or the costs of prescribing, for a sample of 90 service users with depression or schizophrenia, whose medication was managed by a mental health nurse supplementary prescriber or by an independent medical prescriber for a period of at least 6 months.

There was also no significant difference in the safety of prescribing between the two groups using National Institute for Health and Clinical Excellence audit parameters – although the quality of documentation was generally poor, with a substantial amount of information relevant to safe prescribing practice absent from the records of patients in both groups. Thus, there can be cautious optimism.

Nevertheless, what is paramount is the need for the planning of MHN prescribing to be clear and resourced appropriately. The potential change of role of the MHN towards prescribing needs to be considered thoroughly: whether it is needed, what would it change in service provision for the better, do nurses fully understand what is involved, will they be able to accept the responsibility? Prescribing is a powerful concept; to utilize the power nurses need to be competent, confident and, above all, aware that it is only one of the many reasons why service users' recovery takes place.

REFERENCES

1. Daniels NM, Williams GB. Medication in nursing practice: the psychiatric nurse and prescribing authority. In: Barker P (ed.). *Psychiatric and mental health nursing: the craft of caring.* London, UK: Arnold, 2003: 488–94.

2. Norman IJ, While A, Whittlesea C *et al. Evaluation of mental health nurse supplementary prescribing: final report to the Department of Health (England).* Kings College London, UK: Division of Health & Social Care Research, 2007.

3. Nolan P. *A history of mental health nursing.* London, UK: Chapman and Hall, 1993.

4. Rogers A, Pilgrim. D. *Mental health policy in Britain.* Basingstoke, UK: Palgrave, 1998.

5. Ramcharan P, Hemingway S, Flowers K. A client centred case for nurse supplementary prescribing. *Mental Health Nursing* 2001; **21** (5): 6–11.

6. Gournay K, Grey R. Should mental health nurses prescribe? Maudsley Discussion Paper No. 11. London, UK: Institute of Psychiatry, Kings College.

7. National Prescribing Centre. *Improving mental health services by extending the role of nurses in prescribing and supplying medication: a good practice guide.* London, UK: National Prescribing Centre, National Institute for Mental Health, Department of Health, 2005.

8. Luker K, Austin L, Ferguson B, Smith K. *Evaluation of nurse prescribing: final report.* The University of Liverpool, The University of York, 1997.

9. Department of Health. *Review of prescribing, supply of, and administration of medicines.* London, UK: HMSO, 1999.

10. Department of Health. *Nurses will prescribe for chronic illness.* Press release 2002/0488, 21 November. London, UK: DoH, 2001.

11. British Medical Association and the Royal Pharmaceutical Society of Great Britain. *British national formulary.* London, UK: British Medical Association and the Royal Pharmaceutical Society of Great Britain, 2008.

12. Department of Health. *Improving patients' access to medicines. A guide to implementing nurse and pharmacist prescribing within the NHS in England.* London, UK: DoH, 2007.

13. Department of Health. *From values to action: the Chief Nursing Officer's review of mental health nursing.* London, UK: DoH, 2006.

14. Department of Health. *Mental health: new ways of working for everyone. Developing a capable and flexible workforce.* London, UK: DoH, 2007.

15. Grant G, Page D, Maybury C. Introducing nurse prescribing in a memory clinic: staff experiences. *Mental Health Nursing* 2006; **27**: 9–13.

16. Jones M, Jones A. Delivering the choice agenda as a framework to manage adverse effects: a mental health nurse perspective on prescribing psychiatric medication. *Journal of Psychiatric and Mental Health Nursing* 2007; **14**: 418–23.

17. Hemingway S, Harris N. The development of mental health nurses as prescribers: quantifying the emergence. *Mental Health Nursing* 2006; **26** (6): 14–15.

18. Jones M. Case report. Nurse prescribing: a case study in policy influence. *Journal of Nursing Management* 2004; **12** (4): 266–72.

19. Nolan P, Haque S, Badger F *et al.* Mental health nurse perceptions of nurse prescribing. *Journal of Advanced Nursing* 2001; **36** (4): 527–34.

20. Bailey K, Hemingway S. Psychiatric/mental health nurses as non-medical prescribers: validating their role in the prescribing process. In: Cutliffe JR, Ward M (eds). *Key debates in psychiatric/mental health nursing.* London: Churchill Livingstone, 2006: 220–35.

21. Harrison A. Mental health service users' views of mental health nurse prescribing. *Nurse Prescribing* 2003; **1** (2): 78–85.

22. McCartney W, Tyrer S, Brazier M, Prayle D. Nurse prescribing: radicalism or tokenism? *Journal of Advanced Nursing* 1999; **29** (2): 348–54.

23. James V, Shepard E, Rafferty AM. Nurse prescribing: essential practice or political point? In: Jones M (ed.). *Nurse prescribing: politics to practice.* London: Ballière Tindall, 1999: 129–48.

24. McCann T, Baker M. Community mental health nurses and authority to prescribe medication: the way forward? *Journal of Psychiatric and Mental Health Nursing* 2002; **9**: 175–82.

25. Keen T. Gently applying the brakes to the beguiling allure of psychiatric/mental health nurse prescribing. In: Cutliffe J, Ward M (eds). *Key debates in psychiatric/mental health nursing.* London: Churchill Livingstone, 2006: 206–19.

26. Bridge J, Hemingway S, Murphy K. Implications of non-medical prescribing of controlled drugs. *Nursing Times* 2005; **101** (44): 32–3.

27. Jones S, Hemingway S, Williams B. Mental health nurses as prescribers: entering unchartered territory. *Mental Health Nursing* 2007; **27**: 14–17.

28. Clibbens R. *The implementation of independent non-medical prescribing framework.* Wakefield: South West Yorkshire Mental Health Trust, 2007.

29. Mills V, Firth J, Ross A. An evaluation of extended independent and supplementary prescribing in West Yorkshire. Unpublished report by the University of Huddersfield and West Yorkshire Workforce Development Confederation, 2006.

30. Avery AJ, Pringle M. Developing nurse prescribing in the UK. *BMJ* 2005; **335**: 316–17.

31. Cressey D. Nurses are floundering in their new prescribing role. *Pulse* 2007; **67**: 3.

32. Skingsley D, Bradley E, Nolan P. Neuropharmacology and mental health nurse prescribers. *Journal of Clinical Nursing* 2006; **15**: 989–97.

33. Wright K, Jones S. Delivering a non-medical prescribing module for mental health practitioners. *Mental Health Practice* 2007; **10** (5): 36–8.

34. Elsom S, Happell B, Mathias E. Mental health nurse practitioner: expanded or advanced? *International Journal of Mental Health Nursing* 2005; **14**: 190–5.

35. Snowden A. Why mental health nurses should prescribe. *Nurse Prescribing* 2007; **5** (5) 193–8.

SECTION 8

LEGAL, ETHICAL AND MORAL ISSUES

Preface to Section 8

Revolutions begin by some people living them; experiencing different and more integrative feelings about their relations to the outside world. They happen by some people giving up their cherished personal comfort and taking risks. If I desire real change, I must first be prepared for change in myself.

David Brandon

The 'mental health' field has become an increasingly contested ideological arena. At one pole lies the reductionist accounts of 'mental illness' as a genetically determined, biological disorder, and, at the other, an equally radical perspective, framing all so-called 'mental' problems as symptoms of social malaise, life crisis, poverty and disadvantage. Although talk about 'mental health nursing' has been around for decades, it remains an emergent concept; still trying to clarify its identity; still trying to establish where, if anywhere, it fits on the 'illness–social malaise' continuum. Will 'mental health nursing' remain a health-based discipline, retaining its powerful attachment to medicine; or will it become more of a social care discipline, relating to a wider range of social and community-based organizations? Perhaps the answer will lie somewhere else, in a radically new departure, involving the splintering or subdivision of the discipline into a range of 'caring' roles, all focused on nurturing human development.

Whatever the future holds, clearly there will be plenty of challenges. In this section, we consider some of the issues that challenge us today, and look likely to continue to tax us in the immediate future.

Mental health law and legislation differ from one country to the next, but all have common origins, concerning society's responsibility to contain and control its members. What are the challenges in fulfilling this responsibility?

This is linked strongly to issues of morality and ethics, which are discussed specifically in relation to the practice of psychiatric and mental health nursing. What are the core ethical challenges presented to nurses in the course of their working lives, and where do these ethical and moral dilemmas come from?

People who become psychiatric patients are men and women, with differing or changing sexual preferences. To what extent is their sexuality and gender relevant to their status as patients or clients or people in care?

As has been noted throughout this book, psychiatry is a powerful institution, and people in care often feel the effects of that power on an acutely personal level. In a democratic society, how do we begin to understand the concepts of freedom and consent, as they might apply in mental health care?

We return to our roots, metaphorically, to consider how mental health care might be delivered in a culturally meaningful way. In an increasingly multicultural society, what are the important considerations for the development of culturally appropriate care?

Finally, we return to the root meaning of psychiatry and psychotherapy – the study and attempt to heal the 'spirit'. What does spirituality mean in twenty-first century mental health care? How do nurses relate to something as vague, abstract and personal as the notion of our spiritual selves?

CHAPTER 68

Mental health, the law and human rights

Michael Hazelton* and Peter Morrall**

INTRODUCTION

Mental health problems and disorders affect a large number of people throughout the world. For some time now, supranational organizations such as the World Health Organization (WHO) have been warning that mental disorder is fast becoming one of, if not the, most serious health problem globally. Even a brief look at the relevant statistics highlights this as a major area of health concern. For instance, hundreds of millions of people worldwide are affected by mental, neurological or behavioural problems at any point in time. Each year almost 900 000 people die by suicide. Approximately one in four patients visiting a health service has at least one mental, neurological or behavioural disorder, but in the majority of cases these are neither detected nor treated. There is considerable cross-over between mental illness and chronic physical conditions such as cancer, cardiovascular diseases, diabetes and HIV/AIDS – such mental and physical health co-morbidities have become one of the most important treatment challenges in the mental health field internationally; contributing to unhealthy behaviour,

non-compliance with prescribed medical regimens, diminished immune functioning and poor prognosis.

Cost-effective treatments are now available for most mental disorders, which if correctly applied would enable most of those affected to function more effectively in society. However, there are many barriers to effective treatment, including lack of recognition of the seriousness of mental illness and poor appreciation of the benefits associated with providing effective mental health services. There are also ongoing problems of stigma and discrimination. In various ways, policy-makers, insurance companies, health and workplace policies and the public at large discriminate between physical and mental health problems. Moreover, there are important differences in the priority that different countries place on the provision of mental health care. While many wealthy countries underfund mental health services,[1] the situation is much worse in middle and low-income countries, where less than 1 per cent of health expenditure is allocated to mental health. In most countries today, mental health policies, legislation, community care services and facilities and treatments for people with mental illness are not given the priority they deserve.[2]

*Michael Hazelton is Head of the School of Nursing and Midwifery and Professor of Mental Health Nursing at the University of Newcastle, Australia. He published widely on mental health and mental health nursing, is a past Editor of the International Journal of Mental Health Nursing and is currently a member of the editorial boards of the International Journal of Mental Health Nursing, The Australian and New Zealand Journal of Psychiatry, Nursing and Health Sciences and Mental Health and Substance Use: Dual Diagnosis. He has been the recipient of a number of awards for mental health nursing research, and in 2003 was made a Life Member of the Australian College of Mental Health Nurses, the highest honour awarded by that professional organization.

**Peter Morrall has been in the business of 'madness' for 30 years. His latest publications include Murder and Society (2006; Wiley); Madness and Murder (2000; Whurr); Mental Health: Global Policies and Human Rights (edited with Mike Hazelton, 2004; Wiley); The Trouble with Therapy (2008; Open University Press). He lives in York and likes fiddling with the saxophone.

This chapter addresses the ways in which the political and legal systems make provision for the care, treatment and control of people with mental health problems and disorders. The chapter describes the development of mental health policy and legislation in two countries – England and Australia – as examples of how mental health issues and challenges have been addressed within broader social–political contexts. England has been selected as a nation state with origins in the 'old world', while Australia is included for its 'new world' or post-colonial status. Importantly, both countries have placed considerable political emphasis on mental health reform in recent decades. The chapter includes a consideration of the contents and operation of current mental health legislation in both countries, including discussion of the extent to which recent reforms have been undertaken against a background of human rights concerns and the public's right to safety.

ENGLAND

England, although a very old country, is thoroughly embedded in today's global society. Bygone and contemporary social contexts of England are indicative of its age, *and* of the Western-inspired cultural and economic 'new world order' that proliferates today. English 'madness' has also a particular history and a present that make it an exemplary case study with reference to mental health, the law and human rights. England's management of the mad (both care and control) was transported (literally and conceptually) to many parts of the world, as was its legal system. However, England has been rather less proactive over human rights, and in the twenty-first century it has still not enshrined in law a balance between personal liberty and social control.

History

The management of madness has a long history. Protecting the human rights of the mad has a relatively short history.

Whether by 'amateurs' (families and communities) or 'professionals' (principally psychiatry and psychiatric nursing), those perceived to be mentally deviant have been admonished, denigrated, restrained, secluded, excluded and medicalized. Troublesome and troubled people (the disturbed, dangerous and disruptive) have succumbed to all manner of management, involving a fantastic array of implements and impositions aimed at, but only rarely achieving, changes to their human performance (their thoughts, behaviours and emotions). Examples include whips; shackles; water; exercise; work; electricity; an ever-expanding range of pharmaceuticals; and latterly a plethora of psychotherapies.[3] The realities of having to control the most disturbed, disruptive and

dangerous of the mad was to affect the nature of policies and practices of the 'professionals', and was the main reason for their creation. That is, without a society being troubled by madness then the amateurs will remain in charge of the management of madness.

Medical management of madness has been in existence, either bubbling in the background or fermenting in the foreground, for thousands of years.[4] In the Greco-Roman Empires, madness was considered a disease and thereby the province of those practising medicine. During medieval times in Europe and in the Middle East, medical opinion existed alongside, although dominated by, religious and folk notions of madness. But by the end of the nineteenth century in the West, medical domination of madness had become virtually absolute. Notwithstanding challenges from other disciplines and epistemologies purporting to deviate from the medicalized management of madness, this remains the case today. Furthermore, advances in medical diagnostic technology, psychopharmacology and psychosurgery, the embracing by psychiatry of talking therapies, together with the de facto if resentful compliance of psychiatric nursing, and the capitulation of clinical psychologists and psychotherapists to the 'power of psychiatry' (because they do not offer radical alternatives), medical control over madness and the mad business is once again in the ascendancy.

The law has been, compared with medicine, a relative latecomer to the management of madness. Indeed, it has been medical involvement in madness that has necessitated the expansion of legalized control. Moreover, it was the surge in the formal and institutionalized segregation of the mad during the nineteenth century that necessitated an expansion of medical and legal collusion to control this form of social deviance. Specific legislation was then enacted rather than relying on local convention or criminal law.

Although most mad people were cared for by families if not troublesome, or simply roamed from place to place, community-based segregation had been advocated for troublesome mad people in ancient society. For example, Plato advised that 'if a man is mad' (no mention is made of mad women) his family must prevent injury to himself, to others, and to property by keeping him at home.[5]

European laws in the Middle Ages were not consistent within a country and were influenced substantially by religious beliefs and decrees. This meant that madness was vulnerable to being perceived as witchcraft.[6] Such a label could have far worse consequences for the accused (torture, damnation and execution) than being left to roam or being confined.

Before the seventeenth century in England the troublesome mad, if not controlled by their families, were sent to bridewells (Tudor 'houses of correction'), common gaols and workhouses. The legislation that impelled this type of incarceration was not designed to deal with madness, but to punish the 'indolent' sections of the working class and serve as a warning to others that life would be hard if work was not found.[7] The building of workhouses began in the 1630s. The Poor Law Act of 1601 gave the responsibility to every English parish for the elderly, sick, idiots and lunatics within its borders. The Act of Settlement 1662 restricted what was already very limited support for only those who were bona fide residents. If such social deviants could not be encouraged to leave a parish, then they were sent to the workhouses along with the unemployed.

Institutional segregation began in England in the thirteenth century when the religious order St Mary of Bethlehem of London ('Bedlam'), which was already providing care for the physically sick, began to accept the mad.[8] Other institutions were set up in continental Europe by the beginning of the Renaissance in the fifteenth century. For Michel Foucault,[9] the seventeenth century was the age of the 'Great Confinement'. For example, 6000 mad people were incarcerated in the Hôpital Général de Paris, and incarceration of the mad was then to spread throughout France.[5]

But the 'Great Confinement' came later in England. Apart from Bedlam, there were commercially run madhouses in the seventeenth century, but these were in the main for the 'wealthy mad'. By the eighteenth century the 'poor mad' might enter one of the newly created charitable voluntary asylums. John Perceval, son of the only British Prime Minister to be assassinated (Spencer Perceval), was incarcerated in a private asylum near Bristol from 1830 to 1832 having been diagnosed with schizophrenia. He wrote a remarkable account of his loss of liberty in a book titled *Perceval's narrative*:[10]

> Now with regard to my treatment, I have to make at first two general observations … First, the suspicion and the fact of being incapable of reasoning correctly, or deranged in understanding, justified apparently every person who came near me, in dealing with me also in a manner contrary to reason and contrary to nature … Secondly, my being likely to attack the rights of others gave these individuals license, in every respect, to trample upon mine … Instead of great scrupulousness being observed in depriving me of any liberty or privilege … on the just ground, that for the safety of society my valuable rights were already taken away, on every occasion, in every dispute, in every argument, the assumed premise immediately acted upon was, that I was to yield, my desires to be aside, my few remaining privileges to be infringed upon for the convenience of others.

Reflection

Describe the ways in which John Perceval's liberty would have been restricted within this nineteenth century asylum. How is the liberty of patients residing in a twenty-first century mental health ward/unit restricted?

It was, however, not until the nineteenth century that confinement ('asylumdom'[11]) of not just the troublesome mad but as a potential option for anyone troubled by psychological distress became widespread. The 1845 Lunacy Act in England forced local authorities to provide for the mad through a massive public building programme. Asylums were to house more than 100000 inmates by 1900. Moreover, these public asylums were given wide legal powers to compulsorily detain the mad.[7]

The designation of insanity had, ever since the Middle Ages, caused a dilemma for the law. The notion that the mad were not 'human', but essentially 'beasts', was common. As such, they should logically be treated differently by the courts from other social deviants (for example, criminals). But, for much of the period prior to asylumdom there is no or little specialist mental health policy let alone legislation.[12]

In England asylumdom was not instigated by the medical profession. Doctors were not regarded as having effective remedies for madness. They were, as local notables, invited by the local authorities to act as administrators. Incarceration was perhaps for years if not life, and inmates were exposed to horrendously callous treatments (cold baths, hot baths, rotating machines, bloodletting, purges and emetics). Today such lengthy confinement and bizarre managing of the mad seems to be an inexcusable abuse of human rights. But the asylums had been built not only to separate the mad from the 'normals' but also to provide what was considered at the time humane care. In comparison with how the majority of the population lived in the nineteenth century, those in the asylum (usually) received food, shelter and medical attention (all be it rather primitive). Philanthropy and kindness co-existed with eugenics and cruelty.

The Victorian asylums, and those of the twentieth century, were an enormous financial investment, which could not be replicated today. They reflected high ideals. The mad could partake of fresh air in rural surroundings, in the extensive grounds and gardens that most of the asylums had procured.[13] Food and water was comparatively fresh, clean and nutritious. Recreation and rest were encouraged.

The profession of medicine had by the end of the nineteenth century monopolized the market in madness, having successfully neutralized the challenge from the Quakers who had set up alternative institutions based on 'moral therapy'. Psychiatry was well established as a medical area of expertise, and madness had become as much an 'illness' or 'disorder' as pneumonia or malaria. Legislation for the control of the mad had become highly specialized to authenticate the mass segregation of the mad. Institutional segregation and the law provided a captive audience on whom doctors could experiment and thereby develop their subspecialty of psychiatry.

Present

By the middle of the twentieth century, various social, technological and economic changes were affecting where and how the mad were to live. The discovery of anti-psychotic drugs, the unsustainable financial burden of running what were now 'mental hospitals', along with a general shift in Western culture towards more tolerance and liberty, and a score of reports about cruelty inflicted on the residents of these institutions, heralded widespread de-carceration.[11,14] While not articulated as such, mental health law was supporting the human rights of the mad to live in mainstream society, and this trend for legislation to emphasize respect for the mad was occurring throughout Europe, North America and Australasia.

Psychiatry's dominant position in the management of madness was undermined at this stage. The anti-psychiatry movement, social work, psychology, psychotherapy and psychiatric nursing were all vying for the top position in the hierarchy of disciplines managing madness. However, the power of psychiatry has since been boosted considerably by the arrival of new psycho-pharmacological products, the development of sophisticated diagnostic technology, improvements in psychosurgery, and the accomplishment of the genome map. Moreover, psychiatry was able to manoeuvre the management of madness to its benefit by maintaining its dominance in inpatient services, laying claims to the technical outpourings of new scientific developments, and establishing dominance of 'community mental teams' and their organizational offshoots.[15]

Community care in England, however, has been a disaster for the human rights of the mad. Government financial obligations to the large institutions were not effectively transferred to local authorities to fund community care facilities. Despite the growth of empowerment and advocacy movements, and 'consumer' representation within the mad industry, along with proclaimed extra funding, the setting up of a national mental health institute to oversee mental health policy and practice and the installing of a 'mad' tsar, institutional care and care in the community continues to be inadequate, inefficient and inexplicable.

Furthermore, inpatient services had been run down so there was no longer 'asylum' available for many of the troublesome and troubled mad.[16] The large number of mad people who have ended up in prison during the era of community care should be considered a human rights issue. In a paradoxical reversal of history more and more of the mad are nowadays becoming criminalized.

Human rights abuses are no longer hidden within the walls of institutions, but are apparent in the streets of cities. Homelessness, poor housing, unemployment and inadequate supervision are human rights abuses that match the cruelties of the asylums. This abuse and neglect is ongoing:[17]

> Tens of thousands of people [in England] going through a severe mental health crisis are being deprived of the NHS treatment and support that was promised by the government, parliament's spending watchdog disclosed today.
> The National Audit Office said many people with psychosis, severe depression or anxiety could avoid the stress and stigma of being admitted to a psychiatric ward if they were provided with appropriate care at home.

Fifty years after the Universal Declaration of Human Rights and the European Convention on Human Rights, England (and the rest of the United Kingdom) compiled its human rights legislation,[18] therein providing for qualified human rights of the mad.

Reflection

If you were the 'mad tsar' of the English mental health system, what policies would you eradicate and install?

First, the act contains a principle of 'limited rights', meaning that 'persons of unsound mind' can be detained as long as the procedures used are legal. Second, there is a principle in the Act of 'qualified rights'. This determines that a person's private life can be interfered with 'for the protection of the rights and freedoms of others'. Compulsorily removing an individual from his or her home to enforce psychiatric treatment is therefore a possibility if he or she was determined to be a risk to others or himself/herself. Third is the principle of 'proportionality'. This principle allows human rights to be interfered with providing such interference is not arbitrary or unfair. That could result in the use of restraint and seclusion where this is viewed as necessary by the psychiatric disciplines. A fourth principle of the Act is that of 'incompatibility'. All present and future legislation has to be in accord with the Human Rights Act (1998). Given that the Human Rights Act is already extremely 'flexible' with regard to the management of the mad, the designers of new mental health legislation should not have too much difficulty formulating compatible 'exclusion' clauses.

Furthermore, the Human Rights Act states that before an individual can be compulsorily detained a 'true' mental disorder must be established by 'objective' medical experts (Article 5). However, the act omits to define mental disorder in any detail, and the inadequate defining of mental disorder also occurs in previous, present and impending mental health legislation. Moreover, it tautologically posits that the mental disorder must be of a kind or degree warranting compulsory confinement and that the validity of continued confinement depends on the persistence of such a mental disorder. There are also a number of exceptions to these specific conditions. For example, compulsory admission can occur in emergencies, and discharge may be deferred where there is 'public danger'.

But, under Article 3 of the Human Rights Act there are no exclusions relating to the mad. This Article states that there must be 'freedom from torture and inhuman or degrading treatment or punishment'. However, it remains contentious whether or not compulsory detention, restraint, seclusion, enforced treatment and electro-convulsive therapy are inhuman and degrading or therapeutically necessary.

The old mental health laws (the 1983 Mental Health Act and the 1995 amendment Mental Health Patients in the Community Act) have long been discredited. They do not deal adequately with the practicalities of contemporary management, nor with human rights. But the form that new legislation should take has been contested vigorously by the psychiatric disciplines' representative organizations along with mental health support and lobby groups. It has taken nearly 10 years for the mental health legislation of England to be given Royal assent. At the beginning of 2008, however, it had still not been implemented.

Demands for the replacement of the 1983 Act began early in the 1990s following public, media and political outcries at homicides committed by people with a mental disorder and the apparent lack of responsibility for such incidents being displayed by the psychiatric disciplines.[19] The social context for such demands, however, was much wider: the development of post-liberal society.[1,19]

Western liberal democracies have, since the 1980s, moved towards the formation of a new social contract between government and the governed based on rights and responsibilities.[20] Citizens, having been given more personal freedoms and civic duties, are expected to be self-controlled rather than controlled by the hegemonies and agencies of the State. However, those who do not regulate themselves have become susceptible to 'risk' appraisal, regulation and severe social condemnation. Certain groups are demonized: paedophiles, criminal recidivists, prostitutes, drunks, noisy neighbours, school truants and religious extremists. Post-liberal social control increased markedly (for example, detention without trial or for long periods before judicial review) following the bombing of the New York World Trade Center on 11 September 2001, and terrorist atrocities in Bali (2002), Madrid (2004) and London (2005).

Post-liberal laws also apply to the troublesome mad. Risk assessment is de rigueur in all mental health provision, supervision registers for 'severely mentally ill' living in the community is recommended policy, electronic surveillance is common within inpatient facilities, and seclusion and restraint are not only accepted practices but on the increase.

Although mental health law has long been associated with control (for example, much of the 1983 Mental Health Act is designed to deal with compulsory detention of those who are a risk to themselves or others), the Mental Health Act of 2007 is specifically attempting to resolve the tension between post-liberal personal liberty and post-liberal social control. On the one side is the assumed need to protect society from 'risky' mad people living in the community (especially those who refuse to take their medication). On the other is UK and European human rights and related legislation such as the 2005 Mental Capacity Act.[21] Since the introduction of the 1998 Human Rights Act, case law at the European Court of Human Rights has indicated that compulsory admission into institutional care can be considered a 'deprivation of liberty' and thereby to contravene European human rights legislation.

But as the World Health Organization (WHO) realizes,[22] the law does not necessarily safeguard the liberties of the mad:

> People with mental disorders are, or can be, particularly vulnerable to abuse and violation of rights. Legislation that protects vulnerable citizens (including people with mental disorders) reflects a society that respects and cares for its people. Progressive legislation can be an effective tool to promote access to mental health care as well as to promote and protect the rights of persons with mental disorders. The presence of mental health legislation, however, does not in itself guarantee respect and protection of human rights.

However, the 2007 Mental Health Act, although ostensibly containing many safeguards against abuse in terms of inappropriate detention and treatment (especially through the Mental Health Review Tribunal, and independent advocates), has swung more towards control than liberty. For instance, in adopting a single definition of mental disorder to avoid the confusion of different categories evident in earlier legislation, madness is able to be ascribed by the psychiatric disciplines; by allowing long-term detention according to the availability of 'appropriate treatment' for a particular patient, decisions regarding what constitutes 'appropriate treatment' fall to the psychiatric disciplines; and, highly significant within the context of post-liberalism, is the introduction of supervised community treatment (SCT), a similar mechanism to community treatment orders provided for in recent Australian mental health legislation.

Patients who have been detained in hospital may be placed on SCT when they return home. These patients will have to accept that the prescribed treatment (mainly medication) must be taken. The Act is attempting to stop the 'revolving door' of patients leaving hospital psychologically stable but then discontinuing their treatment and being readmitted. Others may 'fall through the net' of management altogether. In extreme cases, some patients may commit suicide or murder.[19,23]

AUSTRALIA

Australia was born modern – the political and institutional arrangements that were the antecedents of the modern Australian state were transported from the UK along with the convicts during the early colonial period. Present-day Australia is an advanced industrialized nation with a culturally diverse population of approximately 21 million. Average life expectancy is in the early eighties for women and the late seventies for men. Indigenous Australians constitute about 2 per cent of the population and have a much lower life expectancy: on average, approximately 20 years less than for their non-indigenous counterparts.[24] The Australian political system is federated, with a national government and eight state/territory governments.

History

European colonization commenced in 1788 and almost immediately it became necessary to provide for those requiring treatment for insanity. Initially, this might be provided in a local gaol or other 'safe place'. Later, special asylums were established.[25] The asylums of the colonial period were usually located away from main population centres, and concentrated on providing a controlled and sheltered life for the residents.[26–28] The second half of the nineteenth century was a period of considerable development in mental health care, especially in New South Wales. Visits by mental health experts to the UK resulted in the introduction of moral treatment and the building of new asylums.[25]

The first half of the twentieth century, which included the two world wars and the Great Depression was characterized by a severe shortage of funds, which seriously hampered the development of mental health services. In the mid-1950s a national inquiry into mental health services reported that local services compared unfavourably with similar countries.[27] However, post-war optimism contributed to an increase in social pressure for reform, including the mental health field. Throughout the 1960s and 1970s the now renamed psychiatric hospitals came under increasing public scrutiny as a mental health community care movement emerged, and new developments in social psychiatry and psychopharmacology suggested a treatment revolution.[27] By the late 1970s community mental health services were developing as the old psychiatric institutions were being allowed to run down. While such developments were poorly coordinated and uneven across the country, they nevertheless contributed to a decline in the availability of psychiatric beds – from 281 beds/100 000 in the early 1960s to 40 beds/100 000 by the early 1990s.[29]

The history of Australian mental health services indicates that significant reforms have almost always been accompanied by concerns surrounding the neglect and abuse of patients. In New South Wales alone about 40 inquiries were conducted into psychiatric services between the early colonial period and the late 1980s.[28] This combination of controversies and official inquiries

into mental health care has continued into the present period.

Present

While Australia has a modern, comprehensive mental health system there is nevertheless a high unmet need for treatment among the many Australians who have a mental health problem or disorder.[30] Since the early 1990s a range of mental health-related issues and service shortcomings have been addressed through a National Mental Health Strategy, implemented through successive 5-year plans.[31] The main policy expectations are that those who use mental health services ought to be able to do so close to where they live; that services should be responsive to the needs of users; that effective care ought to be delivered continuously across a range of inpatient and ambulatory services; and that mentally ill persons ought not to have to endure reduced citizenship entitlements and human rights abuses.[32,33]

While the reforms have undoubtedly brought increased resources and operational improvements,[34] there has been little evidence of beneficial impacts on citizenship participation and human rights protections for those with mental illness and their families.[35] Concerns remain as to whether the policy changes of the last decade can be enforced in practice[36] and the extent to which the onus for claiming the rights set down in policy falls on the vulnerable individuals concerned – the users of mental health services.[37] Indeed, recent evidence suggests that membership of a 'caring' profession such as nursing is insufficient to safeguard against the likelihood of discrimination in the workplace on the basis of mental illness.[38] An area of ongoing concern has been the provision of the rehabilitation, housing and support services necessary for life in the community, all of which remain seriously underdeveloped.[39]

Reflection

Commentators such as Watchirs and Johnstone have suggested that it can be very difficult to enforce the reforms set out in mental health policy in practice. Can you think of six reasons why this might be so?

Sadly, the recently highly publicized cases of Cornelia Rau and Vivian Alvarez (Solon), women with histories of mental illness who were treated as illegal immigrants by Australian immigration officials, have raised concerns regarding the efficacy of deinstitutionalization as public policy and highlighted the ongoing human rights abuses to which those who have mental illness may be exposed.[30] It is ironic that in an era in which the policy aim is to liberalize mental health services, the experience of being in 'care' may be more restrictive than in the past. Inpatient mental health facilities have become much more security conscious. Risk management often seems to take precedence over therapeutic concerns – often in response to workplace health and safety requirements. Closed circuit television monitoring, locked windows and doors, the use of 'high-dependency' (i.e. seclusion) rooms, staff duress alarms, and the use of security guards are widespread in Australian inpatient mental health facilities.[24] There has also been an increasing reliance on the use of 'no tolerance' polices in dealing with patient aggression and violence. This development has recently been criticized for taking the therapeutic initiative away from healthcare practitioners, thus removing opportunities for building client engagement with care.[40,41]

One important aspect of the Australian mental health reforms has been the revision of mental health legislation. At the most basic level mental health law is concerned with finding a balance between safeguarding the rights of individuals with mental illness and also the public's right to safety. As part of the National Mental Health Strategy, a number of initiatives have sought to review and redirect Australian mental health legislation,[37,42] which operates within separate State and Territory jurisdictions. A recent example of revised Australian mental health legislation is the Mental Health Act 2007 (New South Wales), an outline of which is provided in Table 68.1.

While the 2007 Act continues many of the features of the 1990 Act, important new features include: a focus on providing care and treatment in the community; assistance for those affected by mental illness to live and work as active citizens; increased emphasis on involving patients in treatment planning; acknowledgement and support of the role of carers of people with mental health problems and disorders. Other new developments include authorization of ambulance officers to transport persons to mental health facilities; removal of the requirement for inpatient admission in making community treatment orders; extension of duration of community treatment orders to 12 months; prohibition of psychosurgery; and limiting Mental Health Review Tribunal approvals for electroconvulsive therapy to 12 treatments.[43]

TABLE 68.1 Mental Health Act 2007 (New South Wales)

Chapter 1: Preliminary	Outlines the name of the Act, specifies the date of commencement and defines key terms
Chapter 2: Voluntary admission to facilities	Outlines types of voluntary admission to mental health facilities, including children and persons under guardianship. Outlines procedures for discharge, review and detention. Specifies procedures pertaining to refusal of voluntary admission
Chapter 3: Involuntary admission and treatment in and outside facilities	Outlines procedures for involuntary detention and treatment in mental health facilities, including admission to and initial treatment; continuing detention; and leave of absence. Specifies procedures for involuntary treatment in the community using community treatment orders
Chapter 4: Care and treatment	Outlines principles and procedures pertaining to the care and treatment of persons under the Act and the use of mental health treatments including pharmacological and electroconvulsive treatments. Provides for consideration of the rights of patients detained under the Act and their primary carers, including requirements for notification and information sharing regarding medication and rights surrounding detention. Specifies procedures for the transfer of patients to or from mental health facilities and/or other health facilities
Chapter 5: Administration	Outlines administrative procedures for the governance of public and private mental health facilities. Specifies procedures governing responsibilities and powers of official visitors, accredited persons and powers of inspection
Chapter 6: Mental Health Review Tribunal	Outlines the constitution, membership, responsibilities and procedures of the Mental Health Review Tribunal, including the use of legal representation, determination of whether a person is a 'mentally ill person' or a 'mentally disordered' person and the use of interpreters
Chapter 7: Jurisdiction of Supreme Court	Outlines rights of appeal to the Supreme Court, including considerations of jurisdiction
Chapter 8: Interstate application of mental health laws	Outlines procedures for the transfer of patients between NSW and other Australian States and Territories. Specifies procedures for the interstate implementation of NSW community treatment orders; the recognition of and provision of services in respect of interstate orders; and the apprehension of persons under the powers of an interstate Act
Chapter 9: Miscellaneous	Outlines restrictions, limitations and regulations pertaining to the Act

An important feature of the 2007 Act is that more formal consideration will now be given to the role that carers play in providing ongoing emotional and material support for people with mental illness. There will now be provision for appointing 'primary carers' for each patient of a mental health facility. This may be a guardian, where one has been appointed, or a parent, if the patient is under 18 years of age. Most often, however, a spouse or other person primarily responsible for providing care and support for the patient will be nominated. Primary carers will have rights to certain types of information in respect of a patient, such as notification within 24 hours that a person has been involuntarily detained in a mental health facility.[43]

Reflection

Look up the mental health act or similar legislation that operates in your state or country and compare it with the Mental Health Act 2007 (New South Wales). In what important ways is your local mental health legislation similar to and different from the NSW Act?

While the 2007 Act undoubtedly reflects the ongoing liberalization of mental health legislation in Australia and overseas, cases such as those of Cornelia Rau and Vivian Alvarez (Solon) highlight the ongoing serious vulnerabilities of people with mental health problems and disorders, and the extent to which widespread public perceptions in this area continue to be influenced by age-old fears surrounding madness. Following Turner[44] we can note the ontological vulnerabilities and social precariousness associated with mental illness and question the extent to which the policy and legislative reforms of the last decade have made real progress in addressing these.

A key aspect of the recent mental health reform directions has been an attempt to transform the mental patient into the mental health consumer. While the aim has been to elevate the status of those with mental illness as citizens, the form of citizenship envisaged is based on an economic model – a kind of health consumerism.[24,30,35] However, the application of health consumerism to mental health care is by no means straightforward. The life experiences of people with mental illness are difficult to reconcile with the idea of 'consumer choice'. We need only think of what it might be like to face involuntary admission to a psychiatric facility; or to be the subject of a community treatment order requiring treatment with powerful psychiatric drugs to raise concerns about the nature of 'mental health consumerism'. Indeed, even 'voluntary' patients can find it difficult to manage the structures and procedures found in mental health services.[42]

In the end, it may be that the notion of mental health consumerism is contrary to other forms of citizenship which operate more on the basis of 'grass roots' activism. Many users of mental health services prefer to be thought of as survivors, or activists rather than consumers. Increasingly, such people are entering into social and political alliances which seek to challenge and reshape the institutional structures and arrangements that govern mental health care.[30] While there have undoubtedly been significant changes in mental health policy and mental health legislation in the last decade, it is not yet apparent that the new directions have brought clear improvements to the lives of those who are the users of mental health services.

SUMMARY

The relationships among mental health, the law and human rights have been and remain those of complex tension. In both 'old world' England and 'new world' Australia, issues of fear and control coexist with structural and attitudinal changes regarding, for example, citizenship and consumer choice. To understand this complex tension, what has to be appreciated is the historical background to the management of 'madness' in both countries *and* the present seismic social transformations originating from economic and cultural globalization that are affecting every country.

In *Mental health: global policies and human rights*[1] we explored the historical and present contexts of mental health from a range of countries: China, Russia, the USA, Italy, India, Brazil, Egypt, Mozambique, and England and Australia. In this chapter, we have included an additional list of relevant websites containing information about the tense complexity of balancing such factors as the liberty of, and understanding towards, people with mental disorder, the legitimate requirement to protect society, and the abuse of mentally disordered people by society and psychiatry.

REFERENCES

1. Morrall PA, Hazelton MJ (eds). *Mental health: global policies and human rights*. London, UK: Whurr, 2004.

2. World Health Organization. *Mental health: the bare facts*. 2008. Available from: www.who.int/mental_health.

3. Morrall P. *The trouble with therapy: sociology and psychotherapy*. Maidenhead, UK: Open University Press/McGraw-Hill, 2008.

4. Porter R. *A social history of madness: stories of the insane*. London, UK: Weidenfeld & Nicolson, 1987.

5. Porter R. *Madness: a brief history*. Oxford, UK: Oxford University Press, 2003.

6. Gibson M. *Reading witchcraft: stories of early English witches*. London, UK: Routledge, 1999.

7. Busfield J (ed.). *Rethinking the sociology of mental health*. Oxford, UK: Blackwell, 2001.

8. Andrews J, Porter R, Tucker P, Waddington K. *The history of Bethlem*. London, UK: Routledge, 1997.

9. Foucault M. *Histoire de la folie à l'âge classique* [translated as *Madness and civilization*]. Paris, France: Plon, 1961.

10. Perceval J. *Perceval's narrative* (edited by G Bateson). London, UK: Hogarth Press, 1962: 119–20; original 1840.

11. Scull A. *Decarceration: community treatment and the deviant: a radical view*, 2nd edn. Cambridge, UK: Polity Press, 1984.

12. Robinson DN. *Wild beasts & idle humours: the insanity defense from antiquity to the present*. Cambridge, MA: Harvard University Press, 1996.

13. Gittins D. *Madness in its place. Narratives of Severalls Hospital*. London, UK: Routledge, 1998.

14. Miller P, Rose N (eds). *The power of psychiatry*. Cambridge, UK: Polity Press, 1986.

15. Morrall PA. *Mental health nursing and social control*. London, UK: Whurr, 1998.

16. Hill A. The mental health units that shame the NHS. *The Guardian* 2008; **29 June**.

17. Carvel J. Patients in mental crisis not getting help promised. *The Guardian* 2007; **7 December**.

18. Home Office. *Human Rights Act 1998*. London, UK: Stationery Office, 2000.

19. Morrall PA. *Madness & Murder*. London, UK: Whurr, 2000.

20. Rose N. Government and control. *British Journal of Criminology* 2000; **40**: 321–39.

21. Department of Health. *Mental Health Act 2007 – overview*. Updated 16 November 2007, 2008. Available from: www.dh.gov.uk/en/Policyandguidance/Healthandsocialcaretopics/Mentalhealth/DH_078743.

22. World Health Organization. *Resource book on mental health: human rights and legislation*. Geneva, Switzerland: WHO, 2005: 21.

23. Morrall P. *Murder and society*. Chichester, UK: Wiley, 2006.

24. Hazelton M, Clinton M. Mental health, human rights and citizenship in Australia. In: Morrall P, Hazelton M (eds). *Mental health policy: global policies and human rights*. London, UK: Whurr, 2004: 43–60.

25. Crichton A. *Slowly taking control?* Sydney, Australia: Allen and Unwin, 1990.

26. McDonald D. Hospitals for the insane in the young colony. In: Pern J, O'Carrigan J (eds). *Australia's quest for colonial health. Some influences on early health and medicine in Australia*. Brisbane, Australia: Department of Child Health, Royal Children's Hospital, Brisbane, 1983: 183–90.

27. Lewis M. *Managing madness: psychiatry and society in Australia 1788–1980*. Australian Institute of Health. Canberra, Australia: Australian Government Publishing Service, 1988.

28. Human Rights and Equal Opportunity Commission. *Human rights and mental illness. Report of the National Inquiry into the Human Rights of People with Mental illness*. Canberra, Australia: Australian Government Mental Publishing Service, 1993: 5.

29. Australian Institute of Health and Welfare. *Australia's health 2000: the seventh biennial health report of the Australian Institute of Health and Welfare*. Canberra, Australia: Australian Institute of Health and Welfare, 2000.

30. Hazelton M. Mental health reform, citizenship and human rights in four countries. *Health Sociology Review* 2005; **14** (3): 230–41.

31. Australian Health Ministers. *National Health Plan 2003–2008*. Canberra, Australia: Australian Government Publishing Service, 2003.

32. Australian Health Ministers. *Mental health statement of rights and responsibilities*. Canberra, Australia: Australian Government Publishing Service, 1991.

33. Australian Health Ministers. *National mental health policy*. Canberra, Australia: Australian Government Publishing Service, 1992.

34. Whiteford H, Buckingham B, Manderscheid R. Australia's national mental health strategy. *British Journal of Psychiatry* 2002; **80**: 210–15.

35. Hazelton MJ, Clinton M. Mental health consumers or citizens with mental health problems and disorders? In: Henderson S, Petersen A (eds). *Consuming health: the commodification of health care*. Oxford, UK: Routledge, 2001: 88–101.

36. Johnstone M. Stigma, social justice and the rights of the mentally ill: challenging the status quo. *Australian and New Zealand Journal of Mental Health Nursing* 2001; **10** (4): 200–9.

37. Watchirs H. *Application of rights analysis instrument to Australian mental health legislation. Report to the Australian Health Ministers Advisory Council National Mental Health Working Group*. Canberra, Australia: Commonwealth Department of Health and Aged Care, 2000.

38. Joyce T, Hazelton M, McMillan M. Nurses with mental illness: their workplace experiences. *International Journal of Mental Health Nursing* 2007; **16** (6): 373–80.

39. Jablensky A, McGrath J, Herrman H *et al*. Psychotic disorders in urban areas: an overview of the study on low prevalence disorders. *Australian and New Zealand Journal of Psychiatry* 2000; **34**: 221–36.

40. Wand T, Coulson K. Zero tolerance: a policy in conflict with current opinion on aggression and violence management in health care. *Australian Emergency Nursing Journal* 2006; **9**: 163–70.

41. Stone T, Hazelton M. An overview of swearing and its impact on mental health nursing practice. *International Journal of Mental Health Nursing* 2008; **17**: 206–12.

42. Centre for Health Law, Ethics and Policy. *Model mental health legislation. a discussion paper*. Newcastle, Australia: Centre for Health Law, Ethics and Policy, The University of Newcastle, 1994.

43. New South Wales Health. *Information bulletin: Mental Health Act 2007*. Document No. IB2007_053. NSW, Australia: Department of Health, 2007. Available from: www.health.nsw.gov.au/policies/.

44. Turner B. Outline of a theory of human rights. In: Turner B (ed.) *Citizenship and Social Theory*. London, UK: Sage, 1993: 162–90.

WEBSITES FOR MENTAL HEALTH, THE LAW AND HUMAN RIGHTS FROM SELECTED COUNTRIES

China

Amnesty International: *People's Republic of China: Amnesty International Report 2007*. Available from: www.amnesty.org/en/region/asia-and-pacific/east-asia/china

Mental health in China: And now the 50-minute hour. *The Economist* 16 August 2007. Available from: www.economist.com/world/asia/PrinterFriendly.cfm?story_id=9657086

India

Center for Advocacy in Mental Health. *Appeal to health professionals and human rights activists against the use of electroconvulsive therapy in India's mental health institutions*. 2008. Available from: www.sacw.net/2002/wamhicAppeal120403.html

Mental health care needs help. *India Together* 10 January 2008. Available from: www.indiatogether.org/2005/jun/hlt-mental.htm

USA

Advancing Science, Serving Society. *Science and human rights program psychology and human rights: the Ignacio Martin-Baro Fund in review*. 2005. Available from: http://shr.aaas.org/report/xxv/baro.htm

Amnesty International. *United States of America: Amnesty International Report 2007*. Available from: http://thereport.amnesty.org/eng/Regions/Americas/United-States-of-America

Russia

Gay Russian wins employment discrimination case in landmark ruling: court rules homosexuality is not a mental disorder. 2005. Available from: www.ukgaynews.org.uk/Archive/2005sept/2201.htm

Jenkens J. Mental health in post-communist countries. *BMJ* 2005; **331**: 173–4. Available from: www.bmj.com/cgi/content/full/331/7510/173

South Africa

Advancing Science, Serving Society. *The legacy of apartheid: mental health: human rights and mental health*. 2008. Available from: http://shr.aaas.org/loa/recsg.htm

Citizens Commission on Human Rights. *Investigating and exposing psychiatric human rights abuse* [South Africa]. Available from: www.cchr.co.za/message.html

Chile

Center for Mental Health and Human Rights (CINTRAS). *Psychological damage as a consequence of torture and other forms of political repression* [in Spanish – translatable through Google]. 2008. Available from: www.cintras.org

World Health Organization. *Mental Health: Chile*. 2008. Available from: www.who.int/mental_health/policy/country/chile/en/index.html

Vietnam

Amnesty International. *Viet Nam: Fear for safety/torture/ill-treatment/arbitrary detention. Amnesty International urges sending appeals to free lawyer Bui Thi Kim Thanh*. 2006. Available from: www.vietnamhumanrights.net/website/AI_112406.htm

Human Rights Watch. *Testimony on the human rights situation in Vietnam*. 2007. Available from: http://foreignaffairs.house.gov/110/ric110607.htm

Zimbabwe

Knight ZG, Wallace K. *The experience of two displaced white women Zimbabwean farmers: the impact of organised political violence*. 2008. Available from: www.btinternet.com/~psycho_social/Vol5/JPSS5-ZL1.htm

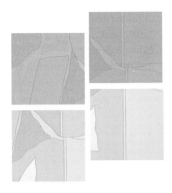

CHAPTER 69

Ethics and nursing

Richard Lakeman*

INTRODUCTION

At the heart of psychiatric–mental health nursing lies the interpersonal relationship between the nurse and a person experiencing some form of distress. Both are part of a web of relationships encompassing family, friends, colleagues, organizations, communities and wider society. All these groups have an interest in and expectations about the nature of the relationship between the nurse and person. Individuals often find themselves in relationships with nurses at a time of extreme powerlessness, distress, vulnerability and estrangement from others, and this is compounded by the stigmatizing effects of being labelled and treated as mentally ill. How the nurse exercises power, behaves in relation to the person, and balances the expectations and wishes of all interested parties have profound ethical implications.

Ethics is concerned with human action, what one ought to do, and forms of belief about right and wrong human conduct.[1] Ethics may also be viewed as the basis for choosing the kind of professional life we believe we should lead, so that we need not look back with regret in the future.[2] The practical purpose of ethics should be to provide guidance to the nurse on the 'right' course of action in a given situation. Nurses are involved in ethical enquiry whenever they spend time considering what they

should do in relation to others and may be said to be practising ethically when they choose to do the right thing and can provide an ethical justification for their actions. In the field of psychiatric–mental health nursing, uncertainty about the right course of action or ethical problems are encountered on a day-to-day basis and hence nurses require highly developed skills in ethical reasoning and ethical problem-solving.

ETHICAL THEORY

An **ethical problem** may be said to arise when moral principles conflict in a given situation. An **ethical dilemma** may be likened to an **avoidance–avoidance** conflict in which there may be several alternative courses of action but each one of them is negative or in some way punishing. Examination of conflicting principles can alert one to a problematic ethical situation. However, the solution to the problem may not be readily apparent. Seedhouse[3] suggests that a willingness by health workers 'to do the right thing' or 'to be moral' is insufficient to ensure ethical practice. People need tools in the form of an understanding of ethical theory and philosophy to guide and justify their actions. It is beyond the scope of this chapter to provide more than a sketch of some of the key features of a few theories of ethics.

*Richard Lakeman is a Lecturer in Mental Health at Dublin City University, Ireland. He has worked across the spectrum of mental health service settings, most recently setting up a homeless outreach team and acting as clinical nurse consultant on a mobile intensive treatment team in North Queensland, Australia. Currently, he has a general interest in helping people to realize recovery and in how people live with extraordinary experiences such as hearing voices and suicidal thinking.

Deontological theories

Deontological theories are concerned with 'duty' and beg the question 'What is my duty in a given situation?' Many people believe it their moral duty to obey God. However, this can be problematic as there are irreconcilable differences between people regarding the will of God and many people who deny the existence of a divine voice of authority. An influential alternative to theological ethics was proposed by Kant, who suggested a universal law, which demands '... that we should only act in accord with a given principle or set of principles if we can, at the same time, reasonably will that it should be binding on all others through space and time'.[4] In many instances Kant's 'categorical imperative' prescribes a very clear duty to act. For example, it would be unconscionable to lie to anyone regardless of the consequences because of the chaos and damage caused if all people were permitted to lie in all circumstances. The ability to reason is central to Kantian notions of morality, and, without the capacity to reason, one cannot enjoy full status as a moral citizen.

Consequentialist (teleological) theories

A broad range of theories hold that actions may be judged good or bad depending on the consequences they produce, i.e. the ends justifies the means. Contention exists over what counts as good consequences (e.g. material gain, happiness, freedom, dignity) and whose good should be promoted (e.g. self, the in-group, the profession, society, or all people equally). Utilitarianism is a theory that proposes that an act may be judged good or bad depending on whether it promotes the greatest balance of good over bad, happiness over unhappiness, and pleasure over pain. The world tends to be viewed in terms of peoples' collective and overall interests. When considering where to invest scarce health resources a utilitarian perspective would require an investment to ensure the greatest good for the greatest number. Whilst at face value this appears appealing, it may also serve as a justification to discriminate and alienate minority groups, or minority points of view.

Moral principles

When people make statements such as 'it isn't fair' or 'do no harm' they are perhaps unwittingly appealing to moral principles. Whilst there may be disagreement about which principle might carry the most weight in a given situation, or how principles might be used, there is general agreement that the principles of autonomy, non-maleficence, beneficence and justice underpin ethical behaviour in health care.

Autonomy is a principle that implies that people ought to be free to choose and act any way they wish providing their actions do not violate or impinge on the moral interests of others. Autonomy means having respect for the self-determination or decision-making of others. Maintaining or promoting people's autonomy and some form of equitable partnership poses one of the greatest ethical problems for psychiatric nurses in their relationships with people in distress.[5–8] In psychiatric–mental health nursing, autonomy is frequently overridden in the interest of promoting the principle of **beneficence** or 'doing good'. Unfortunately, what counts as good and who should be the arbiter of what is good are contentious questions. For example, some people argue that suppression of symptoms through medication is a hindrance to real recovery and that the adverse effects of psychotropic drugs are often worse than experiencing the illness itself.[9] Forcibly administering medication against a person's will is a clear breach of a person's autonomy, yet may be justified by the health professional as being in the person's best interests. Such actions are always ethically problematic and require a legal mandate to act.

'Madness', more latterly 'mental illness', has long been recognized as a class of experience which may profoundly affect the capacity of people to make free and rational choices. Plato is credited with saying 'A man ... either in a state of madness, or when affected by disease, or under the influence of old age, or in a fit of childish wantonness, himself no better than a child ...' could not be held accountable for his crimes.[10] The Kantian notion of morality is focused on the rational being,[11] and someone who is unable to reason from this point of view is unable to possess free moral agency or be held to account for their actions. However, people's reasoning is rarely totally impaired.

Mental health professionals are often called upon to make judgements about a person's **capacity** to make autonomous choices for official purposes (e.g. to determine whether a person requires civil commitment under a Mental Health Act) and during their everyday encounters with people. Even when people are deemed to be severely mentally ill, with some degree of impaired judgement, they are likely to continue to possess intact decision-making capacity in at least some areas. Health professionals therefore require skill in recognizing the person's current strengths or 'ablement' in order to protect and promote a person's autonomy.

Non-maleficence means to do no harm and has long been claimed as 'the first' principle of ethical health care. The meaning of harm is open to interpretation but certainly extends to psychological, social or spiritual harm or suffering. The principle of non-maleficence would provide justification to condemn any act, which might cause another avoidable suffering. The principle of non-maleficence requires nurses to take heed of the experience of patients and first recognize the potential suffering that illness and treatment may cause. For many people the experience of treatment and hospitalization is fraught with traumatic and harmful experiences as illustrated by an extract from Susie's story:[12]

> … Nothing compared with the horror of this psychiatric unit. It was the most traumatic experience I have ever had … It was just total madness, twenty four hours a day, no privacy, all my personal belongings were stolen. I was sexually abused by another patient. I was assaulted. I had no safe space. They were trying to de-stim [sic] me in a very unsafe environment … using punishment.

As well as considering Susie's story in terms of non-maleficence, one may also consider that she had been treated unjustly and did not deserve to be exposed to abuse in any circumstances. **Justice** is a term that may be considered in many ways. For example, justice may be considered as fairness, as revenge (retributive justice), as an equal distribution of benefits (distributive justice) or as equality. Justice in its various forms is a central ethical concept, is used as a justification for action and breached in a myriad of ways in relation to people with mental illness.

The various conceptions of justice can come into play in any given situation. Often, this is a recipe for conflict as illustrated here:

> John is a person who went without treatment for a psychotic disorder because he lived in a rural area where services were not available. He shot and killed a family member, believing him to be possessed by a devil. He was found not guilty of murder because of insanity and was remanded in a psychiatric forensic unit for treatment. He responded quickly to treatment but was not released for some years for fear of the public reaction to a 'murderer' not serving a reasonable sentence. On discharge he was unable to find reasonable accommodation because of the publicity surrounding the case and was unable to find employment because of a history of mental illness.

That John went without early recognition, treatment or care is an issue of distributive justice. Despite responding to treatment, and presumably posing no great risk to others if adequately supported, his continuing incarceration became an issue of retributive justice (or punishment). This in itself was unfair as he was found 'not guilty' because of insanity. Neither was his experience of discrimination 'fair' when he was discharged. The principles of retributive justice and justice as fairness conflicted in John's situation and no doubt impeded his recovery.

Sometimes the ethical principles at stake in a given situation may be vague but they may be refined further into **moral rules**. For example, the rule 'tell the truth' (**veracity**) arises from the principle of autonomy, which recognizes that rational people ought to be free to

choose. Telling a lie therefore would deprive a person of the information needed to make a rational choice and so nurses are obliged to be truthful towards people they care for. While telling a blatant lie may be ethically indefensible in many situations, telling the 'whole truth' can sometimes be destructive. Lawler[13] coined the term **'minifism'** to describe '… verbal and/or behavioural techniques which assist in the management of potentially problematic situations by minimising the size, significance, or severity of an event involving a patient'. 'Good' health professionals are likely to modify their 'gut responses' or manage their self-presentation in their interactions with people in order to minimize the harmful impact of revealing their responses. For example, a nurse may be disgusted by a person's incontinence or body odour. However, being brutally honest about their feelings may shame the person or otherwise cause them a loss of dignity. To prevent such harm, the nurse may sensitively prompt or assist the person to attend to self-care. The person may ask 'This must be really disgusting?' or state 'I'm disgusting', but sensitive nurses will modify their response to minimize the incident and maintain the person's dignity.

Reflection

- Which ethical principles do you value the most and why?
- When considering an ethical course of action do you primarily consider the consequences of the action or the action itself?
- What ethical theory do you identify with and why?

Virtues

A virtue approach to ethics emphasizes the moral character of the person through the question 'What sort of person should I be?' In practice, the resolution of ethical problems commences from a sensitivity to situations as ethically problematic[14] or that the person is vulnerable.[15] In the example outlined above, a nurse may be said to have acted compassionately by minimizing his or her response to the person's incontinence. Virtues provide the disposition that enables a person to reason well and to act according to the right reasons.[16,17] Virtues may also provide an intuitive choosing of the right course of action when moral principles conflict.

The virtues that nurses need depend on the roles they choose or are required to assume.[18] Early nurse education stressed obedience and loyalty to the doctor; however, contemporary nurses are likely to require other virtues, for example courage to realize roles such as advocate. Some virtues which are most useful for psychiatric nursing include:[17,19]

- *Compassion*: the capacity to share another person's suffering and appreciate their humanity and vulnerability.
- *Humility*: remembering that we do not possess all the answers. Humility inclines us towards listening and learning from others.
- *Fidelity*: which provides a commitment to help other people and reminds us that clients have a claim on us that endures even when they refuse the treatment we offer.
- *Justice and courage*: provide not only an inclination to do what is right and fair, but also provide a motivation to act to protect others' interests even at some personal cost.

Virtues may not be learned in the same way as principle-based theories of ethics. They are necessary, but insufficient to ensure ethical behaviour. However, virtues may be developed through practices such as reflection, good mentorship and supervision.

Reflection

Consider a nurse or person you work with whom you consider to be a virtuous person. How does he or she demonstrate virtue?

Criticisms of traditional approaches to ethics

Traditional Western philosophical ethics has failed to provide an account of, or prescribe, a unifying morality that has utility in all situations. The impartiality and detachment associated with traditional ethical decision-making approaches is also at odds with the lived experience of psychiatric nurses, which is characterized by involvement and value-laden clinical judgement. Spreen Parker[20] suggests that dialogue between people concerning their individual needs, desires and values is seen to threaten the impartiality required to make principle-based decisions and '... moral reasoning is confined to an abstract monologue, rather than a relational, embodied dialogue between human beings struggling to make sense of deeply perplexing situations'. At least some nurses have suggested that traditional approaches to ethical problems are antithetical to the practice of nursing founded on an ethos of care, which stresses involvement and the highly contextualized nature of human relations.[21,22]

Further criticisms of traditional approaches to ethics centre on the failure of ethics to address the systematic and systemic oppression of whole peoples, cultures and groups such as the mentally ill. Johnstone[23] suggests that mainstream bioethics is ethnocentric and sexist in nature and has '... only limited practical value and application in the realms of clinical practice in the health care arena'.

An evolving **ethic of care**[24] and feminist approaches to ethics[25] offer different lenses to examine the nature of ethical problems, and prescribe factors other than principles, for example relationships and institutionalized oppressive structures that require consideration in ethical enquiry.

Reflection

Principle-based and ethics of care approaches to ethical problems may lead to different outcomes or decisions depending on particular contextual factors. Consider the issue of preventing someone from attempting suicide. Ordinarily depriving someone of their liberty on the basis of something they might do could not be condoned from a principle-based approach.

- What factors might justify intervening to prevent suicide from a principle-based and ethics of care approach?

THE MANY ETHICAL DIMENSIONS OF PSYCHIATRIC NURSING

Culture and moral pluralism

Globalization facilitated by communication technologies, ease of travel and news media have made it increasingly obvious that people can and do have vastly different world views including conceptions of what is good or proper conduct. All people exist within and are inextricably part of a culture which colours the way they see, make sense of and interact with the world. **Culture** consists of the values or abstract ideals held by members of a given group, and the norms or definite rules and principles people are expected to follow.[26] Culture exists prior to ethics, not the other way round.[4] A cursory review of cultural differences reveals a **moral pluralism**, which must be explored and negotiated if nurses are to claim ethical sensitivity or practice. It is not enough to rely on tradition, appeal to authority, adherence to the law, or to simply follow instructions to ensure ethical practice. To act ethically requires as a starting point an awareness of factors that colour and shape our view of the world.

The traditions and practice of Western psychiatry and psychiatric nursing arise largely from Western values and views of health and wellness. These views are value laden. They are embedded in institutional processes and are often taken for granted by health professionals. For example, most health professionals would accept the 'holistic' notion of people being biological, psychological, social and spiritual beings, although in recent years biogenetic models of distress have been loudly championed within psychiatry.[27] Western psychiatry and psychiatric institutions tend to view the origins of mental distress as biological, which might in turn manifest as psychological or social symptoms. Treatment is primarily biological (i.e. drug treatments) with adjunctive psychological (e.g. psychotherapy) or social (e.g. family education or therapy) interventions. In contrast (as illustrated in Figure 69.1), people from traditional indigenous cultures such as Australian Aboriginal or New Zealand Maori are likely to conceive of distress quite differently, viewing the root cause of distress as being of spiritual or social origin, giving rise to psychological or biological symptoms. The problem itself may be located in the family group or community rather than the individual.

In traditional cultures, when a person manifests with what may appear to be symptoms of psychosis or depression, the problem may be viewed as arising from some spiritual or social transgression possibly of a family member or an ancestor. Treatment may involve prayers or rites, or 'making good' the perceived wrongdoing. In such circumstances a biological deterministic view and treatment of the person may not merely reflect a difference of opinion or a benign approach to care but may cause irreparable damage to the person through removing hope of recovery or causing estrangement from those who might best be able to help.

The importance of respect for cultural difference and culture as fundamental to understanding and promoting health is being recognized (see the *ICN code of ethics for nurses*[28]). Respect for cultural difference requires as a starting point examining one's own values, and the 'taken for granted values and assumptions' that guide everyday behaviour. Culture permeates every facet of human understanding, and provides the threads of the moral fabric upon which may be woven the many relationships which psychiatric–mental health nurses enjoy.

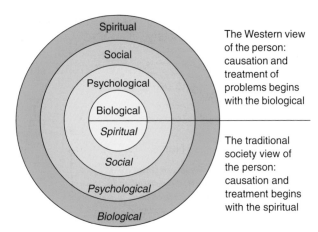

Figure 69.1 The Western holistic view and the traditional cultural view of the person

Reflection

- What do you value?
- What is your personal understanding of the term mental health?
- Contrast your values and ideas about mental health with someone from a different cultural background.

Power and discourse

It has already been suggested that people experiencing mental illness often engage in relationships with psychiatric nurses at times when they have diminished power. A practical purpose of ethics is to guide the use of power by health professionals. This power is often made invisible, or legitimized through the use of language, and often reflects the world view of the dominant culture. Foucault[29] described the formulation of communicative processes on the basis of power as 'discourse'. The world of clinical practice has its own language and logic, which is self-sustaining, in that it serves as a justification for action.[30]

The particular world view – or '**ideology**' – to which clinicians are aligned in practice is founded on assumptions about what it means to be a person, what it means to be distressed, and what it means to nurse the distressed person. These assumptions are never value neutral. Almost invariably they are bound by culture and often serve to subjugate or take away the power of others. The psychiatric discourse shapes people's stories, which are invariably stories of dysfunction and pathology. This is not to say that psychiatric discourse is bad per se. However, it is wrong to assume that psychiatry has the only story to tell in relation to people who are distressed. Indeed, 'narrative therapy' acknowledges that the stories that communities of persons negotiate and engage in give meaning to their experience. Narrative therapy aims to assist people to tell alternative stories, or 're-author' their lives according to preferred stories of strength and courage.[31] In considering the moral lives of psychiatric nurses in relation to communities, groups and individuals, the nurse must be mindful of the power of language, attuned to the various discourses that shape reality, and be open to alternatives.

Psychiatric nurses and society

It may be useful to think of the moral lives of psychiatric nurses as having many dimensions and encompassing a number of key relationships (Figure 69.2). At the 'macro' level nursing is part of society and reflects, maintains and promotes certain interests of society. Governments are concerned with the best way to tackle societal problems and dictate what is considered proper conduct towards others through the passing of laws and regulations.

People diagnosed mentally ill have been and continue to be poorly served by societies and have often experienced abuse, infringement of **human rights** and discrimination. Most Western countries have now adopted the United Nations resolution on the protection of persons

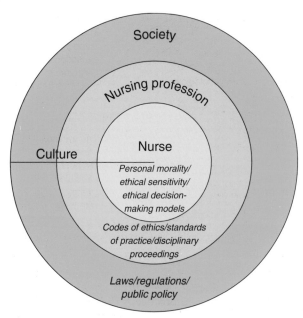

Figure 69.2 The moral lives of psychiatric nurses

In the best possible world one might safely rely on the laws of society as the framework required to behave ethically. Unfortunately, blindly following the law is perhaps the lowest level of moral comportment. Nurses who colluded in the extermination of the mentally ill in Nazi Germany and the labelling as mentally ill and forced medication of political dissidents in the former Soviet Union might claim that they were acting lawfully. However, few (at least from a position of detachment) would conclude that they were acting ethically. At best the law can provide only a crude guide to ethical behaviour in the nurse–person relationship through providing negative sanctions for extreme forms of immoral behaviour, e.g. assaulting another, and defining the circumstances under which certain rights may be breached in the provision of treatment.

Reflection

- Make a list of rights
- For each right identified consider what duty a nurse may have in relation to those rights

with mental illness and the improvement of mental health care.[32] This is an international agreement, which requires member countries to ensure that people diagnosed with mental illness are able to exercise all the civil, political, economic, social and cultural rights enjoyed by others. It also sets out standards for care and treatment and articulates the right for people to be treated in the **least restrictive environment**.

In contemporary Western societies the criminal justice and mental health systems have a mandate for **social control**, i.e. legally mandated and defined roles to contain, control or modify certain types of behaviour deemed undesirable. The threshold for interfering with or restricting a person's liberty in order to assess or treat mental illness involuntarily has typically been raised to diminished rationality, lack of insight and imminent and serious risk of harm to oneself or others.[5] Social control functions involving surveillance, observation and managing difficult behaviours continue to be observed and described in nursing practice.[33] However, even if involuntarily assessment is legally mandated people continue to be entitled to claim other **rights**. Some rights claims require a clear legal and ethical duty of the nurse (e.g. the right to information requires that people be told of their legal status). However, in some instances it may be uncertain where the nurse's duty lies in relation to rights claims. For example, people may claim a right to legal advice or an alternative medical opinion. Nurses have a clear duty not to impede the person from seeking such advice but they may not be bound to facilitate it. The right to be treated with **respect** appears to be foundational, but like notions of beneficence it is open to interpretation.

Particular discourses may be taken up, promoted and shaped by social movements. **Social movements** are loose networks of people who share assumptions about particular problems and who cooperate, in various ways, to address those problems.[34] There have been sustained criticisms of the coercive practices of psychiatry since the anti-psychiatry movement developed in parallel with human rights movements in the 1960s. The most famous advocates such as Szasz[35,36] challenged the existence of mental illness and maintained a critique of psychiatric authority that is often dismissed but has not been comprehensively refuted. More recently, a **critical psychiatry** movement has emerged[37] that is critical of coercive treatment and overemphasis on biological explanations of mental distress. Critical psychiatry seeks to reform psychiatry rather than challenge its authority. There might also be said to be a recovery movement – an offshoot of self-help, survivor movements and anti-psychiatry which aims to promote the idea of personal recovery. The **evidence-based practice** movement promotes a view that the practice of psychiatry and nursing should be based on the best available evidence. Reform and change in the labelling and treatment of people with mental illness has largely been a product of pressure from social movements. They often serve to illustrate problematic areas of taken-for-granted practice or contradictory philosophy and illustrate the social nature of the psychiatric project. The nurse needs to consider the assumptions underpinning these movements, the questions they raise and how compatible they are with each other.

Reflection

A person is diagnosed with schizophrenia and compelled to receive a medication which is known to play a causative role in diabetes and is likely to lead to irreversible movement problems. From the perspective of the social movements outlined above, what questions are raised by this scenario?

- What social movements do you identify with?
- Who are the heroes of that movement?
- What values bind people together?
- What action or change is sought by members?

The nursing profession

Nurses are also part of a profession, which implies a body of knowledge and set of values held by its members. Professions exist in the context of society and reflect many of the values of that society. **Codes of ethics** and standards of practice reflect the publicly declared values of professions. Theories, while less publicly accessible, provide professionals with some framework to understand and guide their work. Watson[38] has described nursing as a 'moral ideal'. Certainly 'grand' nursing theories paint an ideal picture of the nurse's work. No 'grand' nursing theory adequately deals with the problem or the role of nursing in compulsory treatment. Nevertheless, nurses can look to their profession for more specific guidance on how to be and behave in relation to other people.

Reflection

- Review the *ICN code of ethics for nurses*[28] and study the standards under each element of the code.
- Reflect on what each standard means to you. Think about how you can apply ethics in your nursing practice.
- Use a specific example from experience to identify ethical dilemmas and standards of conduct as outlined in the code. Identify how you would resolve the dilemma.

The nursing profession through regulatory bodies is able to **censure** members for behaving in an unprofessional manner, or acting beyond the boundaries of professional conduct. At a less formal level nurses may regulate their own conduct through discourse about professional **boundaries**. A boundary marks out territory, or the margins of an entity. A boundary violation in relation to nursing practice implies that someone is not behaving as a nurse should, and that they are being something else. Boundary discourse appeals to elements of principle-based, rule-based and virtue ethics as well as etiquette. There are a number of potential areas of boundary violation:

- **competency**: practising beyond one's competency or training
- **roles**: practising outside of institutional roles or assuming roles with competing interests
- **physical contact**: inappropriate touching or sexual contact
- **space and place**: undertaking therapeutic interventions outside of usual hours of work or in an inappropriate geographic space (e.g. in someone's bedroom)
- **remuneration**: receiving or soliciting gifts or favours for work done
- **dress and appearance**: dressing provocatively or in an intimidating manner
- **communication**: using inappropriate, derogatory or overfamiliar language
- **intimacy**: becoming 'too close' to clients; disclosing too much about oneself.

Some boundary violations unequivocally reflect a wrongdoing. For example, most professional bodies take a dim view of practitioners having sexual relationships[39] with clients, in part because the client is always more vulnerable in a professional relationship. However, the margins of professional boundaries are often blurred. Nurses experience an ongoing tension between the need to maintain distance from clients and the desire to establish therapeutic relationships.[5] Distance may play a role in maintaining a sense of safety but a degree of intimacy is almost always needed to develop trust and identification with the helper. Physical contact may be an important communicative device that can convey compassion, and at times institutional roles may be unhelpful and confining. Nevertheless, consideration of professional boundaries is an everyday issue for most nurses.

Reflection

Consider each of the boundary areas described above, and for each identify behaviour which is:

- outside of the boundaries of professional nursing practice
- safely within the boundaries of practice
- on the margins.

Nurse and patient

The nurse is in the centre of the circle and must perform activities in relation to people that are instrumental to the profession of nursing, wider society and in the direct interests of the person in care. This causes problems when the interests and demands of different parties conflict. The language of 'patients' rights' has come to permeate discourse in psychiatric services.[4] Such rights and remedies are enshrined in legislation. However, nurses are challenged to consider 'how' they might promote and protect rights (e.g. choice and autonomy) at a time when society also demands that rights are subjugated, under the umbrella of protecting itself from the perceived threat of those with mental illness. Many of the ethical problems that arise within the psychiatric nurse–person relationship are a reflection of the tension which comes when the demands of society and of medicine conflict with the ideals of nursing.

As has already been discussed, a frequently encountered problem in psychiatric practice is balancing the principles of personal autonomy with beneficence. Another concept to consider is that of paternalism. Beauchamp and Childress[18] define **paternalism** as 'the intentional overriding of one person's known preference or actions by another person, where the person who overrides justifies the action by the goal of benefiting or avoiding harm to the person whose will is overridden'. Compulsory treatment is a dramatically paternalistic practice. However, far more frequent and subtle paternalistic practices include rationing a person's cigarettes, refusing someone permission to go for a walk or attempting to bend the will of another through coercive methods. Paternalistic acts are often justified by suggesting that the person has a limited capacity to act in an autonomous manner because of 'mental illness'.[40]

The method by which others try and influence or directly control another's behaviour may vary in terms of the gravity of the ethical problems that arise. MacKlin[11] described a continuum of interpersonal **behaviour control** methods:

- **coercion**: involving a threat of force or bodily harm
- **manipulation**: involving deception to change behaviour; a lesser threat or covert threat
- **seduction/temptation**: involving the offer of enticements; playing to the 'weak will' of another
- **persuasion**: involving reason and argument
- **indoctrination/education**: involving the provision of education or activity (e.g. role modelling).

The use of, or threat of, force is considerably more ethically problematic than weaker methods of influence, but all attempt to override a person's free will and interfere with their autonomy. Lützén[41] described 'subtle coercion' as a common practice which may be conceptualized as an interpersonal and dynamic activity, involving one person (or several) exerting his or her will on another. This requires judging patients' competency, acting strategically, modifying the meaning of autonomy, justifying coercive strategies and ethical reflection. The following incidents create conflicts in decision-making and require the nurse to assess the person's capacity for autonomy and sometimes engage in subtle coercion:

- patient's refusal of treatment, food or self-care
- searching through and keeping a patient's belongings
- patient wanting to leave the hospital

- self-destructive behaviour
- patient being unable to communicate his or her own needs.

Whenever coercive methods are used there is a potential breach of ethics, in that the person's autonomy is compromised. O'Brien and Golding[42] suggest that there should be a prima facie ban on coercive practices. That is, every instance of coercion should be justified and a principle of 'least coercive intervention' should prevail.

Sometimes people are controlled in covert and subtle ways; for example, a person is admitted voluntarily to an inpatient psychiatric unit but comes to appreciate that if he or she chooses to leave they will be prevented by nurses from doing so. In other instances, nurses may use force (e.g. physically restraining a person), or otherwise more profoundly limiting a person's autonomy through the use of seclusion (preventing a person from interacting with others). The use of **physical restraint** and **seclusion** may be legally sanctioned within some psychiatric hospitals in order to prevent harm to the person or others. However, people often experience these practices as coercive, frightening, punishing and harmful.[43,44] In response to behaviour from patients that engenders fear in others, nurses are often constrained by a lack of knowledge about non-coercive alternatives to restraints or seclusion.[4] The ongoing development of **intrapersonal skills** to deal with one's own fear and anxiety, as well as the development interpersonal skills to diffuse the anxiety and allay the fear of others, is an ethical imperative for nurses.

Reflection

- How do you respond to fear and anxiety?
- How might your responses affect the care that you provide?
- What might you do to allay the fear of others?

A further area of ethical tension arising from balancing autonomy with beneficence is the maintenance of **privacy**. The two areas of privacy related to mental health care include access to personal information and access to personal space. Privacy allows one to express characteristics and desires that one would not wish to reveal to others *and* the freedom to control one's self-presentation.[45] People within acute psychiatric inpatient services are frequently under close observation or video surveillance and have severely limited opportunities to control self-presentation. People under the care of **assertive outreach** teams or receiving intensive psychiatric follow-up in their homes also experience an invasion of privacy. This can engender a sense of shame, embarrassment and violation. Surveillance can cause harm, and nurses must balance the potential harm of close monitoring and breaching an individual's privacy with the potential harm that may arise if the person's privacy is maintained.

Technologies such as computerized databases and risk registers pose particular ethical problems and risks. Most jurisdictions have laws or regulations governing how information is collected, stored and shared. In practice, many people may have little awareness of what information is collected and stored about them. In electronic form such information may persist for years and be used for unintended purposes. Information about people's mental health status may be particularly stigmatizing. Nurses are often the collectors of information and as such are ethically obliged to inform the person what information is collected, for what purpose and with whom it will be shared.

Reflection

- Imagine how it might feel to have your behaviour constantly observed by others.
- If you have the opportunity, request colleagues or tutors to place you in a seclusion room or in physical restraints for an undisclosed period of time. Discuss the experience with others.

ETHICAL DECISION-MAKING

In practice, people rarely employ a formal ethical reasoning process when choosing how to act in relation to others. Benner[46] proposed that an ethic of care must be learned through experience, because it is dependent on recognition of '… salient ethical comportment in specific situations located in concrete specific communities and practices, and habits'. However, there will be dilemmas and problems which emerge in everyday practice that are perplexing or require nurses to highlight, negotiate and justify solutions to others, solutions to ethical problems. In such circumstances a problem-solving process may be usefully employed. It is beyond the scope of this chapter to provide a detailed account of any one ethical decision-making process (for further study, see references 3 and 4). All nurses, however, will be familiar with a basic problem-solving process which involves assessment, diagnosing, planning, implementing and evaluating. Assessment involves identifying and describing the relevant ethical elements in a situation. The following questions may be useful to consider in assessment:

- What is the situation (provide a rich description)?
- Who has an interest in the outcome of the decision and what are their views on the right course of action?
- What are the choices you have?

- What may be the possible consequences of each choice?
- What resources are required for each course of action?
- How might each choice affect relationships with others?
- What principles or values stand to be compromised by each choice?
- What principle or value should take precedence in this situation?
- What are the rights of the parties involved?
- What duties arise from these rights?
- What are the legal requirements in the situation?
- Who ought to be involved in decision-making?

After careful examination of a situation it may be found that there is no ethical problem at all, but rather there is a problem of communication, law or policy that can be resolved through means other than ethical reasoning. If it appears that a dilemma or ethical problem remains, goals need to be set and a plan of action made. The plan may involve compromise, negotiation, further consultation, education or mediation. Lastly, the plan needs to be carried out and evaluated. Teams or groups may undertake this process. Indeed, when faced with a dilemma it is generally better not to carry the burden alone, but to seek advice or supervision from others.

Limited moral agency of nurses

Nurses may possess exceptional skills in ethical reasoning, but this does not necessarily confer the freedom to undertake an ethical course of action. Nurses are frequently constrained from exercising free moral agency.[47] In part this is because of the instrumental nature of nursing to medicine and the status of nursing within the healthcare system.[48,49] Quite simply nurses are often legally required to do the bidding of medicine, 'the team' or others. Profoundly ethical decisions relating to a person's rationality, insight, competency, or risk are couched as 'diagnostic' decisions or 'clinical judgements' which according to psychiatric discourse and frequently the law are the purview and territory of medicine. Nurses are often legally required to carry out 'doctor's orders' to administer drugs, contain people under court orders, restrain, seclude and otherwise restrict people's liberty. Nurses are often required to be the enforcers of compulsory treatment orders and contain the responses of people to being treated against their will. Yet, nurses are sometimes ancillary to 'clinical' and treatment decisions, or when decisions are made in 'teams' psychiatric discourse tends to dominate.

In a recent study, Lützén and Shreiber[50] found that the '… nature and resolution of ethical decisions about patient care were contingent on whether or not the cultural or management milieu of the workplace was supportive of nursing practice, that is, a place in which personal and professional growth was encouraged or not'. They suggest that nurses working in some contexts have limited choices because they work in a system that does not provide opportunities to challenge assumptions and work towards changing non-therapeutic environments, without risking personal sanctions. Nursing ethics must contend with the problem of many nurses having little if any voice in ethical decision-making, and the problems of negotiating ethically problematic situations where the contributions and concerns of nursing are rendered invisible.[48,51]

Exposure to the ethical problems of practice can and ought to cause some **moral distress**. However, the power of discourse, the security of tradition and deference to psychiatric authority can lull the nurse into **moral complacency**, or the discarding of once cherished values. Moral discomfort may be functional if channelled into solving the problems of institutionalized oppression and hegemonic discourse which inhibit nurses from acting freely and creating a truly collaborative healthcare ethic.[49] Barker[52] suggests that '… we face a major ethical dilemma in choosing between our faith in biomedical explanations of ill-health, on the one hand, and listening to, and learning from, the people in our care … on the other'. It may be that a greater challenge is accommodating and valuing different points of view, multiple realities and above all not abandoning those people who find themselves in situations that provoke our own moral distress or discomfort.

A pressing and ongoing ethical problem that psychiatric nurses face is realizing the purpose of nursing in relation to people who are distressed or suffering. It is easy and at times enticing to reduce nursing to a set of discrete roles or tasks such as 'managing risk', assessment or administering treatments. However, whilst helpful, such tasks do not necessarily address what the person most needs, which may be to find meaning in suffering. As Frankl observed,[53] 'Suffering ceases to be suffering in some way at the moment it finds a meaning.' Assisting people to grow, find meaning in experience, connect with others and reconnect with self reflect elements of true caring which are constantly threatened by competing discourses and human nature which compels one to flee from suffering. A fruitful starting point for ethical practice regardless of the context is for nurses to reflect on and refine their own philosophical basis of nursing care.

Psychiatric–mental health nursing is an ethical undertaking. The psychiatric nurse is often involved in complex messy situations, involving real people who hold differing accounts of a situation and have different and conflicting interests. Above all, psychiatric nursing practice involves a relationship with people who experience suffering. Ethical practice is more likely when the nurse has knowledge of ethical theory, the possession of clinical knowledge and skill and possesses virtues such as compassion, an awareness of one's own values and the values of others, and an awareness of the ethical dimensions of everyday psychiatric discourse.

REFERENCES

1. Beauchamp TL. *Philosophical ethics: an introduction to moral philosophy*, 2nd edn. New York, NY: McGraw-Hill, 1991.

2. Barker P. Where care meets treatment: common ethical conflicts in psychiatric care. In: Barker P (ed.). *The philosophy and practice of psychiatric nursing*. Edinburgh, UK: Churchill Livingstone, 1999: 199–212.

3. Seedhouse D. *Ethics: the heart of health care*. Chichester, UK: John Wiley & Sons, 1988.

4. Johnstone M-J. *Bioethics: a nursing perspective*, 3rd edn. Sydney, Australia: Harcourt Saunders, 1999.

5. Fisher A. The ethical problems encountered in psychiatric nursing practice with dangerously mentally ill persons. *Scholarly Inquiry for Nursing Practice* 1995; **9** (2): 193–208.

6. Forchuk C. Ethical problems encountered by mental health nurses. *Issues in Mental Health Nursing* 1991; **12** (4): 375–83.

7. Garritson SH. Ethical decision making patterns. *Journal of Psychosocial Nursing* 1988; **26** (4): 22–9.

8. Lützén K, Nordin C. Benevolence, a central moral concept derived from a grounded theory study of nursing decision making in psychiatric settings. *Journal of Advanced Nursing* 1993; **18**: 1106–11.

9. Coleman R. *Recovery an alien concept*. Gloucester, UK: Handsell Publishing, 1999.

10. Conrad P, Schneider JW. *Deviance and medicalization: from badness to sickness*. St Louis, MO: C.V. Mosby, 1980.

11. MacKlin R. *Man, mind and morality: the ethics of behavior control*. Englewood Cliffs, NJ: Prentice-Hall, 1982.

12. Crooks S. Susie's story. In: Leibrich J (ed.). *A gift of stories*. Dunedin, NZ: University of Otago Press, 1999: 9–15.

13. Lawler J. *Behind the screens: nursing, somology, and the problem of the body*. Melbourne, Australia: Churchill Livingstone, 1991.

14. Lakeman R. Commentary on 'Where care meets treatment: common ethical conflicts in psychiatric nursing'. In: Barker P (ed.). *The philosophy and practice of psychiatric nursing*. Edinburgh, UK: Churchill Livingstone, 1999: 213–16.

15. Lützén K, Evertzon M, Nordin C. Moral sensitivity in psychiatric practice. *Nursing Ethics* 1997; **4** (6): 472–82.

16. Armstrong AE, Parsons S, Barker PJ. An inquiry into moral virtues, especially compassion, in psychiatric nurses: findings from a Delphi study. *Journal of Psychiatric and Mental Health Nursing* 2000; **7**: 297–306.

17. Lützén K, Barbarosa da Silva A. The role of virtue ethics in psychiatric nursing. *Nursing Ethics* 1996; **3** (3): 202–11.

18. Beauchamp T, Childress J. *Principles of biomedical ethics*, 4th edn. New York, NY: Oxford University Press, 1994.

19. Christensen RC. The ethics of treating the 'untreatable' (Editorial). *Psychiatric Services* 1995; **46** (12): 1217.

20. Spreen Parker R. Nurses' stories: the search for a relational ethic of care. *Advances in Nursing Science* 1990; **13**: 31–40.

21. Kurtz RJ, Wang J. The caring ethic: more than kindness, the core of nursing science. *Nursing Forum* 1991; **26**: 4–8.

22. van Hooft S. Acting from the virtue of caring in nursing. *Nursing Ethics* 1999; **6** (3): 190–201.

23. Johnstone M. Keynote address. Health care ethics: opening up the debate. Unpublished. Massey University, Palmerston North, NZ, 1995: 1–18.

24. Simms LM, Lindberg JB. *The nurse person: developing perspectives for contemporary nursing*. New York, NY: Harper & Row, 1978.

25. Sherwin S. *No longer patient: feminist ethics and health care*. Philadelphia, PA: Temple University Press, 1993.

26. Giddens A. *Sociology*, 2nd edn. Oxford, UK: Polity Press, 1993.

27. Pilgrim D. The biopsychosocial model in Anglo-American psychiatry: past, present and future? *Journal of Mental Health* 2002; **11** (6): 585–94.

28. International Council of Nurses. *The ICN code of ethics for nurses*. 2000. Available from: www.icn.ch/ethics.htm. Accessed 13 December 2001.

29. Foucault M. *The birth of the clinic: an archaeology of medical perception*. New York, NY: Pantheon, 1973.

30. Goffman E. *Asylums: essays on the social situation of mental patients and other inmates*. Harmondsworth, UK: Pelican Books, 1961.

31. Lobovits D, Epston D, Freeman J. narrativeapproaches.com. 2001. Available from: www.narrativeapproaches.com/. Accessed 24 December 2001.

32. United Nations. *The protection of persons with mental illness and the improvement of mental health care*. 1991. Available from: www.un.org/documents/ga/res/46/a46r119.htm. Accessed 27 December 2001.

33. Hall JE. Restriction and control: the perceptions of mental health nurses in a UK acute inpatient setting. *Issues in Mental Health Nursing* 2004; **25** (5): 539–52.

34. Crossley N. Mental health, resistance and social movements: the collective–confrontational dimension. *Health Education Journal* 2002; **61** (2): 138–52.

35. Szasz T. Psychiatric diagnosis, psychiatric power and psychiatric abuse. *Journal of Medical Ethics* 1994; *20*: 135–8.

36. Szasz T. *The myth of mental illness: foundations of a theory of personal conduct*. New York, NY: Harper Collins, 1974.

37. Double D. *Critical psychiatry*. 2007. Available from: www.critpsynet.freeuk.com/antipsychiatry.htm. Accessed 4 July 2007.

38. Watson JK. *A handbook for nurses*, 6th edn. London, UK: The Scientific Press, 1921.

39. Campbell RJ, Yonge O, Austin W. Intimacy boundaries between mental health nurses and psychiatric patients. *Journal of Psychosocial Nursing & Mental Health Services* 2005; **43** (5): 33–41.

40. Roberts M. Psychiatric ethics; a critical introduction for mental health nurses. *Journal of Psychiatric and Mental Health Nursing* 2004; **11** (5): 583–8.

41. Lützén K. Subtle coercion in psychiatric practice. *Journal of Psychiatric and Mental Health Nursing* 1998; 5: 101–7.

42. O'Brien AJ, Golding CG. Coercion in mental healthcare: the principle of least coercive care. *Journal of Psychiatric and Mental Health Nursing* 2003; **10** (2): 167–73.

43. Johnson ME. Being restrained: a study of power and powerlessness. *Issues in Mental Health Nursing* 1998; **19** (3): 191–206.

44. Mohr WK, Mahon MM, Noone MJ. A restraint on restraints: the need to reconsider the use of restrictive interventions. *Archives of Psychiatric Nursing* 1998; **12** (2): 95–106.

45. Olsen DP. Ethical considerations of video monitoring psychiatric patients in seclusion and restraint. *Archives of Psychiatric Nursing* 1998; **12** (2): 90–4.

46. Benner P. The role of experience, narrative and community in skilled ethical comportment. *Advances in Nursing Science* 1991; **14** (2): 1–21.

47. Yarling RR, McElmurry BJ. The moral foundation of nursing. *Advances in Nursing Science* 1986; **8** (2): 63–73.

48. Liaschenko J. Ethics and the geography of the nurse–patient relationship: spatial vulnerabilities and gendered space. *Scholarly Inquiry for Nursing Practice* 1997; **11**: 45–59.

49. Lakeman R. Nurses are more than tools: instrumentality and implications for nursing ethics. In: King J (ed.). *Proceedings of the 26th International Conference of the College of Mental Health Nurses: Mental health nurses for a changing world: not just surviving, 3–7 September 2000, Broadbeach, Queensland*. Australian and New Zealand College of Mental Health Nurses, 2000: 204–12.

50. Lützén K, Shreiber R. Moral survival in a nontherapeutic environment. *Issues in Mental Health Nursing* 1998; **19** (4): 303–15.

51. Liaschenko J. The shift from the closed to the open body: ramifications for nursing testimony. In: Edwards SD (ed.). *Philosophical issues in nursing*. London, UK: MacMillan Press, 1998: 11–30.

52. Barker P. Patient participation and the multiple realities of empowerment. In: Barker P(ed.). *The philosophy and practice of psychiatric nursing*. Edinburgh, UK: Churchill Livingstone, 1999: 99–116.

53. Frankl V. *Man's search for meaning: an introduction to logotherapy*. New York, NY: Pocket Books, 1963.

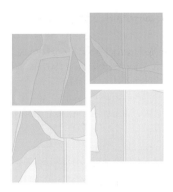

CHAPTER 70

Sexuality and gender

Agnes Higgins*

> It is like we expect clients to be kind of non sexual objects or people.
>
> **Psychiatric–mental health nurse**

INTRODUCTION

In these apparent sexually liberated times people are considered to be more informed and more willing to discuss sexual issues in an open and mature manner. Wherever we go we are bombarded with sexual images – in newspapers, magazines, television and billboards. Consequently, one could be fooled into thinking that inhibitions and prejudices are a thing of the past. In a psychiatric and mental health context sexuality continues to be shrouded in misinformation, taboos, fear and embarrassment. At a time when people's rights are increasingly emphasized, evidence in the area of mental health nursing suggests that the sexual dimension and sexual rights of people experiencing mental health problems continue to be either pushed into the proverbial closet or considered within a pathological or deviant paradigm.[1,2]

Mental illness affects men and women to different degrees, some of this is related to social mores or cultural conventions. Some psychiatric drug treatments have a massive impact on people's sexuality, a factor that, traditionally, has not been properly addressed. At the same time, gay, lesbian, bisexual and transgender persons have been marginalized, if not actively persecuted by psychiatry. This chapter explores some of these issues around sexuality and the implications for the psychiatric–mental health nurse (PMHN).

Reflection

- What do the terms sexuality, sex and gender mean to you?
- How frequently do you consider, within the horizon of your nursing practice, the sexuality of the people you care for?
- Within the service you work in, how open is the multidisciplinary team to discussing issues of sexuality?

TERMINOLOGY: SEXUALITY, SEX AND GENDER

Sexuality can and does mean many different things to different people; consequently, a single understanding is difficult to reach. The literature abounds with definitions of sexuality from many different perspectives with no singular agreed definition. Webb[3] cautions us to remember that sexuality is not located between the umbilicus and the kneecaps, but is a symbol for a complex attribute that goes beyond the confines of copulation and gender designation. Sexuality, therefore, is much more than anatomy and physiology, more than sexual intercourse. Sexuality is an integral factor in the uniqueness of every person and, to a large extent, determines who we are. It is intimately bound up with our self-concept, self-esteem, body image and total self-image. It is rooted in

*Agnes Higgins is an Associate Professor of Mental Health Nursing at Trinity College, Dublin. She has nearly three decades of experience working in mental health, in both clinical practice and education. Her research interest is in the area of sexuality and gender and her PhD study focused on sexuality and mental health.

the human need to relate to others, to give and receive affection, tenderness, intimacy and respect. The Pan American Health Organization and World Health Organization (PAHO/WHO) state that:[4,p.6]

> Sexuality refers to a core dimension of being human which includes sex, gender, sexual and gender identity, sexual orientation, eroticism, emotional attachment/love and reproduction. It is experienced or expressed in thoughts, fantasies, desires, beliefs, attitudes, values, activities, practices, roles, [and] relationships. Sexuality is a result of the interplay of biological, psychological, socio-economic, cultural, ethical and religious/spiritual factors. While sexuality can include all of these aspects, not all of these dimensions need to be experienced or expressed.

The term sexuality is sometimes synonymously used with the term sex, yet their meanings are different. *Sex* is the 'sum of biological characteristics that defined the spectrum of humans as females and males'.[4,p.6] Sexuality, therefore, is a much broader concept, incorp-orating the biological as well as the cultural, social and psychological aspects, whereas the term sex relates more to the biological state or the sexual act.[5] The other term that requires some clarification is *gender*. While sex refers to biological differences between men and women, gender is the 'sum of cultural values, attitudes, roles, practices and characteristics based on sex'.[4,p.7] Differentiating between sex and gender is important to highlight that differences between men's and women's behaviours do not automatically derive from differences in biological sex (biological determinism). In the vast majority of situations gender differences are shaped and influenced by cultural mores and norms. Men and women are socialized from an early age into different gendered behavioural patterns.

GENDER, SEXUALITY AND MENTAL ILLNESS: THE HISTORICAL CONTEXT

There is a tendency to dismiss the past as being 'unscientific' and view current practice as more humane, informed and 'evidence based'. However, we must look to the past if only to ensure that we are not condemned to repeat it. The history of sexuality and people diagnosed with mental illness is a history of misunderstanding, control and abuse, frequently served up in the guise of medical science.

Throughout the nineteenth century, gender differences in mental illness were strongly linked to reproductive biology, with women's reproductive biology being subjected to a more pathologizing discourse than men's.[6] Generally, insanity in women was thought to be related to a defect or irritation in their reproductive system, especially their uterus. In what is often termed the 'ovarian model' of female behaviour, physicians saw women as driven by the tidal current of their reproductive system,

which was bounded by puberty and the menopause. Gynaecologists such as Henry, when asserting the relationship between mental illness and female reproductive organs, insisted that eventually,[7,p.1001]

> … nerve centres in the uterus, and possibly the tubes, would be found, which [would] have an important influence on mental equilibrium.

On this premise, he argued that mental disorder in women could be prevented and cured through radical hysterectomies. Cautioning against conservative surgery, and stressing the fact that 'many insane women who have pelvic trouble do not complain of it', he urged the eradication of 'all [pelvic] irritation by what ever means necessary, no matter how radical the [surgery] work required'.[7,p.1001] Others argued that it was plain to 'the casual observer that women become insane during pregnancy, after parturition, and during lactation' and testified to the fact that sudden cessation of menstruation was undoubtedly the cause of some manic episodes.[8,p.479] Subsequently, the concepts of puerperal mania and puerperal insanity gave formal expression to the link between birth and mental disorder.

The concept of involutional melancholia, first introduced by Kraeplin in 1896, served as an important mechanism to link the menopause with mental disorder. Involutional melancholia was said to occur in both men and women; however, because of its link to the female menopause the diagnosis was more frequently assigned to women.[6] Busfield[6] noted that *hysteria*, with its etymological roots in the Greek term 'hysteron' meaning the womb, was considered to be primarily a female condition. The terms 'feminine' and 'hysterical' became almost synonymous.

Drawing on theories of conservation of energy, physicians also asserted that educating women would threaten their reproductive function, with the consequent results of atrophy of the breasts, interruption to the menstrual cycle, sterility, mental breakdown or the bearing of sickly, neurotic children.[6,9] Such views helped to confine women to their domestic roles and helped sow the seed that any desire, with its potential to interfere with mothering and the domestic role, was unfeminine, 'abnormal' and had the potential to damage the mental health of the next generation. It also helped to construct and reinforce images of women as hapless victims of biology, passive agents in life and more biologically predisposed to higher rates of mental illness.[6]

While men's reproductive system was given far less attention in the psychiatric literature, it did not completely escape attention. In explaining why the male reproductive system did not exercise a parallel control over men's mental health, medical wisdom believed that, although men experienced developmental changes, they were less difficult to negotiate because of the absence of a uterus.[9] This view was supported and reinforced by Freud's theory of sexual development, which emphasized the difficulties experienced by women in negotiating sexual development. According to Freud, a woman's negotiation of sexual development was more difficult, since she must both change her desire from mother to father and shift the site of sexual pleasure from the 'inferior' clitoris associated with mother/female body to vaginal pleasure associated with father/male body.[10]

Throughout the eighteenth and indeed part of the nineteenth century, masturbation was understood to be a cause of insanity in men and a special form of masturbatory insanity was identified.[6] Benjamin Rush, considered the father of American psychiatry, claimed that male masturbation produced seminal weakness, impotence, tabes dorsalis, pulmonary consumption, hypochondriasis, loss of memory, dementia and death.[9] Although women were swelling the ranks of the institutions, only a few physicians commented on female masturbation. When commented upon, female masturbation was considered to be the antithesis of Freud's view on mature female sexuality and a contradiction to the prevailing notion of women as passionless and passive sexual beings. Consequently, female masturbation was considered a symptom of illness as opposed to causing mental illness.[8] As hardly any other condition among people with mental illness was considered as deplorable, the mentally ill were subjected to a range of treatments including: concocted food products; physical restraint in straightjackets; bandaging of the genitals; the application of leeches to the genitals; cold baths and sedation.[11] In more extreme situations women were subjected to clitoridectomies.[9,12]

Since the formal classification of mental illness, in the form of the *Diagnostic statistical manual* (DSM) in 1952 and the *International classification of diseases and related health problems* (ICD) in 1900, over the years numerous other mental illnesses have been constructed as a consequence of their link to sexual behaviour. Based on a belief that sexual attraction to the opposite sex was the desired norm and an indisputable fact of nature, a view that was reinforced by theological, evolutionary and biological theories of the time, the American Medical Association, in conjunction with the American Psychiatric Association, included homosexuality as a psychopathic personality disorder in the first DSM published in 1952.[13] Subsequently, many aetiological theories were put forward. Early ideas suggested that homosexuality was a congenital anomaly caused by exposure to hormonal deficits or hormonal excess in utero. Other theories included atypical brain structure, genetic predisposition and environmental influences.[14]

To conceive homosexuality as a manifestation of 'ill health' rather than a sin was held to be a more liberal approach, as people were not seen as personally and morally responsible for their sickness.[15] However, considering the treatment given to people, the practical consequences of being judged sick instead of sinful were not always that different. Mental healthcare professionals, in an attempt to modify the person's behaviour, acted as agents of social control through the use of aversion therapy, psychotherapy, libido-reducing drugs and electroconvulsive therapy.[11] As a consequence of sustained protests, by the Gay Liberation Movement in the USA, as opposed to some scientific insight, homosexuality was removed from DSM III in 1987 and *The international classification of diseases* in 1992.[11] Despite this, as recently as 1994 a doctor writing in the British medical press urged the Department of Health in the UK to 'devote more attention to the risk factors that lead to homosexuality' and described homosexuality as 'biologically destructive'.[16,p.854]

The eugenics movement (a science devoted to improving the human race and derived from the Greek word for 'well born') was strongly influenced by Darwin's work on evolutionary theory and Spencer and Galton's theory on inheritance and moral degeneracy. Eugenics had followers within psychiatry.[17] Premised on beliefs that mental illness had a strong genetic component and procreation among people with mental health problems would lead to social degeneracy and 'race suicide', social hygienists campaigned for restrictions on people's right to reproduce.[17] Adherents to the eugenics movement frequently cited evidence that people with mental illness were hypersexual, immoral and governed by animalistic sexual urges.[12]

To prevent reproduction, 'eugenicists recommended that measures should be taken to detect and isolate people likely to become insane, and to segregate them so as to prevent their breeding'.[18,p.38] Staff in institutions were instructed to maintain gender segregation between the mentally ill, and guard against any 'illicit' associations between men and women.[17] The possibility that the mentally ill would marry each other was met with disapproval by families and healthcare professionals alike. For example, in 1903, Dr Carr, a superintendent of the Omagh Asylum in Ireland, beseeched both Protestant and Catholic clergy to refuse to consecrate marriages between people with a family history of insanity.[19]

Taken to the extreme, in the early 1900s in some countries, degeneracy theory gave rise to such radical measures as the adoption of laws that authorized sterilization without informed consent. In some cases arguments were made for the beneficial effects to people's mental health of the complete removal of testes and ovaries such as the following comment from Barr:[20]

> As sexual impulses dominate their lives, the removal of this excitation, as has been proven, not only makes them more tractable, as does gelding for the ox, but the general health improves, and nervous disorders, to which many are subject, become more amenable to treatment, therefore far from being an injury, the

slight and nearly painless operation required, improves physical vigor and they become contented and happy … It is not always essential that testicles and ovaries be removed, but I prefer it, as it gives absolute security … If, for sentimental reasons, the removal of the testes and ovaries will not be considered, ligation of the spermatic cord or vasectomy in the male and fallectomy or tuberectomy in the female, may be performed through the vagina.

Although degeneracy theory has been discounted within the scientific literature, disapproval of people with mental health problems marrying each other and bearing children continues to be met with disapproval within society.[21,22] Vandereycken[21] suggested that the image of people having no control over their sexual drives, especially people experiencing psychosis, supported the use of drugs to suppress sexual desire. In today's context it could be argued that the drug-induced suppression of sexual desire and the production of hyperprolactinaemia in women, which has a contraceptive effect and is found to be a primary cause of sexual dysfunction in women,[23] is another more subtle way of maintaining old power relations and enforcing reproduction control, under the guise of therapy.

Reflection

- When a person is prescribed medication, how frequently do you inform them, or enquire about, the side-effects that affect sexuality and sexual function?
- If a woman told you that she wants to stop taking medication because she wants to get pregnant, how would you respond?
- If you were prescribed medication that affected your sexuality, what help and advice would you like?

PRESCRIBED DRUGS AND SEXUALITY

The biological paradigm of mental illness still casts a significant shadow on psychiatric–mental health nursing. Its focus is on the classification and elimination of symptomatic behaviours and experiences, through the use of medication or other biological interventions. Mental distress is seen as *illness*, with treatment remaining within the expertise of the medical profession, which espouses to know what is best for the person. In keeping with this view, there is an expectation that service users conform to Parsons'[24] idea of the sick role: they seek help and, in an unquestioning manner, accept and conform to the advice of the medical professional, whether it be the doctor or the doctor's representative – the PMHN.

The use of antidepressant and anti-psychotic drugs continues to be a central pillar of this paradigm. However, these drugs have many adverse side-effects, which severely

affect the person's quality of life. Evidence suggests that drug-induced iatrogenic sexual dysfunction is more prevalent than healthcare professionals think. Research[25,26] in this area indicates that between 40 and 65 per cent of service users have reported some form of sexual dysfunction, with some service users likening the impact of the drugs to 'sexual suicide'.[27,p.22]

Our current scientific knowledge regarding sexuality cannot fully explain the neurophysiology, neuroendocrinology and psychological mechanism induced by drugs. In most cases, side-effects that affect sexual function are idiosyncratic and unpredictable with no apparent relationship between the type of drug used, dose and the incidence of a specific sexual dysfunction. It is generally thought that drugs that enhance serotonin or decrease dopamine tend to diminish sexual function and desire. In addition, drugs that block the cholinergic and alpha-adrenergic receptors also induce sexual dysfunction.[28]

Sexual dysfunctions reported by women include desire and arousal problems, poor vaginal lubrication, diminished organism or anorgasmia, and menstruation changes (irregular menses, amenorrhoea or menorrhagia). While many of the traditional anti-psychotics induce hyperprolactinaemia in women, with the resulting loss of reproductive capacity, cases of unplanned pregnancy in women who had been changed from older, typical oral or depot anti-psychotics to atypical drugs have also been reported. Men have reported erection difficulties (difficulty in achieving or maintaining an erection, including morning erections) and ejaculatory difficulties (reduced ejaculatory volume, retrograde ejaculation, delayed ejaculation or total inhibition of ejaculation). In addition, both men and women have reported incidents of gynaecomastia, galactorrhoea and breast discomfort.[23,28] All of these side-effects can severely affect the person's sense of body image, self-esteem, intimacy and relationship needs. In some cases, they may deprive the person of their right to sexual expression and pleasure by making them fearful of initiating or engaging in an intimate relationship.[27]

There is a tendency among PMHNs to ignore the sexual rights of service users when it comes to their role in drug administration and education.[29,30] Sexual rights include the rights to:

- express one's full sexual potential
- sexual autonomy, privacy, equity and pleasure
- make free and responsible reproductive choices
- comprehensive sexual health education
- sexual health care.[4]

The following quote from a PMHN, about side-effects of drug treatments that affect sexuality, illustrates the obvious ethical issues related to consent, sexual rights and service user involvement in their own care.

I didn't feel I could say it [side-effects that affect sexual function] to him, so it was pushed aside, you *know, not spoken of … you would list off some, you will get dry mouth, blurred vision, those … Sexual function or loss of libido they are down the bottom of the list, but you didn't get to the bottom … The sexual side effects are just absent.*

Psychiatric–mental health nurse

When asked, nurses offer a number of reasons for their unwillingness to engage service users in collaborative discussions about the possibility of iatrogenic sexual dysfunction. These include:

- lack of knowledge about sexual effects
- lack of comfort in talking about sexual issues
- a failure to see service users as sexual beings.

There is also an erroneous belief that there is an inverse relationship between education on sexual dysfunction and compliance with medication, a belief that has assumed mythical status within mental health nursing.[30,31] Nurses do not appear to be aware of, or are ignoring, the evidence suggesting that the provision of information about drugs simply increases service users' knowledge and understanding of their treatment in the short term (up to 1 year), and does not have a significant impact on compliance or relapse.[32,33]

Even when service users have the courage to report these side-effects, there is a tendency to ignore or minimize the impact of them on the person, with nurses opting to emphasize the importance of 'drug compliance' and symptom reduction, regardless of the emotional and sexual cost to the person. Service users may even be advised that iatrogenic sexual dysfunction will disappear with time and to continue with the drugs, although all the evidence suggests that spontaneous resolution of iatrogenic-induced sexual dysfunction rarely occurs.[30]

Reflection

Within your service:

- How are services developed to ensure the needs of gay, lesbian, bisexual and transsexual people are addressed?
- How are services developed to ensure gender-sensitive care?

GAY, LESBIAN, BISEXUAL AND TRANSSEXUAL

Despite the diversity of sexual expression in the world, heterosexuality has always been the dominant sexuality and consequently the desired social norm. All other sexualities have been constructed as 'other', with 'other' coming to mean abnormal or deviant. Being gay, lesbian, bisexual or transsexual (GLBT) is not in itself a mental health problem. However, coping with the effects of discrimination can be detrimental to the mental health of GLBT people. Like many other minorities in society, they face many forms of prejudice, harassment and discrimination, which are rooted within the heterosexist structures of society and societal homophobic attitudes.[14] The invisibility of lesbian and gay identity in mainstream culture can damage people's self-esteem and make it hard for people to feel a sense of belonging to a society that seems not to recognize that they exist. The negative internalization of society's attitudes may also adversely affect the person's self-esteem and sense of security. The possible consequence of ostracism, stigma and reprisal, in a homophobic culture, can make 'coming out' extremely difficult for people.[14]

Whether mental healthcare professionals are aware of it or not, they are not immune to the discriminatory attitudes held within society. Several research studies, which have explored gay and lesbian and bisexual (GLB) people's experience of the mental health services, suggest that GLB people can experience the same discrimination within the mental health service as they do in wider society.[34–36] Many service users do not feel safe to be 'out' in the mental health service and report frequently experiencing insensitivity, prejudice and discrimination from staff and other service users in the form of homophobia, biphobia and heterosexism.[34,35] Although participants in King and McKeown's study[36] did identify sensitive practices and indicated that things were improving, a number cited examples of overt homophobia and subtle forms of discrimination, ranging from lack of empathy, through the presumption of heterosexuality, to an unwillingness to discuss sexuality. Service users who did discuss their sexuality often received 'clumsy and ill informed responses' and reported that mental health professionals often assumed that their sexuality was the main cause of their problem. Consequently, service users had a deep distrust of the psychiatric service and feared that healthcare professionals would focus on treating their homosexuality rather than their anxiety or stress.[37] The presumption of heterosexuality and the use of heterosexist language by nurses was also criticized, as not only did this reinforce the invisibility of GLB people within the service but it may have forced some service users to lie about their sexuality for fear of stigmatization.[36,37]

The dominance of heterosexuality, as normative sexuality, is also reflected in organizational rules that emphasize limiting the opportunities for members of the opposite sex to be together unobserved, and prohibiting service users from entering bedrooms of the opposite sex for fear of service users engaging in a sexual relationship, while these same rules allow complete freedom to people of the same sex. The construction of sexual relationships in terms of the traditional heterosexual relationships no doubt results in a lack of awareness of the need to protect service users from making poor decisions around same sex relationships or the need to protect service users from the risk of sexual exploitation from people of the same sex.[2]

IMPLICATIONS FOR PSYCHIATRIC–MENTAL HEALTH NURSING

Since the World Health Organization first identified the need for health professionals to be educated in the area of sexuality,[38] sexuality has gradually become a legitimate area of concern for nurses across all nursing disciplines. PMHNs are now considered to have a clinical and professional responsibility to address sexuality issues with service users.[39] That said, there were a number of authors, within other disciplines, who critiqued the medicalization of everyday life and the inclusion of activities, such as 'expressing sexuality' within the 'gaze' of healthcare professionals.[40,41] Viewed through the lens of these writings, it could be argued that the formal recognition of sexuality as a dimension of the nurse's role is a reflection of the 'rise in surveillance medicine',[41,p.112] or a form of 'governmentality' and colonization,[40] with the nurse being charged with the tasks of assessing, monitoring and intervening in matters relating to intimate aspects of people's lives.

However, despite these arguments if PMHNs want to be truly responsive to people they need to challenge their attitudes and beliefs around the sexuality of people who experience mental health problems. PMHNs need to include sexuality as a dimension of assessment, and include a discussion on sexuality and intimate and sexual relationships at the initial stages of care. In this way, nurses can act as role models, educating service users that sexuality and sexual relationships can be openly discussed without shame or guilt.

Although the literature on the sexual health dimension of assessment is sparse, what is available suggests that mental health staff do not perceive service users as having sexual and relationship needs and generally ignore the sexual domain in assessment.[42,43] Even when records had identified sections related to sexuality, such as contraception, sexual abuse and sexual risk behaviour, they were not completed. This is of concern for a number of reasons; for example, without information on contraception it is possible that women will miss doses and be discharged at increased risk of pregnancy, or women are not advised about the possible impact of psychotropic medication on a fetus. It is also of concern that PMHNs are not assessing service users' risk to sexual exploitation or providing education on issues such as relationship development, negotiating safe sexual relationships or prevention of pregnancy. By developing education programmes that assist people to develop intimacy skills and healthy sexual relationships, PMHNs may assist service users who experience long-term mental health problems to overcome some of the social isolation and loneliness they experience.[44]

If PMHNs wish to work within the recovery model of mental health care and respect people's right to make an informed choice, as well as their right to make self-defeating choices, there is a need for some fundamental changes in nurses' approach to their role with medication. Nurses need to be more proactive in informing service users and enquiring about all side-effects of drugs, including those that affect sexuality. There is a need to move from a paternalistic model of care to one that focuses on meaningful collaborative discussions about choice of treatment, which respects decisions even if in conflict with professional perspectives. The introduction of standardized side-effect assessment tools and the regular formal questioning of service users about experiences of side-effects have the potential to reduce the side-effect burden as medication can be changed or reduced. In addition, as some drugs are unsafe to take during pregnancy, there is a need for nurses to discuss and advise on options available, such as contraception.

The promotion of mental health among gay and lesbians is a legitimate area of work for the PMHN. Mental health professionals need to educate themselves about gay and lesbian issues and create an environment where disclosure can take place. To do this nurses need to be aware of their own assumptions and prejudices that may marginalize GLBT service users and challenge the current heterosexual biases within service delivery. To ensure that the heterosexual assumptions of society are not reinforcing, thus exacerbating, isolation, the use of heterosexual language in nurses' interview style needs to be avoided, information and advice on recourses that are relevant to gay, lesbian and bisexual people needs to be an integrated part of service provision, and there needs to be development of education programmes that encompass sexual diversity as opposed to being based on the normative assumption of heterosexuality.

Sexuality also needs to be actively acknowledged and foregrounded within nursing curricula at all levels. In addition, nurse managers play an important role in setting the organizational culture and leading change in this area of practice by communicating a clear message of the relevance and importance of service users' sexuality and rights. If the predominant management ethos is one that values the control of service users' sexuality through surveillance and medication as opposed to dialogue, autonomy, participation and education, then a culture that ignores the wider issues in relation to the sexual dimension of the service users' lives is likely to be fostered. Individual practitioners also need space to think aloud about the sexual issues that occur in practice. This can be created through the introduction of a model of clinical supervision for nurses whereby staff will be enabled to engage in the self, theoretical and relational reflection necessary to relate with service users in an intimate and therapeutic manner. The professional and personal awareness required to respond to service users' sexuality in an open and empowering manner is not a one-off event, but a life-long professional journey.

Reflection

Within your service:

- How is sexual health included within education/rehabilitation programmes?
- How are residential services developed to enable sexual expression of the people who live there?

SUMMARY

Sexuality is a quality of life issue for all people and a healthy enjoyment of one's sexuality is an integral part of the human experience and a basic right of all. Indeed, the inclusion of sexuality as part of health care is crucial if the holistic ideology espoused in all healthcare and mental health literature is to be realized. However, sexuality as it relates to people with mental health problems continues to be problematic for PMHNs. This chapter set out to explore some of the issues around sexuality and people who experience mental health problems, and to advocate for PMHNs to acknowledge the presence of sexuality in all nurse–service user encounters, and to respect the sexual rights of people experiencing mental distress. Hopefully, this chapter will enable PMHNs to address sexuality and begin to undo some of the 'silent omission' that has surrounded the sexuality of people who access the mental health services.

REFERENCES

1. McCann E. Exploring sexual and relationship possibilities for people with psychosis – a review of the literature. *Journal of Psychiatric and Mental Health Nursing* 2003; **10** (6): 640–9.

2. Higgins A. Veiling sexualities in a psychiatric nursing context: a grounded theory study. PhD Thesis. Dublin, Ireland: The University of Dublin Trinity College, 2007.

3. Webb C. *Sexuality, nursing and health*. Chichester, UK: John Wiley & Sons, 1985.

4. Pan American Health Organization/World Health Organization. Promotion of sexual health: recommendations for action. *Proceedings of a regional consultation convened by the Pan American Health Organization (PAHO) and the World Health Organization (WHO) in collaboration with the World Association of Sexology*. Antigua, Guatemala: Pan American Health Organization/World Health Organization, 2002.

5. Van Ooijen E, Chranock A. *Sexuality and patient care: a guide for nurses and teachers*. London, UK: Chapman & Hall, 1994.

6. Busfield J. *Men, women and madness: understanding gender and mental disorder*. London, UK: Macmillan Press, 1996.

7. Henry WO. To what extent can the gynaecologist prevent and cure insanity in women. *Journal of American Medical Association* 1907; **48** (12): 997–1003.

8. Barrus C. Gynaecological disorders and their relationship to insanity. *American Journal of Insanity* 1895; **51**: 475–91.

9. Showalter E. *The female malady: women, madness and English culture 1830–1980*. London, UK: Virago, 1985.

10. Appignanesi L, Forrester J. *Freud's women*. London, UK: Virago Press, 1992.

11. Kutchins H, Kirk S. *Making us crazy. DSM: the psychiatric bible and the creation of mental disorders*. London, UK: The Free Press, 1997.

12. Whitaker R. *Mad in America: bad science, bad medicine, and the enduring mistreatment of the mentally ill*. Cambridge, MA: Perseus Publishing, 2002.

13. American Psychiatric Association. *The diagnostic and statistical manual of mental disorder*. Washington, DC: American Psychiatric Association, 1952.

14. Wilton T. *Sexualities in health and social care: a textbook*. Buckingham, UK: Open University Press, 2000.

15. O'Connell-Davidson J, Layder D. *Methods, sex and madness*. London, UK: Routledge, 1994.

16. Rayner P. *Doctors and homosexuality*. BMJ 1994; **308** (6932): 854.

17. Shorter E. A history of psychiatry: from the era of the asylum to the age of prozac. New York, NY: John Wiley & Sons, 1997.

18. Nolan P. *A history of mental health nursing*. London, UK: Chapman & Hall, 1993.

19. Nolan P, Sheridan A. In search of the history of Irish psychiatric nursing. *International History of Nursing Journal* 2001; **6** (2): 35–43.

20. Barr M. The asexualization of the unfit. *The Alienist and Neurologist* 1912; **xxxiii**.

21. Vandereycken W. Shrinking sexuality: the half known sex life of psychiatric patients. *Therapeutic Communities* 1993; **14** (3): 143–9.

22. National Disability Authority. *Public attitudes to disability in the Republic of Ireland*. Dublin, Ireland: National Disability Authority, 2002.

23. Higgins A, Barker P, Begley C. Neuroleptic medication and sexuality: the forgotten aspect of education and care. *Journal of Psychiatric and Mental Health Nursing* 2005; **12** (4): 439–46.

24. Parsons T. Illness and the role of the physician: a sociological perspective. *American Journal of Orthopsychiatry* 1951; **21** (3): 452–60.

25. Rothschild A. Sexual side effects of antidepressants. *Journal of Clinical Psychiatry* 2000; **61** (Suppl 11): 28–36.

26. Smith S, O'Keane V, Murray R. Sexual dysfunction in patients taking conventional antipsychotic medication. *British Journal of Psychiatry* 2002; **181**: 49–55.

27. Deegan P. Human sexuality and mental illness: consumer viewpoints and recovery principles. In: Buckley P (ed.). *Sexuality and serious mental illness*. Amsterdam, The Netherlands: Harwood: 1999, 21–33.

28. Higgins A. The impact of psychotropic medication on sexuality. *British Journal of Nursing* 2007; **16** (9): 545–50.

29. Happell B, Manias E, Roper C. Wanting to be heard: mental health consumers' experiences of information about medication. *International Journal of Mental Health Nursing* 2004; **13** (4): 242–8.

30. Higgins A, P Barker, Begley CM. Iatrogenic sexual dysfunction and the protective withholding of information: in whose best interest? *Journal of Psychiatric and Mental Health Nursing* 2006; **13** (4): 437–46.

31. Cort E, Attenborough J, Watson JP. An initial exploration of community mental health nurses' attitudes to and experience of sexuality-related issues in their work with people experiencing mental health problems. *Journal of Psychiatric and Mental Health Nursing* 2001; **8** (6): 489–99.

32. Gray R, Wykes T, Gournay K. From compliance to concordance: a review of the literature on interventions to enhance compliance with antipsychotic medication. *Journal of Psychiatric and Mental Health Nursing* 2002; **9** (3): 277–84.

33. Fernandez RS, Evans V, Griffiths RD *et al.* Educational interventions for mental health consumers receiving psychotropic medication: a review of the evidence. *International Journal of Mental Health Nursing* 2006; **15**: 70–80.

34. McFarlane L. *Diagnosis homophobic: the experience of lesbians, gay men and bisexuals in mental health services.* London, UK: PACE, 1998.

35. Golding J. *Without prejudice: Mind lesbian, gay and bisexual mental health awareness research.* London, UK: Mind, 1997.

36. King M, McKeown E. *Mental health and social wellbeing of gay men, lesbians, and bisexuals in England and Wales.* London, UK: Mind, 2003.

37. Robertson A. The mental health experiences of gay men: a research study exploring gay men's health needs. *Journal of Psychiatric and Mental Health Nursing* 1998; **5**: 33–40.

38. World Health Organization. *Education and treatment in human sexuality: the training of health professionals.* Geneva, Switzerland: World Health Organization, 1975.

39. Royal College of Nursing. *Sexuality and sexual health in nursing practice.* London, UK: Royal College of Nursing, 2000.

40. Foucault M. *The birth of the clinic.* London, UK: Tavistock, 1973.

41. Armstrong D. The rise of surveillance medicine. In: Nettleton S, Gustafsson U (eds). *The sociology of health and illness reader.* Cambridge, UK: Polity Press, 2002: 112–18.

42. Cole M. Out of sight, out of mind: female sexuality and the care plan approach in psychiatric inpatients. *International Journal of Psychiatry in Clinical Practice* 2000; **4** (4): 307–10.

43. McCann E. The sexual and relationship needs of people with psychosis living in the community. Unpublished PhD Thesis. London, UK: City University, 2004.

44. Higgins A, Barker P, Begley C. Sexual health education for people with mental health problems: what can we learn from the literature? *Journal of Psychiatric and Mental Health Nursing* 2006; **13** (6): 687–97.

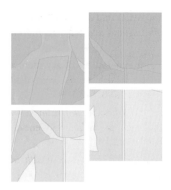

CHAPTER 71

Freedom and consent

Alec Grant*

INTRODUCTION

I hope in this chapter to challenge some conceptual sacred cows within psychiatric–mental health nursing. Drawing primarily on the British experience and literature, I aim to encourage readers to engage productively in relatively *unspoken* aspects of the area of freedom and consent. There is much that is good and useful practised in the name of psychiatric–mental health nursing. However, like Glenister,[1] I believe that it may, at worst, be characterized by institutional and professional denial around specific areas of user freedom. Although knowledge of mental health law is essential to nursing practice,[2–9] as both symptom of and defence against such denial, nurses frequently displace disturbing aspects of users' freedom onto more comfortable areas such as 'capacity' and other legal concerns.

I invite psychiatric–mental health nurses to begin to combat the above trend by seriously engaging in three related challenges.

- First, the rhetoric of empowerment needs to be questioned. At worst, this can seduce student nurses into imagining service users are genuinely situated at the centre of their care, with psychiatric–mental health nurses free to co-facilitate this process.
- Second, how users' need around freedom and consent is constructed in the literature needs to be considered. There are multiple influences on, and possibilities for, the identity construction of service users. Dominant

mainstream constructions vie with alternatives proposed by users who contest, for example, diagnosis- or problem-based identities. Nurses may need to think about where they stand in this debate.
- Finally, nurses must engage with problems endemic to the environmental and cultural conditions which 'set the scene' for the services that users receive and nurses deliver.

In large part, these conditions – whether in residential or community settings – give rise to fundamental difficulties around users' freedom and consent. Nurses may fail to recognize these if their ethical attention is focused only on the legal literature.

THE RHETORIC OF EMPOWERMENT

For service users to experience increased freedom and equality in participating in their own care and treatment, they must harness their power positively. The emerging concept of *empowerment* is problematic and needs to be considered across several contexts. The growth of the user movement,[10] taken at face value, envisions an increasingly vocal collective promoting the need for nurses and other mental health workers to *seriously and meaningfully* listen to users and engage with them in collaborative decision-making;[10,11] to involve them in nursing educational programmes;[12] and to enable them to take more control than has hitherto been the case over their own care

*Alec Grant is a Principal Lecturer at the University of Brighton, UK. His key interests are in clinical supervision, cognitive–behaviour therapy and the impact of organizational issues on practice.

I Justine Fonsong, a year one mental health nursing student from Sept 2017 intake at John Moors University hereby express the interest and passion to request for a transfer into adult nursing. I have taken into consideration many reasons before arriving at this decision. I strongly believe that adult nursing is for me because I like to work not only with people who have mental health conditions but also in a vibrant environment where people are treated with a variety of physical health conditions and making positive contribution regarding to the quality of care provided to patients. This will give me the opportunity to use my nursing skills and also develop new skills especially as I will be working in an environment that is diverse with other problems. I understand the volume of workloads and pressure that goes with this commitment. However, i pride myself in my commitment and attitude towards my work. There is no doubt I will be up to the task.

I have work with mental health nurses during placement. This has helped me to have a clearer view of what their roles and responsibilities are as a mental health nurse. In most instances they barely deal with clinical task and this is one of the areas I am so passionate about in nursing. I love to work in a ward that I can administer drips and other forms of medication. I also like to care for elderly patients who may be bed bound, collect blood when needed and carry out continuous observation using all the necessary equipments as required. These skills can only be fully achieved in adult nursing.

Also, adult nursing have lots of areas of specialities which I am passionate about, thus providing me with lots of experience and opportunities to further develop my profession. Examples include accident and emergency, intensive care unit, acute medical unit, respiratory problems, neurology, oncology and renal. I will be so please to have the opportunity in exploring the various branch of healthcare as listed above. I started my first adult placement on the 14/05/2018 in a respiratory unit and I have so far enjoyed every minutes of it. I provided care to patient with different respiratory conditions with support from my mentor. Within the ward I have also care for patient with some sort of mental health problems. My experience in mental health has also been very valuable in this situation. I think my performance in this placement is actually outstanding given the fact that is my first placement in adult nursing. I have achieved lots of clinical skills already and I am looking forward to achieve more before the end of my placement. Some of the clinical skills I have gained include communication skills, administering drips, injecting patient, wound caring, monitor fluid intake, urine output and stool type.

Adult nurses have higher degree of flexibility to transfer from one area of speciality to another. They benefit from continuing personal and professional development. This help to enhance the knowledge and skills they need to deliver care to patient in a wider area of health within our community. Adult nurses are easily employed in a mental health services which is not the case with mental health nurses. Even in a situation where a mental health nurse may wish to divert into adult nursing, they will have to complete at least a 2 years adult nursing program in the university. Meanwhile an adult nurse will only need to study a mental health adaptation program for 6 month in order to divert into mental health nursing.

In conclusion, I am a reliable and flexible person willing to bring about and accept change. I can work as part of a team or autonomously and have the ability to use my own initiative for problem solving. Finally, I am a team player with skills in team bonding. I have always enjoyed all my duties/placements, this has improved my skills and ability so far. This includes being able to communicate verbally in a competent manner to individuals and groups, being able to produce sound written reports to a high standard, being able to relate to children, young people, adults and those in distress. I have an awareness of anti-discriminatory practice and commitment to working in a way that promotes anti-discriminatory practice. I have the ability to manage a varied workload and effectively prioritise demands. I am a non judgemental person, always willing to listen to other's opinions but can be assertive when required. I have developed all these skills in my previous employments as Health Care Assistant, recent placements and academic task. These skills are vital for adult nursing, coupled with my desire to care and protect patients, an adult nursing offer will fulfil my long term aspiration and do what i desire most.

management.[10,13] However, this rosy view needs to be balanced by an awareness of the institutionally endorsed order and control characteristic of inpatient and community settings,[1,10,14,15] and by what Morrall[15] described as a thinly disguised tokenism:

> … it can be viewed as politically naïve to believe that this will empower … those suffering from chronic mental illness. The impression that [they] are being offered an opportunity to participate in the organization of their care and treatment may well serve to give a token illusion of empowerment, which is in itself disempowering. It can be said that it is not in the interests of the state or professionals to dilute their influence by investing power in … any … service user or carer group.

What empowerment means in practice for nurses will also hinge on them taking a position in regard to the supposed ethical demands of their role.[16] This is by no means straightforward, as a range of possible future ethical and professional identities seduces nurses. They are invited to choose, for example, between the comforting certainties promised by so-called evidence-based mental health practice;[17] a humanly 'ordinary and decent' view of their future role;[18] or a more esoteric view of psychiatric–mental health nursing as a unique and essentially spiritual form of engaging with the humanity of those in psychic distress.[19] However, nurses may discover that, in practice, their professional role socialization is shaped more by institutional[1] and organizational[20] factors than either they or psychiatric–mental health nursing luminaries would care to admit.

Reflection

Consider the influences on the development of your own identity as a psychiatric–mental health nurse. To what extent do you feel that you have been free to choose this as opposed to constrained by 'external' forces?

IMPLICATIONS FOR NURSES AND SERVICE USERS

Identity construction

The rhetoric of empowerment exists within a broader force field of *identity* and *relational politics* in mental health in twenty-first century Britain.[21] A cacophony of voices declare the meaning of being a nurse or service user. In addition to the demands upon nurses to actively work at ethical and professional identity construction, user needs articulated around issues of freedom and consent will vary as a function of ethnicity,[22–24] cultural and religious diversity,[23–25] gender,[26–30] sexuality,[31,32] resistance to representation,[10,33] and the increased tendency for individual[10,33] and corporate[10,11,13] self-definition.

This picture of active identity shaping is in turn inseparable from the broader context of an information society saturated with ever-increasing forms of textual representation. In a positive sense, the psychiatric nursing discussion list[34] has facilitated the emergence of an international psychiatric–mental health nursing identity.[20,35,36] Nurses and, increasingly, users enthusiastically engage in hyper-real dialogue, in which problems around user empowerment, freedom and consent are vigorously discussed – sometimes intelligently, sometimes defensively.

Notwithstanding institutional factors constraining development, in a postmodern vision of psychiatric–mental health nursing, possibilities thus exist for psychiatric–mental health nurses to combine multiple approaches to, and skills in, developing their craft.[21] However, existential angst accompanies this plethora of choices. Because of this, it is not really surprising that psychiatric–mental health nurses characteristically display a tendency towards binary logic with regard to what constitutes the proper focus of psychiatric–mental health nursing on both the psychiatric nursing discussion list and in the literature, and align themselves with often polarized practice and philosophy 'camps'.[37–45] A consistently negative effect of this may be the relegation of the lived experiences and needs of service users around freedom and consent in favour of privileging the dominant agenda of any one particular camp.[21,46–48]

In terms of the capacity of nurses to meaningfully engage with user empowerment, a further and related problem with the rhetoric of empowerment is the continued *overinvestment* in humanistic principles in psychiatric–mental health nursing curricula.[18,20,47,49]

Their uncritical acceptance serves to conceal or marginalize several problems around user freedom and consent. First, in terms of the broader contemporary psychotherapy dialogue, assuming users are free to make informed choices about what they need or want when they may be lacking in sufficient control,[50] readiness to change,[51] self-esteem,[52] hope that change is possible,[53,54] or in the belief in a successful outcome to such an intervention to make those choices in the first place,[54,55] may amount to unwitting abuse on the nurse's part.

There is a further contemporary difficulty with the modernist notion of the coherent 'growing person', from the social constructionist perspective.[56] This notion makes little sense within a postmodern interdisciplinary world view, which envisions and articulates the experiences of multiple, fractured and distributed selves, reflected in service users' perspective and related literature.[57–59]

It may be timely for psychiatric–mental health nursing to challenge the cosy overemphasis of caring enshrined in person-centred curricular approaches and give more attention to considering what they need to do to avoid fulfilling their future institutional capacity to engage in 'violence, coercion and control'.[1] The notion of the self-actualizing user also seems fatuous in the light of environmental and organizational problems in inpatient[10] and community mental health care.[14] These serve to disadvantage users and will be addressed more specifically later.

Soft cop or nurse?

Consider the view of Simpson (A. Simpson, personal communication, 2001), a community psychiatric–mental health nurse researcher, with recent clinical experience of assertive outreach work targeted at homeless mental health clients. He described a bleak and invidious picture of today's British community psychiatric–mental health nurse trapped between two worlds:

> … [despite the sense of the need to maintain a therapeutic role] the supervision register brought in alongside CPA [Care Programme Approach] increased the sense of the CPN [community psychiatric–mental health nurse] as soft cop … the soft police control role is experienced by many nurses as shifting the emphasis towards monitoring people – making sure you keep in contact with people … this results in a blame culture … organizational blame and avoiding risk. All emphasis is in maintaining contact and being seen to do that. If someone commits suicide or kills someone then the finger of blame points at the CPN.
>
> The supervision register didn't work and has been scrapped in line with refinements to the CPA … CPNs are taking on the care coordinator role … having to do more case management and overseeing, with less time to have hands on care with the client … some would say that's okay … employing more community support workers … that respond to a clients' need for a far more accessible, more practical, less talking in jargon worker. The argument against is that to be effective as a CPN you have to have a close relationship with a client.
>
> There's a lot of good stuff in the NSF [National Service Frameworks for Mental Health] … plans for very positive stuff for when things go wrong. However, alongside of that are proposals for the new law (new Mental Health Act) with the emphasis on risk … with more involvement in sectioning. The argument for: good relationship means a better person to section. The argument against: that this is relationship destroying.

Misery without tears

A question emerging for nurses from the above quotation is 'To what extent do existing constructions of service users enhance or inhibit empowerment?' For a broader and more detailed response to this question, readers of this chapter may wish to consult the excellent work of both Parker and his colleagues[60] and Barker and Stevenson.[61] For the moment it is useful to give a specific example of how users' freedom and consent may in reality be enhanced or undermined by assumptions prevalent in the research literature. The 'compliance therapy'

research of Gray *et al.*[62] illustrated the tendency of some British nurse researchers to make (arguably) morally unacceptable, absolutist 'truth claims' from the results of their quantitative paradigm research.[63] Gray *et al.*[62] have been charged with ignoring the issues of social control implicit in their work, where some patients may not have the choice of opting out of a medicosocial structure and where:

> Power is built into the social fabric of mental illness of which we are all a part. It is difficult to compete with the power of money and the new-found knowledge that money can generate.[64]

Long,[64] with support from major qualitative researchers,[63] argued that it behoves quantitative psychiatric–mental health nursing researchers to abandon the fallacy of considering their approach the most *superior* and *only* window in the world worth looking through, and of being above consideration of the ethical and philosophical implications of their methods. Similarly, Gergen[65] highlighted the 'cultural imperialist' position taken by those who fail to attend to the power-imbued, socially constructed nature of what passes for 'neutral' science, in which statistical outcomes portray 'human beings with the tears wiped off'.

In contrast, user-focused research may offer an additional empirical approach to enable individuals with mental health problems to articulate their needs in ways less distorted and influenced by what many regard as a thinly disguised social control and economic agenda. In the early years of this decade, users from the so-called severe and enduring end of the mental health spectrum were trained to conduct research among others with the same severity of problem.[13] Emerging conclusions were that users are perfectly capable of making balanced judgements on the services they receive, and indeed are more likely to open out to researchers who have been through similar experiences.

To conclude this section, it seems apparent that, to accord users adequate respect, psychiatric–mental health nurses need to grapple with the problems around user freedom and consent, in the context of *both* user and nurse identity construction *and* the rhetoric of empowerment.

I will now discuss ways in which acute inpatient and community cultures and environments undermine user freedom. More attention will be paid to problems in acute inpatient environments, because of the overwhelming evidence – at least in Britain – of their intrinsically abusive nature. My aims are to focus the reader's critical awareness of some problem areas and highlight possible solutions emerging from contemporary research.

ACUTE PSYCHIATRIC WARDS

> … acute wards resemble jails and by extension, the nurses jailors.[66]

> I have been discounted both as an agent in my own life … recently, I was told 'Just remember who you are. You're only a patient'.[10]

A reduction over the years in long-stay facilities, and the failure to provide adequate community services, has led to increased pressures on the use of acute psychiatric services. The general picture of acute inpatient wards in England is bleak: although costly in accounting for two-thirds of mental health budgets,[67] there is little evidence that inpatient stays are clinically effective[68] or cost-effective interventions across the range of mental health crises,[69] providing little more than custodial care.[70]

Patients admitted on a voluntary basis often experience the admission as coercive, with many subsequently attempting to leave, only to be compulsory admitted to prevent them from doing so.[71] Patients may want to leave because psychiatric inpatient units are, generally speaking, unpleasant environments. There seems to be a consensus across the user, carer and professional literature that acute inpatients often feel deprived of therapeutic activity and sufficient contact with nurses, and at times feel unsafe and at risk of physical and sexual assault.[1,28,72,73] Patients on acute wards also report boredom because of the limited recreational activity available. They have limited participation in, and information about, their care, which may often be poorly planned and coordinated.[74] Further research, which seems to have established reasonably well that high emotion is a significant factor in worsening the experience of false beliefs and voice hearing,[75] suggested, somewhat paradoxically, that acute inpatient environments may often be likely to provoke a worsening of the symptoms they purport to manage and reduce.

A frequent reason given for trained nursing staff being unable to use their psychotherapeutic skills in acute settings is that they are overworked, spending a disproportionate amount of time on administrative and coordination duties, and managing time-limited crises, at the expense of ongoing, in-depth patient care.[76,77] Nurses have reported decreasing work satisfaction and poor morale, with recruitment, retention and staff sickness as associated problems.[77] Consequently, agency nurses staff many wards. Given the above, it is unsurprising that the nursing of service users in inpatient settings emerges as a site of struggle over client freedom.[10]

Alternatives to acute care are few however, and acute inpatient nurses in Britain today are, in the main, set up for failure. The introduction of clinical governance[78] into the National Health Service aims to increase clinical accountability within trusts and improve on the delivery of patient-centred, evidence-based practice. Jarring with this expectation, and in keeping with the general picture of problems in acute inpatient care described above, Flanagan's[79] small-scale qualitative research of acute inpatient psychiatric–mental health nursing suggested that nurse–patient contact was both limited and usually informal. Overstretched nurses focused most of their energies on a minority of more difficult to manage clients at the expense of less troublesome ones. These nurses were unable to identify specific interventions drawn from research or underpinned by a clear theoretical rationale. Only a small percentage felt that they had sufficient and appropriate training to prepare them for working with psychotic individuals and, equally, few admitted to reading about or discussing recent research or developments in practice.

SECLUSION, RESTRAINT AND SPECIAL OBSERVATION

Without suggesting that it is acceptable practice, it is understandable from the above picture that seclusion and restraint are much used interventions. A systematic review carried out for the Cochrane Library[80] on the empirical status of seclusion and restraint for people deemed as suffering from serious mental illnesses concluded that there are no controlled studies in existence that evaluate the usefulness of seclusion or restraint among those people. Indeed, in support of Sallah,[81] there are potentially serious adverse effects for the use of these techniques, described in the qualitative studies included in the review. The review concludes with the recommendation that alternative ways of dealing with unwanted or harmful behaviours need to be developed.

One method of controlling and containing the most disturbed patients, considered imminently at risk of harming themselves or others, is through observation. Observation has, however, recently been described as a 'woefully weak intervention whose limited effectiveness can be judged by the one-third of people who commit suicide while inpatients'.[82] Bowers and Park[83] in their review of the literature on special observation (SO), while conceding that the procedure is based on clinical pragmatism and traditional custom and practice rather than evaluative research, take a more balanced view. They argue that there is little agreement between healthcare areas about what nurses should do during SO, but report that under certain circumstances the practice can be therapeutic. Conversely, they summarize evidence to suggest that in other circumstances nurses find it stressful and patients dislike it.

Nurses who find the process stressful do so because, among other reasons given, it is frequently regarded as a low-status activity, thus delegated to junior or untrained staff, and because the paternalistic process tends to influence styles of nurse–patient interactions which infantilize the patient receiving SO. Perhaps a more fundamental reason for nurses finding the procedure difficult is the problem of SO placing nurses in a position where patients' rights to privacy and human dignity are temporarily suspended for safety reasons.

From the perspective of the service user, the evidence is equivocal. Inpatients may either feel isolated, degraded, policed, coerced and lacking in interaction with their observer, or understood and accepted.[83] Jones *et al.*[84] reported the findings of a pilot study from the perspective of the patient, in which the experience was predominantly described by most clients as negative. What made observation more palatable was the observing nurse interacting more with the client and providing information about the observation process.

Bowers and Park[83] soberly conclude that SO may be effective for some types of patients and not others, and that different levels of SO may have differing efficacy in different circumstances. For example, a highly intrusive level of SO might be an effective strategy in preventing the suicide, in the short term, of users with severe depression, but completely counterproductive with the violent, paranoid patient. The degree of efficacy might also depend upon what observers do during SO, and how skilled or otherwise they are.

Re-focusing

Partly triggering a vigorous psychiatric nursing list dialogue entitled 'engagement versus obs' in the spring of 2001,[34] Dodds and Bowles[66] provided an alternative to 'formal observation' in re-focused nurse activity. This work builds on the research of Barker and Cutcliffe,[85] who argued that clinical risk in acute psychiatric–mental health inpatient nursing merited engagement rather than observation strategies. In a case study of radical changes to the management of inpatients in an acute English inner city male admission ward, Dodds and Bowles[66] took the view that, arising from a culture of acute psychiatry characterized by medical dominance, formal observation undermines and violates patients' rights and inhibits the development of satisfying supportive relationships between nurses and inpatients.

The objective of their 're-focusing' project was to reclaim nursing control over care in order to reduce formal observations, replacing 'control'-oriented with 'care' interventions, progressing from an individual to a group basis over time. The incidence of formal observation was gradually reduced over a 6-month period, with nurses spending increasingly more time with patients in one-to-one settings, 'enabling alternative nursing interventions to be collaboratively developed with the patients'. Eighteen months into the project, one-to-one observations were totally discontinued, a change which

… has released a significant amount of nursing time. Within the first year of the project, nurses began to provide a weekly programme of activities for patients that continues presently; a programme is published which informs patients what to expect in the coming week … community meetings introduced with an agenda determined by patients and staff.

The authors also reported, among other improvements in the general area of client freedom, reductions in inpatient suicide rates, in deliberate self-harm, in absence without leave, in violent incidents on the ward and in staff sickness. They described a major change in the characteristics of patient care, with

… patients … more engaged with their named nurses, better informed and more involved in their care. All patients now hold their own copies of care plans and discuss them before and after their review with medical staff, on a minimum of a weekly basis.

The most important benefit for clients arising from this project was described as the 'gift of time', which the authors argue is one of the key elements of psychiatric–mental health nursing, valued more highly than any other intervention experienced while in hospital.[86]

In summary, acute inpatient environments present considerable challenges to overstretched psychiatric–mental health nurses keen to enhance client freedom in, and consent for, the inpatient experience. Building on earlier research,[85] the promising work of Dodds and Bowles[66] does, however, suggest a radical, successful and empirically supported alternative to more traditional custodial responses.

THE COMMUNITY EXPERIENCE

The care programme approach (CPA)[87] governs the psychiatric management of people with mental health problems living in the community. However, Rose[13] found that the majority of users in her study did not know what the CPA was for; were clearly not, as advocated, involved in drawing up their care plan; did not know that they had a plan; did not know who their CPA contacts were, or who to contact in a crisis. Mental health professionals were found to assess service users according to their needs, often interpreted as 'problems'. Rose argued that most users in her study felt that their strengths and abilities had not been considered, and reported that what was missing from their care was a 'sympathetic ear and the chance to talk about ordinary things'. This report indicates that, despite the rhetoric of empowerment, and despite locating users in the community at the centre of their care, at least some may not feel meaningfully involved in making collaborative decisions at any level or stage of the process.

Skulduggery

With Rose's findings in mind it is useful at this point to turn to the work of Morrall,[14] who studied the professional context and practice among community psychiatric–mental health nurses (CMHNs). Although his work was local and qualitative, thus by no means generalizable to all community settings, it speaks to the overall problem of users' freedom and consent. It suggests the probability that at least some groups of CMHNs contribute to practice conditions which may undermine the expressed and actual needs of service users around empowerment.

Morrall found that CMHNs in his study organized their caseloads on an arbitrary basis, while being unable to clearly articulate their role. Moreover, they did not in the main receive or accept guidance on the form of intervention appropriate for their clients. Clients were often discharged without an adequate objective evaluation of how ready they were for this.

Supporting previous observations of the behavioural strategies CMHNs use in managing their caseloads, Morrall argued that the group he studied would not in the main openly disagree with the unwelcome control exerted upon them by consultant psychiatrists. Instead, they used in his words 'skulduggerous contrivances' to combat this:

> One CPN stated that when given an 'inappropriate' referral by the psychiatrist, one or two visits are made to the client before she or he is discharged, rather than simply refusing to accept the client in the first place.

Morrall reported the trend of CMHNs either resisting or not having clinical supervision, and adopting sometimes covert techniques to manipulate caseload size. They also exhibited a reluctance to discuss clients on a regular basis with referring agents, including the basis and rationale for their decisions to discharge clients.

The work of Rose and Morrall may help readers of this chapter to consider the extent to which local community psychiatric–mental health nursing practice resembles or deviates from the authors' findings. It might also help preparation of a more acceptable future ethical identity. The key issue is the extent to which aspects of users' freedom and consent is undermined by professionals who actively conceal their practices, and employ covert tactics to avoid engaging with some clients. The major challenge for readers attracted to community psychiatric–mental health nursing as their chosen field is for them to manage their future professional and ethical identities in such a way as to avoid being socialized into skulduggerous practice.

My own experience of teaching on BSc courses in community psychiatric nursing at the University of Brighton does suggest that CMHN students are, in the main, unaccustomed to regular, effective and meaningful clinical supervision. Indeed, most seem resistant to, and defended against, the concept. This trend must be considered in the broader phenomenon of the relative failure of clinical supervision to impact significantly on the work of psychiatric–mental health nurses. In large part, this can be at least partly explained in terms of resistance among psychiatric–mental health nurses, their managers, and writers on clinical supervision in nursing to consider the impact of, or seriously engage with, crucial organizational factors.[88]

THE FUTURE

It is clear that mental health workers and mental health service users are talking and listening together more. What is open to question is both the quality of discussion and the boundaries of debate.[10]

All professions constituting the future mental health service workforce will need to be trained to respond to the needs of service users more effectively.[13] It follows that students must receive adequate and appropriate education and training to do so.[10] A major challenge for lecturers, users, carers and psychiatric–mental health nursing students in the future is to prepare for this while striving to retain and – in the interests of users and carers – ethically enhance a nursing identity.[10,21,48] The dialogue must become more open, and less characterized by professional and institutional forms of denial. Educators must therefore abandon an anachronistic *overinvestment* in humanistic assumptions and principles and take on board strategies for helping nurses respond helpfully to the multiple identities and needs of twenty-first century mental health users. This process must include some attention in curricula to the ways in which organizational factors in mental healthcare settings reduce the likelihood of classroom learning producing effective organizational change and practice.[1,15,89,90]

Nurse educators must also recognize that both clinical and educational areas will probably continue to function for the foreseeable future as blame cultures.[91] Such cultures are, theoretically at any rate, likely to work against liberating professional education agendas. For the foreseeable future, many psychiatric–mental health nurses, like their teachers, will continue to be socialized into an agenda of avoiding creative risk-taking, and are likely to fall back on the kind of established custom and practice, ultimately undermining clients' freedom and consent, favoured in many acute and community settings.[21,89,90]

To balance the above problems, the future will also hopefully see the burgeoning of an already established community of multi-identity psychiatric–mental health nurses and service users, including mental health nurse practitioners and educators who have 'outed' their mental health difficulties.[20,21,34,59] There are, at least for some readers, unfulfilled ongoing dialogic possibilities for solving ethical issues around freedom and consent by participation in the psychiatric nursing discussion list.[34] To some degree, this may fulfil the need expressed by the users' movement in Britain to improve on the 'quality of discussion and the boundaries of debate' between users and psychiatric–mental health nurses.[10]

SUMMARY

In this chapter I have tried to broaden the dialogue on the problems of freedom and consent for psychiatric–mental health nurses and service users, moving away from a myopic focus on legal issues only. With an eye to the future, I hope to have helped readers develop their conceptual, theoretical and empirical vocabulary to begin to meaningfully combat professional and institutional denial and selective attention around important aspects of user freedom and consent. The overarching challenge for psychiatric–mental health nurses of the future is to give much more attention than has hitherto generally been the case to listening to, and taking seriously, the experiences and concerns of the people they purport to empower.[10] In this regard, the last word must go to Dunn,[11] who has recently reminded us that

> … wherever the mentally ill and their loved ones … try and make their voices heard, there is such an overwhelming catalogue of misery reported that I do not have the slightest doubt that there is very considerable cause for concern about their treatment. If I had to sum it up in one brief sentence, I would say that the overwhelming complaint made by the mentally ill and their families is that of not being listened to or not being taken seriously.

The key points of this chapter are:

- Psychiatric–mental health nurses should question the rhetoric of empowerment, where service users are assumed to be at the centre of their care and psychiatric–mental health nurses free to co-facilitate this process.
- Nurses should also consider how users' needs around freedom and consent are constructed in the literature and where they stand on these sets of issues.
- Finally, nurses need to engage with problems in the environmental, cultural and organizational conditions within which they work, which may constrain the possibilities around true freedom and consent.

REFERENCES

1. Glenister D. Coercion, control and mental health nursing. In: Tilley S (ed.). *The mental health nurse: views of practice and education*. Bodmin, UK: Blackwell Science, 1997.

2. Department of Health and Welsh Office. *Code of practice: Mental Health Act 1983*. London, UK: The Stationery Office, 1999.

3. Mind: The Mental Health Charity. *Mind the law: capacity*. London, UK: Mind, May 2000.

4. Applebaum PS, Griiso T. The MacArthur treatment competence study. 1. Mental illness and competence to consent to treatment. *Law and Human Behaviour* 1995; **19**: 105–26.

5. Department of Health. *Reference guide to consent for examination or treatment*. London, UK: Department of Health, March 2001 (copies available free from: Department of Health, PO Box 777, London SE1 6XH; or from NHS Response Line 0541 555 455; or from the Department of Health website www.doh.gov.uk).

6. Department of Health. *12 key points on consent: the law in England*. Available from: www.doh.gov.uk. Accessed March 2001.

7. Green C. When is a patient capable of consent? *Nursing Times* 1999; **95** (7): 50–1.

8. Grisso T, Appelbaum PS. *Assessing competence to consent to treatment: a guide for physicians and other health professionals*. New York, NY: Oxford University Press, 1998.

9. Lord Chancellor. *Making decisions: the government's proposals for making decisions on behalf of mental incapacitated adults*. London, UK: HMSO, 1999.

10. Campbell P. Listening to clients. In: Barker P, Davidson B (eds). *Psychiatric nursing: ethical strife*. London, UK: Arnold, 1998.

11. Dunn C. *Ethical issues in mental illness*. Aldershot, UK: Ashgate, 2000.

12. English National Board. *Regulations and guidelines for the approval of institutions and programmes*. London, UK: ENB, 1996.

13. Rose D. *Users' voices: the perspectives of mental health service users on community and hospital care*. London, UK: The Sainsbury Centre for Mental Health, 2001.

14. Morrall P. *Mental health nursing and social control*. London, UK: Whurr, 1999.

15. Morrall P. Clinical sociology and empowerment. In: Barker P, Davidson B (eds). *Psychiatric nursing: ethical strife*. London, UK: Arnold, 1998.

16. Barker P, Davidson B (eds). *Psychiatric nursing: ethical strife*. London, UK: Arnold, 1998.

17. Newell R, Gournay K (eds). *Mental health nursing: an evidence-based approach*. London, UK: Churchill Livingstone, 2000.

18. Clarke L. *Challenging ideas in psychiatric nursing*. London, UK: Routledge, 1999.

19. Barker P. *The philosophy and practice of psychiatric nursing*. London, UK: Churchill Livingstone, 1999.

20. Grant A. Psychiatric nursing and organizational power: rescuing the hidden dynamic. *Journal of Psychiatric and Mental Health Nursing* 2001; **8**: 173–88.

21. Grant A. Knowing me knowing you: towards a new relational politics in 21st century mental health nursing. *Journal of Psychiatric and Mental Health Nursing* 2001; **8**: 269–75.

22. The Sainsbury Centre for Mental Health in collaboration with the University of Central Lancashire, Health and Ethnicity Unit. *Improving care for detained patients from black and minority ethnic communities*. National Visit 2. A visit by the Mental Health Act Commission to 104 Mental Health and Learning Disability Units in England and Wales. London, UK: The Sainsbury Centre for Mental Health, 2000.

23. Jennings S. *Creating solutions: developing alternatives in black mental health*. London, UK: King's Fund Publishing, 1997.

24. Warner L, Nicholas S, Patel K *et al. Improving care for detained patients from black and minority ethnic communities. Preliminary report*. National Visit 2. A visit by the Mental Health Act Commission to 104 mental health and learning disabilities units in England and Wales. London, UK: The Sainsbury Centre for Mental Health in association with The University of Central Lancashire, 2000.

25. Copsey N. *The provision of community mental health services within a multi-faith context.* London, UK: The Sainsbury Centre for Mental Health, 1997.

26. Newton S-A. Women and mental health nursing. In: Tilley S (ed.). *The mental health nurse: views of practice and education.* Bodmin, UK: Blackwell Science, 1997.

27. Thilbert D. Working with women. In: Barker P, Davidson B (eds). *Psychiatric nursing: ethical strife.* London, UK: Arnold, 1998.

28. NHS Executive. *Safety, privacy and dignity in mental health units: guidance on mixed sex accommodation for mental health services.* London, UK: NHS Executive, 2000.

29. Orme J. *Gender and community care: social work and social care perspectives.* New York, NY: Palgrave, 2001.

30. Kohen D (ed.). *Women and mental health.* London, UK: Routledge, 2000.

31. Golding J. *Without prejudice: MIND lesbian, gay and bisexual mental health awareness research.* London, UK: MIND Publications, 1997.

32. McFarlane L. *Diagnosis: homophobic – the experiences of lesbians, gay men and bisexuals in mental health services.* London, UK: PACE (the Project for Advice, Counselling and Education), 1998 (email: pace@dircon.co.uk).

33. Coleman R. The politics of the illness. In: Barker P, Stevenson C (eds). *The construction of power and authority in psychiatry.* Oxford, UK: Butterworth Heinemann, 2000.

34. Psychiatric Nursing List. Homepage. Available from: www.city.ac.uk/sonm/psychiatric-nursing/.

35. Lakeman R. Psychiatric nursing. The Internet: facilitating an international culture for psychiatric nurses. *Computers in Nursing* 1996; **16** (2): 87–9.

36. Bowers L. Constructing international professional identity: what psychiatric nurses talk about on the Internet. *International Journal of Nursing Studies* 1997; **34** (3): 208–12.

37. Clarke L. Nursing in search of a science: the rise and rise of the new nurse brutalism. *Mental Health Care* 1999; **21**: 270–2.

38. Cannon B, Coulter E, Gamble C *et al.* Personality bashing. *Mental Health Care* 1999; **21**: 319.

39. Ritter S. Insulting distortion. *Mental Health Care* 1999; **21**: 319.

40. Rogers P. Persecution complex. *Mental Health Care* 1999; **21**: 319.

41. Barker P. Arrested development. *Mental Health Care* 1999; **21**: 393.

42. Stevenson C. Power and control. *Mental Health Care* 1999; **21**: 393.

43. Duncan-Grant A. Misrepresentation, stereotyping, and acknowledging bias in science: responses to Liam Clarke. *Mental Health Care* 1999; **21**: 336–7.

44. Gournay K. What to do with nursing models. *Journal of Psychiatric and Mental Health Nursing* 1996; **2**: 325–7.

45. Barker PJ, Reynolds B. Rediscovering the proper focus of nursing: a critique of Gournay's position on nursing theory and models. *Journal of Psychiatric and Mental Health Nursing* 1995; **3**: 75–80.

46. Repper J. Adjusting the focus of mental health nursing: incorporating service users' experiences of recovery. *Journal of Mental Health* 2000; **9** (6): 575–87.

47. Dallard D. What does counselling do? A critical re-examination of Rogers' core conditions. *Mental Health Care* 1999; **21**: 383–5.

48. Rolfe G, Gardner L. The possibility of a genuine mental health nursing. In: Barker P (ed.). *Psychiatric and mental health nursing: the craft of caring.* London, UK: Arnold, 2003.

49. Grant A. Tales from the order of received wisdom (or some contemporary problems with mental health nurse education in Britain). *Journal of Psychiatric and Mental Health Nursing* 2002; **9**: 622–7.

50. Rotter JB. Generalized expectancies for internal versus external control of reinforcement. *Psychological Monographs* 1966; 80.

51. Diclemente CC, McCounnaughy EA, Norcross JC, Prochaska JO. Integrative dimensions for psychotherapy. *International Journal of Eclectic Psychotherapy* 1986; **5** (3): 256–73.

52. Fennell M. *Overcoming low self-esteem: a self-help guide using cognitive–behavioural techniques.* London, UK: Robinson, 1999.

53. Snyder CR, Ilardi SS, Cheavens J, *et al.* The role of hope in cognitive behaviour therapies. *Cognitive Therapy and Research* 2000; **24** (6): 747–62.

54. Grant A, Townend M, Mills J, Cockx A. *Assessment and case formulation in CBT.* London, UK: Sage Publications, 2008.

55. Bandura A. *Social learning theory.* London, UK: Prentice-Hall, 1977.

56. Rogers CR. *On becoming a person: a therapist's view of psychotherapy.* London, UK: Constable, 1988.

57. Wetherell M, Maybin J. The distributed self: a social constructionist perspective. In: Stevens R (ed.). *Understanding the self.* London, UK: Sage, in association with The Open University, 1997.

58. Holstein JA, Gubrium JF. *The self we live by. Narrative identity in a postmodern world.* New York, NY: Oxford University Press, 2000.

59. Short N, Grant A, Clarke L. Living in the Borderlands; writing in the margins: an autoethnographic tale. *Journal of Psychiatric and Mental Health Nursing* 2007; **14**: 771–82.

60. Parker I, Georgaca G, Harper D *et al. Deconstructing psychopathology.* London, UK: Sage, 1999.

61. Barker P, Stevenson C (eds). *The construction of power and authority in psychiatry.* Oxford, UK: Butterworth-Heinemann, 2000.

62. Gray R, Gournay K, Taylor D. New drug treatments for schizophrenia: implications for mental health nursing. *Mental Health Practice* 1997; **1**: 20–23.

63. Denzin NK, Lincoln YS (eds). *Handbook of qualitative research*, 2nd edn. Thousand Oaks, CA: Sage, 2000.

64. Long A. Have we the right to deny people their right to embrace their emotional pain? *Journal of Psychiatric and Mental Health Nursing* 2001; **8**: 85–92.

65. Gergen KG. *An invitation to social construction.* London, UK: Sage Publications, 1999.

66. Dodds P, Bowles N. Dismantling formal observation and refocusing nursing activity in acute inpatient psychiatry: a case study. *Journal of Psychiatric and Mental Health Nursing* 2001; **8**: 183–8.

67. Kennedy P. Mental health: implementing the national service framework (Editorial). *Health Policy Matters* 2000; **1**: 1.

68. The Sainsbury Centre for Mental Health. *Acute problems: a survey of the quality of care in acute psychiatric wards.* London, UK: The Sainsbury Centre for Mental Health, 1998.

69. Minghella E, Ford R, Freeman T *et al. Open all hours: 24-hour response for people with mental health emergencies.* London, UK: The Sainsbury Centre for Mental Health, 1998.

70. Mental Health Act Commission and the Sainsbury Centre for Mental Health. *The national visit: a one-day visit to 309 acute psychiatric admission wards by the MHAC in collaboration with the Sainsbury Centre for Mental Health.* London, UK: Sainsbury Centre for Mental Health, 1997.

71. Fanham FR, James DV. Patients' attitudes to psychiatric hospital admission. *The Lancet* 2000; **335**: 594.

72. The Sainsbury Centre for Mental Health. *Acute problems: a survey of the quality of care in acute psychiatric wards.* London, UK: The Sainsbury Centre for Mental Health, 1998.

73. Department of Health. *Modernising mental health services.* London, UK: HMSO, 1998.

74. Moore C. Acute psychiatric wards: what do patients get? *Mental Health Practice* 1998; **1**: 12–13.

75. The British Psychological Society. *Understanding mental illness: recent advances in understanding mental illness and psychotic experiences.* A report by the British Psychological Society Division of Clinical Psychology. Leicester, UK: The British Psychological Society, 2000.

76. Gijbels H. Mental health nursing skills in an acute admission environment: perceptions of mental health nurses and other mental health professionals. *Journal of Advanced Nursing* 1995; **21**: 460–5.

77. Higgins R, Hurst K, Wistow G. Nursing acute psychiatric patients: a quantitative and qualitative study. *Journal of Advanced Nursing* 1999; **29**: 52–63.

78. Department of Health. *The new NHS.* London, UK: HMSO, 1997.

79. Flanagan T. Mental health nursing in the acute inpatient setting: unravelling the chaos. Research paper presented at *Developing evidence to enhance practice,* 6th Annual INAM Research Conference. University of Brighton, 2001.

80. Sailas E, Fenton M. Seclusion and restraint for people with serious mental illnesses. *Cochrane Database of Systematic Reviews* 2001; Issue 2. Available from: www.update-software.com/abstracts/ab001163.htm.

81. Sallah D. Alternatives to seclusion. In: Tilley S (ed.). *The mental health nurse: views of practice and education.* Bodmin, UK: Blackwell Science, 1997.

82. Barker P, Cutcliffe J. Hoping against hope. *Open Mind 101* 2000; **Jan/Feb**: 18–19.

83. Bowers L, Park A. Special observation in the care of psychiatric inpatients: a literature review. *Issues in Mental Health Nursing* 2001; **22**: 769–86.

84. Jones J, Lowe T, Ward M. Inpatients' experiences of nursing observation on an acute psychiatric unit: a pilot study. *Mental Health and Learning Disabilities Care* 2000; **4** (4): 125–9.

85. Barker P, Cutcliffe J. Clinical risk: a need for engagement not observation. *Mental Health Practice* 1999; **2** (8): 8–12.

86. Jackson S, Stevenson C. The gift of time from the friendly professional. *Nursing Standard* 1998; **12**: 31–3.

87. Department of Health. *National Health Service and Community Care Act.* London, UK: HMSO, 1990.

88. Grant A. *Clinical supervision among mental health nurses: a critical organizational ethnography.* Portsmouth, UK: Nursing Praxis International, 2001.

89. Morgan G. *Images of organization.* Thousand Oaks, CA: Sage, 1997.

90. Grant A, Mills J. The great going nowhere show: structural power and mental health nurses. *Mental Health Practice* 2000; **4**: 6–7.

91. Department of Health. *An organisation with a memory: report of an expert group on learning from adverse events in the NHS Chaired by the Chief Medical Officer,* 2000. Available from: www.doh.gov.uk.

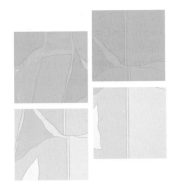

CHAPTER 72

Providing culturally safe care

Anthony J. O'Brien,* Erina Morrison**
and Ruth DeSouza***

INTRODUCTION

The encounter between a nurse and a service user may involve an interaction between two people with multiple and very different identities. For both the nurse and the service user, a wide range of beliefs, experiences, norms and values will influence perceptions of mental health and mental health care. The therapeutic relationship is influenced by a multiplicity of cultural beliefs and values – those of the nurse and those of the service user. The role of the nurse is to develop a relationship which recognizes and respects the service user's cultural and religious identities, and the influence of cultural identity on the therapeutic encounter. We wish to affirm the shifting and multiple nature of cultural identity, rather than propose a model of identity as fixed and unchanging.

Here, we shall discuss the issue of *culture* as it relates to mental health nursing. We have included reference to religious identity, given the increasing religious diversity of many Western countries, and the recognition of the need for psychiatry to develop partnerships with faith-based organizations.[1] Global population movements challenge our traditional views of culture and require new responses from mental health nurses.[2] We aim to provide a basis for mental health nurses to reflect on their own cultural identities and those of the people they care for. We *do not* prescribe how you should engage with people from cultural backgrounds different from your own. Rather, we suggest that you think about cultural and religious identity; what impact cultural difference has on the interactions between nurse and service user. Although the term 'culture' is most frequently used to refer to ethnic culture, it can usefully be applied to a range of differences, including those of gender, sexuality, physical ability, age and religion.[3] Here, 'culture' refers to ethnic culture, although it is recognized that the discussion may also have relevance to various forms of group *belonging*, such as social class, religion and gender.

Research and theory on the 'need for nursing'[4,5] provides a theme which integrates this chapter with other

*Tony O'Brien is a Senior Lecturer in Mental Health Nursing at the University of Auckland, and a Nurse Specialist in Liaison Psychiatry at Auckland City Hospital, New Zealand. He is interested in social issues in mental health nursing and in ways of reducing coercion in mental health care. He is a fifth generation Pakeha New Zealander of Irish and Scots ancestry.

**Erina Morrison is of Te Arawa, Ngati Whakaue and Ngati Kahunungu, Rakaipaaka descent, with affiliation to Tainui. Erina has a clinical background in acute assessment and care, inpatient therapeutic programmes. She has lectured in undergraduate and postgraduate programmes, teaching in cultural safety, Maori health and advanced practice. Research has included clinical indicators for standards of practice, and Maori mental health nursing. Erina is passionate about quality nursing service provision, and safe work environments with happy nurses.

***Ruth DeSouza is a Senior Research Fellow and Coordinator of the AUT Centre for Asian and Migrant Health Research. She has worked as a nurse therapist, clinician, educator and researcher and is a passionate advocate for inclusion. Ruth originates from Goa, but was born in Tanzania then moved to Kenya before her family migrated to New Zealand.

sections of this book. Embedded in the three levels of need identified by this body of work is the need for cultural respect and affirmation. As with other human needs, cultural needs do not immediately show themselves to the nurse, and should not be identified independently by the nurse. Instead, the service user should identify those needs. The need for engagement as a basis for providing culturally safe care recognizes the relationship between nurse and service user as central to the process of providing appropriate care. Without a relationship of empathy and trust, service users are unlikely to identify cultural needs, and so will be unlikely to avail themselves of ways of meeting them.

We draw on New Zealand and other international experiences in developing the concept of cultural safety. Consistent with the view that reflection on cultural identity is the basis for providing culturally safe care to others,[6] the chapter should be seen in the light of the authors' cultural identities and context.

- *Tony O'Brien*, is a Pakeha[a] male academic and clinical practitioner.
- *Erina Morrison-Ngatai*, is a Maori[b] female academic.
- *Ruth DeSouza* is a researcher who is an East African, Goan, New Zealander.

We work in a postcolonial New Zealand society that is meeting the challenges of restoration and redress for its indigenous people, and of the neocolonization processes of globalization. While the model of cultural safety we outline is applicable beyond New Zealand, like models of nursing and mental health care, it needs interpretation in local contexts, if it is to fully acknowledge the realities of individual nurses and service users.

Reflection

How would you define yourself, in 'cultural' terms? Would you give priority to ethnicity, religious beliefs, gender, or some other aspect of 'culture'?

RACE, ETHNICITY AND CULTURAL IDENTITY

The concept of race has its origins in anthropologists' attempts to classify human beings based on observable differences in physical attributes. Many early writings on race, including those of prominent theorists of psychiatry, reflect views of the innate superiority of white people over other races.[6,7] Because of these associations, use of the term 'race' is in decline.[8] 'Race' refers to human groupings based on physical markers,[6] and a set of associated social and political processes sometimes termed

'racialization'.[9] In the health sciences it is now more common to speak of 'ethnicity', a term that implies a sense of *group belonging*, which is self-claimed and not imposed on the basis of observable physical attributes.[10] However, the concept of ethnicity recognizes the biological basis of physical characteristics of ethnic groups. The terms 'race' and 'ethnicity' are sometimes used interchangeably.

Culture can be defined as a set of traditions, beliefs, values and practices shared by members of a social group.[10] While it is commonly thought that culture and ethnicity are synonymous, the concepts are not identical. A person is born with particular characteristics, some of which are attributable to ethnicity, in the biological sense discussed above. Frequently, individuals are influenced by characteristics of more than one ethnic group. For instance, a person's physical characteristics may reflect Chinese and Caucasian ancestry. Recent research using DNA technology shows that individuals may not be aware of all the influences on their ancestry.[9] Physical markers are also subject to interpretation and so do not have fixed or stable meanings.[6] If we wish to understand a person's beliefs, values and behaviour, we need to know about the group affiliations of that person, or their culture.

Members of a single ethnic group will have different experiences of what it means to be a member of that group. However, the language used to describe ethnicity reflects the tendency to make generalizations, which have the potential to become stereotypes. The term 'Asian' has been criticized for its tendency to obscure differences between specific ethnic groups[11] in the United States, Canada, Britain,[12] Australia[13] and New Zealand.[14] Differing uses of 'Asian' within Britain include or exclude ethnic Indians or Chinese in different surveys and do not always reflect individuals' self-perceived ethnic identities.[12] A similar issue is found in New Zealand, where two differing constructions of 'Asian' are employed.[14] Popular discourse and the media employ a racially based construction that includes only East and Southeast Asian peoples, while the other construction, increasingly used in health research, includes peoples from East, South and Southeast Asia, but excludes peoples from the Middle East and Central Asia. In health, such broad categories can mask high health needs of groups within the category, resulting in services being targeted inappropriately. In clinical practice, service users may not identify with broad categories such as 'Asian', leading to potential for miscommunication. To make sound clinical decisions about the mental health needs of members of this group, it is necessary to recognize its diversity.[12,13]

Within ethnic groups other forms of group belonging will influence individuals' perceptions of health. As Pilgrim and Rogers[8] note, within different cultures there are differences in the experience of mental distress, for example

---

[a] The term 'Pakeha' is used in New Zealand to refer to people of Anglo, Celtic or Caucasian ancestry.
[b] Maori people are the indigenous people of Aotearoa/New Zealand.

those based on gender. Furthermore, for some people religion represents a world view that is a more defining marker of identity than ethnicity. Nurses need to recognize that identification of 'culture' can be a form of imposition, in which a nurse classifies a service user, based on the nurse's beliefs or expectations about that person's cultural identity.[15] This is especially so if the nurse's classification is based solely on characteristics such as name, skin colour or facial features, rather than on the person's expressed cultural identity. Box 72.1 summarizes the results of New Zealand research documenting clinical nursing practice in the area of identification of cultural needs.

Box 72.1: Identification of cultural needs

Legal, ethical and moral issues

In a recent audit of case notes in 11 out of 22 mental health services in New Zealand[16] it was found that, in 65 per cent of cases, service users were not given the opportunity to identify their cultural needs. In addition, 28 per cent of service users were not offered support for those cultural issues they did identify. Encouragingly, in 65 per cent of cases, Maori cultural advisors were consulted regarding the care of Maori service users. However, only 23 per cent of Maori service users were offered cultural assessment, in accordance with the requirement of the New Zealand Mental Health Standard.[17] For the purposes of this study, identification of ethnicity by the nurse was not considered to represent an opportunity to identify cultural needs. Assessment is a key aspect of nursing care, and is crucial to planning appropriate care. Without an opportunity to identify cultural needs, service users are not able to access cultural support, and this is likely to adversely affect their engagement with and response to care. Providing an opportunity to identify cultural needs is dependent on the establishment of rapport, and should be negotiated with the service user.

Reflection

Which 'ethnic' groups do you belong to?
How does this differ from your 'cultural identity'?
How easy, or difficult, is it for you to define your 'ethnicity' and 'cultural identity'?
What does that mean for you?

CULTURAL DIFFERENCES IN CLINICAL PRACTICE

Western psychiatry is highly influenced by culture, and it is here that we must begin. The illness model of mental distress is a construct developed by Western psychiatry, but which contrasts sharply with collectivist ways of thinking, e.g. of Indian, African, Asian and Polynesian cultures.[8,18] Also, Western models of mental health care are based on the ideal of disengagement of the self, so that the search for mental health becomes a search for an ideal individual self. This is reflected in models of psychotherapy and treatment, which assume a *universal self*, free of the influences of culture.[19] This ignores the paradigms of collectivist cultures. For example, Maori cultural beliefs see good mental health as an outcome of *harmony* with oneself, one's family, community, ancestors, creator and the environment.[20] Within Western models of mental health, culture and religion provide the *content* (thoughts, perceptions, feelings) associated with mental illness, while the *form* (depressed mood, psychosis) is considered to be culture free. Leff[21] presents evidence from studies in a wide range of countries, which suggests that functional psychosis is a universal human experience. However, he cautions that this conclusion should be interpreted carefully, as the instruments used in the studies 'were constructed in the West and may have imposed a cultural stereotype on the patient populations examined'.[21,p.42]

Whatever the influence of culture on the content or form of mental illness, when people come into contact with mental health services, culture plays a significant role. Evidence suggests that ethnicity influences presentation to services, assessment and decisions about care and treatment.[22] Ethnicity has also been found to influence pathways to care, diagnosis, prescribing patterns and use of ECT.[8,23] While there are many factors that may mediate the influence of ethnicity (such as age, social isolation, gender, socioeconomic status, severity of illness), it seems that ethnicity is a significant factor in service users' involvement in mental health care. It is also possible that aspects of a person's presentation, ascribed to culture, are actually related to other aspects of their identity, such as religion.[24] While ethnicity may be evident to an observer, religious beliefs are not usually obvious. Both cultural and religious identity will influence the acceptability and appropriateness of mental health services.

Working at the 'care face'[25] of mental health brings nurses into close contact with service users, in situations where ethnic difference may play a crucial role in shaping relationships. One area of nursing practice that has been influenced by ethnicity is nurses' perceptions of *dangerousness*. When behaviour is perceived to be dangerous there are a number of responses available. These range from 'one-to-one' intervention and supported time out, through to coercive measures such as seclusion and restraint. Nurses' responses to acts of violence may be influenced by the ethnicity of the service user. In a study of violence in inpatient units there was no difference, based on ethnicity, in rates of compulsory detention.[26] However, the same study reported that non-violent black[c] patients were four times more likely than non-violent whites to be admitted to a locked unit. Another study found that restraint was almost four times more likely to be used following violence by black than by white service users,[27] suggesting that nurses may have a lower tolerance of violence by blacks than by whites.

While there is clear evidence that rates of diagnosis and decisions about treatment and care are influenced by clinicians' perceptions of ethnicity, there is also concern that insufficient attention may be given to the influence of biological differences between different ethnic groups. Metabolism of psychoactive medications, development of side-effects and adverse effects, and thresholds of effectiveness have all been shown to have some variability related to ethnicity.[28] The effects of these differences may be further compounded by cultural differences in help-seeking, expression of symptoms and patterns of communication.[28] Nurses need to be familiar with the specific effects of psychoactive medications on different ethnic groups, and of cultural differences in patterns of response.

Developing effective responses to cultural difference

Nurses learn, through therapeutic relationships, to respond to the emotional distress of service users. Part of this process involves reflection on the experiences, assumptions and skills the nurse brings to the therapeutic relationship. The increasing ethnic diversity of countries in which mental health nursing is practised suggests a need for reflection on cultural identity as part of the process of development of nursing skills.[6] Reflection should include consideration of power differences in the nurse–patient relationship, placing the onus for recognizing and responding to cultural difference with the nurse rather than the service user.[29] Clinical supervision can provide opportunities to reflect on the influence of cultural identity on clinical practice.[30]

The diverse cultural needs of users of health services require that nurses develop approaches to care that recognize and respect the cultures of service users.

- Cultural *sensitivity* is 'an ongoing awareness of cultural differences and similarities among populations'.[31] It involves awareness of cultural difference and knowledge of some of the culturally specific beliefs and practices that may influence service users' engagement with care.
- Cultural *competence* is defined as 'respect for, and understanding of, diverse ethnic and cultural groups, their histories, traditions, beliefs and value systems'.[32] This recognizes the need for nurses to be sensitive to the culture of service users, and to respond to cultural diversity within the service user group. Wells[33] has identified

the need for cultural competence to extend beyond the individual, and embrace institutional change.
- Cultural *proficiency* begins with examination of cultural biases, those 'cultural values and beliefs that are internalized through the socialization process',[33,p.193] and includes organizational change within the educational institutions and health services.
- Cultural *safety* meets Wells' criteria for cultural proficiency, but also requires reflection on the particular history and social context of the society in which health care is provided.

Reflection

How does the 'cultural background' of a person influence how you relate to that person?

CULTURALLY SAFE CARE

Cultural safety differs from cultural sensitivity, cultural competence and cultural proficiency by envisaging a *process of change:* from sensitivity, through awareness, to safety. Although it originated in New Zealand, cultural safety has been applied to a range of social contexts.[3,34,35]

Cultural safety has been defined as:

> The effective nursing of a person/family from another culture by a nurse who has undertaken a process of reflection on her/his own cultural identity and recognizes the impact of the nurse's cultural identities on his/her own nursing practice.[15,36]

Although cultural safety was originally developed as a response to the disproportionate health problems of Maori, the concept is applicable to all cultures.[37] Within a dominant culture, indigenous peoples, and those seen as different by the dominant culture, are potentially at risk and require culturally safe care. This is also important for immigrant groups,[38,39] for example Pacific Island people in New Zealand, Vietnamese in Australia, West Indians in the UK or North African immigrants to European countries.

Cultural safety begins with analysis of the historical relationships between the different groups that make up a society.[40] The focus of cultural safety is on the social positions of these groups rather than solely on their distinctive cultural beliefs or practices as a basis for developing culturally safe relationships with service users.[37] On this basis, health is placed in a political and historical context. Cultural safety focuses on the social, economic, political and historical influences on health, and on providers of health services.[35] Because the political and

---

^cWhile 'black' does not refer to a particular ethnicity, it is a term used to refer to non-white minorities, particularly in Britain.[11]

historical context of each society is unique, cultural safety needs to be given specific meaning within local contexts. The principle of recognition of the histories of different cultures within different societies, the historical relationships between different cultures, and, in particular, issues of power differences between cultures is a significant extension of concepts such as cultural sensitivity and cultural competence.

Nurses learning to be *culturally safe practitioners* begin with reflection on their own cultural identity and history, and move, through guided education, to commitment to personal and political change. Woods and Schwass[34] depict this process of change as occurring in three stages: *dualism*, *relativism* and *evolving commitment*. The model of change is outlined in Figure 72.1, with examples of development of cultural safety in the process of assessment.

Stage 1: dualism	*Clinical example*
At this stage, nurses rely on authority to provide answers to questions of cultural difference. They look to literature and expert opinion to guide their thinking, although their own beliefs are strongly held. A characteristic statement at this stage is 'Culture doesn't matter to me. I treat everyone the same regardless of their culture'. Nurses are not aware that they cannot step outside their own culture, and that their interactions are, in part, culturally determined.	A nurse conducts an assessment interview and records the service user's ethnicity after asking the patient to select ethnicity from a list. There is no discussion of whether the categories available reflect the person's cultural identity. The nurse believes that while it is important to acknowledge cultural identity, this can be achieved on the basis of ethnicity. There may be an assumption that the person will make any special needs known, and so no inquiry about special cultural needs is undertaken. Any requests regarding cultural needs are responded to on the basis of the same treatment to all patients regardless of particular cultural needs.
Stage 2: relativism	*Clinical example*
Here, nurses are aware of the diversity of cultural perspectives, but may feel that all views have equal validity. Authorities, including cultural authorities, are simply one more opinion. No one action appears better than another. A nurse might say, 'We all have our own views, but none of us can claim to be right. Even members of the same culture might have different views. We should try to respect them all.' This recognizes diversity both between and within cultures. However, that diversity is seen as invalidating actions that are committed to a particular cultural perspective.	As part of the assessment interview the service user is asked to identify his or her ethnicity, but also asked if the available categories accurately reflect the service user's cultural identity. Additional comments or issues are recorded after discussion with the service user. The nurse is aware that ethnicity does not determine cultural beliefs, and asks if there are any particular cultural needs. Specific needs will be addressed if the resources for doing this are immediately available. If there are no resources immediately available this is simply recognized as a limitation of the system.
Stage 3: evolving commitment	*Clinical example*
The nurse at this stage is able to both recognize diversity of cultural perspectives, and commit themselves to a course of action. The action is informed by the realities of the nurse's culture, his place in the power relationships of health care, and the realities of the culture of the service user. Commitment is demonstrated in the statement: 'People don't always feel safe to identify their cultural needs. We need to create a safe environment in which needs can be expressed, and provide the right supports so that those needs can be met'. The nurse making this statement is aware that factors outside the individual nurse–patient relationship influence the health care encounter, and consciously uses the power of her position to benefit the patient.	The nurse creates a safe environment for the assessment interview, perhaps by involving members of the service user's family, with the consent of the service user. The service user self-identifies his or her ethnicity, and is given an opportunity to identify any specific needs or concerns. When specific needs are identified by the service user, the nurse talks to colleagues and members of the service user's cultural group to establish ways of providing appropriate cultural support. Support is provided only in consultation with the service user. The nurse reflects on the impact of social processes on the healthcare encounter and uses the experience to further his or her own knowledge of resources and supports available, and to make that knowledge available to other nurses in the service.

Figure 72.1 Developing cultural safety in the process of assessment. Adapted from Woods and Schwass[34]

Cultural safety and collaborative care

The process of psychiatric–mental health nursing involves establishing collaborative therapeutic relationships with service users on the basis of their need for nursing care.[5] Barker's *Tidal Model* of mental health nursing[5] stresses the need for the person's experience of mental distress or illness to be understood by the nurse. It also emphasizes provision of 'support and services a person might need to live an ordinary life'.[5,p.234] However, development of understanding between nurses and service users is influenced by differences that must be negotiated by the nurse.[29] In cross-cultural encounters the paradoxical nature of nursing is apparent. After researching nurses' experiences of cross-cultural caring, Spence[41] concluded that 'Trying to be oneself in a way that enables others to be themselves, under circumstances that are intrinsically never fully knowable, is unlikely to be free of tension.'

Nurses who are focused on establishing a therapeutic relationship will consider both their own cultural identities and those of the service user. Making sense of the experience of mental distress or illness requires understanding of the influence of culture on that experience. Because of the sheer diversity of service users' cultural identities in relation to that of the nurse, it will not be possible for nurses to understand all the possible cultural influences the nurse and service user bring to the therapeutic relationship. Such an approach, while demonstrating culturally sensitivity, assumes that racism is the product of ignorance and that, by learning about other cultures, people will be educated out of their prejudices.

Nurses also need to provide opportunities for service users to make their cultural needs known. Additional strategies include developing partnerships with cultural intermediaries or developing ethnic support worker roles.[42] Collaborative care relies on therapeutic communication, which reflects the cultural backgrounds of nurses and service users. Communication patterns are influenced by culture, with many communication patterns being culture bound. In a study of Chinese service users' communications patterns with nurses, unique cultural influences were identified.[43] While the nurses were aware that Chinese culture had a significant effect on therapeutic communication, their communication strategies tended to reflect the Western models of their nursing education. The researchers recommended that Chinese service users would benefit from nurses' improved understanding of culturally bound communication strategies. As discussed previously in this chapter, understanding the culture of others does not involve becoming an expert or authority on those cultures.

In New Zealand Morrison-Ngatai[20] has discussed a Maori model of communication, which, while consistent with principles of therapeutic communication, respects the cultural identity of Maori service users. We discuss the *Te Niho-Mako* model here not to suggest that it should be adopted by others, but as an exemplar of how general theory on therapeutic communication can be reinterpreted to take account of the needs of a specific cultural group.

The *Te Niho-Mako* model 'fosters the inherent need for Maori, of connecting, linking and bonding'.[20] The three concepts which form the model are *tata*, *kupu* and *tika*. Their nearest equivalents in Pakeha terms are *attending*, *listening* and *etiquette*. While the first two concepts are familiar, the third refers to rightness of the situation: feelings and thoughts are expressed in ways that are sometimes verbal, sometimes physical. Within the *Te Niho-Mako* model spontaneity, rather than reserve, is valued. The model is recommended to nurses caring for Maori service users, although it is regarded as being of particular value in situations where Maori care for Maori (see Culturally specific services).

The dominant *interpersonal model* of mental health nursing is a Western construct, developed within a North American cultural context and adopted in other Western and non-Western countries. However, the practice of mental health nursing needs to be responsive to the realities of the diverse cultures in which it takes place, in order to provide care that service users experience as culturally safe.

Service user involvement

It can be useful to consider issues of culture in the context of moves to involve users of services in planning, provision and evaluation of mental health services. Mental health services have traditionally been organized around the needs of service providers, rather than service users,[44,45] and have reflected the cultural values of the provider group. However, users of services are disproportionately members of minority cultures, whose values are not always recognized in the services provided.

Involvement of service users has meant that nurses have had to consider how their practice best meets the needs of the people they care for.[44,45] One way of meeting the needs of culturally diverse groups is to involve those groups in the provision of services. Service users can be involved in direct care roles or in advisory roles aimed at promoting the cultural safety of the service. Nurses can expect to work alongside service users and can learn from both the service experience and cultural experience this group has to offer.

Involvement in services can extend to managing service provision. Pierre[46] describes the role of a company formed by service users to provide services to ethnic minority service users in Liverpool, UK. In providing services the company seeks to create a non-racist environment which challenges institutional processes encountered by ethnic minorities in mainstream services. Pierre concludes that 'user involvement is not an impossible dream, but a necessary possibility and a desirable antidote to the uncaring, unhelpful and unwanted image of psychiatry currently portrayed among black users'.[46]

The cultural safety model calls for changes at an institutional level in order that mental health services are safe for members of all cultures. It also draws attention to issues of power in the provision of mental health services. Service users from under-served ethnic groups can be involved in the provision of mainstream services (those which are available to all members of the community), or in the development of culturally specific services to members of their own communities.

Reflection

What cultural factors would you want to be 'taken into consideration' to ensure your emotional security/safety?

Culturally specific services

Another response to the over-representation of service users from minority cultures is the development of services provided by members of those cultures for service users of their own culture.[47,48] Culturally specific services aim to overcome the problem of cultural domination often experienced in mainstream services, and to meet the needs of service users in ways that are consistent with their cultural beliefs. New Zealand has developed a model of *kaupapa Maori* services for Maori service users.[18] While the same range of treatment options available in mainstream services is available in Maori services, the staff are all Maori, and committed to observing Maori protocol in providing services.

Staff of culturally specific services may be nurses or other health professionals, or they may be employed especially for their cultural knowledge and skills. This will include traditional and contemporary cultural knowledge. Culturally skilled staff work alongside clinical staff, providing treatment programmes that are likely to include cultural activities and incorporate cultural protocols within standard forms of treatment.

While culturally specific services may be useful for members of over-represented minorities, caution needs to be exercised in offering service users choice in participating in culturally specific services. We have already discussed the important issues of choice in cultural identity, and the same caution needs to be exercised in offering culturally specific care. If clinicians ascribe culture on the basis of ethnicity, then there may be misunderstandings in offering culturally specific care.

Culturally specific services have the potential to offer a real alternative to service users, which challenges the dominant Western values of mental health services. Nurses from marginalized ethnicities need educational opportunities aimed at developing the unique combination of cultural and clinical skills necessary to provide culturally

specific care. They need to recognize that culturally safe care requires structural change supported by allocation of resources in order to address the effects of historical processes.

Huarahi Whakatu: recognition of cultural competencies

Since 2004 nurses in New Zealand have been required to demonstrate clinical competency in order to retain their licence to practise. This requirement has led to the development of competency recognition programmes that have enabled nurses to document their clinical practice and professional development. For Maori nurses, competence represents more than clinical skills and participation in standard professional development activities. Maori nurses value their cultural skills, and are expected by Maori consumers to bring knowledge of Maori culture to their professional practice. This means that Maori nurses are required to develop dual cultural and clinical competencies. Huarahi Whakatu[49] is a professional recognition programme developed by Maori nurses as a pathway for recognition of these dual competencies.

The need to recognize Maori cultural competencies was first recognized by nurses working in non-government organizations, especially kaupapa Maori services where Maori cultural values are integral to care and treatment. However, the competencies of Huarahi Whakatu are considered to be transferable to mainstream services, which provide care for both Maori and non-Maori consumers. Huarahi Whakatu recognizes that culturally safe care requires specific Maori cultural skills to enable Maori to work safely with Maori. It also recognizes that standard recognition programmes, while ensuring generic skills of cultural safety, may not be adequate to meet the needs of specific cultural groups. Huarahi Whakatu has been endorsed by Te Ao Maramatanga (New Zealand College of Mental Health Nurses) and is currently being trialled in a range of services. The programme will be subject to an application for endorsement to the Nursing Council of New Zealand in 2008.

Reflection

How do you – or your colleagues – take account of 'cultural difference' in providing mental health care?

FUTURE DEVELOPMENTS

Ethnic diversity in Western countries is increasing at an unprecedented rate.[2] In addition, minority ethnic groups have become more vocal about maintaining their cultural identity and practices. Global political events have led to religious diversity becoming more visible in Western countries. Combined with increased immigration from non-traditional source countries this has led to increased societal anxiety and the desire to address issues of cohesion and national identity. Increasing diversity is likely to continue, through continuing population movements throughout the twenty-first century. This will place demands on individual nurses to reflect on the nature of their own cultural identities and the implications of cultural differences for their encounters with service users.

Nurses will also need to develop a broad range of cultural skills and knowledge, although they cannot be expected to become experts in the cultures of service users. Services will need to consider how to recruit and retain nurses from marginalized ethnic groups, and may need to provide culturally specific services for some populations. The value of mental health services working with faith-based organizations has been signalled as something with great potential in mental health care.[1] Individual, institutional and social change is necessary to meet the challenges of cultural diversity.

While much of the responsibility for addressing issues of providing culturally safe care rests with service managers and funders, individual nurses can also take action to improve their responsiveness to service users from cultures different from their own. *Clinical supervision* offers an opportunity for reflection on cultural issues, including cultural identity, power and the nurse's ability to respond to cultural needs. Supervision with nurses from different cultures is one way of facilitating this, either as supervisors or as participants in group supervision.[30]

Opportunities to develop cultural knowledge and skills may also present themselves in the form of service development and education, liaison with cultural services and discussion with colleagues and service users. Nurses need to focus on development of cultural awareness and skills as part of their professional development, and as part of their commitment to meeting the full range of needs of service users.

The continued relevance of interpersonal models of mental health nursing will depend on their capacity to respond to the demands of increasing cultural diversity. The nursing relationship has been described as frequently 'one way traffic'.[5] Concepts such as collaborative care mark nursing's commitment to know and respond to the other, recognizing that the capacity to know another person is limited by the nurses' perceptions of 'otherness'. For nurses to more fully offer themselves to service users, the cultural dimension of the nursing relationship needs to be acknowledged and explored.

REFERENCES

1. Leavey G, King M. The devil is in the details: partnerships between psychiatry and faith-based organizations. *British Journal of Psychiatry* 2007; **191**: 97–8.

2. Kelly BD. Globalization and psychiatry. *Advances in Psychiatric Treatment* 2003; **9**: 464–74.

3. Endrawes G, O'Brien L, Wilkes L. Mental illness and Egyptian families. *International Journal of Mental Health Nursing* 2007; **16**: 178–87.

4. Barker P. The Tidal Model: developing an empowering, person-centred approach to recovery within psychiatric and mental health nursing. *Journal of Psychiatric and Mental Health Nursing* 2001; **8**: 233–40.

5. Barker P, Jackson S, Stevenson C. The need for psychiatric nursing: towards a multidimensional theory of caring. *Nursing Inquiry* 1999; **6**: 103–11.

6. Gustafson DL, White on whiteness: becoming radicalized about race. *Nursing Inquiry* 2007; **14**: 153–61.

7. Fernando S. 'Race', criminality and forensic psychiatry. A historical perspective. In: Kaye C, Lingiah T (eds). *Race, culture and ethnicity in secure psychiatric practice. Working with difference.* London, UK: Jessica Kingsley, 2000: 49–54.

8. Pilgrim D, Rogers A. *A sociology of mental health and illness*, 2nd edn. Buckingham, UK: Open University Press, 1999.

9. Skinner D. Racialized futures: biologism and the changing politics of identity. *Social Studies of Science* 2006; **36**: 459–88.

10. Fernando S. *Race, culture and psychiatry*. London, UK: Tavistock/Routledge, 1988.

11. Bhopal RS, Phillimore P, Kohli HS. Inappropriate use of the term 'Asian': an obstacle to ethnicity and health research. *Journal of Public Health Medicine* 1991; **13** (4): 244–6.

12. Aspinall PJ. Who is Asian? A category that remains contested in population and health research. *Journal of Public Health Medicine* 2003; **25**: 91–7.

13. Paradies YC. Beyond black and white. Essentialism, hybridity and indigeneity. *Journal of Sociology* 2006; **42** (4): 355–67.

14. Rasanathan K.. The novel use of 'Asian' as an ethnic category in the New Zealand health sector. *Ethnicity and Health* 2006; **11** (3): 211–27.

15. Bourke L, Sheridan C, Russell U *et al*. Developing a conceptual understanding of rural health practice. *Australian Journal of Rural Health* 2004; **12**: 181–6.

16. O'Brien AP, O'Brien AJ, Hardy DJ *et al*. The New Zealand development and trial of mental health nursing clinical indicators – a bicultural study. *International Journal of Nursing Studies* 2003; **40**: 853–61.

17. Standards New Zealand. *National mental health sector standard*. Wellington, New Zealand: Standards New Zealand, 2001.

18. Durie M. Mental health and Maori development. *Australian and New Zealand Journal of Psychiatry* 2000; **33**: 5–12.

19. Carnevale FA. Towards a cultural conception of the self. *Journal of Psycho-social Nursing* 1999; **37** (8): 26–31.

20. Morrison-Ngatai L. Communication in practice. An insight into the dynamics of communication for Maori. Implications for mental health nurses. Paper presented at 23rd Annual Conference of the Australian and New Zealand College of Mental Health Nurses, Adelaide, South Australia, October 20–23, 1997.

21. Leff J. *Psychiatry around the globe. A transcultural view*. London, UK: Gaskell, 1988.

22. Spector R. Is there racial bias in clinicians' perceptions of the dangerousness of psychiatric patients? *Journal of Mental Health* 2001; **10**: 5–15.

23. Morgan C, Mallett R, Hutchinson G, Leff J. Negative pathways to psychiatric care and ethnicity: the bridge between social science and psychiatry. *Social Science & Medicine* 2004; **58** (4): 739–52.

24. Bhui K, Stansfield S, Hull S *et al.* Ethnic variations in pathways to and use of specialist mental health services in the UK. *British Journal of Psychiatry* 2003; **182**: 105–16.

25. Barker P, Whitehill I. The craft of care: towards collaborative caring in psychiatric nursing. In: Tilley S (ed.). *The mental health nurse. Views of education and practice.* Oxford, UK: Blackwell, 1997: 15–27.

26. Noble P, Rogers S. Violence by psychiatric inpatients. *British Journal of Psychiatry* 1989; **155**: 384–90.

27. Bond CF, DiCandia CG, McKinnon JR. Responses to violence in a psychiatric setting: the role of patients' race. *Personality and Social Psychology Bulletin* 1988; **14**: 448–58.

28. Mohr W. Cross-ethnic variations in the care of psychiatric patients. A review of contributing factors and practice considerations. *Journal of Psycho-social Nursing* 1998; **36** (3): 16–21.

29. Walsh C. Negotiating difference in mental health nursing in New Zealand. In: Tilley S (ed.). *The mental health nurse. Views of education and practice.* Oxford, UK: Blackwell, 1997: 172–85.

30. DeSouza R. Multicultural relationships in supervision. In: Wepa D (ed.). *Clinical supervision in the Aotearoa/New Zealand. A health perspective.* Auckland, New Zealand: Pearson Education, 2007: 96–109.

31. Majumdar B, Browne G, Roberts J, Carpio B. Effects of cultural sensitivity training on health care provider attitudes and patient outcomes. *Journal of Nursing Scholarship* 2004; **36** (2): 161–6.

32. Bush CT. Cultural competence: implications of the Surgeon General's report on mental health. *Journal of Child and Adolescent Psychiatric Nursing* 2000; **13**: 177–8.

33. Wells MI. Beyond cultural competence: a model for individual and institutional cultural development. *Journal of Community Health Nursing* 2000; **17**: 189–99.

34. Woods PJ, Schwass M. Cultural safety: a framework for changing attitudes. *Nursing Praxis in New Zealand* 1993; **8**: 4–15.

35. Brown AJ, Fiske J-A. First Nations women's encounters with mainstream healthcare services. *Western Journal of Nursing Research* 2001; **23**: 126–47.

36. Nursing Council of New Zealand. *Guidelines for cultural safety in nursing and midwifery education.* Wellington, New Zealand: Nursing Council of New Zealand, 1996.

37. Polaschek NR. Cultural safety: a new concept in nursing people of different ethnicities. *Journal of Advanced Nursing* 1998; **27**: 452–7.

38. Bhugra, D. Migration, distress and cultural identity. *British Medical Bulletin* 2004; **69**: 129–41.

39. DeSouza R. Working with refugees and migrants. In: Wepa D (ed.). *Cultural safety.* Auckland, New Zealand: Pearson Education, 2004: 122–33.

40. Richardson S. Aotearoa/New Zealand nursing: from eugenics to cultural safety. *Nursing Inquiry* 2004; **11**: 35–42.

41. Spence DG. Hermeneutic notions illuminate cross-cultural nursing experiences. *Journal of Advanced Nursing* 2001; **35**: 624–30.

42. Fuller JD, Martinez L, Muyambi K *et al.* Sustaining an Aboriginal mental health service partnership. *Medical Journal of Australia* 2005; **183**: S69–72.

43. Arthur D, Chan HK, Fung WY *et al.* Therapeutic communication strategies used by Hong Kong clients with their Chinese clients. *Journal of Psychiatric and Mental Health Nursing* 1999; **6**: 29–36.

44. Epstein M, Orr AM. An introduction to consumer politics. In: Clinton M, Redmond S (eds). *Advanced practice in mental health nursing.* Oxford, UK: Blackwell, 1999: 1–16.

45. Repper J. Adjusting the focus of mental health nursing: incorporating service users' perspective of recovery. *Journal of Mental Health* 2000; **9**: 575–87.

46. Pierre SA. Psychiatry and citizenship: the Liverpool black mental health users' perspective. *Journal of Psychiatric and Mental Health Nursing* 2000; **7**: 249–57.

47. Bhui K, Sashidharan SP. Should there be separate psychiatric services for ethnic minority groups? *British Journal of Psychiatry* 2003; **182**: 10–12.

48. Sheikh A. Should Muslims have faith based services? *BMJ* 2007; **334**: 74.

49. Maxwell-Crawford KM. *Huarahi Whakatu. Maori mental health nursing career pathway.* Palmerston North, New Zealand: Te Rau Matatini. Available from: www.matatini.co.nz/publications/series4/Huarahi%20Whakatu%20Nursing%20Career%20Pathway.pdf. Accessed 2 October 2007.

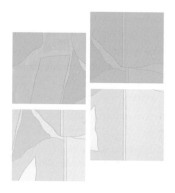

CHAPTER 73

Spirituality, nursing and mental health

Stephen G. Wright*

INTRODUCTION

I was 10 years old and playing football in the street; snotty nosed kids in dirty T-shirts and worn old shorts. Brian stood on the pavement alone, just watching with a lonely, longing look on his face. Nobody spoke to him, and he spoke to no one. He had come from a few streets away and wandered into our patch, an odd thing to do in those days – kids kept pretty much to the streets near home. He might just as well have wandered over from a foreign country. He went to the same school as me, but was in a different year. One of my teammates called out his name together with a dirty word and told him to 'Get lost'.

They put me in goal, the place where the least useful player could be safely stored, there being no skill required but to stand around a lot and (hopefully) block the ball anyway you could if it came your way.

I was always useless at football, and so I learned an early lesson about exclusion in my working class childhood – always being the last to be picked for a team. I remember feeling some sympathy for Brian, for I too had the feeling for much of my childhood of being left out, not wanted. I can see him now as I write this as clearly as I could see him then, his grey pullover with a hole at the elbow, his dull brown hair all spiky and unkempt, his muddy shoes with socks rolled down to his ankles. The

backdrop, of red brick council houses and ranks of factory chimneys pushing into the blue summer sky, frames the picture memory of him I keep.

I was bored in goal and all the action seemed to be taking place at the far end. I sat down on the pile of clothes that marked one goalpost and the next thing I knew Brian was beside me offering a stick of chewing gum. 'Ta', I said, and smelled the spearmint as I took it from the silver wrapper. He was about to speak when I caught an expression of alarm on his face. He was looking at something behind me but before I could turn I felt the slap across the back of my head. I whirled round in pain and tears to find my older brother reaching over me and shouting 'Get inside!' It was only a few yards to our front door, but by then the salt water had created long lines through the dirt on my cheeks and my cries of protest. He banged the door behind us, 'Mam told you to stay away from him.'

When I looked out the window everyone had gone, except Brian leaning by himself against the lamppost.

I never quite understood then why I was supposed to avoid him. The words used by grown-ups to express disapproval were assumed to mean something to me, but they did not. Brian lived alone with his mother, who had 'gone mental'. Whatever that was it was clearly a serious thing, and obviously worse than measles or mumps because I knew when I had had these things you were

*Stephen G. Wright is Chairman and co-founder of the Sacred Space Foundation (www.sacredspace.org.uk). He is the founding editor of the journal Spirituality and Health International, and Associate Professor with the Faculty of Health and Social Care at the University of Cumbria, UK, and patron of the Manchester Area Bereavement Forum.

not allowed to play with anybody. So I thought maybe 'mental' was something you could catch. As far as I knew, Brian was a perfectly 'normal' kid like me, but, whatever it was his mother had got, then it seems there was a risk that he could have it too and could even pass it on to me.

I never saw him again. Older neighbours muttered words like 'fostered' and 'nervous breakdown' and somehow these seemed to be linked to his disappearance. Perhaps they were something to do with death, for I knew that when Mr Haworth up the street died he went away and I never saw him again either. But I did not dwell too much on these mysteries; there were long summer days to enjoy before it was back to school.

Decades later I sat in nursing school where I was introduced to the sociological concepts of 'stigma' and 'disabling the normal' and I remembered Brian and how his mother's mental illness not only stigmatized her but spread out across the family. I was left with uncomfortable feelings about just what it was to be 'normal' – who or what had defined the parameters. Caught up in the tendency towards binary opposition in our culture where *good–bad*, *sane–mad* seemed so clear-cut I was in conflict. The *mad–sane* paradigm came to be meaningless in my progress through nursing as I met the disturbed souls fitting no diagnostic label (much as we, with breathtaking certainty, made sure they had them!). Most disturbed people seemed to me to be having a perfectly understandable response to the madness of their situation; a reflection of the horror of their reality. Faced with all this existential angst, why not go crazy, get drunk, take drugs or shop till they dropped? Maybe I was the insane one because I could not see what was wrong with life?

VANITY, BADNESS AND THE FAMILIAR

In Durham Cathedral a line of black stones is inlaid across the aisle stretching from one wall to the other. In the Middle Ages this was the limits to which women could proceed. Beyond that, it was men only; women were unworthy of drawing close to the holy of holies. In some schools of thought they still are deficient in some way, not quite up to the 'normal'; a standard set by men and, some believe, by God too. Where has the line been drawn in mental health, and what happens when we cross it? Currently, psychobiological models of what is normal mental health prevail. When the line is crossed – when we cannot function or relate 'normally' to others – a diagnosis rapidly follows, often serving in some way to keep you forever beyond the line.

A spell working in a secure unit for profoundly disturbed women led me to encounter the deepest and darkest shadows of the human psyche. All 16 women had committed terrible crimes of violence, including murder, and were judged to be not just bad but mad. All had been abused as children; all had histories of deprivation, drug and alcohol abuse, criminality and violence (towards themselves and others). I was both fearful and awestruck by these women. In the face of their reality, or what they had been told or learned *was* reality, they had kept it together and stayed behind the line for so long. Under the sorrow and hurt of their years, they had sometimes found happiness and joy. Yet, they had crossed this line of normality drawn by forces beyond their control and were forever condemned. When their reality crossed into the reality of the normal, catastrophe was the only outcome.

These two worlds vie for authority, and at the fluctuating boundary is the grist for the mill of modern mental health care. The line between is rarely clear, although we invest huge legal, financial, personal and organizational energy in making it otherwise. Nurses and patients meet on this messy frontier in the giving and receiving of effort to hold the imaginary line, for here we find the unfolding and infinite crisis of meaning; here, people struggle to make sense of themselves and the world.

The prophet wails at the transitory emptiness of life. 'Vanity of vanities! All is vanity' (Ecclesiastes), for in Hebrew vanity is *hevel* – meaning vapour, wind, things transient and impermanent. The passing nature of ordinary reality has led many in all spiritual traditions into the quest for the possibility of a non-ordinary reality (arguably the 'real' reality), the landscape of the soul, the absolute, *God*. The writer of Ecclesiastes seems to have been a mystic; having looked through the doors of perception beyond material reality, he saw another reality. Such shifts in boundaries, such spiritual emergence, from our established way of seeing the world can produce a profound transformation in the way we live our lives. We can become more fully human, or we can crash into mental chaos.

There is much scholarly discussion on the line between madness and mysticism, but for nurses in the field of psychiatry this is no mere theoretical debate. We are pushed into engaging with our own inner struggle over the rights and wrongs of the approaches and treatments on offer. Some manage this conflict by accepting the status quo, others seek to work from within but try to change things, and others escape the profession (coping strategies, defined decades ago in Marlene Kramer's[1] seminal nursing study). A fourth way has unfolded in my experience – that of nurses *internalizing* the conflict and becoming sick. The commonest form of that sickness is *burnout*, when the energy invested in shoring up the defences against conflict fails, and we collapse into an inability to function.[2,3] Such a crisis is spiritual.

SPIRITUALITY, RELIGION AND HEALTH

There is growing evidence that a major cultural shift towards matters spiritual is under way,[4] and a knock-on effect is found in the expectations of patients seeking spiritual support from nurses. Yet the evidence suggests that there is still much confusion, among nurses especially, over what spirituality and religion are and what relevance if any they have to health care.[5]

Everybody seeks meaning, purpose, direction and connection in life. We all at some point, perhaps continually, seek answers to all those great existential questions such as 'Who am I?', 'Why am I here?', 'Where am I going?' and 'How do I get there?' We all pursue love, joy, relationships, work and activities that nurture and feel 'right' to us, and this pursuit may or may not be God centred. This is spirituality, and it lies at the very roots of our being. Religion can be seen as the ritual, liturgy, doctrines and practices that we collectively bring to our spiritual life, to codify and unify it with others, and which may provide answers to those existential questions. Everybody is spiritual but only some are religious.

While spirituality for most people embraces some form of deity or transcendent realm, this is not universal. What matters is that we *believe* in something and that we feel we *belong* to something, not least because there are direct health benefits.[6] On balance, those committed to spiritual practice and/or religious connection are more likely to live longer, healthier and happier lives than those who do not. There is no evidence that one belief system is superior to any other and there may be downsides; for example, some ill people can get worse because they think God has deserted or is punishing them.[7] Curiously, the healthiest and happiest people in one study were not those *getting* support from their religious community, but those who felt they were *giving* most.[8] What seems to be going on is that the spiritual–religious paradigm offers people a sense of centre, of focus, of meaning in an often meaningless and chaotic world.[9] Without this, the distress may not only cause physical ailments[10] but also project us into all manner of mental disturbance from depression to psychosis. Spirituality, until recently largely ignored by the field of psychiatry, seems to be a connecting factor as it directly affects our well-being – both patients and staff.[11,12]

Religion can be seen as the conduit through which we channel and express our 'way of seeing'. This 'seeing' can also change as we encounter beliefs and experiences that challenge our status quo – sudden insight, trauma or the presence and parables of great spiritual beings, such as the Buddha or Jesus, can change our way of seeing joyfully but can also leave us feeling chaotic and confused. Transformational experiences – or intimations of the absolute – can easily be dismissed as madness or delusion,[13–17] and when linked to God can be dismissed as the need for an 'opium' to dull the pain of an unjust world and an instrument to keep people under control (Marx), a sign of neurosis arising from the need for a father figure (Freud), or consolation in the sorrow of the world (Feuerbach). Others, such as Sartre, put the desire for God down to our own desire to *be* God and find our own meaning in the world.

Recent studies suggest our brains are 'wired' for God,[18] or that we may be genetically programmed to connect with the divine[19] – the outcome of an evolutionary process that advantaged a religious tendency because it helped people survive and find meaning in a distressing world. Physiologists place the mystic, ineffable experience as an effect of an outpouring of serotonin or endorphins, or a product of electrical discharges in temporal lobe epilepsy, whereas others have shown that it can be drug induced.[20] Is religiosity therefore just some kind of mental illness or deficiency, which with the right treatment we can cure or with the right education grow out of? Or maybe it is just good health insurance?

MAD OR MYSTICAL?

Underhill's[21] classic text on mysticism describes five distinct stages, moving from the purgation of old ways of seeing to union with the divine. Many people report such mystical union, and it is probably far more common than is generally believed as indicated by the work of the Alister Hardy Trust.[22] Modern research[23] is increasingly supporting what many spiritual traditions have always claimed – that consciousness is more than the product of the brain and that the absolute is not a delusion but reality. Is the madman drowning in these boundless waters in which the mystic swims? Is our mental health system packed with people whose underlying distress is spiritual but not recognized as such?

The pain of the mystical/spiritual crisis or emergence may be confused with psychosis, but 'emergence' (if nurtured rightly) changes us positively – we tend to be more whole, more loving, more forgiving, more functional in the world and not less. Our compassion extends to ourselves and others, reducing the risks. We become more accepting, inclusive and embracing of others and ourselves, more discerning rather than judgemental. We are also more likely to be more trusting and able to work collaboratively with others, fostering a sense of humility and the possibility that we are not always right, that we do not always have to be in control. Through all these 'mores' – which are all about 'becoming' – a spiritual experience ultimately enhances rather than diminishes our humanity. And mystics eventually learn who it is safe to talk to so that they do not get branded insane!

SOUL AND SPIRIT

The notion that we might have *souls* – that we are not so much human beings having a spiritual journey as *spiritual beings* having a human journey (de Chardin[24]) – runs against the grain of much of modern scientific health care. Reduced to our ego/personhoods, 'Who I am' becomes the plaything of multiple attachments to countless roles and identities and functions. A spiritual emergence may shift us out of this limited way of seeing, but we can find ourselves being seen as crazy in some quarters. Into this unknown landscape the soul now emerges, for a spiritual emergence is all about the birthing of the soul. Our culture is now deeply rooted in the possibility that human beings can be happy and healthy with ever more scientific advances, material comforts and designer bodies and babies. The pain of that birthing happens when the soul punches through these limited perceptions. Much of our healthcare system strains with this perspective. In studious efforts to keep religion and spirituality and their downsides and uncertainties out of health, a whole swathe of the human spiritual experience has been sidelined, restricting the possibility of helping patients draw upon their spiritual and soul resources in time of need.

A full exploration of the concept of *soul* here is beyond the scope of this chapter, and many would deny that such a thing exists. This material view of human beings prevails in our healthcare system. But briefly, known as the real, true or highest Self, soul, that 'of God' in everyone, the Essence – it suggests a quality of consciousness, presence and being that is in but not of the ordinary or 'false' self as the Hindu tradition describes it. The personhood, or ego – that conglomeration of ways in which we find our place in the world – is a very useful thing to have for getting around, relating, separating, connecting but according to these world views (held by the great majority of people in the world) it is not all that we are.[25] In the soul, in our essence, which is both personal and transpersonal, found in all things yet contained by none, we not only find our individuality, we also find unity, with all that is.

In his poem *The Waste Land* TS Eliot[26] captures the disjointed conversations, the disconnected relationships, the sterility of language and the dark and dull existence of community, the purposelessness, nihilism and *ennui* in a landscape without soul. Three great unconscious forces – the fears of death, separation and meaningless – govern much of human existence. The possibility of Essence may help us overcome these. Our unwillingness or inability to deal with these dark fearful forces in ourselves may spill over into neglect or abuse of ourselves or others. The impact of unresolved unconscious stuff among healthcare staff is harmful to them and those they care for, which is well summarized in Obholzer and Roberts'[27] survey.

However, calls for change in the dominant materialist paradigm in mental health care are getting louder, from both patients and professionals.[28,29] The reduction of human beings to biological processes where who *we are* is relegated to the outcome of a bunch of neurones and neurochemicals is being challenged. The idea that, when we break down, we can be 'fixed', by tweaking with the right chemical or psychotherapeutic spanners, is increasingly seen as simplistic.

In the play *Equus*[30] we see despair and spiritual pain writ large when the psychiatrist must confront honestly, in himself and his profession, the terrible limitations to his understanding of the complexity and intricacy of the human psyche, and his (in)ability to help. One 'case' finally breaks through his efforts to convince himself that as a psychiatrist he knew what he was doing. He comes to recognize that sometimes in his treatments he may not be helping but dulling and deadening the life force in his patients:

> … passion, you see, can be destroyed by a doctor. It cannot be created …

and later he cries in despair

> In an ultimate sense I cannot know what I do in this place – yet I do ultimate things. Essentially I cannot know what to do – yet I do essential things. Irreversible, terminal things. I stand in the dark with a pick in my hand, striking at heads! … I need … a way of seeing in the dark. What way is this? What dark is this? I cannot call it ordained of God; I can't get that far.

KNOW YOURSELF

If nurses are to revitalize the care of people with mental health problems and refresh it with the integration of spirituality, what about the spirituality of the nurses themselves? Studies suggest that nurses are reticent about spirituality, not just because they are unsure what it is but also because they are unsure of their own spirituality.[5]

It is relatively easy to learn the instrumental things of nursing – the practical and theoretical know-how of problem-solving. It is a much tougher call to know oneself and others so that we can relate more fully, more meaningfully – for such expressive skills touch the very depths of us and what it is to be human. Our effectiveness, or otherwise, falls upon our willingness and ability to connect with others, and that in turn is dependent on our knowing of ourselves. Thoreau[31] wrote:

> It is something to be able to paint a picture, or carve a statue, and so to make a few objects beautiful. But it is far more glorious to carve or paint the atmosphere in which we work, to affect the quality of the day – this is the highest of arts.

How nurses affect the quality of the patient's day – how they imbue it with meaning, purpose, direction, wholeness, relationship – is the very stuff of spirituality and of spiritual care. Spiritual care is not just about that delivered by the 'expert' chaplain, but is integral to nursing care. Every time we 'come alongside' another, listen deeply and open our hearts to the suffering of the other so that he or she may find a way through it is spiritual care and I will explore some of these concepts in more detail later. While the maturing nurse moves along the trajectory from novice to expert, as Benner[32] in her classic study so richly illuminated, there may be yet another level beyond excellence. It is the level of *art form (or craft)*, when there is a synthesis of knowledge and experience, of inner and outer connection, of seeing patterns beyond conscious thought that transcends reduction by rational analysis. Such a way of caring costs no less than the presence of our whole, aware and healed self to the healing opportunity of the other. It is the 'manifestation of the nurse's fundamental self and source of being through the mastery of acts of caring.'[33]

There is much talk in therapeutic circles of the 'wounded healer'.[34,35] We come into nursing with all the personal baggage of our wider world experience and need to explore more deeply what this baggage, usually in our unconscious, is like so that we can become healed ourselves and not risk projecting this onto others or causing further suffering to ourselves.

'Know yourself' was inscribed in the forecourt of the temple at Delphi. To know ourselves we must plunge deep into the unknown realms of our interior castle, as Theresa of Avila called it. And it seems we have two choices. We can go there willingly, that is consciously, to explore and become more whole, or we can bumble along through life hoping and trusting that somehow we will get it all together and learn to be a better person and nurse. Through approaches such as counselling, psychotherapy, retreat time, insight tools such as the Enneagram and so on, those of us drawn to this strange and wonderful world of nursing can consciously seek insight – *In*-sight – to inform and understand, to clarify and to heal (and *none* of us is unwounded) so that we may transform from wounded healers into the healed. There is a way up to a higher level of being as a person and a nurse – more whole, more loving, more aware, more compassionate, more at ease with the world with more equanimity. These 'mores' and others like them are the very stuff of becoming a fulfilled human being. To get this high we must also descend lower, to unpick the ties that bind and restrict us, our fears and angers and resentments and hatreds, many of which are lurking away in our unconscious, limiting us from being more at ease with the world, catching us in ping-pong reactions over which we seem to have no control and which hurt ourselves and others.

For some the possibility of infinite exploration is thrilling and inspiring, to others it is profoundly scary. Yet, if nurses and nursing might well profit from a more explicit and conscious attention to the being of nurses as well as our doing, how can we do this safely? I suggest four key principles for safe spiritual awakening. These may be applied to both patients and nurses.[36]

1 *Soul friends*. In the Celtic Christian tradition this is the *Anam Cara*. This is not a safe journey if undertaken alone. What is needed is the support of one or more wise spiritual counsellors or mentors to whom we can turn for guidance. These gurus, therapists, teachers, mentors, guides are people who have walked the path before us and know how to support us in times of need.

2 *Soul communities*. Groups of people with whom we feel at home and who lovingly nourish our ongoing spiritual awakening. It might be a fellow group of meditators, a church group and so on; there are many possibilities. The community adds to the checks and balances that can keep us safe in the almost crazy time when one way of seeing ourselves is replaced by another.

3 *Soul foods*. Sources of inspiration that refresh, renew and revitalize us. Everything from, literally, good food that nourishes our body or therapies that nurture it, to the arts, scripture, being in environments of peace and beauty, listening to words and music that have heart and meaning for us.

4 *Soul works*. Developing spiritual practices which keep us on track and take care of us and foster deepening insight – meditation, prayer, yoga, retreat time, sacred dance, ta'i chi, exploring our Enneagram, labyrinth walking – there is an enormous range of possibilities.

These four elements together make for a safer evolution of our consciousness and a safer passage through spiritual crisis, helping us to take care of ourselves, to discern the true from the false and to awaken us to the even grander potential of our humanity in nursing.

SPIRITUAL CRISIS: A NURSING RESPONSE

Few people I have met have had the sudden, blinding, life-changing awakening to Truth that St Paul experienced on the road to Damascus. For most of us, it is the steady plod up the mountain with many an apparent slip along the way. Often, there is a sudden shake that comes with a great trauma – loss of a loved one, illness, burnout. A patient with cancer I recently met told me that she had learned to love the (terror) of her cancer because 'without it I would have stayed asleep. My cancer was my spiritual awakening'. Thus, plunged into spiritual crisis, the muddy waters of the wasteland are perturbed. We are shaken out of our way of seeing things or some echo within keeps calling us to the surface, through the shadow, to find the light.

Spiritual pain and spiritual crisis are tough experiences, and there are signs that paradigms of help beyond the psychobiological are gaining ground. A recent (2007) search of the Internet revealed over 8.5 million references to *spiritual crisis*. Numerous organizations (e.g. www.spiritualcrisisnetwork.org.uk) and individuals are offering more imaginative approaches than a diagnosis of psychosis. Many of the websites of religious organizations seem more willing to acknowledge its existence, but where they have pulled back the void has been filled by nurses, psychiatrists, counsellors, psychotherapists and numerous new age therapists.

Nursing help has curious parallels with the spiritual help offered by priests. Hearing the person's story (the 'confession') unburdens them; suggesting actions to put things right (penance) and expressions of support and acceptance (forgiveness) often follow to restore well-being. In offering that one-to-one support, we add a further dimension from the section above – the nurse can become a 'soul friend'. This is the principle of *accompaniment* – the one who is well and skilled guiding the person through the interior crisis (the same principle as spiritual direction in religious settings), nourishing them with sound guidance (soul food) and suggesting ways to take better care of themselves (soul works) and offering help in groups (soul communities) even if only temporary ones.

A key skill here in which the mental health nurse helps is with the quality of discernment – helping the patient sort out the true from the untrue, the nourishing from the harmful. The analogy to priestly ministry is not so far fetched, for in helping people make sense of their world, to move through crisis and into a new equilibrium and perhaps making significant life changes in the way they are and the way they see themselves, is this not soul care, is this not spiritual care? And is it not also a crisis of the soul for the nurse (judging by the numbers who burn out) when the inability or lack of opportunity or resources to deliver what we know is needed drags us down? Further parallels can be seen in Guenther's[37] concept of 'spiritual midwifery' in spiritual direction. To midwife is a different way of working from the disease-orientated medical model. The midwife helps something to be born, invariably painfully, something that is already present and seeking naturally to come into the world, something that is not 'ill' but deeply healthy. Is not the most effective psychiatric nurse one who 'midwifes' that state of being which is healed and whole waiting within the person in crisis to come into the world?

Part of this midwifery process in relation to spirituality is finding out what the patient's spiritual needs are. For example, some nurses have developed tools for spiritual assessment, which interestingly we can use for patients as well as ourselves.[38] However, it could be argued that if a tool is needed should we be asking the questions at all? Personally, on this latter subject, I have noted mature nurses tend to move well away from the questionnaire format and can elicit information about the patient's spiritual needs through sensitive discussion around a number of themes such as identifying the patient's spiritual practices, beliefs, sources of help, traditions and so on.

The discovery process is also dependent upon critical ability to listen to and connect deeply to the other. In the fraught world of modern health care, and restricted by our own limitations of insight and skill, often our capacity to hear and fully be with the other is profoundly limited. In the book of Job in the Old Testament, Job is assailed by just about every imaginable form of suffering. Friends constantly come along to advise and console, telling him that it will be all right – 'Job's comforters'. In exasperation, he tells them to stop, and 'listen to what I am saying' for that is all the comfort he wants of them. Listening deeply – without leaping in with a desire to fix things or without taking on board the other's anguish in a kind of faux compassion – is an art of nursing. The distractions of the environment are not the only thing that get in the way of listening deeply; our own inner chorus of mental processes drowns things out too, arising from that fearful place in ourselves that wants to solve and fix and be sure.

Listening at this deep level does not come easy and is rarely arrived at simply by life experience. It takes courage and awareness to set aside ourselves and all our 'stuff' and to be fully present for, and attentive to, the other. The solution is to encourage the evolving of more aware nurses who can see beyond the masks that we present to each other. This can only be done in the view of many spiritual teachers, by adopting a commitment to spiritual practice and expansion of our consciousness that connects us to the deep peace and safety that lies in our very essence, our hearts, our souls – enabling us to let go of the fear that binds us to the masks we wear.

When we can confidently switch off our ego agendas, we can get ourselves out of the way and give our total attention to the other and thus 'have a brand new experience: by not interrupting or arguing he will hear things that he has never heard before. The speaker too will have a brand new experience. He will be aware that he is being heard by someone who is not going to come back to him with a reply, criticism or opposition. And not only is he heard, he hears himself.'[39] Thus, we learn to 'pay attention, to listen to what is not being said (or to what is being said but minimised)' and to learn the art of 'waiting' and 'asking the right questions' rather than having the right answers. The use of silence, waiting, getting the self out of the way and ensuring the space for the other to speak enable a deeper quality of listening to take place that can truly promote healing, understanding, compassion and connection. Deep listening, a natural part of the repertoire of nursing, helps the other, but in so doing we hear ourselves as well.

Reflection

The territory of spirituality is fraught with difficulty for mental health nurses, but also great opportunities. Ask yourself:

- How far have you explored and integrated your *own* spirituality?
- How safe do you feel at the edge of professional boundaries, where spiritual care slips across into religious care?
- Can you pray with patients and support them in other religious practices associated with spiritual expression?
- To what extent can you be sure of the spirituality of another person, if you are not sure of our own?

SUMMARY

I have explored my views on these topics in the previous paragraphs, and now it is your turn to explore these possibilities. It is indeed an ethical and practical minefield, perhaps explaining why so many nurses have steered clear of it. But, as I have suggested above, the landscape is changing and it seems nurses have no choice but to respond; the status quo does not appear to be an option.

The renewal of *soul* in the wasteland of health care, and our culture more widely, will arise paradoxically from the very newness which helped to set it aside. The Essence will be the same, but its form and manifestation will be different and unique to its time. We see it now in the shifting sands of the reordering of the religions, the movements in our understanding of the nature of consciousness, the ecology movement, and the rise of 'integrated' or holistic health care. These and other signs suggest that the wasteland may also be the fertile ground for a renewal and reintegration of Essence, of Soul, into health and healing. The alternatives are there, becoming more known and drawing greater allegiance. For those in the field of mental health care, perhaps excitedly, perhaps with fear, the re-spiriting of health holds out the prospect of a completely different vision for mental health care of the future, where the old paradigms are challenged, broken down and reformed and ways of alleviating spiritual pain renewed and discovered. The tension between the material and the spiritual is an unnecessary one, for a truly holistic way of seeing is able to embrace the paradox of opposites, the challenge of diversity. It does not have to be a case of science or spirit, but maybe science *and* spirit, and mental health nurses willing to venture out into this way of seeing may yet reap immeasurable benefits for those we seek to serve, and ourselves.

REFERENCES

1. Kramer M. *Reality shock*. St Louis, MO: Mosby, 1974.

2. Snow C, Willard P. *I'm dying to take care of you*. Redmond, UK: Professional Counsellor Books, 1989.

3. Wright S. *Burnout: a spiritual crisis*. Nursing Standard Essential Guide. Harrow, UK: RCN Publications, 2005.

4. Heelas P, Woodhead L (with Seel B, Szerszynski B, Tusting K). *The spirituality revolution: why religion is giving way to spirituality*. Oxford, UK: Blackwell, 2005.

5. McSherry W. *Making sense of spirituality in nursing practice*. Edinburgh, UK: Churchill Livingstone, 2000.

6. Koenig H, McCullogh M, Larson B. *Handbook of religion and health*. New York, NY: Oxford University Press, 2002.

7. Pargament K, Koenig H, Tarakeshwar N, Hahn J. Religious struggle as a predictor of mortality among medically ill elderly patients. *Archives of Internal Medicine* 2001; **161**: 1881–5.

8. Krause N. Church based social support and mortality. *Journal of Gerontology* 2006; **61** (3): S140-6.

9. Tillich P. *The courage to be*. Yale, CT: Yale University Press, 2000.

10. Pert C. *Molecules of emotion*. New York, NY: Scribner, 1997.

11. Goleman D. *Emotional intelligence*. New York, NY: Bantam, 1995.

12. Wright S. *Reflections on spirituality and health*. Chichester, UK: Wiley, 2005.

13. Wright SG. And let the darkness … . *Spirituality and Health International* 2006; **7** (4): 175–80.

14. Grof S, Grof C (eds). *Spiritual emergency: when personal transformation becomes a crisis*. New York, NY: Putnam, 1989.

15. Dennet D. *Breaking the spell*. London, UK: Penguin, 2006.

16. Dawkins R. *The God delusion*. London, UK: Bantam, 2006.

17. Hitchens C. *God is not great*. London, UK: Atlantic, 2007.

18. Newberg A, D'Aquili E, Rause V. *Why God won't go away*. New York, NY: Ballantine, 2001.

19. Hamer D. *The God gene*. New York, NY: Doubleday, 2004.

20. Schultes RE, Hofmann A. *Plants of the Gods*. Rochester, NY: Healing Arts Press, 1992.

21. Underhill E (first published 1910). *Mysticism*. Oxford, UK: Oneworld, 1993.

22. Maxwell M, Tschudin V. *Seeing the invisible*. London, UK: Arkana, 1990.

23. Dossey L. PEAR lab and the nonlocal mind: why they matter. *Explore* 2007; **3** (3): 191–6.

24. de Chardin PT. *The phenomenon of man*. London, UK: Collins, 1959.

25. Almaas A. *The diamond heart*. London, UK: Shambhala, 2000.

26. Eliot TS. *The four quartets*. London, UK: Harcourt Brace Jovanovich, 1944.

27. Obholzer A, Roberts V (eds). *The unconscious at work*. London, UK: Brunner-Routledge, 2003.

28. Powell A. Spirituality, healing and the mind. *Spirituality and Health International* 2005; **6** (3): 166–72.

29. Barker P, Buchanan-Barker P (eds). *Breakthrough: spirituality and mental health*. London, UK: Whurr, 2005.

30. Schaffer P. *Equus*. London, UK: Penguin Classics, 2006.

31. Donahue M. *Nursing: the finest art*. St Louis, MO: Mosby, 1985.

32. Benner P. *From novice to expert: excellence and power in nursing practice*. New York, NY: Addison Wesley, 1984.

33. Gaydos H. The art of holistic nursing and the human health experience. In: Dossey B, Keegan L, Guzzetta CE (eds). *Holistic nursing: a handbook for practice*, 3rd edn. Gaithersburg, MD: Aspen, 2000.

34. Nouwen H. *The wounded healer*. London, UK: Darton Longman & Todd, 1994.

35. Wright SG, Sayre-Adams J. *Sacred space: right relationship and spirituality in health care*. Edinburgh, UK: Churchill Livingstone, 2000.

36. Wright SG. Survivors of the system. *Nursing Standard* 2005; **19** (42): 32–3.

37. Guenther M. *Holy listening: the art of spiritual direction*. London, UK: Darton Longman & Todd, 1992.

38. Burkhardt M, Jacobsen M. Spirituality and health. In: Dossey BM, Keegan L, Guzzetta C (eds). *Holistic nursing: a handbook for practice*, 3rd edn. Gaithersburg, MD: Aspen, 2000.

39. Pinney R. Creative listening. Personal publication. Cited in Pym J. *Listening to the light*. London, UK: Rider, 1999.

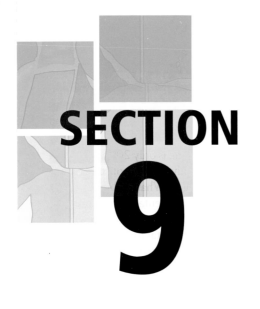

recovering from illness', the people concerned may be thinking more about 'recovering their lives', either after or even as a part of the process of being 'mentally ill'.

O'Hagan developed this concern, noting that service users in New Zealand had

> Other concerns about recovery that went deeper than semantics or uninformed criticism: first, that recovery is an import from America; second, that the Americans, in emphasising recovery as an individual process, have seemed to overlook that it is a social process as well; and third, that recovery in America evolved out of psychiatric rehabilitation and was perhaps driven more by professionals than by service users.[11]

Perhaps because of the distinct cultural context of Aotearoa/New Zealand O'Hagan and her colleagues were keen to establish a recovery model that did not simply ape the US original, but was more social, or sociocultural in emphasis. However, the New Zealand recovery philosophy also had some philosophical 'teeth'.

> Much of the American recovery literature accepted, at least implicitly, the biomedical model of 'mental illness'. It did not place a great deal of emphasis on challenging the veracity or the dominance of the biomedical model in mental health services. We wanted the recovery approach in New Zealand to signal that there are many ways of understanding and responding to mental health problems and that no one way should dominate at the expense of others.[11,p.2]

O'Hagan's reservations about pasting a recovery philosophy over traditional 'mental illness' values is well stated.

What is recovered?

People may well be 'ill at ease' with themselves or others, or 'ill-fitted' for the challenges that life presents. However, as O'Hagan's colleagues noted, many reject the idea that they are 'mentally ill', in any traditional medical sense.[12] This is neither a theoretical nor a semantic dispute. When people locate their problems within the world of their lived experience,[13] the metaphorical nature of their 'illness' becomes clear, with implications for the 'recovery journey'.

'Recovery' of physical health appears more straightforward. People 'recover' from, for example, a cold, heart attack, stroke or a malignancy. In each case, the person recovers (fully or partly) from the disturbed or abnormal physical state, either because of the body's natural defences or because of treatment or rehabilitation which specifically targets the affected organ or system. Since there is no manifest 'pathology' associated with 'mental illness', the concept of 'recovery' is bound to be different. Since there are no tests for 'mental illness', we can never identify, specifically, what has 'gone wrong', as

might be the case with leukaemia or diabetes. Instead, when people experience 'mental illness', their *life* – and how they live it – is affected. Consequently, in mental health it seems more appropriate to talk about 'recovering one's life'.

Recovery roots

As O'Hagan noted, the definition of mental health recovery is often traced to Anthony's work:[14,p.15]

> A person with mental illness can recover even though the illness is not 'cured'. Recovery is a way of living a satisfying, hopeful, and contributing life even with the limitations caused by illness. Recovery involves the development of new meaning and purpose in one's life as one grows beyond the catastrophic effects of mental illness.

However, the earlier writings of Pat Deegan[15] provide the origins for the all-important metaphor of the 'recovery journey'.[16] Although little acknowledgement is paid to the influence of Alcoholics Anonymous (AA), the contemporary mental health recovery literature differs little from the philosophical assumptions of AA and Narcotics Anonymous (NA) from over 60 years ago.[17] These groups first developed the ideas of empowerment, mutual support and self-help that are commonly found in today's mental health recovery literature, especially the *Blueprint*[18] developed in New Zealand by O'Hagan and her colleagues. In particular, AA and NA recognized that, however useful professional help might be, recovery had to be pursued actively by the person and the person would need the help of others, especially people who knew the 'problem territory'. Most notably, AA acknowledged that 'alcoholism' was a disease, which could never be 'cured', but from which recovery was possible.

Since the end of the 1970s, recovery has been proposed as an alternative to mainstream ideas of psychiatric care, especially for people with so-called 'serious' and/or 'enduring' forms of mental illness.[14,19–21] A significant change in language has accompanied this change in philosophy. The passive 'patient' role has been transformed into a more active 'user/consumer' of services,[22,23] which Manos[24] appropriately called the 'prosumer' – someone directly influencing the help they required.

Notably, most of the significant descriptions of recovery were developed by people who either had been or still were psychiatric 'patients and who professed a more optimistic, empowering, approach to identifying the help people might need to deal with problems of human living'.

There are a few formal studies of recovery, from a psychiatric–medical perspective[25,26] in the professional literature. However, what is commonly called the 'recovery *movement*' is based more on philosophical *conviction* than scientific evidence.

The original proponents of recovery argued that people with 'serious mental illness' *could* recover and described some of the social and interpersonal processes that appeared to aid or enable recovery.[27] These accounts, which emphasize *personal* experience, echo Samuel Smiles' ideas about 'living by example' when he first coined the term 'self help' in the nineteenth century:[28,p.57]

> The great results in life are usually attained by simple means and the exercise of ordinary qualities.

How such views fit with the objective, unworldly 'evidence' beloved by researchers, politicians and professionals is not at all clear[29] because mainstream services often assimilate alternative concepts, if only to become more 'consumer-friendly'.[30] This is nowhere more obvious than in the current situation in which government departments espouse recovery while promoting ideas of 'compulsory treatment' or 'compliance'. Conflicts are, therefore, inevitable.[31,32] Clearly, this derives from the philosophical tension between the *person* focus of the concept of recovery and the *patient* (or illness) focus of traditional psychiatric medicine.

Reflection

What does 'recovery' mean to you? What have you 'recovered' from in your own life?

The story of recovery

Almost a decade ago, Barker *et al.*[33,p.xxiii] noted that:

> For generations, it has been assumed that the stories told by people in mental distress are somehow inaccurate, flawed or downright invalid. The role of psychiatry has been to judge the validity of patients' accounts and to correct them, via therapy. A prevailing problem even of 'modern' psychiatry has been the reluctance to accept stories … as valuable in their own right. … We recognise that the storytellers are the story.

Sally Clay is a mental health advocate and psychiatric survivor with a 35-year-long experience of psychiatric 'care and treatment'. She has helped many people appreciate the complex nature of the concept of recovery through the telling of her story. She has no illusions about the ephemeral nature of concepts such as 'recovery' and especially how they might be used to meet political agendas. Sally wrote:[34]

> Recovery is the latest buzz word in the mental health field. For the last year or so, I have been labelled 'recovered from mental illness'.

When invited to discuss her 'recovery' with psychiatrists in New York State, Sally noted that there was *no* discussion of

> the nature of mental illness itself. … If we are recovered, what is it that we have recovered from? If we are well now and were sick before, what is it that we have recovered to? … The psychiatrists in our dialogue become visibly uneasy when the subject arises, and they divert the discussion to less threatening lines of thought. 'Coping mechanisms' are just such a diversion, an attempt to regard the depth of madness as something that can be simply 'coped' with.[34,pp.26–7]

As an American, Sally Clay anticipated the concerns of O'Hagan and her colleagues in New Zealand. She recognized that it was inappropriate to think about 'recovery' in the same context as 'cure' or 'rehabilitation'. Indeed, the concept of recovery is so deeply personal for many people that it defies definition. However, it has also become an important social construct, meaning different things to different people. Not surprisingly, there is a tension between 'professional' and 'user–consumer' constructions of 'recovery'.

RECOVERY VALUES

Recovering from 'mental illness'

Ramon *et al.*[35] recently compared the 'emergence' of the concept of recovery in Australia and the UK. They noted that, among other things, this 'emergent' concept of recovery[35]

- is *not* about going back to a previous pre-illness state
- is about forging a new way of living controlled by the newly found *self-agency* of users
- focuses on 'recovering' from the trauma of psychosis, treatment, stigma, lack of skills and opportunities for valued activities
- encourages interdependency and self-help
- requires systematic effort, with risk taking *and* risk avoidance, with the 'right to fail'
- entails a move from a deficit model of living with mental illness to a strengths perspective, where the person might live 'outside of illness'.

However, a key problem with this overview is that it continues to be framed by the concept of 'mental illness', which has long outlived any usefulness.

Recovering the experience of life

The *Tidal Model of mental health recovery*[3,36,37] was launched in the mid-1990s and, since then, has generated over 100 projects in the UK, Ireland, Canada, Japan, Australia and New Zealand, ranging from outpatient addictions, through acute and forensic units, to the care of older people with dementia.[38] Nurses in palliative care have also explored the use of the Tidal Model as an alternative philosophy for death and dying.

Although there are numerous models of 'recovery', Tidal is probably the first mental health recovery model to be developed by nurses in practice,[39] drawing mainly upon nursing research.[3,40,41] Tidal's original focus was on developing a specific way of 'thinking' about the kind of care and support that people might need to begin the voyage of recovery:

> [H]ow do we tailor care to fit the specific needs of the person and the person's story and unique lived experience, so that the person might begin, or advance further on the voyage of recovery?

In that sense, Tidal focuses on the 'problems in living' which people experience and how they might live a more *constructive life*, albeit under difficult circumstances.

The person is, obviously, the key driver within the recovery process, but the practitioner can offer vital help to unlock the person's potential for recovery.

Six key philosophical assumptions are embraced by the Tidal Model:[3]

1 A belief in the *virtue of curiosity*: the person is the world authority on her or his life and its problems. By expressing genuine curiosity, professionals can learn something of the 'mystery' of the person's story.
2 Recognition of the *power of resourcefulness*. Rather than focusing on problems, deficits and weaknesses, Tidal seeks to reveal the many resources available to the person – both personal and interpersonal – that might help on the voyage of recovery.
3 Respect for the *person's wishes*, rather than being paternalistic, and suggesting that we might 'know what is best' for the person.
4 Acceptance of the *paradox of crisis* as opportunity. Challenging events in our lives signal that something 'needs to be done'. This might become an opportunity for a change in life direction.
5 Acknowledging that all goals must, obviously, *belong to the person*. These will represent the small steps on the road to recovery.
6 The virtue in *pursuing elegance*. Psychiatric care and treatment is often complex and bewildering. The simplest possible means should be sought which might bring about the changes needed for the person to move forward.

Practice-based evidence

Tidal developed from practice-based research conducted in the mid-1990s in England, Northern Ireland and the Republic of Ireland into what people *needed* nurses *for*; what people and their families *valued* in nursing; and what nurses *did* that appeared to make a difference. Over the past decade a wide range of mental health professionals

and users–consumers have helped further develop the model. Tidal is committed to compassionate caring and genuine 'nursing' – *providing the conditions necessary for growth and development*. However, this is not restricted to the professional discipline of nursing. People with experience of psychiatric care, both in hospital and in the community, helped in the design, evaluation and development of the original model. Over the past 5 years, other 'user–consumer–consultants', from different countries, have helped refine the philosophical basis of Tidal, by helping to clarify its value base: what Tidal 'stands for'.

Reflection

How is 'recovery' relevant to nursing practice? What kind of things might nurses do that would actively enable this?

The 10 Tidal commitments

The Tidal Model embraces specific assumptions about people, their experience of problems of human living and their capacity for change. From these assumptions we have developed a set of related values that provide practitioners with a philosophical focus for helping people make their own life changes, rather than trying to manage or control 'patient symptoms'. The 10 commitments remind us that although rules come from the head, reflecting our masculine selves (*animus*), commitment comes from the feminine heart (*anima*). To help practitioners, in any setting, employ the 10 commitments, a set of 20 Tidal competencies[42] were developed that have been used to audit recovery practice in several projects, notably in England[43] and Scotland.[44]

1 *Value the voice*: the person's story represents the beginning and endpoint of the helping encounter, embracing not only an account of the person's distress but also the hope for its resolution. The story is spoken by the voice of experience. We seek to encourage the true voice of the person – rather than enforce the voice of authority. Traditionally, the person's story is 'translated' into a third person, the professional account, by different health or social care practitioners. This becomes not so much the person's story (my story) but the professional team's view of that story (history). Tidal seeks to help people develop their unique narrative accounts into a formalized version of 'my story', through ensuring that all assessments and records of care are written in the person's own 'voice'. If the person is unable, or unwilling, to write in their own hand, then the nurse acts as secretary. Recording what has been agreed, conjointly, is important – writing this in the 'voice' of the person.
2 *Respect the language*: people develop unique ways of expressing their life stories, representing to others

that which only they can know. The language of the story – complete with its unusual grammar and personal metaphors – is the ideal medium for illuminating the way to recovery. We encourage people to speak their own words in their distinctive voice.

Stories written about patients by professionals are, traditionally, framed by the arcane, technical language of psychiatric medicine or psychology. Regrettably, many service users and consumers often come to describe themselves in the colonial language of the professionals who have diagnosed them.[45] By valuing – and using – the person's natural language, the Tidal practitioner conveys the simplest, yet most powerful, respect for the person.

3 *Develop genuine curiosity*: the person is writing a life story but is in no sense an 'open book'. No one can know another person's experience. Consequently, professionals need to express genuine interest in the story so that they can better understand the storyteller and the story.

Often, professionals are only interested in 'what is wrong' with the person, or in pursuing particular lines of professional enquiry, e.g. seeking 'signs and symptoms'. Genuine curiosity reflects an interest in the person and in the person's unique experience, as opposed to merely classifying and categorizing features, which might be common to many other 'patients'.

4 *Become the apprentice*: the person is the world expert on the life story. Professionals may learn something of the power of that story, but only if they apply themselves diligently and respectfully to the task by becoming apprentice minded. We need to learn from the person what needs to be done, rather than leading.

No one can ever know another person's experience. Professionals often talk 'as if' they might even know the person better than they know themselves. As Thomas Szasz noted:[46]

How can you know more about a person after seeing him for a few hours, a few days or even a few months, than he knows about himself? He has known himself a lot longer! ... The idea that the person remains entirely in charge of himself is a fundamental premise.

5 *Use the available toolkit*: the story contains examples of 'what has worked' for the person in the past or beliefs about 'what might work' for this person in the future. These represent the main tools that need to be used to unlock or build the story of recovery. The professional toolkit – commonly expressed through ideas such as 'evidence-based practice' – describes what has 'worked' for other people. Although potentially useful, this should be used only if the person's available toolkit is found wanting.

6 *Craft the step beyond*: the professional helper and the person work together to construct an appreciation of what needs to be done 'now'. Any 'first step' is a crucial step, revealing the power of change and potentially pointing towards the ultimate goal of recovery. Lao Tzu said that the journey of a thousand miles begins with a single step. We would go further: any journey begins in our *imagination*. It is important to imagine – or envision – moving forward. Crafting the step beyond reminds us of the importance of working with the person in the 'me now': addressing what needs to be done now, to help advance to the next step.

7 *Give the gift of time*: although time is largely illusory, nothing is more valuable. Time is the midwife of change. Often, professionals complain about not having enough time to work constructively with the person. Although they may not actually 'make' time, through creative attention to their work, professionals often find the time to do 'what needs to be done'. Here, it is the professional's relationship with the concept of time which is at issue, rather than time itself.[47] Ultimately, any time spent in constructive interpersonal communion, is a gift – shared by both parties.

8 *Reveal personal wisdom*: only the person can know himself or herself. The person develops a powerful storehouse of wisdom through living the writing of the life story. Often, people cannot find the words to express fully the magnitude, complexity or ineffability of their experience, invoking powerful personal metaphors to convey something of their experience. A key task for the professional is to help the person reveal and come to value that wisdom, so that it might be used to sustain the person throughout the voyage of recovery.

9 *Know that change is constant*: change is inevitable for change is constant. This is the common story for all people. However, although change is inevitable, growth is optional. Decisions and choices have to be made if growth is to occur. The task of the professional helper is to develop awareness of how change is happening and to support the person in making decisions regarding the course of the recovery voyage. In particular, we help the person to steer out of danger and distress, keeping on the course of reclamation and recovery.

10 *Be transparent*: if the person and the professional helper are to become a team then each must put down their 'weapons'. In the story-writing process the professional's pen can all too often become a weapon: writing a story that risks inhibiting, restricting and delimiting the person's life choices.

Professionals are in a privileged position and should model confidence by being transparent at all times, helping the person understand exactly what is being done and why. By retaining the use of the person's own language, and by completing all assessments and care plan records together (in vivo), the collaborative nature of the professional–person relationship becomes even more transparent.

Reclamation: in our own voice

Many areas of mental health practice have developed 'professional' forms of language that are awkward to use and confusing for the uninitiated. The Tidal Model avoids the use of jargon, valuing instead the ordinary, everyday language that people use to talk about themselves or with family or friends.

Traditionally, psychiatry devalued the person's voice, by promoting the use of diagnostic jargon.[48] Given the power imbalance between professionals and their 'patients' many people end up describing their own experience in the technical language of psychiatry and psychology, as if their own story were 'not good enough'.[49] The Tidal Model emphasizes the importance of understanding the 'lived experience' through use of natural language, allowing people to express themselves using their own metaphors and grammar. In that sense, Tidal aims to help people *reclaim* the story of their distress and, ultimately, their whole lives.

The dictionary tells us that *reclamation* means 'the efforts necessary to *seek the return of one's property*'. In the psychiatric context, reclamation means '*the return of personhood and its accompanying story*'. The Latin root of reclamation (*reclamare*) means 'to cry out against'. The story of the development of the 'user–consumer' voice over the past 30 years represents one of the most powerful developments in mental health worldwide. All such groups are *reclaiming* their story and personhood through the act of 'speaking up' or 'speaking out', both of which are central to the act of reclamation within Tidal.

The reclamation metaphor

In Tidal terms *reclamation* refers to the pursuit of a productive use of something that was either *lost* or considered *worthless*. Across the estuary from my home in Scotland lies the landing strip of Dundee airport. This land was once submerged beneath the estuary but, over many years, was gradually drained and protected from further flooding by a sea wall. What once was lost from view – and was literally *useless* – was brought into view, and transformed into something of great value. This work was accomplished slowly, with great effort and skill, not to mention at some considerable risk to the people involved.

This is a fitting metaphor for the process of reclamation that is possible for those whose lives have been submerged, metaphorically, by the experience of madness.[a] The old English term *madness* evokes the range and depth of the disruption involved. It is far more evocative of 'what happens' to people than the technical babble of psychiatric diagnosis, or the political correctness of expressions such as 'mental health problems'. In reclaiming their lives from the waters of madness, people

bring back to the surface a person who has, to large extent, been lost from view: lost from the sight of family and friends if not also from themselves.

In reclaiming their lives, people need to undertake the lengthy, difficult and often threatening process of draining the effects of madness from their lives; transforming something that once was thought to be both *meaningless* and *worthless* into something of great value if not priceless.

Reflection

What have you 'reclaimed' in your own life that was 'lost from view?' How did you 'reclaim' this part of yourself or your life story?

BEYOND RECOVERY

The reclamation *attitude* contrasts strongly with the traditional idea of rehabilitating the so-called 'mentally ill' found in some, though not all, recovery models. Indeed, reclamation reminds us that we are all in recovery. Everyone – whether high-flying professional or temporarily laid-low 'service user' – is struggling with something – perhaps a variety of things – that haunts us, limiting our capacity for becoming fully human.

As Ann Helm writes (Chapter 8):

> The complexity of early relationships provides in itself much for some of us to recover from. Add to that the difficult adolescent voyage towards self-identity and the uncertainty of adult life and it could be asked of anyone reading this chapter, has he/she recovered? Recovery is not a destination, but the journeying task of making sense of life itself, … We are all in recovery.

The first Tidal step in facilitating reclamation is to write all the main assessment 'stories' and subsequent descriptions of necessary care *in the person's own voice*, rather than translate these into professional note-taking. This focus on 'my story' validates users and consumers. It also shows how willing the practitioner is to work actively *with* the person. Again, Sally Clay wrote:[50]

> The Tidal Model makes authentic communication and the telling of our stories the whole focus of therapy. Thus the treatment of mental illness becomes a personal and human endeavour, in contrast to the impersonality and objectivity of treatment within the conventional mental health system. One feels that one is working with friends and colleagues rather than some kind of 'higher-up' providers. One becomes connected with oneself and others rather than isolated in a dysfunctional world of one's own.

---

[a] Many of my colleagues from the user–consumer–survivor community favour use of the old expression *madness* as a meaningful alternative to the medical expression 'mental illness'.

Reclamation: finding meaning in drowning

The person's story describes not only the circumstances that led to the person's need for help but also holds the promise of what needs to be done to begin the process of recovery. Although influenced by different schools of psychotherapy, Tidal emphasizes *ordinary conversation* in a way that differs greatly from most other 'therapeutic approaches'. People are natural 'story-tellers'[51] and the more 'everyday'[52] the nature of the 'narrative', the more meaningful the story becomes.[53] In the same way, the kinds of *questions* we might want to ask people are 'extraordinarily ordinary':

- What is it like to feel *as if* you are being followed?
- What is it like to feel that life is no longer worth living?
- What is it like being you?

It is important to recognize that the person is living with the experience of distress and difficulty, day in and night out. Professionals risk being patronizing when they talk about how 'badly' people are coping. When someone spends 24 hours a day with their 'demons', the most obvious, curious question is:

- *How* do they do that?

How do people manage to keep going, when the going is so obviously hard? It is high time that we forgot about 'teaching patients skills' through 'psychoeducation'. The person already has developed a way of living with distress, *however imperfect* that might be. The next question is:

- How might we help you to develop this into something more effective, for you?

This perspective casts the professional in a very different light. Instead of offering 'tried and tested' remedies, or teaching new skills, the professional does 'genuine nursing of the mind' by helping:

- to nurture the person's existing talent for dealing with problems of living
- the person grow through adversity
- the person become more aware that she or he is already on the path to recovery.

Reclamation: what lies beneath

As I have noted, within the professional literature there has always existed the risk that 'recovery' is seen as a euphemism for 'cure'. However, as the AA model soberly illustrated, there can be no cure, but life can be reclaimed. From the depths of drunken desperate dependency might emerge a new, reclaimed identity – sober, *inter*dependent and hopeful. That identity is deeply conscious of what lies beneath – the dangerous depths of despair and personal inadequacy. That new identity is fully aware of how fragile are the defences against the ever-threatening sea. However, such knowledge – gained through the hard and dangerous work of reclamation – supports the lifelong process of becoming human, especially through helping others to do the same.

AA provides another example for contemporary mental health care. People who have experienced human 'breakdowns' and who have reclaimed their personal identity can consolidate their journey of recovery by helping others do likewise. Like the best education, we learn best by trying to help others learn. The simple notion of the buddy system and the recovering community embrace a vital moral for us all. Despite our recent infatuation with the notion of individuality, as Mary O'Hagan and her colleagues pointed out, humans are inherently social. We are at our noblest when we are helping others to *be* and to *become* their own person.

Discovering new land: rediscovering ourselves

Although I talk a lot about 'mental health' it remains largely a mystery to me, and I think to most of us. I need to make an effort, to struggle to work out what, exactly, *is* mental health. It is something I need to discover for myself.

Across the Tay estuary from my home is moored Captain Scott's ship *Discovery*, on which he first sailed to the Antarctic. His second – and ill-fated – voyage of discovery was made on the *Terra Nova*. *Discovery* and *Terra Nova* symbolize for me the hopeful, yet demanding, voyages people make, as they find meaning in their near-drowning experiences in the waters of madness. Here, they reclaim themselves. Here, they bring back to the surface the person who was, for so long, lost from sight.

The landing strip of Dundee airport is *Terra Nova* – new land reclaimed from the depths. But the *discovery* of that new land lay in the ambition and imagination of those who first dreamt that this was possible. We all need to hold on to a hopelessly optimistic view of people if we are ever to help them reclaim their full personhood. Surely, such a 'hopelessly optimistic' attitude is what we would want to be expressed towards us, if we were drowning in despair?

Reflection

How do you help people with mental health problems find meaning in their experiences of distress or disturbance?

SUMMARY

The commonest thing that people say about the Tidal Model is that 'it's just common sense'. This is what I would call an honest fiction. It feels like 'commonsense', because there are no complex words or ideas within it. However, look around and the idea of helping people reclaim their personhood, and their lives, by simple, ordinary forms of help does not appear to be all that common. Instead, we have lots of professional, political and bureaucratic jargon, and mountains of paper 'care/treatment' plans, coordinated by a growing number of 'therapeutic agencies'. In my view, Tidal is *one example* of 'uncommon sense'.[38]

Another common thing which people say about Tidal is:

> It doesn't feel as if I am being treated; it just feels as if someone is listening to me, hearing what things are like for me.

A couple of years ago, a woman with a history of psychiatric services recognized how this 'ordinary' Tidal experience could become 'extraordinary'. She wrote:

> Tidal has made room for my voice. I'm not just another patient who is mentally ill. I am a person with goals and dreams and a life worth living. I get to discover and learn and make changes. Now I can think, decide and act for myself. I don't need someone else to save me anymore, because I have been given the opportunity to save myself.

In making her own 'discovery' she learned the power of reclamation at first hand. She learned that she had to 'take back' herself and her story, before she could begin the long voyage of recovery.

REFERENCES

1. Barker P, Whitehill I. The craft of care: towards collaborative caring in psychiatric nursing. In: Tilley S (ed.). *The mental health nurse: views of practice and education.* Oxford, UK: Blackwell Science, 1997.

2. Barker P. The Tidal Model: a radical approach to person-centred care. *Perspectives in Psychiatric Care* 2001; **37** (3): 79–87.

3. Barker P, Buchanan-Barker P (eds). *The Tidal Model: a guide for mental health professionals.* New York, NY: Brunner Routledge, 2005.

4. Davidson L, Strauss J. Sense of self in recovery from severe mental illness. *British Journal of Medical Psychology* 1992; **65**: 131–45.

5. Mental Health Commission New Zealand. *Recovery competencies for New Zealand mental health workers.* Wellington, New Zealand: MHC, 2002.

6. Repper J. Adjusting the focus of mental health nursing: incorporating service users' experiences of recovery. *Journal of Mental Health* 2000; **9**: 575–87.

7. Scottish Executive. *Rights, relationships and recovery – the report of the National Review of Mental Health Nursing in Scotland.* Edinburgh, UK: Scottish Executive, 2006.

8. Mental Health Commission. *A vision for a recovery model in Irish mental health services*: Discussion paper. Dublin, Ireland: MHC, 2006.

9. Department of Health. *From values to action: the Chief Nursing Officer's review of mental health nursing.* London, UK: Department of Health, 2006.

10. Lapsley H, Nikora L, Black R. *Kia Mauri Tau! Narratives of recovery from disabling mental health problems.* Wellington, New Zealand: Mental Health Commission, 2002.

11. O'Hagan M. Recovery in New Zealand: lessons for Australia. *Australian e-Journal for the Advancement of Mental Health* 2004; **3**: 1–3.

12. Buchanan-Barker P, Barker P. Lunatic language. *Openmind* 2002; **115**: 23.

13. Barker P. The Tidal Model: the lived experience in person-centred mental health care. *Nursing Philosophy* 2000; **2** (3): 213–23.

14. Anthony WA. Recovery from mental illness: the guiding vision of the mental health service system in the 1990s. *Psychosocial Rehabilitation Journal* 1993; **16**: 11–23.

15. Deegan PE. Recovery: the lived acceptance of rehabilitation. *Psychosocial Rehabilitation Journal* 1988; **11**: 11–19.

16. Deegan PE. Recovery as a journey of the heart. *Psychiatric Rehabilitation Journal* 1996; **19**: 91–7.

17. Frank D. *The annotated AA handbook: a companion to the Big Book.* Fort Lee, NJ: Barricade Books, 1996.

18. Mental Health Commission. *Blueprint for mental health services in New Zealand.* Wellington, New Zealand: Mental Health Commission, 1998.

19. Chamberlin J. *On our own: patient controlled alternatives to the mental health system.* New York, NY: Hawthorn Books, 1978.

20. Deegan P. Recovery: the experience of rehabilitation. *Psychosocial Rehabilitation Journal* 1988; **11** (4): 11.

21. Fitzpatrick C. A new word in serious mental illness: recovery. *Behavioural Healthcare Tomorrow* 2004; **August**: 2–5.

22. Barham P, Hayward R. *From the mental patient to the person.* London, UK: Routledge, 1991.

23. Deegan P. Recovering our sense of value after being labelled. *Journal of Psychosocial Nursing* 1993; **31**: 7–11.

24. Manos E. Speaking out. *Psychosocial Rehabilitation Journal* 1993; **16** (4): 117–20.

25. Harding CM, Brooks GW, Ashikaga T et al. The Vermont longitudinal study of persons with severe mental illness. 1. Methodology, study sample and overall status 32 years later. *American Journal of Psychiatry* 1987; **144**: 718–26.

26. Harrison G, Hopper K, Craig T et al. Recovery from psychotic illness: a 15 and 25 year follow-up study. *British Journal of Psychiatry* 2001; **178**: 506–17.

27. Fisher D. Hope, humanity and voice in recovery from mental illness. In: Barker P, Campbell P, Davidson B (eds). *From the ashes of experience: reflections on madness survival and growth.* London, UK: Whurr, 1999.

28. Smiles S (original 1859). *Self help: with illustrations of conduct and perseverance.* London, UK: IEA Health and Welfare Unit, 1996.

29. Goode CJ. What constitutes the 'evidence' in evidence-based practice? *Applied Nursing Research* 2000; **13** (4): 222–5.

30. Barker P, Buchanan-Barker P. Death by assimilation. *Asylum* 2003; **13** (3): 10–13.

31. McLean A. Recovering consumers and a broken mental health system in the United States: ongoing challenges for consumers/survivors and the New Freedom Commission on Mental Health. *International Journal of Psychosocial Rehabilitation* 2003; 8: 47–68.

32. Neuberger J. *The moral state we're in.* London, UK: Harper/Collins, 2005.

33. Barker P, Campbell P, Davidson B (eds). *From the ashes of experience: reflection on madness, survival and growth.* London, UK: Whurr, 1999.

34. Clay S. Madness and reality. In: Barker P, Campbell P, Davidson B (eds). *From the ashes of experience: reflection on madness, survival and growth.* London, UK: Whurr, 1999: Chapter 2.

35. Ramon S, Healy B, Renouf N. Recovery from mental illness as an emergent concept and practice in Australia and the UK. *International Journal of Social Psychiatry* 2007; **53**: 108–22.

36. Barker P. It's time to turn the tide. *Nursing Times* 1998: **18** (94): 70–2.

37. Barker P. The Tidal Model: the healing potential of metaphor within the patient's narrative. *Journal of Psychosocial Nursing and Mental Health Services* 2002; **40** (7): 42–50.

38. Buchanan-Barker P. Uncommon sense: the Tidal Model of mental health recovery. *Mental Health Nursing* 2004; **23**: 12–15.

39. Brookes N. Phil Barker: the Tidal Model of mental health recovery. In: Tomey AM, Alligood MR (eds). *Nursing theorists and their work*, 6th edn. New York, NY: Mosby, 2006: Chapter 32.

40. Barker P, Jackson S, Stevenson C. The need for psychiatric nursing: towards a multidimensional theory of caring. *Nursing Inquiry* 1999; **6**: 103–11.

41. Vaughn K, Webster D, Orahood S, Young B. Brief inpatient psychiatric treatment: finding solutions. *Issues in Mental Health Nursing* 1995; **16**: 519–31.

42. Buchanan-Barker P, Barker P. The Tidal Commitments: extending the value base of recovery. *Journal of Psychiatric and Mental Health Nursing* 2008; **15**: 93–100.

43. Gordon W, Morton T, Brooks G. Launching the Tidal Model: evaluating the evidence. *Journal of Psychiatric and Mental Health Nursing* 2005; **12**: 703–12.

44. Lafferty S, Davidson R. Person-centred care in practice an account of the experience of implementing the Tidal Model in an adult acute admission ward in Glasgow. *Mental Health Today* 2006; **March**: 31–4.

45. Barker P. The Tidal Model: psychiatric colonization, recovery and the paradigm shift in mental health care. *International Journal of Mental Health Nursing* 2003: **12** (2): 96–102.

46. Szasz TS. Curing the therapeutic state: Thomas Szasz on the medicalisation of American life. Interviewed by Jacob Sullum. *Reason* 2000; **July**: 27–34.

47. Jonsson B. *Ten thoughts about time.* London, UK: Constable and Robinson, 2000.

48. Kirk SA, Kutchins H. *Making us crazy: The psychiatric bible and the creation of mental disorders.* New York, NY: Free Press, 1997.

49. Furedi F. *Therapy culture: cultivating vulnerability in an uncertain age.* London, UK: Routledge, 2003.

50. Clay S. A view from the USA. In: Barker P, Buchanan-Barker P (eds). *The Tidal Model: a guide for mental health professionals.* New York, NY: Brunner Routledge, 2005: Foreword.

51. Fisher WR. *Human communication as narration: toward a philosophy of reason, value, and action.* Columbia, SC: University of South Carolina Press, 1987.

52. Zeldin T. *Conversation: how talk can change our lives.* Mahwah, NJ: Paulist Press, 2000.

53. Brunner J. *Acts of meaning.* Cambridge, MA: Harvard University Press, 1990.

SECTION
10

THE FUTURE OF PSYCHIATRIC AND MENTAL HEALTH NURSING IN CONTEXT

Preface to Section 10

Illnesses are almost always spiritual crises in which older experiences, and phases of thought, are cast off in order to permit positive changes.

Josef Beuys

The language of nursing is very similar throughout the world. However, its practice varies greatly from one country to the next. Nursing has, traditionally, been a vocation, based on traditional notions of human service. More recently, it has aspired to be a profession, with its standards and regulatory bodies for the control and monitoring of 'good practice'. Now it seeks to become a discipline, with its own knowledge base, which although unique might complement and enable the work of other members of the multidisciplinary mental health team.

In this final section I invited some colleagues in the major countries of the developed world to offer a brief description of 'where' psychiatric and mental health nursing stood, in the light of their country's social and cultural context. What events are occurring, locally and internationally, which will affect the future development of psychiatric and mental health nursing? Nurses are, increasingly, a mobile workforce. Many nurses migrate, temporarily or permanently, to work in other countries. Hopefully, an appreciation of what psychiatric and mental health nursing *means* in different countries will be useful, even to those nurses who decide to 'stay home'.

It has been my good fortune to visit and work with nursing colleagues in many different countries. The old adage 'travel broadens the mind' is true. If one has experience of only one work setting in one country to draw upon, one's understanding of the profession of nursing will be limited indeed. I hope that by gaining at least a small insight into 'what is happening' and the possible reasons for particular developments, in different countries, readers will gain a deeper insight into their own working practice and its likely future development.

As the reader will find, although there exists some common human ground, what is deemed to be important for the immediate future of mental health nursing is changeable when crossing continents.

In drawing the book to a close I reflect on what I choose to call the 'politics of caring'. After almost 40 years in the mental health field, I have had the privilege of witnessing, often at first hand, many major developments both in nursing and across other disciplines. In this final chapter, I look into my own hand-crafted crystal ball, and consider what are the key challenges that face psychiatric and mental health nursing and how these relate to the continuing development of the human race.

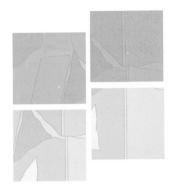

CHAPTER 78

The United Kingdom context

Jon Allen*

INTRODUCTION

Why do we no longer care for the mentally ill in hospital? Why does the government not spend more on people with mental illness? Why do we have all this bureaucracy and form filling? What do people in the health authority and in the Department of Health know about my job and what it is like on the front line? Why cannot the government just trust us to get on with it? Why does it have to keep moving the deckchairs but never actually make any meaningful changes?

These questions and concerns circulate through every health service setting every day, and each of them is fundamentally a question about healthcare policy. Most of us training to be or practising as clinicians of one sort or another get frustrated by politics interfering in the business of health care. After all, we are the professionally trained people, and we know what the people who use our services need. Left to our own devices without politicians, professional managers and administrators, we might have a decent chance of sorting it all out.

This may be true if we had perfect infrastructure to support us; if we had enough resources to deal with all the demand for our services that the country's population could throw at us; and if our work premises were 'state of the art'.

Unless we live in a world of heavily rose-tinted spectacles, we know that the challenge of setting healthcare strategies and policies and managing their delivery effectively and fairly, with limited resources, is huge. Furthermore, it is not getting any easier. As research discovers new treatments, the world becomes smaller, inequalities appear greater, and global threats to health and well-being emerge.

This chapter challenges readers to step outside their box as clinicians with just the patients they see in mind, and begin to think about health care from a wider perspective. It aims to help readers think about the purpose, the challenges and impact of healthcare policy-making. It will demonstrate how effective government policy increases the health and well-being of populations, even if in the process it upsets practitioners by making us change the way we have always done things.

MACROECONOMICS AND HEALTH

In a World Bank discussion paper Hauk et al.[1] stated the two key aims of health policy-makers:

1 to get the most health gain for the limited budget they have available for health
2 to eradicate or minimize any inequalities in the health status of the population.

*Jon Allen has been a mental health nurse for over 20 years ago and is presently Director of Nursing in Oxfordshire and Buckinghamshire Mental Health NHS Trust, UK. He was the founding chairman of the National Forum of Mental Health and Learning Disability Nurse Directors and Leads.

The importance of achieving these aims is not just because health is good and important in its own right. It is pretty well established that the poor health of a population affects the economic wealth of a country. So the relationship is not just that the poorer a country is, the poorer is the health of its population. The poorer the health of a country, the poorer economically the country is likely to be overall.[2]

Importantly, the wealth of a country and the level of its gross domestic product (GDP) that it *invests* in health does not show a perfect correlation with health *outcomes*. For example, a regression analysis of mortality of children under five and percentage of GDP spent on health for all countries demonstrates an adjusted r^2 (coefficient of determination) of only 0.11. This suggests that only 11 per cent of the variance in under-five mortality rates can be explained by the percentage of GDP invested in health. A practical example is that in 2003 Luxembourg spent $3680 per person on health and Portugal spent only $1791 (both amounts are expressed in terms of purchasing power parity, thus removing any local pricing differences); however, both countries had similar rates of under-five mortality per 1000 live births and overall life expectancy (www.who.org).

This is important because it helps us to understand that even if a country spends a lot on health, and associated services, it does not necessarily achieve better health for its population. There must be factors other than money that explain how much health improvement a country gets for the amount of money it invests in health.

These other factors might be manifold. However, some researchers have tried to isolate some of them. Reidpath and Allotey[3] identified a broad set of measures on the governance of a country and were able to demonstrate an r^2 of 0.72 (p = 0.001) between the healthy life expectancy measure for each country and the scores calculated for governance in each country. This suggests that 72 per cent of the variance in healthy life expectancy might be explained by the quality of countries' governance. The composite measure of governance used included measures on voice and accountability, political stability, government effectiveness, regulatory quality, rule of law and control of corruption.

Although these are broad measures, the specific measures of government effectiveness which will determine how much value it gets in terms of health gain from its health expenditure will include areas such as prioritization of services and treatments to be provided; approaches to equity of access and distribution of services; ability to handle political pressure and tensions; the effectiveness of workforce planning; how effectively and efficiently services are managed; and how services are financed. Each of these areas represents key areas of policy, and is relevant across all areas of health care.

In the four countries of the UK, as decision-making regarding health policy is devolved to each country's government, there are increasing differences in the decisions being taken by each government. Government policy, as well as spending, affects health outcomes. Consequently, it will be important for practitioners in each country to be informed about how policies are diverging, and what that might mean for their practice and for the care, treatment and support for the people they are working with.

Reflection

In what ways do you think ineffective government and government corruption could lead to poor health outcomes?

MENTAL HEALTH CARE IN THE FOUR COUNTRIES OF THE UK

The four countries of the UK (England, Wales, Scotland and Northern Ireland) differ in several ways. For instance, each country has a different level of GDP, and each has grown at different rates over the last decade or more. In 2005, England had a GDP per person of £18 097 per head, which had grown at a rate of 2.8 per cent (after inflation) on average over the last 15 years. In Wales, the GDP was only £13 813 and had grown on average by only 2.1 per cent. Scotland's GDP was £16 944 and had grown at 2.6 per cent and Northern Ireland's was £14 196 and had grown at 3.3 per cent.

While this variance may not seem large, a difference of over £4000 per person may be significant in terms of what can be afforded to invest in health. Also, the higher rate of growth in Northern Ireland demonstrates that it is converging in terms of wealth with Scotland and England more quickly than Wales. Until 1998, Wales had a slightly larger GDP per capita than Northern Ireland; since then, Northern Ireland's economy has grown at a higher rate than that of Wales. This may be important for thinking about the health and wider policy moves of a government and why it might diverge from other areas of the UK. If Wales is becoming the poor man of the UK, how is this reflected in health status and health policy and are their any differential impacts in the area of mental health care?

Can we pick out these macroeconomic differences in health and well-being in these countries, particularly in data indices that are related to mental health? Clearly, there are differences, but they do not readily match the differences in GDP. If we look at the suicide rate in 2001 (Welsh statistical service) we can see that Scotland had the highest rate in the UK at 17 per 100 000; Wales was second with a rate of 12 per 100 000; England was third with 9 per 100 000; and Northern Ireland lowest with 7 per 100 000. There are also differences reflected in the recorded incidence of common mental disorders. Wales has the highest rate with an incidence of 19 per cent, i.e. 19 out of 100 people will, at some point in their life, suffer from a common mental illness such as depression or anxiety. England has a rate of 16.5 per cent and Scotland 14 per cent.[4] Mortality from alcohol use is another reasonable proxy indicator for mental health. Scotland again has the highest rate, with a standardized mortality ratio of 38 per 100 000, Northern Ireland has the second worst rate at 19.9, followed by Wales with a rate of 16.5 and England with a rate of 15.[4]

So far, we can see that the countries in the UK have different levels of wealth, and on average they have different health status and outcomes in terms of some high-level indicators of mental health. Wales appears to be turning into the poorest country of the UK, but we can also see that Scotland appears to be the sickest.

Government policy and effectiveness will be part of creating this scenario, but they will also be part of dealing with the specific health issues that lead to ill health and premature mortality. For example, a country which has malaria cannot be wholly blamed for having a higher rate of malarial deaths than a country that does not have malaria. But questions might be asked if its death rate is higher than neighbouring countries that also have malaria, or if it does little to deal with malaria in terms of its health policies and investments.

Reflection

How might poor health outcomes influence a country's economic output?

UK OVERALL HEALTH POLICY

Having established the importance of health policy and how it affects the health outcomes of a country, it is time to think more specifically about the UK's health policy. Before we explore the specifics of mental health and mental health nursing, we need to consider some bigger questions, such as how is health care paid for and how is it organized and managed?

In the UK, the majority of health care is free at the point of use, and paid for through general taxation. A major review of the future funding needs and mechanisms for health care in the UK, conducted by the former chief executive of the National Westminster Bank, Sir Derek Wanless, supported that this was the most efficient way to fund health care.[5] However, out of this review came an increasing focus on the need to further empower people to take more responsibility for their own health and well-being, and to invest in more preventative and primary health care, thus reducing the need for hospitalization. Furthermore, the Wanless review heralded the introduction of a more market-orientated approach to

the delivery of health services. This led the NHS in England to move from being a provider of services to a purchaser of services from a range of organizations accredited by the NHS in terms of quality and price.

This has further developed in health and social care policy and reform by taking the NHS to a position where people are increasingly given choice of service providers and, for those with longer term health and social care support needs, having individualized budgets to purchase directly the support services and help they need. These may result in radically different choices from those services that health and social care professionals might have chosen.

These big policy movements, explained all too briefly here, provide the backdrop to other, more specific, policy developments. It is at this level that policy has its most fundamental level of divergence among the four UK countries.

England is pursuing a policy which brings in market-like competition between service providers. All health service organizations are moving towards existing as independent commercially viable entities in competition with the private and 'not for profit' sector to provide NHS services.

However, Scotland, Northern Ireland and Wales have increasingly moved towards a system which has large planning and commissioning health boards, buying health services *on behalf* of local populations from large NHS provider organizations. There is no significant agenda on plurality of provision, competition or service users' choice of health service provider.

These differences are emergent, and it is too early too tell which will serve people with mental health problems better. However, they will increasingly lead health services in England to operate very differently from services elsewhere in the UK.

In England, it is still not clear how far the agenda of choice and plurality of provision will roll out for mental health service users. However, service commissioners are already using their new market freedoms to ask other service providers to bid to provide services when they are not happy with their current local provision. As a result, many service users are benefiting from direct payments, using their allocated budgets to meet their own support needs. All these interventions remove the advantages or monopoly power from service providers. Free marketeers would argue that this alone will improve the quality and efficiency of services. The less optimistic argue that these improvements will happen only if the market is well managed.

These different operating frameworks may also lead to noticeable differences for nurses in practice. These might include for those working in England:

1 The increasing availability to choose between different employing organizations, offering different career opportunities and benefit packages.

2 If the market works well, opportunities may exist for nurse entrepreneurs to establish independent alternative nurse-led mental health services, providing service users and commissioners with increased choices of support and treatment services.

3 As healthcare organizations are exposed to disciplines of a more market-orientated economy, employers should have higher expectations of the staff to be 'customer focused', working effectively with service users, their carers and the general practitioners who refer them.

Reflection

What might be the advantages and disadvantages for mental health service users of being able to choose from a range of service providers?

MENTAL HEALTH POLICY AND MENTAL HEALTH NURSING

While the health policy discussed above sets the operating framework for how services are planned and funded, more specific policy is being developed to help health service commissioners and providers determine the types of services they should purchase, and the level of quality they should expect. This element of policy is important as it distils the evidence of what type of services and interventions are effective. This enables commissioners to effectively prioritize their limited financial resources, and helps providers invest appropriately in facilities and workforce to meet commissioners' expectations. For mental health in England and Wales these take the form of *national service frameworks*, and in Scotland and Northern Ireland they are *national strategies*.[6-9]

The recommendations of these strategic documents are broadly similar. This is not surprising when the evidence base for effective mental health care is reasonably robust, and the demographic, cultural and historical patterns of service delivery in each of the counties are not too different.

The recommendations from these strategies include:

- improving mental health promotion
- better primary mental healthcare services for common mental health problems
- increasing availability of psychological therapies
- improving access to specialist services for people with more serious mental illnesses, especially in crises and in the early stages of illness
- improving the quality of acute inpatient care services
- reducing stigma and discrimination
- improving services for people from ethnic minority groups
- improving the physical health and well-being of people with serious mental health problems

- promoting recovery from serious mental illness by improving social inclusion for people with mental health problems, e.g. access to employment, housing and recreation
- improving the integration of health and social services and coordination of services for individuals
- improving involvement of service users and their carers in the planning, delivery and evaluation of services
- improving information relating to the delivery of mental health services
- developing and improving services for specific groups, e.g. people with personality disorders and people in the criminal justice systems.

The next level of policy is provided in the form of increasingly specific guidance or strategies. These documents provide guidance and advice to commissioners and service providers on how they might best set up specific services and implement particular treatments. In the case of mental health nurses, this involves how to make the most effective use of a particular element of the workforce.

Both England[10] and Scotland[11] have recently reviewed mental health nursing in light of the priorities within their national mental health strategies. In developing these strategies, both countries consulted widely with nurses and their representative bodies, service users and carers and employers of nurses.

Workforce strategies relating to professional groups are a peculiar form of guidance. They have to reconcile the needs and aspirations of people who use the services, the profession's own aspirations for its own development, and employers' needs for a cost-effective competent workforce, appropriately targeted at the issues for which it employs that workforce.

There are significant similarities between the English and the Scottish reviews[10,11] of mental health nursing. Both emphasized the need for mental health nursing to focus on the following areas:

- working with the more severely ill
- embracing the recovery approach
- improving skills and abilities in promoting and supporting physical well-being
- increasing the number of nurses trained to deliver psychological therapies
- increasing the amount of time qualified nurses spend directly with patients in inpatient care
- developing the role of nurses in line with changing legislation, e.g. nurse prescribing, new roles under reformed mental health legislation.

Importantly, both reviews recognize that mental health nurses are a key resource in the effective delivery of modern mental health services. Both reviews embed themselves in the wider strategic and policy framework, and see the role of the nurse extending across medical and psychological practice and taking increasingly sophisticated roles in the management and leadership of care delivery and services.

Reflection

How does guidance from your Department of Health and other national health bodies influence you and your colleagues' practice?

SUMMARY

This chapter has provided a broad overview of the relevance and the importance of healthcare policy to the overall health and well-being of a country. It has provided an insight into how high-level issues such as how wealthy a country is and how effective its government is can influence the health policy and health outcomes in a country.

An overview of high-level differences in wealth and health data for the four countries of the UK has been looked at, and this was followed by a discussion of the emerging difference in high-level operating policies for health service planning and financing in England and the rest of the UK. Some potential implications of these changes for service and care delivery were discussed.

Finally, mental health policy for the four countries of the UK was considered, and its role in supporting effective and efficient health services was highlighted. The policies of all four counties were found to focus on similar priorities for the development of mental health services.

The English and Scottish reviews of mental health nursing were also considered and demonstrated to be closely tied into their respective country's mental health policies. Both reviews demonstrated an increasing recognition of the value of the mental health nursing workforce to the delivery of clinically effective and cost-effective services. In both reviews, there is a desire to increase the focus of the areas of practice where mental health nurses should be used, and an increasing expectation of nurses extending their skill sets to take on increasing responsibilities that were once the sole domain of other professional groups.

Effective governments use their country's resources to generate welfare for the population as a whole. Each government should continually try to increase the welfare for all of its population, minimizing the inequalities that exist in society. Health and well-being is one of the key elements of welfare. Effective policy-making ensures that an appropriate amount of money is being spent on health and that the mechanisms for planning, organizing, financing and delivering health care are effective and efficient. This includes supporting health services to spend money wisely on evidence-based services. It also includes supporting the effective use of limited skills and competence in the workforce by removing unnecessary restrictions and barriers, which create inefficient professional monopolies.

REFERENCES

1. Hauk K, Smith P, Goddard M. *The economics of priority setting in healthcare: a literature review.* Health Nutrition and Population. Washington, DC: The World Bank, 2004.

2. World Health Organization. *World health report 2000: health systems improving performance.* Geneva, Switzerland: WHO, 2000.

3. Reidpath D, Allotey P. Structure (governance) and health; an unsolicited response. *BMC International Health and Human Rights* 2006; **6** (12): 1–7.

4. Singleton N, Bumpstead R, O'Brien M. *Office for National Statistics: psychiatric morbidity among adults living in private households, 2000.* London, UK: Stationery Office, 2001.

5. Wanless D. *Securing our future health: taking a long term view.* London, UK: HMSO, 2002.

6. Department of Health. *National service framework for mental health: modern standards and service models.* London, UK: DoH, 1999.

7. The Bamford Review of Mental Health & Learning Disability (N. Ireland). 2005. Available from: www.rmhldni.gov.uk/amh_contents.pdf.

8. Welsh Assembly Government. *Commissioning adult mental health services, 2005.* Available from: www.wales.nhs.uk/sites3/home.cfm?orgid=438.

9. NHS Scotland. *Delivering for mental health.* Edinburgh, UK: Scottish Executive, 2006.

10. Department of Health. *From values to action: the Chief Nursing Officer's review of mental health nursing.* London, UK: The Department of Health, 2006.

11. NHS Scotland. *Rights, relationships and recovery: the report of the national review of mental health nursing in Scotland.* Edinburgh, UK: Scottish Executive, 2006.

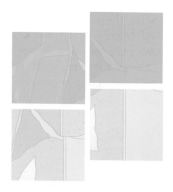

CHAPTER 79

The European context

Seamus Cowman*

INTRODUCTION AND BACKGROUND

In healthcare ministries across Europe, the realization is dawning that European Union (EU) law has profound consequences for the organization of healthcare systems. In some countries, there are public and private partnerships, and across many countries there are serious concerns being expressed about the availability and level of publicly funded healthcare systems. Duncan[1] suggests that there is a paradox in European terms in that for years there was pressure from many interest groups for the EU to be 'doing something' about health. Yet health is so high on national political agendas that most governments do not want the EU interfering with it. The EU was given powers to spend money on European-level health projects but, to date, has not passed laws harmonizing public health measures in member states.

The professional role and the scope of practice for all professions have evolved and developed in line with the individual healthcare policies of each country. A significant factor across countries is professional regulation through various forms of authority. In the more established EU member states, such as the UK and Ireland, regulation is conducted through a statutory body in the form of a Nursing Board; however, in the most recently joined member states from Eastern Europe there is an absence of statutory nursing bodies and such a function is most often undertaken within the Ministry of Health.

Given the diverse circumstances influencing care of the mentally ill, there is much variance in the education and

training and role of the psychiatric nurse in Europe. Unlike general nursing, there is a lack of specific European Directives governing the education and training of the psychiatric nurse. In the 1970s the introduction of Sectoral Directives for general nursing created a European identity for general nurses and facilitated freedom of movement for general nurses to practice in all European member states including reciprocal recognition of qualifications. The lack of such a system for psychiatric nurses has resulted in them not enjoying the same freedom of movement and right to practise across the health services of European countries. The enlargement in the number of countries in the EU in recent years has further exacerbated the lack of commonality in the education and training and role of the psychiatric nurse across Europe.

This chapter will review the significant historical developments as they have influenced the evolution of psychiatric nursing in Europe. The different and changing perspectives on the role of the nurse in Europe will be examined. A prospective view on the role of the nurse in mental health care in the years ahead is presented, and the case is made for European agreement on the education and training of the psychiatric nurse and the essential elements that constitute the essence of psychiatric nursing.

HISTORICAL REFLECTIONS

There are distinctive differences between Western and Eastern Europe in terms of development, and indeed the

*Seamus Cowman is Professor and Head of Nursing at the Royal College of Surgeons in Ireland. He has worked in psychiatric nursing as a clinical practitioner, educator and researcher. His current research focus is violence in mental health services.

historical discourse and available literature on psychiatric nursing. The literature on psychiatric nursing in Western Europe provides a strong sense of the role of the nurse as it evolved in the traditional mental hospital setting. In those early days, a major element of the nursing role involved the enforcement of rules, and psychiatric nursing was the cornerstone of service delivery.[2] During the latter part of the twentieth century there was a major shift in mental healthcare policy away from institutional care to a more community-based service. Taylor[3] contends that psychiatric nursing was a major health profession when most people with mental illness were cared for in large institutions, and the suggestion is made that the value of psychiatric nursing is now being questioned as the large mental hospitals are closing.

In the past little was known about the practice of psychiatric nursing in Central and Eastern Europe. In recent times there have been major changes and social upheaval in Central and Eastern Europe with social and political revolutions leading to radical changes in healthcare systems. The resulting greater transparency has focused attention on levels of abuse and misuse of the mental healthcare systems, including its use to discipline and punish social dissidents.[4] Such was the environment for the practice of psychiatric nursing, which was delivered by individuals who were lacking specialist education and training and with an impoverished ability to provide any meaningful therapeutic engagement with clients of the system. The recognition of the importance of mental health nursing as a force in enhancing service delivery led to the World Health Organization's (WHO) Nursing in Action project.[5] Primarily because of the influence of initiatives by the WHO, a number of Eastern European countries have engaged in a process of review of their education programmes for the preparation of psychiatric nurses. Countries such as Romania and Poland are in various stages of policy development with phased implementation of new and reformed education programmes for psychiatric nursing. It may be expected that, once such countries become more established within the EU, educational and practice developments will be accelerated in an attempt to harmonize mental healthcare services across Europe.

A predominant feature of psychiatric nursing history in all of Europe is the extent to which the role was prescribed by medical staff and included participation in many questionable interventions with no scientific basis. Such roles included warm and cold baths, malaria treatment, insulin coma, lobectomy, lobotomy and more recently electroconvulsive therapy. Domestic manual and farm work was undertaken by patients and supervised by nurses. In the early days, the nursing role, which was carried out with little autonomy, was eloquently captured in an Irish context by a resident physician:[6,p.23]

> The idea of a keeper [psychiatric nurse] comprehends a person constantly supervising the madmen.

> In this institution therefore the apartments, where the patients are confined during the day should never be without keepers. They should be locked in with the patients and the porter should let them out only at times stated by the regulations. They should be considered as sentinels and be constant to their post and vigilant on duty.

With the exception of the Eastern European block, in the early 1970s governments across Europe became increasingly concerned about the large mental institutions and the custodial nature of mental health services. In the Federal Republic of Germany there was concerted government effort to establish smaller psychiatric units and to introduce therapeutic and rehabilitative psychiatry, as had occurred in the UK in the 1950s, the USA in the 1960s and Italy in the 1970s. Weurth[7] described it as being 'like a wave of liberation'. Following this the picture of psychiatry in Germany changed considerably. For example, in 1961 a newly admitted patient expected to stay in a psychiatric hospital for 6–9 years; by 1985, half the patients left the facility after less than 4 weeks. Only one of 100 stays was longer than 1 year.[7]

The earliest days of mental health care and the evolutionary pathways of Eastern and Western Europe are not dissimilar, except that the early mental health history of Western Europe is reflective of a more recent history of Eastern Europe, which is now undergoing rapid change.

EUROPEAN STRUCTURES

The concept of a EU commenced with the Treaty of Rome in 1957, and applied to 15 member states of Europe and the three Economic Area States (EEA). In 2004, the EU expanded to admit 10 new countries and another three countries – Bulgaria, Romania and Turkey – are working towards joining the EU. The EU now includes 25 member states of Europe. One of the challenges in bringing about reform in the new EU member states is that for 45 years they have been under communist control and lacking in independent governance. The isolation of the Eastern bloc[8] disguised and distorted technical and cultural progress during the period of the cold war. This distortion led to a lack of progress in mental health care which has resulted in an outdated mental health system across the region by way of legacy. The task to reform mental health across the EU member states is immense and will require global and Europe-wide initiatives.

A *Mental health declaration for Europe*[9] and a *Mental health action plan for Europe*[10] was endorsed by the ministers of health of the 52 member states in the European region of the WHO in 2005. The declaration favours community-based mental healthcare settings, with social inclusion and reduced discrimination. The action plan recommends a series of actions in five key areas to:

1 foster awareness of mental well-being
2 tackle stigma
3 implement comprehensive mental health services
4 provide a competent work force
5 recognize the experience and importance of service users and carers in planning and developing services.

In the final analysis it is likely that progress will be determined by the level of committed financial resources given that the average EU spend on mental health is about 5 per cent whereas the lowest mental health budget levels reported are less than 2 per cent in some countries of the former Soviet Union.[11]

The relationships among economic integration, migration and welfare were some of the basic ideas behind the European Community, and such principles having been established in the Treaty of Rome they were extended in the Treaty of Maastricht in 1992. Notably, the original Treaty of Rome did not include health nor did it enhance greater movement of people in Europe through mutual recognition of qualifications. It was only in the early 1970s that the necessary procedures and directives were first established which facilitated freedom of movement and reciprocal recognition of qualifications across the EU. Today, professional recognition within the EU occurs by means of two different regimes:

- sectoral directives
- general systems directives.

Sectoral directives bestow a rather privileged position on certain individual health professions, including medical doctor, dental practitioner, pharmacist, general care nurse and midwife. The directives provide for minimum harmonization of training and automatic recognition of title throughout the EU. Their operation is strongly supported by the intensive work of EU advisory committees for each individual profession. The advisory committees comprise representation of each member state, and exchange information, develop documentation and suggest change. The sectoral directives[12,13] for general nursing were introduced in 1977 and allowed general nurses to enjoy freedom of movement and automatic recognition of their nursing qualification across EU member states. Most significantly psychiatric nurses were not included in the sectoral directives.

The *general systems directives*[14] were introduced in 1994 in an attempt to harmonize a greater number of academic and professional qualifications. They apply across a wide range of professions, and follow varying levels and durations of education and training. Unlike the sectoral directives they do not guarantee immediate and automatic recognition of different qualifications and the host country may require additional training and testing and supervised practice as part of the recognition process. Psychiatric nursing falls within the control of the general systems directive.

Primarily because of the application of sectoral directives general nursing has a much stronger identity in Europe than does psychiatric nursing. General nurses enjoy greater privileges and rights to practise across EU member states than do psychiatric nurses. The lack of a sectoral directive for psychiatric nursing means that there is no minimum stated education and training requirement for psychiatric nursing in Europe, with resultant implications for psychiatric nursing practice.

There is an increasing need for mobility among health professions in Europe. Some countries such as Germany educate more professionals than they need whereas others are in need of certain professionals. It is also the case that an increasing need for health services along with service imbalances may lead to increased movement of nurses in years to come. This requires that the EU political, legal and administrative systems put in place to facilitate such movement are improved and perfected.[15] The right of every European citizen to live and work in other member states is fundamental, and a basic assumption is that freedom of movement will give EU citizens opportunities to develop their skills and experiences.

Recent efforts in Europe have been focused on simplifying EU rules in order to facilitate the free movement of qualified people between member states, particularly in view of an enlarged EU.[16] The proposed changes include greater liberalization of the provision of services and more automatic recognition of qualifications. It is important that psychiatric nursing qualifications are part of the changes to the recognition of evidence of training. In looking to the future and in a European context, much work needs to be done to ensure that psychiatric nurses:

- are better informed about EU documentation and its importance to them
- across Europe are agreed in principle on the minimum acceptable education and training requirements for psychiatric nursing in Europe
- recognize the importance and potential influence of the EU agenda generally in strengthening the care of the mentally ill and in particular the practice of psychiatric nursing in Europe
- create a forum and proactive agenda in pursuance of common goals in the best interest of psychiatric nursing in Europe.

NURSING EDUCATION

There are many differences in psychiatric nursing education across Europe. In the newer EU member states from Eastern and Central Europe, regulated education and training for psychiatric nursing is in its infancy, whereas in Western

Europe regulation through a national nursing board is well established. In 1995, Welch[17] described the limitations in Eastern and Central Europe, in particular a lack of regulatory structures and significantly the lack of clinical experiences in education programmes for psychiatric nursing.

Psychiatric nursing education commenced as a certificated training programme in a hospital-based school of nursing in the early 1900s. Across most of Europe nursing education has now been integrated into or linked to the third-level university-based education system of member states, with nursing students receiving their education alongside other university students. It should be noted that the integration of psychiatric nursing education into the third-level education system exists in various forms ranging from full integration into third-level education to rather tenuous links. The removal of students from the nursing labour force of mental health services is a significant factor in the changes that have taken place in nursing education in some EU countries.

MODELS OF NURSING EDUCATION

Across Europe three different models of psychiatric nursing registration education programmes are discernible with different types and levels of professional regulation and academic awards. The three models are:

1 specialist model
2 generic core and specialist pathway
3 generic programme.

Specialist model

The specialist model represents the earliest formalized approach to psychiatric nursing education. Students had direct entry to a programme of training which was entirely focused on psychiatric nursing and, when completed, it entitled the nurse to work exclusively in the psychiatric setting. For the training programme, psychiatric nursing students were recruited by hospitals and they formed an essential part of the nursing workforce. Students therefore had to fulfil the requirements of dual roles as employee and student. Such a model having commenced in the early twentieth century was implemented widely across countries such as The Netherlands, the UK and Ireland. Today, Ireland remains as the only EU country to have maintained a specialist entry programme for psychiatric nurses. This programme is now totally integrated into the third-level education sector and, in Ireland since September 2002, has been conducted as a 4-year degree psychiatric nurse registration programme.

Generic core and specialist pathway model

The recognition and acceptance that there are central tenets of a clinical and theoretical nature underpinning nursing education irrespective of clinical setting led to the establishment of a core programme for nursing education. Such a programme was introduced into the UK in the latter part of the 1980s and remains as the predominant model of nursing education in the UK. The UK model involves a common foundation programme of 18 months' duration, followed by a second 18 months that is focused on psychiatric nursing and is much more practice based.

Generic model

The generic model is the most common educational model for the preparation of psychiatric nurses across Europe. In this model, which is promoted through the WHO, all nursing students including psychiatric nursing students enter a similar programme of registration, usually of 3 years' duration. The generic model is well established in EU member states such as Italy, Norway, Sweden and Spain. Internationally, there is a move towards the generic model; for example, in the late 1980s Australia replaced the specialist model with a generic model. In more recent years, The Netherlands changed from a traditional specialist programme to a generic model. In The Netherlands, all students obtain psychiatric nursing experience but there is no specialist qualification. Students in the final 6 months may, if they wish, choose a psychiatric specialist element. During the programme, students gain experience in many clinical settings.

There are many criticisms of the core/specialist and generic models of psychiatric nurse education as the most appropriate approach to the educational preparation of psychiatric nurses. Bowers et al.[18] point to the implications for the skill and expertise of graduating nurses and highlight the need for specific action to safeguard psychiatric nursing skills within the generic curriculum. In an Australian context, a similar concern was expressed[19] about the movement of psychiatric nursing education to a generic model in Victoria, Australia, and in particular a devaluing of the skills and practice of psychiatric nursing to the extent that the very survival of the specialist branch of nursing is in serious jeopardy. A position paper from the Australian and New Zealand College of Mental Health Nurses[20] highlighted the constraining effects on the practice of generic nurse training. The paper suggested that the generic programme resulted in minimal clinical experiences for psychiatric nurses, and the regulation of mental health nursing is seriously undermined.

In looking towards a future agenda, it is important that the concerns of some psychiatric nurse leaders about the suitability of the generic model of psychiatric nursing education be taken seriously. Therefore, a European study to examine and evaluate the impact of the different models of psychiatric nursing education in Europe must be commissioned with the aim of ensuring the best educational approaches in the preparation of psychiatric nurses into the future.

IDEOLOGICAL POSITIONS

There is a strong tradition of institutional care in Europe and, primarily because of this, it may be argued that nurses are trapped within a medical and institutional model that adversely affects the type and level of service that they provide. In particular, psychiatric nursing has been dominated by therapeutic shifts within the discipline of psychiatry. On the other hand, the scope of psychiatric nursing practice expanded. Significantly, it has been identified[21] that primarily because of the wide-ranging role, psychiatric nurses now occupy a pivotal and central role in services for mentally ill people in many care and treatment locations.

Given the strong historical association between psychiatric medicine and psychiatric nursing, the challenging question is to what extent can the psychiatric nursing role develop outside of medicine. In Europe, psychiatric nursing remains strongly institutionally based and medically dominated. Psychiatric nurses in Western Europe, much more so than in Eastern or Central Europe, have achieved a level of autonomous practice and have in a significant way diversified their practice into settings outside of the institution, including the community and the home.

The reduced reliance on custodial care, changing mental healthcare legislation and the requirement for multidisciplinary patterns in the care of the mentally ill have profound implications for the role of the nurse. Psychiatric nurses will be expected to provide care to different groups, with whom they have had minimal contact in the past. There is a new emphasis on health promotion, early intervention, community development and on nursing being provided closer to where people live and work, as well as making access to services easier for vulnerable groups of the population.

The search for a universal ideology to guide nursing practice has been raised, and, in terms of practice, psychiatric nurses are involved in all forms of treatment from merely monitoring medication to introducing psychotherapeutic modalities. There is clearly a lack of a single unifying ideological approach to psychiatric nursing in Europe; indeed, ideological eclecticism may represent a core foundation for the practice of nursing. However, the lack of an agreed understanding and a single ideology for psychiatric nursing in Europe introduces serious limitations, and it is suggested that psychiatric nurses are hard pressed to define or predict the outcomes of nursing.[22]

Across Europe there is a lack of authoritative information on psychiatric nursing roles. However, there is general agreement that mental health problems require patterns of care which draw on psychological, spiritual and social well-being as well as the physical aspects of the person. The juxtaposition between traditional custodial roles and the evolving therapeutic role of the nurse is eloquently summed up by Peplau[23] when she suggests that there is a significant difference between taking responsibility for the care of people and being therapeutically responsive to each person.

A number of studies have been undertaken to describe the role of the psychiatric nurse in different Europe countries. In one of the earliest UK studies, Altschul[24] concluded that it had proved impossible to obtain any picture of the treatment ideologies that prevailed among nurses. Cormack[25] found little evidence of therapeutic activity. In another study,[21] nine categories of the psychiatric nursing role were identified. These included assessing patients' needs and evaluating care, planning care, nurse–patient interactions, pharmaceutical interventions, education, documenting information, coordinating the services of nurses and other professionals for patients, communicating with other professionals and grades of staff, and the administration and organization of clinical work. Importantly, psychiatric nurses performed independent functions as well as collaborating with other professional groups to provide patient/client care. The study[21] identified that psychiatric nurses considered the central tenet of psychiatric nursing to be that of the caring relationship between patient and nurse. It was reported that psychiatric nurses cared for patients at different levels; for example, for patients with greater dependency levels nursing meant *doing for* patients those activities that they could not do for themselves. In other cases, the nurse's role involved care at a level of *doing with* individuals, which meant supporting, supervising and working alongside patients in a way that recognized their strengths. At another level, nurses at times provided a presence, *being with* patients, when other more active interventions were not possible, not required or inappropriate.

Clearly, the psychiatric nursing role is evolving and it is important that the future role of the psychiatric nurse develops in a centrally coordinated way across Europe.

THE PRACTICE OF PSYCHIATRIC NURSING IN EUROPE

As previously indicated, across the EU region there is much variance in the level of investment and the environment for care, and this directly affects psychiatric nursing. Across the EU, psychiatric nursing environments range from outdated, overcrowded dickensian institutions to purpose-built modern units. High staff turnover and problems with recruitment and retention are a salient feature of psychiatric nursing in Europe. In a recent study, it has been shown that greater levels of job satisfaction exist among nurses working in community care rather than institutional care.[26] Factors related to autonomy, choice of work location and work environment were perceived as significant factors influencing job satisfaction. It is therefore important that there are concerted EU efforts to make psychiatric nursing more attractive so as to stabilize the psychiatric nursing workforce across Europe.

There have been no dramatic scientific discoveries that provide an understanding of the nature and aetiology of mental illness. The lack of discoveries in cures for the major illnesses of schizophrenia and depression at this point in history distinguishes the mental health branch of health care from other branches of health care. In Western Europe the major advances in the past 20 years have been in terms of social and economic conditions, which have contributed to greater community integration for the mentally ill and an active agenda of deinstitutionalization. The psychiatric nursing role since its inception has had the mentally ill as its prime concern in spite of constraints placed on it by an archaic institutional system with often draconian policies leading to stagnation in the mental healthcare system.

Stagnation and a lack of future direction led to the establishment of a WHO expert committee on psychiatric nursing as far back as 1956.[27] One of the main activities of the expert committee was to determine the skills required for psychiatric nursing practice in the future. The committee also provided guidance on nursing education and in particular the content of the curriculum. The report of the expert committee exerted a seminal influence as it provided the necessary stimulus for discussion and analysis on psychiatric nursing across different countries. In highlighting the interpersonal role of the nurse and the preventive and health promotion role in redirected health services the report was insightful and futuristic in its time.

PSYCHIATRIC NURSING PRACTICE AGENDAS

In looking to the future, the establishment of formal and informal EU forums to share common understandings of the care of the mentally ill is essential to a strong psychiatric nursing profession in Europe. In spite of different types and levels of mental health service in Europe, there is an identified core set of values to be pursued.

Community psychiatric nursing

It remains the situation that the majority of psychiatric nursing work is carried out in mental healthcare institutions, yet the majority of policy documents from individual countries espouse community mental healthcare approaches. The establishment of integrated community mental healthcare teams and the introduction of a seamless service between institution and home is a major challenge. Psychiatric nurses are pivotally poised to be team leaders in mental healthcare teams and in directing and developing the services. Community psychiatric nursing services have developed over the past 40 years; however, across Europe they have been poorly planned with no

rational basis on which community psychiatric nursing manpower needs are planned.[28] From a EU perspective it is important that a concerted effort is made to develop the community psychiatric nursing role in terms of assessment, diagnosis, therapist and liaison between primary and secondary care. In developing the role of therapist there are opportunities for psychiatric nurses to specialize in a particular therapeutic approach, e.g. family therapy and behavioural therapy.

There has been concern expressed that the move towards primary care has deskilled nurses in relation to patients with enduring mental illness. However, new initiatives such as the Thorn programme has prepared nurses for problem-orientated care management, assertive outreach and psychological interventions with psychotic patients and their families.[29]

Transcultural issues

Freedom of movement, conflicts and complex emergencies have created a large number of refugees and asylum seekers across Europe. Such migrants include vulnerable people who are at an increased risk of psychosocial trauma following acts of ethnic cleansing, murder, sexual violence, torture and mutilation. During the course of the last century, two world wars took place and as a result we should now have a greater understanding of the long-term negative traumatic effects that conflict has on the social well-being of people.

Clearly, durable solutions to the mental health problems of displaced people remain elusive. It is suggested[30] that displaced people suffer from a series of psychosocial assaults summarized by the 'four Ds':

1 disintegration of the psyche as a result of torture and other abuse
2 dispossession of property, and position in society, family and friends
3 dislocation from homes, countries and cultures
4 disempowerment as aliens in the new country.

It may be argued that all psychiatric syndromes are culture bound, e.g. attitudes to medication and the medical model vary with ethnicity.[31] The culturally bound presentation of mental disorders is a salient feature in our lack of understanding of causation. The relationship between migration and mental illness is interesting. For example, schizophrenia is six times more common in African Caribbeans living in the UK[32] than in the native population and four times more common among migrants to The Netherlands than in the native population.[33]

In dealing with the current plight of immigrants more attention must be given to mental health and psychosocial well-being. The WHO[34] has recognized the need for a rapid response to the mental health needs of refugees and displaced populations. In supporting the WHO's position, psychiatric nurses can be centrally involved in leading and directing initiatives such as providing training in basic mental health skills for humanitarian workers and ensuring community empowerment and cultural sensitivity.

Autonomous practice and forces for change

There has been much debate on establishing new roles outside the conventional role of the psychiatric nurse. There are many driving forces for change in nursing, with the underlying impetus arising from pressures within society. The WHO[35] recognized the driving forces as being:

- population changes – older, diversity in ethnicity, structure, culture and expectations
- health problems are changing – including diseases, work patterns, lifestyle and the environment
- our understanding of what causes good and poor health is rapidly developing as we uncover more of the links between poor health and social circumstances
- new knowledge, techniques and approaches
- research is improving our insight into what is effective care
- the location of care is moving nearer to and into people's homes with hospitals reserved for the most acute cases
- the demands on government and private resources are rising and health will have to compete.

As European harmonization continues the EU will become one large community of people whose healthcare needs will be more and more influenced through EU policy initiatives. Diversity in healthcare needs will require a shift in responsibility for all healthcare professionals. Psychiatric nurses are well positioned to become clinical leaders primarily because as first-line professionals they have continuous contact with other agencies and service users and a good understanding of how communities function and the problems they face. How can psychiatric nurses be best positioned to work in multidisciplinary environments in the hospital and community care setting and inculcate change on an ongoing basis?

The extension and expansion of the role of the psychiatric nurse and the scope of practice must be developed within a structured EU framework which builds on existing practice and, in particular, different levels of practice. The WHO[35] in particular offers an interesting perspective on nursing roles as:

- care provider – who considers the patient/client holistically as an individual and as an integral part of a family, the community and the culture
- decision-maker – who identifies relevant health- and illness-related needs or problems and chooses what interventions to use
- communicator – who is able to promote healthy lifestyles by effective collaboration, explaining, teaching and advocacy

- community leader – who, having won the trust of people among whom he/she works, ideally can identify and reconcile individual and community health requirements
- manager – who can make appropriate use of available data and work harmoniously with individuals and organizations both inside and outside the healthcare system.

There are many opportunities for the development of specialist and advanced nursing roles in psychiatric nursing; however, such opportunities have been unevenly applied across the EU. To date, advanced and specialist nursing roles have been implemented in areas of psychiatry such as behavioural therapy, counselling, family therapy, challenging behaviours, forensic, child and adolescent, substance abuse, suicide prevention, eating disorders and sexual abuse.

The available research is very supportive of advancing the scope of psychiatric nursing. In one of the earliest accounts, it was shown that aftercare provided by community psychiatric nurses was as effective as aftercare by a psychiatrist.[36] The highly effective and efficient role of the psychiatric nurse in primary care has also been demonstrated.[37] More recently, the development of the role of psychiatric nurse consultant has been perceived very positively.[38] A primary aim of the psychiatric nursing profession in Europe must be an expansion/extension of the scope of practice in line with mental health service requirements.

European forums

There is a tendency for psychiatric nurses in Europe to look towards the USA for ideas, rather than develop a common understanding which can be shared by nurses across Europe. There is also a tendency towards insular thinking, with few links between individual countries, little sharing or comparisons of practices, or little collaborative research. There is an urgent need for EU psychiatric nursing forums that focus on the many challenging nursing issues, such as suicide, drug and alcohol abuse. Best practice EU guidelines and standards must arise from within the discipline of psychiatric nursing and should be developed through EU research collaborations.

One the very few successful EU groups in this regard is the European Violence in Psychiatry Research Group (EViPRG),[39] which was formed in 1997 to promote sharing of expertise and knowledge among researchers into violence in psychiatry. Other important aims of the group are to identify, share and disseminate good practice on the prevention and management of violence in psychiatry and to bring together the different psychiatric disciplines. The membership of EViPRG includes Belgium, Denmark, Finland, France, Germany, Greece, Republic of Ireland, Italy, The Netherlands, Norway, Portugal, Slovenia, Spain, Sweden, Switzerland, UK,

Turkey and Poland. EViPRG is a model of EU collaboration that has served to generate a common understanding of the problems, challenges and solutions to violence in psychiatry.

Horatio[40] (European Association of Psychiatric Nurses) is another example of a collaborative group. Horatio was established in 2006 and includes psychiatric–mental health nursing organizations and individual nurses in the association. The specific aims of the group are twofold: to advocate the interests of the members by providing input into the decision-making processes on issues relevant to psychiatric–mental health nurses in Europe; to promote the development of psychiatric–mental health nursing practice, education, management and research.

It is important that EU collaborations be enhanced in nursing and that a greater level of EU funding be available to facilitate such developments.

SUMMARY

In most countries of Europe there is now a greater awareness and recognition of the potential benefits of a strong nursing profession. It is important that the high regard given in some countries is translated into a common EU agenda for psychiatric nursing and the establishment of minimum acceptable standards for the education and training of psychiatric nurses. A greater understanding of the mental health challenges common to all countries must serve to drive developmental initiatives to determine the scope of psychiatric nursing practice in Europe. This must be done with limitless imagination to envision a preferred future for psychiatric nursing in Europe.

Patients/clients and their family members as advocates and consumers of the services are putting pressure on service providers to provide a wider and more diverse range of services. In responding to this agenda service providers are placing a greater emphasis on skill mix and a requirement for more diverse and flexible approaches in the delivery of services. This will present new opportunities for the psychiatric nursing profession in Europe, including interdisciplinary work and autonomous nursing roles at specialist, advanced practitioner and consultant nurse level. The requirement for evidence-based practice will necessitate a paradigm shift in the nursing profession with the establishment of a strong nursing research culture and in particular research utilization.

Psychiatric nursing across Europe is fragmented and there are few links, with little sharing, comparisons or collaborative research. Language differences are a reality and may have contributed to insular thinking; however, it must not be seen as a barrier to sharing best practice. There is a growing communication network in Europe, as, for example, the work of EViPRG and Horatio. However, in Europe there are major challenges ahead in terms of common agendas, communications and labour mobility in psychiatric nursing.

REFERENCES

1. Duncan B. Health policy in the European Union: how it's made and how to influence it. *BMJ* 2002; **324**: 1027–30.

2. Nolan P. *A history of mental health nursing.* London, UK: Chapman & Hall, 1993.

3. Taylor CM. Advertising psychiatric nursing. *Archives of Psychiatric Nursing* 1994; 8 (3): 143–4.

4. Lader M. *Psychiatry on trial.* London, UK: Penguin, Harmondsworth, 1977.

5. World Health Organization. *Health for all.* Nursing Series 1–6. Copenhagen, Denmark: Regional Office for Europe, 1992.

6. Reynolds J. *Grangegorman; psychiatric care in Dublin since 1815.* Dublin, Ireland: Institute of Public Administration, 1992.

7. Weurth V. A comparison: an open psychiatric unit in the US and Germany. *Journal of Psychosocial Nursing* 1993; **31** (3): 29–33.

8. Tomov T. Mental health reforms in Eastern Europe. *Acta Psychiatrica Scandinavica* 2001; **104** (s410): 21–6.

9. World Health Organization. *Mental health declaration for Europe.* Copenhagen, Denmark: WHO, 2005.

10. World Health Organization. *Mental health action plan for Europe.* Copenhagen, Denmark: WHO, 2005.

11. Knapp MJ, McDaid D, Mossialos F, Thornicroft G. *Mental health policy and practice across Europe.* Buckingham, UK: Open University Press, 2005.

12. Council of the European Community. *Council Directive (77/452EEC) concerning the mutual recognition of diplomas and certificates and other evidence of the formal qualifications of nurses responsible for general care: including measures to facilitate the effective exercise of the right of establishment and freedom to provide services.* Brussels, Belgium: Council of the European Community, 1977.

13. Council of the European Community. *Council Directive (77/453EEC) concerning the coordination of provisions laid down by law, regulation or administrative action in respect of the activities of nurses responsible for general care.* Brussels, Belgium: Council of the European Community, 1977.

14. Council of the European Union. *A second general system for the recognition of professional education and training to supplement Directive 89/48/EEC. Directive 92/51/EEC.* Brussels, Belgium: Council of the European Union, 1992.

15. Skar M. *Mobility in the European health sector. The role of transparency and recognition of vocational qualifications.* CEDEFOP. Luxembourg: Office for Publications of the European Communities, 2001.

16. EU Document 2002/0061. *Proposal for a directive of the European Parliament and of the Council on the recognition of professional qualifications.* Brussels, Belgium: Commission of the European Communities, 2002.

17. Welch M. Recent developments in psychiatric nurse education in the countries of Central and Eastern Europe. *International Journal of Nursing Studies* 1995; **32** (4): 366–72.

18. Bowers L, Whittington R Almvik R *et al*. A European perspective on psychiatric nursing and violent incidents: management, education and service organisation. *International Journal of Nursing Studies* 1999; **36**: 217–22.

19. Happel B. Psychiatric nursing in Victoria, Australia. A profession in crisis. *Journal of Psychiatric and Mental Health Nursing* 1997; **4**: 417–22.

20. Australian and New Zealand College of Mental Health Nurses. *Regulatory practices for mental health nursing*. Canberra Australia: Australian and New Zealand College of Mental Health Nurses, 1996.

21. Cowman S, Farrelly M, Gilheaney P. An examination of the role and function of the psychiatric nurse in clinical practice in Ireland. *Journal of Advanced Nursing* 2001; **34** (6): 745–53.

22. Peplau H. Tomorrows world. *Nursing Times* 1987; **7 January**: 29–32.

23. Peplau H. Psychiatric mental health nursing: challenge and change. *Journal of Psychiatric and Mental Health* 1994; **1**: 3–7.

24. Altschul AT. *Patient–nurse interaction*. London, UK: Churchill Livingstone, 1972.

25. Cormack D. *Psychiatric nursing described*. London, UK: Churchill Livingstone, 1983.

26. Ward M, Cowman S. Job satisfaction in psychiatric nursing. *Journal of Psychiatric and Mental Health Nursing* 2007; **14**: 454–61.

27. World Health Organization Expert Committee on Psychiatric Nursing. *First report*. Geneva, Switzerland: WHO, 1956.

28. Royal College of Psychiatrists. *Community psychiatric nursing*. Occasional paper OP40. London, UK: Royal College of Psychiatrists, 1997.

29. Gournay K. Mental health nurses working purposefully with people with severe and enduring mental illness: an international perspective. *International Journal of Nursing Studies* 1995; **32**: 341–51.

30. Silov D, Tarn R, Bowles R, Reid J. Psychosocial needs of torture survivors. *Australian and New Zealand Journal of Psychiatry* 1991; **25**: 482–90.

31. Lefley HP. Culture and chronic mental illness. *Hospital and Community Psychiatry* 1990; **41** (3): 277–85.

32. Harrison G. Searching for the causes of schizophrenia: the role of migrant studies. *Schizophrenia Bulletin* 1990; **16**: 663–71.

33. Selten JP, Slaets JP, Khan RS. Schizophrenia in Surinamese and Dutch Antillean immigrants to the Netherlands: evidence of an increased incidence. *Psychological Medicine* 1997; **27**: 807–11.

34. World Health Organization. *Rapid assessment of mental health needs of refugees, displaced and other populations affected by conflict and post-conflict situations*. Geneva, Switzerland: WHO, 2001.

35. World Health Organization. *Nursing and midwives for health: a WHO European strategy for nursing and midwifery education*. Copenhagen, Denmark: Regional Office for Europe, 1999.

36. Paykel T, Griffiths J. *Community psychiatric nursing for neurotic patients*. London, UK: RCN Publications, 1983.

37. Gournay K, Brooking J. The community psychiatric nurse in primary care: an economic analysis. *Journal of Advanced Nursing* 1995; **22**: 769–78.

38. Jones P. Consultant nurses and their potential impact upon health care delivery. *Clinical Medicine* 2002; **2** (1): 39–40.

39. The European Violence in Psychiatry Research Group. Available from: www.liv.ac.uk/eviprg.

40. Horatio, the European Association for Psychiatric Nurses. Available from: www.horatio-web.eu/index.html.

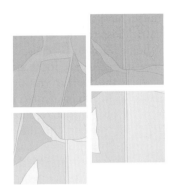

CHAPTER 80

The Japanese context

Mami Kayama*

SOCIAL HOSPITALIZATION AND THE NEW LAW

A law designed to integrate welfare services for individuals physically, mentally or intellectually impaired was enacted in 2006. The result of several years of policy changes and deliberation, it has had profound effects on the physical and mental healthcare system. In 2002 the Japanese Council on Public Health, a governmental body, disclosed the existence of 72 000 psychiatric hospital inpatients, whom it termed 'social hospitalization' patients. These patients had symptoms that would not prevent them from living in the community but lacked the support services and community acceptance to enable them to do so. Support services were available under four different laws, which covered people with physical, mental and intellectual disabilities as well as juvenile delinquents. Under the new law, facilities and services are provided according to the degree of disability. This epoch-making integration was expected to change the perception of mental disorder, defining it as one disability among others.[1]

The 2002 Japanese Council on Public Health report defined 'social hospitalization' as hospitalization of patients whose symptoms and social functioning are adequate for living in the community. The major reason for their continued hospitalization is the shortage of social resources to support their community life. Traditionally in Japan, the family is expected to support and care for the patient. This custom may persist because many people blame families for mental illness. Public opinion is changing, however, and people increasingly believe that families of mentally disabled people should receive the services of professional caregivers and be free from the heavy responsibility of care.

CHANGING THE ROLE OF PSYCHIATRIC NURSING

For the past 30 years, Japanese psychiatric nurses have provided inpatient bedside care, in which the nurse's first priority is to restore the patient's rhythm of daily life. Nurses encourage patients to get up in the morning, to eat meals regularly, to be groomed and to sleep at night. This requires much time and good communication, especially with psychotic patients. The traditional inpatient service will not have prepared nurses or patients for the services which will be present under the new system, such as short-term hospitalization. Nurses now have to learn about the new system, deliver the information to patients, and encourage them to assert their right to use various services.[2] The new system requires patients themselves to decide what kind of services they want to use and apply for them. Nurses can only help them realize their preferences.

SETTING TO WORK

The new law requires the disabled to shoulder 10 per cent of the charges for welfare services they receive,

*Mami Kayama is a Professor of Nursing in the Department of Psychiatric and Mental Health Nursing, St Luke's College, Tokyo, Japan. She was previously Associate Professor at the University of Tokyo and has studied the development of community care and the role of families in different countries.

although naturally a ceiling would be set. Also, those with a low income, which accounts for the majority among the disabled, would receive special reductions in payment or even exemptions.

But the framework of this reduction and exemption, which the Health, Labor and Welfare Ministry says is the 'result of meticulously taking into account the low-income earners', is complex, increasing anxiety among the disabled. The ministry needs to explain the framework to the public more thoroughly. There is little public resistance to the idea of integrating the systems and extending support to help the disabled secure jobs.

RESEARCHING THE EFFECTS OF NURSES' HOME VISITS

The Japanese system of nursing licence: RN and PHN

A brief description of the Japanese system of nursing licensure provides the necessary background for understanding contemporary Japanese psychiatric nursing. Home visits have become an essential component of psychiatric care. There are two kinds of certification for making home visits. These are registered nurse (RN) and public health nurse (PHN). All PHNs have a RN licence; there is a national examination for the PHN licence. RNs without baccalaureate degrees take the examination after receiving a further 6–12 months of special education. The home visiting roles of RNs and PHNs are different. Most PHNs work at public health centres as civil servants. In contrast, many RNs work at private hospitals. PHNs are expected to be coordinators or supporters of RNs, but today the rapid increase in the ageing population has led to a change of roles for RNs and PHNs in home visiting.

In 1992 a revised health and medical insurance system launched a system of visiting nurses service stations (VNSSs). A VNSS may be sponsored by a psychiatric hospital, other types of hospitals, a physicians association, the Japanese Nursing Association or by the private capital of a nurse manager or other private company. VNSSs chiefly provide home visits to the elderly but also provide care for mentally disabled people. VNSSs employ *home-helps*. There are various kinds of home-helper's licence. Many of these are based on a 6-month period of communication education. The home-helpers do not have an educational background in medicine.

In general most staff of VNSSs do not have practice experience in psychiatric nursing. They are often fearful about caring for people with mental illness and seek special skills to enhance their home visiting work. As mentioned, many of them were trained as care providers for elderly people; thus, VNSS staff often ask psychiatric nurses to lecture on psychiatric care.

Nurses and public health nurses have a long history of home visiting. Some psychiatric hospital nurses were aware of the effectiveness of home visits to psychiatric patients before health insurance started to pay for these visits. From the late 1970s, when the fee for visiting nurse services was not reimbursed by health insurance in Japan, some considerate nurses in hospitals started to visit discharged or pre-discharged patients in their homes in order to meet their needs. As a result of their efforts, the Health and Medical Service for the Elderly Law, passed in 1982, provided health insurance reimbursement for nurses' home visits. In 1992, a revision of this law launched the system of VNSSs directed by nurses. In 2005, the insurance system was changed to improve community care. Home visits were a major issue. Today, a nurse can visit a patient's home five times before discharge from the hospital to help prepare the patient for community life. For 3 months after discharge, the nurse can visit the patient five times a week with insurance reimbursement. On these visits, nurses can cooperate with psychiatric social workers, occupational therapists and physical therapists.[3]

Length of hospitalization

The visiting care service records for 138 patients with a diagnosis of schizophrenia at one public hospital were reviewed. All had received the service for more than 2 years since visiting care service began in 2003. The total length of inpatient stay, before and after the introduction of visiting care service, was calculated. The difference between population means of the groups – before and after the introduction of home visiting – was also calculated. This study showed a change in the number of hospital stays 2 years before and after the commencement of visiting care service (Figure 80.1).

Data from a 1998 report on hospital management showed that the average length of hospital stay in Japan was 419.1 days. After the home visiting care service started, this was reduced to 97.5 days. There was, however, no change in the number of admissions.

In another study, visiting nurses looked for signs of major difficulties in patients. When these signs were noted, the nurses encouraged patients to go to a psychiatrist. It was

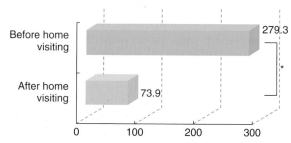

Figure 80.1 Average length of hospital stay ($N = 134$). **$P < 0.01$

found that if patients received consultation early, the length of admission became much shorter.[4]

The preventive care function

A study we conducted showed that nurses' preventive home visiting shortened the length of admission. Based on the effectiveness of this service, visiting nurses are now regarded as a specialist support to psychiatric patients at home. The strength of home visiting seems to be in the details of their interpersonal relationships. Based on a qualitative analysis of data from the study, nurses' behaviour in response to patients' symptoms was characterized along five dimensions, as shown in Box 80.1.

Box 80.1: Care given on exacerbation of symptoms

- Symptom monitoring
- Compensatory care for patient's self-care deficit
- Perceiving patients' failure in their activities of daily living
- Making judgement on present condition
- Suggesting visit to outpatient department

---

1 *Symptom monitoring*. This was the most frequently occurring care behaviour among nurses in our study. There were two aspects to symptom monitoring: one was monitoring symptoms that were characteristic of schizophrenia such as hearing voices, inappropriate laughter, persecution feelings and delusions; the other was the monitoring of patients' emotional expressions, such as anxiety and anger that accompanied patients' daily living. The visiting nurses monitored these behaviours as indicators of patients' symptom exacerbation.

2 *Compensatory care for patient's self-care deficit*. When a patient's condition worsened, several activities of daily living that became difficult for him or her to do were observed. These included taking medications, going to hospital and eating meals. In such cases, the nurses accompanied patients to eat out, administered medication, or made unscheduled visits in order to encourage the patient to go to hospital.

3 *Assessing patient's ability to perform activities of daily living (ADLs)*. It was also noted that nurses were able to observe changes in patients' ADL. When patients became unable to carry out their ADLs – for example, when they could no longer cope with daily activities, ate almost nothing or did not take medication at all – the nurse's visiting care could no longer meet the patient's needs.

4 *Disposition of patients*. On perceiving a patient's failure regarding his or her ADLs, visiting nurses reported directly to the patient's doctor, and then decided how to support the patient as a team from then on. The decision involved a choice between supporting the patient continuously on an outpatient basis, or admitting the patient to hospital so that he or she could regroup.

5 *Suggesting hospital visits or admission*. Visiting nurses tried to help patients become aware of their own symptoms, so that they could recognize the development of breakdown in their daily living activities. In such circumstances, the nurses suggested that a visit or admission to a hospital might be necessary for them. When the nurses thought it would be difficult for the patient to transfer from home to hospital, they would consider accompanying the patient.

FORENSIC PSYCHIATRY AND PSYCHIATRIC NURSING

In 2005, the government also enacted a law titled 'Lunatics medical observation method'. Under this new law, every prefecture was required to have a forensic ward that meets special standards governing ward construction and staffing. The purpose of this law was to provide medical care to mentally ill persons alleged to have engaged in criminal activity. Implementation has just begun in inpatient settings. However, it will be a challenge for nursing staff to improve forensic nursing care.

THE EXPANDING ROLE OF HUMAN COMMUNICATION

Japanese nurses are now encountering technological and policy and social changes at an increasing rate. We need enough knowledge to empower patients to take advantage of the new social resources. Nurses must change their attitudes about hospital admission and community care.

The philosophy of nursing that we have learned is human centred. Every new law or new system appears to be approaching this philosophy. Japanese psychiatric nurses are aware of this point and will take steps to expand the role of human communication in this effort.

REFERENCES

1. *The Japan Times Weekly* 28 May, 2005.

2. Kayama M, Zerwech J, Thornton K, Murashima S. Japanese expert public health nurses empower clients with schizophrenia living in the community. *Journal of Psycho-social Nursing and Mental Health Services* 2001; **39**: 40–5.

3. Murashima S, Nagata S, Magilvy J *et al.* Home care nursing in Japan: a challenge for providing good care at home. *Public Health Nursing* 2002; **19** (2): 94–103.

4. Kayama M, Matsushita T, Funakoshi A *et al.* Effectiveness of home visits by psychiatric nurses: an empirical study using psychiatric length of stay as an outcome measure (in Japanese). *Seishin-Igaku* 2005; **47** (6): 647–53.

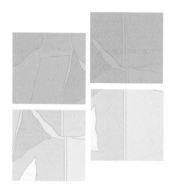

CHAPTER 81

The United States context

Shirley A. Smoyak*

INTRODUCTION

Change is rarely embraced with open arms, even when there is acknowledgement that something needs fixing. Although the clinical practice of psychiatric nursing is based solidly on communication skills, reframing difficult situations, systems thinking and being articulate, nurses can be as resistant to change as any other group. In my half-century, plus, as a professional nurse, I never cease to be amazed by how we manage to ignore or resist good ideas, common sense and golden opportunities. For this chapter, I have selected three changes which I believe are not only inevitable but will dramatically affect, in a positive way, the practice of psychiatric nurses and the care received by our consumers. These are:

1 The professional practices of nurses will be re-examined, and what they do will be organized by the skills and knowledge needed, not by artificial boundaries. More attention will be paid to answering the question 'How do you know?', as innovations in clinical practice are considered.

2 Consumers will become more knowledgeable about their health needs and demand a collaborative working model with their healthcare providers. Psychosocial rehabilitation models will provide the groundwork for nurses and consumers designing working partnerships.

3 Public health and mental health will again be partners, thus providing the bedrock needed for working in communities. With this realignment, prevention and population-based strategies will be possible.

NEW DIMENSIONS OF PROFESSIONAL PSYCHIATRIC NURSING PRACTICE

In the USA, in the late 1950s and early 1960s, physicians, nurses and patients or clients were distressed with the dysfunctional healthcare system. Several nationally funded studies documented the animosity between the professions and the reasons for nurses leaving the field. In the 1970s, the National Joint Practice Commission (NJPC), comprising eight physicians appointed by the American Medical Association (AMA) and eight nurses appointed by the American Nurses Association (ANA), worked to repair the discord and attempted to institute collaboration and colleagueship in primary care settings. Problems in educational systems and service delivery settings were addressed. Advanced practice nurses were at the centre of the debates. New strategies were developed

Shirley A. Smoyak was a psychiatric nurse before chlorpromazine (Thorazine; Largactil). This says it all – that she had only her wits to deal with the people on the wards of the state mental hospitals where she worked. She currently is Professor II (Distinguished Professor) at the Rutgers University Division of Continuing Education and Outreach, and also teaches at the University of Medicine and Dentistry of New Jersey, School of Public Health. She has been Editor of the Journal of Psychosocial Nursing and Mental Health Services since 1981.

and promulgated by co_____ces and publications. Many lessons were learned in ___t decade and the following years. Ironically, there was never a psychiatrist on the NJPC, so I had no partner to talk to and plan with during this decade.

New ways of relating to each other can be realized when basic questions about assumptions and beliefs are placed squarely on the table. 'Who owns what?' and 'Who has the knowledge and/or skills to do what?' are basic questions to begin the dialogue. The fact that no one can 'own' knowledge, in the sense that this is licensed or controlled, is critical. The needed negotiations are then more clearly seen as dialogues about time, place, populations and politics. As psychiatric nurses expand their practices to include prescriptive authority, such dialogue will be very important.

The legacy of Hildegard E. Peplau

How and why advanced practice nurses developed as they did in the USA is a story that takes more space than allotted here. It is a fascinating tale, and one which could offer some direction to countries just setting out to incorporate this level of nursing into the healthcare arena.

Hildegard E. Peplau is the acknowledged leader of the movement to prepare psychiatric nurses with Masters degrees. In the late 1950s at Rutgers, the State University of New Jersey, College of Nursing, Newark, NJ, she developed a Master of Science programme, which prepared clinical specialists in psychiatric nursing. The 2-year academic programme required 16–20 hours of work each week with severely ill patients with mental illness in state hospitals. Her seminars about the interpersonal relationships were conducted at the hospitals. Before this, Masters degrees had an administrative or education focus, not clinical. This change to a clinical focus was met with great scepticism by many.

Dr Peplau managed to secure the clinical settings for these Masters students by explaining to the physician superintendents that what they were doing was 'group work'. If the word 'therapy' had been used, the programme would not have had a clinical site. Fifty years later, the words 'therapy' and 'psychotherapy' are used easily and forthrightly to describe what these nurses do. Barbara Callaway captured the dimensions of Dr Peplau's groundbreaking work in her biography *Hildegard Peplau: psychiatric nurse of the century*.[1]

The new emphasis in psychiatric nursing is basing one's practice on evidence. Throughout her teaching career, Dr Peplau repeated the message that psychiatric nurses needed to pay attention to the effects of what their words and actions were. She spent endless hours encouraging her students, both basic learners and those in continuing education settings, to be as aware of what they said and did as they were of their observations of patients' behaviours. While she never used the term 'evidence-based practice', this is what she practised, herself, and encouraged others to do.

The interest in evidence-based practice has had a slower start in psychiatric nursing than in medical–surgical practice areas, in which randomized clinical trials (RCTs) are considered the gold standard for any proposed clinical intervention. The admonition to, first, do no harm was the main point in an editorial I wrote for the *Journal of Psychosocial Nursing and Mental Health Services*.[2] Lilienfeld, a psychologist, is considered, in the USA, to be the champion of bringing to the attention of professionals and their clients that talk therapies should be scrutinized carefully to ensure that harm is not being done.[3] In psychiatric nursing, we have paid attention to providing the least restrictive settings during hospitalizations, cautioning against the use of restraints and not using medications to subdue troublesome behaviours of clients. But there has been only silence about measuring the effectiveness or potential harm of talk therapy of any kind. This needed change is long overdue. Professional practice choices and decisions will continue to change as patients and consumers become full partners.

CONSUMERS AS PARTNERS

Even in mid-century, as Dr Peplau was teaching graduate students and nurses in the continuing education workshops across the USA, the notion that psychiatric patients needed to be considered as people with full citizenship rights was emphasized. This was a time before patient advocates, usually lawyers, became a part of the government system at the federal and state levels. Ward staff were not pleased when they were reminded that patients had rights and that their wishes needed to be appreciated and implemented wherever possible.

In the USA, consumers began to make it clear that they expected to be treated as partners, and not just as recipients of care when the psychosocial rehabilitation movement began in the late 1970s. The National Alliance for the Mentally Ill (NAMI) was founded in 1979 by a group of parents championing the cause for their mentally ill sons and daughters.[4] Today, this group is a significant factor in congressional decisions about funding for mental illness, including insurance requirements. Many nurses are members of, and partners with, NAMI.

Consumers share strategies with each other about identifying and accessing professional providers who are resonant with their needs. They know, for instance, that, although they may find many psychiatrists in the yellow pages of the phone book, only a small minority of these actually practise in ways that the consumers find useful. Consumers may also find it difficult to locate a psychiatric nurse, who may be their preferred provider. Advanced practice nurses are fewer in number than psychiatrists.

Psychosocial rehabilitation is regarded as a fairly new concept, with William Anthony regarded as its founder.[5] Its principles dictate that strengths and goals be considered as more important than illness, deficits and symptoms, and that persons affected by mental illness be included actively in any treatment planning.

Possibilities, not deficits, need the attention of nurses and patients, working together. Bear in mind that these principles, which emphasize that normality be the focus, were practised in the oldest of the asylums. Work, especially farming, was considered essential to assure that cure would be the outcome. Some hospitals, such as those run by Quakers, used religion as an adjunct to work. It was not unusual to have patients in classroom settings, studying language or geography. The fact is that many practices that we consider to be new, today, are actually rooted in history.[6]

Interestingly, Anthony[5] spoke and wrote in the 1970s about psychosocial rehabilitation needing a model, or agreed-upon set of practices. While the concept was clear, putting the actual actions into words and practice was a challenge. Its ideology is very much like the earlier emphasis on moral treatment, whose credo was the same.

Anthony presented his psychosocial rehabilitation model at the Rutgers University Institute for Health, Health Care Policy and Aging Research. During his seminars several nurses would point out that his process bore many similarities to the process of nursing: identifying a problem, designing an intervention, taking action and evaluating the outcome.

The new field of psychosocial rehabilitation attracts many psychiatric nurses, since its model affirms what they do in their practice settings. It is difficult to provide a definitive number documenting how many psychosocial rehabilitation practitioners are first nurses, or psychiatrists, or other mental health professionals. There are now training programmes from the associate of arts degree to the doctorate whose focus is psychosocial rehabilitation.

The 15 330 Masters-prepared psychiatric nurses are a minority in the mental health field. We are a tiny group compared with 40 731 psychiatrists, 77 456 psychologists, 31 278 school psychologists, 96 407 social workers and 44 225 marriage and family therapists. Perhaps the most startling statistic is that there are now 100 000 professionals with Masters degrees in psychosocial rehabilitation.[7] This group is the newest addition to the ranks of mental health professionals and a significant number of people are graduating.

NEW DATA ON MENTAL HEALTH PRACTITIONERS

The World Health Organization (WHO), in collaboration with the International Council of Nurses (ICN), published the latest statistics in the *Atlas, 2007, Nurses in mental health*.[8] It is the latest addition to the *Atlas* series of publications from the Department of Mental Health and Substance Abuse of the WHO. This new *Atlas* presents the results of a global survey on the availability, education, training and role of nurses in mental health care. The findings are significant, although not entirely unexpected. The most consistent, and not unexpected, finding is the severe shortage of mental health nurses in most low and middle income countries. Charts and graphs show the lack of adequate opportunities for education and training in mental health both during the initial preparation periods and during continuing education.

In the Executive Summary, the statement is made:[8,p.1]

> To the best of our knowledge, there are no published estimates of the numbers of nurses in mental health settings nor is there any information about the quantity or quality of mental health training for nurses. This lack of information is particularly problematic for low and middle income countries, as nurses are often the primary providers of care for people with mental illnesses in those countries.

The project began in 2004; the original questionnaire was made available in six languages and distributed in a manner to assure global representation. Completed questionnaires came from 171 member states of the WHO, associate members and five territories. The percentage of completed questionnaires by WHO region was: Africa, 100 per cent; the Americas, 83 per cent; Southeast Asia, 91 per cent; Europe, 77 per cent; Eastern Mediterranean, 95 per cent; and Western Pacific, 93 per cent.

Recommendations emerging from this report are grouped into three main categories:

1 recognize nurses as essential human resources for mental health care
2 ensure that adequate numbers of trained nurses are available to provide mental health care
3 incorporate a mental health component into basic and post-basic nursing training.

This survey is essentially a counting document, providing data on where nurses work (mental health settings, mental hospitals, psychiatric units in general hospitals, community settings and so on) organized by the WHO regions. There are data about their education and involvement in policy and legislation. Much more work needs to be done on what the nurses actually do as they practise. In Chapter 10,[8,p.43] there are some initial analyses of what nurses do – but the categories are large rather than specific (e.g. psychological services, independent consultation, primary health, management of services). Worldwide, 14.2 per cent of psychiatric nurses can prescribe psychotropic medications, but the manner in which they do this as well as constraints and regulations were not studied.[8,p.45]

COLLABORATION AMONG PROFESSIONAL GROUPS AND CLIENTS

Professionals from all disciplines will need to learn how to collaborate fully with people for whom they are offering care. Frances Hughes, a Commonwealth Fellow, has also forecast this projected change.[9] She adds a type III to the practice models identified by the National Joint Practice Commission in the 1970s.[10]

- Type I describes work that is highly specific, with practitioners undergoing rigorous training for the specialty.
- Type II work can be accomplished by generalist practitioners from different backgrounds.
- Type III work is accomplished in a collaborative mode, with patients and practitioners sharing in the assessment and decision-making about treatment strategies (Box 81.1).

Box 81.1: Types of work

Type I work (highly specific)

- Workers are highly specialized and have considerable technical training.
- Few clashes or conflicts among workers.
- Workers know their places and what they have to do.
- Examples:
  baseball – pitchers and catchers
  health care – operating suites or emergency centres.

Type II work (general)

- Workers from different backgrounds can do the work equally well.
- Many conflicts over jurisdictions and relationships.
- Competition, rivalry, blaming.
- Examples:
  baseball – the outfield (left, centre, right)
  health care – primary care settings.

Data presented in a document produced by the US Department of Health and Human Services (USDHHS) reflect information only on nurses with graduate degrees in psychiatric–mental health nursing.[11] Many psychiatric nurses are in hospital and community settings where their titles may not even indicate a nursing degree (e.g. manager, coordinator, specialist, discharge planner). Some nurses are Masters prepared, but the majority are not. Such is the case in clinical settings across the country. It is impossible to produce accurate accounting of the educational background and post-graduation training for the nurses in psychiatric settings who had their basic preparation in diploma, associate degree or baccalaureate degree programmes. The good news is that, in the actual clinical settings, a spirit of collegiality and team

building is the case in most instances. Clinical specialists and the newer psychiatric nurse practitioners serve as mentors and guides for the other nurses. My guess would be that in settings where there are no Masters-prepared nurses, the nurses there rise to the challenge of care delivery for their patients. The bad news is that we do not have the data to address the question of how academic preparation affects care delivery. In this age of outcome measures, we are handicapped by not having basic statistics on our entire workforce.

There are some interesting comparative statistics in the area of gender and race.[12] Nurses are still overwhelmingly women (6 per cent men). Even social workers, also a predominantly female occupation historically, now have proportionately more men (about 23 per cent). Female members of the American Psychiatric Association in 1999 totalled 29 per cent, whereas nearly half (48 per cent) of psychologists were women. Nurses have the highest proportion reporting their race as white (94.6 per cent), with psychologists next at 91.7 per cent and social workers at 89 per cent. Psychiatrists, on the other hand, report 73.8 per cent as white, with 13.3 per cent as Asian/Pacific Islander. There is more diversity in their ranks than in the other three.

Less than 5 per cent of female graduate-prepared nurses are younger than 35 years today. In 1988, 18 per cent were under 35. The ageing trend continues, with the current average age at 48 years. Regionally, the greatest percentage of advance practice nurses reside in the South Atlantic, East North Central and Middle Atlantic. More than 50 per cent of the nurses received their highest degree more than 10 years ago. Employment practices indicate that 65 per cent of the nurses hold just one position, while the others report two or more practice positions.

While the nurse practitioner movement is more than 35 years old, psychiatric nursing has just recently moved in this direction. Issues and debates about certification mechanisms and boards continue. The current three types of preparation, clinical nurse specialist (CNS), nurse practitioner (NP) and combined, present dilemmas for those who write the certification examinations. Further, while other disciplines/professions reserve certification processes for those with advanced preparation, nursing has muddied the waters considerably by certifying generalists.

As consumers become stronger advocates for themselves, and are joined by family members and professionals who value accountability, the outcome will surely be closer scrutiny about how practices are conducted. The bottom line will be: are things better for the client? Ways to measure outcomes in psychiatric practice, when the consumer–professional relationship is the focus, need to be developed. When consumers and nurses are equally knowledgeable about medications, side-effects, alternative approaches to therapy, the value of dialogue and action-orientated treatment, mental illness will surely lose considerable stigma. Nurses and consumers will enjoy new respect at work and in communities.

INTEGRATING PUBLIC HEALTH AND MENTAL HEALTH

Americans like convenience, and they like to have what they need or want instantly. In the USA, we have grouped materials and services in interesting ways. For instance, we can fill our car with fuel and fill ourselves with coffee and a doughnut at the same time. We can shop for almost anything in grander and grander shopping centres, and eat at the same time (sitting down or walking around). Some new shopping centres even have exercise spas. Banks used to have one focus per institution; now we have one-stop banking in most urban settings where we can cash cheques, save for a rainy day, arrange a mortgage and get a loan all in one visit. Grocery stores have become mini-shopping centres and include pharmacies (with blood pressure checking devices), flower shops and photography centres.

And we apparently believe that providing good health care requires that it also be integrated. The advent of primary care a quarter of a century ago was heralded as the way to ensure accessible, affordable, appropriate services. Fragmentation was supposed to end when practitioners adopted the new ways of organizing care. The associated frustrations with various barriers to care were supposed to become history. Ironically, parallel to this new interest in providing one-stop shopping for patients, the old fragmentation and animosity between nurses and physicians continued. As noted above, the NJPC attempted to address these problems, and turned its attention to primary care settings and how the practitioners arranged their work.

When I tried to engage nurses in a discussion then about why 'primary nursing' was used in a different way from 'primary care', the positions taken were very clear. Nurses believed that they had to strengthen their own profession and image first, before engaging in any new collaboration with physicians. They saw MDs as the enemy, and they were acting on a need to draw the wagons around and keep their territory safe from invasion. Of course, MDs were also feeling attacked by the articulate, uppity, new breed of nurse practitioner who 'didn't know her place'.

Now, more than 25 years later, we are supposed to be working on integrating mental health in primary health. Surgeon General David Satcher convened a meeting in late 2000 'to advance the integration of mental health services and primary health care'.[11] This meeting was an outgrowth of the 1999 Surgeon General's report on mental health.[12] A nurse, Brenda Reiss-Brennan, MS, APRN, CS, President of Primary Care Family Therapy Clinics, served as the consultant and meeting organizer, conducting over 90 interviews in preparation for the deliberations among the participants representing healthcare professionals, consumers, families, foundations and government agencies. Included among the interviewees were experts representing businesses, researchers, employers, economists, epidemiologists, providers, healthcare consultants and payors, as well as the participants listed above.

Among the group's recommendations were the following:

1. Convene a group under the auspices of the USDHHS to develop a framework for the integration of mental health care and primary care, including a focus on comorbidities, diverse modalities and diverse populations. (Note that this is very similar to the mission of the NJPC, but including mental health.)
2. Incorporate a list of skills, knowledges, attitudes and simple tools that reflect evidence-based 'best practices' and treatment management, leading to improved outcomes. (Note that the providers of such services are not named. The NJPC's idea of 'those who learn together earn together'[13] might yet be a reality.)
3. Design education and training standards for the integration of mental health care and primary care with all stakeholders, including accreditation bodies, and promote implementation of those standards by schools of health and behavioural health. (Note that you should stay tuned to see how these new schools evolve. Will we be talking about a 'fifth profession' again? With a primary care twist or spin?)

Those among us who have vested interests in keeping identities intact, and are resistant to change, will not have an easy time of what is to come. On the other hand, we could adopt John Gardner's position, 'Life is full of golden opportunities carefully disguised as irresolvable problems' (Satcher's opening remarks on 30 November 2000;[11] from a reflection by John Gardner, who was Secretary of Health, Education and Welfare in the 1960s).

REFERENCES

1. Callaway BJ. *Hildegard Peplau: psychiatric nurse of the century.* New York, NY: Springer Publishing Co., 2002.

2. Smoyak S. Primum non nocere (first, do no harm). *The Journal of Psychosocial Nursing and Mental Health Service* 2007; **45** (9): 8–9.

3. Lilienfeld S. Psychological treatments that cause harm. *Perspectives on Psychological Science* 2007; **2**: 53–70.

4. Smoyak S. Specialization: challenges for psychiatric nurses. *The Journal of Psychosocial Nursing and Mental Health Service* 2007; **46**: 8–9.

5. Anthony W. Psychosocial rehabilitation: a concept in need of a method. *American Psychologist* 1977; **32**: 658–62.

6. Smoyak S. What's new is really old. *The Journal of Psychosocial Nursing and Mental Health Service* 2007; **45** (10): 7–8.

7. Center for Mental Health Services, Manderscheid RW, Henderson MJ (eds). *Mental health, United States, 2000*. DHHS Publication No. (SMA) 01-3537. Washington, DC: Supt. of Docs, US Government Printing Office, 2001. Available from: www.samhsa.gov. Free single copies may be requested from the National Mental Health Services Knowledge Exchange Network.

8. World Health Organization. *Atlas, 2007, Nurses in mental health*. Geneva, Switzerland: WHO, 2007.

9. Hughes F. *Healthcare delivery issues: key lessons from the United States*. Paper prepared for the Commonwealth Fund, Harkness Fellowship, April 2002, at the University of Pennsylvania, Philadelphia, PA, 2002.

10. Smoyak S. Problems in interprofessional relationships. *Bulletin of the New York Academy of Medicine* 1977; **53**: 51–9.

11. US Department of Health and Human Services (DHHS). *Report of a Surgeon General's working meeting on the integration of mental health services and primary health care, 30 November to 1 December 2000, Atlanta, Georgia (Carter Center)*. Rockville, MD: USDHHS, Public Health Service, Office of the Surgeon General, 2001.

12. US Department of Health and Human Services (DHHS). *Mental health: a report of the Surgeon General*. Rockville, MD: Substance Abuse and Mental Health Services Administration, Center for Mental Health Services, National Institute for Mental Health Substance Abuse and Mental Health Services Administration, Center for Mental Health Services, National Institute for Mental Health, 1999.

13. Hoekelman R. *Nurse–physician relationships: problems and solutions*. Commencement address to graduates of the Pediatric and Medical Nurse Associate Training Programmes, Rush-Presbyterian, St Luke's Medical Center, Chicago, Illinois, 26 June 1974.

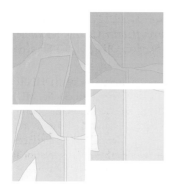

CHAPTER 82

The Canadian context

Nancy Brookes,* Margaret Tansey**
and Lisa Murata***

INTRODUCTION

Here, we provide a brief overview of the Canadian context for psychiatric and mental health nursing. Canada is a federation consisting of 10 provinces and three territories, the world's second largest country in total area. Our perspective is from Ontario and in particular Ottawa, Canada's capital. We shall share one story of our experience with psychiatric and mental health nursing, the *craft of caring* at the Royal Ottawa Mental Health Centre.

THE CANADIAN HEALTHCARE SYSTEM: A WORK IN PROGRESS

Canadians are very proud of their healthcare system. In a television contest in 2004, Canadians voted Tommy Douglas as 'The Greatest Canadian', no doubt because of his most memorable achievement – North America's first government-run hospital and medical care insurance plan. He saw the birth of public hospitalization and Medicare, universal insurance for hospital and physician

care.[1] A second phase, not yet realized, would extend Medicare to home, community, long-term care and pharma-care. In the early 1980s Tommy Douglas reiterated his vision 'Let's not forget that the ultimate goal of Medicare must be to keep people well rather than just patching them up when they get sick.'[1] In 1997, a national forum called for Medicare to include home care, pharma-care and an end to physicians' fees for services. Now a more contemporary view would also include the need to focus on social and environmental determinants of health and social justice.

THE CANADA HEALTH ACT

The principle of universal heath care for all is entrenched in the Canada Health Act, often called 'Medicare'. The Canada Health Act is the federal insurance legislation that covers the criteria and conditions for national healthcare services. Under the 1984 Canada Health Act, the provincial and territorial health plans must provide basic standard healthcare services in order to receive

*Nancy Brookes is the Nurse Scholar with the Royal Ottawa Health Care Group and an Adjunct Professor at the University of Ottawa. She contributed the chapter on the Tidal Model of mental health recovery in Nursing theorists and their work (Tomey AM, Alligood MR (eds). Nursing theorists and their work, 6th edn. St Louis, MO: Mosby, 2006).
**Margaret Tansey is Vice President, Professional Practice and Chief of Nursing at the Royal Ottawa Health Care Group. She maintains a practice with older adults. She is also Academic Consultant, University of Ottawa. Nancy and Margaret were graduate students together in the nursing programme at McGill University in Montreal, Canada.
***Lisa Murata is the Clinical Nurse Educator at the Royal Ottawa Mental Health Centre. She is also a certified Solution Focused Therapist.
All three have their Canadian certification in psychiatric and mental health nursing.

full federal funding. The governments of the provinces and territories administer and deliver the healthcare services. There are five main principles in the Canada Health Act:[2]

1 *Public administration*: non-profit public authorities administer provincial health insurance. The public authority is accountable to the governments of the province or territory, and the records and accounts are subject to public audits.
2 *Comprehensiveness*: all insured health services provided by hospitals and physicians are covered. The services of other healthcare practitioners and services may be covered at the discretion of the province or territory.
3 *Universality*: all insured Canadians are entitled to basic healthcare services.
4 *Portability*: Canadians moving between provinces or territories in essence take their coverage with them and coverage is continuous.
5 *Accessibility*: all insured persons have access to medically necessary insured services without direct charges.

It is interesting that in Canada health care is federal but not nationalized, as in Britain for example. So, while there is universal access to hospital, physicians and some preventive programmes, there are some inconsistencies from province to province. It is still necessary to have a provincially issued health card that entitles insured Canadians to medically necessary coverage. Basic services are covered throughout Canada, and, above that, different provinces may cover different services, e.g. eye examinations and non-hospital physiotherapy services are no longer covered in Ontario. Also about 30 per cent of all healthcare expenditures are paid for outside the public health system.[1]

The 1988 national document *Mental health for Canadians: striking a balance*[3] offers a frequently used definition of mental health: 'the capacity of the individual, the group and the environment to interact with one another in ways that promote subjective well-being, the optimal development and use of mental abilities (cognitive, affective and relational), the achievement of individual and collective goals consistent with justice and the attainment and preservation of conditions of fundamental equality.'

The Canadian Mental Health Association, in collaboration with others, has moved away from a biomedical model and provided direction for mental health care through the evolution of *A framework for support*.[4] This has evolved since the 1980s, when it called for the involvement of consumers and families in mental health systems that are community focused and recovery orientated. Partnerships redefined consumers and families as key players and change agents with a wealth of practical and experiential knowledge. The *framework* includes three resource bases, community, knowledge and personal. The goal of the project is to ensure that people with serious mental health problems live fulfilling lives in the community.

PSYCHIATRIC AND MENTAL HEALTH NURSING STANDARDS

The Canadian Federation of Mental Health Nurses developed *Canadian standards of psychiatric and mental health nursing practice*[5] based on Benner's domains of practice. The practice of psychiatric and mental health nursing is founded on the therapeutic use of self, where nurse–person interactions are purposeful and directed at the promotion of mental health and fostering the functional status of persons experiencing problems in living. This was the first step towards national certification in the specialty. We adopted these standards for the Royal Ottawa Mental Health Centre and they are useful in framing the work of nurses as well as with students.

PSYCHIATRIC AND MENTAL HEALTH CERTIFICATION

The national psychiatric and mental health nursing community chose to create and participate in a specialty certification programme, and the first psychiatric and mental health nursing examination was in 1995. This is a basic certification: there is no advanced psychiatric and mental health nursing certification. Psychiatric and mental health nursing is described as a specialized area of nursing, which has as its focus the promotion of mental health, the prevention of mental illness, and the care of persons experiencing mental health problems and mental disorders.[5] Benner's domains of nursing practice framed the process for the psychiatric and mental health nursing certification. Interestingly, for all 17 specialties, in order to sit the initial examination the diploma-prepared registered nurse must have 2 years experience in the specialty within the 5 preceding years. For registered nurses with baccalaureate preparation, only 1 year of specialty experience is required. This is odd as students may complete their baccalaureate education without having any experience in a particular specialty. It is also interesting to note that psychiatric and mental health certification is one of the most popular specialties. Since 2001, the numbers of nurses achieving psychiatric and mental health certification is consistently among the top three.

While various post-basic mental health nursing education programmes have been developed across the country, in Canada there is no common formation or foundation. The requirement for basic certification is a particular length of experience, but, although expected, no content is prescribed and programmes are not necessarily accredited.

NURSING EDUCATION: A SELECTIVE HISTORICAL PERSPECTIVE

The report *Nursing education in Canada: historical review and current capacity*[6] details the education and history for the three regulated nursing professions: registered nurses, licensed/registered practical nurses and registered psychiatric nurses. Like the history of Canada, nursing education has two roots, English speaking and French speaking.

In French Canada in 1639 three French nuns from the Order of Augustine de la Misericorde de Jesus arrived in what is now Quebec City. There they established and ran the Hotel-Dieu hospital. Jeanne Mance, a laywoman, also arrived in Canada in the 1600s. She set up the Hotel-Dieu hospital in Montreal, and a different order of nuns from France came to assist her. In both cases they established schools of nursing. Religious orders were the backbone of the system in Quebec until the 1960s.

In English Canada, schools were established based upon Nightingale's principles. However, Nightingale's critical principle that schools should be financially independent of hospitals was not economically feasible and nursing students were pushed into service. Hospital boards of directors – until later in the twentieth century – dominated the schools.

University-based education enjoyed a different beginning. Several universities were approached to establish schools of nursing, but they declined. Only the president of the University of British Columbia supported the establishment of a school of nursing in 1919.

Two struggles dominated the first half of the twentieth century. One involved moving the control of diploma nursing education from hospitals. The other related to developing the structure for baccalaureate nursing degree programmes. Community college systems developed across Canada and many schools moved from hospitals to community colleges. The debate about whether nurses required degrees raged for much of the twentieth century. However, by 1989 all provinces and the Canadian Nurses Association endorsed the 'entry to practice' as a baccalaureate degree. In the 1990s, entry to practice became a reality, each province enjoyed a unique journey to the degree entry to practice and some continue in progress, e.g. Quebec.

The National Nursing Competency project, a Canadian Nurses Association initiative through the 1990s, recommended that the baccalaureate degree is required to meet these competencies. In Ontario, as of 1 January 2005, the baccalaureate entry to practice for registered nurses became a reality and the last graduates of diploma programmes graduated by 31 December 2004.

Registered psychiatric nurses

In Canada psychiatric nurses are registered only in the four western provinces. A Canadian nurse – Effie Jane Taylor – trained as a nurse at Johns Hopkins University, Baltimore, MD, USA, and went on to become dean of nursing at Yale University, New Haven, CT, USA. She introduced the first psychiatric nursing component into the curricula of general nursing programmes and this trend continued and consolidated in the USA and Eastern Canada in 1913. In western Canada, a programme in Brandon, MB, was the first to prepare psychiatric nurses at psychiatric hospitals and, in around 1930, in the other three western provinces. Programmes were developed and taught by British-trained medical superintendents. Psychiatrists influenced the design and future of psychiatric nursing programmes in the absence of any nursing input. They were based explicitly on the British system of training psychiatric nurses. In the early 1970s, a shift in every province for all nursing programmes moved from hospitals to community colleges and/or universities. Currently, in Canada there are also two psychiatric nursing options, a diploma or a degree. However, registered nurses and their organizations[6] dominate the Canadian nursing system.

ISSUES IN NURSING EDUCATION

The Canadian psychiatric and mental health nursing community has significant concerns about basic nursing education. Many programmes no longer have dedicated psychiatric and mental health nursing within their programmes. Rather, the content called psychosocial nursing is integrated throughout the curricula. There are also fewer and fewer hours of clinical placement in programmes that continue to offer them, around 60 psychiatric and mental health nursing clinical hours in total. Students can conceivably leave a generic baccalaureate programme without ever having set foot in psychiatry or interacting with persons living with mental illness. This is a particular concern as one effective way to decrease stigma is to actually connect with persons living with a mental illness or connect with their family.

Psychiatric and mental health nursing student study

Like most places there are practical challenges in nursing education. These include limitations in clinical placements in the community and in acute and mental health care. We also experience limitations in the ability to recruit faculty, clinical teachers and preceptors. Retention of students is also a concern.

In our community, students who come to the Royal Ottawa Mental Health Centre for their basic psychiatric and mental health nursing placement are invited to participate in a study. Although the data are saturated within the study of students' experience of their psychiatric and mental health clinical placement, they tell us it is an honour to be the focus of study. We see this as a recruitment tool.

THE ROYAL OTTAWA STORY

The Royal Ottawa Mental Health Centre is the largest provider of specialized mental health services for people with serious and complex mental health problems in eastern Ontario. It is a teaching hospital affiliated with the University of Ottawa and provides a number of different clinical programmes across the care continuum.

The complex interplay among societal, consumer and professional forces led to us starting the twenty-first century with a newly created position of Chief of Nursing. This followed with a vision for nursing at the Royal Ottawa: to become an internationally recognized centre of excellence for psychiatric and mental health nursing that has at its core committed, person-centred professional practice and scholarship. It provided and still provides our direction. We were recovering from the losses of the previous decade, deep cuts in the nursing workforce, massive hospital restructuring and bed reductions and significant cuts to hospital budgets. However, we had a strong foundation upon which to build.

Several factors helped us begin our journey towards excellence. Ivy Dunn, who had been the Director of Nursing for 19 years, left a legacy of primary nursing, advanced practice roles and advocacy for nurses and for patients. We knew that Ivy herself was a trailblazer and a culture carrier. There is her story of her early days working at a psychiatric hospital in Montreal with Dr Heinz Lehmann when he introduced the 'miracle' drug chlorpromazine to North America. She had just been promoted to Supervisor of Nursing. She was responsible for 100 female patients who sat or lay on the floor all day, refused to wear clothes, were incontinent and were fed pureed food. Knowing that medication alone would never resolve all the problems, she developed the 'I expect' nursing approach to patient care. She conducted daily morning rounds, greeting each person by name and stating her expectation that they would, for example, dress and eat with a knife and fork or use the toilet. Amazingly, within 6 months, 98 per cent of the women were clothed, continent and the hospital doors were opened (I. Dunn, personal communication, 7 November 2003). We have actually found the 'I expect' model particularly helpful in working with our staff!

In the autumn of 2001, we came across Barker's Tidal Model of psychiatric and mental health nursing.[7,8] It had a powerful impact on us and we immediately went to the website and became the first North American site. Later, we realized that the reason Barker's work resonated with us was that we were steeped in the McGill Model.[9] The McGill Model, developed using grounded theory, postulates that the fundamental task of nursing is to assist persons and families in developing their potential for health. The salient features are health, family, collaboration and learning. It is also person centred and strengths based. Nursing has a distinct and unique role within health care – that of complementing the work of the interprofessional team. We implemented Tidal across the Royal Ottawa Mental Health Centre and we are currently rolling it out at our Brockville Campus. Our nurses began to reap the rewards of practising collaborative, person-centred, strength-based nursing. Now, we hear nurses discussing patients and patient care instead of complaints and union issues. On the units, we see nurses actively engaging with patients rather than sitting in the back offices. The Royal Ottawa Mental Health Centre has become the hub of the Canadian Tidal community.[10] We have enjoyed the opportunity to connect with colleagues from across the country, Newfoundland to British Columbia, and internationally around the globe.

> ### Reflection
>
> Compare the Canadian mental health nurse education context with your own country's context. How does the education of the psychiatric and mental health nurse differ? How is it similar?
>
> How can direct clinical experience with persons living with mental illness benefit the nursing student?

SUMMARY

We live in interesting times. A number of initiatives promise to improve mental health care within the province and across Canada – and nursing is poised to make its contribution. We lag behind most other provinces, but recently in Ontario there has been a move towards regionalization. Fourteen local integrated health networks have been established across the province. A Canadian Collaborative Mental Health Initiative (CCMHI) funded by the Canadian Council on Learning promises to increase awareness and the interprofessional practice of collaborative, person-centred mental health care. This direction is echoed in the provinces and territories and at the local level. Canada remains one of the only developed countries without a mental health strategy. On 31 August 2007 the federal government officially launched the new Canadian Mental Health Commission. There are three main objectives: to launch a 10-year campaign against discrimination faced by many who live with mental illness; to create a national knowledge exchange centre; and to develop a national mental health strategy for Canada.[11] The commission will be housed in part at our University of Ottawa Institute of Mental Health Research.

As Sister Elizabeth Davis, Chair, Canadian Health Services Research Foundation, said in 2005, 'We're in a new place; we're not on the edge of the old place. We're not pushing the envelope; we're in a completely new envelope. So the rules have changed. Every fundamental premise of the old way of thinking no longer applies.'

REFERENCES

1. Silversides A. *Conversations with champions of Medicare*. Ottawa, Canada: Canadian Federation of Nurses Unions, 2007.

2. Government of Canada, Health Canada. *Canada health act: overview*. Available from: www.hc-sc.gc.ca/hcs-sss/medi-assur/overview-apercu/index_e.html. Accessed 16 July 2007.

3. Health and Welfare Canada. *Mental health for Canadians: striking a balance*. Ottawa, Canada: Ministry of Supply and Services Canada, 1988.

4. Trainor J, Pomeroy E, Pape B. *A framework for support*, 3rd edn. Toronto, Canada: Canadian Mental Health Association, 2004.

5. Buchanan J, Harris D, Greene A *et al*. *Canadian standards of psychiatric and mental health nursing practice*, 2nd edn. Toronto, Canada: Canadian Federation of Mental Health Nurses, 1998.

6. Pringle D, Green L, Johnson S. *Nursing education in Canada: historical review and current capacity*. Ottawa, Canada: The Nursing Sector Study, 2004.

7. Barker P, Buchanan-Barker P. *The Tidal Model: a guide for mental health professionals*. New York, NY: Brunner Routledge, 2005.

8. Brookes N. Phil Barker: Tidal Model of mental health recovery. In: Tomey AM, Alligood MR (eds). *Nursing theorists and their work*, 6th edn. St Louis, MO: Mosby, 2006.

9. Gottlieb L, Rowat K. The McGill Model of nursing: a practice derived model. *Advances in Nursing Science* 1987; **9** (4): 51–61.

10. Brookes N, Murata L, Tansey M. Guiding practice development using the Tidal Commitments. *Journal of Psychiatric and Mental Health Nursing* 2006; **13** (4): 460–3.

11. Curry B. Mental health panel aims to stamp out discrimination. *Globe and Mail* 2007; **31 August**: A1 and A8.

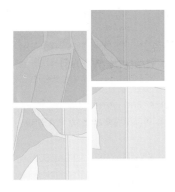

CHAPTER 83

The Australian and New Zealand context

Jon Chesterson,* Michael Hazelton**
and Anthony J. O'Brien***

INTRODUCTION

This chapter provides an overview of mental health nursing in Australia and New Zealand, noting the significant historical, political and cultural affinities between the two countries as well as the differences marked by *Te Tiriti o Waitangi* (The Treaty of Waitangi) in Aotearoa, New Zealand. Mental health nursing continues to face significant professional and workforce challenges. In the last 5 years strategic opportunities for professional governance and practice development have been generated by the profession and through mental health policy reforms in both countries. How the profession responds to these challenges will determine the extent to which mental health nursing is able to meet its obligations to people with mental illness and their families, and in promoting mental health and well-being in our two societies.

AUSTRALIAN POLICY CONTEXT

Australia's federal system of government involves close cooperation between a national government and eight state and territory governments, Council of Australian Governments (COAG). In health, the role of national government is to respond to national healthcare issues, coordinate national health policy priorities and reform, manage a national healthcare system through Medicare and funding for GP services, and distribute funds to states and territories for public health services. It is the responsibility of states and territories to provide public hospital and community health services at local level. By contrast, health policy in New Zealand is determined by one central government through the Ministry of Health, and implemented locally through 21 district health boards.

Australia's first, second and third national mental health plans have been implemented over 16 years since

*Jon Chesterson works in promotion and prevention for Hunter New England Mental Health (NSW Health) Newcastle, Australia, and Chairs the NSW Branch and Board of Credentialing, Australian College of Mental Health Nurses. He is a Past Board Director for Lifeline (Newcastle-Hunter) and PRA (Psychiatric Rehabilitation Association); past president of the Australian & New Zealand College of Mental Health Nurses; and a founding member of the Mental Health Council of Australia.
**Michael Hazelton is Head of the School of Nursing and Midwifery and Professor of Mental Health Nursing at the University of Newcastle, Australia. He published widely on mental health and mental health nursing, is a past Editor of the International Journal of Mental Health Nursing and is currently a member of the editorial boards of the International Journal of Mental Health Nursing, The Australian and New Zealand Journal of Psychiatry, Nursing and Health Sciences and Mental Health and Substance Use: Dual Diagnosis. He has been the recipient of a number of awards for mental health nursing research, and in 2003 was made a Life Member of the Australian College of Mental Health Nurses, the highest honour awarded by that professional organization.
***Anthony J. O'Brien is a Senior Lecturer, School of Nursing, University of Auckland, and Nurse Specialist, Liaison Psychiatry, Auckland District Health Board, New Zealand.

1992 under the National Mental Health Strategy. This involved a joint statement by the health ministers of the Commonwealth, states and territories for the direction and future development of mental health services and to ensure access for all Australians with mental health problems and disorders.[1] During the first plan (1992–7), significant improvements were reported in the range, quality, responsiveness and community orientation of mental health services and integration with mainstream health care. Improvements were less than expected in some areas. Consumers and carers reported difficulties with access; quality of services remained uneven within and across jurisdictions; primary care providers reported continuing insularity of mental health services; and stigma and discrimination remained high for people with a mental illness. During the second plan (1998–2003), priority was given to reforms in mental health promotion and prevention; building partnerships in service reform; and enhancing service quality and effectiveness. Studies commissioned in the first stage of the strategy including a national survey of mental health and well-being in 1997 indicated high levels of unmet need for mental health care.[2–4] The initial policy focus on the long-term needs of people with a mental illness was expanded to give greater emphasis on population health issues. The third plan (2003–8),[5] continues with greater emphasis on combating stigma and discrimination; staff training initiatives to establish and consolidate evidence-based practice; widespread adoption of routine outcome measurement; protection of consumer rights; and closer collaboration between specialist mental health and primary care services.[6] Box 83.1 summarizes key components in the current phase of the National Mental Health Strategy in Australia.

The Strategy has been received positively and viewed as a policy success, but doubts have been raised about the extent to which the reforms have resolved the historical marginalization and exclusion of people with mental illness. Studies indicate that people with long-term mental disorders live marginal lives characterized by severe disability, stigma and discrimination, social isolation, unemployment, homelessness and poverty. There remains a serious lack of community-based rehabilitation services, behavioural and psychosocial treatments, social support and community integration.[2–4]

NEW ZEALAND POLICY CONTEXT

The National Mental Health Strategy in New Zealand has been implemented over 14 years. The Second New Zealand Mental Health and Addiction Plan (Te Tahuhu) was released in 2005.[7] Where the previous plan emphasized development of a greater range of specialist mental health services and mental health workforce, Te Tahuhu has taken a broader focus. There are now no stand-alone

---

> **Box 83.1: National Mental Health Strategy in Australia 2008[1,5]**
>
> ### National Mental Health Strategy (NMHS) – Australia
>
> **A commitment by Australian and state and territory governments to improve the lives of people with a mental illness.**
>
> - *National Mental Health Policy 1992*: Joint statement by Health Ministers (COAG)
> - *Statement of Rights and Responsibilities 1992*
> - *3rd National Mental Health Plan 2003–8*: (1) Mental health promotion and prevention; (2) responsiveness to consumers and carers; (3) strengthen quality of service delivery; (4) foster research, innovation and sustainability
> - *Australian Health Care Agreements 2003–8*: $331 million allocated to states and territories to facilitate mental health reform plus $66 million for national reforms on safety, quality, improved patient outcomes, increased responsiveness of MHS
> - *COAG National Action Plan 2006–11*: Strategic framework of coordination and collaboration between government, private and non-government sector to deliver support care systems for people with mental illness to participate in the community
> - *National Strategic Framework for Aboriginal and Torres Strait Islander Peoples' Mental Health and Social and Emotional Well Being 2004–9*: OATSIH
> - *National Suicide Prevention Strategy*
> - *Towards Better Health for Veteran Community*: MHS blueprint
>
> ### Specific programme initiatives
>
> - Mental health services in rural and remote areas programme
> - Mental health support for drought affected communities
> - Mental health nurse incentive programme (MHNIP)
> - Better outcomes in mental health care – better access initiatives
> - Support for day-to-day living in the community: personal support programmes and additional non-government organization sector funding

---

psychiatric hospitals in New Zealand; mental health care is predominantly community based; and there is an increasing range of services provided by non-government organizations (NGOs). The community focus of mental health services is reflected in Te Tahuhu's 10 leading challenges for mental health and addictions services, to be met this decade (2005–15). These challenges include mental health promotion, supporting a recovery focus among mental health service providers, and development of mental health initiatives in primary care. The mental health needs of the indigenous Maori population are recognized in current policy and New Zealand's increasing ethnic diversity, with a commitment to improving responsiveness to the Asian population. The broader focus on mental health reflects a commitment to collaboration across health, disability and social service sectors and has become a mainstream issue in New Zealand health care.

Another major influence on mental health policy in New Zealand is the Mental Health Commission. The principal document guiding the work of the Commission is the *Blueprint for mental health services*.[8] The Commission has been the primary driver of the recovery focus of mental health services, for example through development of recovery competencies for mental health workers.[9] More recently, *Te Hononga, connecting for greater well-being*[10] is directed at the mental health and addiction sectors and the wider community, providing a guide for development until 2015. Particular concerns are to address stigma and discrimination, which has been the focus of the government-funded 'Like minds like mine' media campaign.[11] Box 83.2 summarizes key components in the current phase of the National Mental Health Strategy in New Zealand.

Despite policy commitments and development of a greater range of services over the past decade, there remain concerns around availability of mental health services, especially psychological services,[12] and continued development of mental health in primary care.[13] Forensic mental health services have grown considerably in the past decade, amidst concerns about unmet mental health need throughout the New Zealand prison population.[14] The Mental Health Commission concludes that achievement of mental health goals over the next decade will depend on development of a more inclusive society, in which the issues of people with mental illness gain greater acceptance within and beyond the mental health sector.

Reflection

How does the national mental health policy in your country affect your practice?

Box 83.2: National Mental Health Strategy in New Zealand 2008[7,8,10]

National Mental Health Strategy – MOH, New Zealand
To decrease prevalence of mental illness/problems in the community and increase health status, reduce impact of mental disorders.
Looking forward: strategic directions for MHS 1994

- *Te Rau Hinengaro New Zealand Mental Health Survey 2006*
  - 47 per cent of New Zealanders will experience a mental illness and/or addiction in their lives and one in five people will be affected in any 1 year
- *Te Tāhuhu Improving Mental Health 2005–15*: 2nd New Zealand Mental Health and Addiction Plan – 10 challenges
  - Promotion and prevention
  - Building mental health services
  - Responsiveness
  - Workforce and culture for recovery
  - Maori mental health
  - Primary health care
  - Addiction
  - Funding mechanisms for recovery
  - Transparency and trust
  - Working together
- *Te Kōkiri* Mental Health and Addiction Action Plan 2006–15

Mental Health Commission
Blueprint for MHS in New Zealand 1998 – How Things Need To Be
- *Te Hononga 2015 Connecting for Greater Wellbeing 2007*: A unifying picture of the mental health–addiction sectors and community in 2015

GOVERNANCE, LEADERSHIP AND PARTNERSHIP

The International Council of Nurses (ICN) defines governance as the process of controlling or guiding the profession. Clinical governance provides a framework for how: the profession and its members are defined; its scope and standards of practice, education and ethics are determined; and systems of accountability are established.[15]

In Australia and New Zealand, regulation of mental health nursing is governed by nursing legislation, the Trans-Tasman Mutual Recognition Act (TTMRA) and, to a lesser extent, mental health legislation. In New Zealand the legislation and nurse regulatory authorities operate at national level; in Australia, at state and territory level, except for the TTMRA. At a broader level, sociopolitical and economic forces also exert a regulatory effect, through national mental health standards,[16,17] policy and planning, funding for education and health, workforce planning and industrial relations. In Australia, establishment of a single national regulatory framework for nursing and midwifery is planned for 2010, which may eventually replace state and territory nursing boards.

Codes of nursing conduct and ethics are determined by national nurse regulatory authorities.[18–21] Standards of practice for mental health nursing are regularly reviewed in each country by two professional bodies (Box 83.3).[22,23] The Australian College of Mental Health Nurses (ACMHN) and Te Ao Maramatanga – New Zealand College of Mental Health Nurses (NZCMHN) – have an estimated membership of 18 and 12 per cent, respectively, of the mental health nursing workforce. Both colleges have

Box 83.3: Standards of practice: combined; ACMHN 1995 (in review);[22] Te Ao Maramatanga NZCMHN 2004[23]

Standards of practice for mental health nursing in Australia and New Zealand

1 Culturally safe and sensitive practice
2 Partnership base for therapeutic practice
3 Systematic care, contemporary nursing practice, healthcare/treatment plan
4 Promote health and wellness – individual, family, community
5 Ongoing education, professional growth, practice development, research base
6 Ethical practice – professional identity, independence, authority, partnership

memoranda of understanding and partnerships with other professional bodies such as psychiatrists (Royal Australian and New Zealand College of Psychiatrists), allied health, and national peak bodies in nursing and mental health (NGO) sectors. Both colleges host annual international and local conferences on mental health nursing and the peer reviewed *International Journal of Mental Health Nursing* (IJMHN), published under the auspices of the ACMHN, provides effective forums for dissemination of clinical practice, education and research. The ACMHN and NZCMHN websites are the principal carriers of professional and practice development news in both countries. Three sub-specialty special interest groups have emerged under the auspices of the ACMHN in consultation: psychiatric nurse liaison, private practice and child and adolescence. Other specialist nursing organizations include the Psycho-Geriatric Nurses Association, Drug and Alcohol Nurses Association and Professional Association of Nurses in Developmental Disability Australia. The Australian College has moved towards a shared governance framework and pathway for mental health nursing in Australia incorporating credentialing and underpinned by cross-sector partnerships among the profession, statutory/regulatory authorities, tertiary education and health service provider sectors (Figure 83.1).

Credentialing and accreditation

Credentialing has been defined as the evaluation of an individual nurse's performance against relevant practice standards.[24] Accreditation is a process by which educational programmes and/or education and healthcare providers are evaluated for quality, relevance and performance. In 1998, the ANZCMHN[a] commissioned a literature review on credentialing, recommending a collaborative approach, involving the College and Nursing Board of Tasmania, be piloted in Tasmania.[25] The Royal College of Nursing Australia in 2001 outlined the feasibility of a national approach in relation to advanced and specialist nursing practice.[26]

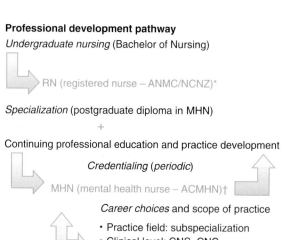

Professional development pathway

Undergraduate nursing (Bachelor of Nursing)
RN (registered nurse – ANMC/NCNZ)*

Specialization (postgraduate diploma in MHN)
+
Continuing professional education and practice development
Credentialing (periodic)
MHN (mental health nurse – ACMHN)†

Career choices and scope of practice
• Practice field: subspecialization
• Clinical level: CNS–CNC
• Health sector: public–private–primary/GP (MHNIP)
• Private practice–consultancy
• Management–education–research

Advanced practice (Masters/NP Masters)
NP (nurse practitioner – ANMC/NCNZ)*

Figure 83.1 Shared governance in mental health nursing: professional development pathway. *Statutory by boards; †self-regulatory specialization by professional body in collaboration with key sectors

[a] The Australian and New Zealand College of Mental Health Nurses was predecessor of the colleges in each country, constituted when a branch of the former ACMHN formed in New Zealand from 1993 to 2004.

Some state nursing boards within Australia have continued to review and accredit postgraduate courses in mental health nursing and endorse mental health nurses, but these arrangements are likely to disappear upon establishment of a national nurse regulatory framework. In New Zealand, there has been no clear indication of the establishment of credentialing by a professional body. The Health Practitioners Competence Assurance Act 2003 requires the Nursing Council of New Zealand to ensure public safety and professional competence of nurses to practice, while new quality assurance provisions require mandatory demonstration of competency, certification and accountability of nurses.

The ACMHN defines credentialing as a key component of professional (clinical) governance in which members of a profession set standards for practice and establish minimum requirements for entry, continuing practice, endorsement and recognition.[27] Credentialing articulates standards of practice at individual practitioner level to:

- improve professional accountability, transparency, autonomy
- focus on evidence-based practice and mental health outcomes
- commit to ongoing education and practice development
- safeguard quality of healthcare delivery
- uphold standards of profession and ethical practice
- protect human rights and choices
- maintain public trust and confidence.

The Credential for Practice Program (CPP) commenced nationally in 2004 and received Commonwealth funding in 2006. Box 83.4 summarizes criteria for the mental health nurse (MHN) credential, renewed periodically every 3 years. Programme enhancement is possible through accreditation of postgraduate and undergraduate courses in mental health nursing from Australian universities.

Box 83.4: MHN credential in Australia, ACMHN 2008

Criteria

- Current licence to practise as RN in Australia
- Postgraduate mental health nursing qualification or equivalent
- Minimum duration of practice in mental health
- Recency of practice in mental health
- Record of ongoing professional development
- Continuing professional education: points system
- Continuing practice development: points system
- Referees and professional declarations

WORKFORCE PLANNING, EDUCATION AND PRACTICE DEVELOPMENT

Serious gaps have emerged in mental health workforce planning at all levels in Australia and New Zealand. Mental health services face serious problems in recruitment and retention, and too few registered nurses currently progress beyond initial nursing qualifications to complete postgraduate studies in mental health nursing. Various reports have indicated low morale in the workforce and a diminishing skills base. A number of solutions have been implemented to improve workforce planning and current mental health policy objectives.[28–30]

1. Maintain comprehensive, reliable data on national mental health workforce.
2. Foster collaborative approaches to workforce planning and service delivery in the healthcare system and programme design in the university sector, based on population needs.
3. Facilitate dissemination of evidence-based practice (EBP) in mental health services, and undergraduate and postgraduate courses in university schools of nursing.
4. Establish and support clinical supervision and mentorship programmes for mental health nurses and other health professionals in mental health services.
5. Build career pathways to support preparation of mental health nurses at both subspecialist and advanced levels.
6. Give priority to clinical effectiveness, multidisciplinary treatment and care in mental health nursing research.

There have been important developments in how mental health nursing is taught at university. In 2006 the Australian government announced funding for 450 new undergraduate places in mental health nursing. This stimulated enhancement of mental health content (including clinical placements) in many undergraduate nursing programmes, with several universities opting to introduce mental health specialization streams. Several models are emerging from the university sector: Majors in mental health within undergraduate comprehensive nursing programmes; a 4-year undergraduate comprehensive nursing programme with integrated honours year in mental health nursing; and a double degree in comprehensive and mental health nursing. Since 2006, government-sponsored scholarships have been made available for postgraduate studies in mental health nursing.

Reflection

What impact does a shortage in supply and skills level of mental health nurses have on patient care and service delivery? How can this be addressed and whose responsibility is it?

Mental Health Nurse Incentive Program

In 2007, the Australian Government introduced the Mental Health Nurse Incentive Program (MHNIP). This initiative funds general practitioners (GPs), psychiatrists in private practice, Aboriginal medical services and other relevant primary healthcare providers to engage mental health nurses. The primary target group are people with low-prevalence mental disorders, focusing on early intervention, relapse prevention, short-term case management and psychosocial interventions. In determining the eligibility requirements for Medicare reimbursement and engagement of mental health nurses, nurses are required to be an RN *and* hold the MHN credential. This initiative creates an entirely new sector and field of practice for mental health nursing in Australia, which up until now has been predominantly in state-based mental health services and a few private psychiatric hospitals. Although no comparable programme has been established in New Zealand, the primary care sector has been identified as a priority for development of a mental health nursing role.[13]

Better outcomes and access

Recent expansion in the Australian government's Better Outcomes in Mental Health Care Initiative[1] has emphasized the importance of closer collaboration between mental health nursing and general practice. Although this initiative opens up exciting opportunities for mental health nursing in Australia, the discipline was largely unprepared for the extensive development of knowledge and skills required to work effectively in general practice service environments.[31] There are a few mental health nurses in private practice who have acquired Medicare provider status under specific conditions; however, these arrangements are not as flexible as the Better Access Initiative[1] introduced in 2006. This initiative is designed to improve GP referral and access to mental health professionals in private practice for people predominantly with high-prevalence disorders, based on previously identified gaps in service use, focusing on early intervention, short-term treatment and psychosocial interventions. This includes psychologists, social workers and occupational therapists. Mental health nurses were excluded from these provisions, ostensibly on account of the Australian government's perception of the impact on implementation of the MHNIP.

Development of nurse practitioner

Mental health nurse practitioners (NP) are established in New Zealand and most Australian States.[32–34] The coming decade will see more widespread introduction of this advanced role in mental health services. This has necessitated development of postgraduate nurse practitioner programs at Masters level in New South Wales and elsewhere in Australia and New Zealand. The advent of the mental health nurse practitioner will augment developments in the population health approach through:

1. stronger alliances between primary health and mental health services, including shared care services with general practitioners;[13]
2. improved services in rural and remote regions;
3. building of mental health promotion and prevention programmes;
4. improved capacity of mental health services to respond to unmet needs in mental health care.

Mental health outcomes

Australia and New Zealand have adopted standardized outcome measurement in mental health services, introduced originally in NSW with whole of workforce training (MHOAT). This involved standardized mental health assessment, documentation, monitoring and evaluation of care on a routine basis in all hospital and community settings and use of validated outcome measures.[35–38] Successful outcomes for people with mental illness depend on many factors: effectiveness of treatment and psychosocial interventions, therapeutic relationships, quality of service delivery, nature of illness, recovery, personal characteristics, resilience and social determinants. Standardized outcome measurement is a systems-based solution to document and evaluate care, but does not provide the substance of care or address social determinants. It is a start in that it establishes minimum standards and resources around a cluster of common processes and procedures, and provides the means to collect outcome data at a population level to evaluate progress.

2020 VISION

The longer term vision for mental health nursing in Australia and New Zealand is emerging in response to recent initiatives and the broad context of national mental health reforms in the two countries. The discipline needs to provide sound professional judgement and leadership within its own ranks and contribute effectively to the broader agendas of the community, government policy and service developments. Building on this foundation we offer the following blueprint.

- **Clinical governance and sustainability**. *Effective system of shared governance, professional recognition and accountability for mental health nursing practice.* Credentialing in Australia provides a solid foundation for mental health nursing as a specialty, a platform for career pathways, and incentives for postgraduate education and professional development. It represents a step towards self-determination and professional autonomy, from which clinical practice and equitable partnerships can be built. Immediate goals and challenges include: adoption by all members of the discipline, build capacity to administer the CPP and be fully self-funding, develop sustainability, and programme enhancement through accreditation of postgraduate and undergraduate courses in mental health nursing from Australian universities.

- **Clinical leadership**. *Sustained, bold, visionary clinical/professional leadership for the discipline.* This has traditionally relied on individual champions and it needs to be mentored in others and embedded in practice. Studies of the mental health nursing workforce have indicated significant gaps in clinical leadership.[28–30] While mental health nurses can identify problems faced by the discipline, most have an expectation that decisions and actions necessary to 'make a difference' will be made by someone else.[39] Nurses in leadership and management roles need to identify with and support the profession as role models, and support and empower other nurses to follow. Clinical leadership needs to be re-envisioned in the clinical setting. Leadership skills and clinical decision-making need to be vested in the role of all mental health nurses, building skills, confidence, competence, trust, professional accountability and autonomy. Continuing education, practice development and clinical supervision need to be fully supported.

Reflection

What are the characteristics of good clinical leadership? Can you identify someone you work with or from the past who showed good clinical leadership in mental health nursing? What was it that he or she did that made a difference?

- **Workforce development**. *Skilled mental health nursing workforce with comprehensive strategy for recruitment, retention, educational preparation and specialization based on the mental health needs of the population.* This is vital for the integrity of the profession, a healthy workforce and quality service delivery. Staff shortages restrict practice, create stressful clinical and workplace environments, lower staff morale, thus limiting capacity for change, practice development and innovation. Inadequate staffing levels and skills mix lock staff out of continuing education and clinical supervision opportunities, and undermine therapeutic relationships and quality time spent with patients and clinical programmes. Despite recent funding improvements for mental health services, the percentage of national and state health budgets allocated to mental health is around 8–9 per cent, significantly below international benchmarks in comparable countries. Health services need to invest in recruitment and retention strategies and incentives; flexible career options; and healthy clinical and workplace environments that are practical, friendly and aesthetic. The university sector needs to develop and maintain collaborative programme

designs based on the needs of the profession, workforce and population.

- **Practice development**. *Quality, sustainable practice development is based on contemporary practice standards, evidence-based practices, research and scholarship in mental health nursing.* The colleges of mental health nursing at national levels have managed research funds and annual research grants, facilitated annual corporate-sponsored mental health and well-being awards, and clinical and research awards. More recently, some health departments have funded practice innovation scholarships.

Reflection

What would be a useful area of practice around which to develop a clinical practice guideline and why? What steps would you take in developing it? Who would you consult with? What elements would be highlighted in your general information to the public and where could they access it?

- **Mental health promotion and prevention**. *Practice is fully integrated at an individual, family, community and population level to promote emotional and social well-being and prevent mental illness, disability and disadvantage.* This is a key area for practice development discussed in Chapter 66 – alignment with World Health Organization goals and national action plans in both countries.[40,41] Social determinants of mental health, it is argued, is currently a missing dimension in mental health nursing.[42]

- **Social inclusion, citizenship and meaningful lives**. *Practice is based on civil rights, citizenship, participation in society and access to community resources required to live a meaningful life.* Societal attitudes have an effect on disability and social disadvantage associated with mental illness. A sense of community belonging is a key to citizenship. To this end mental health nursing ought to become more closely involved in current debates on the relationship between social capital and mental health.[43–45] It is also important for mental health nurses to acknowledge ways in which mentally ill people strive to give meaning to their lives, through personal development, social connection and spiritual beliefs.[46] Social justice and advocacy are key aspects of the philosophy and practice of mental health nursing and a cornerstone for strategic alliances between the discipline and consumer sector.[47]

- **Consumer, carer, NGO sector partnerships**. *Collaborative partnerships are a key focus of the mental health nursing practice at individual, family, community and organizational level.* The New Zealand Mental Health Commission has developed a strong agenda of consumer involvement[48] and the NGO sector has established a national collaborative network called Platform. The

Mental Health Council of Australia is an independent peak national body for the mental health NGO sector, which has produced two recent reports of national significance, Lets Get to Work and Time for Service, which have been instrumental in shaping policy and thinking.[49,50] Non-government organizations are key stakeholders, especially with respect to supported housing, employment, vocational training, social support networks, family and carer support, community access and integration, which play a fundamental role in recovery and social inclusion.

- **Therapeutic optimism and hope.** *The focus of care and therapeutic relationship is based on recovery principles, therapeutic optimism and hope.* A lack of therapeutic optimism remains evident among healthcare professionals. It is not so much mental illness that damages peoples' lives, but the reactions and attitudes of those around them. Hope and encouragement are central to recovery. Mental health nursing has a strong tradition drawing on humanistic values, encouraging individual autonomy, and adopting authoritative rather than authoritarian ways of being with those in care. The focus of the discipline must continue to be based on recovery and engagement. The therapeutic attitude of mental health nursing must reflect warmth, empathy, respect, openness and authenticity.

- **Ethics and social justice.** *Practice and clinical decision-making is founded on fundamental human rights, professional codes of ethics, social justice, dignity and respect for people's cultural and spiritual beliefs.* Decisions that affect people's lives and made on their behalf cannot be based solely on health and clinical grounds, nor on welfare and interests of others around them. Legal and ethical frameworks are required to balance complex rights and responsibilities. While the human rights of people with mental illness have been strongly asserted in mental health policies,[51–53] there is a continued legacy of restrictive practices, services and social control. Mental health nursing has a strong ethical foundation to its practice.[18–21,54,55] Ethical studies have long been a component of university nursing curricula, but this is not yet a cornerstone of practice development in mental health nursing. To date, the 'talk' has not significantly influenced the 'action'.

- **No profession without unity.** *Mental health nurses are inclusive, respect their colleagues, encourage diversity of opinion, and actively engage in the development of professional unity, autonomy, advocacy and partnership.* The profession must be more accepting and optimistic of itself, its place in society, working towards its future, not seeking to displace any other. The principles reflected in professional nursing standards and codes of ethics, how nurses behave to others, must be internalized at an individual and collegial (collective) level. No more horizontal violence, waiting for someone else

to act, submissive or subversive behaviour, opting out, but a professional ethic based on reason. If mental health nurses do not identify and participate in their profession, and feel justly satisfied in their work, it affects their practice, colleagues and patients, and the profession's capacity to develop and resource itself. The greatest capacity for change here is in the hands of the profession. The colleges in both countries have embraced this reality and offer the means to accomplish it.

- **Public visibility and media strategy.** *Public awareness, trust and confidence in mental health nursing is supported by good practice, mental health literacy and professional voice on mental health issues in the media.* Mental health nursing has rarely enjoyed the same degree of public recognition and trust as other fields of nursing. Until recently mental illness was largely hidden from public view and mental health nurses today remain remarkably invisible and low profile. Mental health-related media reports remain largely sensationalized. Good news stories on mental health are growing, often solicited by consumers, carers and mental health staff when they are empowered to do so. The discipline needs to be more 'media-savvy' and involved in the public media.[56] In becoming advocates and sources for news stories on mental health, spokespersons for the discipline need to contribute to public debate on mental health issues, lead by example and publicize the important contribution that mental health nursing makes in the community. The discipline needs to develop a public media strategy, build its professional image and profile, strengthen community relations, and encourage use of existing Mindframe Media training resources developed under the Australian NMHS to empower members of the profession.

SUMMARY

There is no doubt that government-led mental health strategies have brought about opportunities and challenges for mental health nursing. Professionally led initiatives have also taken hold and, where there is congruence between the two, the greatest opportunities arise. It is important to find the correct balance between the two – to remain relevant and connected while maintaining independent authority and voice. Adding to the evidence-based practice literature, contemporary theories of recovery and mental health nursing, such as the Tidal Model,[57] offer up new opportunities to examine the therapeutic substance and relevance of mental health nursing in the twenty-first century. The path ahead will be determined by the capacity to which mental health nurses themselves, individually and collectively as a discipline, respond to change, to emerging national and global issues that affect people's mental health, alliances built at international and local levels, and the generative disciplinary knowledge and expertise brought to bear in solving these problems. Developments in the first decade of the twenty-first century are already rejuvenating and shaping the future of mental health nursing in Australia and New Zealand. The capacity of the discipline to determine its own place in society rests with its members, its practices, the partnerships forged, and the extent to which mental health nursing is able to assertively reach out in relevant and meaningful ways into the communities it serves.

REFERENCES

1. Commonwealth Department of Health and Aged Care. *Mental health and wellbeing Australia.* Available from: www.mentalhealth.gov.au. Accessed January 2008.

2. McLennan A. *Mental health and wellbeing: profile of adults, Australia 1997.* Canberra, Australia: ABS, 1998.

3. Harvey C, Evert H, Herrman H *et al. Disability, homelessness and social relationships among people living with psychosis in Australia.* Canberra, Australia: Commonwealth of Australia, 2002.

4. Frost B, Carr V, Halpin S. *Employment and psychosis.* Canberra, Australia: Commonwealth of Australia, 2002.

5. Australian Health Ministers. *National mental health plan 2003–2008.* Canberra, Australia: Australian Government, 2003.

6. Hazelton M. Mental health reform, citizenship and human rights in four countries. *Health Sociology Review* 2005; **14**: 230–41.

7. Minister of Health. *Te Tāhuhu – improving mental health 2005–2015: the second New Zealand mental health and addiction plan.* Wellington, New Zealand: Ministry of Health, 2005.

8. Mental Health Commission. *Blueprint for mental health services in New Zealand. How things need to be.* Wellington, New Zealand: MHC, 1998.

9. Mental Health Commission. *Recovery competencies for New Zealand mental health workers.* Wellington, New Zealand: MHC, 2001.

10. Mental Health Commission. *Te Hononga. Connecting for greater well-being.* Wellington, New Zealand: MHC, 2007.

11. Vaughan G, Hansen C. 'Like minds, like mine': a New Zealand project to counter the stigma and discrimination associated with mental illness. *Australasian Psychiatry* 2004; **12** (2): 113–17.

12. Peters J. *'We need to talk'. Talking therapies – a snapshot of issues and activities across mental health and addiction services in New Zealand.* Auckland, New Zealand: Te Pou O Te Whakaaro Nui. The National Centre of Mental Health Research and Workforce Development, 2007.

13. O'Brien AJ, Hughes FH, Kidd JD. Mental health nursing in New Zealand primary care. *Contemporary Nurse* 2006; **21** (19): 142–52.

14. Ministry of Health. *Census of forensic mental health services 2005.* Wellington, New Zealand: MOH, 2007.

15. International Council of Nurses. *ICN on regulation: towards 21st century models, 3rd in a series on regulation.* Geneva, Switzerland: ICN, 1998.

16. Ministry of Health Project Team. *The national mental health standards.* Wellington, New Zealand: MOH, Manatu Hauora, 1997.

17. Project Consortium for the Mental Health Branch. *National standards for mental health services.* Canberra, Australia: Commonwealth Department of Health and Family Services, 1997 [under review].

18. Australian Nursing and Midwifery Council. *Code of professional conduct for nurses in Australia.* Canberra, Australia: ANMC, 2003.

19. Australian Nursing and Midwifery Council. *Code of ethics for nurses in Australia.* Canberra, Australia: ANMC, 2002.

20. Nursing Council of New Zealand. *Code of conduct for nurses.* Wellington, New Zealand: NCNZ, 2006.

21. Horsfall J, Cleary M, Jordan R. *Towards ethical mental health nursing practice: monograph.* SA: ANZCMHN, 1999.

22. Australian & New Zealand College of Mental Health Nurses. *Standards of practice for mental health nursing in Australia.* SA: ANZCMHN, 1995 [under review].

23. Te Ao Maratamanga New Zealand College of Mental Health Nurses (NZCMHN). *Standards of practice for mental health nursing in New Zealand,* 2nd edn. Auckland, New Zealand: NZCMHN, 2004.

24. Royal College of Nursing Australia. *Credentialing advanced nursing practice and accreditation of continuing education programs: an exploration of issues and perspectives.* Discussion Paper No. 4. Canberra, Australia: RCNA, 1996.

25. Hazelton M, Farrell G, Biro P. *Self-regulation and credentialing in mental health nursing: report to the nursing board of Tasmania.* SA: ANZCMHN, 1998.

26. Royal College of Nursing Australia. *Feasibility of a national approach for the credentialing of advanced practice nurses and the accreditation of related educational programs; final report.* Canberra, Australia: RCNA; 2001.

27. Chesterson J. *Credential for practice program v1.2 (2003).* Credentialing News 03–04. Canberra, Australia: ANZCMHN. Available from Credentialing Pages Archive, www.acmhn.org; Chesterson J, Jeon Y. Tasmania MHN project: national workshops survey report to council. Unpublished. Canberra, Australia: ANZCMHN, 2004.

28. Clinton M. *Scoping study of the Australian mental health nursing workforce 1999: report from ANZCMHN to Commonwealth Department of Health and Aged Care.* Canberra, Australia: CDHAC, 2001.

29. Australian Health Workforce Advisory Committee. *Australian mental health nursing supply, recruitment and retention.* Canberra, AHWAC, 2003.

30. Hamer H, Finlayson M, Thom K *et al. Mental health nursing and its future: a discussion framework: report to Deputy Director General (Mental Health).* Wellington, New Zealand: Ministry of Health, 2006.

31. Burrows G, Singh B, Grigg M (eds). *Mental health in Australia,* 2nd edn. South Melbourne, Australia: Oxford University Press, 2007: 91–2.

32. Hughes F, Carryer J. *Nurse practitioners in New Zealand.* Wellington, New Zealand: Ministry of Health, 2002.

33. Wand T, White K. Progression of the mental health nurse practitioner role in Australia. *Journal of Psychiatric and Mental Health Nursing* 2007; **14** (7): 644–51.

34. Elsom S, Happell B, Manias E. Mental health nurse practitioner: expanded or advanced? *International Journal of Mental Health Nursing* 2005; **14** (3): 181–6.

35. Coombs T, Meehan T. Mental health outcomes in Australia: Issues for mental health nurses. *International Journal of Mental Health Nursing* 2003; **12** (3): 163–4.

36. Eagar K, Trauer T, Mellsop G. Performance of routine outcome measures in adult mental health care. *Australian & New Zealand Journal of Psychiatry* 2005; **39**: 713–18.

37. Lakeman R. Standardized routine outcome measurement: pot holes in the road to recovery. *International Journal of Mental Health Nursing* 2004; **13** (4): 210–15.

38. Hazelton M, Farrell G. *Evaluating the outcomes of mental health care – an introduction: monograph.* SA: ANZCMHN, 1998.

39. Clinton M, Hazelton M. Towards a Foucauldian reading of the Australian mental health nursing workforce. *International Journal of Mental Health Nursing* 2002; **11**: 18–23.

40. Commonwealth Department of Health and Aged Care. *National action plan for promotion, prevention and early intervention for mental health.* Canberra, Australia: CDHAC, 2000.

41. Ministry of Health. *Building on strengths. A new approach to promoting mental health in New Zealand/Aotearoa.* Wellington, New Zealand: MOH, 2002.

42. Lauder W, Kroll T, Jones M. Social determinants of mental health: the missing dimensions of mental health nursing? *Journal of Psychiatric and Mental Health Nursing* 2007; **14** (7): 661–9.

43. Whitely R, McKenzie K. Social capital and psychiatry: review of the literature. *Harvard Review of Psychiatry* 2005; **13** (2): 71–84.

44. Henderson S, Whiteford H. Social capital and mental health. *Lancet* 2003; **362**: 505–6.

45. De Silva MJ, McKenzie K, Harpham T, Huttly SR. Social capital and mental illness: a systematic review. *Journal of Epidemiology and Community Health* 2005; **59**: 619–27.

46. Barker P, Campbell P, Davidson B (eds). *From the ashes of experience.* London, UK: Whurr Publishers, 1999.

47. Barker P, Chesterson J. The logic of experience: developing appropriate care through effective collaboration. In: Barker P (ed.). *The philosophy and practice of psychiatric nursing.* Edinburgh, UK: Churchill Livingston, 1999: 117–32.

48. Mental Health Commission. *Service user workforce development strategy for the mental health sector, 2005–2010.* Wellington, New Zealand: MHC, 2005.

49. Mental Health Council of Australia. *Let's get to work – a national mental health employment strategy for Australia.* Canberra, Australia: MHCA, 2007.

50. Mental Health Council of Australia. *Time for service: solving Australia's mental health crisis.* Canberra, Australia: MHCA, 2006.

51. Commonwealth Department of Human Services and Health. *Mental health statement of rights and responsibilities.* Canberra, Australia: Commonwealth of Australia, AGPS, 1991.

52. Human Rights and Equal Opportunity Commission. *Human rights and mental illness (Burdekin) report of national inquiry into human rights of people with mental illness.* Canberra, Australia: AGPS, 1993.

53. Commonwealth Department of Health Housing and Community Services. *Social justice for people with disabilities.* Canberra, Australia: Commonwealth of Australia, AGPS, 1991.

54. Barker P, Davidson B (eds). *Psychiatric nursing. Ethical strife.* London, UK: Arnold, 1998.

55. Barker P, Baldwin S (eds). *Ethical issues in mental health.* London, UK: Chapman & Hall, 1991.

56. Farrow TL, O'Brien AJ. Discourse analysis of newspaper coverage of the 2001/2002 Canterbury, New Zealand mental health nurses' strike. *International Journal of Mental Health Nursing* 2005; **14**: 196–204.

57. Barker P, Buchanan-Barker P. *The Tidal Model: a guide for mental health professionals.* Hove, UK: Brunner-Routledge, 2005.

WEBSITES

Australian College of Mental Health Nurses (ACMHN): www.acmhn.org

Australian Nursing and Midwifery Council: www.anmc.org.au

Commonwealth Mental Health Well-being Australia: www.mentalhealth.gov.au

EPPIC: www.eppic.org.au

Headroom AUS – Mental Health for Young People: www.headroom.net.au

Headspace NZ – Mental Health for Young People: www.headspace.org.nz

Like Minds NZ – Reducing stigma of mental illness: www.likeminds.govt.nz

Mental Health Association Australia: www.mentalhealth.asn.au

Mental Health Commission NZ: www.mhc.govt.nz

Mental Health Council of Australia: www.mhca.org.au

Mental Health Foundation of Australia: www.mhfa.org.au

Mental Health Foundation of New Zealand: www.mentalhealth.org.nz

Mental Illness Foundation of Australia (MIFA): www.mifa.org.au

Ministry of Health NZ – Mental Health: www.moh.govt.nz/mentalhealth

Multicultural Mental Health Australia: www.mmha.org.au

NSW Health – Mental Health: www.health.nsw.gov.au/living/mental.html

Nursing Council of New Zealand: www.nursingcouncil.org.nz

Platform NZ – NGO Mental Health Sector: www.platform.org.nz

Schizophrenia Fellowship NZ: www.sfnat.org.nz

Te Ao Maramatanga – New Zealand College of Mental Health Nurses: www.nzcmhn.org.nz

VicHealth – Mental Health: www.vichealth.vic.gov.au/Content.aspx?topicID=17

Working Well NZ – Mentally Healthy Workplaces: www.workingwell.co.nz

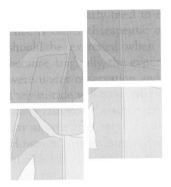

CHAPTER 84

The politics of caring

Phil Barker*

WHO CARES ANY MORE, ANYWAY?

Confusion and optimism

If you have studied carefully the preceding 83 chapters of this book, I suspect that by now you are a little confused. At least, I *hope* that you are confused. There is nothing more uncertain than certainty.[a] However, as shall see later, at times, being too certain of something can be dangerous.

Confusion is useful. It may prompt *you* to ask some intelligent, probing, *curious* questions about the human business called 'caring'. Of course, I am making the bold assumption that you believe that nursing *is* about 'caring' for *people*: as opposed to *policing, containing, managing, secluding, incarcerating, disempowering* or otherwise *invalidating* 'patients/clients'.

I make no apologies for this *radical* (meaning 'fundamental'; from Latin *radix*, root) outlook. Ideology is about being 'too certain' about something and much of what passes for politics is little more than ideology. Both occupy fairly dominant positions in the mental health field. However, these political and ideological factors are subtle, and sometimes sinister. If nurses are not to be swayed by political 'spin' or indoctrinated by the latest propaganda, then they will need to be sure of one thing at least: their professional identity. What does it mean to be a psychiatric–mental health nurse (PMHN) at the beginning of the twenty-first century? How does that professional *raison d'être* translate into practice?

Hence our need to be radical: addressing the *root* of the professional care issue. At certain times in their lives, *everyone* needs help from someone else. The key questions are:

- What kind of help, exactly, do people *need*?
- What kind of help can be *offered*?
- What is likely to *get in the way* of such offers of help?

The myth of mental health nursing

This book provides a comprehensive overview of the theory and practice of psychiatric–mental health nursing. Yet, having read it, you may still be uncertain as to what *exactly* is psychiatric–mental health nursing.

Q: What exactly do nurses do that distinguishes them from social workers, psychiatrists, psychologists or 'ordinary people' who help their friends and family deal with their problems?

This question has been asked in several different ways over the past 50 years and, for some, it is a question that has been 'done to death'.[1] However unfashionable this question might be, it has to be asked. If we cannot say with confidence what nursing 'is', how can anyone be prepared to become a nurse? More importantly, if we cannot tell other people what (exactly) is psychiatric–mental health nursing, then how will we recruit people to the field?

*Phil Barker is a Psychotherapist and Honorary Professor at the University of Dundee, UK.

[a] Philosophers, at least, are wary of certainty. Wittgenstein noted, 'For "I know" seems to describe a state of affairs which guarantees what is known, guarantees it as a fact. One always forgets the expression "I thought I knew"' (Wittgenstein L. *On certainty*. London, UK: Blackwell, 1977: 13).

The nature of *medicine* is self-evident – the 'science or practice of the diagnosis, treatment and prevention of disease' (Oxford English Dictionary; OED). Similarly the essence of *psychology* is easily characterized – the 'scientific study of the human mind and its functions' (OED).

However, most dictionaries offer only the vaguest of indications in attempting to define nursing, reflecting perhaps our professional uncertainty: 'the practice of caring for the sick as a nurse' (OED). Unlike medicine and psychology, no mention is made here of any *art*, far less any *science* of nursing. What the dictionary compilers meant by *caring* is, of course, anyone's guess.

This seems to suggest that mental health nursing is a *myth*: something that many people believe in – both the professional and the layperson; which gives symbolic meaning to their lives; but which cannot be *demonstrated* in any objective sense.

Values: first do no harm

I have been asking nurses to tell me what nursing 'means' for at least 25 years. Most nurses are confident about their various 'roles' but few offer anything resembling a definition of their craft – whether as a 'science' or an 'art'. One of my mentors, Desmond Cormack, made a special study of the 'role and function' of the psychiatric nurse.[2] However, Cormack concluded that what nurses *did* (or rather *said* they did), or the functions they believed to be *important*, might not actually be what they *should* be doing (in either a practical or moral sense).

Q: Is nursing care always *good* for the person who receives it?

Values clearly are important. Nightingale reframed the Hippocratic Oath, stating that the nurse's first responsibility was *to do no harm*. This begs the question: 'do nurses *never* do harm?' Or if they do, is such harmful 'care', in some sense, 'in the patient's best interests?'

I was reminded of these questions when, a couple of years ago, I spoke at a conference in the former Benedictine monastery at Irsee in Bavaria. In 1849 the monastery was converted for use as an asylum, and a full century later many medical and nursing staff were sentenced for their part in sending over 2000 adults and children, from this 'asylum', to their deaths in Nazi extermination camps. All told, more than 70 000 people were considered by the Nazis to be *Lebensunwerten Lebens* – 'lives not worthy of living'. They were 'eliminated' by a social policy, which granted official permission for murder on an industrial scale. At the end of the day, however, the mere fact that the policy was 'official' offered no protection to those who had carried it out. Nurses were among those who were called to account.[3]

During the Third Reich, home care nurses reported disabled Germans to the authorities so that they could be 'dealt with' in line with National Socialist policy.

Some paediatric nurses received bonuses for starving disabled children to death. The Imperial War Museum in London holds chilling film of a uniformed 'nurse' helping a naked man into a gas chamber. Some of the nurses who fulfilled such ghastly roles confessed only to 'following orders', which became the actual words of the Nuremburg defence. Others defiantly repeated the mantra of 'euthanasia' fed to them by the Nazi propagandists, and claimed to have brought a welcome end to miserable lives.

It is tempting to think that this was all a long time ago, in a land far away. However, it is Holocaust Memorial Day (27 January; see www.hmd.org.uk/about/) as I write this chapter. It seems fitting to remind myself, at least, that Africa, the former Soviet Union and China have all witnessed their own 'holocausts'. More specifically, the 'Nuremberg defence' – 'only following orders' – is still used by those charged with abuse or torture, most recently American service personnel at Abu Ghraib in Iraq.

Defining nursing: the 'promotion of growth and development'

Talking specifically about the psychiatric–mental health nursing context, Grant[4] argued that:

> what nurses *do* at any one time, as opposed to what they might like to do (for some at least, influenced by Barker's writing), is likely to generally conform to that which has been established in local custom and practice, and related patterns of expectation and influence.

Does this mean that the nurses who led the unfortunate *Lebensunwerten Lebens* to the gas chambers were just *conforming* 'to that which had been established in local custom and practice, and related patterns of expectation and influence'. This seems to me to be merely a more long-winded way of saying 'only following orders'. And, if the reader protests that the holocaust example is too extreme, where do we draw the line?

I raise this difficult question because I believe that it is important to distinguish between what we call (name) things and what things are (in actuality). Some of the people, at the very least, cooperated in the killing of helpless people during the Third Reich, and some can still be seen, in their nursing uniforms, committing the acts. However, in no way should we ever consider their acts as examples of 'nursing practice'. What people are called, or expected to do, is not always what they end up doing, in practice.

For this reason I believe that we need not a *professional* definition of nursing, but a *functional* definition. I offered a tentative definition in Chapter 1 (trephotaxis; the provision of the necessary conditions for the promotion of growth and development). When people are providing the conditions that appear necessary for others to grow and develop, as persons, in their relationship to life, and its many problems and difficulties, we could say that they are *nursing* that person. When people who are *called* nurses are doing things to or on behalf of others that do not lead to some ostensible growth and development, they may be doing something important, but they are not doing nursing.

The ethics of healing

The Nuremberg defence led, indirectly, to the development of the Nuremberg Code for Ethical Human Experimentation (ohsr.od.nih.gov/guidelines/nuremberg.-html). This ordered that the interests of science should never take precedence over the rights of the human subject. Eli Wiesel, a Holocaust survivor, observed later that 'respect for human rights in human experimentation demands that we see persons as unique, as ends in themselves'.[5] Although such respect should also be extended to everyday practice, this seems to be a forlorn hope.

Robert Whitaker's book *Mad in America*[6] provides a terrifyingly detailed account of the ruthless, megalomaniacal form of scientism that is an important part of the history of contemporary psychiatry. Whitaker described how the Nuremberg Code, on which Wiesel pinned so much hope, was flagrantly breached, almost before the ink was dry. He claimed that this breach continued up until, at least, the late 1990s, as psychiatric researchers worked out clever ways to 'get round' the ethical problems surrounding the development of new drugs, which they called *routine obfuscation*: not telling subjects that they were receiving chemicals that would make their symptoms *worse*, rather than better.[6] However, few nurses ever become involved in such drug development research. So, what relevance does this have for nursing?

It seems clear that 'parallel breaches' of the Nuremberg Code occur regularly in routine psychiatric practice, and many nurses openly admit to their involvement. I know several nurses old enough to have participated in deep insulin coma 'therapy' in the 1960s. I know hundreds more who assisted in unmodified electroconvulsive 'therapy' when there was no 'evidence' as to its usefulness to the patient. Rarely, was 'informed consent' an important part of the procedure.

Several studies illustrate how, even today, many practising nurses 'fail to advise' people taking psychotropic drugs of what might be involved: that they risk becoming diabetic; developing heart problems; losing their libido; and becoming impotent, among various other physical health problems, including death.[7] They know that this is not 'right'. They rationalize their actions on the grounds that it is 'in the best interests' of the patient.

Most PMHNs, worldwide, are now university graduates. However, in my experience few appear to have more than a sketchy appreciation of the history of psychotropic drugs.[b] For many, the idea that the *main* function of 'neuroleptics' is to *induce brain damage* is dismissed as an 'anti-psychiatry scare story'. The facts are there if anyone cares to look. Leaving aside for a moment people deemed to be 'psychotic', psychotropic drugs have been aggressively promoted in the care (and management) of older persons. The available evidence illustrates how such drugs serve only to accelerate the onset of dementia and increase the risk of death.[8]

The original 'chemical cosh' (chlorpromazine; Largactil or Thorazine) replaced the intentional brain-damaging 'therapies' of the 1930s – insulin coma, electroshock and lobotomy (leucutomy) – for one simple reason. Chlorpromazine was more *efficient* in generating the passivity considered desirable by psychiatric professionals or the patients' families.

The original research into Largactil or Thorazine (chlorpromazine) was led by a French surgeon, Henri Laborit, who was looking for a sedative to potentiate barbiturate sleep therapy. Laborit was so impressed by the *effects* of chlorpromazine that he promoted the new drug to his psychiatrist colleagues as a 'veritable medicinal lobotomy'.[9]

The common term 'neuroleptic' was coined by Deniker and Delay – from the Greek, meaning: to 'take hold of the nervous system'. They believed that they had discovered the ideal chemical restraint, and could now dispense with the straightjacket. In their view, when 'disturbed' patients became apathetic, lacked initiative and lost interest in their surroundings, this was 'good news'. Ironically, even today, psychiatric professionals still describe these *intended* effects, disingenuously, as 'side-effects'. The 'neuroleptic' is intended to damage the brain: slowing down its function, shrinking its capacity, as a means of pacifying the 'mad' patient.

Indeed, the early researchers from 50 years ago recognized that chlorpromazine caused deficits, which were eerily similar to *encephalitis lethargica*, which had affected over 5 million people between 1916 and 1927. The only difference was that chlorpromazine made this happen at a much faster pace. This led the original researchers to note that it would be possible to *cause true encephalitis epidemics* with the new drugs.[6]

Sir William Osler, the 'father of modern medicine', famously said that 'The desire to take medicines is perhaps the greatest feature which distinguishes man from animals.' However, clearly there exist some classes of drugs that humans actively *seek*, and others they *avoid*. People pay large amounts of money to access 'psychotropic drugs' such as alcohol and nicotine. In most countries, others risk criminalization to access cannabis, cocaine, heroin, barbiturates, sex hormones, steroids and various other drugs,

---

[b] I am willing to accept that my 'experience' of teaching and working with nurses in several different countries may be limited.

with 'psychotropic properties'. How many people would go out of their way to access (far less to steal) a consignment of chlorpromazine or lithium carbonate?

Coercive care: a contradiction in terms?

Contemporary academic journals continue to publish studies describing how nurses appear to have few ethical qualms about coercing patients to accept neuroleptic medication.[10] In reporting the effect of so-called 'side-effects', Harris and Lovell[11] casually noted how 'sufferers can experience a wide range of distressing, embarrassing, debilitating and *sometimes fatal side-effects'*. Well, there is nothing more distressing than death, I suppose.

Society's enduring affection for psychiatric medical treatment derives from a heady mix of lies and deception,[6,12] which has largely obscured the real story of recovery – especially from the so-called 'serious and enduring disorders' such as schizophrenia. The popular fallacy, accepted and promoted by many psychiatric professionals, mental health charities and government health ministers, is that people with 'serious and enduring mental illness' *need* to take medication *on a lifelong basis*. The corollary is that if they are 'non-compliant' then they may need to be 'obliged' to take such drugs.[13] There is *no scientific basis* for this belief.

On the contrary, it has long been known that at least one-third of people with a diagnosis of schizophrenia recover completely, irrespective of what happened to them. Longitudinal studies of the 'importance of medication' offer intriguing results. The original long-term studies of 'chronic schizophrenics' discharged from hospital showed that the group which 'recovered' involved those who had weaned themselves off their neuroleptic drugs.[14] These findings echo the World Health Organization's description of the much higher recovery rates from schizophrenia in developing nations, where drug treatment is rarely possible, solely on economic grounds. This contrasts greatly with the 'chronicity' common in the affluent West, where psychotropic drug therapy is the norm.[15] Other, experimental, studies have demonstrated the possibility of providing effective 'recovery-focused care', for people with 'serious' forms of psychosis, *without the need for medication*. These studies

are frequently overlooked, or ignored.[16,17] All this is part of the 'politics of mental health care'.

In no way does this critique represent an 'anti-medication' view. If anything, it reflects a human rights perspective. I believe that people should not be coerced into receiving 'treatment' against their wishes. However, if people wish to accept – or even request – psychotropic drugs, or indeed any other 'physical' or 'psychological' intervention, that request should be respected as their choice.

RECLAIMING CARING – REPLACING NURSING?

I have met thousands of PMHNs who are rightly proud of their craft. However, invariably, this was little more than a private expression of pride. Few were connected to any formal organization that could bring *their* understanding of the importance of nursing to a wider, public, audience. Presently, psychiatric–mental health nursing is like a sleeping giant – awaiting some magical event to rouse it.[18] A more unkind metaphor would be to suggest that the discipline is not so much asleep, as invisible. And because of this 'invisibility', few politicians and public bodies take psychiatric–mental health nursing all that seriously, if they consider it at all.

PMHNs need to look beyond their immediate world of work, for the world outside is changing – fast. New 'experiments' in education and practice are exploring alternatives to traditional forms of support for people with mental health problems. For 'alternatives' read 'alternative to nursing'.

Radcliffe[19] noted that:

> Everyone knows that nurses do a lot of things, but there remains some uncertainty as to what defines them as nurses. It may be a capacity to multi-task or to respond effectively to change. It might be organizational brilliance, an ability to coordinate, acting as the glue that holds everything together, keeping everyone safe. But this remains unspecific, almost fuzzy.

In this highly specialist age, having a vague 'fuzzy' job is clearly a disadvantage. In Radcliffe's view:[19]

> Too much of nursing is doing what nobody else gets round to or wants to do. Whatever power nurses might have had to design care, to oppose policy or ideology or to liberalize the post-confinement age was lost in the struggle to hold things together when there was no money – just the slogan of community care and a lot of goodwill. Now nurses often take pride in being jacks of all trades rather than masters of anything. Of course this is a form of mastery, but not a defining one. The days have long passed when a nurse might have said that their uniqueness was the ability to *be with* someone when they were at their most distressed … There appears to be no value any longer for that special

---

Reflection

Some key questions for PMHNs are:

- What are your values?
- What beliefs support the decision-making process, which in turn supports your practice?
- What are the origins of these beliefs?
- Why are they important to your identity as a psychiatric–mental health nurse?

talent. Its absence does more than deskill the nurse – it dislocates care itself. If that special skill – the talent for presence – is not at the heart of what mental health services offer – viz. company, the beginning of understanding, or the lack of fear in the face of the patient's demons – then services stop being about health and become something to do with organization, tolerance or containment.

Radcliffe is a former psychiatric nurse himself, so he knows what he is talking about. Ironically, he views the new breed of 'mental health practitioner' as someone who might be able to do more nursing than nurses do themselves.

In the UK, and increasingly other countries, the professional context is changing, as various 'graduate mental health workers' or 'mental health practitioners'[19] are introduced to the field. Such 'practitioners' are trained specifically to work alongside nurses and other health and asocial care professionals, in an attempt to ensure that the personal, *human needs* of the patient/client/consumer are met. Radcliffe, who is charged with training this new breed of worker, offers a pithy definition:[19]

An MHP is someone who will spend their time helpfully, therapeutically with the patient.

The implication is that no one else is offering such *help* or *therapeutic* support. A worrying situation for nurses, I would have thought, given that these core functions are meant to lie at the heart of nursing care.

Radcliffe[19] added:

Of course they [MHPs] can run shifts, write notes and plans, admit and discharge and help on the drugs round. But the focus of their identity [is] around therapeutic contact. This was what drew them into mental health and also represented what they saw as the greatest need.

As nurses are trapped in the office, fiddling with computers and telephones, the 'new breed' is 'being present' with the 'patient'.

When I ask nurses why they came into the field, almost everyone tells me that they wanted to care for people, not to lock and unlock doors or shuffle mountains of paperwork. Somewhere, along the way, they lost control of their original vocation. Is there a risk that nursing is being pushed into an administrative or supportive role, while other agencies – like the MHPs – take their old place as the purveyor of *presence*?

In the UK and Ireland another new group of 'carer' is emerging called 'support, time and recovery' (STR) workers. In the foreword to a Department of Health (England) publication, a service manager commented:[20]

STRs have proven that the 'recovery model' works with an unstinting commitment and belief that individuals can recover. The future's bright – the future's STR!

This is good news for the people who are the 'patients'. However, the implication is either that there are not enough nurses to provide the time and support to enable 'recovery' or that nurses do not give this time and support. One way or another, a cause for concern for nurses.

Reflection

Some key questions for PMHNs are:

- What do people need nurses for?
- How do you ensure that people get what they need from you, as a nurse?
- How will you promote a wider understanding of what nursing *really* is?
- How will you prevent nursing being sidelined, as an administrative or medical support service?

MENTAL HEALTH SERVICE: LOSING ITS PURPOSE?

Healing or just being helpful?

This book has considered how nurses might help people work towards 'mental health', minimizing their experience of mental distress at the same time. But what is 'mental health' and what is its relationship to the state of being *human*?

A century ago psychiatry and psychology were still interested in, if not fascinated by, the concept of the mind. Not all nations employ the English term 'mind' in their mental health vocabulary, and some, like the Germans, still use *geist* or spirit to refer to what the English-speaking world calls the 'mind'. This is refreshing, since psychiatry originally meant the study of the 'spirit' or 'soul', and psychotherapy meant the 'healing of the spirit'. Today, we have all but abandoned our interest in the 'spirit' or 'soul' of women and men in exchange for trying to tweak the neurotransmitters in their brain as a means of making them happy.

Interest in the 'psyche' or 'soul' has become the province of the human development or 'personal growth' movement, or features in New Age 'self-actualization' workshops. However, the 'personal growth' and New Age movements have little interest in people with serious problems. Personal growth is a euphemism for capitalistic iconography. In Brandon's[21] view this was an exercise in self-diminishment. People who are attracted to the notion of 'improving' themselves must first buy the notion that they are faulty or stunted. Jerome Frank, cited in Dineen,[22] saw the folly of this:

Ironically, mental health education, which aims to teach people how to cope more effectively with life, has instead increased the demand for psychotherapeutic help. By calling attention to symptoms they might otherwise ignore and by labelling those symptoms as signs of neurosis, mental health education can create unwarranted anxieties, leading those to seek psychotherapy who do not need it. The demand for psychotherapy keeps pace with the supply, and at times one has the uneasy feeling that the supply may be creating the demand.

The typical 'personal growth' clients are like characters in a Woody Allen film, trying to 'actualize' all their deeply hidden 'potential'. This ephemeral stuff is a far cry from the hard work of mental health 'recovery', where people struggle with actual problems in human living, if not also with abstract demons that are real in their effects.

Recovery in mental health is hard work and so occupies a very different landscape from the sunny horizons of personal growth psychology. Recovery involves a strenuous journey, taken over very rocky ground. Helping people to 'recover' is an equally daunting task for the helper, who risks being taken to the (metaphorical) edge of their own core humanity. Sometimes, the effort of trying to enable someone else's recovery might even tip the helper over into the abyss of his or her own human incompetence. We realize that we have very little to offer – apart from ourselves.

Whereas the 'personal growth' movement is awash with gurus, 'wise men' and 'wise women', all focused on doing something 'magical', the ordinary world of mental health is full of ordinary people doing extraordinary things. Despite the vain ambitions of the founders of psycho-*therapy*, we realize that we are not healing anything, and certainly not the 'spirit'. In helping people to make their own recovery journeys, we accept that our role is more that of support, confidante and witness, rather than *active healer*. Indeed, we recognize that the healing lies not in the destination but in the taking of the recovery journey itself. When people begin to reclaim their own identity and personhood, they slowly begin to recover their life, and their place in the wider community of souls.

Metaphors and madness

When I ask nurses what, exactly, they are doing with the people in their care, they tell me that they are: *helping* people to *deal with, recover, fix, address, cope with* or otherwise *live with* some problem in their lives – or maybe just life itself. In a very real sense, nursing interest in, and focus upon, 'problems' validates Thomas Szasz's original argument that 'mental illness' was a *myth*. However, Szasz never denied the reality of the human pain or discomfort that people called 'mental illness'.

> In asserting that there is no such thing as mental illness, I do not deny that people have problems coping with life and with each other.[23]

History may well conclude that Thomas Szasz's[24] assertion that mental illness was a myth was finally found to be right, although many would say for all the wrong reasons.

What is called 'mental illness' or 'mental disorder' has many correlates – biological, chemical, psychological and social. However, as Szasz has recently noted, in physics, we use the same laws to explain why planes fly, and why they crash. However, psychiatry uses one set of laws to explain so-called *sane* behaviour, which it attributes to choices (reason). However, it uses a quite different set of laws to explain *insane* behaviour, which it attributes to causes (disease). For Szasz[25] this was akin to the theory of phlogiston, once presumed to be a part of the nature of combustion. What is actually *going on* within and around people when they are described as in states of 'mental illness' is, to say the least, highly complex. However, whatever *it* is, *it* must be predicated on the same laws of choosing and reasoning as other aspects of the person's life.

According to traditional psychiatric wisdom, a person in a state of 'florid psychosis' is 'completely out of touch with reality'. However, this person manages to suspend the psychotic state long enough to beg, light and subsequently smoke a cigarette. Coleman[26] offered similar examples, from his own experience, of how the apparently irrational behaviour of the person in psychosis is a mask for the highly intentional choices of the person. The reality of madness is that others – family, friends, neighbours, professionals – do not appreciate the choices of the 'mad' person. Indeed, on reflection, some people regret the choices they made when in a state of mental distress. However, this does not diminish their status as choices.

It is frequently asserted that people kill themselves, or kill other people, because they are 'under the influence of hallucinations' or some other 'psychotic process'. How often do we hear that someone 'heard a voice' telling the person to go and mow a neighbour's lawn, or accept the blame for some wrongdoing? Why do we never hear actors at the 'Oscars' paying tribute to their 'voices, without whom I would not be standing here today!'

Why do 'psychotic processes' only seem to get people into trouble, and never seem to be a part of anyone's 'success story'. If this was a 'physical law' – like aerodynamics – what makes something go up would also cause something to go down.

Similarly, I have met many people over the past 40 years who claimed that they were 'someone else' – other than who I *thought* the person was. I have never met anyone who claimed – as a function of some 'so-called delusional process' – to be the 'office cleaner' or the 'woman who lives at number 59'. Instead, people who were in this so-called 'delusional' state always claimed to be someone important, or at least interesting. One does not need to be a psychoanalyst to recognize that when someone says 'I am not me, I am someone else' that person is trying to say something very important, at least to them.

Surveys demonstrate that members of the general public believe that, when someone goes 'crazy', this is likely to be related to some upset, trauma, disadvantage or tragedy in their life, either from the past or present.[27] Only professionals cling to the absurdly reductionist idea that all this 'mad talk' is merely a sign of a 'chemical imbalance', or the effect of some as yet *unspecified biological anomaly*. Ordinary people remain in touch with their core humanity, whereas at least some mental health professionals have 'lost the human plot'.

Reflection

Some key questions for PMHNs are:

- Do you need a theory of 'mental illness' to find out what kind of help someone needs?
- Do you need a theory of 'mental illness' to work out how to deliver that help?
- What is the *purpose* of nursing?
- How will you help others know and understand that purpose?

THE CHALLENGE OF CARING

What works?

As we have noted several times already, contemporary health care is dominated by ideas about evidence, and questions about the efficacy and efficiency of interventions. An all too common question is 'Does this or that intervention 'work'?' The question is interesting, but naïve.

Everything 'works' in *some* way. Even when 'nothing' seems to happen, nothing is clearly 'something'. A simpler, yet more profound scientific question is 'What happens?' when we do this, rather than that?

An alternative set of questions might be:[c]

- In *what way* does (intervention 'X') work?
- To *whose specific end*?
- To *what particular purpose* (or outcome)?

Of course, all of this is metaphorical. Things do not *work* in the way people called 'workers' work. We simply cannot find any other way to describe such happenings, without comparing them to something else. Given the context of nursing, in which many of the functions involved in caring involve the manipulation (metaphorically) of abstract elements – *support, platonic love, respect, dignity, power* – it is important that nursing, as a discipline, recognizes that its vocation belongs to a quite different territory of evidence: the world of human experience and, arguably, aesthetics. However, nurses still have a responsibility to *clarify* 'what happens' when they manipulate 'support' or 'platonic love', etc. They need to show what 'use' this might be to the person who is on the receiving end.

Fitness to practise

Apart from *knowing* what we need to do, we need to ask whether we are *capable* of doing it. A sports team can have the best coach, equipped with the best strategy that can be mustered. However, if the team does not possess the highest level of fitness, supporting the highest level of commitment to winning, then it is beaten before the game begins. Sport provides a crude but useful analogy for what is expected of nurses.

In the USA some hospitals hire university students to take over the menial task of observing suicidal patients, asserting that such surveillance is not appropriate for professional nurses. In the UK some Trusts have even employed security firms to do a similar surveillance work on acute wards. These post-psychiatric developments are either a clarion call to re-engage with caring for people in great distress, or a signal that nursing, and those who manage nurses, have abandoned care in favour of physical containment. Arguably, anyone with even a modicum of medical preparation could monitor and advise the psychiatric team of the 'presentation' of the patient – which is often all some psychiatrists ask for in a 'good nurse'. However, the only people who can provide the necessary conditions for the promotion of human growth and development – acknowledging the root definition of nursing: to *nourish* – will be those with a heart big enough for the task.

It is over 100 years since Freud founded psychoanalysis. When someone asked him why he always sat *behind* the patient during the analysis, Freud answered honestly that he was not the kind of person who could sit looking people full in the face for 8 hours a day. What Freud needed, and what his clientele needed, were, clearly, two quite different things. Things have not changed much. Today, we still find it difficult to confront madness. We still find it difficult to stare madness firmly in the face. Instead, we hide behind euphemisms and abstract theories.

We still find it difficult to look at people simply, yet profoundly, as people at the centre of a metaphorical maelstrom, which threatens to engulf and, ultimately, drown them.

- We find it hard to face the young man who had dreams of being an astronaut or maybe just a father or lover, but who ended up as just another 'service user' with a 'serious and enduring mental illness'.
- We find it hard to face the dreamer who will not take his medication, will not fit into this grossly misshapen society, and who has ended up as either a nuisance to

---

[c] I am indebted to my friend Thomas Szasz for helping me appreciate the simple, yet challenging, logic of 'efficacy'.

his family or to the politicians who ultimately direct the mental healthcare traffic.

It is all too commonly said of nursing that 'anyone could do it'. It is 'hardly rocket science'. This is very true. I believe that almost anyone could sit with someone for a few hours, a day maybe, giving support that is responsive to the changing nature of the person experience and its expression though the person's behaviour.

However, I believe that to be able to deliver such flexible, responsive care for hours at a stretch, 5 days a week for 30–40 years, requires a discipline that is truly impressive. Not everyone can do that. Some never actually 'catch alight'. Others, 'burn out' during the process.

Reflection

Some key questions for PMHNs are:

- What challenges does 'caring' present to you?
- How do you deal with those challenges?
- Who do you turn to when you run out of 'solutions'?
- How has your idea of caring changed since you first decided to become a nurse?

KEEP IT SIMPLE – FOR LIFE IS COMPLEX ENOUGH

People and persons

I was an 'accidental nurse'. I planned to work in the old hospital at the top of the hill for only a few months. However, from day 1 I was hooked by the people I met. I was fascinated by who they had been and how they had come to end up here. My fascination with people meant that I always struggled with the idea that they were 'patients' – somehow different from me. It was obvious: I was just a whole lot more fortunate.

Some nurses find it difficult to engage patients as *people*. This is understandable. Why did we, the professions, spend so long trying to figure out what to call those in our care – *patients, clients, users* or *consumers* – when we could just have called them *people*? All this fiddling with language is no more than a clever way of avoiding eye contact. By redefining the 'people' as some 'other' thing, we avoid confronting the fact that their pain is much like ours. My favourite psychiatric quote is from Harry Stack Sullivan,[28] who said 'Everyone is much more simply human than otherwise.' In Scotland we say that 'we are a' Jock Tamson's bairns'. We are all the same under the skin. But, the recognition of that similarity scares us! Over the past few years a wide range of 'health education' projects have attempted to help the general public recognize that people with (for example) 'schizophrenia' are people first and foremost. The irony of these campaigns is that the professionals working with 'people with schizophrenia' have, for so long, struggled to accept

their people status. Professionals still struggle to use ordinary language to talk about *people* and *persons*.

Powering up nursing

I always hoped that nursing would set a good example and dispense with obscure jargon and just 'tell it like it is'. I am still hopeful. In all mental health services – hospital or community – nurses greatly outnumber other disciplines. Generally speaking, nurses are not seen as 'powerful'. (When was the last time you saw a nurse on television, or in the press, discussing contemporary mental health issues?) However, although nurses may have little *overt* power, they have great *covert power*. They can help make things happen or make sure that they do not. My hope is that nurses will use their subtle, near-invisible power to make a real difference within the politics of caring.

They can start doing this by abandoning the absurd professional constructs – such as 'illness', 'suffering', 'lack of coping skills', 'psychoeducation' – which get in the way of human relations. These concepts and constructs are designed to put others at a disadvantage. As Shaw[29] said, 'all professions are a conspiracy against the laity'. Once they have dispensed with the 'baggage' of professionalism, they can begin to discover how easy it is to have a human relationship with a person in human distress.

If you do not believe that it can be that easy try this. The next time you:

- pay someone a 'domiciliary visit', or
- interview someone in a 'consulting room', or
- wrestle someone to the floor, as part of a 'de-escalation manoeuvre'

ask yourself:

- whose mother/daughter/sister/wife/lover/partner/friend is this *woman*?
- whose father/son/brother/husband/lover/partner/friend is this *man*?

If asking yourself, privately, this question does not make your immediate task *more difficult*, then you have not been called to nurse.

After almost 40 years in the mental health field I have learned many things that were interesting, but only one thing that was truly important. I learned that most, if not all, of the people I met had ambitions to be an architect or an astronaut; an angel or an artist. They were all people who dreamed of being somebody, rather than just another mental health 'patient' statistic. I am sure that you have met these people also.

So, the next time that man or woman welcomes you into their home, or bars the door – literally or metaphorically – you will remember reading this chapter.

- You will remember that we all stand in the shadow of dangerous ideologies. Such false ideas risk alienating the man or woman in front of you *as persons*, even if they do not actually advocate sending them to the gas chamber.

- You will remember that you have no idea what kind of help this man or woman needs, but a good place to start would be asking them.
- You will remember that, although you hold a briefcase, syringe or prescription pad in your hand, the only valuable thing you carry is in your heart. How can you let the person know that?
- You will remember that the most 'serious' problems this man or woman possesses are reflections of your own problems, or those close to you. And you see yourself or your loved ones when you look into this man's or woman's eyes.
- You will remember not to look away. You will remember that this look is what the *politics of caring* is all about.

REFERENCES

1. Clarke L. Declaring conceptual independence from obsolete professional affiliations. In: Cutcliffe J, Ward M (eds). *Key debates in psychiatric/mental health nursing.* Edinburgh, UK: Churchill Livingstone, 2006: Chapter 5.

2. Cormack DFS. *Psychiatric nursing observed: a descriptive study of the work of the charge nurse in acute admission wards of psychiatric hospitals.* London, UK: Royal College of Nursing, 1976.

3. McFarland-Icke BR. *Nurses in Nazi Germany: moral choice in history.* Princeton, NJ: Princeton University Press, 1999.

4. Grant A. Psychiatric nursing and organizational power: rescuing the hidden dynamic. *Journal of Psychiatric and Mental Health Nursing* 2001; **8** (2): 173–7.

5. Annas GJ, Grodin MA (eds). *The Nazi doctors and the Nuremburg Code: human rights in human experimentation.* New York, NY: Oxford University Press, 1995.

6. Whitaker R. *Mad in America: bad science, bad medicine and the enduring mistreatment of the mentally ill.* Cambridge, MA: Perseus Books, 2003.

7. Higgins A, Barker P, Begley C. Iatrogenic sexual dysfunction and the protective withholding of information: in whose best interests? *Journal of Psychiatric and Mental Health Nursing* 2006; **13** (4): 437–46.

8. Ancelin MY. Non-degenerative mild cognitive impairment in elderly people and the use of anticholinergic drugs: longitudinal cohort study. *British Medical Journal* 2006; **332**: 455–9.

9. Laborit H. Quoted in Johnson AB. *Out of Bedlam: the truth about deinstitutionalisation.* New York, NY: Basic Books, 1990: 40.

10. Lind M, Kaltiala-Heino R, Suominen T *et al.* Nurses' ethical perceptions about coercion. *Journal of Psychiatric and Mental Health Nursing* 2004; **11**: 379–85.

11. Harris NR, Lovell K, Day JC. Consent and long-term neuroleptic treatment. *Journal of Psychiatric and Mental Health Nursing* 2002; **9**: 475–82.

12. Szasz TS. *Coercion as cure: a critical history of psychiatry.* London, UK: Transaction Publishers, 2007.

13. Lawton-Smith S. *Community based compulsory treatment orders in Scotland.* London, UK: Kings Fund, 2006.

14. Harding C. The Vermont longitudinal study of persons with severe mental illness. *American Journal of Psychiatry* 1987; **144**: 727–34.

15. Jablensky A. Schizophrenia: manifestations, incidence and course in different cultures, a World Health Organization ten-country study. *Psychological Medicine* 1999; **2** (Suppl 20): 1–95.

16. Ciompi LR. The Soteria concept – theoretical bases and practices: 13-year experiences with a milieu-therapeutic approach to acute schizophrenia. *Psychiatrica et Neurologica Japonica* 1997; **9**: 634–50.

17. Fenton WS, Hoch JS, Herrell JM *et al.* Cost and cost effectiveness of hospital versus crisis residential care for patients with serious mental illness. *Archives of General Psychiatry* 2002; **59**: 357–64.

18. Barker P, Buchanan-Barker P. Still invisible after all these years: mental health nursing on the margins. *Journal of Psychiatric and Mental Health Nursing* 2005; **12**: 252–6.

19. Radcliffe M. Meanwhile over in the corner: reclaiming care. *Journal of Psychiatric and Mental health Nursing* 2006; **13**: 453–5.

20. DH/NIMHE National Workforce Programme. *Mental health policy implementation guide: support, time and recovery (STR) workers: learning from the national implementation programme.* Final handbook. London, UK: Department of Health, 2008.

21. Brandon D. *The Tao of survival: spirituality in social care and counselling.* Birmingham, UK: Venture Press, 2001.

22. Dineen T. *Manufacturing victims – what the psychology industry is doing to people.* Quebec, Canada: Robert Davies, 1996.

23. Szasz TS. *The second sin.* London, UK: Routledge and Kegan Paul, 1974: 98–9.

24. Szasz TS. *The myth of mental illness.* New York, NY: Hoeber-Harper, 1961.

25. Szasz TS. Mental illness; psychiatry's phlogiston. *Journal of Medical Ethics* 2001; **27** (5): 297–301.

26. Coleman R. The politics of the illness. In: Barker P, Stevenson C (eds). *The construction of power and authority in psychiatry.* London, UK: Butterworth Heinemann, 2000.

27. Morrison A, Read J, Turkington D. Trauma and psychosis: theoretical and clinical implications. *Acta Psychiatrica Scandinavica* 2005; **112**: 327–9.

28. Sullivan HS. *The interpersonal theory of psychiatry.* New York, NY: WW Norton and Co, 1953.

29. Shaw GB. *The doctor's dilemma*, Act I, 1911.

Index

Page numbers in **bold** indicate figures, tables or boxes.